DIAGNOSTIC PATHOLOGY

SOFT TISSUE TUMORS

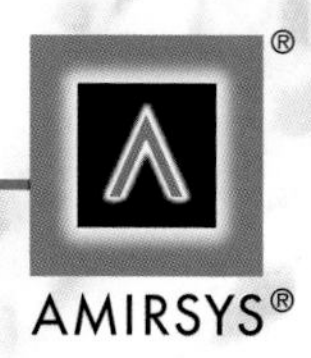

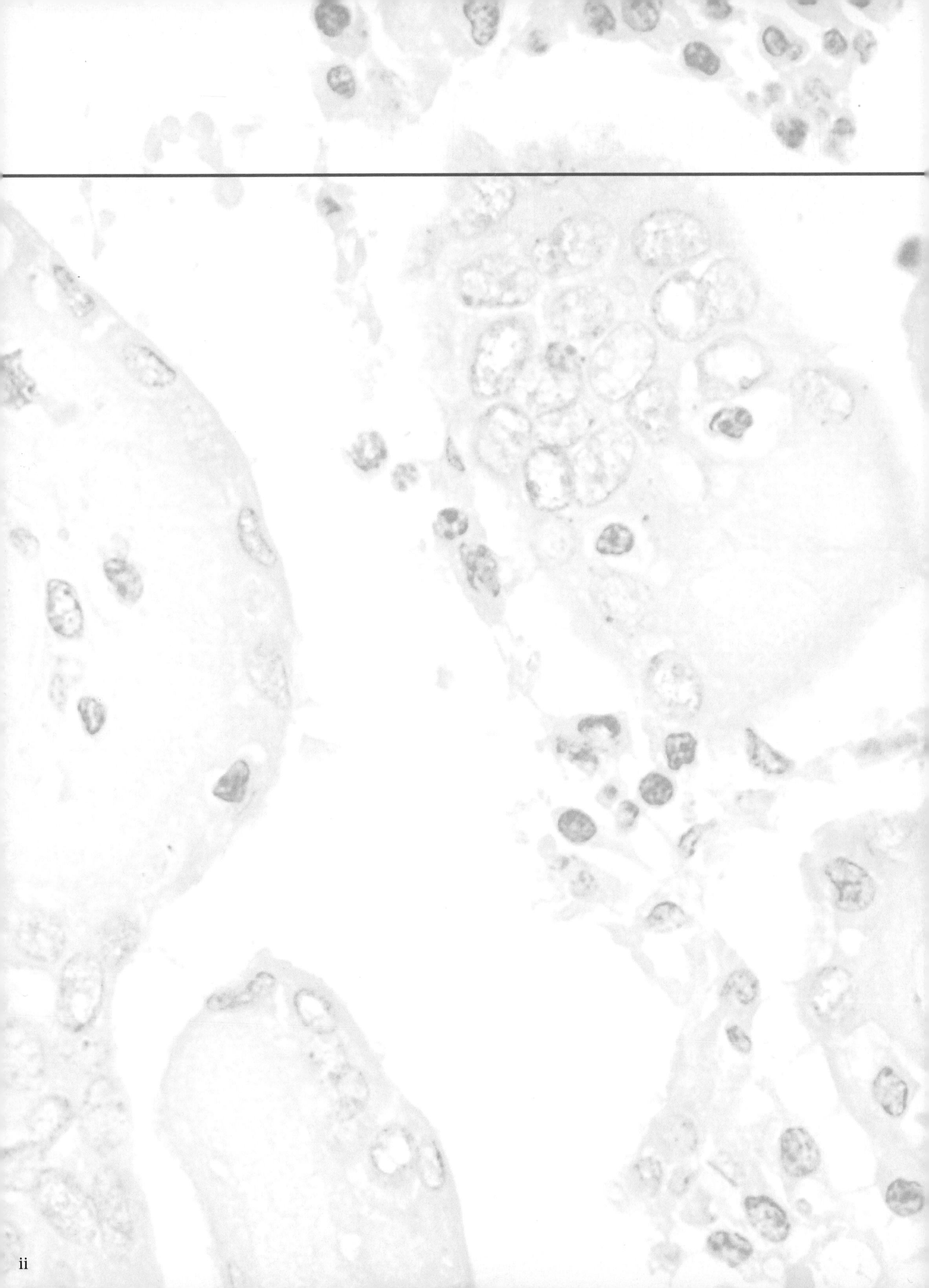

DIAGNOSTIC PATHOLOGY
SOFT TISSUE TUMORS

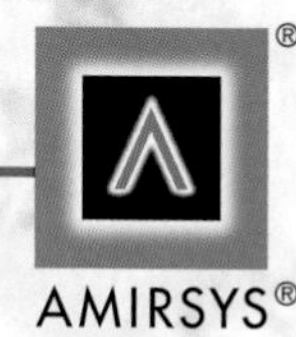

Cyril Fisher, MD, DSc, FRCPath
Consultant Histopathologist
Royal Marsden NHS Foundation Trust
Professor of Tumor Pathology
Institute of Cancer Research
University of London
London, United Kingdom

Thomas Mentzel, MD
Dermatopathologische Gemeinschaftspraxis
Friedrichshafen, Germany
Associate Professor
Department of Pathology
University of Freiburg
Freiburg, Germany

Elizabeth A. Montgomery, MD
Professor of Pathology, Oncology,
and Orthopedic Surgery
Johns Hopkins Medical Institutions
Baltimore, MD

David R. Lucas, MD
Director of Surgical Pathology
Professor of Pathology
Department of Pathology
University of Michigan Medical School
Ann Arbor, MI

Khin Thway, BSc, MBBS, FRCPath
Consultant Histopathologist
Royal Marsden NHS Foundation Trust
London, United Kingdom

David S. Cassarino, MD, PhD
Consultant Dermatopathologist and Staff Pathologist
Southern California Permanente Medical Group
Los Angeles, CA
Clinical Professor
Department of Dermatology
University of California at Irvine
Irvine, CA

Amitabh Srivastava, MD
Assistant Professor
Department of Pathology
Dartmouth Hitchcock Medical Center & Dartmouth
Medical School
Lebanon, NH

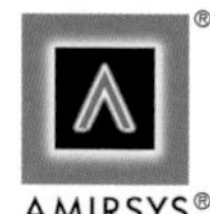

Names you know. Content you trust.®

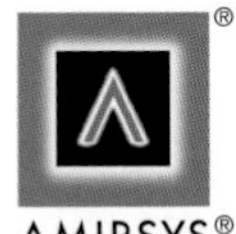

AMIRSYS®
Names you know. Content you trust.®

First Edition

Printed in Canada by Friesens, Altona, Manitoba, Canada

ISBN: 978-1-9318-8450-1

Notice and Disclaimer

Library of Congress Cataloging-in-Publication Data

Diagnostic pathology. Soft tissue tumors / [edited by] Cyril Fisher.
p. ; cm.
Other title: Soft tissue tumors
Includes bibliographical references.
ISBN 978-1-931884-50-1
1. Soft tissue tumors--Diseases--Diagnosis--Handbooks, manuals, etc. 2. Pathology, Surgical--Handbooks, manuals, etc. 3. Soft tissue tumors--Diseases--Diagnosis--Atlases. I. Fisher, Cyril. II. Title: Soft tissue tumors.
[DNLM: 1. Soft Tissue Neoplasms--diagnosis--Atlases. 2. Soft Tissue Neoplasms--pathology--Atlases. WD 375 D536 2011]
RC280.S66D53 2011
616.99'4--dc22
2010023853

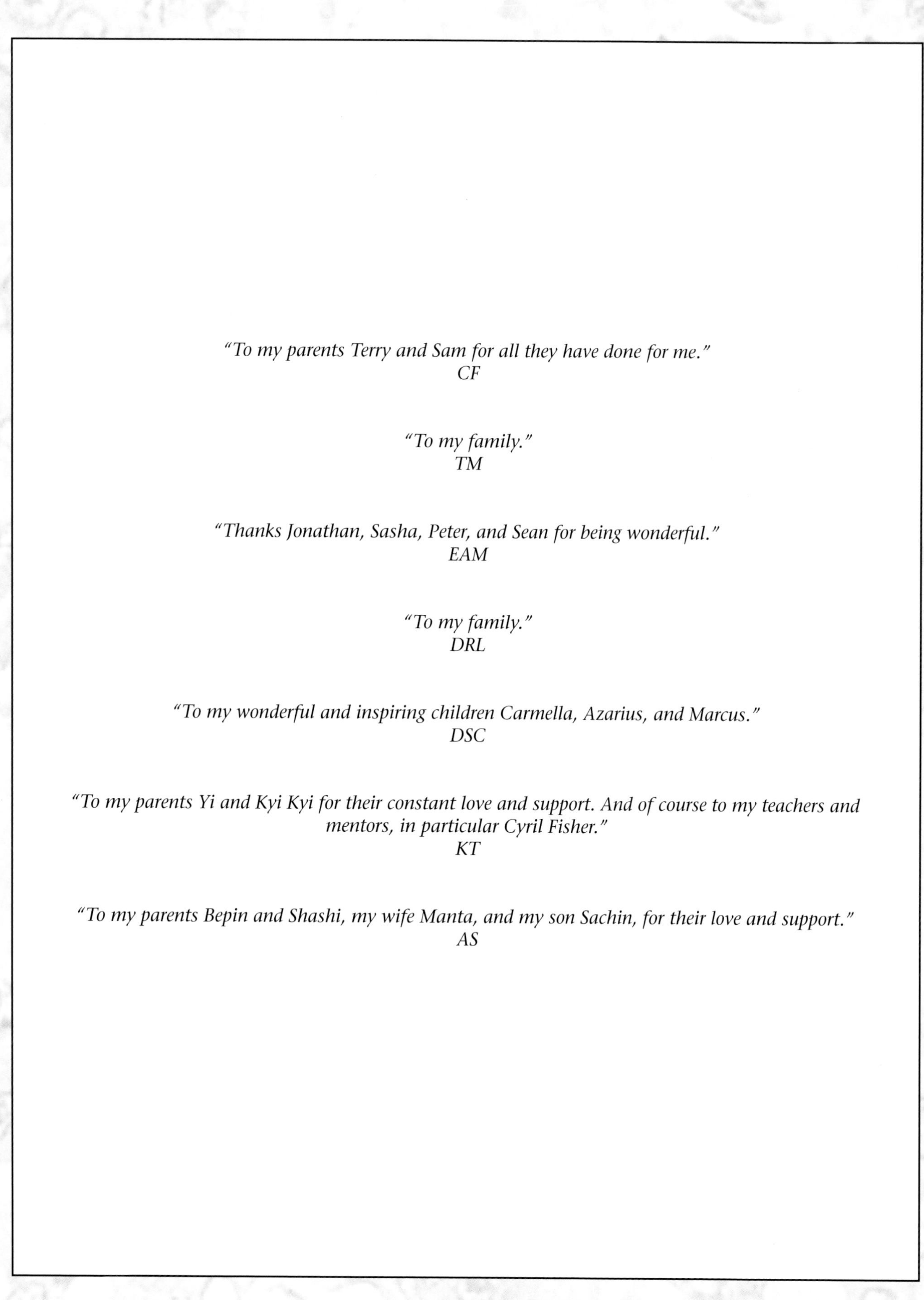

"To my parents Terry and Sam for all they have done for me."
CF

"To my family."
TM

"Thanks Jonathan, Sasha, Peter, and Sean for being wonderful."
EAM

"To my family."
DRL

"To my wonderful and inspiring children Carmella, Azarius, and Marcus."
DSC

"To my parents Yi and Kyi Kyi for their constant love and support. And of course to my teachers and mentors, in particular Cyril Fisher."
KT

"To my parents Bepin and Shashi, my wife Manta, and my son Sachin, for their love and support."
AS

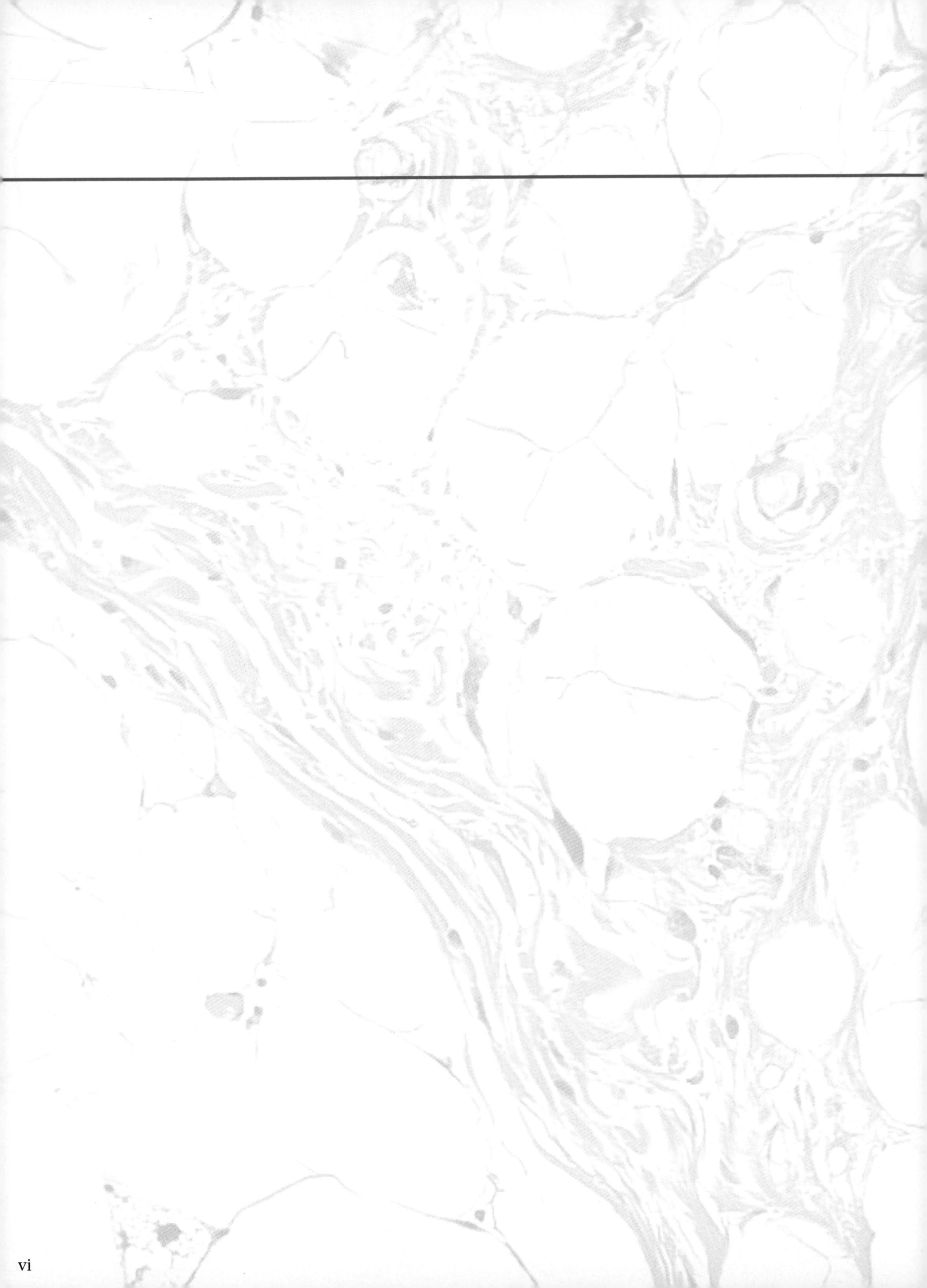

CONTRIBUTING AUTHORS

Jonathan B. McHugh, MD
Assistant Professor of Pathology
Department of Pathology
University of Michigan Medical School
Ann Arbor, MI

Julie C. Fanburg-Smith, MD
Orthopaedic and Soft Tissue Pathology
Deputy Chair and Medical Director
AFIP/AIPL
Washington, DC/Silver Spring, MD

Steven D. Billings, MD
Staff Pathologist
Cleveland Clinic
Cleveland, OH

DIAGNOSTIC PATHOLOGY

SOFT TISSUE TUMORS

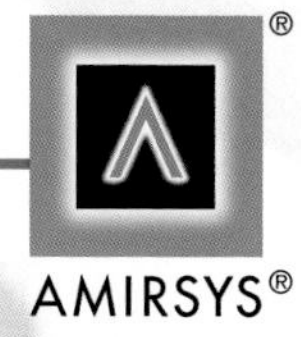

Amirsys, creators of the highly acclaimed radiology series Diagnostic Imaging, proudly introduces its new Diagnostic Pathology series, designed as easy-to-use reference texts for the busy practicing surgical pathologist. Written by world-renowned experts, the series will consist of 15 titles in all the crucial diagnostic areas of surgical pathology.

The third book in this series, *Diagnostic Pathology: Soft Tissue Tumors*, contains over 700 pages of comprehensive, yet concise, descriptions of more than 190 specific diagnoses. Amirsys's pioneering bulleted format distills pertinent information to the essentials. Each chapter has the same organization providing an easy-to-read reference for making rapid, efficient, and accurate diagnoses in a busy surgical pathology practice. A highlighted Key Facts box provides the essential features of each diagnosis. Detailed sections on Terminology, Etiology/Pathogenesis, Clinical Issues, Macroscopic and Microscopic Findings, and the all important Differential Diagnoses follow so you can find the information you need in the exact same place every time.

Most importantly, every diagnosis features numerous high-quality images, including gross pathology, H&E and immunohistochemical stains, correlative radiographic images, and richly colored graphics, all of which are fully annotated to maximize their illustrative potential.

We believe that this lavishly illustrated series, with its up-to-date information and practical focus, will become the core of your reference collection. Enjoy!

Elizabeth H. Hammond, MD
Executive Editor, Pathology
Amirsys, Inc.

Anne G. Osborn, MD
Chairman and Chief Executive Officer
Amirsys Publishing, Inc.

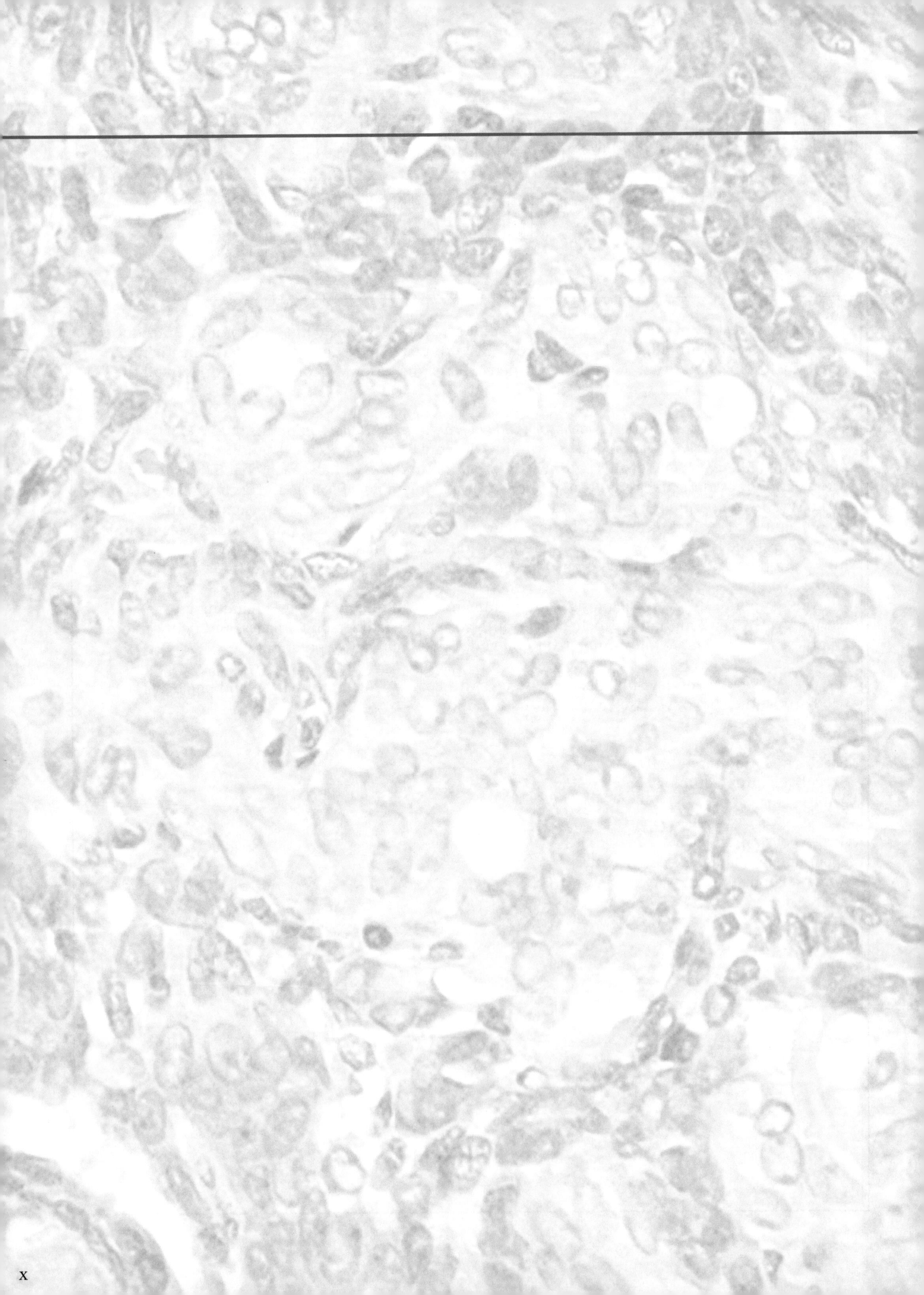

PREFACE

Soft tissue tumors often present difficulties for the surgical pathologist. Such tumors not only are rare and therefore infrequently encountered but also have a wide range of appearances with often subtle differences among entities. This reference aims to provide concise, practical information about each tumor, to illustrate the range of appearances encountered at the microscope, and to facilitate differential diagnosis by allowing comparison with other similar lesions.

Every chapter includes a wealth of information in uniform, bulleted format, including clinical features, pathologic findings, immunohistochemistry, cytogenetic and molecular genetic information where relevant, and differential diagnoses. All are fully illustrated with clinical, radiographic, and microscopic images to show the range of appearances and variations that might be encountered. Additional points and diagnostic tips are included in the detailed legends that accompany each image. The Key Facts about each entity are summarized in a separate box for quick reference, and immunohistochemistry information in many chapters is presented in convenient tabular form.

The content is arranged by differentiation lineage based on the World Health Organization's Consensus Classification, with the addition of other tumors not included therein, such as neural and cutaneous neoplasms, as well as more recently characterized entities. In response to the increasing demand by pathologists and non-pathologists alike for data capture in synoptic or structured form, we have included standard protocols for examination and reporting of soft tissue sarcomas.

A glance at the surgical pathology literature shows that our knowledge and understanding of soft tissue tumor pathology advances with amazing rapidity. New entities are described, familiar ones are reevaluated with clinicopathologic studies, and new investigative techniques and pathology-dependent therapeutic options emerge. No printed book can be fully up to date. The Amirsys eBook Advantage™ included with each printed copy of *Diagnostic Pathology: Soft Tissue Tumors* will provide fully searchable text, a complete listing of antibodies, and regular updates. This will indeed be a practical resource of continuing value.

We hope that *Diagnostic Pathology: Soft Tissue Tumors* will prove to be useful in everyday practice at the bench or microscope to facilitate diagnosis, reporting, and therefore management of soft tissue tumors.

Cyril Fisher, MD, DSc, FRCPath
Consultant Histopathologist
Royal Marsden NHS Foundation Trust
Professor of Tumor Pathology
Institute of Cancer Research
University of London
London, UK

ACKNOWLEDGMENTS

Text Editing
Ashley R. Renlund, MA
Kellie J. Heap
Arthur G. Gelsinger, MA
Katherine Riser, MA

Image Editing
Jeffrey J. Marmorstone

Medical Text Editing
Dora M. Lam-Himlin, MD

Illustrations
Laura C. Sesto, MA
Richard Coombs, MS
Lane R. Bennion, MS

Art Direction and Design
Laura C. Sesto, MA

Assistant Editor
Dave L. Chance, MA

Production Leads
Kellie J. Heap
Melissa A. Hoopes

SECTIONS

TABLE OF CONTENTS

SECTION 1 Soft Tissue Introduction

Introduction and Overview

Molecular Pathology

Examination of Soft Tissue Tumors

Immunohistochemistry

SECTION 2 Adipose Tissue Lesions

Benign

Intermediate

Malignant

SECTION 3 Fibroblastic/ Myofibroblastic Lesions

Benign

Intermediate

Malignant

SECTION 4
Fibrohistiocytic Lesions

Benign

Intermediate

Malignant

SECTION 5
Genital Stromal Tumors

Benign

SECTION 6
Mesothelial Lesions

Benign

Malignant

Examination of Mesothelioma Specimens

SECTION 7
Myoepithelial Lesions

Intermediate

SECTION 8
Nerve Sheath Lesions

Benign

Benign/Malignant

Malignant

SECTION 9
Neural and Neuroectodermal Lesions

Benign

Benign/Malignant

Malignant

Examination of PNET/ Ewing Sarcoma Specimens

SECTION 10
Osseous and Chondroid Lesions

Benign

Intermediate

Malignant

SECTION 15
Lesions of Uncertain Differentiation

Benign

Intermediate

Malignant

SECTION 16
Other Lesions

Benign

Malignant

Examination of GIST Specimens

SECTION 17
Antibody Index

DIAGNOSTIC PATHOLOGY
SOFT TISSUE TUMORS

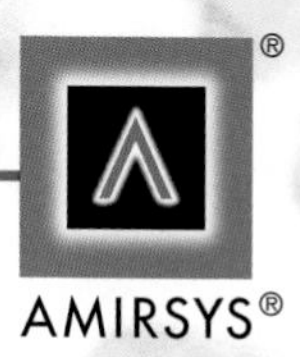

Soft Tissue Introduction

Introduction and Overview

Molecular Pathology

Examination of Soft Tissue Tumors

Immunohistochemistry

OVERVIEW OF GRADING AND STAGING

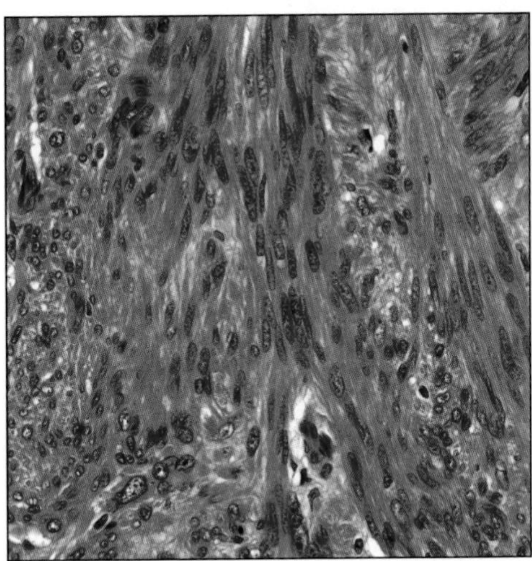

This is leiomyosarcoma with a differentiation score of 1. The tumor is composed of well-organized fascicles of spindle cells with uniform nuclei and abundant cytoplasm, and it resembles normal smooth muscle.

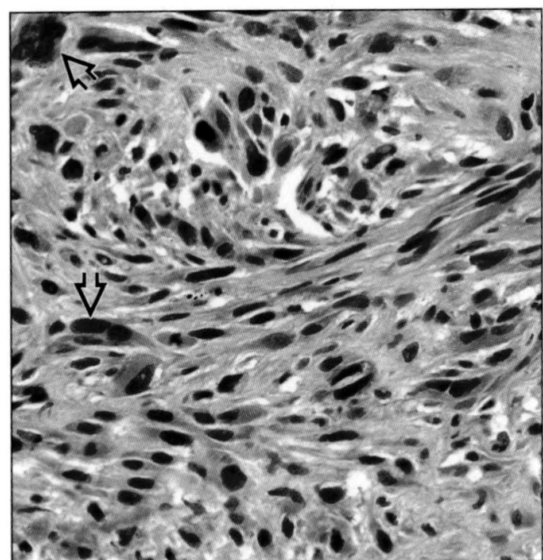

This is leiomyosarcoma with a differentiation score of 3. A fascicular architecture is only focally present. The cells show high nuclear/cytoplasmic ratio and focally marked nuclear pleomorphism ⮚.

GRADING AND STAGING SYSTEMS

Grading System of French Cancer Centers

- Fédération Nationale des Centres de Lutte Contre le Cancer (FNCLCC)

Staging System

- TNM classification of tumors 7th edition (TNM)

HISTOLOGICAL FEATURES EVALUATED IN GRADING (FNCLCC)

Differentiation

- Score 1: Sarcoma histologically very similar to normal adult mesenchymal tissue
  - Well-differentiated examples of liposarcoma, leiomyosarcoma, fibrosarcoma, malignant peripheral nerve sheath tumor (MPNST), chondrosarcoma
- Score 2: Sarcoma of defined histological subtype
  - Myxofibrosarcoma, myxoid liposarcoma, extraskeletal myxoid chondrosarcoma
  - Conventional examples of fibrosarcoma, leiomyosarcoma, MPNST, pleomorphic malignant fibrous histiocytoma with storiform pattern
- Score 3: Sarcoma of uncertain type, embryonal and undifferentiated sarcomas
  - Synovial sarcoma, rhabdomyosarcoma, clear cell sarcoma, epithelioid sarcoma, malignant rhabdoid tumor, epithelioid malignant schwannoma, alveolar soft part sarcoma, malignant Triton tumor, mesenchymal chondrosarcoma
  - Extraskeletal Ewing sarcoma and osteosarcoma
  - Poorly differentiated examples of fibrosarcoma, leiomyosarcoma, MPNST
  - Pleomorphic malignant fibrohistiocytoma (MFH) without storiform pattern; giant cell and inflammatory MFH
  - Undifferentiated sarcoma

Mitotic Index per 10 High-Power Fields (HPF)

- Score 1: 1-9 mitoses
- Score 2: 10-19 mitoses
- Score 3: 20 or more mitoses
  - Total number in 10 successive HPF in most mitotically active areas
  - Avoid ulcerated, necrotic, or hypocellular areas

Percentage of Microscopic Tumor Necrosis

- Score 0: No necrosis
- Score 1: Necrosis < 50%
- Score 2: Necrosis > 50%
  - Tumor necrosis should be evaluated at macroscopic and microscopic levels
  - Macroscopic assessment should always be confirmed by microscopic evaluation

Grade

- Summation of 3 scores indicates grade
  - Grade 1: Total score 2 or 3
  - Grade 2: Total score 4 or 5
  - Grade 3: Total score 6, 7, or 8
- In practice, some tumors are always graded by diagnosis
  - Always grade 1
    - Atypical lipomatous tumor, dermatofibrosarcoma, infantile fibrosarcoma, angiomatoid fibrous histiocytoma
  - Always grade 3
    - Ewing sarcoma/PNET, rhabdomyosarcoma (except spindle cell and botryoid variants), angiosarcoma, pleomorphic liposarcoma, soft tissue osteosarcoma, mesenchymal chondrosarcoma, desmoplastic small round cell tumor, extrarenal malignant rhabdoid tumor
  - Not formally graded but managed as high grade
    - Alveolar soft part sarcoma, clear cell sarcoma, epithelioid sarcoma

OVERVIEW OF GRADING AND STAGING

Soft Tissue Sarcoma Staging

TNM	Description
Primary Tumor (T)	
TX	Primary tumor cannot be assessed
T0	No evidence of primary tumor
T1	Tumor 5 cm or less in greatest dimension
T1a	Superficial tumor (above deep fascia)
T1b	Deep tumor (involves or lies beneath deep fascia or in body cavity)
T2	Tumor > 5 cm in greatest dimension
T2a	Superficial tumor
T2b	Deep tumor
Regional Lymph Nodes (N)	
NX	Regional lymph nodes cannot be assessed
N0	No regional lymph node metastasis
N1	Regional lymph node metastasis
Distant Metastasis (M)	
M0	No distant metastasis
M1	Distant metastasis

Adapted from 7th edition AJCC Staging Forms.

Anatomic Stage/Prognostic Groups

Stage	Tumor	Node	Metastasis	Grade
Stage IA	T1a	N0	M0	G1, GX
	T1b	N0	M0	G1, GX
Stage IB	T2a	N0	M0	G1, GX
	T2b	N0	M0	G1, GX
Stage IIA	T1a	N0	M0	G2
	T1b	N0	M0	G2
Stage IIB	T2a	N0	M0	G2
	T2b	N1	M0	G2
Stage III	T2a, T2b	N0	M0	G3
	Any T	N1	M0	Any G
Stage IV	Any T	Any N	M1	Any G

Adapted from 7th edition AJCC Staging Forms.

IMAGE GALLERY

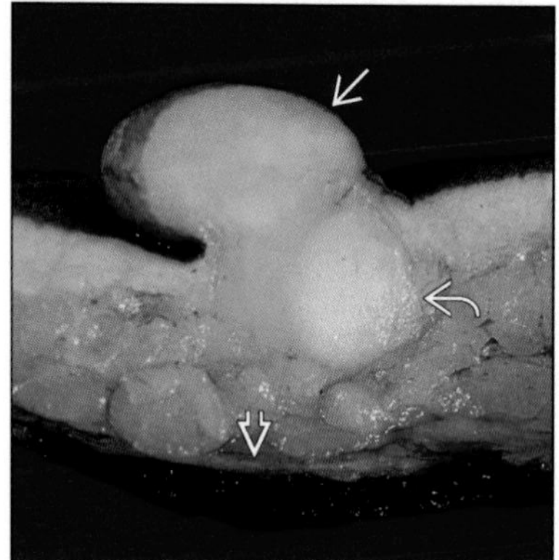

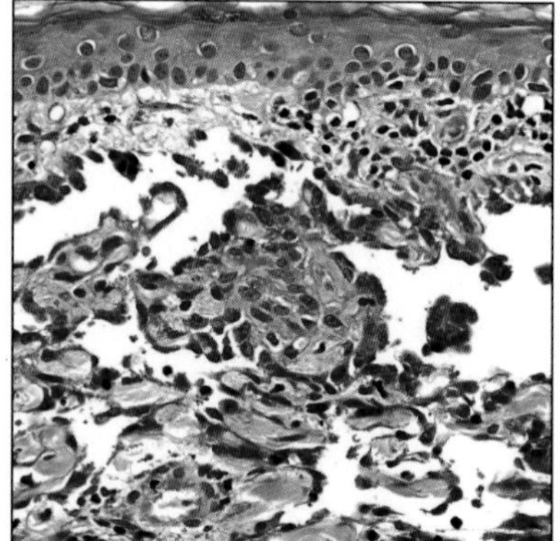

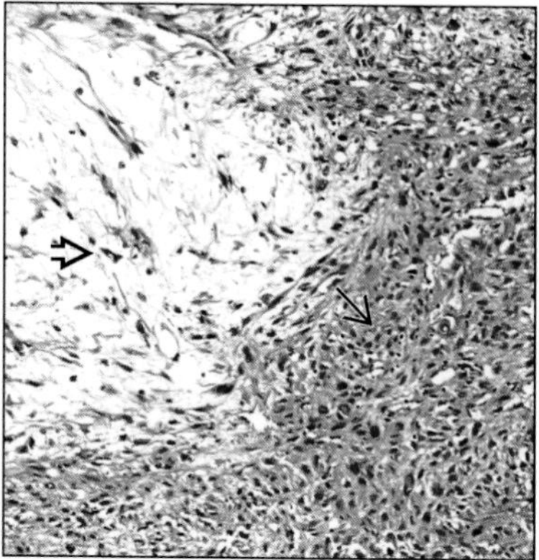

(Left) *This example of dermatofibrosarcoma protuberans involves the skin ➡ and subcutis ➡ but does not extend to deep fascia ➡. It is classified as grade 1, stage T1a.* ***(Center)*** *This cutaneous angiosarcoma is well differentiated but should be managed as a high-grade malignancy.* ***(Right)*** *This shows myxofibrosarcoma with low- ➡ and high-grade ➡ areas. The latter display increased cellularity, pleomorphism, and mitoses.*

TRANSLOCATIONS AND OTHER GENETIC ANOMALIES IN SARCOMAS

Diagnostic Molecular and Cytogenetic Findings in Sarcomas

Histologic Type	Translocation or Rearrangement	Fusion Gene or Other Feature
Alveolar soft part sarcoma	t(X;17)(p11;q25)	*ASPL-TFE3*
Angiomatoid fibrous histiocytoma	t(12;22)(q13;q12)	*EWSR1-ATF1*
	t(12;16)(q13;p11)	*FUS-ATF1*
	t (2;22)(q33;q12)	*EWSR1-CREB1*
Clear cell sarcoma of soft parts	t(12;22)(q13;q12)	*EWSR1-ATF1*
Clear cell sarcoma (gastrointestinal)	t(2;22)(q33;q12)	*EWSR1-CREB1*
Dermatofibrosarcoma protuberans and variants	t(17;22)(q21;q13)	*COL1A1-PDGFB*
	Ring form of chromosomes 17 and 22	
Desmoplastic small round cell tumor	t(11;22)(p13;q12)	*EWSR1-WT1*
	t(21;22)(q22;q12)	*EWSR1-ERG*
Endometrial stroma sarcoma	t(7;17)(p15:q21)	*JAZF1-JJAZ1*
	t(6;7)(p21;p22)	*JAZF1-PHF1*
	t(10:17)(q22;p13)	
Epithelioid hemangioendothelioma	t(1;3)(p36.3;q25)	
	t(10;14)(p13;q24)	Gene for VEGF-related protein at 14q24
Epithelioid sarcoma	Abnormalities of 22q	*INI1* inactivation
Ewing sarcoma/primitive neuroectodermal tumor	t(11;22)(q24;q12)	*EWSR1-FLI1*
	t(21;22)(q12;q12)	*EWSR1-ERG*
	t(2;22)(q33;q12)	*EWSR1-FEV*
	t(7;22)(p22;q12)	*EWSR1-ETV1*
	t(17;22)(q12;q12)	*EWSR1-E1AF*
	inv(22)(q12;q12)	*EWSR1-ZSG*
Extraskeletal myxoid chondrosarcoma	t(9;22)(q22;q12)	*EWSR1-NR4A3*
	t(9;17)(q22;q11)	*TAF1168-NR4A3*
	t(9;15)(q22;q21)	*TCF12-NR4A3*
Fibrosarcoma, infantile	t(12;15)(p13;q26)	*ETV6-NTRK3*
	Trisomies 8, 11, 17, and 20	
Gastrointestinal stromal tumor		*KIT, PDGFRA* mutations
Inflammatory myofibroblastic tumor	2p23 rearrangement	*ALK* fusions with various genes
Leiomyosarcoma	Deletion of 1p	
Liposarcoma		
Well-differentiated	Ring form of chromosome 12	12q13-15 amplicon including *MDM2, CDK4, HMGA2*
Dedifferentiated	Ring forms and complex changes	12q14 amplicon including *MDM2, CDK4, HMGA2, ASK1*, and *JUN* amplification
Spindle cell		*RB1* deletion
Myxoid/round cell	t(12;16)(q13;p11), t(12;22)(q13;q12)	*FUS-DDIT3*
	t(12;22)(q13;q12)	*EWSR1-DDIT3*
Pleomorphic	Complex changes, multiple karyotypes	
Low-grade fibromyxoid sarcoma	t(7;16)(q33;p11)	*FUS-CREB3L2*
		FUS-CREB3L1 (in a small number of cases)
Malignant rhabdoid tumor	Deletion of 22q	*INI1* inactivation
Malignant peripheral nerve sheath tumor	Complex changes	*NF1* inactivation, *INK4A* deletion
Myxofibrosarcoma	Ring form of chromosome 12, complex changes	
Myxoinflammatory fibroblastic sarcoma	t(1;10)(p22;q24), t(2;6)(q31;p21.3)	
Rhabdomyosarcoma		
Embryonal	Trisomies 2q, 8, and 20	Loss of heterozygosity at 11p15
Alveolar	t(1;13)(p36;q14)	*PAX7-FKHR*
	t(2;13)(q35;q14)	*PAX3-FKHR*
Synovial sarcoma	t(X;18)(p11;q11)	*SS18-SSX1, SS18-SSX2*
		SS18-SSX4 (very rarely)
	t(X;20)(p11;q13)	*SS18L1-SSX1*

Genetic Findings in Benign and Intermediate Soft Tissue Tumors

Histologic Type	Translocation of Rearrangement	Fusion Gene or Other Feature
Adipose tumors		
Lipoma	t(3;12)(q27-28;q15), *HMGA2* rearrangements at 12q15	*HMGA2-LPP* fusion
Spindle cell and pleomorphic lipoma	Loss of 13q12, 16q13, polysomy of 12	*RB*/13q14 allelic loss
Hibernoma	11q13 rearrangements	
Lipoblastoma	8q11-13 rearrangements	*PLAG1-HAS2*
Chondroid lipoma	t(11;16)(q13;p12-13)	
Cellular angiofibroma	Loss at 13q	*RB*/13q14 allelic loss
Chondroma of soft tissue	*HMGA2* rearrangements	
Desmoplastic fibroblastoma	t(2;11)(q31;q12)	
Fibroma of tendon sheath	t(2;11)(q31-32;q12)	
Fibromatosis		
Sporadic deep		*CTNNB1* (β-catenin gene) mutations
In familial adenomatous polyposis		Germline *APC* inactivating mutations
Leiomyoma		
Cutaneous hereditary	1q42.3-q43 rearrangements	*MCUL-1* mutations (fumarate hydratase)
Uterine	*HMGA2* rearrangements	
Nerve sheath tumors		
Neurofibroma	9p21-22 rearrangements	*NF1* deletion (17q11) in neurofibromatosis type 1
Perineurioma	22q11.2-12 rearrangements	*NF2* loss
Sclerosing perineurioma	t(2;10)(p23;q24), monosomy 10	
Schwannoma	Changes in 22, 7, X, Y	*NF2* mutations in neurofibromatosis type 2
Mammary-type myofibroblastoma	Partial monosomy of 13q and 16q	Allelic loss at *RB*/13q14 and *FKHR*/13q14
Myoepithelioma	t(1;22)(q23;q12)	*EWSR1-PBX*
	t(19;22)(q13;q12)	*EWSR1-ZNF444*
		EWSR1-POU5F1
Plexiform fibrohistiocytic tumor	t(4;15)(q21;q15)	
Solitary fibrous tumor	12q15 rearrangements	
	t(8;12)(p11.2;q24.3)	
	t(12;17)(q15;q23)	
Tenosynovial giant cell tumor	t(1;2)(2p:13q)	*CSF1-COL6A3*

PROTOCOL FOR THE EXAMINATION OF SOFT TISSUE TUMORS

Soft Tissue: Biopsy

Surgical Pathology Cancer Case Summary (Checklist)

Procedure

___ Core needle biopsy

___ Incisional biopsy

___ Other (specify): ___________________________

___ Not specified

Tumor Site

___ Specify (if known) : ___________________________

___ Not specified

Tumor Size

Greatest dimension: _________ cm

*Additional dimensions: _________ x _________ cm

___ Cannot be determined

Macroscopic Extent of Tumor (select all that apply)

___ Superficial

  ___ Dermal

  ___ Subcutaneous/suprafascial

___ Deep

  ___ Fascial

  ___ Subfascial

  ___ Intramuscular

  ___ Mediastinal

  ___ Intraabdominal

  ___ Retroperitoneal

  ___ Head and neck

  ___ Other (specify): ___________________________

___ Cannot be determined

Histologic Type (World Health Organization [WHO] Classification of Soft Tissue Tumors)

Specify: ___________________________

___ Cannot be determined

Mitotic Rate

Specify: _________ /10 high-power fields (HPF)

(1 HPF x 400 = 0.1734 mm²; x40 objective; most proliferative area)

Necrosis

___ Not identified

___ Present

  Extent: _________ %

___ Cannot be determined

Histologic Grade (French Federation of Cancer Centers Sarcoma Group [FNCLCC])

___ Grade 1

___ Grade 2

___ Grade 3

___ Ungraded sarcoma

___ Cannot be determined

Margins (for excisional biopsy only)

___ Cannot be assessed

___ Margins negative for sarcoma

  Distance of sarcoma from closest margin: _________ cm

  Specify margin: ___________________________

  Specify other close (< 2 cm) margin(s): ___________________________

____ Margin(s) positive for sarcoma

Specify margin(s): ____________________________

*Lymph-Vascular Invasion

*____ Not identified

*____ Present

*____ Indeterminate

*Additional Pathologic Findings

*Specify: ____________________________

Ancillary Studies

Immunohistochemistry

Specify: ____________________________

____ Not performed

Cytogenetics

Specify: ____________________________

____ Not performed

Molecular pathology

Specify: ____________________________

____ Not performed

Pre-biopsy Treatment

____ No therapy

____ Chemotherapy performed

____ Radiation therapy performed

____ Therapy performed, type not specified

____ Unknown

Treatment Effect

____ Not identified

____ Present

*Specify percentage of viable tumor: ________ %

____ Cannot be determined

**Data elements with asterisks are not required. However, these elements may be clinically important but are not yet validated or regularly used in patient management. Adapted with permission from College of American Pathologists, "Protocol for the Examination of Specimens from Patients with Tumors of Soft Tissue." Web posting date October 2009, www.cap.org.*

Soft Tissue: Resection

Surgical Pathology Case Summary (Checklist)

Procedure

____ Intralesional resection

____ Marginal resection

____ Wide resection

____ Radical resection

____ Other (specify): ____________________________

____ Not specified

Tumor Site

Specify (if known): ____________________________

____ Not specified

Tumor Size

Greatest dimension: ________ cm

*Additional dimensions: ________ x ________ cm

____ Cannot be determined

Macroscopic Extent of Tumor (select all that apply)

____ Superficial

____ Dermal

____ Subcutaneous/suprafascial

PROTOCOL FOR THE EXAMINATION OF SOFT TISSUE TUMORS

___ Deep
  ___ Fascial
  ___ Subfascial
  ___ Intramuscular
  ___ Mediastinal
  ___ Intra-abdominal
  ___ Retroperitoneal
  ___ Head and neck
  ___ Other (specify): ___________________________
___ Cannot be determined

Histologic Type (World Health Organization [WHO] Classification of Soft Tissue Tumors)

Specify: ___________________________
___ Cannot be determined

Mitotic Rate

Specify: _________ /10 high-power fields (HPF)
(1HPF x 400 = 0.1734 mm²; x40 objective; most proliferative area)

Necrosis

___ Not identified
___ Present
  Extent: _________ %

Histologic Grade (French Federation of Cancer Centers Sarcoma Group [FNCLCC])

___ Grade 1
___ Grade 2
___ Grade 3
___ Ungraded sarcoma
___ Cannot be determined

Margins

___ Cannot be assessed
___ Margins negative for sarcoma
  Distance of sarcoma from closest margin: _________ cm
  Specify margin: ___________________________
  Specify other close (< 2 cm) margin(s): ___________________________
___ Margin(s) positive for sarcoma
  specify margin(s): ___________________________

****Lymph-Vascular Invasion***

*___ Not identified
*___ Present
*___ Indeterminate

Pathologic Staging (pTNM)

TNM descriptors (required only if applicable, select all that apply)
  ___ m (multiple)
  ___ r (recurrent)
  ___ y (post-treatment)

Primary tumor (pT)
  ___ pTX: Primary tumor cannot be assessed
  ___ pT0: No evidence of primary tumor
  ___ pT1a: Tumor ≤ 5 cm in greatest dimension, superficial tumor
  ___ pT1b: Tumor ≤ 5 cm in greatest dimension, deep tumor
  ___ pT2a: Tumor > 5 cm in greatest dimension, superficial tumor
  ___ pT2b: Tumor > 5 cm in greatest dimension, deep tumor

Regional lymph nodes (pN)
  ___ pNX: Regional lymph nodes cannot be assessed

PROTOCOL FOR THE EXAMINATION OF SOFT TISSUE TUMORS

____ pN0: No regional lymph node metastasis

____ pN1: Regional lymph node metastasis

Specify: Number examined: __________

Number positive: __________

Distant metastasis (pM)

____ Not applicable

____ pM1: Distant metastasis

*Specify site(s), if known: ______________________________

**Additional Pathologic Findings*

*Specify: ______________________________

Ancillary Studies

Immunohistochemistry

Specify: ______________________________

____ Not performed

Cytogenetics

Specify: ______________________________

____ Not performed

Molecular pathology

Specify: ______________________________

____ Not performed

Pre-resection Treatment (select all that apply)

____ No therapy

____ Chemotherapy performed

____ Radiation therapy performed

____ Therapy performed, type not specified

____ Unknown

Treatment Effect

____ Not identified

____ Present

*Specify percentage of viable tumor: __________ %

____ Cannot be determined

**Data elements with asterisks are not required. However, these elements may be clinically important but are not yet validated or regularly used in patient management. Adapted with permission from College of American Pathologists, "Protocol for the Examination of Specimens from Patients with Tumors of Soft Tissue." Web posting date October 2009, www.cap.org.*

PROTOCOL FOR THE EXAMINATION OF SOFT TISSUE TUMORS

Soft Tissue Sarcoma Staging

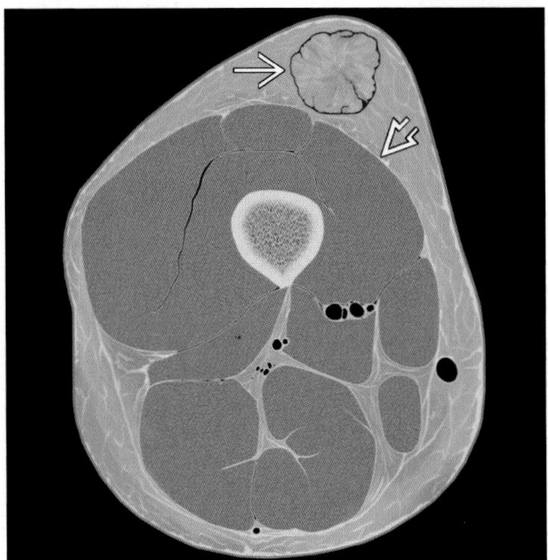

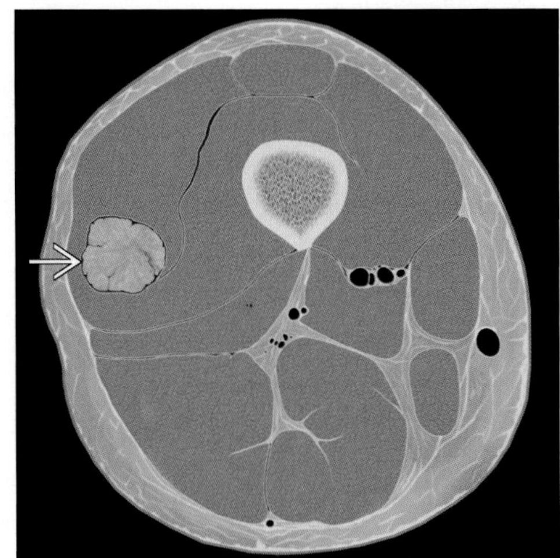

(Left) *Axial graphic shows a T1a soft tissue sarcoma ➡. These tumors are 5 cm or less in greatest dimension. The "a" designation refers to the tumor being located superficial to, and not involving, deep fascia ➡.* ***(Right)*** *Axial graphic shows a T1b soft tissue sarcoma ➡. These lesions are less than or equal to 5 cm in diameter. The "b" designation refers to a deep lesion. Involvement of superficial fascia or a location exclusively deep to the fascia is defined as a deep tumor.*

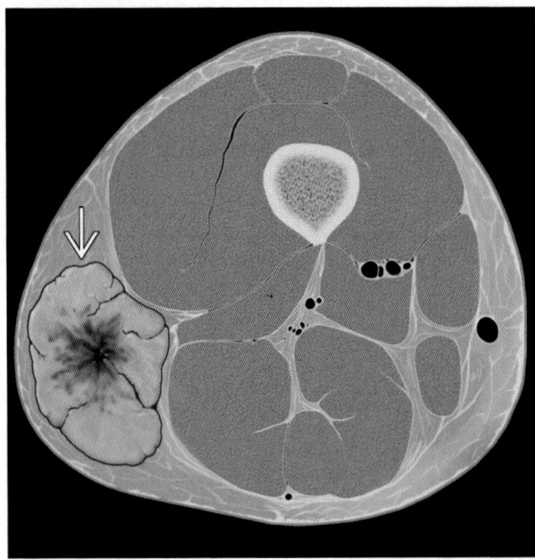

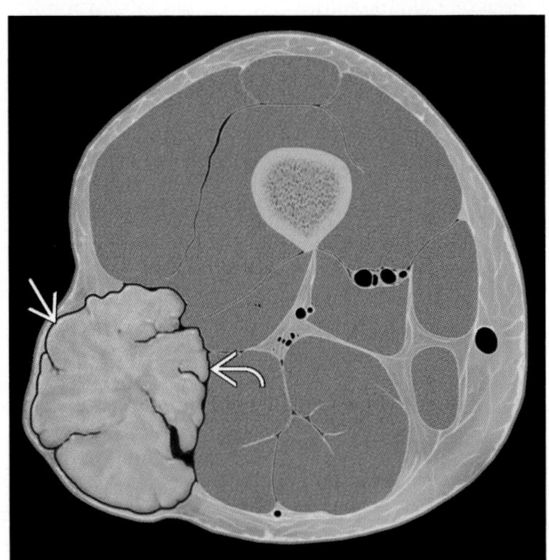

(Left) *Axial graphic shows a T2a soft tissue sarcoma ➡. These tumors are over 5 cm in greatest dimension. The "a" designation indicates that the mass is located superficial to the superficial fascia, without any fascial involvement.* ***(Right)*** *Axial graphic shows a T2b soft tissue sarcoma ➡, > 5 cm. Although it is located superficial to the deep fascia ➡, the absence of fat between tumor and fascia is suspicious for fascial involvement, indicating designation as a deep lesion.*

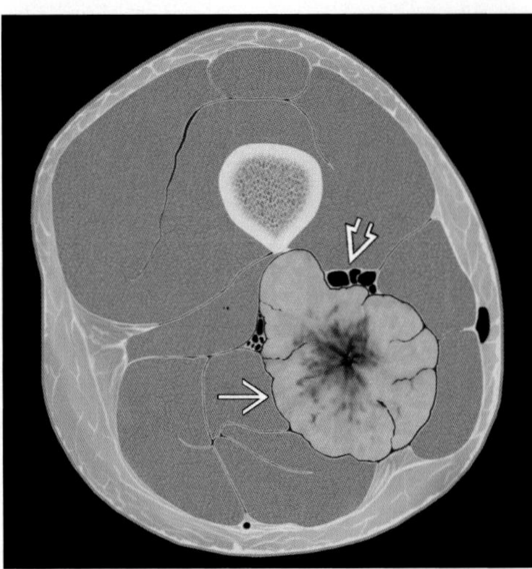

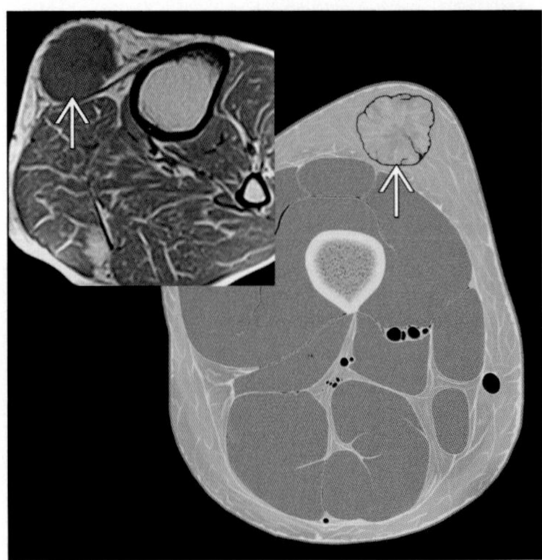

(Left) *Axial graphic shows another type of T2b soft tissue sarcoma ➡. This tumor is > 5 cm and is located beneath deep fascia. Note that this tumor abuts neurovascular structures ➡. Neurovascular involvement is not included in the current staging system.* ***(Right)*** *Axial graphic and MR of stage 1 soft tissue sarcoma. Stage 1 soft tissue sarcoma is always low grade. It can be any size and may be located either superficial or deep to the fascia. A T1a mass ➡ is shown in this example.*

Soft Tissue Sarcoma Staging

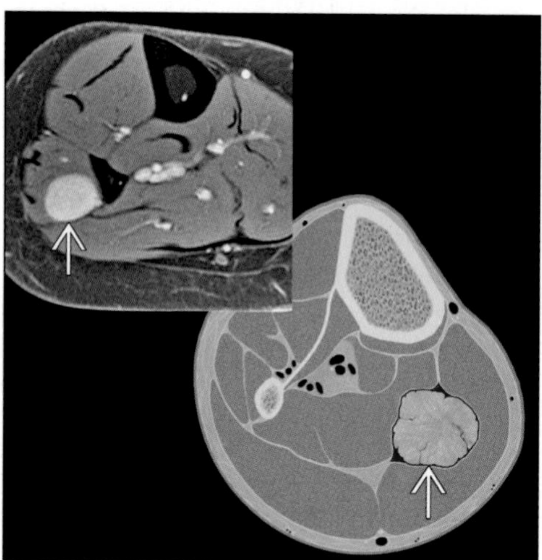

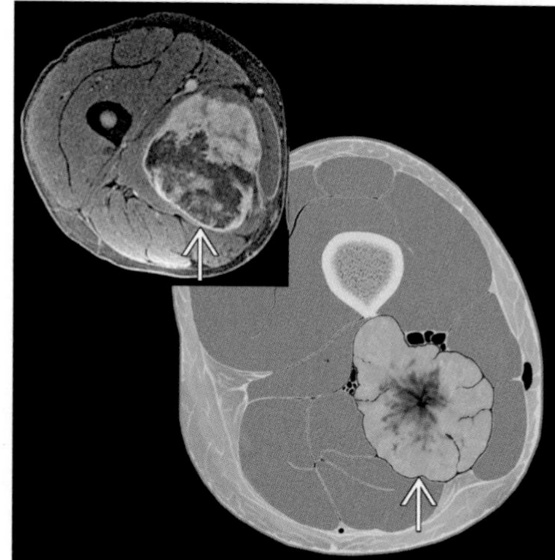

(Left) *Axial graphic and MR show a stage II soft tissue sarcoma. These lesions are all G2 or G3 tumors. If the mass is 5 cm or less, it may be either G2 or G3 and may be located superficial (T1a) or deep (T1b ➡) to the fascia. However, T2 tumors are > 5 cm.* ***(Right)*** *Axial graphic and MR show stage III sarcoma. These tumors are > 5 cm, superficial (T2a) or deep (T2b ➡) to the deep fascia, and high-grade (G3). Nodal metastases, with any lesion size, location, or grade, is also stage III.*

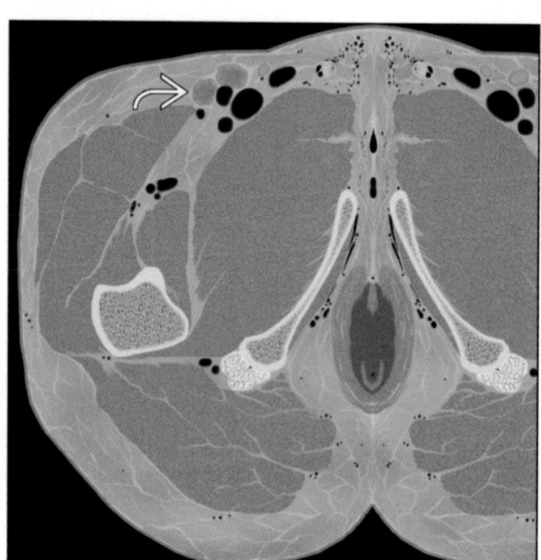

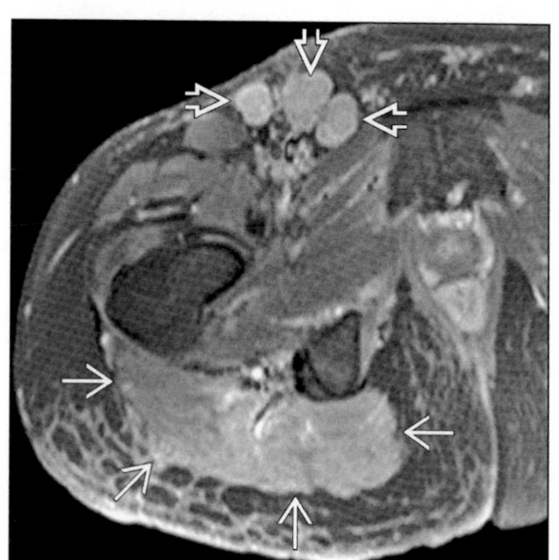

(Left) *Axial graphic through the low pelvis shows inguinal adenopathy ➡. The presence of involved lymph nodes makes this stage III disease. The primary tumor can be any size or grade and at any depth.* ***(Right)*** *Axial MR with contrast shows an abnormal gluteus maximus muscle ➡, which was infiltrated with tumor. Note the prominent inguinal adenopathy ➡.*

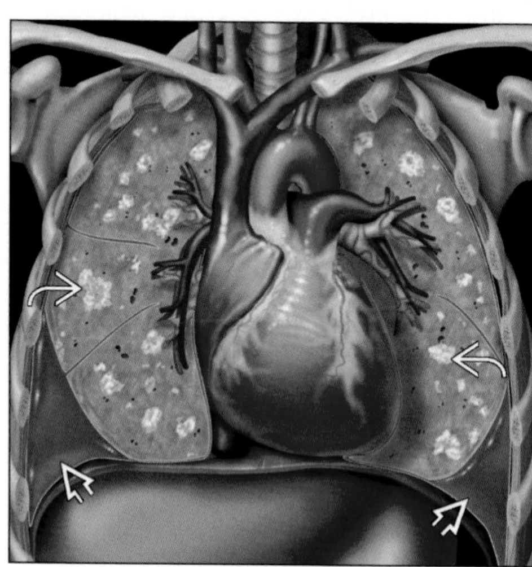

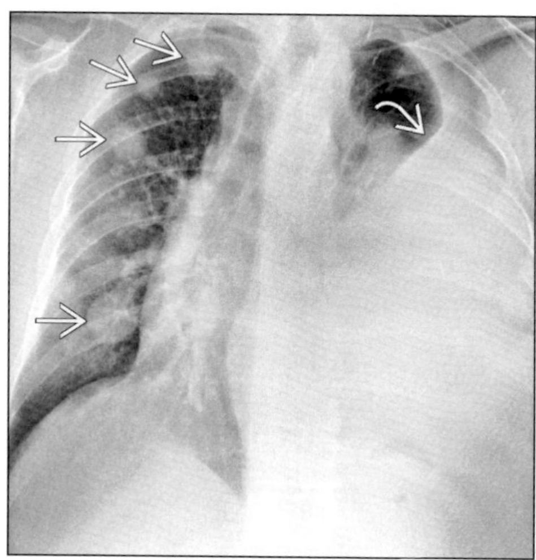

(Left) *Coronal graphic through the lungs demonstrates multiple bilateral pulmonary metastases ➡ and malignant pleural effusions ➡. The presence of distant metastases makes this stage IV disease. Stage IV primary tumors can be any size, have any depth, and have any histologic grade.* ***(Right)*** *Chest radiograph in a patient with a malignant nerve sheath tumor shows multiple pulmonary metastases ➡ and a large malignant effusion ➡ filling the left hemithorax.*

SOFT TISSUE IMMUNOHISTOCHEMISTRY

Immunohistochemistry of Selected Spindle Cell Soft Tissue Tumors

Tumor	CD34	CK	SMA	S100	Desmin	Other Diagnostic Markers
Angiosarcoma	+	±	-	-	-	CD31, FLI-1, FVIIIRAg
Dermatofibrosarcoma	+	-	-	+ (Bednar)	-	
Follicular dendritic cell sarcoma	-	-	-	+	-	CD21, CD23, CD35, fascin, D2-40
Gastrointestinal stromal tumor	+	-	+	-	±	CD117, DOG1, H-caldesmon
Inflammatory myofibroblastic tumor	-	±	+	-	±	ALK (50%)
Kaposi sarcoma	+	-	-	-	-	CD31, HHV8
Leiomyosarcoma	-	±	+	-	+	H-caldesmon, SMM
Myofibrosarcoma	-	-	+	-	±	Calponin, H-caldesmon (-)
Malignant peripheral nerve sheath tumor	±	±	-	±	+ (Triton)	
Solitary fibrous tumor	+	-	-	-	-	Bcl-2, CD99, CD56
Spindle cell carcinoma	-	+	+	-	-	EMA, CK5/6, CK34βE12
Synovial sarcoma	-	+	-	±	-	EMA, TLE1, CD99, CD56

± = Positive in some cases.

Immunohistochemistry of Selected Epithelioid Cell Soft Tissue Tumors

Antibody	Epithelioid Sarcoma	Epithelioid MPNST	Epithelioid Angiosarcoma	Anaplastic Large Cell Lymphoma	Carcinoma	Melanoma
CK-PAN	+	-	+	-*	+	-*
EMA	+	-*	-*	+	+	-
S100	-	+	-	-	±	+
CD34	±	-	±	-	-	-
CD31	-	-	+	-	-	-
Desmin	-	-	-	-	-	-*
SMA	+	-	-	-	-	-
INI1	-	±	+	+	+	+
p63	-	-	-	-	+	-
CD30	-	-*	-	+	-	-
CD45	-	-	-	+	-	-

** Rarely positive. MPNST = malignant peripheral nerve sheath tumor.*

Immunohistochemistry of Selected Small Round Cell Tumors

Antibody	Ewing Sarcoma	Desmoplastic SRCT	Neuroblastoma	Alveolar RMS	PD SS	Small Cell Carcinoma	Lymphoma
CD99	+	-	-	±	-	-	±
NF	±	+	+	-	±	-	-
Desmin	-*	+ dot	-	+	-	-	-
Myogenin	-	-	-	+	-	-	-
CD56	-	+	+	+	+	+	±
Chromogranin	-	-*	+	-	-	±	-
Synaptophysin	±	±	+	-	-	±	-
CK	+*	+ dot	-	-	+	+ dot	-
EMA	-	-	-	-	+	+	-
Bcl-2	-	-	-	±	+	±	±
CD45	-	-	-	-	-	-	+
Other positives	FLI-1	WT1 (C-terminal)	NB84	MYO-D1	TLE1	TTF-1	TdT (lymphoblastic)

** Rarely positive. SRCT = small round cell tumor; RMS = rhabdomyosarcoma; PD SS = poorly differentiated synovial sarcoma.*

Immunohistochemistry of Selected Pleomorphic Soft Tissue Tumors

Tumor	CD34	SMA	Desmin	H-Caldesmon	Myogenin	Cytokeratin
Myofibrosarcoma	-	+	-	-	-	-
Leiomyosarcoma	-	+	+	+	-	-
Rhabdomyosarcoma	-	±	+	-	+	-
Sarcomatoid carcinoma	-	±	-	-	-	+
Pleomorphic undifferentiated sarcoma	±	±	±	-	-	-*

** Rarely positive; any CK positivity should raise suspicion of carcinoma, especially in organ-based tumors.*

Adipose Tissue Lesions

Benign

Intermediate

Malignant

OVERVIEW OF LIPOBLASTS AND MIMICS

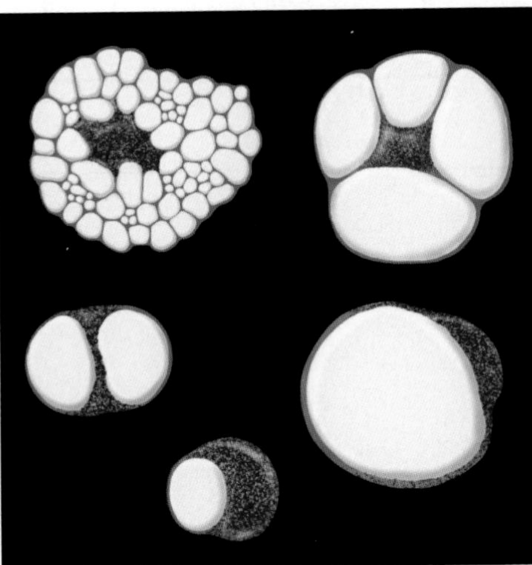

Lipoblasts come in a variety of sizes and shapes. The cytoplasm is filled with lipid that appears as 1 or multiple clean, punched-out vacuoles that indent and scallop the nucleus.

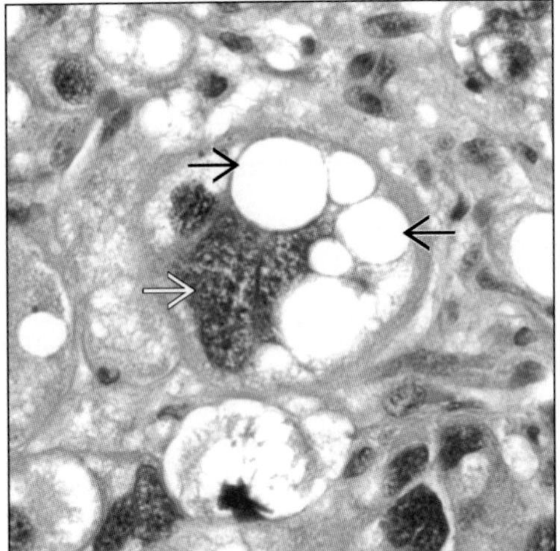

Malignant lipoblasts are required to diagnose pleomorphic liposarcoma. This lipoblast has a large hyperchromatic nucleus ➡ sharply indented by multiple lipid-filled vacuoles ➡.

LIPOBLASTS

Definitions

- Lipoblasts are embryonic mesenchymal cells that develop into fat cells
  - Wide spectrum of cell morphology
    - Primitive spindle cells with small cytoplasmic vacuoles
    - Univacuolated or multivacuolated round cells
    - Signet ring cells
- Neoplastic lipoblasts morphologically recapitulate developmental stages of lipogenesis
  - Malignant lipoblasts characterized by nuclear hyperchromasia and atypia
    - Peripheral crescentic nuclei
    - Multilobated nuclei
    - Multinucleated giant lipoblasts

Background

- Lipoblasts are not required for diagnosing all types of liposarcomas
  - Atypical lipomatous tumor/well-differentiated liposarcoma
    - Lipoblast often present but not required for diagnosis
    - Defined by presence of atypical stromal cells
  - Myxoid/round cell liposarcoma
    - Highly variable numbers of lipoblasts present in a given tumor
    - Wide spectrum in appearance of lipoblasts
    - Univacuolated round cells, multivacuolated cells, signet ring cells
  - Pleomorphic liposarcoma
    - Identification of lipoblasts is required for diagnosis
    - Often contain very large pleomorphic and multinucleated lipoblasts
    - Lipoblasts sometimes sparse
- Lipoblasts are not pathognomonic of liposarcoma
  - Lipoblasts can be found in benign tumors
    - e.g., lipoblastoma
    - e.g., lipoblastic nerve sheath tumor

Criteria for Identifying Malignant Lipoblast

- Nucleus
  - Hyperchromatic
  - Enlarged
  - Indented or sharply scalloped
- Cytoplasm
  - Lipid-forming
  - Clean, punched-out vacuoles
  - Univacuolated or multivacuolated
- Present within appropriate histological milieu

LIPOBLAST MIMICS (PSEUDOLIPOBLASTS)

Background

- Many nonneoplastic and neoplastic conditions have vacuolated cells that mimic lipoblasts
- Cells that mimic lipoblasts
  - Vacuolated and foamy macrophages
  - Foreign-body macrophages
  - Atrophic adipocytes
  - Hydropic cells
  - Lipid-filled cells
  - Glycogen-filled cells
  - Mucin-filled cells
- Important to carefully evaluate cytological features and histological setting to distinguish lipoblast mimics from true lipoblasts

Common Nonneoplastic Conditions with Lipoblast Mimics

- Fat necrosis
- Atrophic fat
- Xanthoma and xanthelasma
- Xanthogranulomatous inflammation
- Silicone granuloma

Morphological Criteria for Identifying Malignant Lipoblasts

Tissue Component	Cytoarchitectural Features
Nucleus	Hyperchromatic, indented or sharply scalloped
Cytoplasm	Lipid-rich with clean, punched-out vacuoles
Histology	Occurring in appropriate histological milieu

- Arthroplasty reaction

Neoplasms with Lipoblast Mimics

- Lipoma with atrophic changes or fat necrosis
- Hibernoma
  - Lipoma-like hibernoma
- Lipofibromatosis
- Myxofibrosarcoma
- Myxoinflammatory fibroblastic sarcoma
- Chondroid lipoma
- Spindle cell hemangioma
- Epithelioid hemangioendothelioma
- Composite hemangioendothelioma
- Angiomyolipoma
- Chordoma (physaliferous cells)
- Undifferentiated pleomorphic sarcoma with phagocytosis or hydropic change
- Rhabdomyosarcoma with glycogenated cells ("spider cells")
- Signet ring cell tumors
  - Carcinoma
  - Melanoma
  - Lymphoma
- Phyllodes tumor
- Solitary fibrous tumor
- Pleomorphic hyalinizing angiectatic tumor
- Pseudomyxoma

SELECTED REFERENCES

1. Coffin CM et al: Lipoblastoma (LPB): a clinicopathologic and immunohistochemical analysis of 59 cases. Am J Surg Pathol. 33(11):1705-12, 2009
2. Rao AC et al: Periductal stromal sarcoma of breast with lipoblast-like cells: a case report with review of literature. Indian J Pathol Microbiol. 51(2):252-4, 2008
3. Plaza JA et al: Lipoblastic nerve sheath tumors: report of a distinctive variant of neural soft tissue neoplasm with adipocytic differentiation. Am J Surg Pathol. 30(3):337-44, 2006
4. Suarez-Vilela D et al: Lipoblast-like cells in early pleomorphic hyalinizing angiectatic tumor. Am J Surg Pathol. 29(9):1257-9; author reply 1259, 2005
5. Oda Y et al: Low-grade fibromyxoid sarcoma versus low-grade myxofibrosarcoma in the extremities and trunk. A comparison of clinicopathological and immunohistochemical features. Histopathology. 45(1):29-38, 2004
6. Cruz J et al: Primary cutaneous malignant melanoma with lipoblast-like cells. Arch Pathol Lab Med. 127(3):370-1, 2003
7. Furlong MA et al: The morphologic spectrum of hibernoma: a clinicopathologic study of 170 cases. Am J Surg Pathol. 25(6):809-14, 2001
8. Nayler SJ et al: Composite hemangioendothelioma: a complex, low-grade vascular lesion mimicking angiosarcoma. Am J Surg Pathol. 24(3):352-61, 2000
9. Meis-Kindblom JM et al: Acral myxoinflammatory fibroblastic sarcoma: a low-grade tumor of the hands and feet. Am J Surg Pathol. 22(8):911-24, 1998
10. Persson S et al: Classical and chondroid chordoma. A light-microscopic, histochemical, ultrastructural and immunohistochemical analysis of the various cell types. Pathol Res Pract. 187(7):828-38, 1991
11. Lodding P et al: Metastases of malignant melanoma simulating soft tissue sarcoma. A clinico-pathological, light- and electron microscopic and immunohistochemical study of 21 cases. Virchows Arch A Pathol Anat Histopathol. 417(5):377-88, 1990
12. Kim H et al: Signet ring cell lymphoma. A rare morphologic and functional expression of nodular (follicular) lymphoma. Am J Surg Pathol. 2(2):119-32, 1978

IMAGE GALLERY

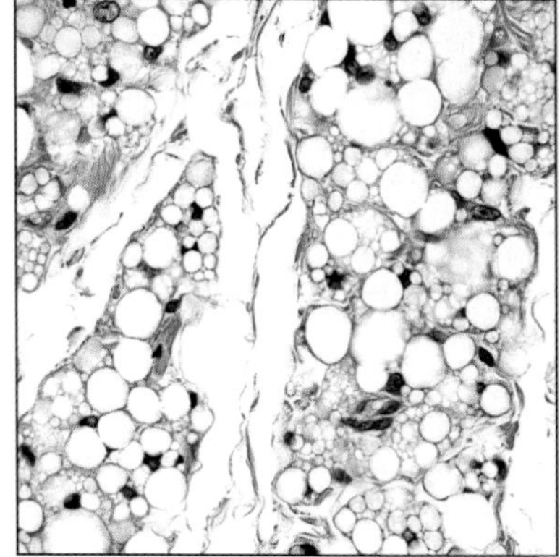

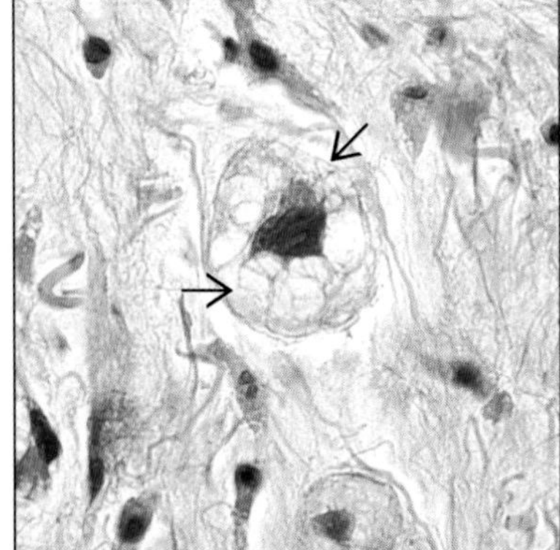

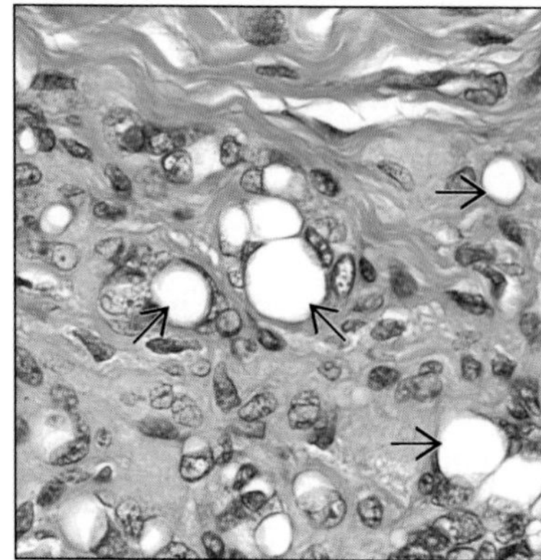

(Left) *Brown fat cells, as in this hibernoma, contain multiple lipid vacuoles and can mimic lipoblasts. These cells, however, lack nuclear atypia.* ***(Center)*** *Pseudolipoblasts are common in myxofibrosarcoma. They differ from true lipoblasts as the vacuoles are not clean and punched-out. Instead, they contain fibrillary mucoid material* →. ***(Right)*** *Vascular neoplasms, such as this composite hemangioendothelioma, have vacuolated endothelial cells* → *that mimic lipoblasts.*

LIPOMA

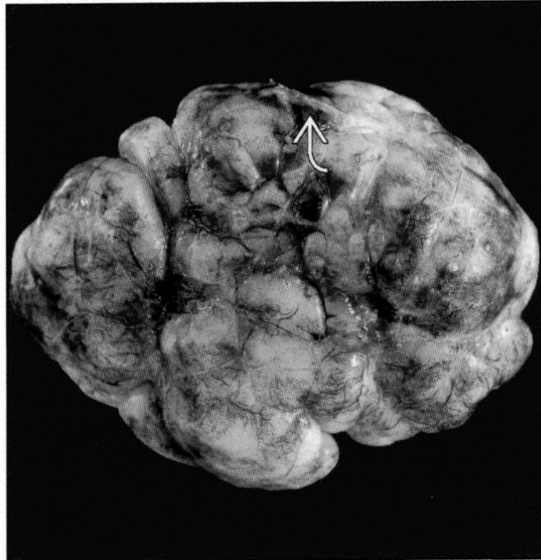

Lipomas are surrounded by a thin, delicate, and transparent capsule ➡ and often show a lobulated appearance.

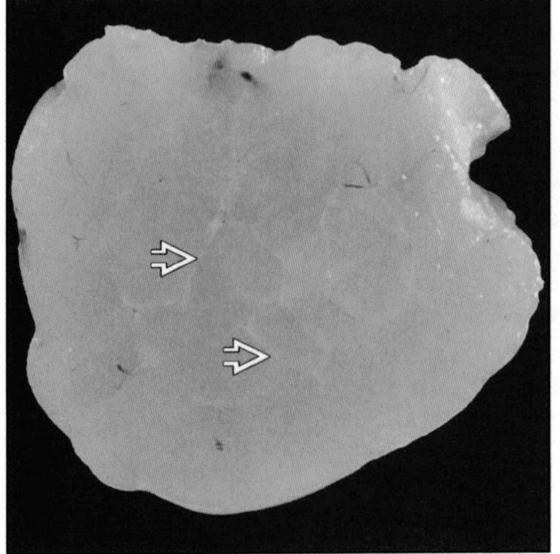

The cut surface of lipomas is homogeneous, yellow, and greasy. Note the delicate fibrous septa ➡, which separate the lesion into lobules.

TERMINOLOGY

Definitions

- Benign tumor of mature white adipocytes

ETIOLOGY/PATHOGENESIS

Unknown

- Although etiology is unknown, lipomas tend to occur more commonly in obese individuals

CLINICAL ISSUES

Presentation

- Painless mass
  - Large lesions may be painful

Treatment

- Surgical excision is curative

Prognosis

- Recurrences in < 5% cases
- Higher recurrence rate in intramuscular lipoma

IMAGE FINDINGS

Radiographic Findings

- Soft tissue mass isodense to subcutaneous tissue
- Delicate fibrous strands may be present, particularly in larger lesions

MACROSCOPIC FEATURES

General Features

- Most common between 40-60 years of age
- Located in subcutaneous or deep soft tissue
- Approximately 5% may be multiple

Gross Features

- Well circumscribed
- Delicate capsule
- Yellow, greasy cut surface
- Myxoid change, bone, or cartilage may be present in some variants
- Infiltrative margins may be present in intramuscular lipoma
- Nodular and papillary appearance seen in lipoma arborescence involving synovium

MICROSCOPIC PATHOLOGY

Histologic Features

- Lobules of mature adipocytes
- Minimal variation in adipocytic size
- Foci of fat necrosis or hemorrhage may be present

Cytologic Features

- Adipocytes with peripheral flattened nucleus
- No nuclear atypia

Variants

- Additional mesenchymal component may be present in some lipomas
  - Abundant fibrous tissue: Fibrolipoma
    - Sclerotic lipoma is variant with predilection for scalp and hands in young men
  - Cartilage: Chondrolipoma
    - Mature hyaline cartilage admixed with adipose tissue
    - Should be distinguished from chondroid lipoma, which is a distinct entity
  - Bone: Osteolipoma
    - Rare
  - Myxoid stromal change: Myxolipoma
    - Some myxolipomas may have prominent vascular component (**angiomyxolipoma**)

Key Facts

Terminology
- Benign tumor of mature white adipocytes

Clinical Issues
- Surgical excision is curative
- Higher recurrence rate in intramuscular lipoma

Macroscopic Features
- Most common between 40-60 years of age
- Approximately 5% may be multiple
- Well circumscribed with delicate capsule
- Yellow, greasy cut surface

Microscopic Pathology
- Lobules of mature adipocytes with minimal size variation
- No nuclear atypia

Ancillary Tests
- Lipomas are cytogenetically heterogeneous

    - Myxolipomas need to be distinguished from myxomas and myxoid liposarcomas
  - Smooth muscle: Myolipoma
    - Considered a distinct entity
- Intramuscular lipoma
  - May have infiltrative margins
  - Entrapped skeletal muscle at periphery
  - Also known as "infiltrating lipoma"
  - Mature adipocytes with no atypia
  - Recurrences may occur in about 15% cases

ANCILLARY TESTS

Immunohistochemistry
- Stain like mature adipocytes (S100 and LEP positive)

Cytogenetics
- Lipomas are cytogenetically heterogeneous
- Common anomalies include
  - Aberrations involving 12q13-15
  - Rearrangements involving 6p21-23
  - Deletions involving 13q

DIFFERENTIAL DIAGNOSIS

Atypical Lipomatous Tumor (ALT)
- Deep-seated intramuscular lipomas may be mistaken for ALT
- Intramuscular lipomas show no nuclear atypia

Myxoid Liposarcoma (MLS)
- Myxolipomas may be mistaken for MLS
- Myxolipomas lack lipoblasts and plexiform vasculature seen in MLS

DIAGNOSTIC CHECKLIST

Pathologic Interpretation Pearls
- Uniform size of adipocytes, delicate fibrous septa, and lack of nuclear atypia are key to diagnosis

SELECTED REFERENCES

1. Gaskin CM et al: Lipomas, lipoma variants, and well-differentiated liposarcomas (atypical lipomas): results of MRI evaluations of 126 consecutive fatty masses. AJR Am J Roentgenol. 182(3):733-9, 2004
2. Tardío JC et al: Angiomyxolipoma (vascular myxolipoma) of subcutaneous tissue. Am J Dermatopathol. 26(3):222-4, 2004
3. Willén H et al: Comparison of chromosomal patterns with clinical features in 165 lipomas: a report of the CHAMP study group. Cancer Genet Cytogenet. 102(1):46-9, 1998
4. Zelger BG et al: Sclerotic lipoma: lipomas simulating sclerotic fibroma. Histopathology. 31(2):174-81, 1997
5. Fletcher CD et al: Intramuscular and intermuscular lipoma: neglected diagnoses. Histopathology. 12(3):275-87, 1988

IMAGE GALLERY

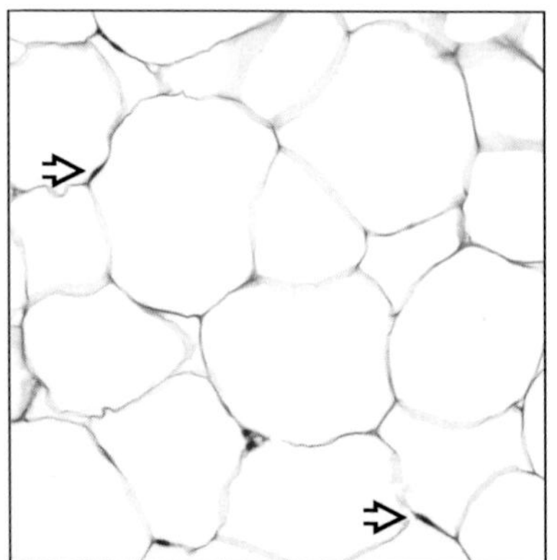

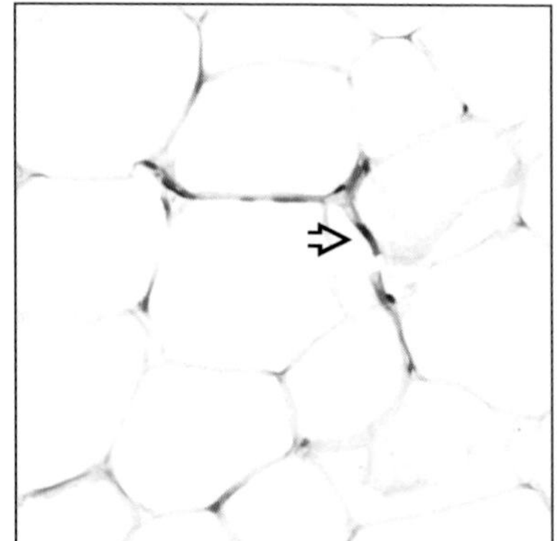

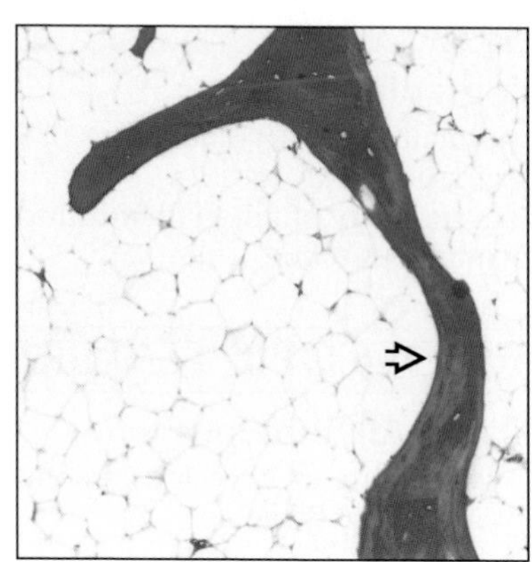

(Left) *Lipomas are composed of mature white adipocytes, which show minimal size variation. The tumor cells show a peripherally flattened nucleus ➢ without any atypia.* ***(Center)*** *The blood vessels in lipomas are delicate and often compressed ➢ between distended adipocytes, making them inconspicuous.* ***(Right)*** *Additional mesenchymal components may be present in some lipomas. Mature lamellar bone ➢ is seen here in this example of an osteolipoma.*

LIPOMATOSIS

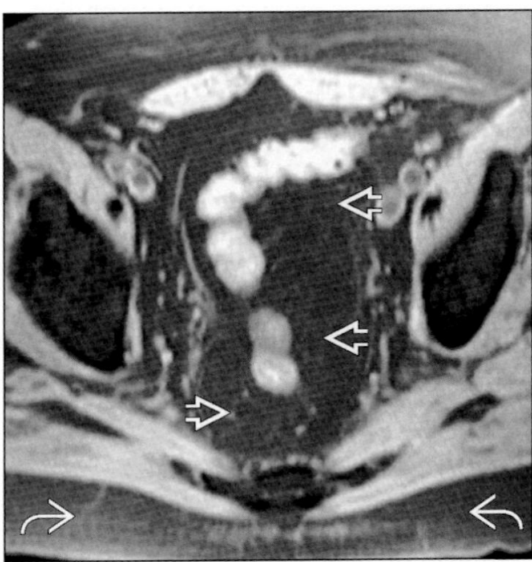

Axial MR shows pelvic lipomatosis ➡ compressing the rectosigmoid colon. Note identical signal intensity of lesional area to subcutaneous fat ➡.

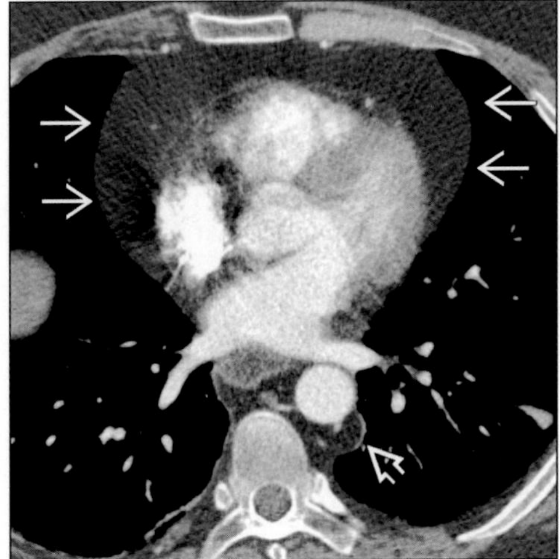

Axial CT shows mediastinal lipomatosis with homogeneous mediastinal fat surrounding the pericardium ➡ and increased fat in the posterior mediastinum ➡.

TERMINOLOGY

Definitions

- Diffuse overgrowth of mature adipose tissue

CLINICAL ISSUES

Presentation

- Painful or painless mass
    - May mimic a neoplasm
- Limb enlargement in extremity lesions
- Laryngeal obstruction, caval compression in mediastinal lipomatosis
- Bowel or bladder obstruction in pelvic lipomatosis

Treatment

- Palliative surgical resection of excessive adipose tissue
- Steroid lipomatosis may regress after source of increased steroids is removed

Prognosis

- Tendency for recurrence due to poor circumscription
- Laryngeal obstruction may prove fatal

IMAGE FINDINGS

Radiographic Findings

- Abnormally large accumulations of fat with poor margination
- Signal intensity of lesion identical to normal subcutaneous tissue

MACROSCOPIC FEATURES

Similar in All Subtypes

- Poorly marginated large accumulations of normal-appearing fatty tissue

Lipomatosis Subtypes

- Diffuse lipomatosis
    - Involves extremity or trunk diffusely
    - Usually affects children in 1st 2 years of life
    - May be associated with macrodactyly and gigantism
- Symmetric lipomatosis
    - Synonyms: Madelung disease, Launois-Bensaude syndrome
    - Massive fat deposition around neck (lipoma annulare colli)
    - Almost exclusively in middle-aged men
        - More common in those of Mediterranean descent
    - May extend around cheek, breast, upper arm
    - Mostly sporadic but may be familial
    - Point mutations in mitochondrial genes reported in symmetric lipomatosis
- Pelvic lipomatosis
    - Perirectal and perivesical regions involved
    - Most commonly affects black men in 3rd-4th decade
    - Rare in women
    - Association with cystitis cystica and cystitis glandularis
- Steroid lipomatosis
    - Source may be endogenous (as in Cushing disease) or exogenous (steroid therapy)
    - Unevenly distributed fatty deposits
        - Face, sternum, or back involved most commonly
- HIV-lipodystrophy
    - Related to use of protease inhibitors
    - Associated with diabetes
    - ↓ facial and extremity fat
    - Increased deposition on back and abdomen

MICROSCOPIC PATHOLOGY

Histologic Features

- Mature adipose tissue in sheets or lobules
- May infiltrate into skeletal muscle or underlying deeper structures

LIPOMATOSIS

Key Facts

Terminology

- Diffuse overgrowth of mature adipose tissue

Clinical Issues

- Presents as painless mass or with obstructive symptoms
- Tendency for recurrence due to poor circumscription
- Diffuse lipomatosis: Limbs or trunk in kids < 2 years
- Symmetric lipomatosis: Fat deposition around neck; middle-aged men of Mediterranean descent
- Pelvic lipomatosis: Typically in black men in 3rd-4th decade
- Steroid lipomatosis: Due to increased exogenous or endogenous steroids

Microscopic Pathology

- Mature adipose tissue in sheets or lobules
- May infiltrate into skeletal muscle or underlying deeper structures
- No nuclear atypia

Cytologic Features

- No nuclear atypia
- No lipoblasts

DIFFERENTIAL DIAGNOSIS

Intramuscular Lipoma (IML)

- IML is confined to muscle
- Nodular rather than diffuse overgrowth of adipose tissue seen in IML
- Entrapped skeletal muscle fibers present in both conditions (more in IML)

Dercum Disease

- Nodular or diffuse deposits of mature adipose tissue
- Confined to subcutaneous region
- Fatty deposits are painful and tender
- Mostly in postmenopausal women around thigh or pelvis

Atypical Lipomatous Tumor (ALT)

- Atypical stromal cells with hyperchromatic nuclei present in ALT
- Atypical multivacuolated lipoblasts present in ALT

DIAGNOSTIC CHECKLIST

Clinically Relevant Pathologic Features

- Gross appearance
    - Diffuse overgrowth of adipose tissue that, on imaging, has same signal as normal subcutaneous tissue

Pathologic Interpretation Pearls

- Morphologically normal adipose tissue that may infiltrate into underlying structures or skeletal muscle

SELECTED REFERENCES

1. Sözen S et al: The importance of re-evaluation in patients with cystitis glandularis associated with pelvic lipomatosis: a case report. Urol Oncol. 22(5):428-30, 2004
2. Klopstock T et al: Mitochondrial DNA mutations in multiple symmetric lipomatosis. Mol Cell Biochem. 174(1-2):271-5, 1997
3. Coode PE et al: Diffuse lipomatosis involving the thoracic and abdominal wall: CT features. J Comput Assist Tomogr. 15(2):341-3, 1991
4. Heyns CF: Pelvic lipomatosis: a review of its diagnosis and management. J Urol. 146(2):267-73, 1991
5. Klein FA et al: Pelvic lipomatosis: 35-year experience. J Urol. 139(5):998-1001, 1988
6. Shukla LW et al: Mediastinal lipomatosis: a complication of high dose steroid therapy in children. Pediatr Radiol. 19(1):57-8, 1988
7. Ruzicka T et al: Benign symmetric lipomatosis Launois-Bensaude. Report of ten cases and review of the literature. J Am Acad Dermatol. 17(4):663-74, 1987
8. Nixon HH et al: Congenital lipomatosis: a report of four cases. J Pediatr Surg. 6(6):742-5, 1971

IMAGE GALLERY

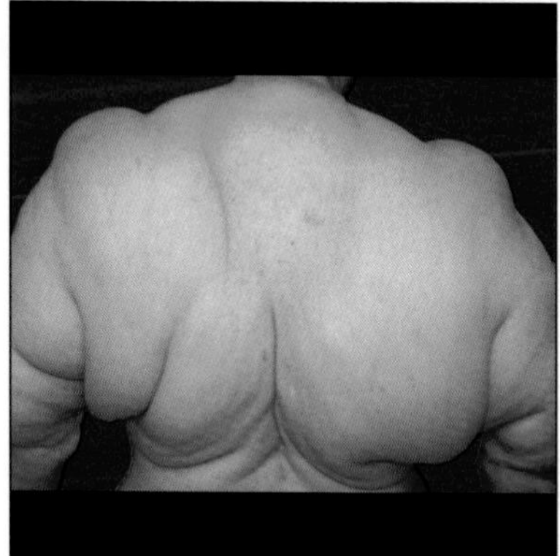

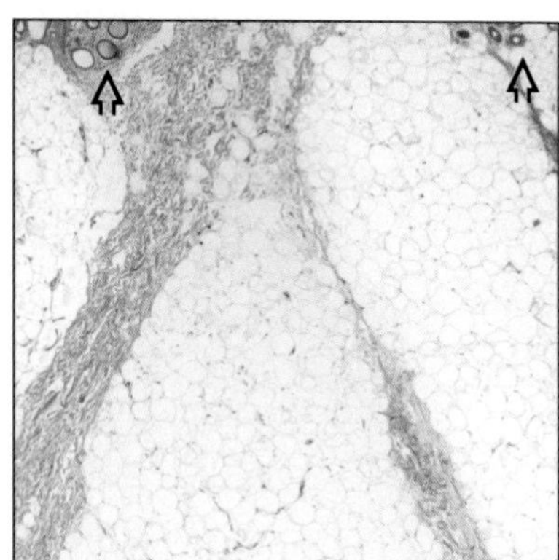

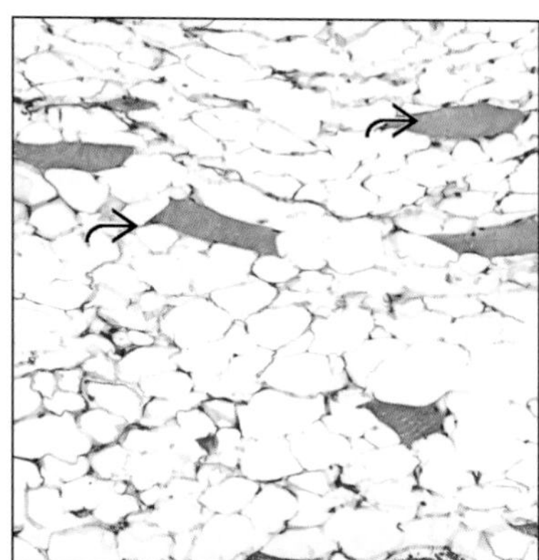

*(**Left**) Diffuse symmetrical lipomatosis with massive accumulation of subcutaneous fat is seen involving the back and upper extremities. (Courtesy C. Demas, MD.) (**Center**) Axillary lipomatosis is shown with massive accumulation of mature adipose tissue in the subcutaneous region. Note dermal appendages at the top ⇨ of the image. (**Right**) The adipose tissue overgrowth in lipomatosis frequently extends into underlying skeletal muscle ⇨ and therefore, mimics an intramuscular lipoma.*

ANGIOLIPOMA

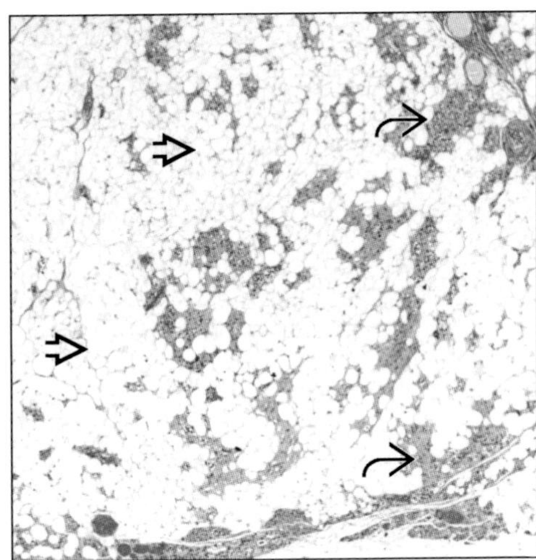

Angiolipomas are biphasic tumors composed of mature adipocytes ⇨ and branching, capillary-sized blood vessels ↗.

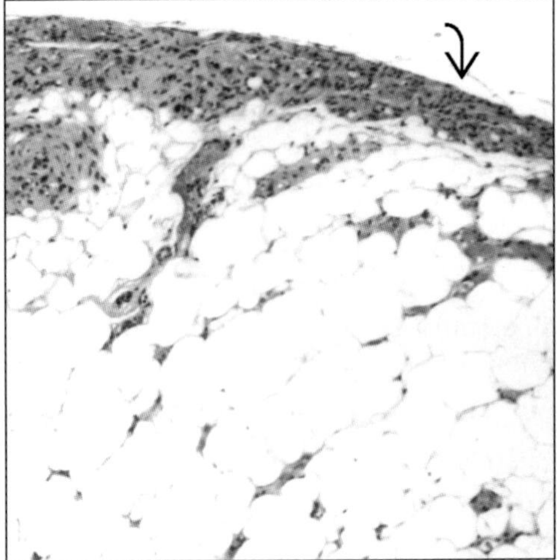

Angiolipomas are surrounded by a delicate capsule ↗, and the vascular component is often most prominent in the subcapsular region.

TERMINOLOGY

Definitions

- Biphasic tumor consisting of mature adipocytes and thin-walled blood vessels with fibrin thrombi

ETIOLOGY/PATHOGENESIS

Familial Predilection

- In a minority of cases (5%)
- Remainder are sporadic

CLINICAL ISSUES

Epidemiology

- Age
  - Common in young adults
- Gender
  - Male predominance

Site

- Forearm, trunk, and upper arm most common sites
- Spinal angiolipomas are considered a distinct entity
  - Infiltrating margins
  - Vascular component mimics arteriovenous malformation or cavernous hemangioma
- Rare instances of visceral involvement (lymph node, duodenum, breast) reported

Presentation

- Painful mass
  - Often present as multiple subcutaneous nodules
  - No correlation between pain and degree of tumor vascularity

Treatment

- Surgical excision

Prognosis

- Always benign
- Do not recur or undergo malignant transformation

MACROSCOPIC FEATURES

Gross Features

- Encapsulated tumor
- Yellow-red nodules
- Typically < 2 cm in size

MICROSCOPIC PATHOLOGY

Histologic Features

- 2 components are present in these tumors
  - Mature adipocytes
  - Branching capillary-sized blood vessels with fibrin thrombi
    - Vascularity and fibrin thrombi often more prominent in subcapsular zone
- Relative proportion of each component is variable
- Variable amount of fibrosis may be present
- Mast cells may be conspicuous in some cases

Cytologic Features

- No nuclear atypia is present in adipocytic or vascular component

Variant Subtype

- Cellular angiolipoma
  - Vascular component predominates in this variant
  - May be mistaken for Kaposi sarcoma or angiosarcoma

ANCILLARY TESTS

Cytogenetics

- Karyotypically normal

ANGIOLIPOMA

Key Facts

Terminology
- Biphasic tumor consisting of mature adipocytes and thin-walled blood vessels with fibrin thrombi

Clinical Issues
- Common in young adults; male predominance
- Painful tender subcutaneous nodule
- May be multiple
- Do not recur or undergo malignant transformation

Macroscopic Features
- Encapsulated, yellow-red nodule
- Typically < 2 cm in size

Microscopic Pathology
- Admixture of mature adipocytes and capillary-sized blood vessels with fibrin thrombi
- Vascular component predominates in cellular angiolipoma

- Translocation t(X;2) has been reported in 1 case

Electron Microscopy
- Transmission
  - Adipocytes and spindle-shaped endothelial cells are seen
  - Fibrin thrombi may be associated with disrupted endothelial cells

DIFFERENTIAL DIAGNOSIS

Lipoma
- Lesions in which adipocytic component predominates may be mistaken for lipoma
- Fibrin thrombi helpful in making diagnosis of angiolipoma

Intramuscular Hemangioma
- Previously known as "**infiltrating angiolipoma**"
- Angiolipomas are small, multiple, and superficial in location, unlike intramuscular hemangioma

Kaposi Sarcoma (KS)
- Cellular angiolipoma may be mistaken for KS
- Endothelial proliferation present in both lesions
- Angiolipomas lack slit-like spaces and PAS(+) hyaline globules seen in KS
- Endothelial cells in KS are HHV8(+)

Angiomyolipoma (AML)
- Spindle cells in AML are HMB-45(+) smooth muscle cells

DIAGNOSTIC CHECKLIST

Pathologic Interpretation Pearls
- Variable admixture of mature adipocytes and branching capillaries with fibrin thrombi

SELECTED REFERENCES

1. Konya D et al: Lumbar spinal angiolipoma: case report and review of the literature. Eur Spine J. 15(6):1025-8, 2006
2. Kazakov DV et al: Primary intranodal cellular angiolipoma. Int J Surg Pathol. 13(1):99-101, 2005
3. Mohl W et al: Duodenal angiolipoma -- endoscopic diagnosis and therapy. Z Gastroenterol. 42(12):1381-3, 2004
4. Sciot R et al: Cytogenetic analysis of subcutaneous angiolipoma: further evidence supporting its difference from ordinary pure lipomas: a report of the CHAMP Study Group. Am J Surg Pathol. 21(4):441-4, 1997
5. Kanik AB et al: Cellular angiolipoma. Am J Dermatopathol. 17(3):312-5, 1995
6. Yu GH et al: Cellular angiolipoma of the breast. Mod Pathol. 6(4):497-9, 1993
7. Dixon AY et al: Angiolipomas: an ultrastructural and clinicopathological study. Hum Pathol. 12(8):739-47, 1981

IMAGE GALLERY

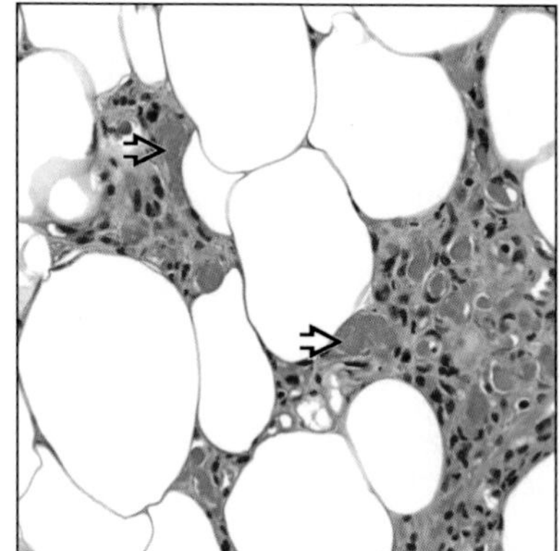

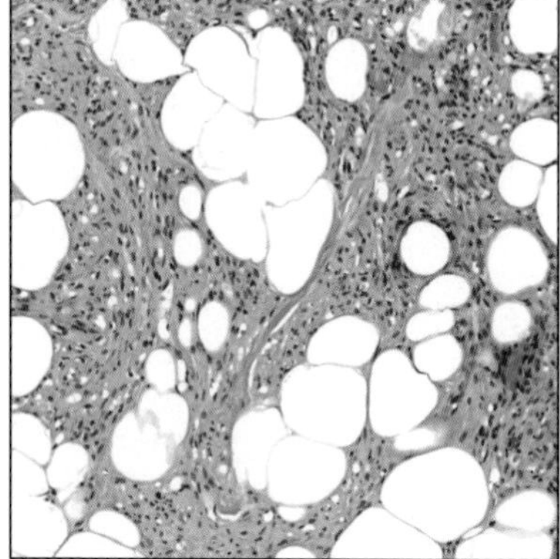

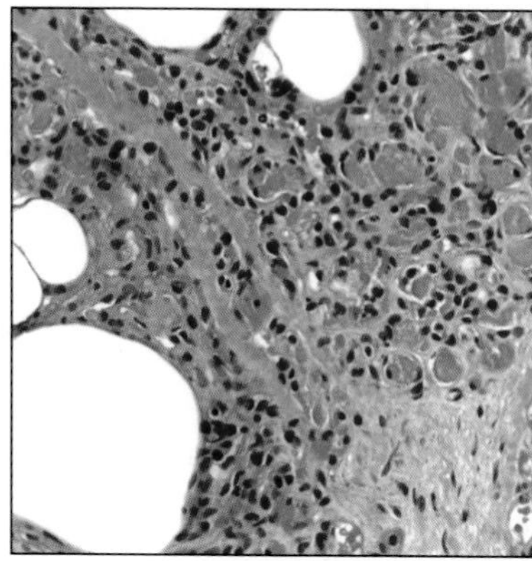

*(**Left**) The vascular component in angiolipomas shows intraluminal fibrin thrombi ⇒. The adipocytic component is benign and shows no nuclear atypia. (**Center**) Cellular angiolipomas show predominance of the vascular component and may be mistaken for Kaposi sarcoma. (**Right**) The presence of intraluminal fibrin thrombi in cellular angiolipomas is helpful in distinguishing them from Kaposi sarcoma or angiosarcoma.*

MYOLIPOMA

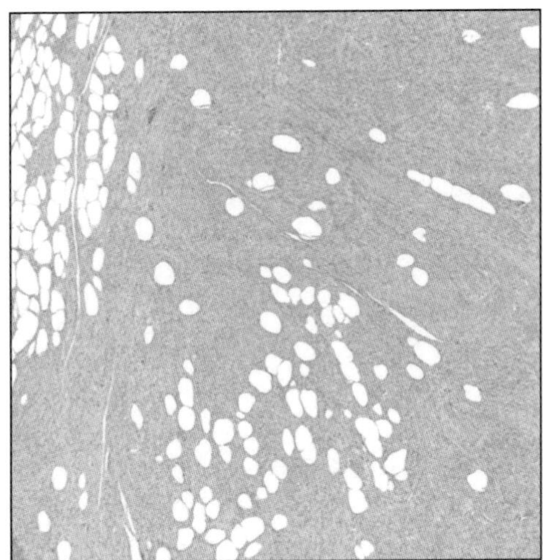

Retroperitoneal myolipoma composed of an admixture of smooth muscle and mature adipose tissue imparts a sieve-like appearance. Most tumors have a predominance of smooth muscle, such as this case.

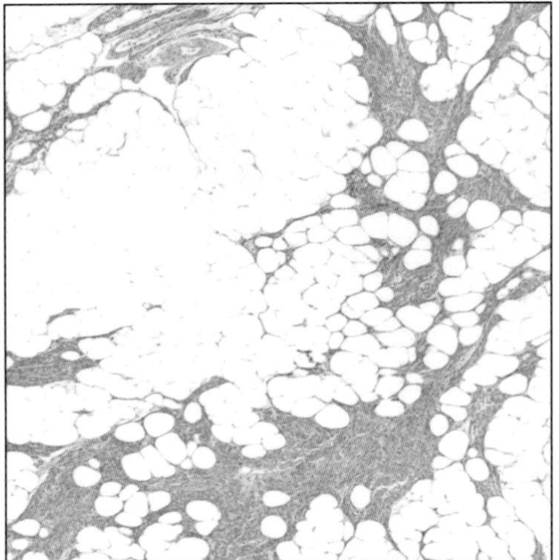

Some myolipomas, such as this pelvic tumor, have a predominance of mature adipose tissue. Note the regular distribution of adipose and smooth muscle, imparting a sieve-like appearance on low power.

TERMINOLOGY

Synonyms

- Extrauterine lipoleiomyoma
- Benign mesenchymoma (nonspecific historical term)

Definitions

- Soft tissue neoplasm composed of mature adipose tissue and smooth muscle

CLINICAL ISSUES

Epidemiology

- Incidence
  - Rare
- Age
  - Adults; peak in 5th-6th decade
- Gender
  - Female predilection

Site

- Most occur in retroperitoneum, pelvis, inguinal canal, and abdominal wall
- Less often occurs in extremities (subcutaneous or deep)
- Rare sites include eyelid, pericardium, tongue, breast, orbit, and intradural

Presentation

- Often found incidentally
- May present with painless or painful soft tissue mass

Treatment

- Surgical approaches
  - Complete excision is treatment of choice

Prognosis

- Excellent prognosis
- Do not recur with complete excision
- No reports of so-called benign metastasizing myolipoma

MACROSCOPIC FEATURES

General Features

- Circumscribed and typically encapsulated
- Yellow to tan-white depending on relative amounts of fat and muscle
- Soft to firm (and whorled) depending on relative amounts of fat and muscle

Size

- Intraabdominal tumors can be quite large
  - Range from 15-26 cm
- Extremity, trunk, and head and neck tumors tend to be much smaller

MICROSCOPIC PATHOLOGY

Histologic Features

- Mixture of mature adipose tissue and smooth muscle
  - Variable amounts of each component in different tumors
    - Majority show smooth muscle predominance
  - 2 components tend to be intermixed throughout tumor, imparting sieve-like appearance
- Smooth muscle component is usually arranged in short intersecting fascicles
  - Smooth muscle cells have oval nuclei with abundant eosinophilic fibrillary cytoplasm
    - May have paranuclear vacuoles
    - Lack cytologic atypia
    - Absent to rare mitotic figures
- Adipose component consists of mature adipocytes
  - No lipoblasts or floret-type giant cells
- Some tumors have patchy chronic inflammation &/or stromal fibrosis
- Scattered thin-walled vessels are often present but lack thick-walled muscular arteries

MYOLIPOMA

Key Facts

Terminology
- Soft tissue neoplasm composed of mature adipose tissue and smooth muscle

Clinical Issues
- Adults; peak in 5th-6th decade
- Female predilection
- Most occur in retroperitoneum, pelvis, inguen, and abdominal wall
- Excellent prognosis

Microscopic Pathology
- Mixture of mature adipose tissue and smooth muscle
- Smooth muscle component is usually arranged in short fascicles
- Adipose component consists of mature adipocytes
- Scattered thin-walled vessels are often present but lack thick-walled muscular arteries

ANCILLARY TESTS

Immunohistochemistry
- Smooth muscle component is positive for smooth muscle markers (actins, desmin, calponin, H-caldesmon)
  - HMB-45 and S100 protein are negative
  - Some tumors express estrogen receptor

DIFFERENTIAL DIAGNOSIS

Spindle Cell Lipoma
- Rare in retroperitoneum and pelvis
- Spindle cells lack smooth muscle differentiation (no eosinophilic fibrillary cytoplasm or paranuclear vacuoles)
  - Myoid markers are negative, but spindle cells are positive for CD34 immunohistochemically

Angiomyolipoma
- Less fascicular growth and less uniform cytology
- Often have more epithelioid cells with vacuolated cytoplasm
  - These cells are positive for HMB-45
- Usually contain thick-walled medium-sized arteries, which are absent in myolipoma

Leiomyoma with Fatty Metaplasia/ Degeneration
- Lack uniform (sieve-like) distribution of fat and muscle throughout tumor that is typical of myolipoma
- Fatty degeneration is relatively common in uterine leiomyomas but is uncommon in soft tissue leiomyomas

Low-Grade Dedifferentiated Liposarcoma
- Diagnostic large hyperchromatic atypical stromal cells will be present in adipocytic component
- Spindle cell component will demonstrate at least mild atypia and increased mitotic activity

SELECTED REFERENCES

1. Takahashi Y et al: Myolipoma of the retroperitoneum. Pathol Int. 54(6):460-3, 2004
2. Fernández-Aguilar S et al: Myolipoma of soft tissue: an unusual tumor with expression of estrogen and progesterone receptors. Report of two cases and review of the literature. Acta Obstet Gynecol Scand. 81(11):1088-90, 2002
3. Michal M: Retroperitoneal myolipoma. A tumour mimicking retroperitoneal angiomyolipoma and liposarcoma with myosarcomatous differentiation. Histopathology. 25(1):86-8, 1994
4. Meis JM et al: Myolipoma of soft tissue. Am J Surg Pathol. 15(2):121-5, 1991

IMAGE GALLERY

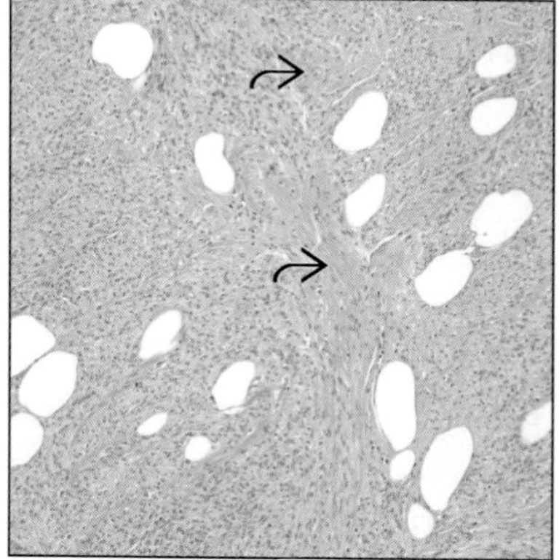

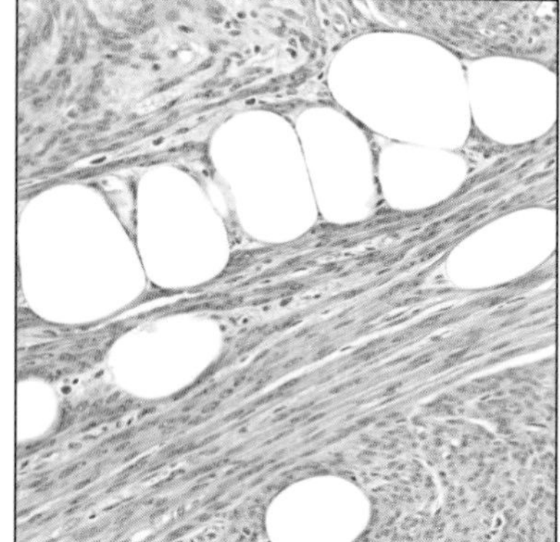

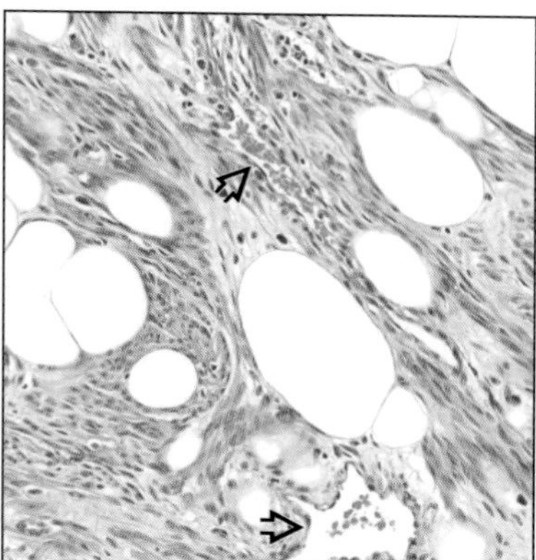

(Left) *H&E shows evenly dispersed adipose tissue and short fascicles of smooth muscle, the typical appearance of myolipoma. Focal areas of sclerosis can be seen ➡ and likely represent a degenerative change.* ***(Center)*** *Short fascicles of elongated spindle cells with oval, cytologically bland nuclei and abundant eosinophilic fibrillary cytoplasm are seen, similar to typical leiomyomas.* ***(Right)*** *Dilated thin-walled vessels ➡ are typical but medium-sized muscular arteries are not.*

MYELOLIPOMA

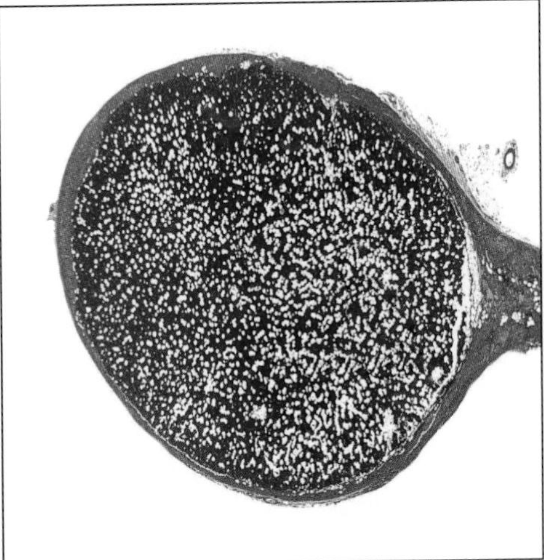

Hematoxylin & eosin shows scanning magnification appearance of myelolipoma. Adrenal glandular tissue is stretched around a circumscribed, nonencapsulated lesion that displays fatty and cellular areas.

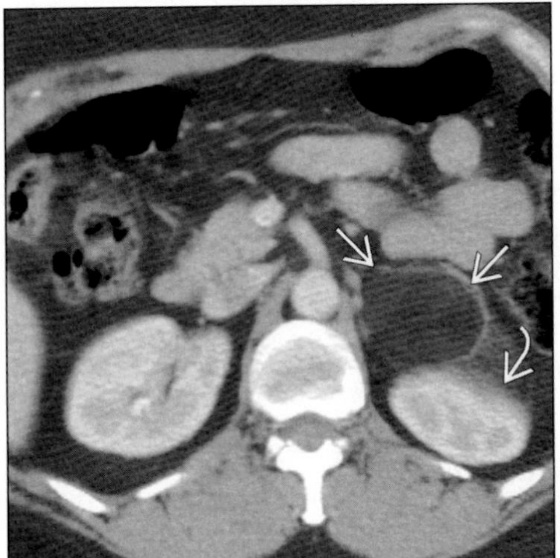

CT shows a predominantly fatty mass ➡ replacing and expanding the left adrenal gland. The left kidney ➡ is displaced. These imaging appearances are characteristic of an adrenal myelolipoma.

TERMINOLOGY

Definitions

- Tumor-like lesion resembling bone marrow composed of hemopoietic tissues, fat, and sometimes bone
- Mostly in adrenal gland
- Rarely other sites

ETIOLOGY/PATHOGENESIS

Associated Conditions

- Cortical adenoma, pheochromocytoma
- Adrenal cortical hyperplasia
  - Possible effect on hemopoietic stem cell rests
- Most are idiopathic

CLINICAL ISSUES

Epidemiology

- Incidence
  - Rare
- Age
  - Older adults, usually after 4th decade
- Gender
  - M = F

Site

- Most common in adrenal gland
- Occasional cases in extraadrenal locations
  - Retroperitoneum, presacral region, mediastinum
  - Lung, liver, spleen, testis

Presentation

- Incidental finding
  - Most cases
- Symptoms of abdominal mass when large
- Massive acute hemorrhage in rare cases

Treatment

- Surgical approaches
  - Excision is curative

Prognosis

- Benign lesion; excellent outcome

IMAGE FINDINGS

Radiographic Findings

- Circumscribed lucent mass
- Adrenal myelolipoma can displace kidney

MACROSCOPIC FEATURES

General Features

- Red-tan circumscribed nodule

Size

- Mostly small, up to about 5 cm
- Rare examples can be very large
  - a.k.a. "giant myelolipoma"

MICROSCOPIC PATHOLOGY

Histologic Features

- Circumscribed, rim of adrenal cortex
- Fat without atypia or lipoblasts
- Hemopoietic elements
  - All 3 cell lines
  - Variable amount, in fatty septa
- Rarely formation of bony trabeculae
  - Peripheral shell or spicules in lesion

Predominant Pattern/Injury Type

- Circumscribed

Predominant Cell/Compartment Type

- Hematopoietic, myeloid

MYELOLIPOMA

Key Facts

Terminology
- Tumor-like lesion resembling bone marrow composed of hemopoietic tissues, fat, and sometimes bone
- Most cases involve adrenal gland
- Rarely other sites

Clinical Issues
- Older adults, usually after 4th decade

Microscopic Pathology
- Circumscribed, nonencapsulated
- Rim of adrenal cortex
- Fat without atypia or lipoblasts
- Hemopoietic elements
  - All 3 cell lines represented

Diagnostic Checklist
- Typically circumscribed adrenal mass

ANCILLARY TESTS

Cytogenetics
- 1 report of t(3;21)(q25;p11) rearrangement
- Some have nonrandom X inactivation

DIFFERENTIAL DIAGNOSIS

Extramedullary Hemopoiesis
- Associated with myeloproliferative disease
  - Multiple deposits
  - Lacks fatty component
- Occasionally seen in primary fatty tumor of soft tissue

Lipoma
- Encapsulated
- Lacks myeloid elements

Well-Differentiated Liposarcoma
- Lacks myeloid elements
- Has scattered enlarged hyperchromatic nuclei
- Can have lipoblasts

Chloroma
- Lacks fatty component
- Only 1 hematopoietic lineage represented
  - Primitive myeloid cells

Pheochromocytoma
- Composed of cords of polygonal cells
- Lacks fat and hemopoietic tissue

Adrenal Cortical Tumor
- Composed of cortical-type cells
- Lacks fat and hemopoietic tissue

DIAGNOSTIC CHECKLIST

Clinically Relevant Pathologic Features
- Typically located in adrenal gland

Pathologic Interpretation Pearls
- Distinct circumscribed mass
- Differentiated fat and marrow elements

SELECTED REFERENCES

1. Vaziri M et al: Primary mediastinal myelolipoma. Ann Thorac Surg. 85(5):1805-6, 2008
2. Kiriakopoulos A et al: Surgical management of adrenal myelolipoma: a series of 10 patients and review of the literature. Minerva Chir. 61(3):241-246, 2006
3. Chang KC et al: Adrenal myelolipoma with translocation (3;21)(q25;p11). Cancer Genet Cytogenet. 134(1):77-80, 2002
4. Sanders R et al: Clinical spectrum of adrenal myelolipoma: analysis of 8 tumors in 7 patients. J Urol. 153(6):1791-3, 1995

IMAGE GALLERY

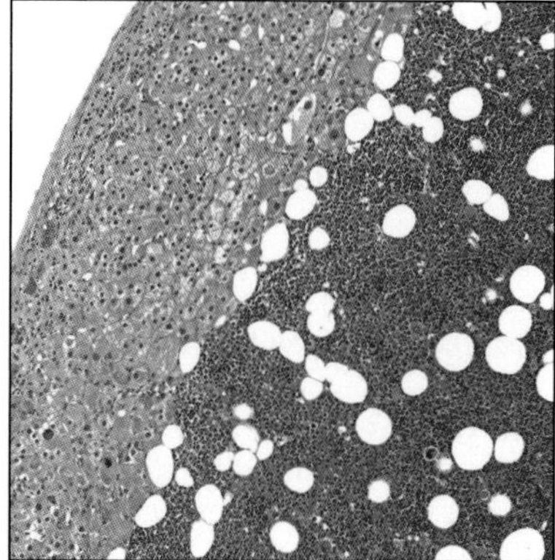

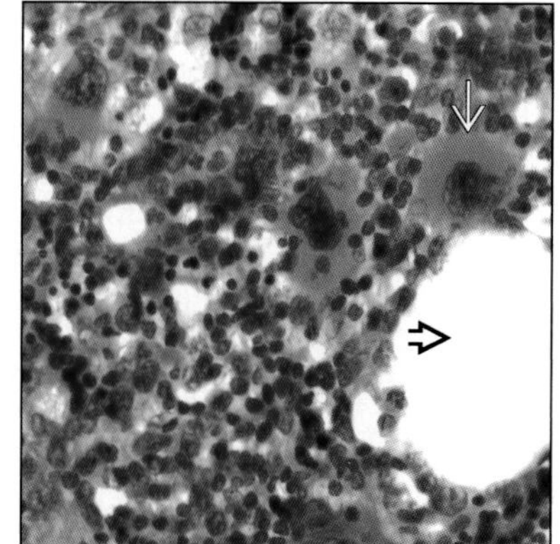

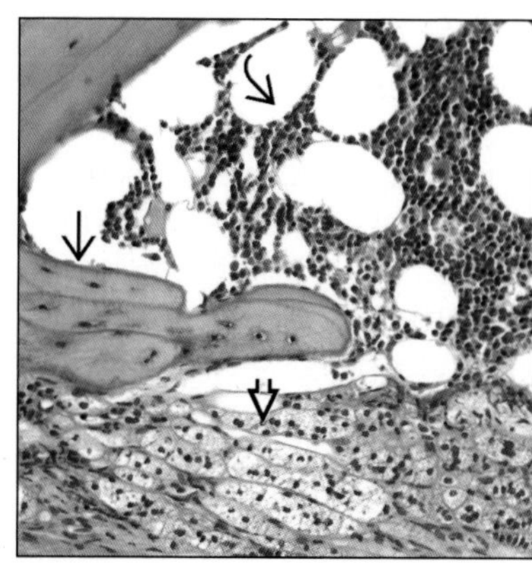

(Left) *Hematoxylin & eosin shows adrenal myelolipoma. The peripheral adrenal cortical tissue is contiguous with a well-demarcated cellular lesion containing fatty spaces.* ***(Center)*** *Hematoxylin & eosin shows cellular hemopoietic tissue in which all cell lines are represented. Megakaryocytes ➡ are prominent. Note fatty space ⇨.* ***(Right)*** *Hematoxylin and eosin shows unusual finding of bone formation in adrenal myelolipoma. Note peripheral adrenal cortical tissue ⇨, mature bone without nuclear atypia →, and fatty marrow-like lesional tissue ↗.*

SPINDLE CELL/PLEOMORPHIC LIPOMA

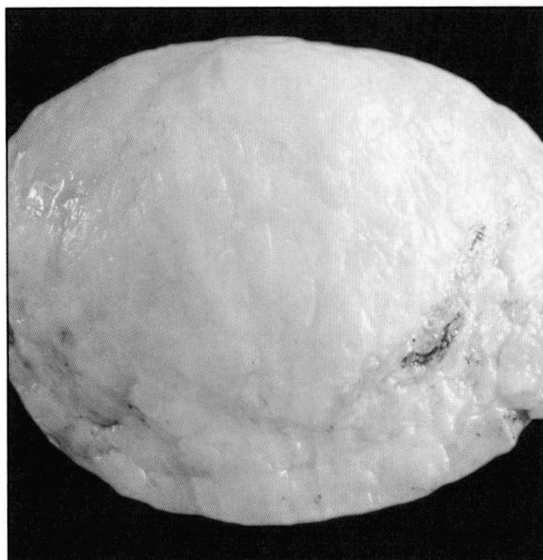

Spindle cell and pleomorphic lipomas are well-circumscribed tumors with a pale yellow, homogeneous appearance that lacks the lobular configuration seen in typical lipomas.

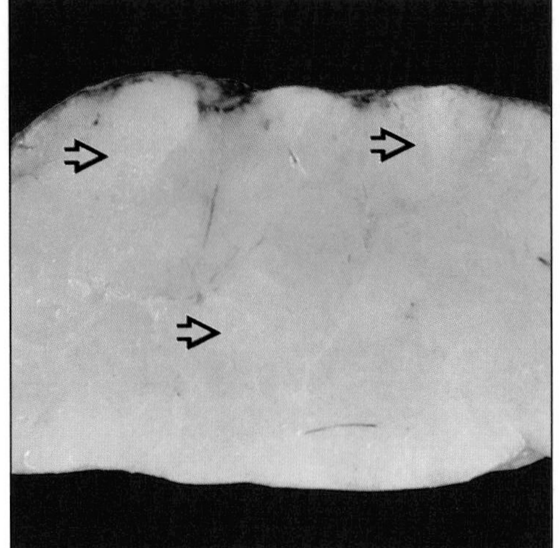

Both spindle cell and pleomorphic lipomas may show gray-white foci ⇨ that are firm in consistency and correlate histologically with spindle cell areas with ropey collagenous matrix.

TERMINOLOGY

Abbreviations

- Spindle cell lipoma (SCL)/pleomorphic lipoma (PL)

Definitions

- Benign adipocytic tumor with variable admixture of spindle cells, ropey collagen, and multinucleated tumor giant cells

CLINICAL ISSUES

Epidemiology

- Age
  - Typically in older age group (> 50 years)
- Gender
  - Predominantly in men; < 10% in women

Site

- Shoulder and posterior neck most common sites of involvement
- Other sites
  - Upper arm
  - Face
  - Oral cavity
- Lower extremity involvement is rare

Presentation

- Painless mass
  - Dermal or subcutaneous nodule
  - Often present for a long duration
  - Rarely multiple or familial

Treatment

- Conservative surgical excision is adequate

Prognosis

- Benign behavior
- Local recurrence is rare

MACROSCOPIC FEATURES

Gross Appearance

- Well-circumscribed tumor
- Yellow/gray-white appearance
- Firm consistency
- Some cases may show myxoid appearance

MICROSCOPIC PATHOLOGY

Histologic Features

- Spindle cell lipoma is composed of a variable admixture of 3 components
  - Mature adipocytes
  - Bland spindle cell proliferation with ropey collagen
  - Myxoid stroma with mast cells
- Pleomorphic lipoma is part of same spectrum
  - In addition to above features, also shows
    - Multinucleated tumor giant cells with peripherally arranged nuclei ("floret cells")
  - Lipoblasts may be present in pleomorphic lipoma

Cytologic Features

- Bland nuclei in spindle cell lipoma
- Hyperchromatic nuclei with multinucleated tumor giant cells in pleomorphic lipoma

Variants

- Pseudoangiomatoid variant
  - Prominent slit-like spaces resembling vascular channels
  - May be mistaken for vascular neoplasm since SCL is also CD34(+)
  - SCL is CD31(-), unlike tumors with true endothelial differentiation
- Fat-free and fat-poor variant
  - Spindle cell proliferation dominates the picture
  - Adipocytes may be scarce or completely absent
  - Similar site predilection as typical SCL/PL

SPINDLE CELL/PLEOMORPHIC LIPOMA

Key Facts

Terminology
- Benign adipocytic tumor with variable admixture of spindle cells, ropey collagen, and multinucleate tumor giant cells

Clinical Issues
- Typically in older (> 50 years) men
- Shoulder and posterior neck most common sites
- Benign behavior

Macroscopic Features
- Well-circumscribed subcutaneous lesions
- Yellow/gray-white, firm with focal myxoid areas

Microscopic Pathology
- Spindle cells with ropey collagen, mature adipose tissue, and myxoid stroma with mast cells
- Spindle cells are diffusely and strongly positive for CD34
- Pleomorphic lipoma is also CD34 positive and shows multinucleated tumor giant cells with peripheral nuclei ("floret" cells)
- Lipoblasts may be present in some PL
- Variants
  - Pseudoangiomatoid variant of SCL shows prominent slit-like spaces resembling vascular channels
  - Spindle cell proliferation dominates the picture in fat-free and fat-poor variant of SCL

Ancillary Tests
- Deletions of 16q and 13q occur in SCL/PL

ANCILLARY TESTS

Immunohistochemistry
- SCL/PL are diffusely and strongly positive for CD34
- Rare cases may stain focally for S100

Cytogenetics
- More complex karyotype than typical lipoma
- Deletions of 16q, usually involving 16q13 region
- Deletions of 13q have also been reported

DIFFERENTIAL DIAGNOSIS

Dermatofibrosarcoma Protuberans (DFSP)
- DFSP occurs in young individuals
- Spindle cells arranged in storiform pattern and infiltrate into subcutaneous tissue
- Shares CD34 positivity with SCL/PL

Peripheral Nerve Sheath Tumors
- Some SCL/PL may show nuclear palisading and mimic peripheral nerve sheath tumors
- S100 and CD34 immunostains useful in making this distinction

Solitary Fibrous Tumor (SFT)
- SFT is also diffusely CD34 positive
- Ectatic branching "staghorn" vascular pattern present in SFT

Sclerosing Well-Differentiated Liposarcoma (WDLPS)
- Unlike WDLPS, SCL/PL are well-circumscribed subcutaneous tumors with diffuse CD34 positivity
- Giant ring chromosomes and MDM2 and CDK4 positivity present in well-differentiated liposarcoma

Spindle Cell Liposarcoma
- Spindle cells arranged in fascicles in spindle cell liposarcoma and lack ropey collagen of SCL/PL
- CD34 positivity present in SCL/PL

Myxoid Liposarcoma
- SCL/PL with prominent vascular proliferation may be mistaken for myxoid liposarcoma

DIAGNOSTIC CHECKLIST

Clinically Relevant Pathologic Features
- Gross appearance
  - Well-circumscribed subcutaneous tumors
- Age distribution
  - Typically occur in older men
- Site of involvement
  - Posterior neck and shoulder

Pathologic Interpretation Pearls
- Spindle cell lipoma
  - Mature adipocytes admixed with bland spindle cells, ropey collagen, and myxoid stroma with mast cells
- Pleomorphic lipoma
  - Hyperchromatic round or spindle-shaped nuclei
  - Multinucleated floret cells with peripheral arrangement of nuclei

SELECTED REFERENCES

1. Billings SD et al: Diagnostically challenging spindle cell lipomas: a report of 34 "low-fat" and "fat-free" variants. Am J Dermatopathol. 29(5):437-42, 2007
2. Fanburg-Smith JC et al: Multiple spindle cell lipomas: a report of 7 familial and 11 nonfamilial cases. Am J Surg Pathol. 22(1):40-8, 1998
3. Dal Cin P et al: Lesions of 13q may occur independently of deletion of 16q in spindle cell/pleomorphic lipomas. Histopathology. 31(3):222-5, 1997
4. Hawley IC et al: Spindle cell lipoma--a pseudoangiomatous variant. Histopathology. 24(6):565-9, 1994
5. Shmookler BM et al: Pleomorphic lipoma: a benign tumor simulating liposarcoma. A clinicopathologic analysis of 48 cases. Cancer. 47(1):126-33, 1981
6. Enzinger FM et al: Spindle cell lipoma. Cancer. 36(5):1852-9, 1975

SPINDLE CELL/PLEOMORPHIC LIPOMA

Microscopic Features

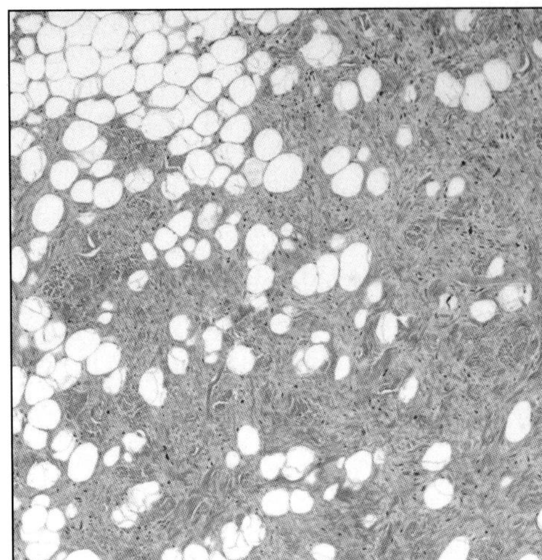

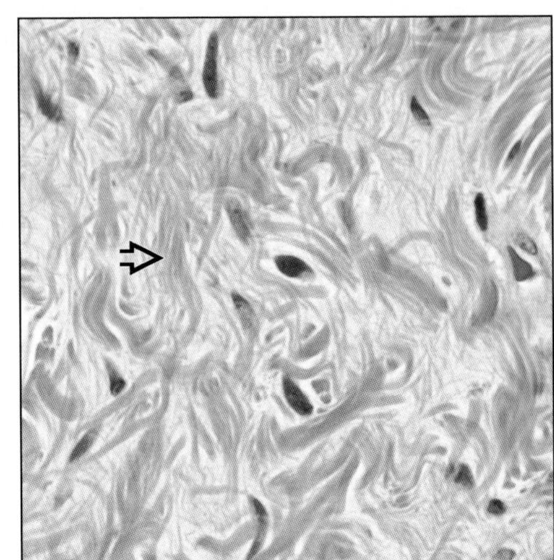

*(**Left**) Spindle cell lipomas show mature adipocytes admixed with bland spindle cell proliferation. (**Right**) The spindle cells in the tumor show no nuclear atypia and are present in a background of a ropey collagenous matrix ➡.*

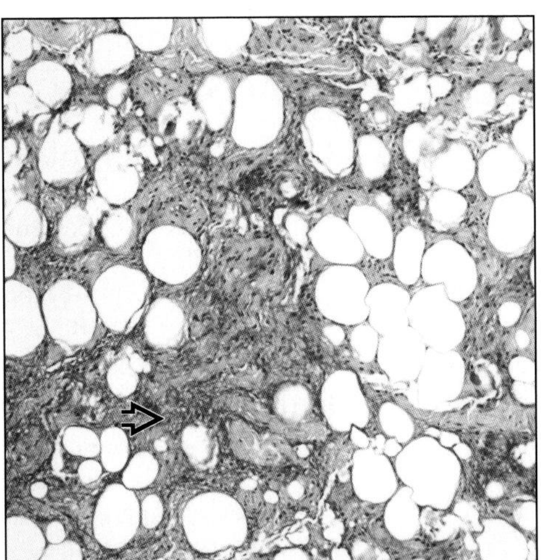

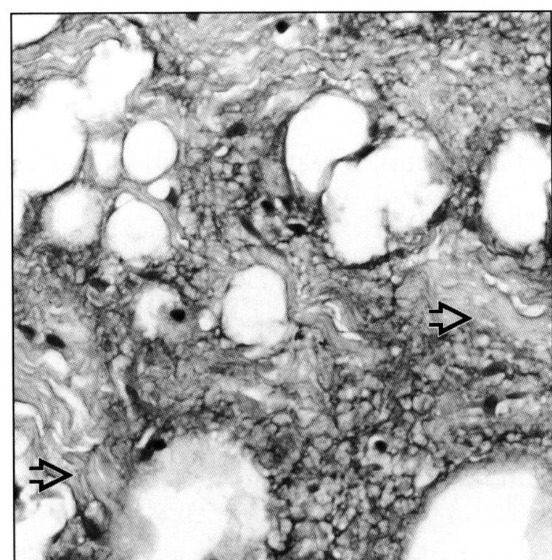

*(**Left**) Myxoid stromal change can be prominent ➡ in some examples of SCL. These cases may be mistaken for myxolipomas or myxoid liposarcomas. SCL are diffusely and strongly CD34 positive. (**Right**) Myxoid zones in spindle cell lipoma are also devoid of any nuclear atypia. The background of thick collagen bundles ➡ points toward the correct diagnosis of spindle cell lipoma in these cases.*

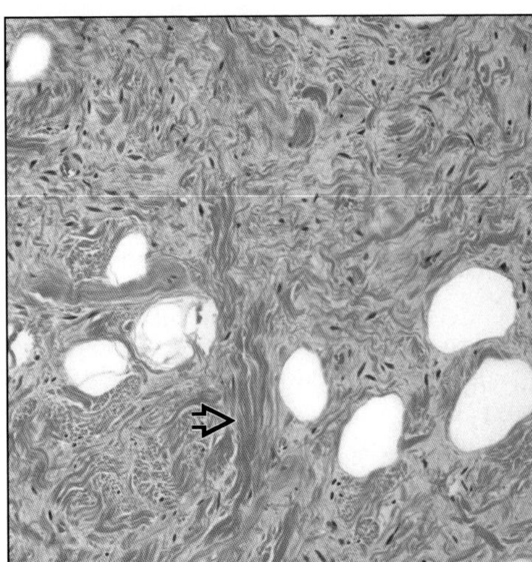

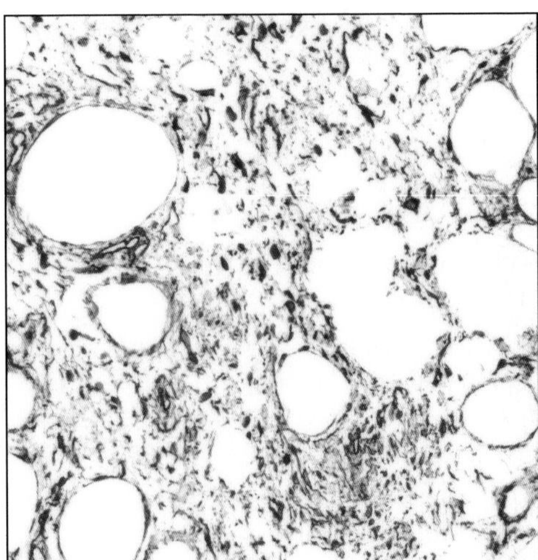

*(**Left**) In some cases, the spindle cell proliferation with ropey collagen ➡ may dominate the overall picture. These tumors are recognized as fat-poor or fat-free variants of spindle cell lipoma. (**Right**) Both spindle cell and pleomorphic lipoma share a diffuse and strong positivity for CD34.*

Microscopic Features

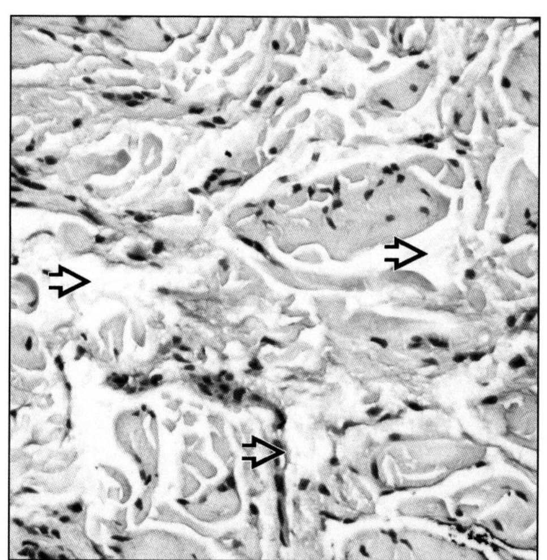

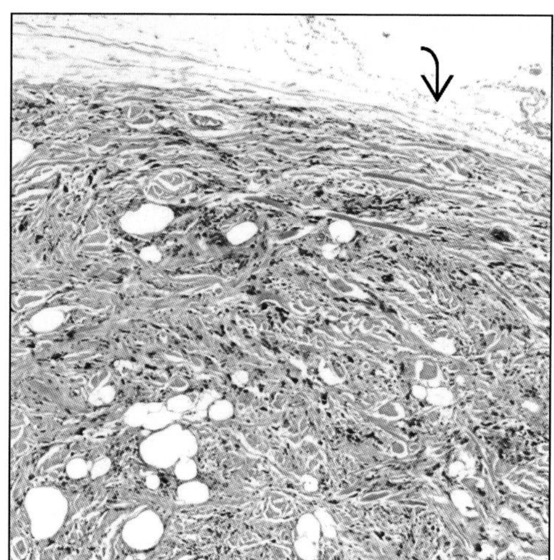

(Left) *Exaggerated slit-like spaces* ⇨ *are present in the pseudoangiomatous variant of SCL, which may be mistaken for a vascular neoplasm.* **(Right)** *Pleomorphic lipomas are well-circumscribed tumors* ⇨ *with hyperchromatic spindle-shaped and round nuclei and a variable number of multinucleated tumor giant cells.*

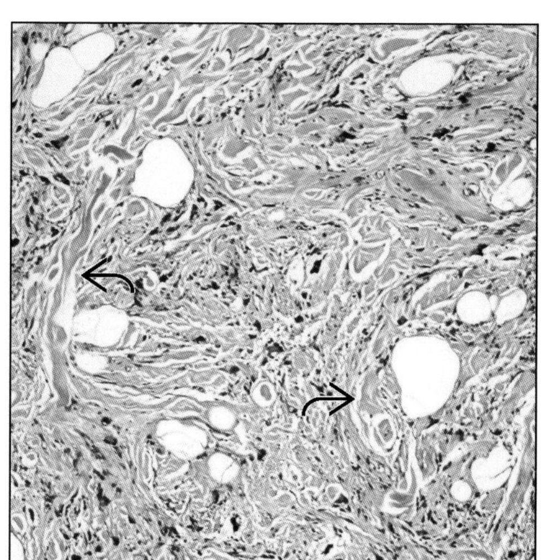

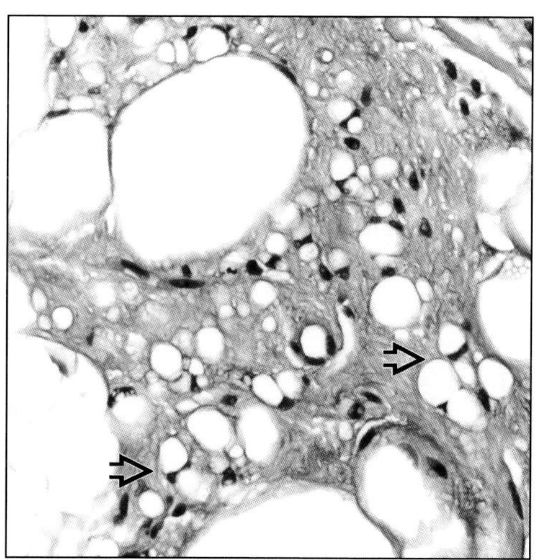

(Left) *The ropey collagen* ⇨ *that is characteristic of SCL is also present in pleomorphic lipomas, suggesting that the 2 lesions are part of the same spectrum.* **(Right)** *Scattered lipoblasts* ⇨ *may be present in pleomorphic lipoma. The presence of lipoblasts or mitotic activity does not affect prognosis in pleomorphic lipoma.*

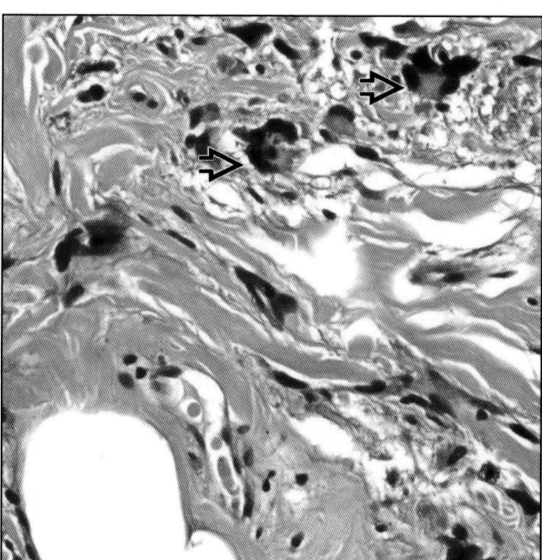

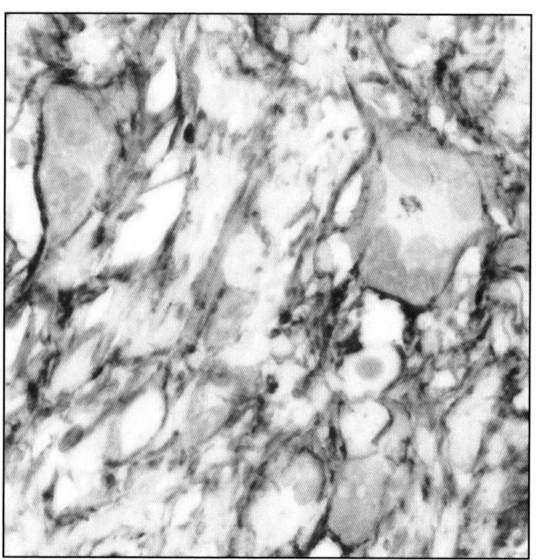

(Left) *The multinucleated tumor giant cells in pleomorphic lipoma have peripherally arranged nuclei* ⇨ *and are described as "floret cells."* **(Right)** *CD34 immunostain is strongly positive in spindle cells and multinucleated floret cells in pleomorphic lipoma.*

HIBERNOMA

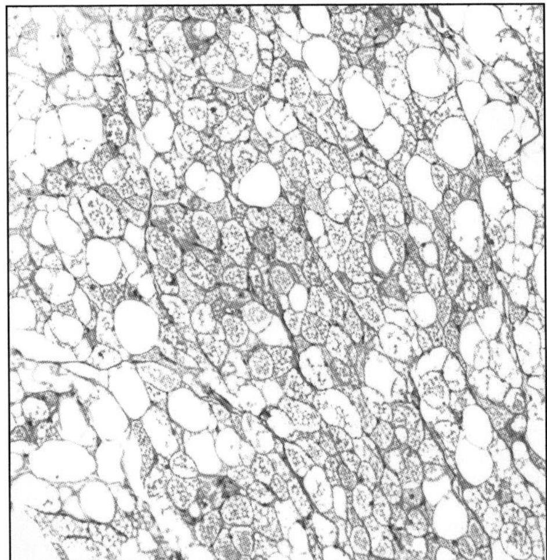

Hematoxylin & eosin shows low-power view of hibernoma, composed of well-defined lobules of polygonal cells. Cells with the appearance of brown fat are mixed with mature adipocytes. No atypia is present.

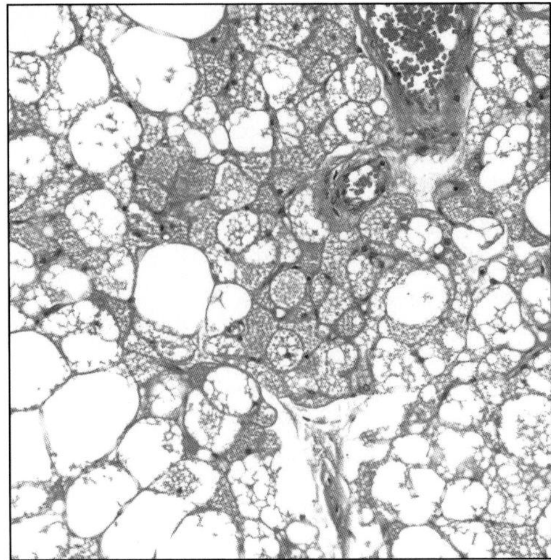

Hematoxylin & eosin shows hibernoma at higher magnification, composed of an admixture of polygonal cells with granular eosinophilic or multivacuolated cytoplasm. Univacuolated adipocytes are also seen.

TERMINOLOGY

Synonyms

- Fetal lipoma, lipoma of embryonic fat

Definitions

- Benign tumor most frequently occurring in younger adults, with differentiation toward brown fat
  - Tumor has characteristic cytogenetic aberrations, mainly involving 11q13-21

ETIOLOGY/PATHOGENESIS

Developmental Anomaly

- Etiology unknown
  - Many occur at sites of normal brown fat in fetuses and newborns
  - Genetic changes in some

CLINICAL ISSUES

Epidemiology

- Incidence
  - Rare; approximately 1% of all adipocytic tumors
- Age
  - Peak incidence: 3rd decade
  - Rare in children
- Gender
  - M = F

Site

- Most tumors subcutaneous; approximately 10% intramuscular
- Thigh is most common site
- Shoulder, back, trunk, abdomen, retroperitoneum

Presentation

- Painless mass
- Slow enlargement

Treatment

- Surgical approaches
  - Simple complete excision

Prognosis

- Excellent; excision is curative
- Does not recur or metastasize

MACROSCOPIC FEATURES

General Features

- Circumscribed, lobulated lesions
- Tan to brown, greasy, sometimes mucoid cut surface

Size

- Range: 1-24 cm (mean: 9.3 cm)

MICROSCOPIC PATHOLOGY

Histologic Features

- Lobulated tumor composed of sheets of cells of varying types
  - Polygonal cells with granular eosinophilic cytoplasm
  - Multivacuolated cells with lipid droplets
  - Univacuolated adipocytes
- Small, bland, central nuclei
- Mitotic figures exceptional
- Myxoid variant
  - Predominantly occurs in males, head and neck region
  - Constituent cells separated by acellular myxoid stroma
- Lipoma-like variant
  - Most common in thigh
  - Mostly univacuolated adipocytes, few hibernoma cells
- Spindle cell variant
  - Rare; found in posterior neck or scalp

HIBERNOMA

Key Facts

Terminology
- Benign tumor with differentiation toward brown fat, most frequently seen in younger adults

Clinical Issues
- Peak incidence in 3rd decade
- Most tumors subcutaneous
- Thigh is most common site
- Can occur in abdomen and retroperitoneum

Microscopic Pathology
- Variable differentiation towards brown fat
- Cells are granular, multivacuolated or univacuolated adipocytes
- Myxoid, lipoma-like, and spindle cell variants
- Cellular atypia unusual, mitoses exceptional

Ancillary Tests
- Variable, sometimes strong positivity for S100

  - Hibernoma cells, thick collagen bundles, mast cells, mature fat

Predominant Pattern/Injury Type
- Lobulated

Predominant Cell/Compartment Type
- Adipose

ANCILLARY TESTS

Immunohistochemistry
- Variable, sometimes strong positivity for S100 protein
- Spindle cell variant may show CD34 positivity

Cytogenetics
- Rearrangements of 11q13-21 in several cases
  - t(9;11)(q34;q13) in 1 case

Electron Microscopy
- Transmission
  - Numerous mitochondria, lipid droplets

DIFFERENTIAL DIAGNOSIS

Residual Brown Fat
- Upper chest and neck, no mass lesion
- Associated with reactive lymph nodes

Lipoblastoma
- Usually in 1st 3 years of life
- Spindle cells, myxoid stroma, vascular pattern

Adult Rhabdomyoma
- Large polygonal cells, abundant cytoplasm
- Cross striations
- Immunoreactive for desmin and myogenin (in nuclei)

Chondroid Lipoma
- Clusters of vacuolated cells
- Chondromyxoid stroma

Atypical Lipomatous Tumor/Well-Differentiated Liposarcoma
- Atypical cells in fibrous septa
- Lipoblasts with hyperchromatic scalloped nuclei
- Immunoreactivity for MDM2 and CDK4

Myxoid Liposarcoma
- Plexiform vascular pattern, lipoblasts
- Round cell component
- Characteristic translocations t(12;16), t(12;22)

SELECTED REFERENCES

1. Chirieac LR et al: Characterization of the myxoid variant of hibernoma. Ann Diagn Pathol. 10(2):104-6, 2006
2. Furlong MA et al: The morphologic spectrum of hibernoma: a clinicopathologic study of 170 cases. Am J Surg Pathol. 25(6):809-14, 2001
3. Mertens F et al: Hibernomas are characterized by rearrangements of chromosome bands 11q13-21. Int J Cancer. 58(4):503-5, 1994

IMAGE GALLERY

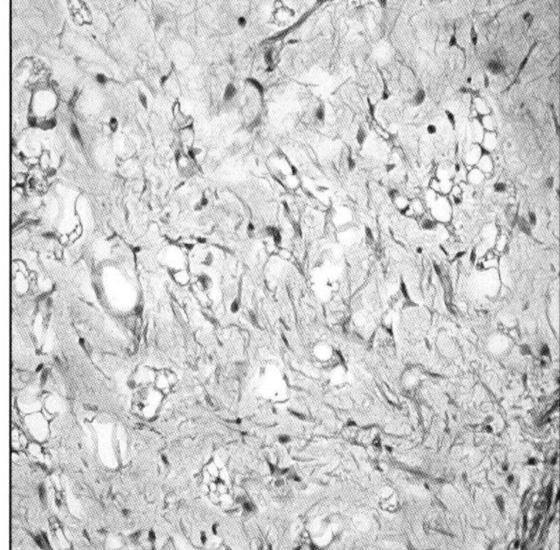

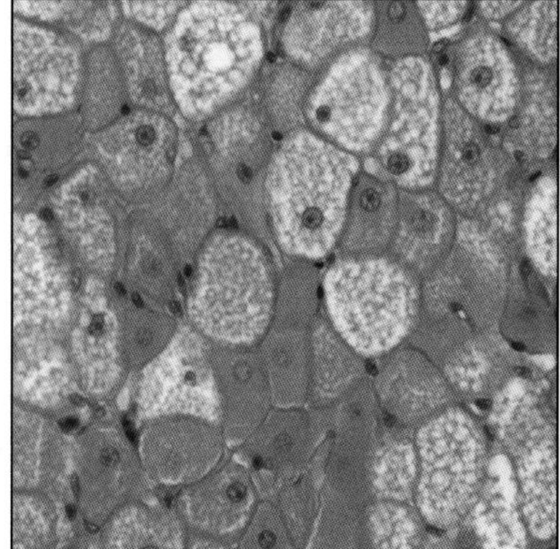

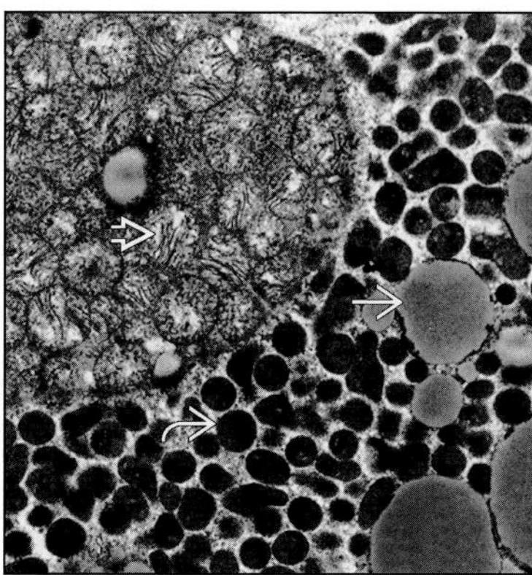

(Left) *Hematoxylin & eosin shows myxoid variant of hibernoma. Small foci of brown fat cells and mature adipocytes are dispersed in myxoid stroma.* ***(Center)*** *Hematoxylin & eosin shows sheets of polygonal cells with well-defined cell borders and abundant cytoplasm containing finely granular eosinophilic cytoplasm or numerous lipid vacuoles.* ***(Right)*** *Electron micrograph of hibernoma shows numerous tightly packed mitochondria displaying transverse cristae ➔. There are also small electron-dense lysosomes ➔ and lipid droplets ➔.*

LIPOBLASTOMA AND LIPOBLASTOMATOSIS

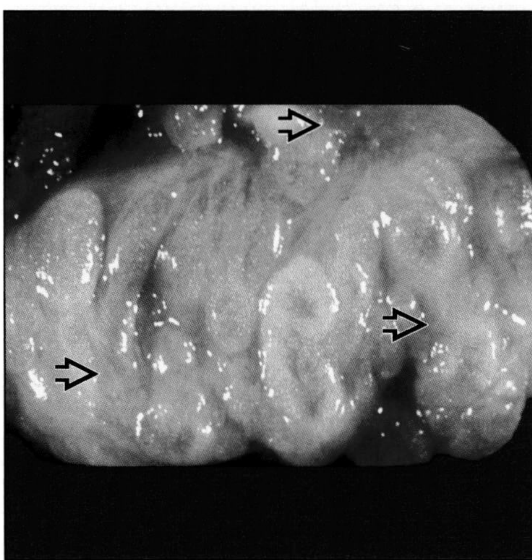

Lipoblastomas have a glistening, pale yellow, lobular appearance with interlobular fibrous septation ⇨, which may also be apparent on gross examination.

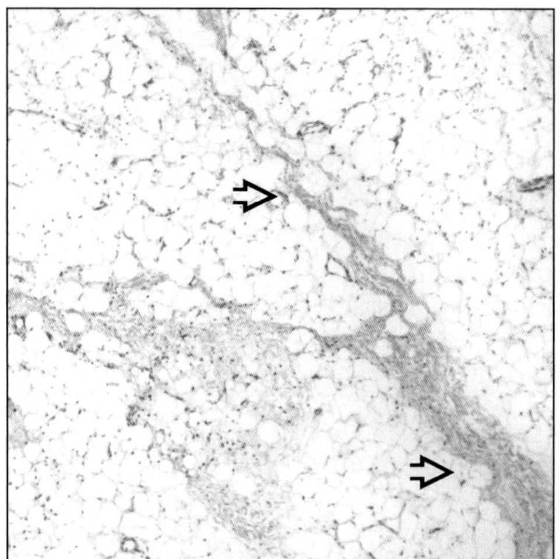

Lipoblastomas are characterized on low power by variably thick fibrous septa ⇨ that impart a lobular configuration to the tumor.

TERMINOLOGY

Synonyms

- Fetal lipoma
- Infantile lipoma
- Embryonic lipoma

Definitions

- Benign tumor resembling fetal adipose tissue
  - Localized tumors designated lipoblastoma
  - Diffuse tumors designated lipoblastomatosis

CLINICAL ISSUES

Epidemiology

- Incidence
  - Rare tumors
- Age
  - Most common in 1st 3 years of life
  - Rare in older children
- Gender
  - More common in males

Site

- Extremities are most common site of involvement
- May involve head/neck or trunk, mediastinum, retroperitoneum, or even visceral sites

Presentation

- Painless mass
  - Slow-growing subcutaneous lesion
  - Deep infiltration in lipoblastomatosis

Treatment

- Surgical excision is curative in most cases

Prognosis

- Benign tumor with no risk for malignant transformation
- Recurrence in up to 20% of tumors; mostly in lipoblastomatosis

MACROSCOPIC FEATURES

Size

- Usually less than 5 cm in greatest dimension

Gross Appearance

- Pale and lobulated
- Myxoid or gelatinous areas often present

MICROSCOPIC PATHOLOGY

Histologic Features

- Lobules of immature adipocytes separated by fibrous septa
  - Admixture of spindle or stellate cells, lipoblasts, and mature adipocytes in varying proportion
  - Degree of adipocytic differentiation is variable
  - Recurrent tumors may show greater degree of maturation
  - Foci resembling brown fat may be present
- Loose myxoid stroma
- Some cases with plexiform vasculature similar to that seen in myxoid liposarcoma
- Lipoblastomatosis
  - Lacks circumscription
  - Less pronounced lobular pattern
  - Entrapped skeletal muscle present in deeper aspects of tumor

Cytologic Features

- No nuclear atypia

ANCILLARY TESTS

Cytogenetics

- Rearrangement of 8q11-13 most common

LIPOBLASTOMA AND LIPOBLASTOMATOSIS

Key Facts

Terminology
- Benign tumor resembling fetal adipose tissue
  - Lipoblastomas are well circumscribed
  - Lipoblastomatosis is deeply infiltrative

Clinical Issues
- Presents in infancy and early childhood

Macroscopic Features
- Pale, lobulated, and myxoid appearance

Microscopic Pathology
- Lobules of immature adipocytes separated by fibrous septa
- Myxoid stroma with plexiform vasculature resembling myxoid liposarcoma

Ancillary Tests
- Rearrangement of 8q11-13 most common cytogenetic anomaly

- Rearrangements involve *PLAG1* gene on 8q12
- *HAS2* on 8q24 and *COL1A2* on 7q22 have been reported as fusion partners for *PLAG1*
- *PLAG1* rearrangement by FISH present in both adipocytic and stromal components of lipoblastoma

Electron Microscopy
- Immature mesenchymal cells
- Lipoblasts in varying stages of development

DIFFERENTIAL DIAGNOSIS

Myxoid Liposarcoma (LPS)
- Rare in 1st 10 years of life
- Less lobulated than lipoblastoma
- Hypercellular round cell areas with nuclear atypia present in myxoid LPS
- Myxoid LPS is characterized by t(12;16)
- Lipoblastomas show rearrangements of 8q11-13 region

Lipoma/Hibernoma
- Lipoma- or hibernoma-like foci may be present in lipoblastoma
- Lipoblasts are not present in typical lipomas or hibernomas
- Myxoid stromal areas with plexiform vasculature are not seen in lipoma or hibernoma

DIAGNOSTIC CHECKLIST

Clinically Relevant Pathologic Features
- Age distribution

Pathologic Interpretation Pearls
- Lobulated tumor with univacuolar or multivacuolar lipoblasts and myxoid stroma
- No nuclear atypia

SELECTED REFERENCES

1. Hicks J et al: Lipoblastoma and lipoblastomatosis in infancy and childhood: histopathologic, ultrastructural, and cytogenetic features. Ultrastruct Pathol. 25(4):321-33, 2001
2. Chen Z et al: Evidence by spectral karyotyping that 8q11.2 is nonrandomly involved in lipoblastoma. J Mol Diagn. 2(2):73-7, 2000
3. Hibbard MK et al: PLAG1 fusion oncogenes in lipoblastoma. Cancer Res. 60(17):4869-72, 2000
4. Collins MH et al: Lipoblastoma/lipoblastomatosis: a clinicopathologic study of 25 tumors. Am J Surg Pathol. 21(10):1131-7, 1997
5. Mentzel T et al: Lipoblastoma and lipoblastomatosis: a clinicopathological study of 14 cases. Histopathology. 23(6):527-33, 1993
6. Chung EB et al: Benign lipoblastomatosis. An analysis of 35 cases. Cancer. 32(2):482-92, 1973

IMAGE GALLERY

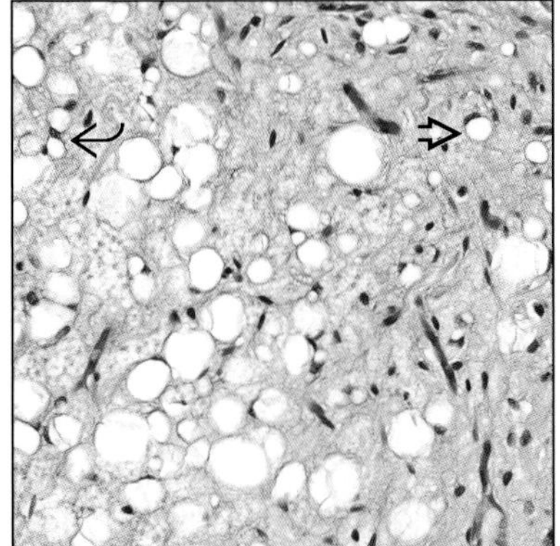
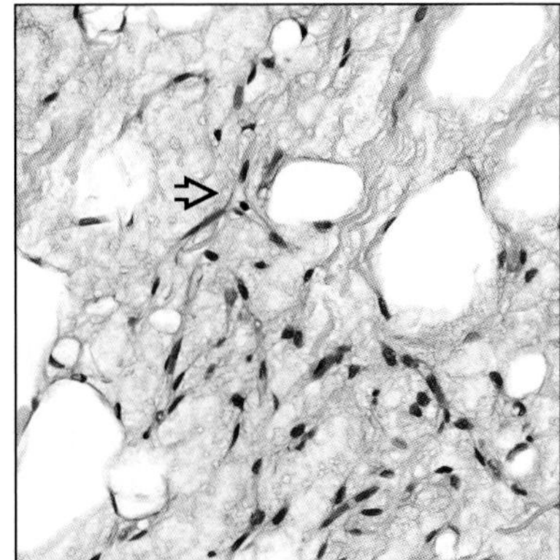
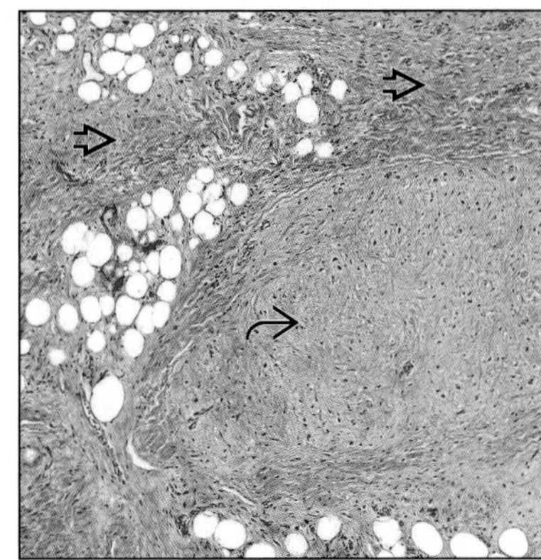

(Left) *Lipoblastomas show univacuolar ➡ and multivacuolar ➡ lipoblasts in a myxoid stromal background and adipocytes in various stages of development.* ***(Center)*** *Some lipoblastomas show a prominent plexiform vasculature ➡, which may be mistaken for a myxoid liposarcoma.* ***(Right)*** *The stroma may be collagenous ➡ or show nodular myxoid areas ➡. This corresponds to the gelatinous nodules seen on gross examination. (Courtesy A. Rosenberg, MD.)*

CHONDROID LIPOMA

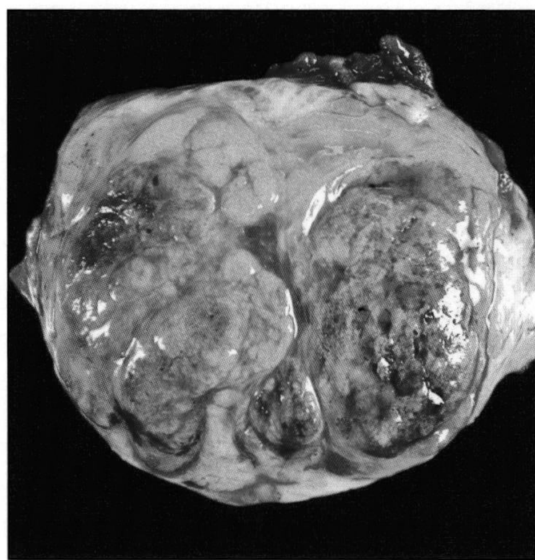

Gross photograph of chondroid lipoma shows a circumscribed lesion with a multilobulated, yellow to tan cut surface and prominent hemorrhage.

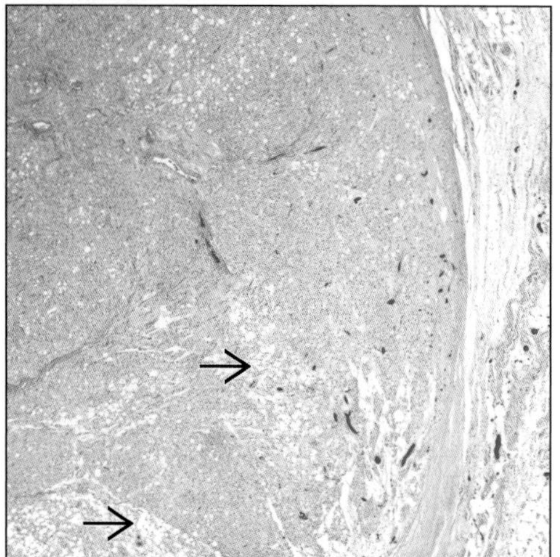

Hematoxylin & eosin shows a well-demarcated, encapsulated lesion within the subcutis. Sheets of cells with eosinophilic granular cytoplasm are admixed with mature adipocytes ⇒.

TERMINOLOGY

Definitions

- Uncommon benign neoplasm with features of embryonal fat and embryonal cartilage
  - Most frequently affects proximal limbs and limb girdles of adult women
- Often mistaken for sarcomas

ETIOLOGY/PATHOGENESIS

Developmental Anomaly

- Etiology unknown

CLINICAL ISSUES

Epidemiology

- Age
  - Adults; peak incidence = 3rd and 4th decades
- Gender
  - M:F = 1:4

Site

- Predominantly proximal limbs and limb girdles
- Trunk, head and neck (especially oral cavity)
- Both superficial and deep locations

Presentation

- Painless mass
  - Recent enlargement in 1/2 of cases

Treatment

- Surgical approaches
  - Simple complete excision

Prognosis

- Excision is curative
- Does not recur locally or metastasize

MACROSCOPIC FEATURES

General Features

- Frequently encapsulated, with yellow to tan, sometimes hemorrhagic cut surface

Size

- 1.5-11 cm (median = 4 cm)

MICROSCOPIC PATHOLOGY

Histologic Features

- Lobulated
- Nests and cords of rounded cells
- Cytoplasm is eosinophilic and granular with intracytoplasmic glycogen or with lipid vacuoles, consistent with lipoblastic differentiation
- No significant atypia or mitotic activity
- Variable mature adipose tissue component
- Prominent myxoid to hyalinized chondroid matrix, containing Alcian blue(+), hyaluronidase-resistant chondroitin sulphate
- Interspersed thick- and thin-walled vessels
- Variable hemorrhage, hemosiderin deposition, fibrosis, and calcification

Margins

- Circumscribed
- Encapsulated

Predominant Cell/Compartment Type

- Adipose

ANCILLARY TESTS

Immunohistochemistry

- Variable positivity for S100 protein in lipoblasts
- Occasional focal cytokeratin positivity, but EMA negativity

CHONDROID LIPOMA

Key Facts

Terminology

- Uncommon benign neoplasm with features of embryonal fat and embryonal cartilage
- Balanced translocation t(11;16)(q13; p12-13) in 2 cases, thought to be specific for lesion

Clinical Issues

- Peak incidence in 3rd and 4th decades
- Female preponderance
- Occurs in superficial and deep locations
- Most frequently affects proximal limbs and limb girdles

Microscopic Pathology

- Nests and cords of rounded cells with granular eosinophilic cytoplasm or multivacuolated cytoplasm containing lipid
- Prominent myxohyaline stroma
- Variable amount of mature adipose tissue
- S100 protein and CD68 positive

- Focal CD68 positivity in vacuolated cells

Cytogenetics

- t(11;16)(q13;p12-13) in 2 cases, which appears characteristic for this lesion

Electron Microscopy

- Spectrum of cellular differentiation
  - Primitive cells sharing features of prelipoblasts and chondroblasts
  - Lipoblasts and mature adipocytes
- Abundant intracytoplasmic lipid and glycogen
- Characteristic knob-like cytoplasmic protrusions

DIFFERENTIAL DIAGNOSIS

Soft Tissue Chondroma

- Hands and feet
- True hyaline cartilage matrix
- No adipocytic component

Myoepithelial Tumor

- Usually superficial
- Ductal/epithelial structures often present
- More pronounced and uniform cytokeratin positivity
- Positive: SMA, EMA, calponin

Myxoid Liposarcoma

- Deep location, can reach large size
- Spindle cell component
- Plexiform vascular pattern
- Round cell liposarcoma has larger cells, few vacuoles
- Characteristic translocations t(12;16), t(12;22)

Extraskeletal Myxoid Chondrosarcoma

- Slowly growing infiltrative tumor
- Multilobulated with fibrous septa
- Can reach large size
- Cells form anastomosing cords
- Cytoplasmic vacuoles usually absent
- No fatty component
- Characteristic translocations t(9;17), t(9:22)

SELECTED REFERENCES

1. Ballaux F et al: Chondroid lipoma is characterized by t(11;16)(q13;p12-13). Virchows Arch. 444(2):208-10, 2004
2. Thomson TA et al: Cytogenetic and cytologic features of chondroid lipoma of soft tissue. Mod Pathol. 12(1):88-91, 1999
3. Kindblom LG et al: Chondroid lipoma: an ultrastructural and immunohistochemical analysis with further observations regarding its differentiation. Hum Pathol. 26(7):706-15, 1995
4. Nielsen GP et al: Chondroid lipoma, a tumor of white fat cells. A brief report of two cases with ultrastructural analysis. Am J Surg Pathol. 19(11):1272-6, 1995
5. Meis JM et al: Chondroid lipoma. A unique tumor simulating liposarcoma and myxoid chondrosarcoma. Am J Surg Pathol. 17(11):1103-12, 1993

IMAGE GALLERY

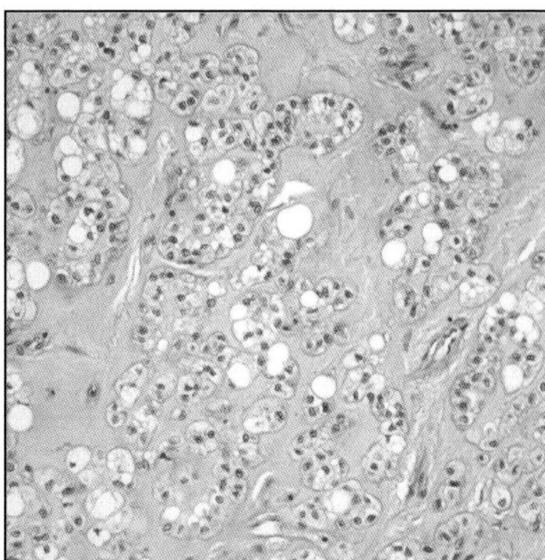

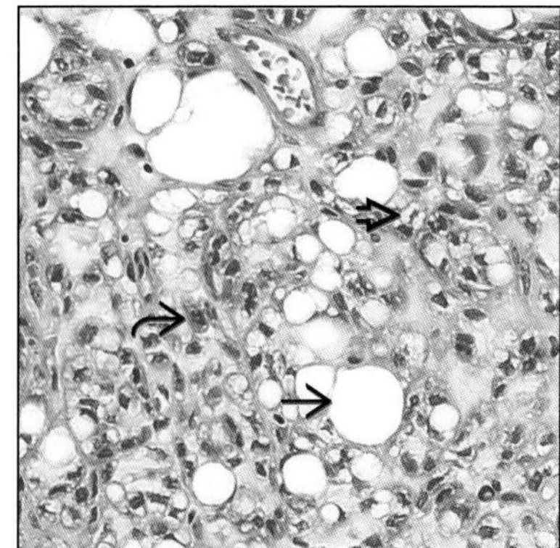

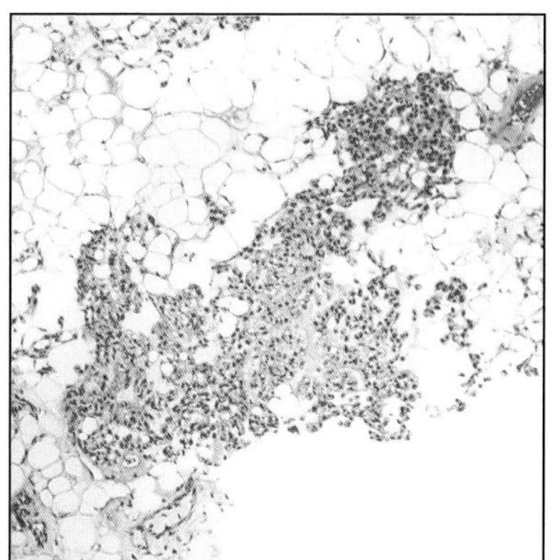

(Left) *Hematoxylin & eosin shows islands of rounded cells in a hypocellular chondroid-like stroma. The cells are lipoblastic-like, with multivacuolated, lipid-containing cytoplasm. Mature adipocytes are present.* ***(Center)*** *Hematoxylin & eosin shows cells with eosinophilic granular cytoplasm ⇗ admixed with lipoblast-like cells ⇨ and mature adipocytes →.* ***(Right)*** *Hematoxylin & eosin shows chondroid lipoma in a core biopsy fragment. Cellular proliferation of rounded cells within myxoid stroma can lead to an erroneous diagnosis of myxoid liposarcoma.*

ATYPICAL LIPOMATOUS TUMOR/WELL-DIFFERENTIATED LIPOSARCOMA

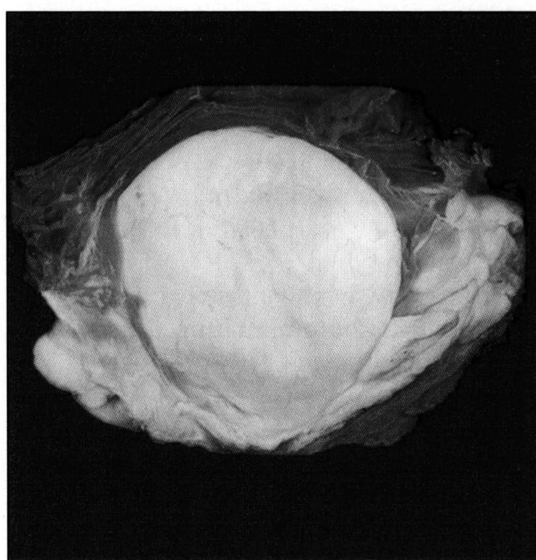

Gross pathology photograph shows a well-circumscribed neoplasm of deep soft tissues with indurated, yellow-white cut surfaces.

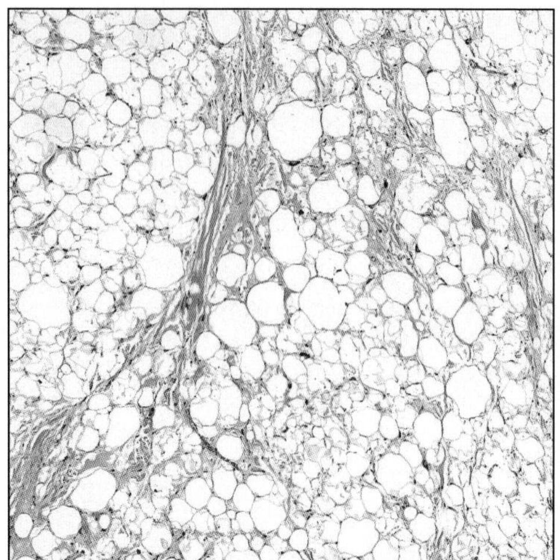

Hematoxylin & eosin shows striking variations in size and shape of lipogenic cells, as well as scattered enlarged cells with enlarged hyperchromatic nuclei.

TERMINOLOGY

Abbreviations

- Atypical lipomatous tumor (ALT)

Synonyms

- Well-differentiated liposarcoma (WDLS)

Definitions

- Intermediate (locally aggressive, nonmetastasizing) lipogenic neoplasm composed of atypical adipocytes

CLINICAL ISSUES

Epidemiology

- Incidence
  - Accounts for 40-45% of all liposarcomas
  - Most frequently in deep soft tissues
    - Retroperitoneum, abdominal cavity, paratesticular region, mediastinum
    - Limbs
  - May also arise in subcutaneous tissue and very rarely in skin
- Age
  - Middle-aged to elderly adults
  - Extremely rare in childhood
- Gender
  - M = F

Presentation

- Deep-seated, painless, and slowly enlarging tumor mass

Treatment

- Complete surgical excision

Prognosis

- In surgically amenable site
  - Recur only rarely after complete excision
- Intraabdominal, retroperitoneal, mediastinal, or paratesticular lesions
  - Often recur locally and may be fatal
- Variable risk of dedifferentiation in extremities (< 2%) and in retroperitoneum (> 20%)

IMAGE FINDINGS

General Features

- Best diagnostic clue
  - Circumscribed lobular mass
- Location
  - Deep soft tissues
- Size
  - Variable
  - Usually > 5 cm
- Morphology
  - Circumscribed lipomatous lesion

MACROSCOPIC FEATURES

General Features

- Well-circumscribed lobular neoplasms
- Color varies from yellow to white
- Fat necrosis may be seen in large lesions

Sections to Be Submitted

- Sample margins and representative sections of tumor
- Look for indurated, firm areas

Size

- May attain very large size

MICROSCOPIC PATHOLOGY

Histologic Features

- Lipoma-like subtype
  - Adipocytes show significant variation in size and shape

ATYPICAL LIPOMATOUS TUMOR/WELL-DIFFERENTIATED LIPOSARCOMA

Key Facts

Terminology

- Intermediate (locally aggressive, nonmetastasizing) lipogenic neoplasm composed of atypical adipocytes

Clinical Issues

- Accounts for 40-45% of all liposarcomas
- Occurs most frequently in deep soft tissues of limbs followed by retroperitoneum, abdominal cavity, paratesticular region, and mediastinum
- Usually presents as deep-seated, painless, and slowly enlarging tumor mass
- Lesions located in surgically amenable soft tissues recur only rarely after complete excision
- Neoplasms arising intraabdominal, retroperitoneum, mediastinum, or spermatic cord often recur repeatedly and may cause death
- Variable risk of dedifferentiation in extremities (< 2%) and retroperitoneum (> 20%)
- May also arise in subcutaneous tissue and very rarely in skin
- Middle-aged to elderly adults
- Intermediate (locally aggressive but nonmetastasizing) malignant mesenchymal tumor

Microscopic Pathology

- Atypical adipocytes, atypical stromal cells, lipoblasts
  - Adipocytes show striking variations in size and shape
  - Enlarged hyperchromatic nuclei
- Lipoma-like subtype
- Sclerosing subtype
- Inflammatory subtype
- Spindle cell subtype

  - Enlarged hyperchromatic nuclei
  - Hyperchromatic and multinucleated stromal cells
  - Lipoblasts may be seen but are not essential for diagnosis
  - Involvement of large vessel walls by atypical tumor cells
  - Prominent myxoid stromal changes may be present
  - Rare chondroid stromal changes
- Sclerosing subtype
  - Scattered bizarre stromal cells with hyperchromatic nuclei
  - Rare atypical lipogenic cells and multivacuolated lipoblasts
  - Fibrillary, collagenous stroma
- Inflammatory subtype
  - Prominent inflammatory infiltrate (lymphocytes, plasma cells)
  - Scattered atypical lipogenic cells/lipoblasts
  - Often edematous stroma
- Spindle cell subtype
  - Atypical lipogenic cells
  - Slightly atypical neuroid spindle cells
  - Fibrous, fibromyxoid stroma
- Heterologous differentiation rarely seen
  - Smooth or striated muscle
  - Cartilage, bone

Predominant Pattern/Injury Type

- Circumscribed

Predominant Cell/Compartment Type

- Adipose
  - Atypical adipocytes, atypical stromal cells, lipoblasts

Grade

- Intermediate (locally aggressive but nonmetastasizing) malignant mesenchymal tumor

ANCILLARY TESTS

Cytogenetics

- Supernumerary ring and giant marker chromosomes
  - Contain amplified sequences originating from 12q14-15 region
  - MDM2, CDK4, SAS, HMGIC are amplified

In Situ Hybridization

- MDM2 and CDK4 amplification can be identified by FISH technique

DIFFERENTIAL DIAGNOSIS

Lipoma

- Lobular growth
- No or only slight atypia of adipocytes
- No increased number of enlarged and hyperchromatic nuclei
- No lipoblasts
- No amplification of MDM2 &/or CDK4

Spindle Cell/Pleomorphic Lipoma

- Usually in elderly male patients
- Arises usually in subcutaneous tissue of neck, shoulder, or upper back
- No or only slight atypia of adipocytes
- Bland CD34(+) spindled &/or multinucleated giant cells ("floret-like giant cells")
- Rope-like collagen bundles; often myxoid stromal changes; scattered mast cells
- No amplification of MDM2 &/or CDK4

Pseudolipoblastic Granulomatous Foreign Body Reaction

- Multivacuolated CD68(+) histiocytes
- No atypical lipogenic cells

Angiomyolipoma

- Myogenic tumor cells expressing myogenic and melanocytic markers
- Thick-walled blood vessels
- Predominantly renal/perirenal tissues

Inflammatory Myofibroblastic Tumor

- Fascicles of myofibroblastic spindled cells

ATYPICAL LIPOMATOUS TUMOR/WELL-DIFFERENTIATED LIPOSARCOMA

Immunohistochemistry

Antibody	Reactivity	Staining Pattern	Comment
CDK4	Positive	Nuclear	Focal expression; may be negative; reactive histiocytes may be positive as well
MDM2	Positive	Nuclear	Focal expression; may be negative; reactive histiocytes may be positive as well

- No atypical lipogenic tumor component
- Expression of ALK in a number of cases (especially in children and adolescents)

Sclerosing Lipoma

- Dermal neoplasms
- No atypical lipogenic tumor cells

Dedifferentiated Liposarcoma

- Abrupt or gradual transition from atypical lipomatous tissue to nonlipogenic component
- Atypical nonlipogenic tumor component with variable morphologic features
- Strong expression of MDM2 and CDK4

Angiolipoma

- Subcutaneous nodules in young adults
- Often multiple lesions
- Often tender to painful lesions
- Forearm represents most common site
- Mature fat separated by small blood vessels
- Vascular channels contain fibrin thrombi

DIAGNOSTIC CHECKLIST

Clinically Relevant Pathologic Features

- Gross appearance
- Organ distribution
- Age distribution

Pathologic Interpretation Pearls

- Atypical lipogenic cells
- Atypical stromal cells
- Often focal nuclear expression of MDM2 &/or CDK4
- Amplification of MDM2 and CDK4 detected by FISH analysis

SELECTED REFERENCES

1. Evans HL: Atypical lipomatous tumor, its variants, and its combined forms: a study of 61 cases, with a minimum follow-up of 10 years. Am J Surg Pathol. 31(1):1-14, 2007
2. Sirvent N et al: Detection of MDM2-CDK4 amplification by fluorescence in situ hybridization in 200 paraffin-embedded tumor samples: utility in diagnosing adipocytic lesions and comparison with immunohistochemistry and real-time PCR. Am J Surg Pathol. 31(10):1476-89, 2007
3. Binh MB et al: MDM2 and CDK4 immunostainings are useful adjuncts in diagnosing well-differentiated and dedifferentiated liposarcoma subtypes: a comparative analysis of 559 soft tissue neoplasms with genetic data. Am J Surg Pathol. 29(10):1340-7, 2005
4. Folpe AL et al: Lipoleiomyosarcoma (well-differentiated liposarcoma with leiomyosarcomatous differentiation): a clinicopathologic study of nine cases including one with dedifferentiation. Am J Surg Pathol. 26(6):742-9, 2002
5. Micci F et al: Characterization of supernumerary rings and giant marker chromosomes in well-differentiated lipomatous tumors by a combination of G-banding, CGH, M-FISH, and chromosome- and locus-specific FISH. Cytogenet Genome Res. 97(1-2):13-9, 2002
6. Nascimento AF et al: Liposarcomas/atypical lipomatous tumors of the oral cavity: a clinicopathologic study of 23 cases. Ann Diagn Pathol. 6(2):83-93, 2002
7. Dei Tos AP et al: Coordinated expression and amplification of the MDM2, CDK4, and HMGI-C genes in atypical lipomatous tumours. J Pathol. 190(5):531-6, 2000
8. Mentzel T: Biological continuum of benign, atypical, and malignant mesenchymal neoplasms - does it exist? J Pathol. 190(5):523-5, 2000
9. Pedeutour F et al: Structure of the supernumerary ring and giant rod chromosomes in adipose tissue tumors. Genes Chromosomes Cancer. 24(1):30-41, 1999
10. Dei Tos AP et al: Primary liposarcoma of the skin: a rare neoplasm with unusual high grade features. Am J Dermatopathol. 20(4):332-8, 1998
11. Kraus MD et al: Well-differentiated inflammatory liposarcoma: an uncommon and easily overlooked variant of a common sarcoma. Am J Surg Pathol. 21(5):518-27, 1997
12. Fletcher CD et al: Correlation between clinicopathological features and karyotype in lipomatous tumors. A report of 178 cases from the Chromosomes and Morphology (CHAMP) Collaborative Study Group. Am J Pathol. 148(2):623-30, 1996
13. Mentzel T et al: Lipomatous tumours of soft tissues: an update. Virchows Arch. 427(4):353-63, 1995
14. Nilbert M et al: Characterization of the 12q13-15 amplicon in soft tissue tumors. Cancer Genet Cytogenet. 83(1):32-6, 1995
15. Dal Cin P et al: Cytogenetic and fluorescence in situ hybridization investigation of ring chromosomes characterizing a specific pathologic subgroup of adipose tissue tumors. Cancer Genet Cytogenet. 68(2):85-90, 1993
16. Weiss SW et al: Well-differentiated liposarcoma (atypical lipoma) of deep soft tissue of the extremities, retroperitoneum, and miscellaneous sites. A follow-up study of 92 cases with analysis of the incidence of "dedifferentiation". Am J Surg Pathol. 16(11):1051-8, 1992
17. Azumi N et al: Atypical and malignant neoplasms showing lipomatous differentiation. A study of 111 cases. Am J Surg Pathol. 11(3):161-83, 1987
18. Bolen JW et al: Liposarcomas. A histogenetic approach to the classification of adipose tissue neoplasms. Am J Surg Pathol. 8(1):3-17, 1984
19. Kindblom LG et al: Atypical lipoma. Acta Pathol Microbiol Immunol Scand [A]. 90(1):27-36, 1982
20. Evans HL et al: Atypical lipoma, atypical intramuscular lipoma, and well differentiated retroperitoneal liposarcoma: a reappraisal of 30 cases formerly classified as well differentiated liposarcoma. Cancer. 43(2):574-84, 1979

Gross and Microscopic Features

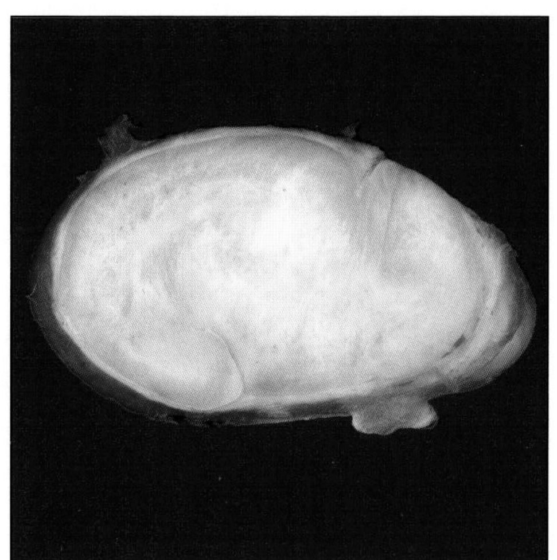
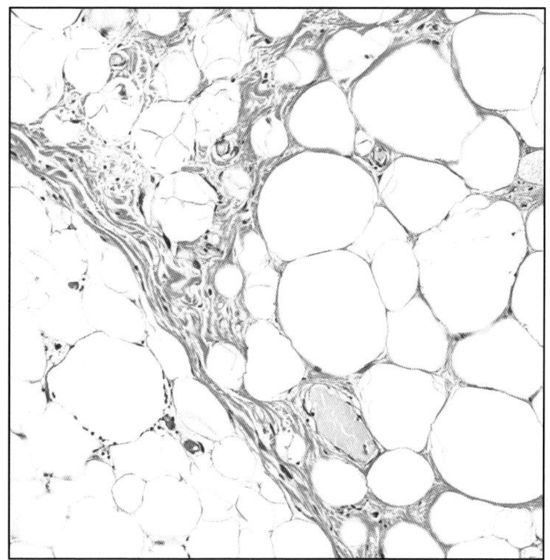

(Left) *Gross pathology photograph shows indurated, gray-white cut surface in this example of an atypical lipomatous tumor.* ***(Right)*** *Hematoxylin & eosin shows the lipoma-like subtype of an atypical lipomatous tumor with variation in size and shape of lipogenic tumor cells and scattered cells with enlarged hyperchromatic nuclei.*

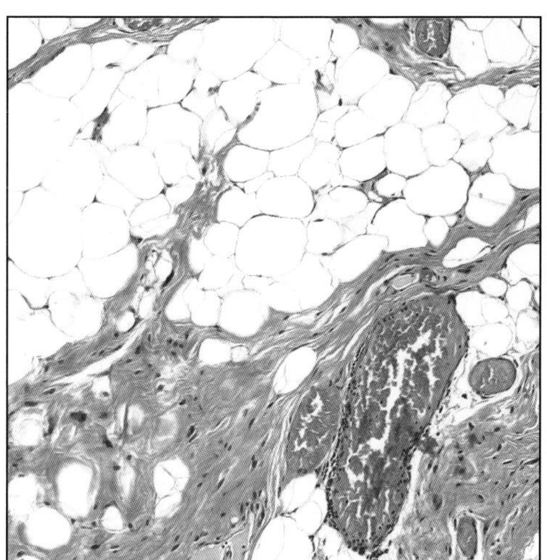
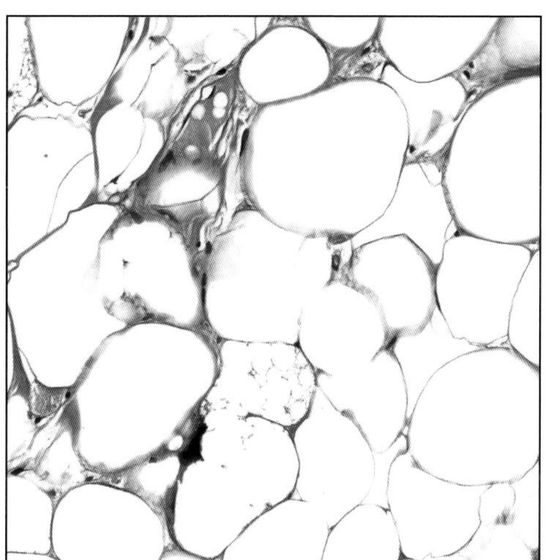

(Left) *Hematoxylin & eosin shows fibrous septa with enlarged cells containing irregularly shaped, hyperchromatic nuclei.* ***(Right)*** *Hematoxylin & eosin shows multivacuolated lipoblasts containing hyperchromatic nuclei. Note the indentation of the hyperchromatic nuclei.*

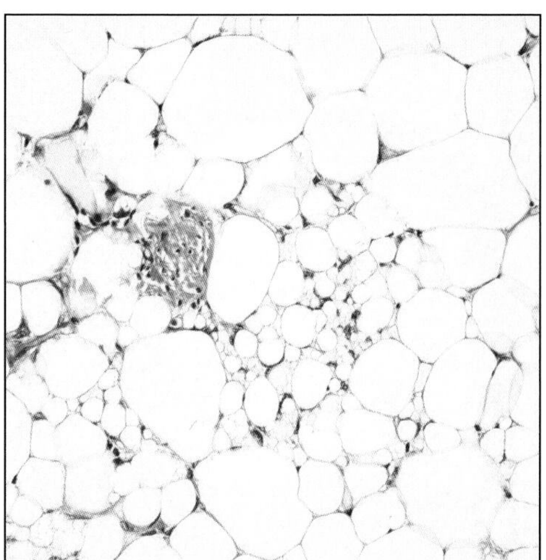
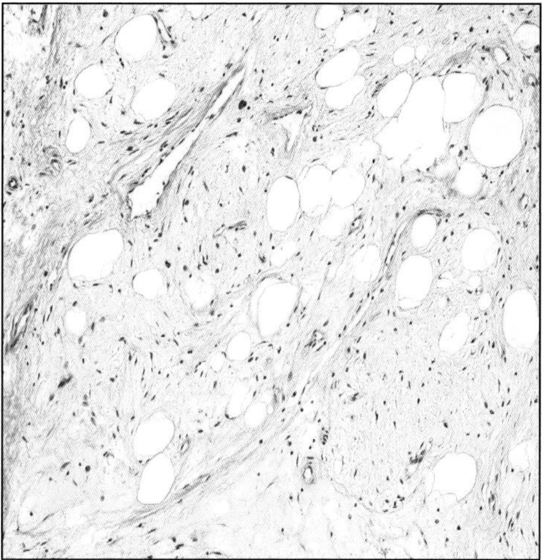

(Left) *Hematoxylin & eosin shows scattered lipoblasts in a perivascular location.* ***(Right)*** *Hematoxylin & eosin shows the lipoma-like subtype of an atypical lipomatous tumor with myxoid stromal changes.*

ATYPICAL LIPOMATOUS TUMOR/WELL-DIFFERENTIATED LIPOSARCOMA

Microscopic and Immunohistochemical Features

*(**Left**) Hematoxylin & eosin shows the lipoma-like subtype of an atypical lipomatous tumor with a focus of chondroid metaplasia. The cartilaginous tissue appears histologically benign. (**Right**) S100P immunostain shows lipogenic cells of variable size and shape and multivacuolated lipoblasts.*

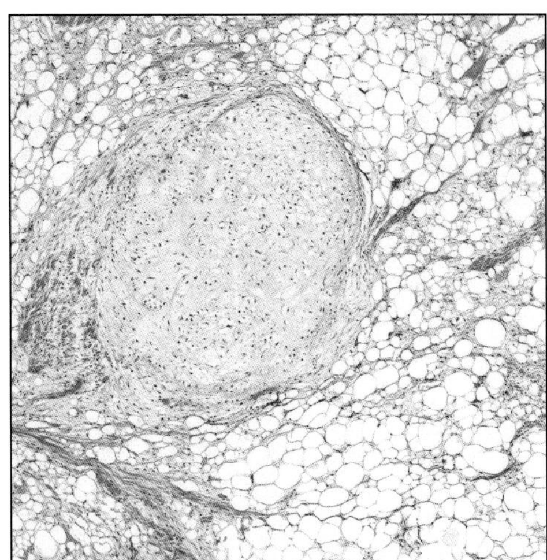

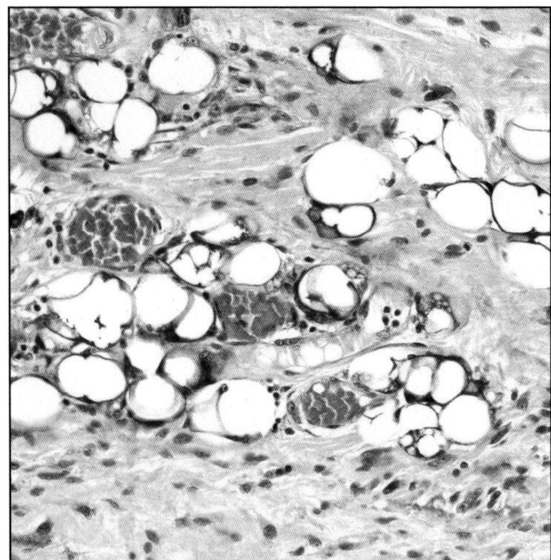

*(**Left**) MDM2 immunostain shows focal nuclear expression. (**Right**) CDK4 immunostain shows focal nuclear expression.*

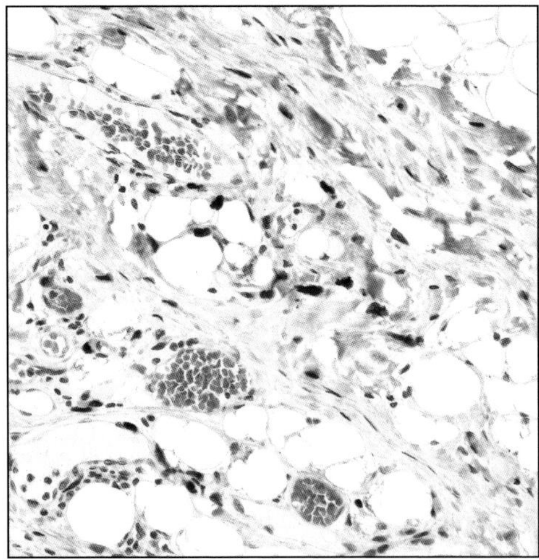

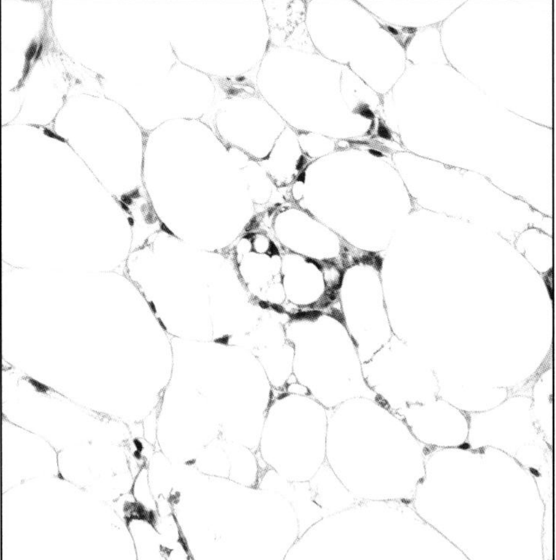

*(**Left**) Hematoxylin & eosin shows scattered lipogenic cells including bivacuolated lipoblasts ➔ set in a prominent collagenous stroma in this example of the sclerosing subtype of an atypical lipomatous tumor. (**Right**) Hematoxylin & eosin shows an example of the inflammatory subtype of an atypical lipomatous tumor with a prominent inflammatory infiltrate, edematous stroma, and only scattered atypical lipogenic tumor cells ➔.*

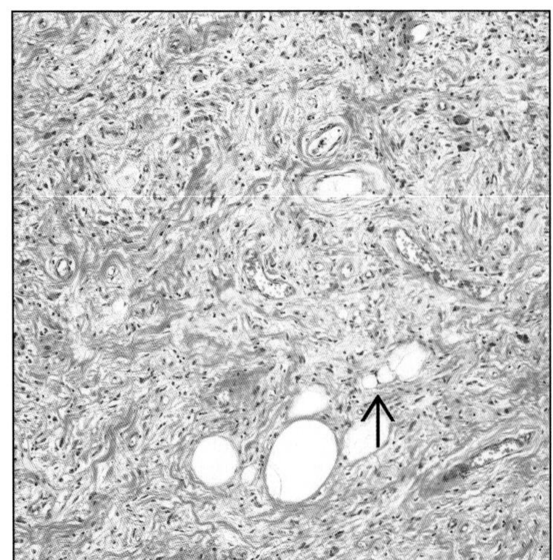

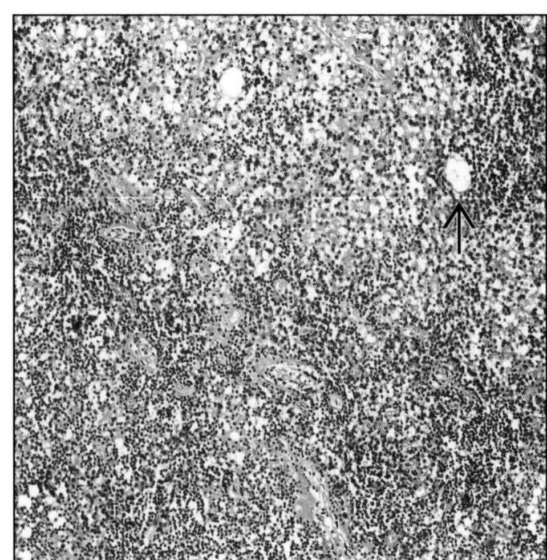

Microscopic Features and FISH Analysis

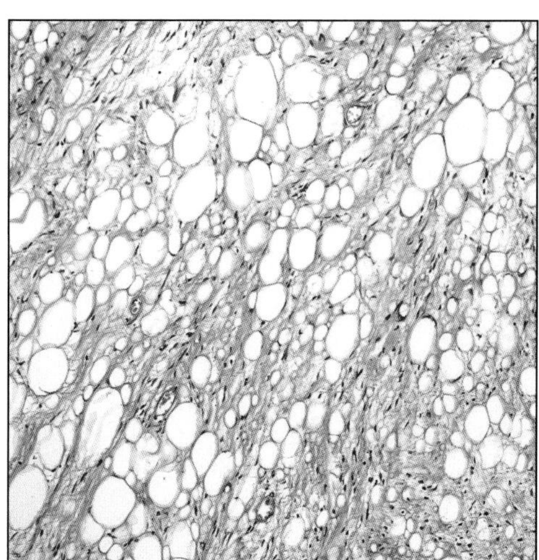

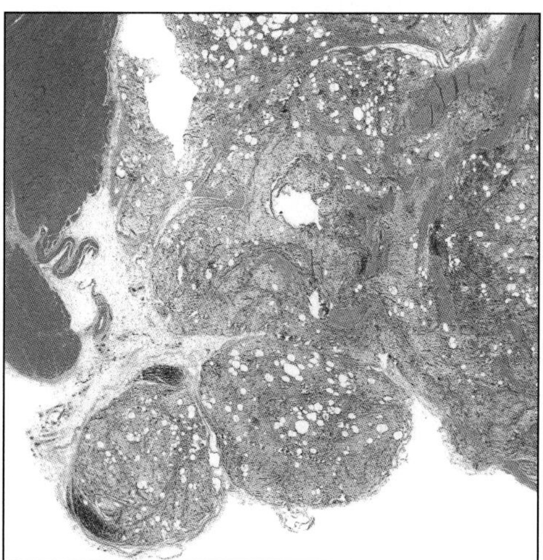

(Left) *Hematoxylin & eosin shows an atypical lipomatous tumor of the spindle cell subtype with atypical lipogenic cells admixed with slightly enlarged spindled tumor cells.* ***(Right)*** *Hematoxylin & eosin of this spindle cell subtype of an atypical lipomatous tumor shows a deep-seated lobular neoplasm.*

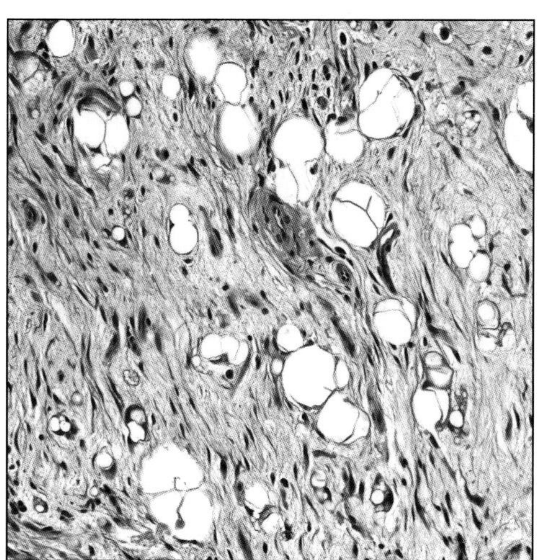

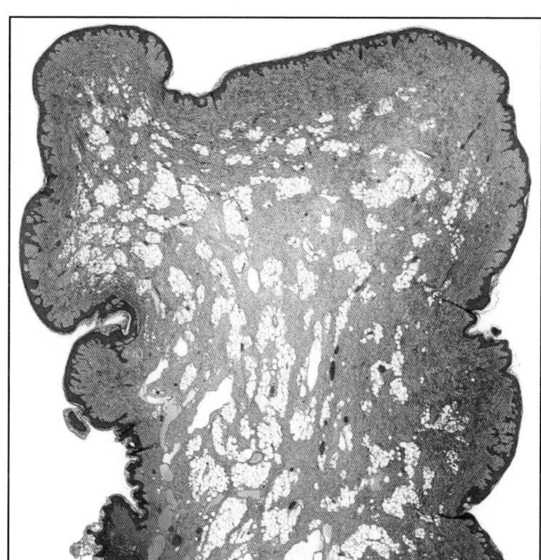

(Left) *Hematoxylin & eosin shows a neoplasm composed of atypical lipogenic and spindled tumor cells with enlarged and hyperchromatic nuclei.* ***(Right)*** *Hematoxylin & eosin shows a low-power view of a rare cutaneous atypical lipomatous tumor.*

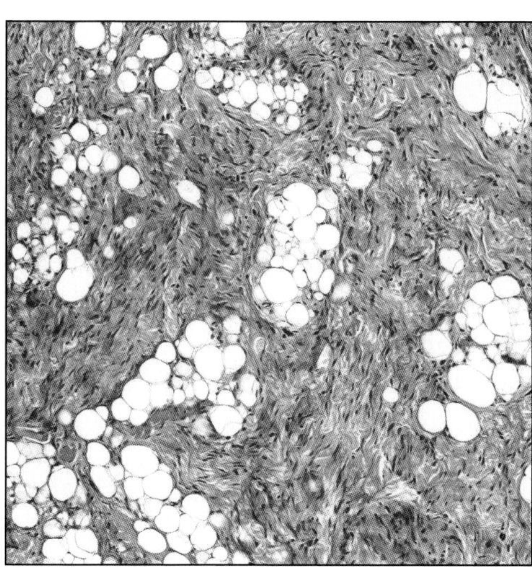

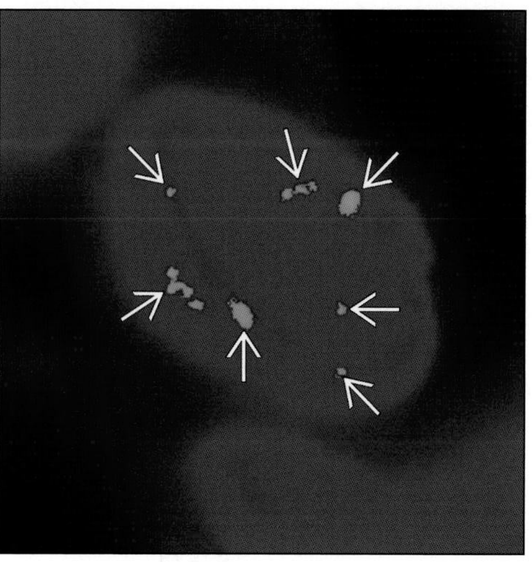

(Left) *Hematoxylin & eosin shows a cutaneous atypical lipomatous tumor as an ill-defined dermal neoplasm composed of atypical lipogenic cells with enlarged and hyperchromatic nuclei.* ***(Right)*** *In situ hybridization FISH analysis shows MDM2 amplification. Note numerous signals* ➡ *in an analyzed tumor cell nucleus.*

DEDIFFERENTIATED LIPOSARCOMA

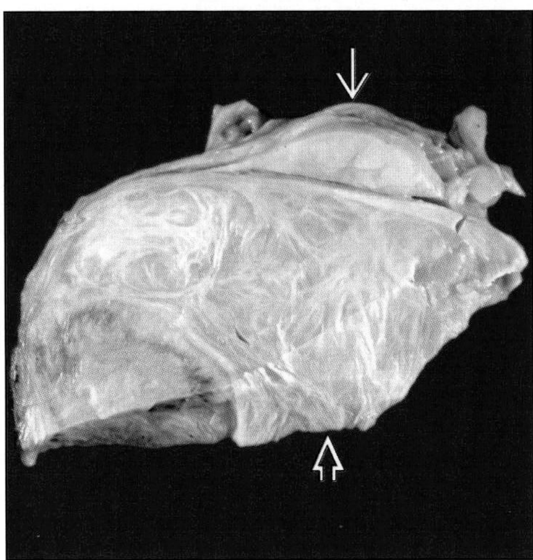

Gross pathology photograph shows an abrupt transition from atypical lipomatous tissue ➡ to a larger, nonlipogenic sarcomatous component ⇨.

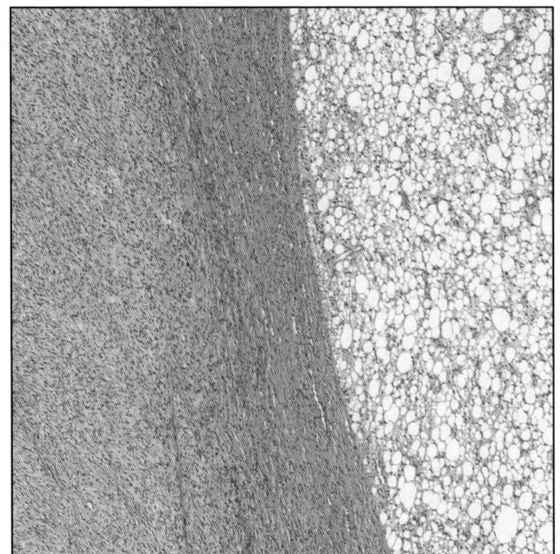

Hematoxylin & eosin shows dedifferentiated nonlipogenic sarcoma (left) with an abrupt transition from atypical lipomatous tumor (right). Note the sharp demarcation between the 2 components.

TERMINOLOGY

Abbreviations

- Dedifferentiated liposarcoma (DDLS)

Definitions

- Malignant lipogenic neoplasm with abrupt or gradual transition from atypical lipomatous tumor to nonlipogenic sarcoma of variable histology

CLINICAL ISSUES

Epidemiology

- Incidence
  - Occurs in ~ 10% of cases of atypical lipomatous tumor
  - 90% arise de novo, 10% in local recurrences
  - Retroperitoneum, intraabdominal cavity are more frequently involved than extremities, spermatic cord, head/neck region, trunk
  - Mainly in deep soft tissues
  - Very rare in subcutaneous and dermal tissues
  - Probably represents time-dependent phenomenon
- Age
  - Middle-aged to elderly patients
- Gender
  - M = F

Presentation

- Large, painless mass
- Slowly growing neoplasm
- Often longstanding mass exhibiting recent increase in size

Treatment

- Surgical approaches
  - Complete excision with tumor-free margins

Prognosis

- Recurs locally in ≥ 40% of cases
- Distant metastases observed in 15-20% of cases
- Overall mortality 25-30% at 5-year follow-up
- Anatomic location is most important prognostic factor
- Retroperitoneal, intraabdominal lesions exhibit worst clinical behavior
- Superficial neoplasms have good prognosis
- Amount and morphological grade of nonlipogenic areas not of prognostic importance

IMAGE FINDINGS

General Features

- Best diagnostic clue
  - Coexistence of fatty and non-fatty-solid components
- Location
  - Retroperitoneum, intraabdominal cavity, deep soft tissues
- Size
  - Large size, usually > 5 cm
- Morphology
  - Circumscribed

MACROSCOPIC FEATURES

General Features

- Large, multinodular yellow mass with solid, often tan-gray or gray-white nonlipomatous areas

Sections to Be Submitted

- Sections of both components must be sampled carefully

Size

- May reach large size, especially in abdomen and retroperitoneum

DEDIFFERENTIATED LIPOSARCOMA

Key Facts

Terminology

- Malignant lipogenic neoplasm showing abrupt or gradual transition from atypical lipomatous tumor to nonlipogenic sarcoma of variable histology

Clinical Issues

- Retroperitoneum, intraabdominal cavity more frequently involved than extremities, spermatic cord, head/neck region, trunk
- Recurs locally in at least 40% of cases
- Distant metastases observed in 15-20% of cases
- Anatomic location represents most important prognostic factor
- Dedifferentiation most probably represents time-dependent phenomenon
- Dedifferentiation occurs in ~ 10% of cases of atypical lipomatous tumor
- Amount and morphological grade of nonlipogenic areas not of prognostic importance

Microscopic Pathology

- Atypical lipogenic tumor cells
- Nonlipogenic sarcoma cells
- Broad variation of nonlipogenic component
- Nonlipogenic component may show low- or high-grade sarcomatous changes
- Abrupt or gradual transition from atypical lipomatous tumor (of any subtype) to nonlipogenic sarcoma
- Heterologous differentiation in ~ 10% of cases

Ancillary Tests

- Amplification of 12q13-21 region similar to changes in atypical lipomatous tumor
- MDM2 and CDK4 overexpression

MICROSCOPIC PATHOLOGY

Histologic Features

- Abrupt or gradual transition from atypical lipomatous tumor (of any subtype) to nonlipogenic sarcoma
- Varying size and shape of lipogenic tumor cells
- Presence of enlarged and hyperchromatic nuclei in lipogenic component
- Nonlipogenic sarcoma component shows broad morphologic variation
- High-grade nonlipogenic sarcoma component (pleomorphic sarcoma, intermediate- to high-grade myxofibrosarcoma-like areas)
- Often presence of multinucleated giant cells
- Increased proliferative activity
- Low-grade nonlipogenic component (uniform fibroblastic spindle cells with mild nuclear atypia)
- Heterologous differentiation in ~ 10% of cases
  - Rhabdomyosarcoma
  - Leiomyosarcoma
  - Osteo- or chondrosarcoma
  - Angiosarcoma
- Rarely neural-like, meningothelial whorling pattern in nonlipogenic areas

Margins

- Clear tumor margins with rim of tumor-free tissue mandatory

Predominant Pattern/Injury Type

- Biphasic
  - Abrupt or gradual transition from atypical lipomatous tumor to nonlipogenic sarcoma areas

Predominant Cell/Compartment Type

- Adipose cell
  - Atypical lipogenic tumor cells
  - Nonlipogenic sarcoma cells

Grade

- Usually grade II of malignancy

ANCILLARY TESTS

Immunohistochemistry

- Useful for recognition of divergent differentiation in nonlipogenic areas

Cytogenetics

- Amplification of 12q13-21 region similar to changes in atypical lipomatous tumor
- MDM2 and CDK4 amplification
- Additional *p53* mutations

DIFFERENTIAL DIAGNOSIS

Atypical Lipomatous Tumor (Spindle Cell Variant)

- Lipogenic neoplasm with atypical adipocytes, lipoblasts, and spindle cells
- No nonlipogenic component

Fibrosarcoma

- No lipogenic component
- No MDM2 &/or CDK4 amplification

Myxofibrosarcoma

- Rarely in retroperitoneal and intraabdominal locations
- No lipogenic component
- No MDM2 &/or CDK4 amplification

Pleomorphic Liposarcoma

- No atypical lipomatous tumor component
- Pleomorphic lipoblasts
- No MDM2 &/or CDK4 amplification

Spindle Cell/Pleomorphic Lipoma

- Clinical features (elderly male patients, back, neck, shoulder)
- Subcutaneous neoplasms
- Encapsulated neoplasms
- No significant atypia of spindle &/or multinucleated giant cell
- No MDM2 &/or CDK4 amplification

DEDIFFERENTIATED LIPOSARCOMA

Immunohistochemistry

Antibody	Reactivity	Staining Pattern	Comment
MDM2	Positive	Nuclear	More positive cells than in ALT
CDK4	Positive	Nuclear	More positive cells than in ALT
Actin-sm	Positive	Cytoplasmic	
Desmin	Positive	Cytoplasmic	
CD34	Positive	Cell membrane & cytoplasm	

DIAGNOSTIC CHECKLIST

Clinically Relevant Pathologic Features

- Organ distribution
- Gross appearance

Pathologic Interpretation Pearls

- Abrupt/gradual transition from atypical lipomatous tumor areas to nonlipogenic sarcoma areas
- Variation of nonlipogenic sarcomatous component
- MDM2 &/or CDK4 amplification
- Most if not all pleomorphic sarcomas in abdomen and retroperitoneum represent DDLS

SELECTED REFERENCES

1. Italiano A et al: HMGA2 is the partner of MDM2 in well-differentiated and dedifferentiated liposarcomas whereas CDK4 belongs to a distinct inconsistent amplicon. Int J Cancer. 122(10):2233-41, 2008
2. Binh MB et al: Dedifferentiated liposarcomas with divergent myosarcomatous differentiation developed in the internal trunk: a study of 27 cases and comparison to conventional dedifferentiated liposarcomas and leiomyosarcomas. Am J Surg Pathol. 31(10):1557-66, 2007
3. Evans HL: Atypical lipomatous tumor, its variants, and its combined forms: a study of 61 cases, with a minimum follow-up of 10 years. Am J Surg Pathol. 31(1):1-14, 2007
4. Singer S et al: Gene expression profiling of liposarcoma identifies distinct biological types/subtypes and potential therapeutic targets in well-differentiated and dedifferentiated liposarcoma. Cancer Res. 67(14):6626-36, 2007
5. Sirvent N et al: Detection of MDM2-CDK4 amplification by fluorescence in situ hybridization in 200 paraffin-embedded tumor samples: utility in diagnosing adipocytic lesions and comparison with immunohistochemistry and real-time PCR. Am J Surg Pathol. 31(10):1476-89, 2007
6. Fabre-Guillevin E et al: Retroperitoneal liposarcomas: follow-up analysis of dedifferentiation after clinicopathologic reexamination of 86 liposarcomas and malignant fibrous histiocytomas. Cancer. 106(12):2725-33, 2006
7. Binh MB et al: MDM2 and CDK4 immunostainings are useful adjuncts in diagnosing well-differentiated and dedifferentiated liposarcoma subtypes: a comparative analysis of 559 soft tissue neoplasms with genetic data. Am J Surg Pathol. 29(10):1340-7, 2005
8. Coindre JM et al: Inflammatory malignant fibrous histiocytomas and dedifferentiated liposarcomas: histological review, genomic profile, and MDM2 and CDK4 status favour a single entity. J Pathol. 203(3):822-30, 2004
9. Hostein I et al: Evaluation of MDM2 and CDK4 amplification by real-time PCR on paraffin wax-embedded material: a potential tool for the diagnosis of atypical lipomatous tumours/well-differentiated liposarcomas. J Pathol. 202(1):95-102, 2004
10. Coindre JM et al: Most malignant fibrous histiocytomas developed in the retroperitoneum are dedifferentiated liposarcomas: a review of 25 cases initially diagnosed as malignant fibrous histiocytoma. Mod Pathol. 16(3):256-62, 2003
11. Adachi T et al: Immunoreactivity of p53, mdm2, and p21WAF1 in dedifferentiated liposarcoma: special emphasis on the distinct immunophenotype of the well-differentiated component. Int J Surg Pathol. 9(2):99-109, 2001
12. Hasegawa T et al: Dedifferentiated liposarcoma of retroperitoneum and mesentery: varied growth patterns and histological grades--a clinicopathologic study of 32 cases. Hum Pathol. 31(6):717-27, 2000
13. Hisaoka M et al: Retroperitoneal liposarcoma with combined well-differentiated and myxoid malignant fibrous histiocytoma-like myxoid areas. Am J Surg Pathol. 23(12):1480-92, 1999
14. Nascimento AG et al: Dedifferentiated liposarcoma: a report of nine cases with a peculiar neurallike whorling pattern associated with metaplastic bone formation. Am J Surg Pathol. 22(8):945-55, 1998
15. Dei Tos AP et al: Molecular abnormalities of the p53 pathway in dedifferentiated liposarcoma. J Pathol. 181(1):8-13, 1997
16. Elgar F et al: Well-differentiated liposarcoma of the retroperitoneum: a clinicopathologic analysis of 20 cases, with particular attention to the extent of low-grade dedifferentiation. Mod Pathol. 10(2):113-20, 1997
17. Henricks WH et al: Dedifferentiated liposarcoma: a clinicopathological analysis of 155 cases with a proposal for an expanded definition of dedifferentiation. Am J Surg Pathol. 21(3):271-81, 1997
18. Pilotti S et al: Distinct mdm2/p53 expression patterns in liposarcoma subgroups: implications for different pathogenetic mechanisms. J Pathol. 181(1):14-24, 1997
19. Yoshikawa H et al: Dedifferentiated liposarcoma of the subcutis. Am J Surg Pathol. 20(12):1525-30, 1996
20. McCormick D et al: Dedifferentiated liposarcoma. Clinicopathologic analysis of 32 cases suggesting a better prognostic subgroup among pleomorphic sarcomas. Am J Surg Pathol. 18(12):1213-23, 1994
21. Weiss SW et al: Well-differentiated liposarcoma (atypical lipoma) of deep soft tissue of the extremities, retroperitoneum, and miscellaneous sites. A follow-up study of 92 cases with analysis of the incidence of "dedifferentiation". Am J Surg Pathol. 16(11):1051-8, 1992

Gross and Histiologic Features

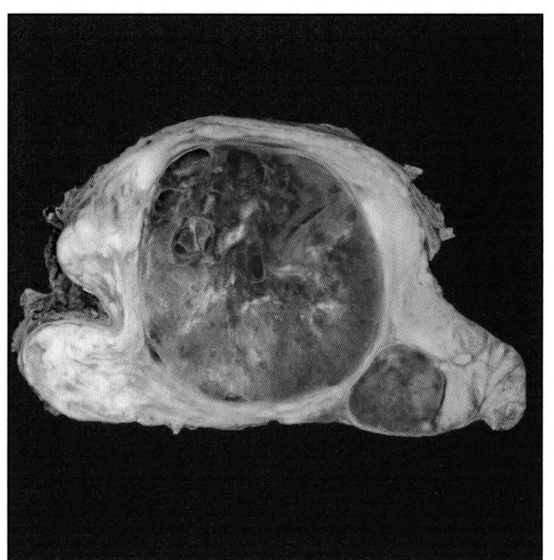

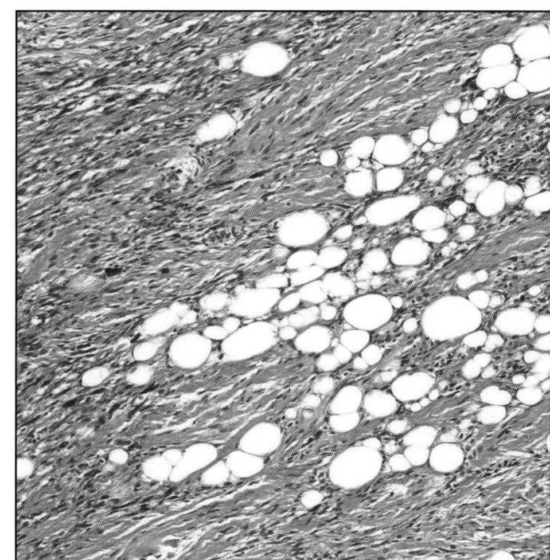

(Left) *Gross pathology photograph shows nodular dedifferentiation. In contrast to lipogenic tumor tissue, nonlipogenic sarcomatous tissue reveals indurated, yellow-brown cut surfaces.* ***(Right)*** *Hematoxylin & eosin shows gradual transition from atypical lipomatous to dedifferentiated areas with some intermingling of the 2 components.*

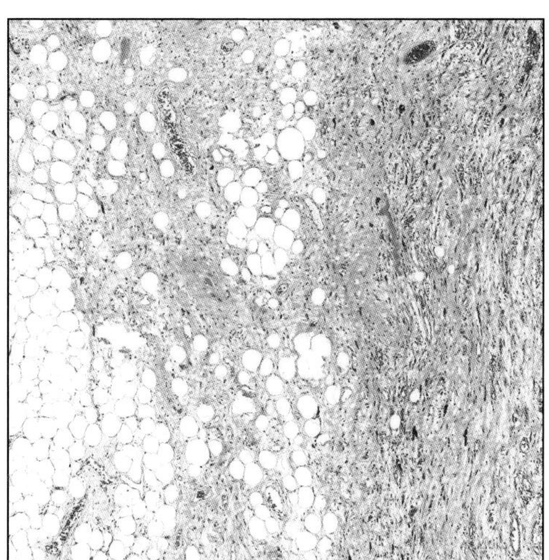

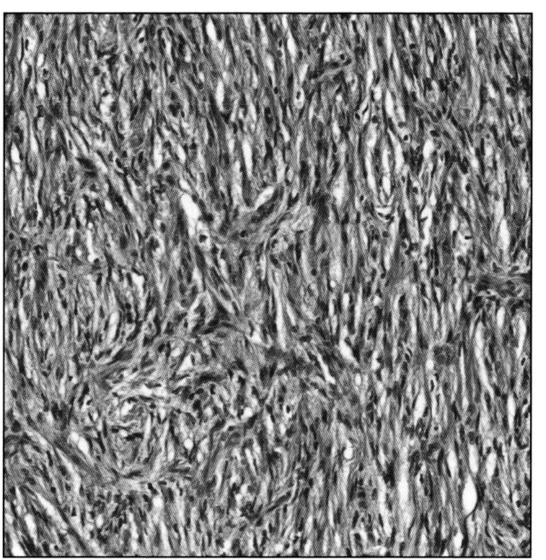

(Left) *Hematoxylin & eosin shows a gradual transition from atypical lipomatous tumor (left) to low-grade dedifferentiated nonlipogenic sarcoma (right).* ***(Right)*** *Hematoxylin & eosin shows low-grade dedifferentiation with a storiform growth of fibroblastic tumor cells.*

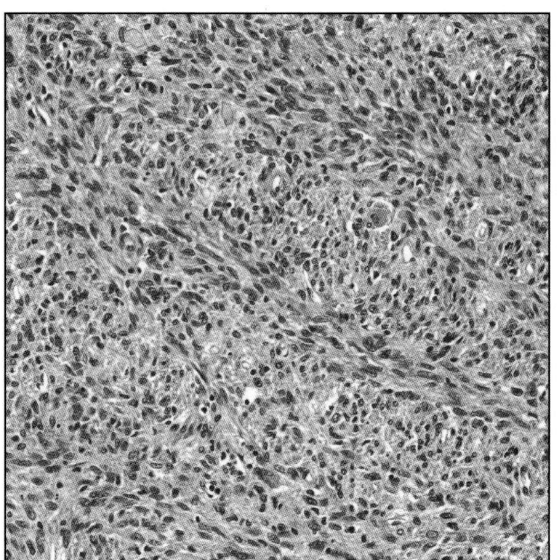

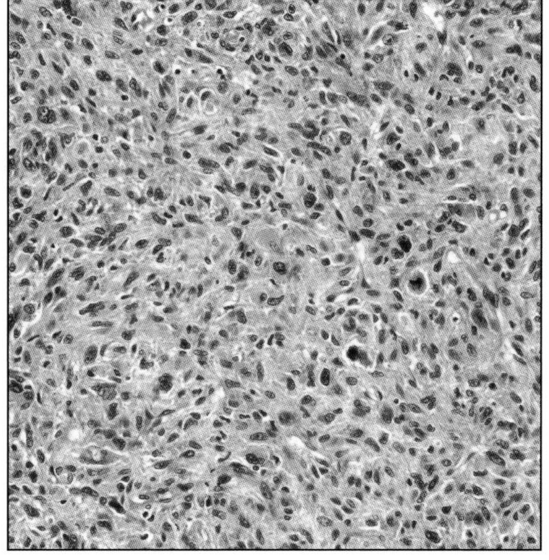

(Left) *Hematoxylin & eosin shows high-grade dedifferentiated liposarcoma resembling fibrosarcoma.* ***(Right)*** *Hematoxylin & eosin shows high-grade malignant malignant fibrous histiocytoma-like dedifferentiation.*

DEDIFFERENTIATED LIPOSARCOMA

Microscopic and Immunohistochemical Features

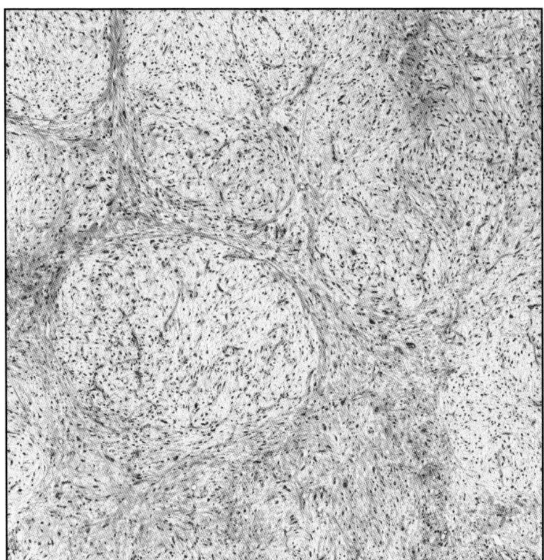
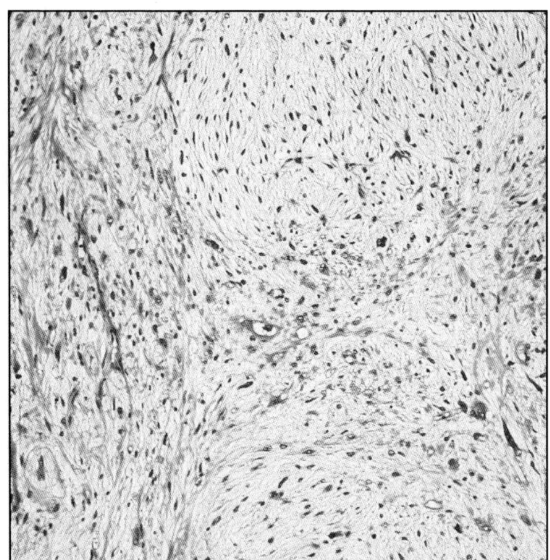

(Left) *Hematoxylin & eosin shows myxofibrosarcoma-like features in the dedifferentiated component. Note the multinodular architecture with atypical cells in the myxoid foci.* ***(Right)*** *Hematoxylin & eosin shows high-power view of myxofibrosarcoma-like dedifferentiated areas. Note enlarged tumor cells with enlarged hyperchromatic nuclei set in a myxoid stroma with elongated vessels.*

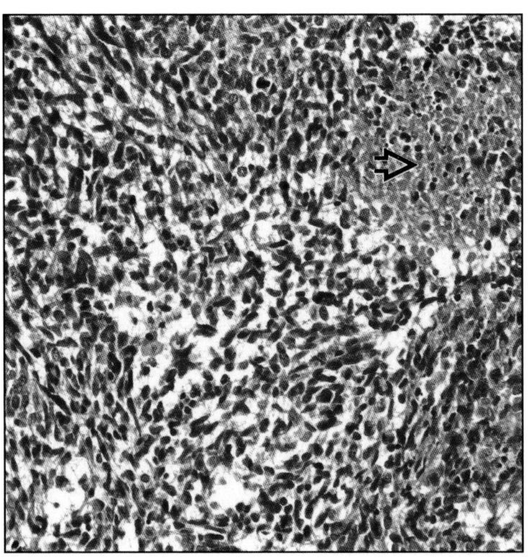
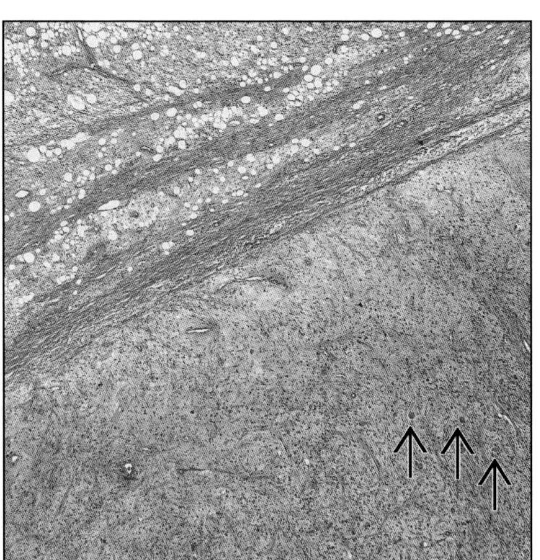

(Left) *Hematoxylin & eosin shows high-grade sarcoma, not otherwise specified, with tumor necrosis ⇨ in the dedifferentiated area.* ***(Right)*** *Hematoxylin & eosin shows transition from atypical lipomatous tumor areas (top) to nonlipogenic sarcomatous tissue with heterologous differentiation. Note the numerous rhabdomyoblasts →.*

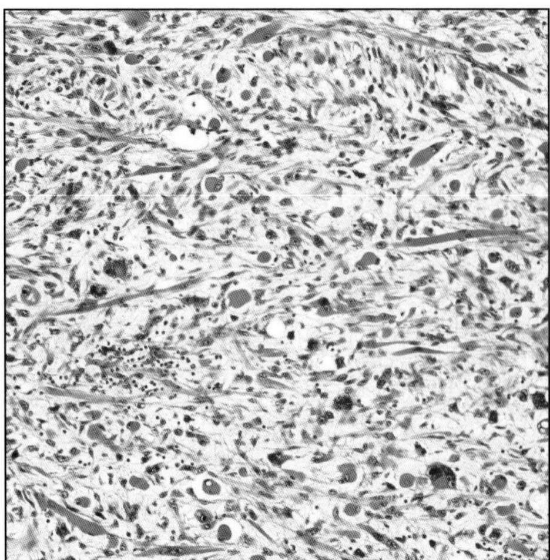
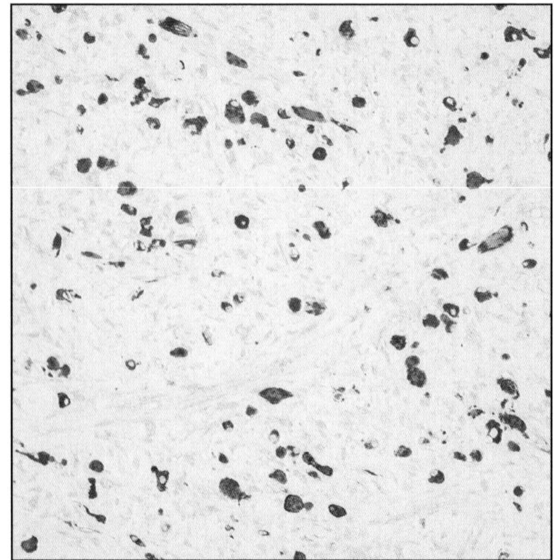

(Left) *Hematoxylin & eosin stain shows numerous rhabdomyoblasts.* ***(Right)*** *Myosin-fast immunostain shows numerous rhabdomyoblasts.*

Microscopic and Immunohistochemical Features

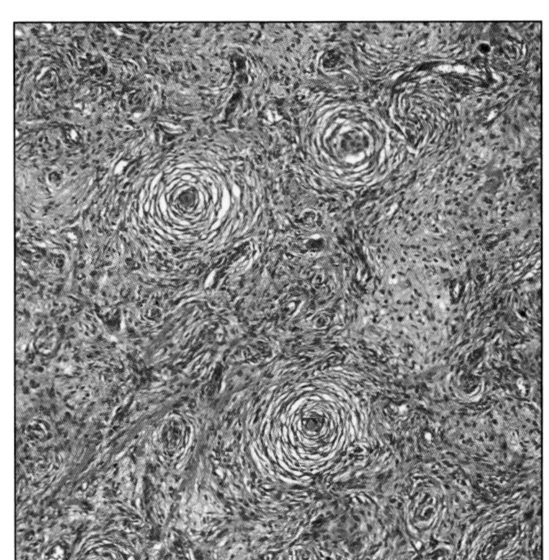

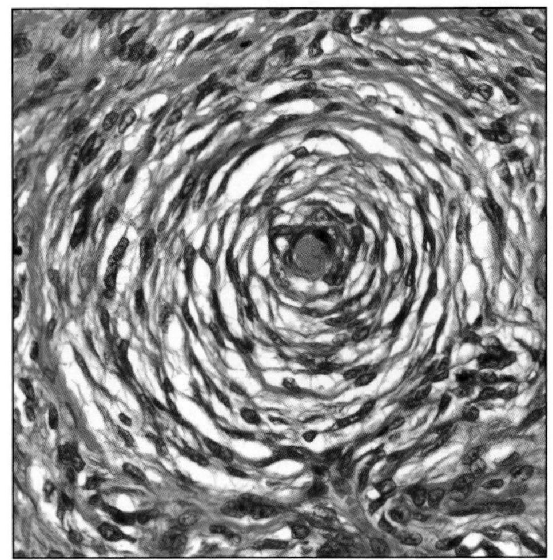

(Left) *Hematoxylin & eosin shows meningothelial-like whorls of spindle cells. This is a rare finding, mostly in nonlipogenic areas, and frequently associated with adjacent metaplastic bone formation.* ***(Right)*** *Hematoxylin & eosin shows higher magnification of spindle cells arranged in concentric whorls. The nature of their differentiation is unknown. Some cases are SMA(+), suggesting myofibroblastic or pericytic differentiation, but electron microscopy does not support this.*

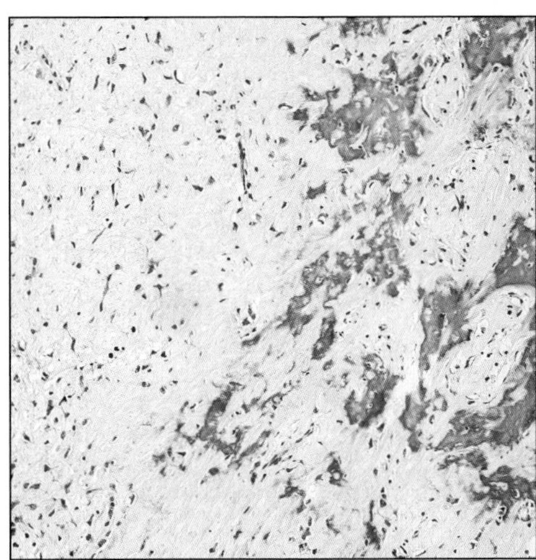

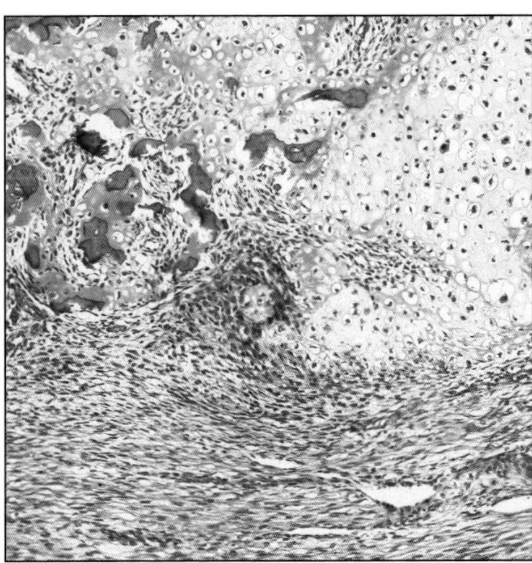

(Left) *Hematoxylin & eosin shows focal metaplastic calcification in the dedifferentiated area.* ***(Right)*** *Hematoxylin & eosin staining shows focal osteocartilaginous heterologous differentiation.*

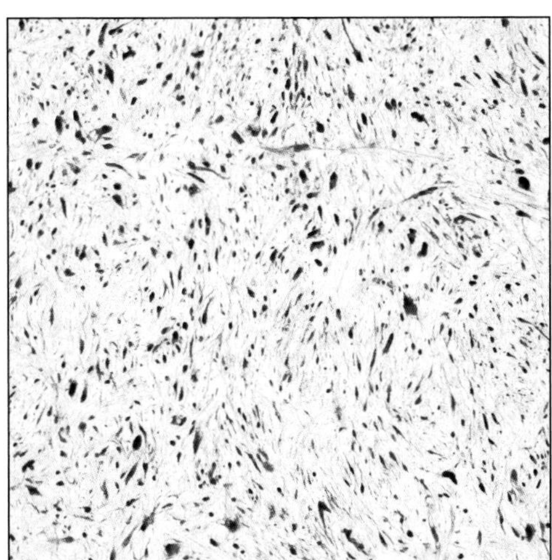

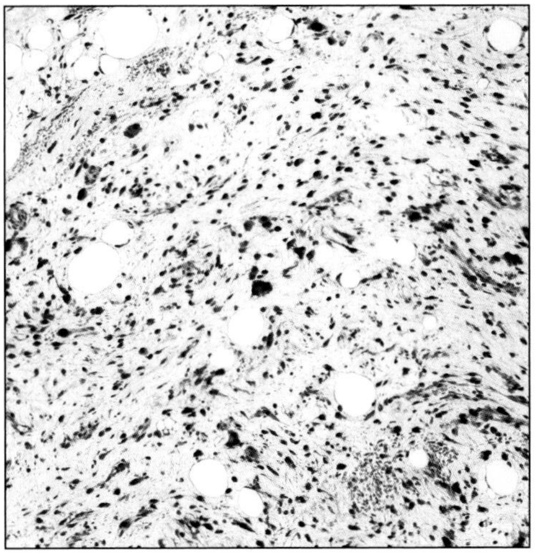

(Left) *CDK4 immunostain shows positivity in numerous tumor cell nuclei. This is a useful diagnostic feature of dedifferentiated liposarcoma.* ***(Right)*** *MDM2 immunostain shows nuclear expression in lesional cells. This is also a useful confirmatory marker for dedifferentiated liposarcoma.*

MYXOID LIPOSARCOMA

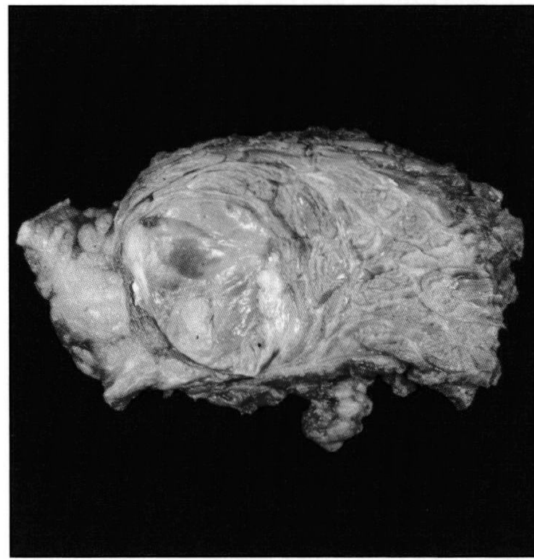

Gross photograph shows a myxoid/round cell liposarcoma with myxoid cut surfaces and small, indurated, gray-white areas corresponding to tumor areas with increased cellularity and round cell morphology.

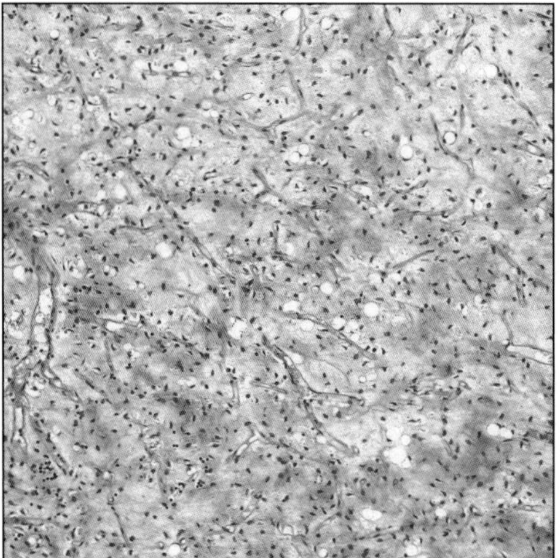

Low-grade myxoid liposarcoma is composed of small, undifferentiated, mesenchymal tumor cells associated with lipoblasts set in a prominent myxoid stroma with thin-walled, branching capillaries.

TERMINOLOGY

Abbreviations

- Myxoid liposarcoma (MLS)

Synonyms

- Myxoid/round cell liposarcoma
- Round cell liposarcoma

Definitions

- Malignant lipogenic neoplasm composed of primitive nonlipogenic mesenchymal cells and a variable number of lipoblasts set in myxoid stroma with characteristic branching blood vessels

CLINICAL ISSUES

Epidemiology

- Incidence
  - 2nd most common type of liposarcoma
  - Accounts for more than 1/3 of all liposarcomas
  - Accounts for ~ 10% of all sarcomas arising in adults
- Age
  - Young adults
  - Peak incidence in 4th and 5th decade
  - Rare in children
  - Commonest form of liposarcoma in patients younger than 20 years
- Gender
  - No gender predilection

Site

- Deep soft tissue of extremities
- 2/3 of cases arise within musculature of thigh
- Rare in subcutaneous location
- Extremely rare in dermal location

Presentation

- Painless mass
- May present initially with synchronous or metachronous multifocal neoplasms
- Deep-seated soft tissue neoplasms

Natural History

- Locally aggressive growth
- Increased rate of local recurrences
- Metastases develop in ~ 30-40% of cases
- Tends to metastasize to unusual soft tissue or bone locations

Treatment

- Surgical approaches
  - Complete excision with wide tumor-free margins

Prognosis

- Presence of round cell areas is of prognostic importance
  - > 5% round cell differentiation is associated with unfavorable outcome
- Large tumor size (> 10 cm) is associated with unfavorable outcome
- Tumor necrosis associated with unfavorable outcome
- p53 overexpression and *p53* mutations associated with unfavorable outcome
- Loss of p27 associated with unfavorable outcome
- Prognosis of multifocal neoplasms is poor independent of morphology
- Molecular variability has no prognostic influence

MACROSCOPIC FEATURES

General Features

- Well-circumscribed, multinodular neoplasms
- Gelatinous cut surfaces in low-grade neoplasms
- Round cell areas correspond to indurated, gray-white tumor areas

MYXOID LIPOSARCOMA

Key Facts

Terminology

- Malignant lipogenic neoplasm composed of primitive nonlipogenic mesenchymal cells and variable number of lipoblasts set in myxoid stroma with characteristic branching blood vessels

Clinical Issues

- 2nd most common type of liposarcoma
- Young adults
- Commonest form of liposarcoma in patients younger than 20 years
- Deep soft tissue of extremities
- May present initially with synchronous or metachronous multifocal neoplasms
- Increased rate of local recurrences
- Metastases develop in ~ 30-40% of cases
- Presence of round cell areas is of prognostic importance
  - > 5% round cell differentiation is associated with unfavorable outcome

Microscopic Pathology

- Uniform, round to oval-shaped, primitive mesenchymal cells
- Small, univacuolated, signet ring lipoblasts
- Prominent myxoid stroma
- Delicate, arborizing, "chicken wire" capillary vasculature

Ancillary Tests

- Most frequently t(12;16)(q13;p11)
- S100 protein can be positive
- MDM2(-) and CDK4(-)

MICROSCOPIC PATHOLOGY

Histologic Features

- Nodular growth pattern
- May show enhanced cellularity at periphery of tumor lobules
- Uniform, round to oval-shaped, primitive mesenchymal cells
- Small, univacuolated, signet ring lipoblasts
- May show "maturation" with lipoma or atypical lipomatous tumor-like areas
- Prominent myxoid stroma
- Mucin pooling
- Delicate, arborizing, "chicken wire" capillary vasculature
- Interstitial hemorrhages
- May contain hibernoma-like cells
- No nuclear pleomorphism
- No significant mitotic activity
- Progression to hypercellular, round cell areas
  - Increased cellularity
  - Nests or solid sheets of back-to-back located round cells
  - Round cells have high nuclear:cytoplasmic ratio
  - Enlarged nuclei that may show overlapping
- Rare hypercellular, spindle cell areas
- Rare heterologous differentiation (cartilaginous, rhabdomyoblastic, leiomyomatous, osseous)
- Reported dedifferentiation may represent rather mixed-type liposarcomas

Predominant Pattern/Injury Type

- Circumscribed

Predominant Cell/Compartment Type

- Adipose
- Lipoblast
- Mesenchymal, adipose cell

ANCILLARY TESTS

Cytogenetics

- Most frequently t(12;16)(q13;p11)
  - In > 90% of cases
  - Fusion of *CHOP* (*DDIT3*) and *FUS* genes
    - Fusion product deregulates some NF-κ-B-controlled genes through interactions with *NFKBIZ*
- More rarely t(12;22)(q13;q12)
  - Fusion of *CHOP* (*DDIT3*) and *EWS* genes

Electron Microscopy

- Lipoblasts in varying stages of maturation are present

DIFFERENTIAL DIAGNOSIS

Chondroid Lipoma

- Encapsulated lobular neoplasms
- Irregular admixture of adipocytes, multivacuolated lipoblasts, small eosinophilic cells
- No delicate, arborizing, "chicken wire" capillaries
- Biologically benign lipogenic neoplasms

Intramuscular Myxoma

- Ill-defined hypocellular neoplasms
- Bland spindled fibroblasts
- No lipogenic component
- No delicate, arborizing, "chicken wire" capillaries

Atypical Lipomatous Tumor

- No immature, primitive mesenchymal tumor cells
- Multivacuolated lipoblasts are more frequent
- May show myxoid stromal changes but no delicate, arborizing, "chicken wire" capillaries
- Nuclear expression of MDM2 &/or CDK4
- Amplification of MDM2 &/or CDK4
- No t(12;16) &/or t(12;22)

Mixed-type Liposarcoma

- Extremely rare neoplasms

MYXOID LIPOSARCOMA

Immunohistochemistry

Antibody	Reactivity	Staining Pattern	Comment
Vimentin	Positive	Cytoplasmic	
CD99	Negative		
CDK4	Negative		
MDM2	Negative		
CK-PAN	Negative		
CLA	Negative		
S100	Equivocal	Nuclear & cytoplasmic	May be useful in round cell neoplasm

- Contains pleomorphic liposarcoma component or atypical lipomatous tumor component

Myxofibrosarcoma

- Dermis, subcutis > deep soft tissue
- Enlarged hyperchromatic tumor cell nuclei
- Significant degree of nuclear atypia
- No lipoblasts
- Pseudolipoblasts (vacuolated fibroblastic tumor cells containing mucin)
- Elongated curvilinear vessels

Extraskeletal Myxoid Chondrosarcoma

- Small eosinophilic tumor cells
- Tumor cells are arranged in clusters and cords
- Only few vessels
- No lipoblasts

Myxoid Dermatofibrosarcoma Protuberans

- Dermal, subcutaneous neoplasm
- Diffuse infiltration of preexisting structures
- No lipogenic component
- No delicate, arborizing, "chicken wire" capillaries
- CD34(+)

Poorly Differentiated, Round Cell Synovial Sarcoma

- No lipogenic component
- No delicate, arborizing, "chicken wire" capillaries
- Focal expression of pancytokeratin and EMA
- Characteristic t(X;18)

Ewing Sarcoma/MPNET

- No lipogenic component
- Membranous CD99 expression
- Characteristic t(11;22) or t(21;22)

DIAGNOSTIC CHECKLIST

Clinically Relevant Pathologic Features

- Organ distribution
- Age distribution

Pathologic Interpretation Pearls

- Primitive mesenchymal tumor cells and signet ring lipoblasts
- Myxoid stroma with arborizing capillaries

SELECTED REFERENCES

1. Göransson M et al: The myxoid liposarcoma FUS-DDIT3 fusion oncoprotein deregulates NF-kappaB target genes by interaction with NFKBIZ. Oncogene. 28(2):270-8, 2009
2. Downs-Kelly E et al: The utility of fluorescence in situ hybridization (FISH) in the diagnosis of myxoid soft tissue neoplasms. Am J Surg Pathol. 32(1):8-13, 2008
3. Fiore M et al: Myxoid/round cell and pleomorphic liposarcomas: prognostic factors and survival in a series of patients treated at a single institution. Cancer. 109(12):2522-31, 2007
4. ten Heuvel SE et al: Clinicopathologic prognostic factors in myxoid liposarcoma: a retrospective study of 49 patients with long-term follow-up. Ann Surg Oncol. 14(1):222-9, 2007
5. Wei YC et al: Myxoid liposarcoma with cartilaginous differentiation: identification of the same type II TLS-CHOP fusion gene transcript in both lipogenic and chondroid components. Appl Immunohistochem Mol Morphol. 15(4):477-80, 2007
6. Oda Y et al: Frequent alteration of p16(INK4a)/p14(ARF) and p53 pathways in the round cell component of myxoid/round cell liposarcoma: p53 gene alterations and reduced p14(ARF) expression both correlate with poor prognosis. J Pathol. 207(4):410-21, 2005
7. Olofsson A et al: Abnormal expression of cell cycle regulators in FUS-CHOP carrying liposarcomas. Int J Oncol. 25(5):1349-55, 2004
8. Antonescu CR et al: Prognostic impact of P53 status, TLS-CHOP fusion transcript structure, and histological grade in myxoid liposarcoma: a molecular and clinicopathologic study of 82 cases. Clin Cancer Res. 7(12):3977-87, 2001
9. Orvieto E et al: Myxoid and round cell liposarcoma: a spectrum of myxoid adipocytic neoplasia. Semin Diagn Pathol. 18(4):267-73, 2001
10. Antonescu CR et al: Monoclonality of multifocal myxoid liposarcoma: confirmation by analysis of TLS-CHOP or EWS-CHOP rearrangements. Clin Cancer Res. 6(7):2788-93, 2000
11. Antonescu CR et al: Specificity of TLS-CHOP rearrangement for classic myxoid/round cell liposarcoma: absence in predominantly myxoid well-differentiated liposarcomas. J Mol Diagn. 2(3):132-8, 2000
12. Oliveira AM et al: p27(kip1) protein expression correlates with survival in myxoid and round-cell liposarcoma. J Clin Oncol. 18(15):2888-93, 2000
13. Tallini G et al: Combined morphologic and karyotypic study of 28 myxoid liposarcomas. Implications for a revised morphologic typing, (a report from the CHAMP Group). Am J Surg Pathol. 20(9):1047-55, 1996
14. Knight JC et al: Translocation t(12;16)(q13;p11) in myxoid liposarcoma and round cell liposarcoma: molecular and cytogenetic analysis. Cancer Res. 55(1):24-7, 1995

Microscopic and Immunohistochemical Features

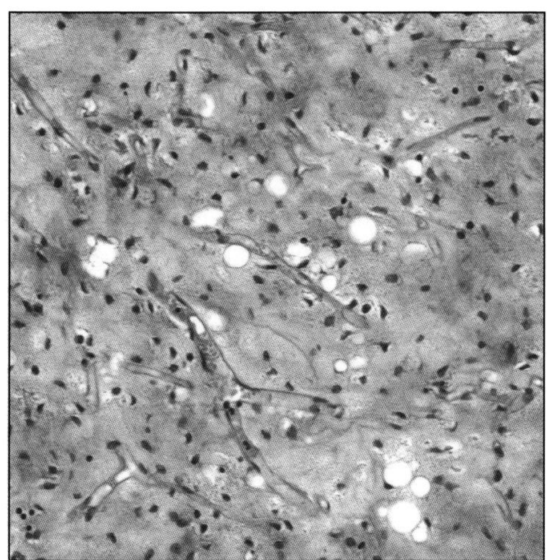

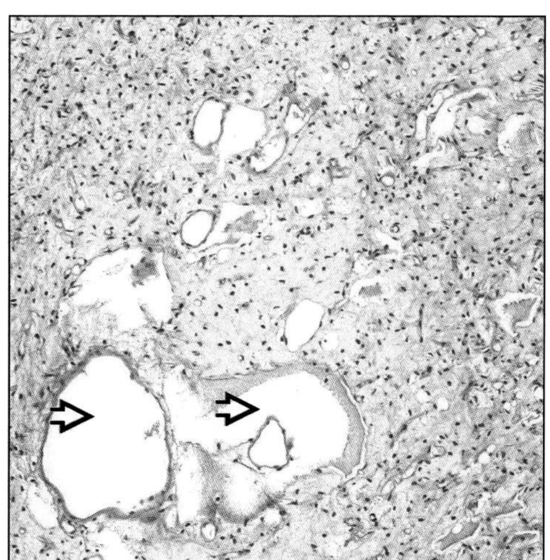

(Left) *Low-grade, purely myxoid liposarcoma contains characteristic thin-walled, branching capillaries. Note uni- and bivacuolated lipoblasts that are often seen in a perivascular location.* ***(Right)*** *The prominent myxoid stroma in cases of myxoid liposarcoma often shows characteristic mucin pooling ⇨.*

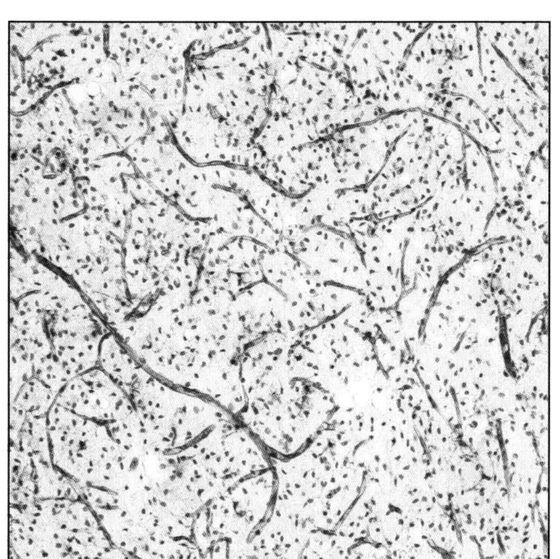

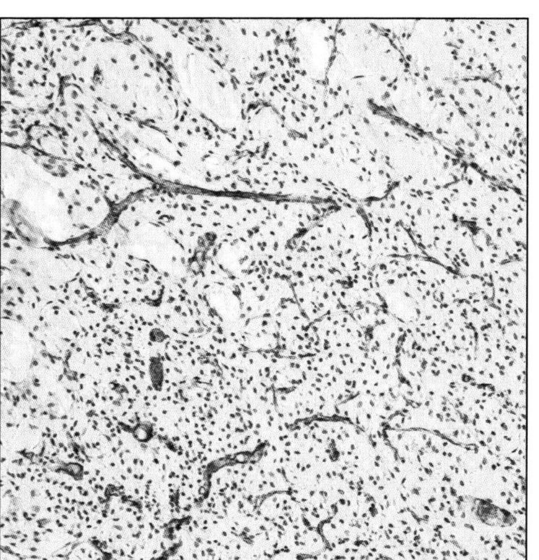

(Left) *CD31 immunostaining highlights the presence of numerous thin-walled, branching capillaries in cases of myxoid liposarcoma.* ***(Right)*** *Numerous thin-walled vessels are detected with actin immunostaining as well, emphasizing that these vessels represent capillaries.*

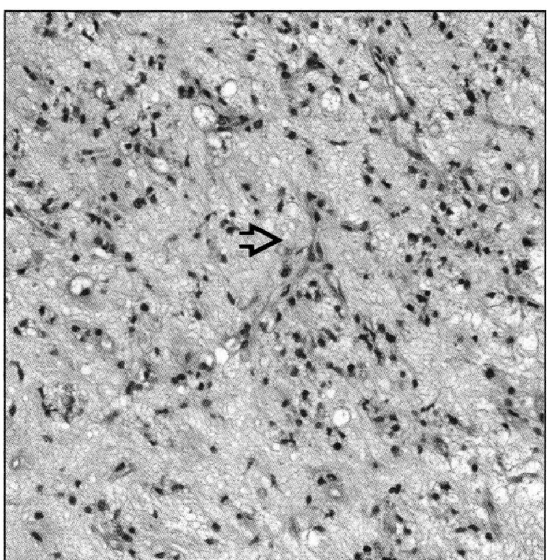

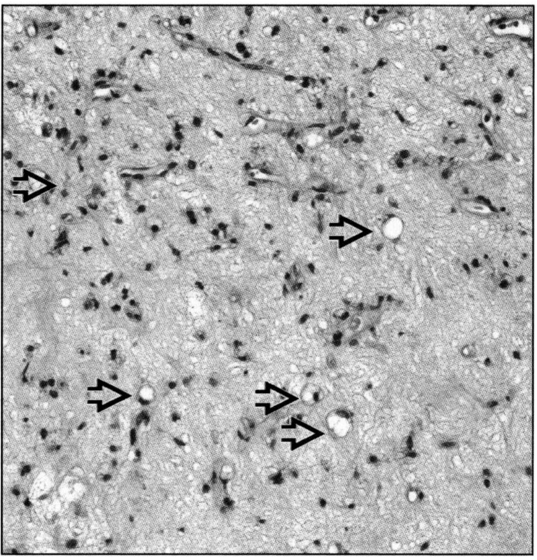

(Left) *An elderly male patient developed this deep-seated, low-grade myxoid liposarcoma composed of numerous small, undifferentiated mesenchymal tumor cells associated with scattered lipoblasts. Note the characteristic branching, thin-walled vessels ⇨.* ***(Right)*** *High-power view reveals scattered uni- and bivacuolated lipoblasts containing hyperchromatic, scalloped nuclei ⇨.*

Microscopic and Immunohistochemical Features

(Left) *A 42-year-old male patient developed a myxoid liposarcoma arising on the thigh. Note the lipoblasts and immature mesenchymal cells set in a myxoid stroma.* **(Right)** *In some tumor areas, an increased cellularity with spindle-shaped tumor cells containing enlarged fusiform nuclei was observed.*

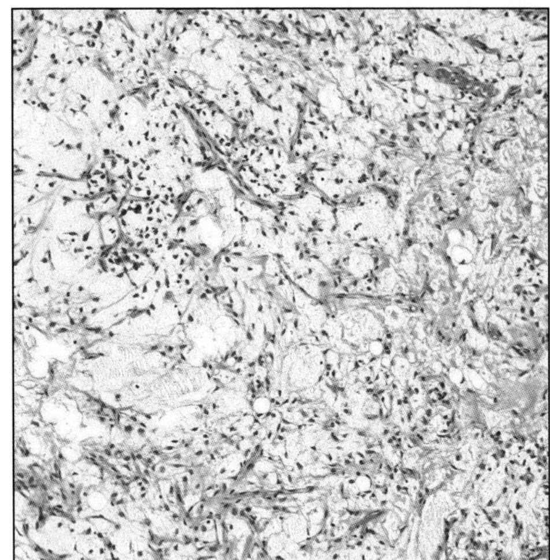

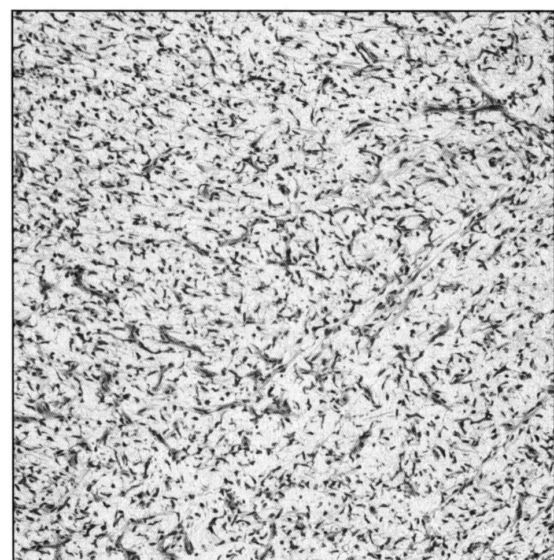

(Left) *In other tumor areas, atypical adipocytic cells as well as multivacuolated lipoblasts were noted, similar to features in an atypical lipomatous tumor ➩. This phenomenon of lipogenic "maturation" may be seen rarely in cases of myxoid liposarcoma.* **(Right)** *No nuclear expression of MDM2 was detected in this myxoid liposarcoma with lipogenic "maturation."*

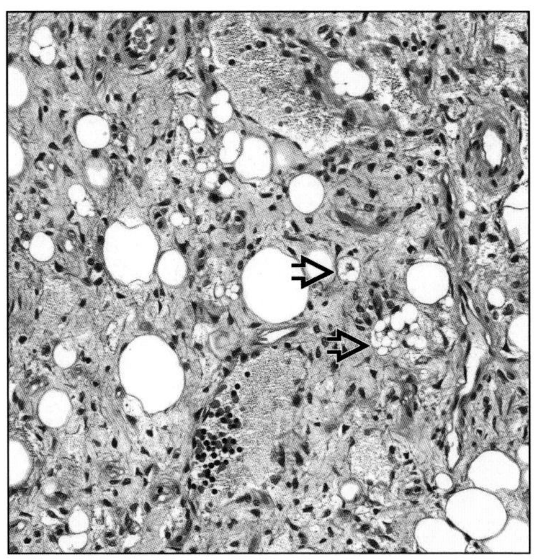

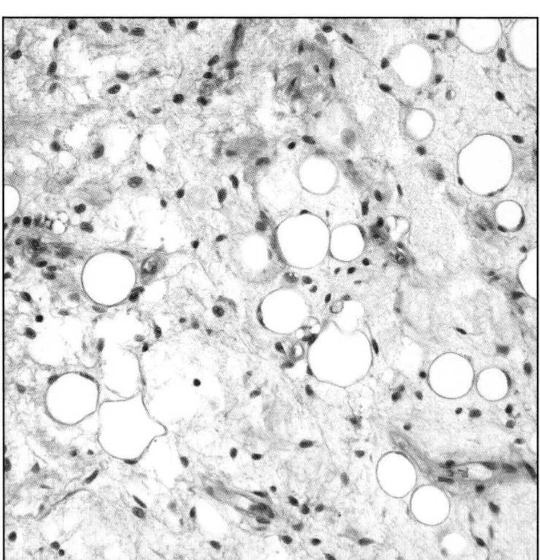

(Left) *Hematoxylin & eosin shows a case of a myxoid liposarcoma with scattered enlarged tumor cells containing enlarged nuclei.* **(Right)** *Interestingly, in a perivascular location, a rim of enlarged round tumor cells with enlarged, round nuclei is seen in this case.*

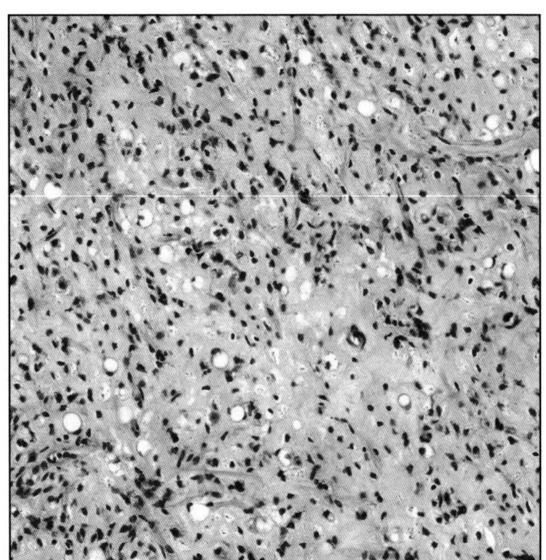

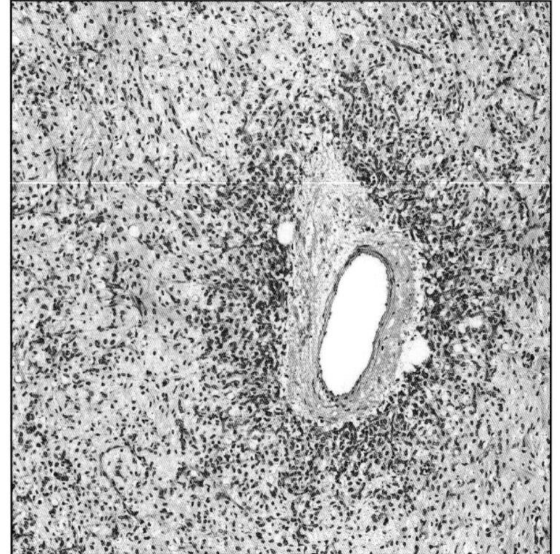

Microscopic and Immunohistochemical Features

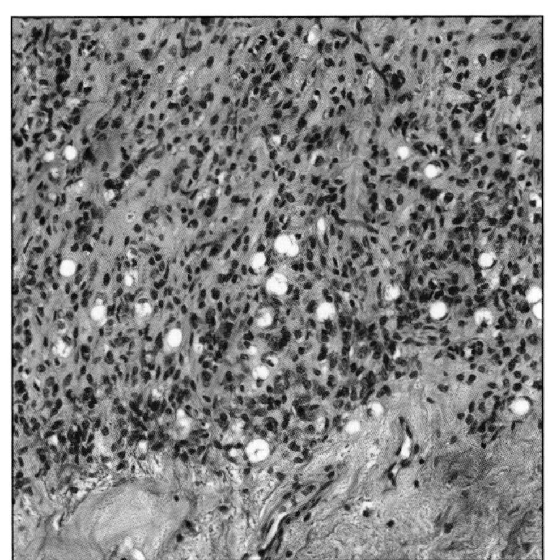

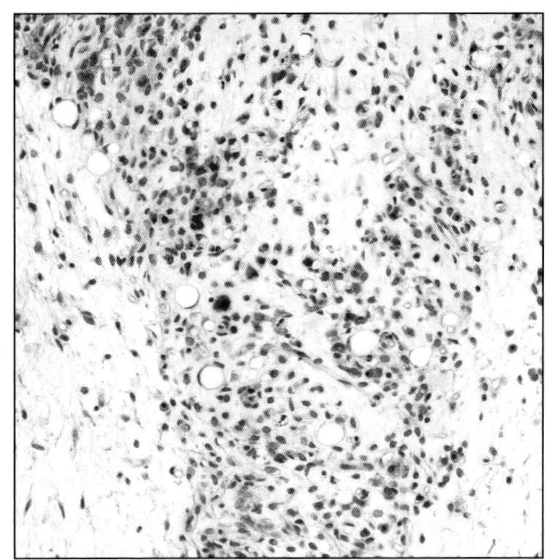

(Left) *Hematoxylin & eosin shows features of low-grade myxoid liposarcoma in the lower part. On the top and center, an increased cellularity with enlarged tumor cells containing enlarged and overlapping round nuclei is observed.* ***(Right)*** *S100 is sometimes helpful in detecting lipoblasts as well as scattered positive round tumor cells, as in this example of myxoid/round cell liposarcoma.*

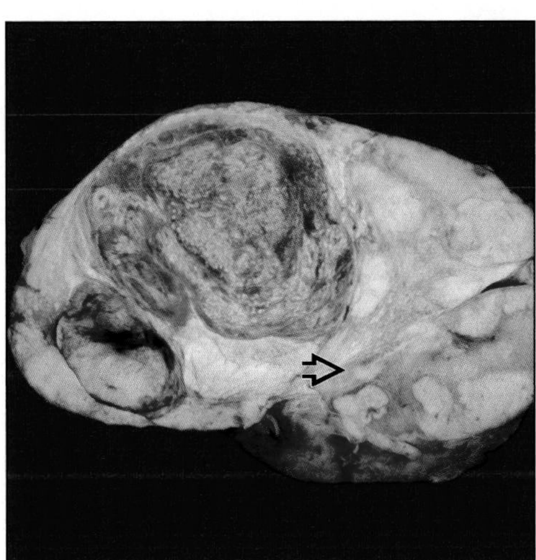

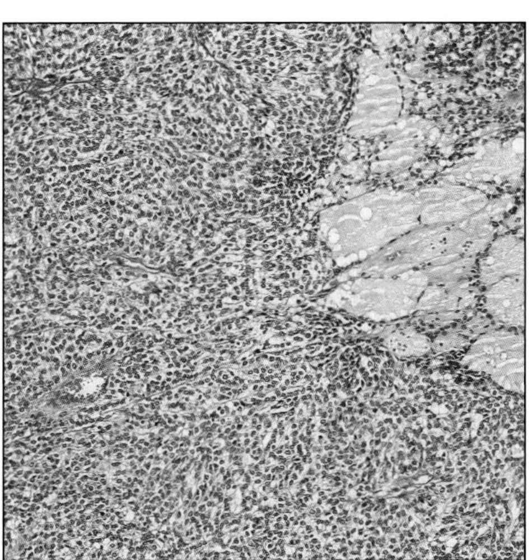

(Left) *Gross photograph of this high-grade round cell liposarcoma shows a deep-seated nodular neoplasm with yellow and gray-white cut surfaces and areas of tumor necrosis. Only small myxoid tumor areas are present ⇨.* ***(Right)*** *Hematoxylin & eosin shows a predominantly high-grade round cell liposarcoma. Only small areas with lower cellularity and myxoid stromal changes are present on the right.*

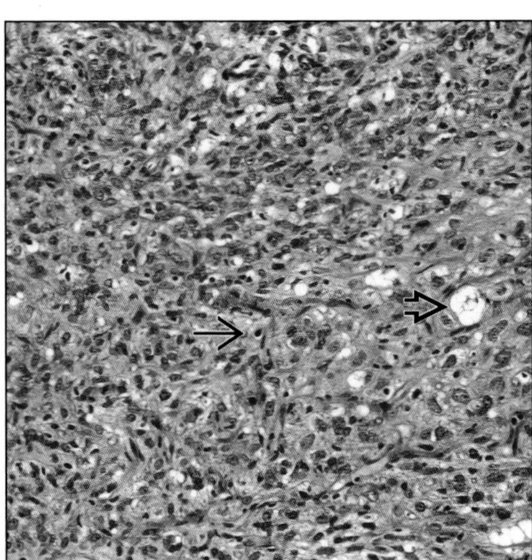

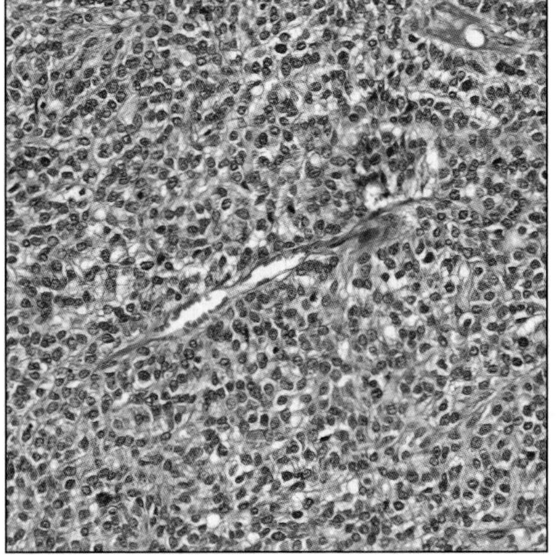

(Left) *High-grade round cell liposarcoma is composed of sheets of enlarged round tumor cells with enlarged round nuclei. Only scattered lipoblasts are seen ⇨. Note the presence of thin-walled, arborizing capillaries →.* ***(Right)*** *Hematoxylin & eosin shows another example of high-grade round cell liposarcoma. In addition to enlarged round tumor cells, scattered enlarged vacuolated tumor cells are present.*

PLEOMORPHIC LIPOSARCOMA

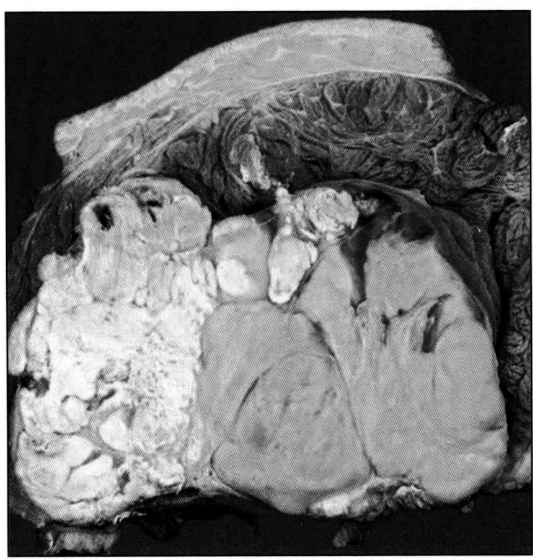

Gross photograph shows an intramuscular, partly necrotic neoplasm with gray-white indurated cut surfaces.

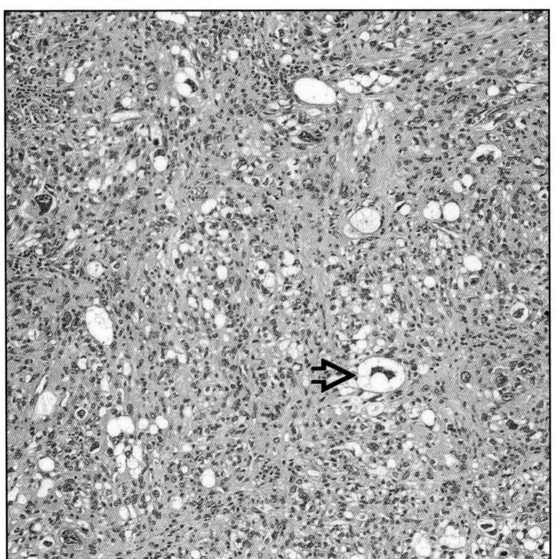

Hematoxylin & eosin shows a high-grade pleomorphic sarcoma containing numerous atypical multinucleated giant cells associated with pleomorphic lipoblasts ➪.

TERMINOLOGY

Abbreviations

- Pleomorphic liposarcoma (PLS)

Definitions

- Pleomorphic high-grade sarcoma containing variable amounts of pleomorphic lipoblasts
- No areas of atypical lipomatous tumor are present
- No sarcomatous component of a different line of differentiation is present

CLINICAL ISSUES

Epidemiology

- Incidence
  - Rarest subtype of liposarcoma
  - Accounts for approximately 5% of all liposarcomas
  - Accounts for approximately 20% of all pleomorphic sarcomas
- Age
  - Most cases arise in elderly patients (> 50 years old)
- Gender
  - Equal sex distribution

Site

- Most cases arise in extremities (lower > upper)
- Trunk and retroperitoneum are more rarely involved
- Rare sites include mediastinum, paratesticular region, scalp, abdominal/pelvic cavities
- Most cases arise in deep soft tissues
- Subcutaneous cases are rare
- Purely dermal cases are very rare but may occur

Presentation

- Deep mass
- Painless mass
- Firm enlarging mass

Natural History

- Many patients have short preoperative history
- Clinically aggressive neoplasm
- 30-50% metastasis rate
- Lung represents preferred site of metastases
- 40-50% overall tumor-associated mortality
- 5-year survival rate of 60-65%

Treatment

- Surgical approaches
  - Complete wide excision with tumor-free margins
- Adjuvant therapy
  - Postoperative radiotherapy may be given for large, incompletely excised neoplasms

Prognosis

- High-grade sarcoma
- Worse prognosis than dedifferentiated liposarcoma
- Better prognosis than high-grade myogenic sarcomas
- Deep-seated large neoplasms are associated with worse prognosis
- > 20 mitoses per 10 high-power fields and necrosis are associated with worse prognosis

MACROSCOPIC FEATURES

General Features

- Firm, often multinodular neoplasms
- White to yellow cut surfaces
- May show myxoid areas
- May show areas of tumor necrosis

MICROSCOPIC PATHOLOGY

Histologic Features

- Well-circumscribed, nonencapsulated, or ill-defined infiltrative neoplasms
- High-grade sarcoma associated with variable number of pleomorphic lipoblasts

PLEOMORPHIC LIPOSARCOMA

Key Facts

Terminology
- Pleomorphic high-grade sarcoma containing variable amounts of pleomorphic lipoblasts

Clinical Issues
- Rarest subtype of liposarcoma
- Accounts for approximately 5% of all liposarcomas
- Most cases arise in elderly patients (> 50 years old)
- Most cases arise on extremities (lower > upper)
- Most cases arise in deep soft tissues
- Clinically aggressive neoplasm
- 30-50% metastasis rate
- 5-year survival rate of 60-65%
- Deep-seated large neoplasms are associated with worse prognosis
- > 20 mitoses per 10 high-power fields and necrosis are associated with worse prognosis
- Surgical approach: Complete wide excision with tumor-free margins
- High-grade sarcoma

Microscopic Pathology
- Well-circumscribed, nonencapsulated, or ill-defined infiltrative neoplasms
- High-grade sarcoma associated with variable amounts of pleomorphic lipoblasts
- Sheets or single pleomorphic lipoblasts
- Pleomorphic lipoblasts contain enlarged, hyperchromatic nuclei scalloped by cytoplasmic vacuoles
- Intermediate- or high-grade myxofibrosarcoma-like areas may be present
- Epithelioid pleomorphic liposarcoma variant

- Sheets or single pleomorphic lipoblasts
- Pleomorphic lipoblasts contain enlarged, hyperchromatic nuclei scalloped by cytoplasmic vacuoles
- Sarcomatous component contains atypical spindled, round, and pleomorphic tumor cells
- Numerous mono- and multinucleated tumor giant cells
- High degree of nuclear atypia
- Numerous mitoses
- Areas of tumor necrosis are often present
- Intermediate- or high-grade myxofibrosarcoma-like areas may be present
- Intra- and extracellular eosinophilic droplets (represent lysosomal structures) are noted
- Rarely prominent inflammatory infiltrate is evident
- Epithelioid pleomorphic liposarcoma variant
  - Contains solid, cohesive sheets of epithelioid tumor cells
  - Foci of atypical lipogenic cells
  - Variable number of pleomorphic lipoblasts
- Small round cell variant
  - Small round tumor cells
  - Variable number of pleomorphic lipoblasts

Predominant Pattern/Injury Type
- Hypercellular

Predominant Cell/Compartment Type
- Lipoblast
- Undifferentiated, pleomorphic

ANCILLARY TESTS

Cytogenetics
- Complex structural chromosomal rearrangements
- High chromosome counts
- May contain ring &/or large marker chromosomes
- No reproducible MDM2 &/or CDK4 amplification

DIFFERENTIAL DIAGNOSIS

Atypical Lipomatous Tumor
- Well-differentiated atypical lipogenic tumor
- No nonlipogenic sarcomatous component
- No pleomorphic lipoblasts
- MDM2 &/or CDK4 amplification

Dedifferentiated Liposarcoma
- Atypical lipomatous tumor component
- Abrupt or gradual transition from atypical lipomatous tumor areas to nonlipogenic sarcomatous tissue
- No pleomorphic lipoblasts
- Prominent MDM2 and CDK4 amplification
- Different genetic profile

High-Grade Myxofibrosarcoma
- More often in subcutaneous location
- Multinodular growth
- No lipogenic component
- No pleomorphic lipoblasts
- Pseudolipoblasts (atypical fibroblastic tumor cells containing cytoplasmic mucin)
- Elongated, curvilinear blood vessels

Pleomorphic Sarcoma, NOS
- No atypical lipogenic tumor cells
- No pleomorphic lipoblasts

Pleomorphic Leiomyosarcoma
- No atypical lipogenic tumor cells
- No pleomorphic lipoblasts
- At least focally smooth muscle differentiation
- Expression of myogenic immunohistochemical markers (actin, H-caldesmon, desmin)

Pleomorphic Rhabdomyosarcoma
- No atypical lipogenic tumor cells
- No pleomorphic lipoblasts
- Presence of rhabdomyoblasts
- Expression of desmin
- Expression of myogenin
- Cytoplasmic expression of WT1 and CD99

PLEOMORPHIC LIPOSARCOMA

Immunohistochemistry

Antibody	Reactivity	Staining Pattern	Comment
Vimentin	Positive	Cytoplasmic	
CK-PAN	Positive	Cytoplasmic	Focal expression in epithelioid variant
Desmin	Negative	Cytoplasmic	Only very rarely focal expression
Actin-sm	Equivocal	Cytoplasmic	Focal expression in half of cases
S100	Equivocal	Cytoplasmic	Positive in half of cases

Metastatic Carcinoma

- No atypical lipogenic tumor cells
- No lipoblasts
- Expression of epithelial immunohistochemical markers

Metastatic Malignant Melanoma

- No atypical lipogenic tumor cells
- No lipoblasts
- Expression of melanocytic immunohistochemical markers

DIAGNOSTIC CHECKLIST

Clinically Relevant Pathologic Features

- Gross appearance
- Organ distribution
- Age distribution

Pathologic Interpretation Pearls

- High-grade sarcoma associated with variable numbers of pleomorphic lipoblasts
- Pleomorphic lipoblasts contain bizarre, enlarged, hyperchromatic nuclei scalloped by cytoplasmic vacuoles
- Pleomorphic lipoblasts contain enlarged, hyperchromatic, scalloped nuclei
- Myxofibrosarcoma-like features may be present
- Rare epithelioid pleomorphic liposarcoma variant

SELECTED REFERENCES

1. Fiore M et al: Myxoid/round cell and pleomorphic liposarcomas: prognostic factors and survival in a series of patients treated at a single institution. Cancer. 109(12):2522-31, 2007
2. Singer S et al: Gene expression profiling of liposarcoma identifies distinct biological types/subtypes and potential therapeutic targets in well-differentiated and dedifferentiated liposarcoma. Cancer Res. 67(14):6626-36, 2007
3. Idbaih A et al: Myxoid malignant fibrous histiocytoma and pleomorphic liposarcoma share very similar genomic imbalances. Lab Invest. 85(2):176-81, 2005
4. Hornick JL et al: Pleomorphic liposarcoma: clinicopathologic analysis of 57 cases. Am J Surg Pathol. 28(10):1257-67, 2004
5. Panoussopoulos D et al: Focal divergent chondrosarcomatous differentiation in a primary pleomorphic liposarcoma and expression of transforming growth factor beta. Int J Surg Pathol. 12(1):79-85, 2004
6. Val-Bernal JF et al: Primary purely intradermal pleomorphic liposarcoma. J Cutan Pathol. 30(8):516-20, 2003
7. Gebhard S et al: Pleomorphic liposarcoma: clinicopathologic, immunohistochemical, and follow-up analysis of 63 cases: a study from the French Federation of Cancer Centers Sarcoma Group. Am J Surg Pathol. 26(5):601-16, 2002
8. Cai YC et al: Primary liposarcoma of the orbit: a clinicopathologic study of seven cases. Ann Diagn Pathol. 5(5):255-66, 2001
9. Downes KA et al: Pleomorphic liposarcoma: a clinicopathologic analysis of 19 cases. Mod Pathol. 14(3):179-84, 2001
10. Meis-Kindblom JM et al: Cytogenetic and molecular genetic analyses of liposarcoma and its soft tissue simulators: recognition of new variants and differential diagnosis. Virchows Arch. 439(2):141-51, 2001
11. Oliveira AM et al: Pleomorphic liposarcoma. Semin Diagn Pathol. 18(4):274-85, 2001
12. Dei Tos AP: Liposarcoma: new entities and evolving concepts. Ann Diagn Pathol. 4(4):252-66, 2000
13. Miettinen M et al: Epithelioid variant of pleomorphic liposarcoma: a study of 12 cases of a distinctive variant of high-grade liposarcoma. Mod Pathol. 12(7):722-8, 1999
14. Dei Tos AP et al: Primary liposarcoma of the skin: a rare neoplasm with unusual high grade features. Am J Dermatopathol. 20(4):332-8, 1998
15. Mertens F et al: Cytogenetic analysis of 46 pleomorphic soft tissue sarcomas and correlation with morphologic and clinical features: a report of the CHAMP Study Group. Chromosomes and MorPhology. Genes Chromosomes Cancer. 22(1):16-25, 1998
16. Schneider-Stock R et al: No correlation of c-myc overexpression and p53 mutations in liposarcomas. Virchows Arch. 433(4):315-21, 1998
17. Zagars GK et al: Liposarcoma: outcome and prognostic factors following conservation surgery and radiation therapy. Int J Radiat Oncol Biol Phys. 36(2):311-9, 1996
18. Klimstra DS et al: Liposarcoma of the anterior mediastinum and thymus. A clinicopathologic study of 28 cases. Am J Surg Pathol. 19(7):782-91, 1995
19. Azumi N et al: Atypical and malignant neoplasms showing lipomatous differentiation. A study of 111 cases. Am J Surg Pathol. 11(3):161-83, 1987
20. Weiss LM et al: Ultrastructural distinctions between adult pleomorphic rhabdomyosarcomas, pleomorphic liposarcomas, and pleomorphic malignant fibrous histiocytomas. Hum Pathol. 15(11):1025-33, 1984

Microscopic Features

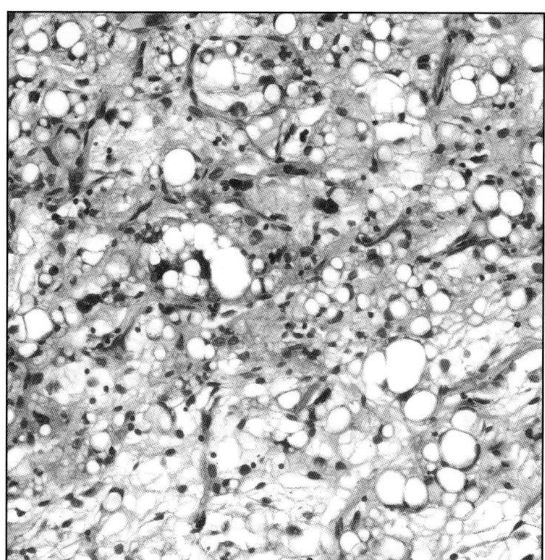

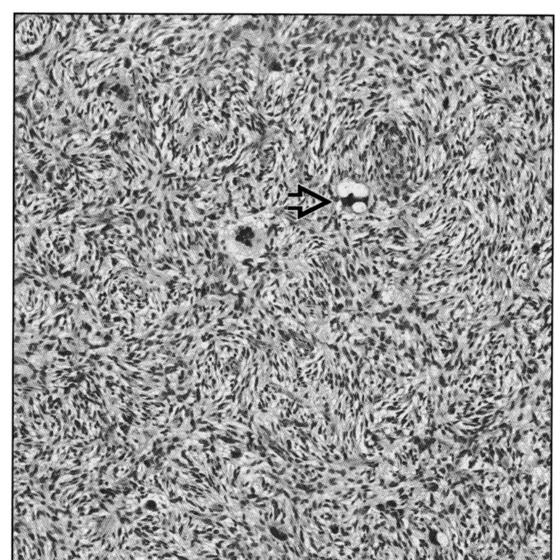

(Left) *Hematoxylin & eosin shows numerous multivacuolated pleomorphic lipoblasts containing enlarged hyperchromatic nuclei scalloped by lipid vacuoles in this pleomorphic liposarcoma.* ***(Right)*** *Hematoxylin & eosin shows a high-grade fibroblastic sarcoma with a storiform growth of atypical spindled and pleomorphic tumor cells. Only scattered pleomorphic lipoblasts are seen ⇨.*

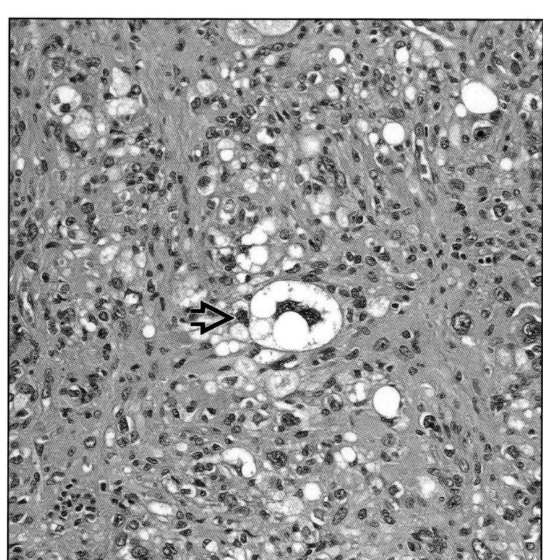

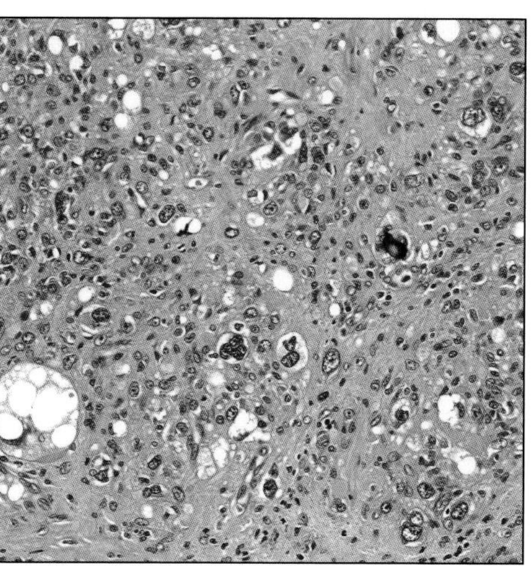

(Left) *Hematoxylin & eosin shows atypical lipogenic tumor cells and pleomorphic lipoblasts ⇨ associated with pleomorphic mesenchymal tumor cells.* ***(Right)*** *Hematoxylin & eosin shows pleomorphic lipoblasts associated with numerous multinucleated giant cells containing enlarged and irregular-shaped nuclei.*

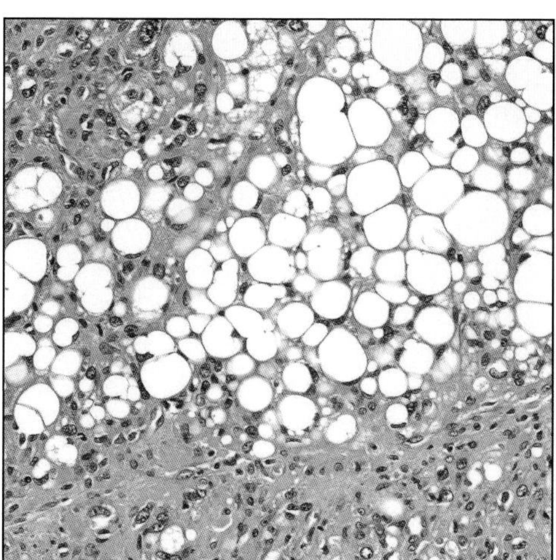

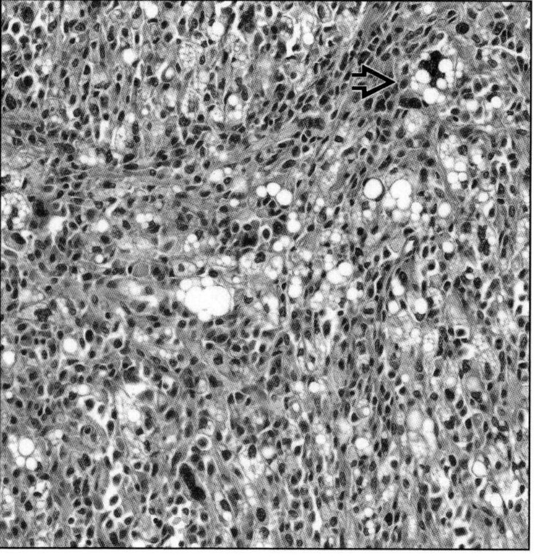

(Left) *Hematoxylin & eosin shows sheets of atypical lipogenic cells and multivacuolated lipoblasts associated with atypical mesenchymal tumor cells.* ***(Right)*** *Hematoxylin & eosin shows pleomorphic tumor cells with enlarged nuclei, atypical lipogenic cells, and multivacuolated pleomorphic lipoblasts ⇨.*

PLEOMORPHIC LIPOSARCOMA

Variant Microscopic Features

*(**Left**) Hematoxylin & eosin shows features of pleomorphic liposarcoma associated with sarcomatous tissue containing numerous osteoclast-like giant cells. (**Right**) Hematoxylin & eosin shows atypical lipogenic tumor cells with striking variations in size and shape and pleomorphic lipoblasts.*

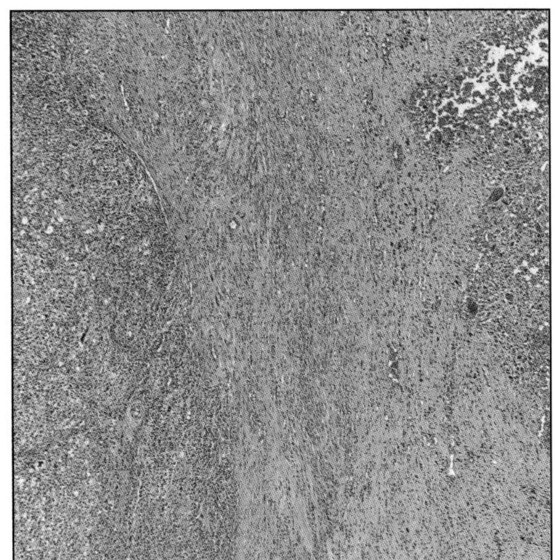

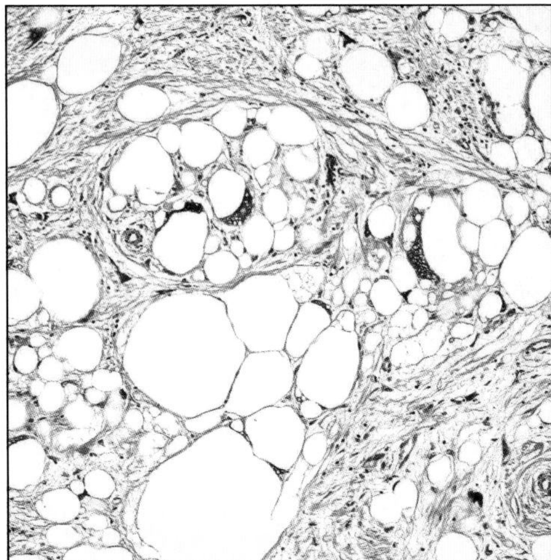

*(**Left**) Hematoxylin & eosin shows pleomorphic lipoblasts containing bizarre, enlarged, hyperchromatic nuclei scalloped by fat vacuoles ➲. (**Right**) Hematoxylin & eosin shows a case of pleomorphic liposarcoma with prominent myxoid stromal changes.*

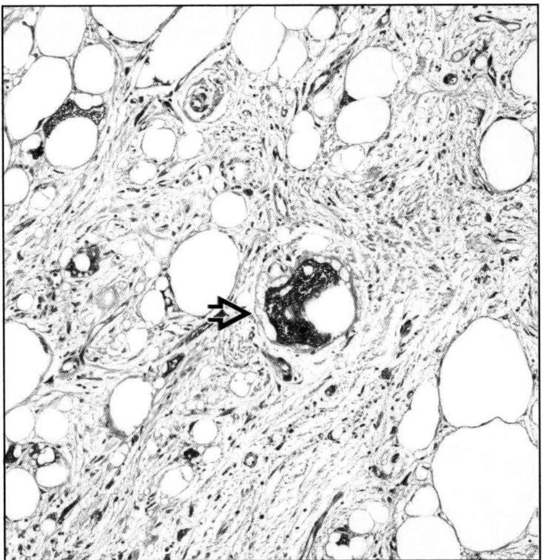

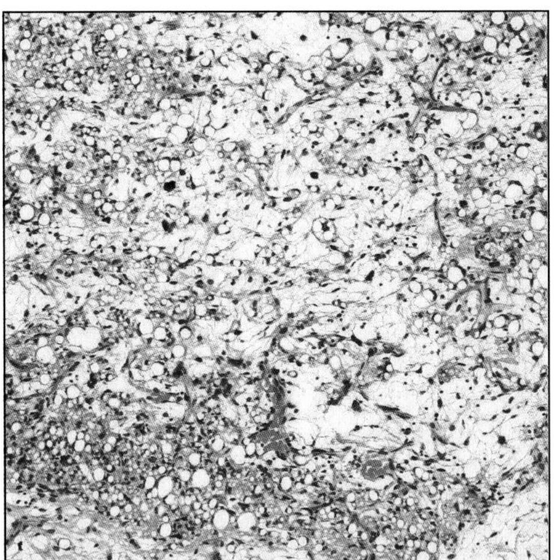

*(**Left**) Hematoxylin & eosin shows high-grade myxofibrosarcoma-like features. Note the scattered pleomorphic lipoblasts ➲. (**Right**) Hematoxylin & eosin shows a rare example of the epithelioid cell variant of pleomorphic liposarcoma. Note the sheets of atypical epithelioid tumor cells.*

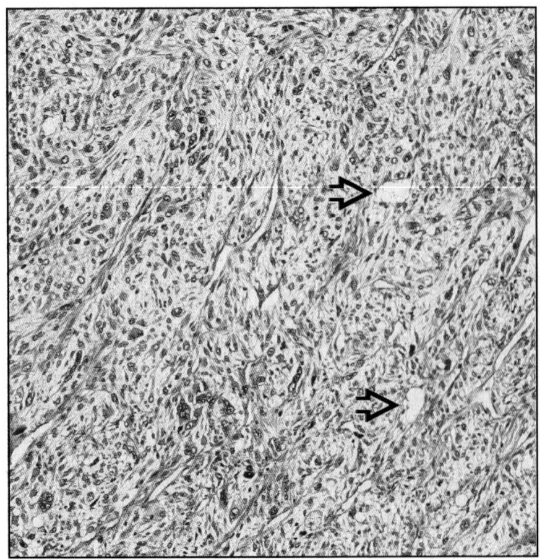

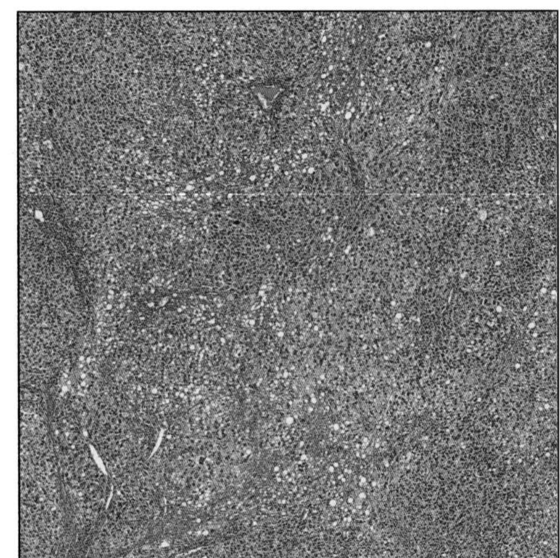

Variant Microscopic and Immunohistochemical Features

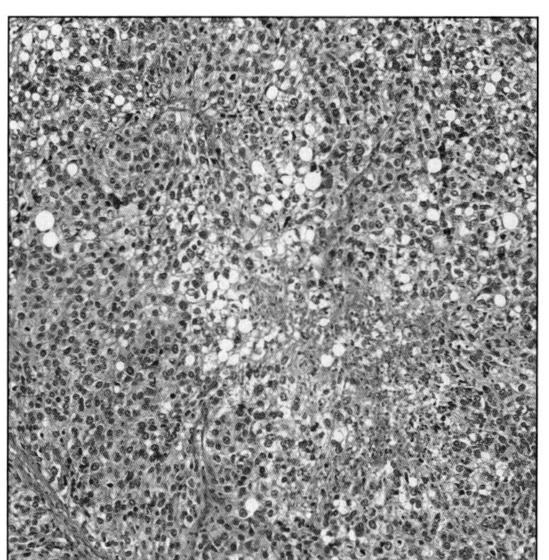

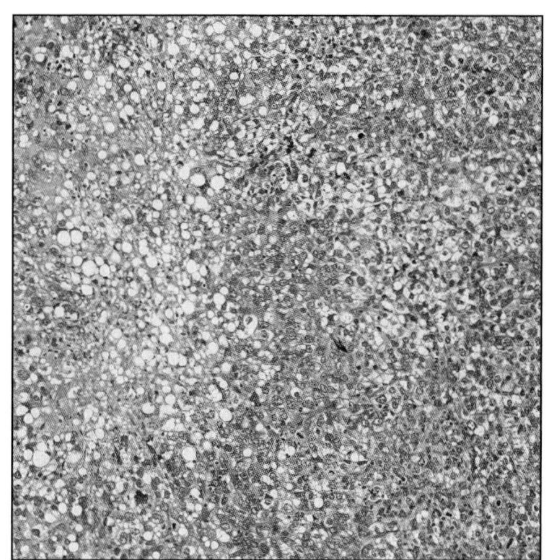

(Left) *Hematoxylin & eosin shows areas of tumor necrosis surrounded by sheets of atypical epithelioid tumor cells.* ***(Right)*** *Hematoxylin & eosin shows atypical epithelioid tumor cells associated with atypical lipogenic cells and numerous lipoblasts.*

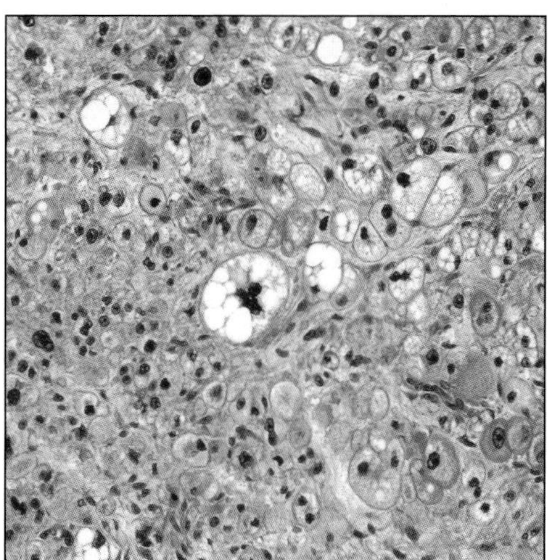

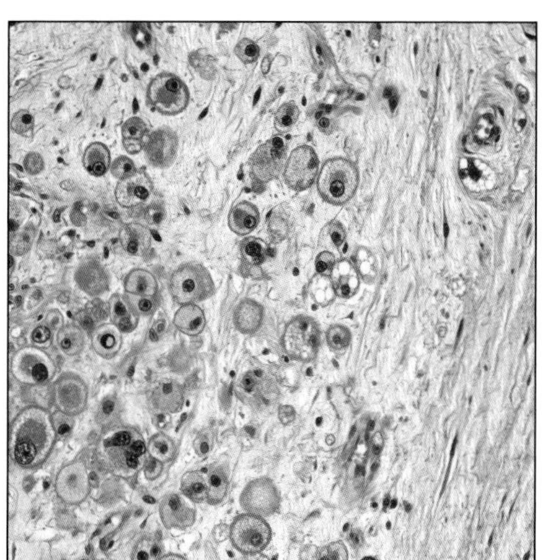

(Left) *Hematoxylin & eosin shows an unusual case of pleomorphic liposarcoma containing scattered pleomorphic lipoblasts and atypical tumor cells containing abundant pale eosinophilic granular cytoplasm.* ***(Right)*** *Hematoxylin & eosin shows atypical tumor cells with abundant pale eosinophilic granular xanthomatous cytoplasm in this unusual pleomorphic liposarcoma.*

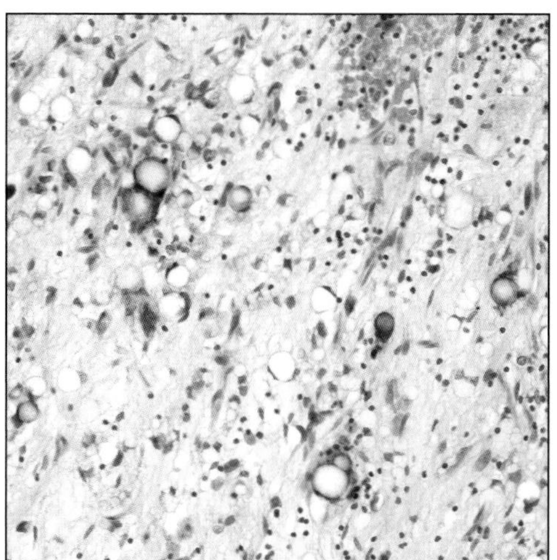

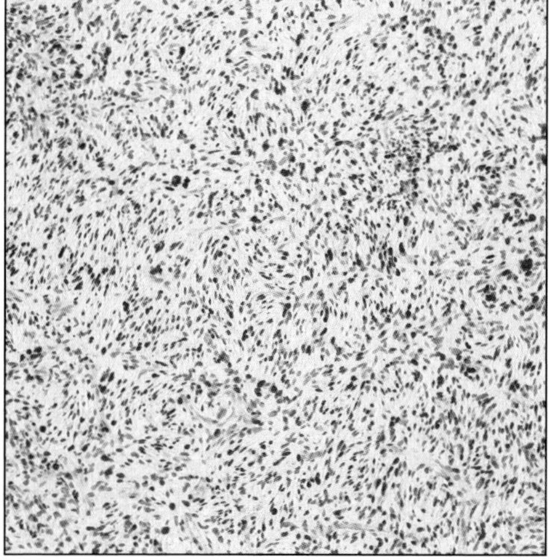

(Left) *S100 shows only scattered positive cells in this pleomorphic liposarcoma.* ***(Right)*** *Ki-67 reveals very high proliferative activity of tumor cells in this pleomorphic liposarcoma.*

MIXED LIPOSARCOMA

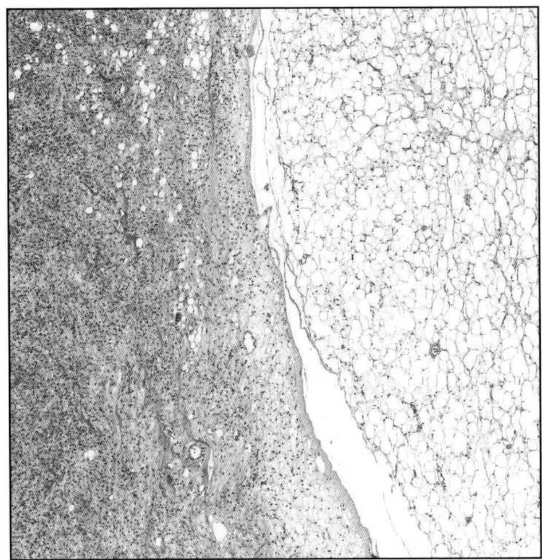

Hematoxylin & eosin shows low-power view of a biphasic lipogenic neoplasm. On the left, features of low-grade myxoid liposarcoma are seen; atypical lipomatous tumor is present on the right.

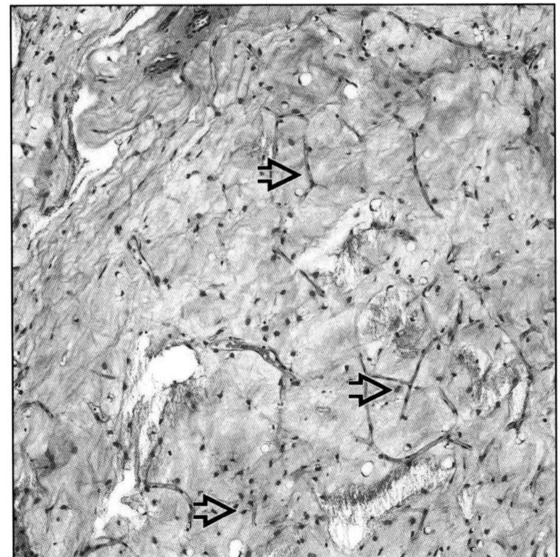

Small undifferentiated cells and univacuolated lipoblasts are set in a prominent myxoid stroma with numerous thin-walled and branching vessels ➢ in the myxoid liposarcoma component.

TERMINOLOGY

Definitions

- Liposarcoma showing morphologic/genetic features of combined myxoid liposarcoma and atypical lipomatous tumor/dedifferentiated liposarcoma, or of myxoid liposarcoma and pleomorphic liposarcoma

CLINICAL ISSUES

Epidemiology

- Incidence
  - Extremely rare
- Age
  - Elderly patients

Site

- Extremities
- Retroperitoneum
- Intraabdominal sites
- Mediastinum

Presentation

- Painless mass
- Slow growing

Natural History

- May show long preoperative duration
- Increased rate of recurrences
- Metastases may occur

Treatment

- Surgical approaches
  - Complete excision with clear margins

Prognosis

- Most malignant component predicts clinical prognosis

MACROSCOPIC FEATURES

General Features

- Large, often multinodular neoplasms
- May contain cystic and solid tumor areas
- Gray-yellow cut surfaces

Sections to Be Submitted

- Numerous sections from different tumor parts

Size

- May reach considerable size

MICROSCOPIC PATHOLOGY

Histologic Features

- Abrupt or irregular admixture of different liposarcoma components
- Combination of atypical lipomatous tumor (ALT)/ dedifferentiated liposarcoma & myxoid liposarcoma
  - Adipocytes with variation in size and shape, enlarged hyperchromatic nuclei, multivacuolated lipoblasts (ALT)
  - Small undifferentiated mesenchymal cells & lipoblasts set in myxoid stroma with "chicken wire" vessels (MLS)
- Combination of myxoid liposarcoma and pleomorphic liposarcoma (PLS)
  - Small undifferentiated mesenchymal cells & lipoblasts set in myxoid stroma with "chicken wire" vessels (MLS)
  - High-grade sarcoma with pleomorphic lipoblasts
- Grading of mixed-type liposarcoma is related to different tumor components

Predominant Pattern/Injury Type

- Circumscribed

Predominant Cell/Compartment Type

- Lipoblast

MIXED LIPOSARCOMA

Key Facts

Terminology
- Liposarcoma showing morphologic/genetic features of combined myxoid liposarcoma and atypical lipomatous tumor/dedifferentiated liposarcoma, or of myxoid liposarcoma and pleomorphic liposarcoma

Clinical Issues
- Extremely rare

Microscopic Pathology
- Abrupt or irregular admixture of different liposarcoma components
- Combination of atypical lipomatous tumor/ dedifferentiated liposarcoma and myxoid liposarcoma
- Combination of myxoid liposarcoma and pleomorphic liposarcoma

ANCILLARY TESTS

Cytogenetics
- Cytogenetic findings of different liposarcoma components are present

DIFFERENTIAL DIAGNOSIS

Atypical Lipomatous Tumor with Myxoid Changes
- Longstanding neoplasms
- Enlarged cells with enlarged, hyperchromatic nuclei also in myxoid tumor areas
- MDM2 &/or CDK4 expression also in myxoid tumor areas
- No thin-walled, branching vessels in myxoid tumor areas
- No genetic findings of myxoid liposarcoma

Dedifferentiated Liposarcoma with Myxoid Changes
- Longstanding neoplasms
- No thin-walled, branching vessels in myxoid tumor areas
- MDM2 &/or CDK4 expression also in myxoid tumor areas
- No genetic findings of myxoid liposarcoma

Dedifferentiated Myxoid Liposarcoma
- Probably represents form of mixed-type liposarcoma

DIAGNOSTIC CHECKLIST

Pathologic Interpretation Pearls
- Abrupt or irregular admixture of different liposarcoma components

SELECTED REFERENCES

1. Mentzel T et al: Mixed-type liposarcoma: clinicopathological, immunohistochemical, and molecular analysis of a case arising in deep soft tissues of the lower extremity. Virchows Arch. 453(2):197-201, 2008
2. Kim JI et al: Gene expression in mixed type liposarcoma. Pathology. 38(2):114-9, 2006
3. Meis-Kindblom JM et al: Cytogenetic and molecular genetic analyses of liposarcoma and its soft tissue simulators: recognition of new variants and differential diagnosis. Virchows Arch. 439(2):141-51, 2001
4. Kato T et al: Case of retroperitoneal dedifferentiated mixed-type liposarcoma: comparison of proliferative activity in specimens from four operations. J Surg Oncol. 72(1):32-6, 1999
5. Mentzel T et al: Dedifferentiated myxoid liposarcoma: a clinicopathological study suggesting a closer relationship between myxoid and well-differentiated liposarcoma. Histopathology. 30(5):457-63, 1997
6. Klimstra DS et al: Liposarcoma of the anterior mediastinum and thymus. A clinicopathologic study of 28 cases. Am J Surg Pathol. 19(7):782-91, 1995
7. Kindblom LG et al: Liposarcoma a clinicopathologic, radiographic and prognostic study. Acta Pathol Microbiol Scand Suppl. (253):1-71, 1975

IMAGE GALLERY

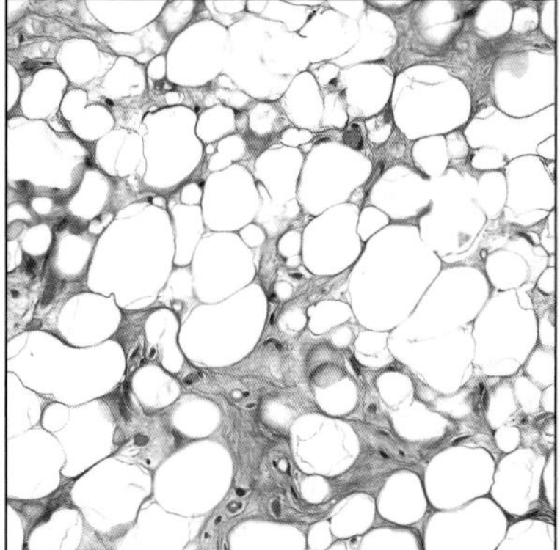

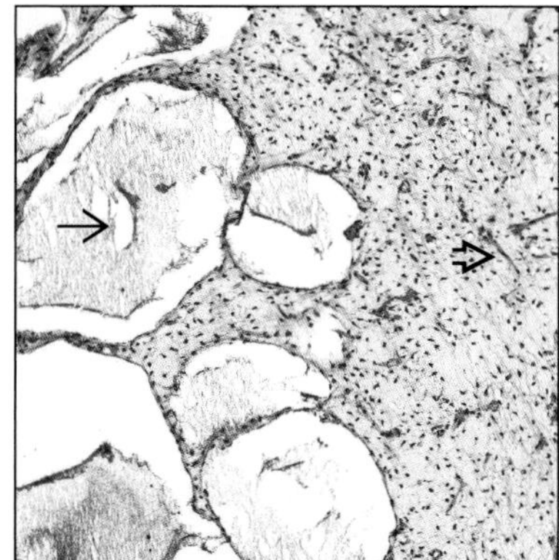

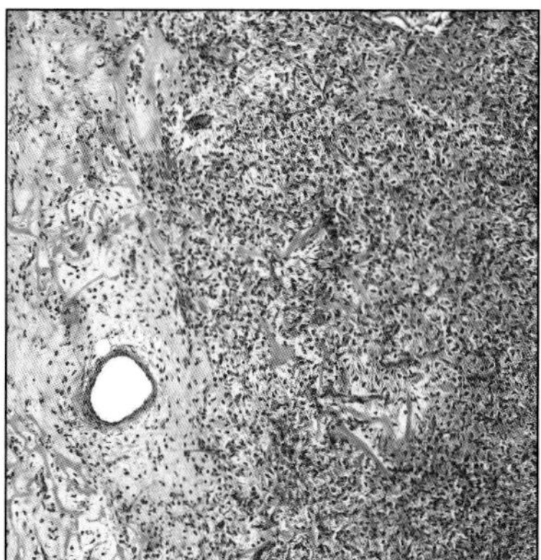

(Left) *Atypical lipomatous tumor areas are composed of adipocytic cells with variations in size and shape, and scattered enlarged and hyperchromatic tumor cell nuclei are seen. Note focal myxoid stromal changes that differ from features in the myxoid liposarcoma areas.* ***(Center)*** *Mucin pools ⇒ and numerous thin-walled, branching vessels ⇨ are seen in the myxoid liposarcoma component.* ***(Right)*** *Focally, progression is seen from low-grade myxoid liposarcoma (left) to more cellular areas with enlarged cells containing overlapping rounded nuclei (right).*

Fibroblastic/Myofibroblastic Lesions

Benign

Intermediate

Malignant

KELOID AND CELLULAR SCAR

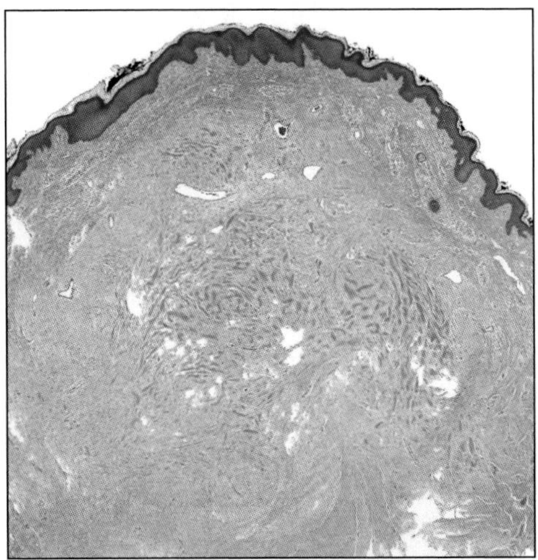

Low-power examination shows a polypoid skin lesion with dense dermal collagen. Note the mild epidermal hyperplasia. Commonly the epidermis overlying a keloid scar is atrophied.

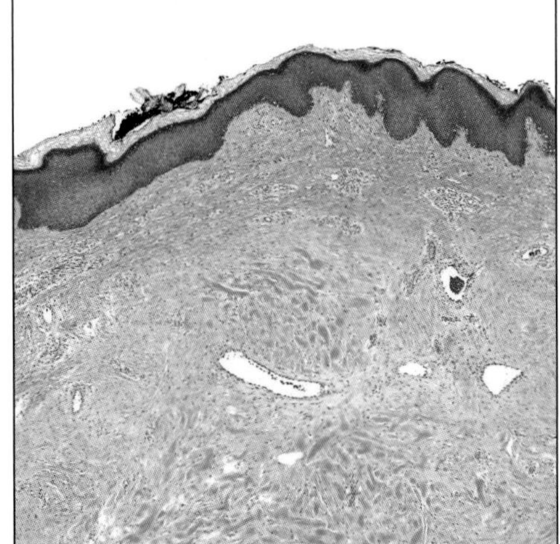

Hematoxylin & eosin shows the superficial aspect of the lesion. Note the dermal scarring with telangiectasia and prominent hyalinized collagen bundles.

TERMINOLOGY

Synonyms

- Scar with keloidal collagen

Definitions

- Scar with prominent thickened and eosinophilic bundles of collagen extending beyond original wound

ETIOLOGY/PATHOGENESIS

Unknown, Possibly Genetic

- Fibroblasts from keloids show decreased apoptosis
- Many cytokines implicated in stimulating fibroblasts, including TGF-β1 and IL-15

CLINICAL ISSUES

Epidemiology

- Age
  - Most common in patients < 30 years
- Ethnicity
  - More common in black patients; least common in Caucasians

Site

- Earlobe is most common site
  - Typically follows ear piercing or other trauma by a few months

Presentation

- Mass is most common
- Scar that grows beyond confines of original wound
- Often erythematous, pruritic lesions with predilection for earlobe in black patients

Treatment

- Options, risks, complications
  - Potentially disfiguring with high risk of recurrence
- Surgical approaches
  - Complete excision, accompanied by concurrent steroid injections or radiotherapy to decrease risk of recurrence
- Drugs
  - Direct injection of steroids is often 1st-line treatment

Prognosis

- Persistence and recurrence are common, but no risk of malignancy

MACROSCOPIC FEATURES

General Features

- Large, nodular, dermal-based lesion with firm white cut surface

MICROSCOPIC PATHOLOGY

Histologic Features

- Dense proliferation of thickened, hyalinized collagen bundles in dermis
- May be background of conventional or hypertrophic scar with smaller collagen bundles and perpendicular vessels
- Decreased vessels compared to conventional and hypertrophic scars
  - Superficial telangiectatic vessels often present
  - Associated with mild chronic inflammation
- Overlying epidermis may show atrophy
- Increased fibroblasts, lymphocytes, and mast cells are usually present

Predominant Pattern/Injury Type

- Fibrosis

Predominant Cell/Compartment Type

- Fibroblast

KELOID AND CELLULAR SCAR

Key Facts

Terminology

- Scar with prominent thickened and eosinophilic bundles of collagen

Clinical Issues

- Persistence and recurrence are common, but no risk of malignancy
- Scar that grows beyond original wound
- Often erythematous, pruritic lesions with predilection for earlobe in black patients

Microscopic Pathology

- Dense proliferation of thickened, hyalinized collagen bundles in dermis
- Decreased vessels compared to conventional and hypertrophic scars
- Increased fibroblasts, lymphocytes, and mast cells are usually present

Top Differential Diagnoses

- Hypertrophic scar

DIFFERENTIAL DIAGNOSIS

Hypertrophic Scar

- Lacks characteristic hyalinized collagen bundles of keloid
- Has more small, perpendicularly oriented vessels; lacks telangiectasia
- Overlapping cases may be seen; may be diagnosed as "hypertrophic scar with focal keloidal collagen"
- Clinically not as elevated as keloid

Desmoplastic Melanoma

- Unlikely, but rarely may enter differential diagnosis if no history of trauma or previous biopsy/surgery
- Re-excision specimens of desmoplastic melanoma may show keloidal collagen
- S100 immunohistochemical stains should be positive
  - Increased numbers of dermal dendritic cells may be seen in scars
  - Should not show spindled morphology of desmoplastic melanoma cells

Nodular Fasciitis

- May rarely show focal keloidal collagen
- Background shows classic features of nodular fasciitis with loose, tissue culture appearance
- Zonation with cellular, myxoid, and more fibrous areas

DIAGNOSTIC CHECKLIST

Pathologic Interpretation Pearls

- Nodular, elevated lesion compared to adjacent skin
- Thickened, hyalinized eosinophilic collagen bundles
- Often see background of hypertrophic scar

SELECTED REFERENCES

1. Wolfram D et al: Hypertrophic scars and keloids--a review of their pathophysiology, risk factors, and therapeutic management. Dermatol Surg. 35(2):171-81, 2009
2. Butler PD et al: Current progress in keloid research and treatment. J Am Coll Surg. 206(4):731-41, 2008
3. Köse O et al: Keloids and hypertrophic scars: are they two different sides of the same coin? Dermatol Surg. 34(3):336-46, 2008
4. Froelich K et al: Therapy of auricular keloids: review of different treatment modalities and proposal for a therapeutic algorithm. Eur Arch Otorhinolaryngol. 264(12):1497-508, 2007
5. Rosen DJ et al: A primary protocol for the management of ear keloids: results of excision combined with intraoperative and postoperative steroid injections. Plast Reconstr Surg. 120(5):1395-400, 2007
6. Thompson LD: Skin keloid. Ear Nose Throat J. 83(8):519, 2004
7. Thompson LD et al: Nodular fasciitis of the external ear region: a clinicopathologic study of 50 cases. Ann Diagn Pathol. 5(4):191-8, 2001
8. Tuan TL et al: The molecular basis of keloid and hypertrophic scar formation. Mol Med Today. 4(1):19-24, 1998

IMAGE GALLERY

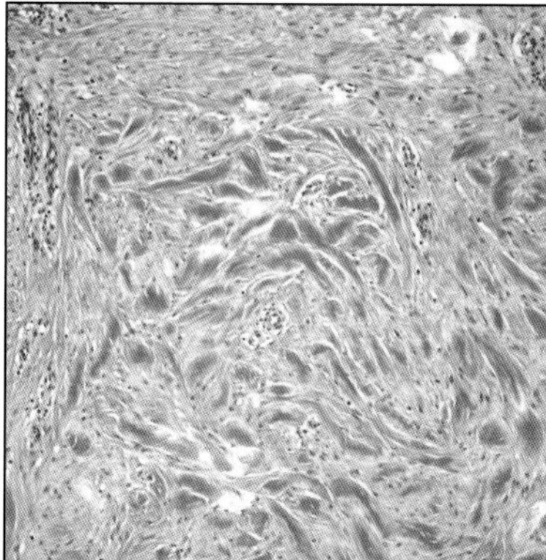

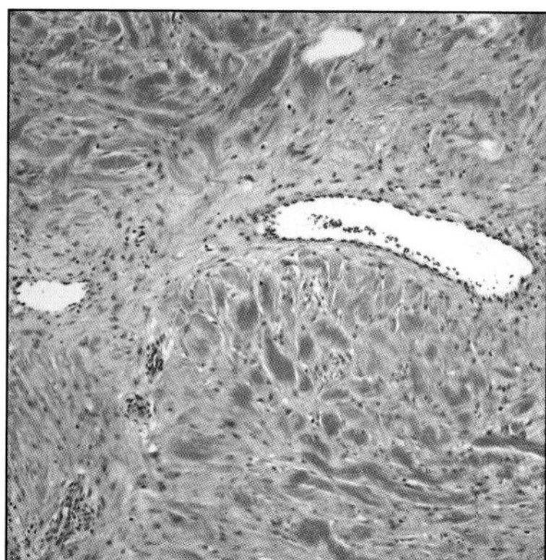

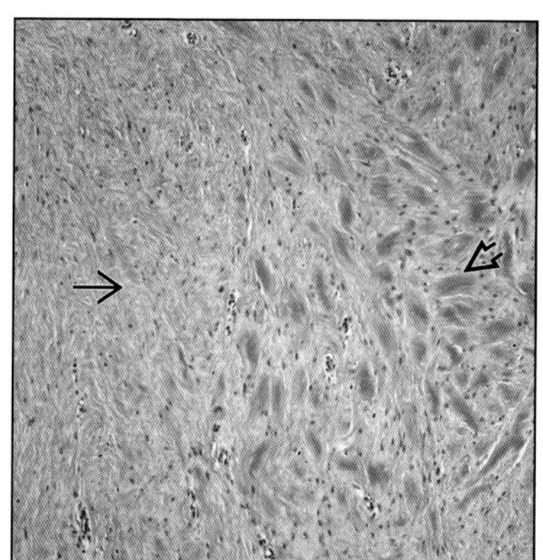

(Left) *Hematoxylin & eosin at higher power examination shows a proliferation of thickened, hyalinized eosinophilic collagen bundles with increased numbers of stromal fibroblasts and scattered lymphocytes. The collagen bundles are randomly orientated and unevenly distributed within the cellular background.* ***(Center)*** *Superficial portion of keloid shows telangiectatic vessels surrounded by thickened collagen bundles.* ***(Right)*** *Hematoxylin & eosin shows comparison between an area of hypertrophic scar → and an area of keloid ⇨.*

ELASTOFIBROMA

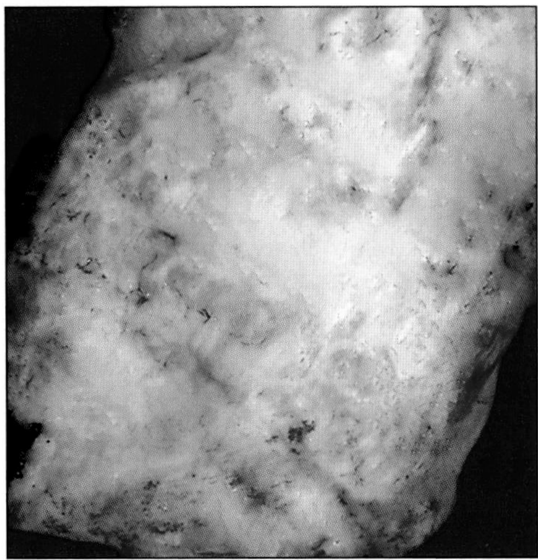

Gross photograph shows a firm white tumor with irregularly infiltrating fat. This formed a firm plaque in the subscapular region; the plaque had been present and slowly enlarging for several years.

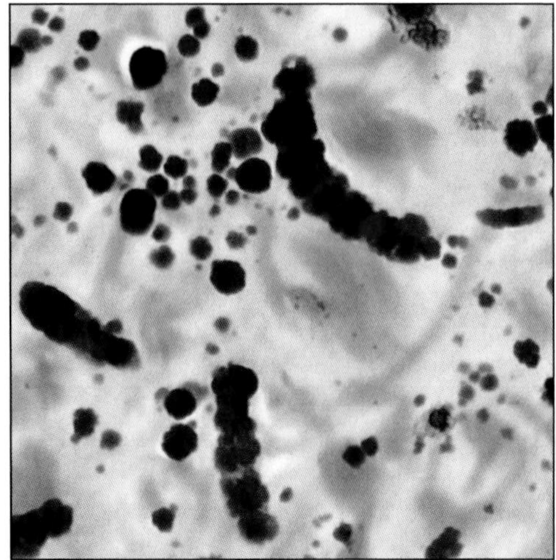

Elastic van Gieson shows elastic fibers at high magnification. Note the "string of beads" appearance with aggregated or separated, variably sized, rounded fragments of black-staining elastic material.

TERMINOLOGY

Synonyms

- Elastofibroma dorsi

Definitions

- Pseudotumor composed of fragmented abnormal elastic fibers in collagenous stroma

ETIOLOGY/PATHOGENESIS

Environmental Exposure

- Some related to trauma or friction
  - Some cases reported in manual workers doing repetitive physical labor
  - Similar microscopic changes are found in 15% of autopsies of older patients

Genetic Predisposition

- Some cases familial
- Examples occur in visceral locations
- Possibly formation of abnormal elastic fibers

CLINICAL ISSUES

Epidemiology

- Incidence
  - Rare
  - Occasionally bilateral
  - Increased incidence in Okinawa, Japan
    - Some familial, genetic component
- Age
  - Mostly over 50 years
- Gender
  - Female predominance

Site

- Typically at inferior margin of scapula on chest wall
  - Deep to muscles of back
  - Can adhere to periosteum
- Also described in other sites
  - Soft tissues
    - Other parts of trunk, arm
  - Visceral locations
    - Oral cavity, stomach, rectum, omentum

Presentation

- Painless mass

Treatment

- Surgical approaches
  - Simple excision

Prognosis

- Excellent

MACROSCOPIC FEATURES

General Features

- Ill-defined, firm, white tissue infiltrating and incorporating fat and skeletal muscle
- Can be adherent to periosteum of rib

Size

- Usually < 5 cm in diameter
- Can be up to 15 cm

MICROSCOPIC PATHOLOGY

Key Microscopic Features

- Infiltrative, ill-defined lesion
- Numerous thickened and fragmented elastic fibers
  - In beaded cords
  - Separate rounded fragments
    - Variable size
- Dense collagenous stroma
- Sparse bland fibroblastic spindle cells
- Infiltrates and entraps fat, skeletal muscle

ELASTOFIBROMA

Key Facts

Terminology
- Pseudotumor composed of fragmented abnormal elastic fibers in collagenous stroma

Etiology/Pathogenesis
- Probably related to trauma or friction

Clinical Issues
- History of manual labor in some cases
- Mostly over 50 years
- Female predominance
- Typically at inferior margin of scapula on chest wall
- Rarely in other locations

Microscopic Pathology
- Infiltrative, ill-defined lesion
- Numerous thickened and fragmented elastic fibers
- Sparse, scattered, bland spindle cells
- Dense collagenous stroma
- Infiltrates fat, skeletal muscle

ANCILLARY TESTS

Histochemistry
- Elastic von Gieson
  - Reactivity: Positive
  - Staining pattern
    - Stromal matrix

Electron Microscopy
- Transmission
  - Irregular rounded masses of electron-dense fibrillary material

DIFFERENTIAL DIAGNOSIS

Nuchal-type Fibroma
- More superficially located (in subcutis)
- Dense collagen
- Sparse; thin elastic fibers

Fibromatosis
- More cellular
- Parallel-aligned spindle cell myofibroblasts
- Mast cells
- Nuclear immunoreactivity for β-catenin

Gardner Fibroma
- Dense collagen
- Sparse elastic
- Associated with familial adenomatous polyposis

Nodular Fasciitis
- Short history, weeks or months
- Cellular, myxoid, and later fibrous areas
- Actin(+)

DIAGNOSTIC CHECKLIST

Pathologic Interpretation Pearls
- Abundant fragmented thickened elastic fibers

SELECTED REFERENCES

1. Mortman KD et al: Elastofibroma dorsi: clinicopathologic review of 6 cases. Ann Thorac Surg. 83(5):1894-7, 2007
2. Hisaoka M et al: Elastofibroma: clonal fibrous proliferation with predominant CD34-positive cells. Virchows Arch. 448(2):195-9, 2006
3. Nishida A et al: Bilateral elastofibroma of the thighs with concomitant subscapular lesions. Skeletal Radiol. 32(2):116-8, 2003
4. Batstone P et al: Clonal chromosome aberrations secondary to chromosome instability in an elastofibroma. Cancer Genet Cytogenet. 128(1):46-7, 2001
5. Nagamine N et al: Elastofibroma in Okinawa. A clinicopathologic study of 170 cases. Cancer. 50(9):1794-805, 1982
6. Peters JL et al: Elastofibroma. Case report and literature review. J Thorac Cardiovasc Surg. 75(6):836-8, 1978
7. Järvi OH et al: Elastofibroma--a degenerative pseudotumor. Cancer. 23(1):42-63, 1969
8. Jarvi O et al: Elastofibroma dorsi. Acta Pathol Microbiol Scand Suppl. 51(Suppl 144):83-4, 1961

IMAGE GALLERY

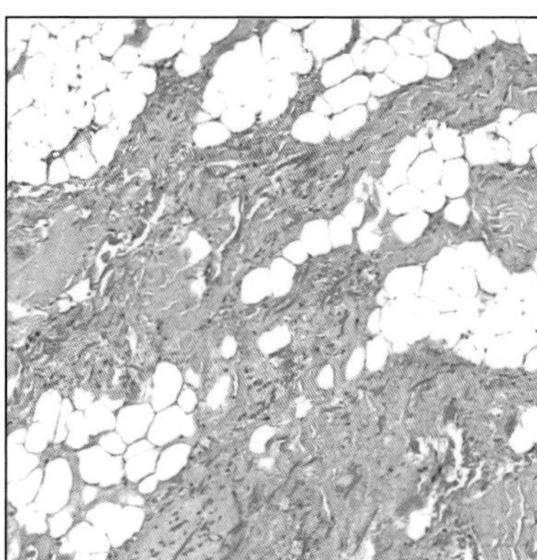

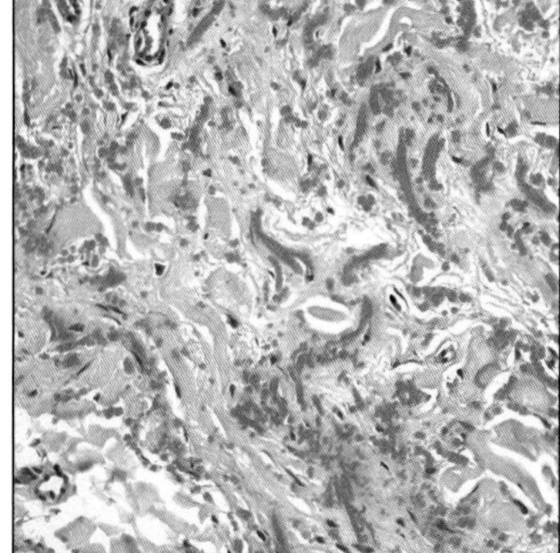

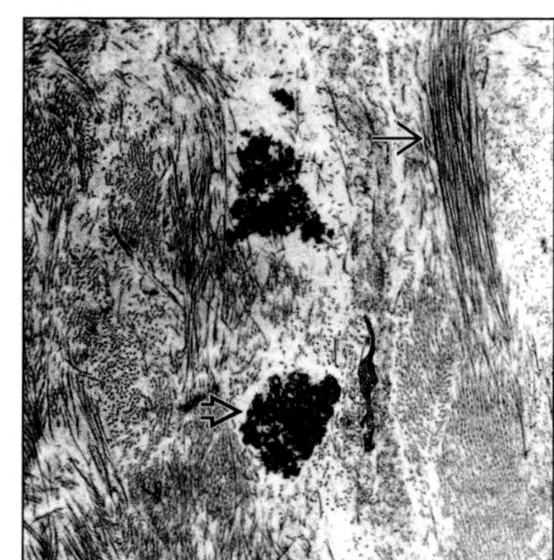

(Left) *Hematoxylin & eosin shows that the tumor is ill defined. Lesional tissue infiltrates as irregular strands into adjacent subcutaneous fat.* ***(Center)*** *Hematoxylin & eosin shows fragments of deeply eosinophilic elastic fibers arranged in wavy cords and numerous spheroids of varying size, dispersed within collagenous stroma.* ***(Right)*** *Electron micrograph shows clumps of electron-dense material ⇨ among collagen fibers →. This is produced in rough endoplasmic reticulum of adjacent fibroblasts and corresponds to the rounded deposits seen by light microscopy.*

NUCHAL AND GARDNER FIBROMA

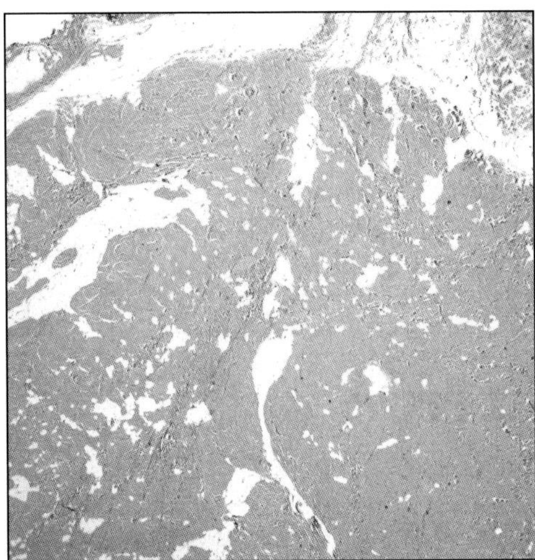

At low magnification, this nuchal-type fibroma is loosely marginated, consisting of dense collagen. The lesion is hypocellular with an admixture of adipose tissue.

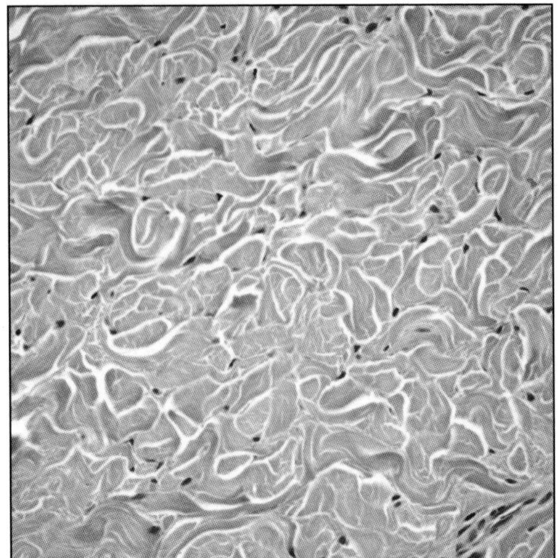

This nuchal-type fibroma is hypocellular, consisting of bland uniform cells. Note the cracked appearance of the dense collagen.

TERMINOLOGY

Synonyms

- Nuchal-type fibroma

Definitions

- Uncommon fibrocollagenous lesion classically arising in cervicodorsal region
  - Not restricted to nuchal region
    - Hence term nuchal-type fibroma
  - Some cases linked to familial adenomatous polyposis (FAP)/Gardner syndrome
    - Germline *APC* gene mutations; colorectal polyposis and fibromatoses

CLINICAL ISSUES

Epidemiology

- Incidence
  - Uncommon
- Age
  - 3rd-5th decades for sporadic lesions
    - Sporadic lesions often nuchal
  - Infants to adolescents for Gardner-associated cases
    - Mostly involve trunk, head and neck, extremities
- Gender
  - Striking male predominance in sporadic cases
  - No gender predominance in Gardner-associated cases

Presentation

- Painless mass
- Sporadic examples associated with diabetes mellitus

Prognosis

- Cured by local excision
  - Occasional recurrences when incompletely excised
- Gardner-associated lesions can be harbingers for colorectal polyposis or fibromatoses

MACROSCOPIC FEATURES

General Features

- Poorly circumscribed subcutaneous masses
- < 1 cm to > 10 cm; median size: 3-4 cm
- Plaque-like rubbery cut surface

MICROSCOPIC PATHOLOGY

Histologic Features

- Formless sheets of densely collagenized tissue with clefts and cracks
- Hypocellular
- Small nuclei
- Variable entrapped adipose tissue and nerves

Predominant Pattern/Injury Type

- Fibrous

Predominant Cell/Compartment Type

- Fibroblast

DIFFERENTIAL DIAGNOSIS

Nuchal Fibrocartilaginous Tumor

- Arises in posterior neck at junction of nuchal ligament and deep cervical fascia
- Probably a reactive process
- Contains prominent cartilaginous tissue

Elastofibroma

- Typically arises in inferior portion of scapula
- Degenerated elastic fibrils forming "chenille" (French for caterpillar) bodies

Fibromatosis

- Usually deep large lesion

NUCHAL AND GARDNER FIBROMA

Key Facts

Terminology

- Uncommon fibrocollagenous lesion classically arising in cervicodorsal region
- Some cases linked to familial adenomatous polyposis (FAP)/Gardner syndrome

Clinical Issues

- Sporadic lesions usually in older men, often nuchal
- Gardner-associated cases often involve trunk, head and neck, extremities of children; no gender predominance

Microscopic Pathology

- Formless sheets of densely collagenized tissue with clefts and cracks
- Hypocellular
- Small nuclei

Immunohistochemistry

Antibody	Reactivity	Staining Pattern	Comment
β-catenin	Positive	Nuclear	Usually accumulates in nuclei of lesions from patients with Gardner syndrome; more often negative in non-Gardner-associated lesions
CD99	Positive	Cell membrane & cytoplasm	Most cases are CD99 reactive
CD34	Positive	Cytoplasmic	
Cyclin-D1	Positive	Nuclear	In keeping with alterations in Wnt pathway
myc	Positive	Nuclear	In keeping with alterations in Wnt pathway

- Associated with familial adenomatous polyposis (FAP)/ Gardner syndrome; mutations in β-catenin or *APC* gene
  - Most are sporadic
- Cellular lesions arranged in sweeping fascicles
- β-catenin staining shows nuclear labeling; CD34 usually negative

Fibrolipoma

- Superficial lesions, usually well marginated or encapsulated
- No entrapped nerves

DIAGNOSTIC CHECKLIST

Clinically Relevant Pathologic Features

- Possibility of familial adenomatous polyposis/ Gardner syndrome should be raised when these are encountered in extranuchal sites in young patients

SELECTED REFERENCES

1. Coffin CM et al: Gardner fibroma: a clinicopathologic and immunohistochemical analysis of 45 patients with 57 fibromas. Am J Surg Pathol. 31(3):410-6, 2007
2. Wehrli BM et al: Gardner-associated fibromas (GAF) in young patients: a distinct fibrous lesion that identifies unsuspected Gardner syndrome and risk for fibromatosis. Am J Surg Pathol. 25(5):645-51, 2001
3. Zamecnik M et al: Nuchal-type fibroma is positive for CD34 and CD99. Am J Surg Pathol. 25(7):970, 2001
4. Michal M: Non-nuchal-type fibroma associated with Gardner's syndrome. A hitherto-unreported mesenchymal tumor different from fibromatosis and nuchal-type fibroma. Pathol Res Pract. 196(12):857-60, 2000
5. Michal M et al: Nuchal-type fibroma: a clinicopathologic study of 52 cases. Cancer. 85(1):156-63, 1999

IMAGE GALLERY

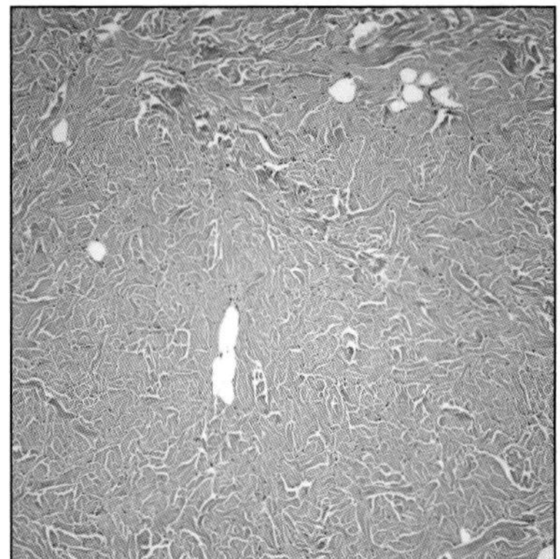

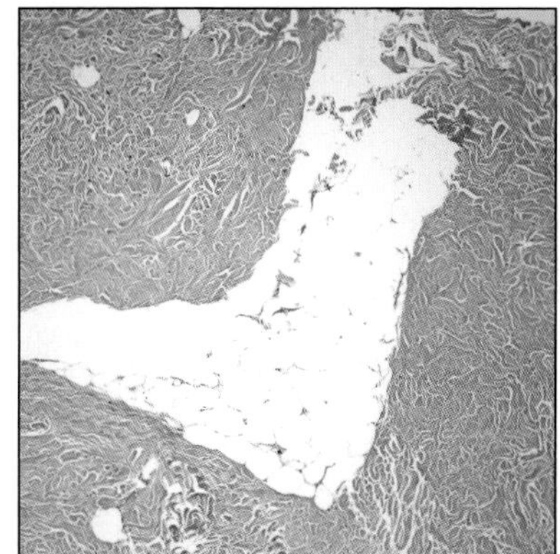

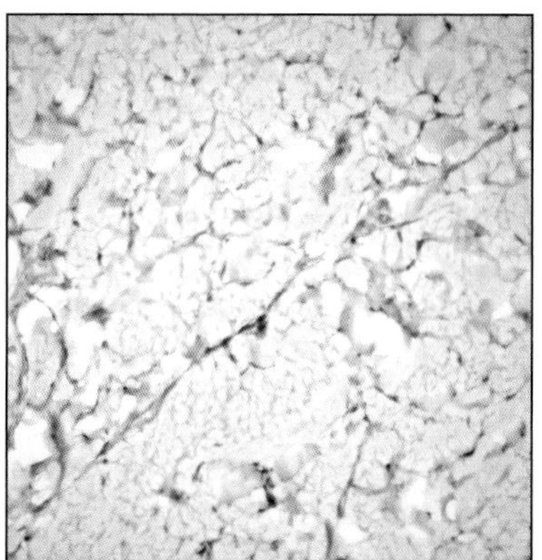

(Left) *Hematoxylin & eosin shows a nuchal fibroma. This lesion was on the neck of an elderly man, the classic presentation. However, identical lesions can be found in extranuchal sites. Such extranuchal lesions can be associated with familial adenomatous polyposis (FAP)/Gardner syndrome.* ***(Center)*** *Nuchal fibromas and Gardner-associated fibromas often display prominent entrapped adipose tissue.* ***(Right)*** *CD99 often labels the proliferating cells in nuchal-type fibromas, including those associated with Gardner syndrome.*

NUCHAL FIBROCARTILAGINOUS PSEUDOTUMOR

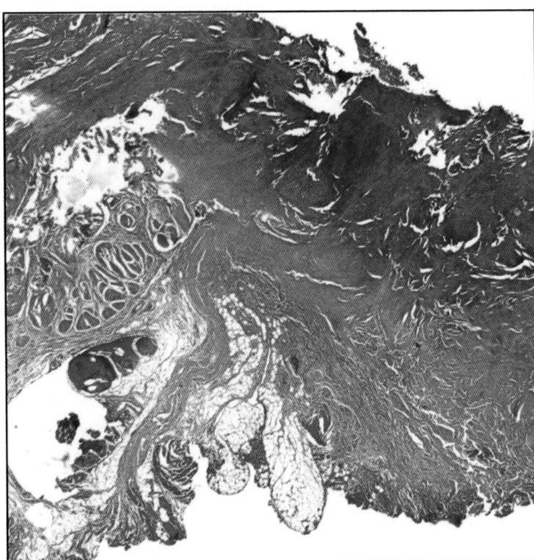

Hematoxylin & eosin shows chondroid metaplasia within dense fibrous tissue of nuchal ligament, shown here at its junction with deep fascia. (Courtesy J.X. O'Connell, MD.)

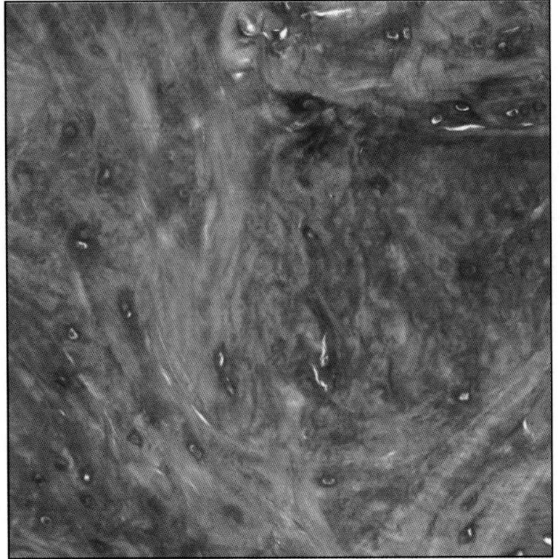

Hematoxylin & eosin shows nuchal fibrocartilaginous pseudotumor with area of cartilaginous metaplasia, which displays variable basophilic staining of chondroid stroma. This area is sparsely cellular.

TERMINOLOGY

Definitions

- Metaplastic (pseudoneoplastic) nodule of fibrocartilage originating within nuchal ligament

ETIOLOGY/PATHOGENESIS

Environmental Exposure

- Nuchal ligament subject during neck flexion to mechanical trauma from spinous processes
  - Sesamoid bone formation might result from fibrocartilaginous metaplasia
- Most patients have history of whiplash or direct trauma, commonly motor vehicle crash
- Rare examples are spontaneous

CLINICAL ISSUES

Epidemiology

- Incidence
  - Very rare
    - < 20 cases reported
- Age
  - Majority in adults
  - Occasional cases in childhood

Site

- In nuchal ligament
  - Fibrous and elastic ligament or band in midline
    - Attached to medial nuchal line and external occipital protuberance of skull
    - Extends to spinous process of C7
    - Anterior border is attached to spinous processes of other cervical vertebrae
  - Lesion is usually at level of vertebrae C4-5 or C5-6
    - At posterior aspect of base of neck in midline
    - At junction of nuchal ligament and deep fascia

Presentation

- Painless mass

Treatment

- Surgical approaches
  - Simple excision

Prognosis

- Excellent
  - Reported examples have not recurred

IMAGE FINDINGS

MR Findings

- Focal thickening of nuchal ligament at C4-5 or C5-6 level

MACROSCOPIC FEATURES

General Features

- Ill-defined yellow-white nodule
  - Within fibrous tissue of nuchal ligament or at junction with fascia
  - Can extend into surrounding tissues
  - Not attached to bone

Size

- 1-3 cm (mean: 2.5 cm)

MICROSCOPIC PATHOLOGY

Key Microscopic Features

- Fibrous tissue
  - Sparsely cellular
  - Cracking artifact
- Nodule of cartilage
  - Scanty bland chondrocytes
- No cytologic atypia
- No inflammation

NUCHAL FIBROCARTILAGINOUS PSEUDOTUMOR

Key Facts

Terminology
- Metaplastic (pseudoneoplastic) nodule of fibrocartilage originating within nuchal ligament

Etiology/Pathogenesis
- Remote or recent history of neck trauma

Clinical Issues
- Majority in adults
- At posterior aspect of base of neck in midline
- At junction of nuchal ligament and deep fascia

Microscopic Pathology
- Hypocellular fibrous tissue and cartilage
- No calcification

Top Differential Diagnoses
- Nuchal fibroma
- Soft tissue chondroma
- Calcifying aponeurotic fibroma

- No calcification
- Elastic fibers fragmented at margin of lesion

ANCILLARY TESTS

Immunohistochemistry
- Chondroid cells
  - Positive for S100 protein
- Fibroblastic cells
  - Express CD34
  - Lack desmin, actin, CD99

Electron Microscopy
- Transmission
  - Cells show features of fibroblasts or chondrocytes

DIFFERENTIAL DIAGNOSIS

Nuchal Fibroma
- In subcutaneous tissue
- Not in midline, nor confined to nuchal region
- Hypocellular collagen bands infiltrate locally
- Lacks cartilage

Soft Tissue Chondroma
- Extremity location
- Related to tendon
- Nodules of cartilage
- Giant cell reaction, calcification

Calcifying Aponeurotic Fibroma
- Most commonly in subcutis of hands and feet
- Calcification in chondroid foci
- Cellular fibroblastic component
  - Often disposed in files

DIAGNOSTIC CHECKLIST

Clinically Relevant Pathologic Features
- Organ distribution

Pathologic Interpretation Pearls
- Benign cartilage in fibrous tissue

SELECTED REFERENCES

1. Nicoletti GF et al: Nuchal fibrocartilaginous pseudomotor. Case report and review of the literature. J Neurosurg Sci. 47(3):173-5; discussion 175, 2003
2. Zamecnik M et al: Nuchal fibrocartilaginous pseudotumor: immunohistochemical and ultrastructural study of two cases. Pathol Int. 51(9):723-8, 2001
3. Luévano-Flores E et al: Nuchal fibrocartilaginous pseudotumor in a 10-year-old girl. Arch Pathol Lab Med. 124(8):1217-9, 2000
4. Laskin WB et al: Nuchal fibrocartilaginous pseudotumor: a clinicopathologic study of five cases and review of the literature. Mod Pathol. 12(7):663-8, 1999
5. O'Connell JX et al: Nuchal fibrocartilaginous pseudotumor: a distinctive soft-tissue lesion associated with prior neck injury. Am J Surg Pathol. 21(7):836-40, 1997

IMAGE GALLERY

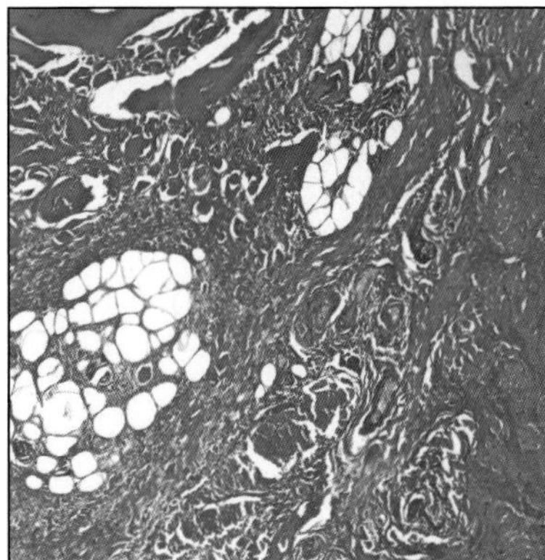
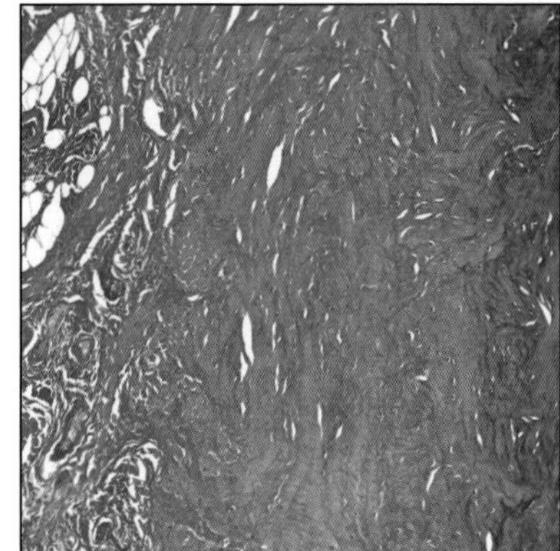
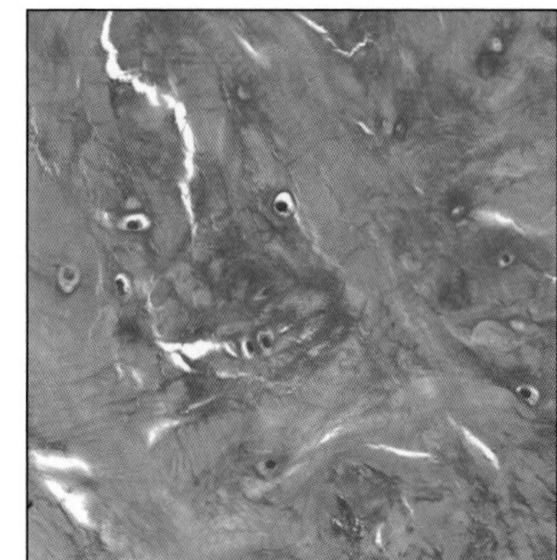

(Left) *Hematoxylin & eosin shows junction of nuchal ligament and deep fascia with reactive fibrous tissue extending into adjacent fat.* ***(Center)*** *Hematoxylin & eosin shows chondroid metaplasia arising with ill-defined margin in fibrous tissue, the latter displaying "cracking" artifact.* ***(Right)*** *Hematoxylin & eosin shows metaplastic cartilage with scattered bland chondrocytes in focally fibrillary stroma. Note sparse cellularity and absence of atypia or pleomorphism, allowing distinction from chondrosarcoma. The chondrocytes are immunoreactive for S100 protein.*

FIBROMA OF TENDON SHEATH

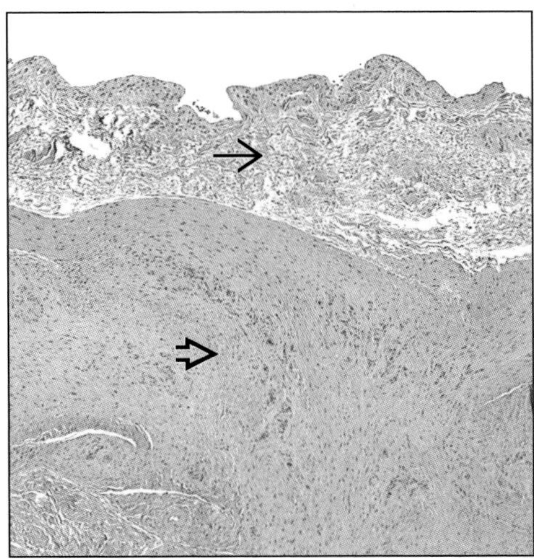

Fibroma of tendon sheath (FTS) typically presents as a small soft tissue nodule in a finger. This micrograph depicts a circumscribed fibroma ⇨ attached to a synovial-lined tendon sheath →.

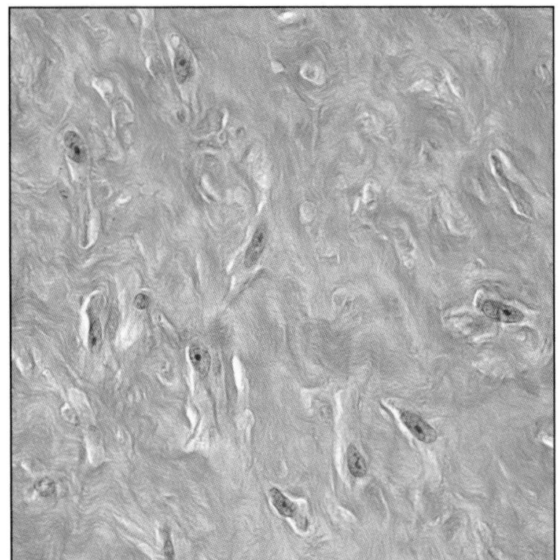

The proliferating cells in FTS are fibroblasts and myofibroblasts characterized by bipolar spindle and stellate cells with abundant amphophilic cytoplasm and vesicular nuclei with solitary nucleoli.

TERMINOLOGY

Abbreviations

- Fibroma of tendon sheath (FTS)

Definitions

- Small benign fibrous nodule typically attached to tendon sheath

ETIOLOGY/PATHOGENESIS

Histogenesis

- Generally regarded as reactive nonneoplastic process
  - Single report of clonal chromosomal aberration t(2:11)
    - Possibly neoplastic process

CLINICAL ISSUES

Epidemiology

- Incidence
  - Uncommon, exact incidence unknown
- Age
  - Median: 30 years (range: 5 months to 70 years)
- Gender
  - Men slightly outnumber women

Site

- Hand (80%)
  - Most common in fingers (50%)
    - Especially thumb, index, or middle finger
- Lower extremities (11%)
  - Anterior knee, ankle, foot, or toe
- Rare sites: Trunk, chest, back, and shoulder
- Rare intraarticular cases

Presentation

- Painless mass
- Slow growing
- Uncommon findings: Nerve impingement, carpal tunnel syndrome

Treatment

- Surgical approaches
  - Simple excision

Prognosis

- Excellent
  - 24% recurrence rate
  - Re-excision usually curative

IMAGE FINDINGS

MR Findings

- Focal nodular mass with decreased signal on all pulse sequences and little or no enhancement

MACROSCOPIC FEATURES

General Features

- Well circumscribed
- Often lobulated
- Hard, rubbery, or gelatinous

Size

- Median: ≈ 2 cm (range: 0.5-5 cm)

MICROSCOPIC PATHOLOGY

Histologic Features

- Well demarcated
- Attached to tendon or tendon sheath
- Benign fibroblasts and myofibroblasts
- Variable fibrous to myxoid stroma
- Slit-like vascular spaces
  - Lined by flattened endothelial cells
  - Most prevalent at periphery
  - Characteristic feature of FTS

FIBROMA OF TENDON SHEATH

Key Facts

Terminology
- Small benign fibrous nodule typically attached to tendon sheath

Clinical Issues
- Most common in fingers

Macroscopic Features
- Median size: ≈ 2 cm (range: 0.5-5 cm)

Microscopic Pathology
- Well demarcated
- Attached to tendon or tendon sheath
- Benign fibroblasts and myofibroblasts
- Slit-like vascular spaces
- Cellular nodular fasciitis-like areas

Top Differential Diagnoses
- Nodular fasciitis
- Superficial fibromatosis

- Cellular nodular fasciitis-like areas
  - Most prevalent at periphery
  - Transition zone between fibrous and nodular fasciitis-like areas
- Storiform areas in some tumors
- Low mitotic rate
- Rare cases with cellular pleomorphism

Cytologic Features
- Abundant finely granular amphophilic cytoplasm
- Bipolar and stellate forms
- Vesicular nucleus with single nucleolus

DIFFERENTIAL DIAGNOSIS

Nodular Fasciitis
- Rare in fingers
- Usually arises from fascia
- Less circumscribed
- More cellular and mitotically active

Superficial Fibromatosis
- Rare in fingers
- Arises from palmar or plantar fascia
- Infiltrates surrounding tissue

Giant Cell Tumor of Tendon Sheath
- Common in fingers
- Arises from tendon sheath
- Round to reniform stomal cells, osteoclastic giant cells, hemosiderin, xanthoma cells

Collagenous Fibroma/Desmoplastic Fibroblastoma
- Rare in fingers
- Arises in subcutis or skeletal muscle
- Larger size
- Stellate-shaped myofibroblasts

Benign Fibrous Histiocytoma
- Rare in fingers
- Typically arises in dermis but can be deep-seated
- More cellular
- Well-defined storiform pattern
- Infiltrative growth with entrapment of dermal collagen
- Multinucleated giant cells common

SELECTED REFERENCES

1. Fox MG et al: MR imaging of fibroma of the tendon sheath. AJR Am J Roentgenol. 180(5):1449-53, 2003
2. Dal Cin P et al: Translocation 2;11 in a fibroma of tendon sheath. Histopathology. 32(5):433-5, 1998
3. Lamovec J et al: Pleomorphic fibroma of tendon sheath. Am J Surg Pathol. 15(12):1202-5, 1991
4. Pulitzer DR et al: Fibroma of tendon sheath. A clinicopathologic study of 32 cases. Am J Surg Pathol. 13(6):472-9, 1989
5. Jablokow VR et al: Fibroma of tendon sheath. J Surg Oncol. 19(2):90-2, 1982
6. Chung EB et al: Fibroma of tendon sheath. Cancer. 44(5):1945-54, 1979

IMAGE GALLERY

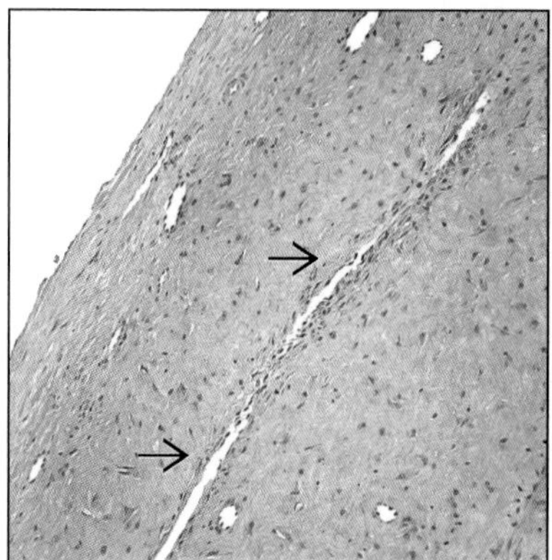

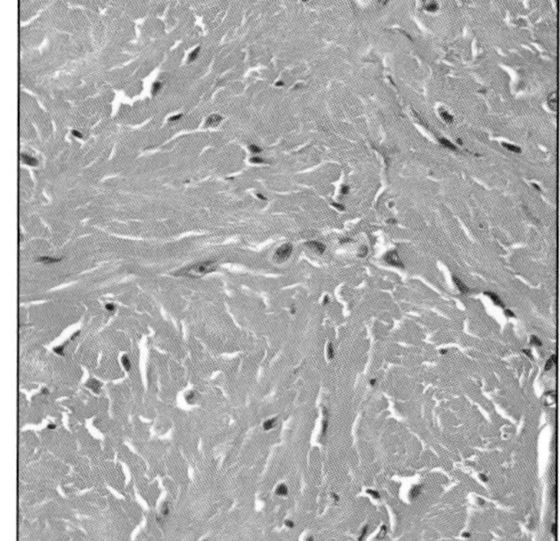

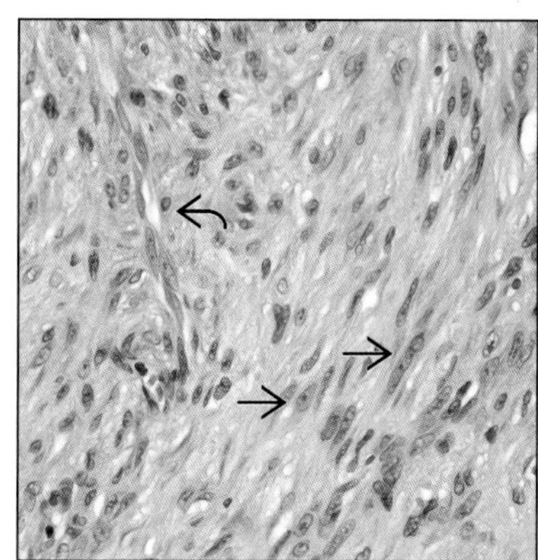

*(**Left**) Long slit-like blood vessels ⇒ located at the periphery are characteristic of fibroma of tendon sheath. The stroma varies from fibrous to myxoid. (**Center**) This micrograph depicts a hypocellular area with dense hyalinizing stromal fibrosis. (**Right**) By contrast, this area has a more cellular nodular fasciitis-like appearance consisting of plump myofibroblasts ⇒, capillaries ⇗, and fibromyxoid stroma. Transitional zones between fibrous and nodular fasciitis-like areas are common.*

PLEOMORPHIC FIBROMA

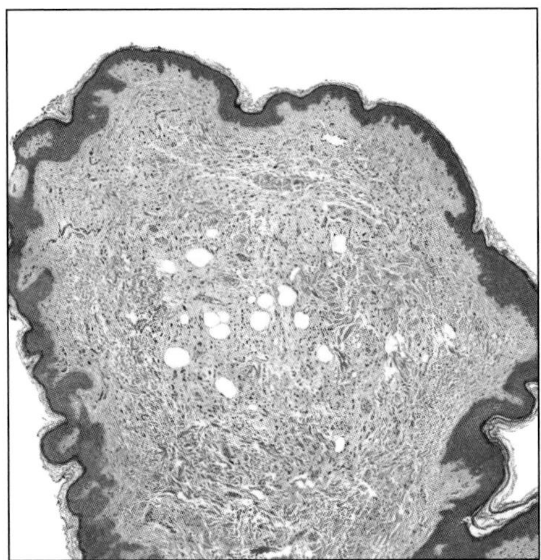

Scanning magnification shows a polypoid (skin-tag-like) lesion with a fibromyxoid stroma. The lesion is usually solitary and occurs on the trunk, head and neck region, or extremities.

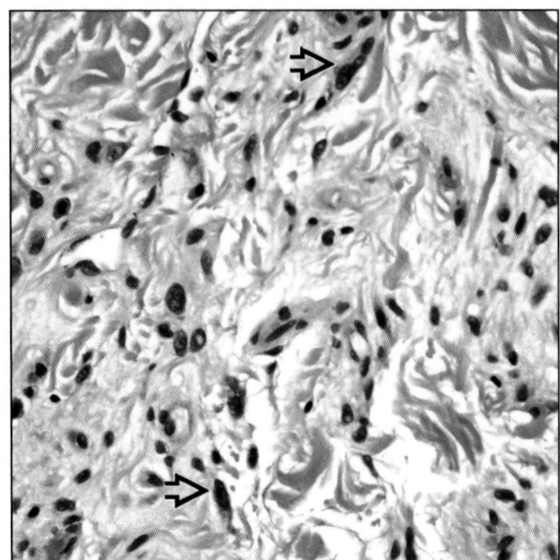

High-power examination shows a population of enlarged, hyperchromatic-staining spindled ➪, stellate, and multinucleated cells set in a fibromyxoid stroma. No mitoses are seen.

TERMINOLOGY

Abbreviations

- Pleomorphic fibroma (PF)

Definitions

- Benign dermal-based neoplasm composed of pleomorphic-appearing myofibroblasts

ETIOLOGY/PATHOGENESIS

Unknown

- Some cases may be related to ischemia, trauma, or degenerative changes

CLINICAL ISSUES

Presentation

- Slow-growing skin nodule
  - Usually dome-shaped or polypoid-appearing
  - Flesh-colored and nonulcerated
- Typically occur on trunk, extremities, or head and neck region

Treatment

- Surgical approaches
  - Complete conservative excision is curative

Prognosis

- Benign tumors with excellent prognosis
- May show local recurrence if incompletely excised

MACROSCOPIC FEATURES

Size

- Range: 0.4-1.6 cm

MICROSCOPIC PATHOLOGY

Histologic Features

- Well-circumscribed, dome-shaped or polypoid hypocellular proliferation of dermal spindle cells
- Lesional cells are predominantly spindle-shaped, also with stellate and multinucleated cells
- Cells show enlarged hyperchromatic nuclei with small nucleoli and scant amounts of eosinophilic cytoplasm
- Mitotic figures are rare or absent
  - No atypical mitoses should be seen
- Stroma typically composed of hyalinized-appearing collagen fibers
  - Some cases show overlapping features with sclerotic fibroma
    - i.e., these cases show storiforming of hyalinized collagen bundles with collagen clefts
- Myxoid areas may be present
  - Can be prominent/diffuse in some cases (myxoid pleomorphic fibroma)

Predominant Pattern/Injury Type

- Fibrous

Predominant Cell/Compartment Type

- Fibroblast/myofibroblast

ANCILLARY TESTS

Immunohistochemistry

- Typically positive for actin-sm, CD34, and vimentin
- FXIIIA variably positive

DIFFERENTIAL DIAGNOSIS

Atypical Fibroxanthoma (AFX)

- Highly cellular and atypical-appearing dermal-based tumor associated with solar elastosis

PLEOMORPHIC FIBROMA

Key Facts

Terminology
- Benign dermal-based neoplasm composed of pleomorphic-appearing myofibroblasts

Clinical Issues
- Slow-growing skin nodule
- Usually dome-shaped or polypoid-appearing
- May show local recurrence if incompletely excised

Ancillary Tests
- Cells are typically positive for actin, CD34, and vimentin; variable positivity for FXIIIA is reported

Diagnostic Checklist
- Cells appear pleomorphic and hyperchromatic but lack mitotic activity
- Hypocellular dermal proliferation of spindled, stellate, and multinucleated cells

- Mitotic figures are easily found, including atypical forms, in most cases
- CD34 is typically negative, and nonspecific markers (including CD68, CD10, and CD99) are usually positive

Dermatofibroma
- Usually does not show degree of pleomorphism seen in PF, although rare cases may ("dermatofibroma with monster cells")
- More typical dermatofibroma areas should be present at periphery of tumor
  - Collagen trapping, histiocytoid cells, and overlying epidermal hyperplasia are usually present
- CD34 is typically negative, unlike PF

Fibrous Papule (Angiofibroma)
- Small, dome-shaped papule, which shows dermal fibrosis and increased blood vessels with telangiectasia
- Scattered enlarged, mildly pleomorphic-appearing fibroblasts may be present
- CD34 should be negative in most cases, and FXIIIA is usually positive

Sclerotic Fibroma
- Shows characteristic storiform pattern of thickened, hyalinized-appearing collagen bundles with clefts between them
- Some cases show overlapping features with PF, with population of enlarged, pleomorphic-appearing spindled cells
  - Therefore, some authors believe that PF is a variant of sclerotic fibroma, but this is not universally accepted

DIAGNOSTIC CHECKLIST

Pathologic Interpretation Pearls
- Hypocellular dermal proliferation of spindled, stellate, and multinucleated cells
- Cells appear pleomorphic and hyperchromatic but lack mitotic activity

SELECTED REFERENCES

1. Mahmood MN et al: Solitary sclerotic fibroma of skin: a possible link with pleomorphic fibroma with immunophenotypic expression for O13 (CD99) and CD34. J Cutan Pathol. 30(10):631-6, 2003
2. García-Doval I et al: Pleomorphic fibroma of the skin, a form of sclerotic fibroma: an immunohistochemical study. Clin Exp Dermatol. 23(1):22-4, 1998
3. Pitt MA et al: Myxoid cutaneous pleomorphic fibroma. Histopathology. 25(3):300, 1994
4. Kamino H et al: Pleomorphic fibroma of the skin: a benign neoplasm with cytologic atypia. A clinicopathologic study of eight cases. Am J Surg Pathol. 13(2):107-13, 1989

IMAGE GALLERY

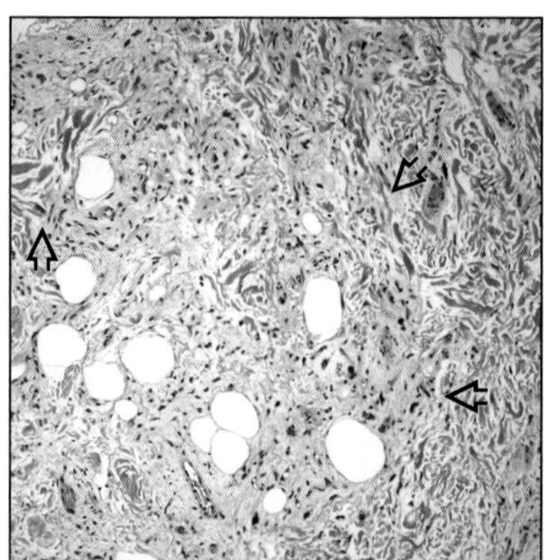

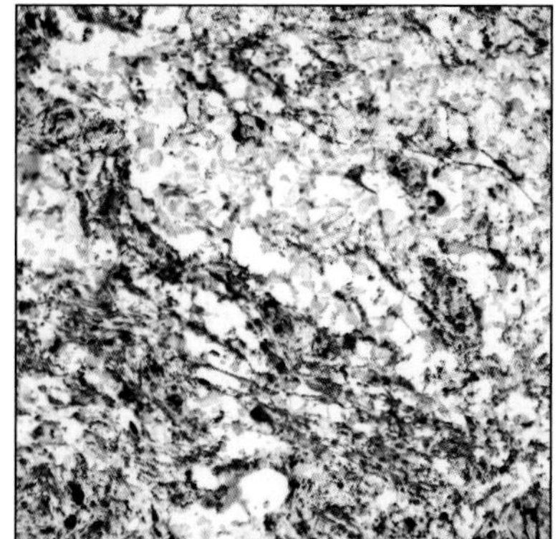

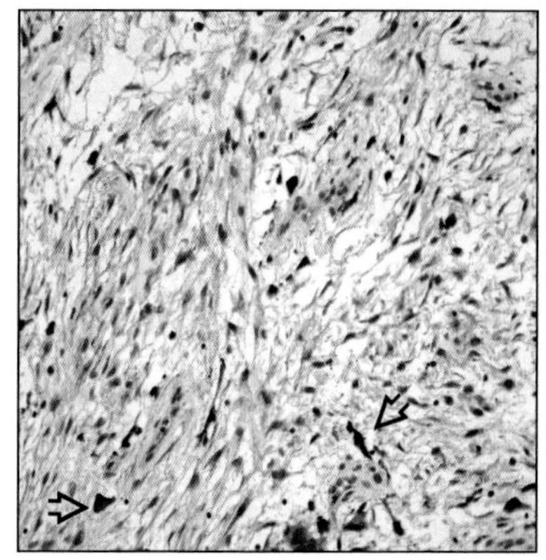

(Left) Intermediate-power examination shows areas of collagenous stroma alternating with more myxoid areas ➢ containing the pleomorphic, hyperchromatic-staining cells. *(Center)* Positive CD34 shows strong and diffuse staining of the spindled and multinucleated cells. *(Right)* Positive FXIIIA staining shows more patchy staining of a subset of the lesional cells ➢.

STORIFORM COLLAGENOMA

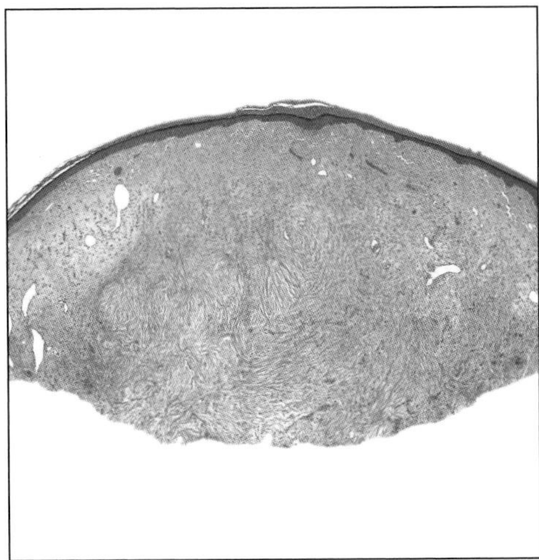

Scanning magnification view shows a dermal-based nodular fibroblastic proliferation with storiforming of collagen.

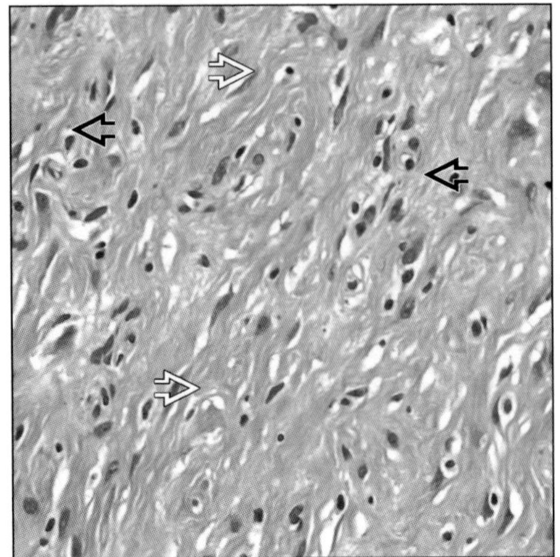

Higher power magnification shows bland fibroblasts ➡ and scattered inflammatory cells ➡ in a dense fibrous stroma.

TERMINOLOGY

Synonyms

- Sclerotic fibroma

Definitions

- Benign, dermal-based fibroblastic proliferation with storiforming collagen

ETIOLOGY/PATHOGENESIS

Unknown

- May be related to trauma
- Some cases may represent regressed dermatofibromas
- Some cases are genetic
  - Multiple lesions are associated with Cowden syndrome, consistent with a genetic influence

CLINICAL ISSUES

Epidemiology

- Age
  - May occur at any age, including infants and elderly
- Gender
  - Occurs in both males and females

Site

- Present most commonly on the face, extremities, and trunk

Presentation

- Slow-growing, flesh-colored papule or nodule

Treatment

- Surgical approaches
  - Complete conservative excision is curative

Prognosis

- Excellent; may locally recur but no metastatic potential

MACROSCOPIC FEATURES

General Features

- Dermal nodule with firm yellow-tan surface

Size

- Typically 0.5-3 cm

MICROSCOPIC PATHOLOGY

Histologic Features

- Circumscribed, unencapsulated dermal nodule
- Composed of thickened, hyalinized-appearing collagen bundles in storiform/whorled pattern
  - Prominent clefts often seen between collagen bundles
- Cells are typically small, bland, spindled to stellate fibroblasts
- Occasional cases may show large, bizarre-appearing cells ("pleomorphic sclerotic fibroma"), similar to pleomorphic fibroma
  - These cells do not show infiltrative features or increased mitotic activity
- Pacinian collagenoma is rare variant with onion skinning, mimicking pacinian corpuscle

Predominant Pattern/Injury Type

- Fibrous

Predominant Cell/Compartment Type

- Fibroblast

ANCILLARY TESTS

Immunohistochemistry

- Generally not necessary, but cells will stain for FXIIIA, CD34 (focally), and vimentin
- Ki-67 staining may highlight a few scattered nuclei, but overall staining is low

STORIFORM COLLAGENOMA

Key Facts

Terminology
- Sclerotic fibroma
- Benign, dermal-based fibroblastic proliferation

Microscopic Pathology
- Composed of thickened, hyalinized-appearing collagen bundles in storiform/whorled pattern
- Occasional cases may show large, bizarre-appearing cells ("pleomorphic sclerotic fibroma"), similar to pleomorphic fibroma

Ancillary Tests
- Immunohistochemistry generally not necessary, but cells will stain for FXIIIA, CD34 (focally), and vimentin

Top Differential Diagnoses
- Dermatofibroma
- Pleomorphic fibroma
- Collagenous fibroma

DIFFERENTIAL DIAGNOSIS

Dermatofibroma (DF)
- Typically does not show prominent storiforming of collagen, although it may be focally present in rare cases
- Areas of conventional DF with collagen trapping and histiocytic cells should be present
  - Some cases may show overlapping features, leading some investigators to believe that sclerotic fibromas are involuting dermatofibromas

Pleomorphic Fibroma
- Clinically resembles a skin tag
- Pleomorphic cells are more prominent, and storiforming pattern of collagen should be absent

Collagenous Fibroma
- Usually subcutaneous tumors with only rare dermal involvement
- Densely collagenous or fibromyxoid stroma; lacks prominent storiforming of collagen

Acral Fibrokeratoma (Subungual and Periungual Fibroma)
- Usually shows overlying hyperkeratosis and acanthosis
- Proliferation of thick collagen bundles, often vertically oriented

DIAGNOSTIC CHECKLIST

Pathologic Interpretation Pearls
- Dermal nodule of thickened, hyalinized-appearing collagen bundles in storiform/whorled pattern

SELECTED REFERENCES

1. Nakashima K et al: Solitary sclerotic fibroma of the skin: morphological characterization of the 'plywood-like pattern'. J Cutan Pathol. 35 Suppl 1:74-9, 2008
2. González-Vela MC et al: Sclerotic fibroma-like dermatofibroma: an uncommon distinctive variant of dermatofibroma. Histol Histopathol. 20(3):801-6, 2005
3. Chen TM et al: Pleomorphic sclerotic fibroma: a case report and literature review. Am J Dermatopathol. 24(1):54-8, 2002
4. Chang SN et al: Solitary sclerotic fibroma of the skin: degenerated sclerotic change of inflammatory conditions, especially folliculitis. Am J Dermatopathol. 22(1):22-5, 2000
5. Martín-López R et al: Pleomorphic sclerotic fibroma. Dermatology. 198(1):69-72, 1999
6. Pujol RM et al: Solitary sclerotic fibroma of the skin: a sclerotic dermatofibroma? Am J Dermatopathol. 18(6):620-4, 1996
7. Requena L et al: Multiple sclerotic fibromas of the skin. A cutaneous marker of Cowden's disease. J Cutan Pathol. 19(4):346-51, 1992
8. Rapini RP et al: Sclerotic fibromas of the skin. J Am Acad Dermatol. 20(2 Pt 1):266-71, 1989

IMAGE GALLERY

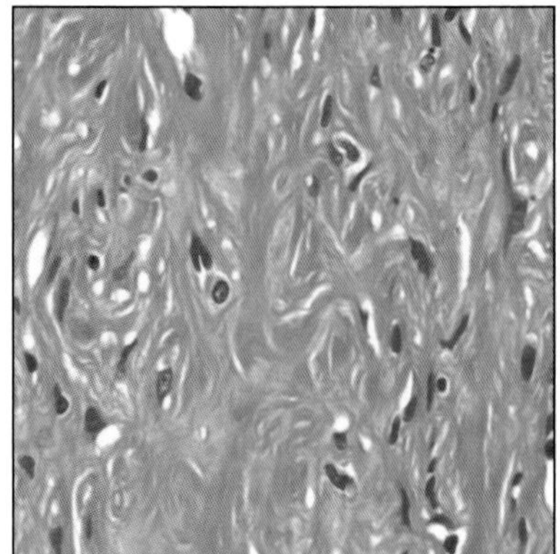

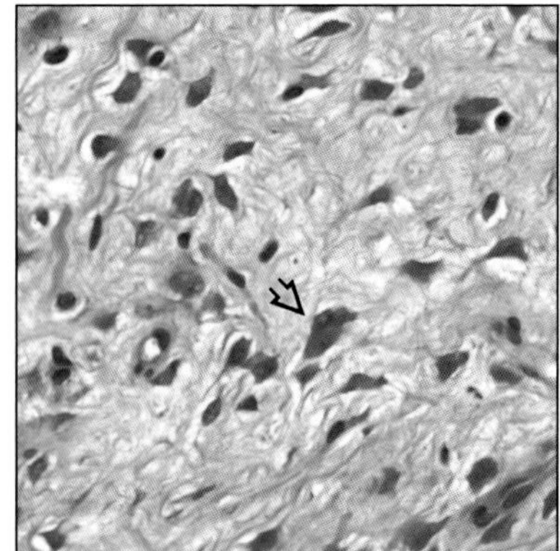

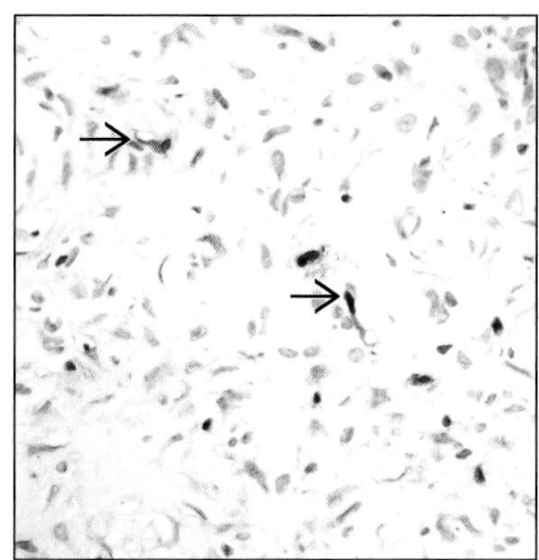

(Left) High-power magnification shows bland fibroblast cells in a dense fibrous stroma. *(Center)* An example with scattered large, pleomorphic stellate fibroblasts ⇨ shows features similar to pleomorphic fibroma (so-called "pleomorphic sclerotic fibroma" or "giant cell collagenoma"). *(Right)* FXIIIA immunohistochemistry shows staining of scattered spindle cells →.

CALCIFYING APONEUROTIC FIBROMA

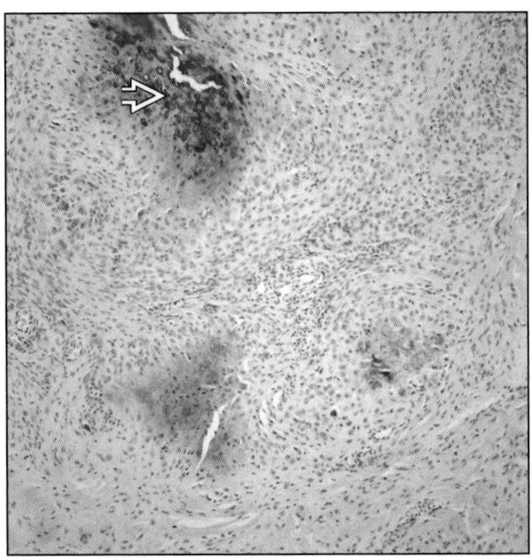

Hematoxylin & eosin shows a classic pediatric calcifying aponeurotic fibroma. There are rounded to spindled cells around islands of poorly delineated matrix, which is focally calcified ⮚.

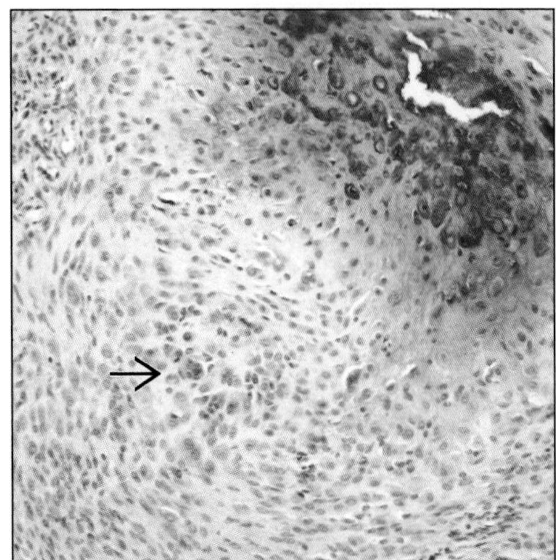

Hematoxylin & eosin shows a higher magnification view. A few giant cells can been seen ⇒.

TERMINOLOGY

Synonyms

- Keasbey tumor
- Juvenile aponeurotic fibroma
- Calcifying fibroma

Definitions

- Lesion consisting of spindled fibroblasts, epithelioid mesenchymal cells, and chondroid foci ± mineralization
  - Typically arises in hands and feet of children

CLINICAL ISSUES

Epidemiology

- Incidence
  - Rare: < 150 examples available in Armed Forces Institute of Pathology repository
- Age
  - Median age: 11-12 years
    - Most arise in 1st decade of life
  - Adult examples known
- Gender
  - Male predominance

Presentation

- Painless infiltrative mass, typically involving hands or feet
  - Usually involves palms and fingers, dorsal hand rare
  - Other anatomic sites: Back, knee, thigh, forearm
  - Usually 2-3 cm

Treatment

- Conservative excision if typical histology (rather than morbid operations)
  - Re-excision of recurrences

Prognosis

- Prone to local recurrences
  - About 40% reported to recur
    - Highly infiltrative
- Rare case reports of metastases
  - Review of illustrations from 1 case suggests lesion was not calcifying aponeurotic fibroma

MACROSCOPIC FEATURES

General Features

- Ill-defined, firm or rubbery, can have gritty areas
- 2-3 cm

MICROSCOPIC PATHOLOGY

Histologic Features

- Fibrous growth with multiple extensions into surrounding tissue
- Centrally located zones of cartilage formation and stippled calcification
  - Associated osteoclast-like giant cells may be present
  - Calcifications range from fine granules to large masses
  - Chondrocyte-like cells can be arranged in linear columns radiating from pockets of calcification
  - True ossification uncommon
- Mitoses scarce
- Calcification increases with age
  - Lesions from infants and small children may lack calcification
- Aneuploidy reported but no characteristic translocation/fusion product

DIFFERENTIAL DIAGNOSIS

Infantile Fibromatosis

- Usually involves proximal extremities of head and neck
- Elongated fibroblasts with myxoid background

CALCIFYING APONEUROTIC FIBROMA

Key Facts

Terminology
- Lesion consisting of spindled fibroblasts, epithelioid mesenchymal cells, and chondroid foci ± mineralization
  - Typically arises in hands and feet of children

Clinical Issues
- Male predominance
- Median age: 11-12 years
  - Most arise in 1st decade of life
- Prone to local recurrences

Microscopic Pathology
- Fibrous growth with multiple extensions into surrounding tissue
- Centrally located zones of cartilage formation and stippled calcification
- Mitoses scarce

- Seldom calcified or ossified

Synovial Sarcoma
- Usually deep soft tissue of more proximal extremity
- Cellular
- Display focal keratin labeling
- Characteristic t(X;18) with associated rearrangements of *SYT* gene
- Can be calcified, but calcified areas usually lack chondroid rim

Palmar and Plantar Fibromatosis
- Multinodular
- Sweeping cellular fascicles of fibroblasts
  - Plantar fibromatosis often has brisk mitotic activity
- Cartilage and calcification rare
- Giant cells can be seen (especially in plantar fibromatosis)

Chondroma
- Usually affects older adults
- Usually involves hands
- Lack spindle cell fibromatosis-like component

SELECTED REFERENCES

1. Kacerovska D et al: Cutaneous and superficial soft tissue lesions associated with Albright hereditary osteodystrophy: clinicopathological and molecular genetic study of 4 cases, including a novel mutation of the GNAS gene. Am J Dermatopathol. 30(5):417-24, 2008
2. Fetsch JF et al: Calcifying aponeurotic fibroma: a clinicopathologic study of 22 cases arising in uncommon sites. Hum Pathol. 29(12):1504-10, 1998
3. Alho A et al: Aneuploidy in benign tumors and nonneoplastic lesions of musculoskeletal tissues. Cancer. 73(4):1200-5, 1994
4. Benichou M et al: [Juvenile aponeurotic fibroma (Keasbey tumor) with metastatic course. Apropos of a case] Ann Pediatr (Paris). 37(3):181-4, 1990
5. Marty-Double C et al: Juvenile fibromatosis resembling aponeurotic fibroma and congenital multiple fibromatosis. One case with pleuropulmonary involvement. Cancer. 61(1):146-52, 1988
6. Lafferty KA et al: Juvenile aponeurotic fibroma with disseminated fibrosarcoma. J Hand Surg [Am]. 11(5):737-40, 1986
7. Allen PW et al: Juvenile aponeurotic fibroma. Cancer. 26(4):857-67, 1970
8. Lichtenstein L et al: The Cartilage Analogue of Fibromatosis. A Reinterpretation of the Condition called "juvenile Aponeurotic Fibroma". Cancer. 17:810-6, 1964
9. Keasbey LE: Juvenile aponeurotic fibroma (calcifying fibroma); a distinctive tumor arising in the palms and soles of young children. Cancer. 6(2):338-46, 1953

IMAGE GALLERY

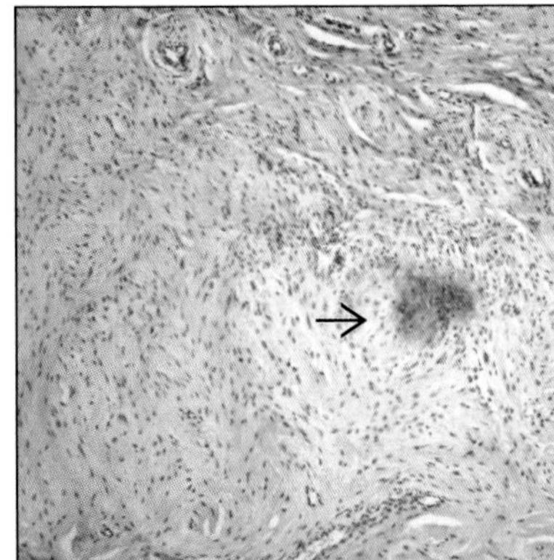

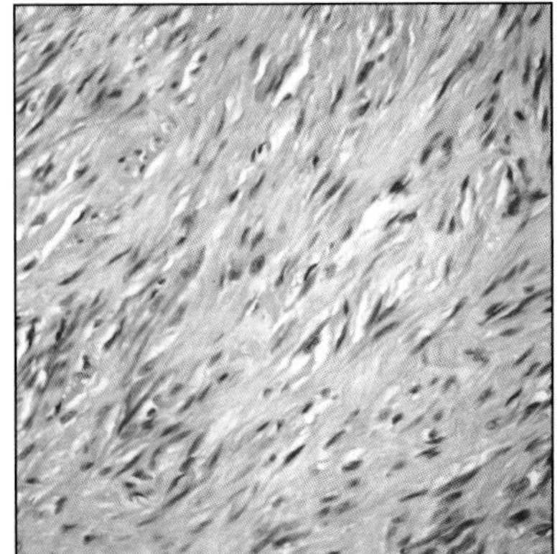

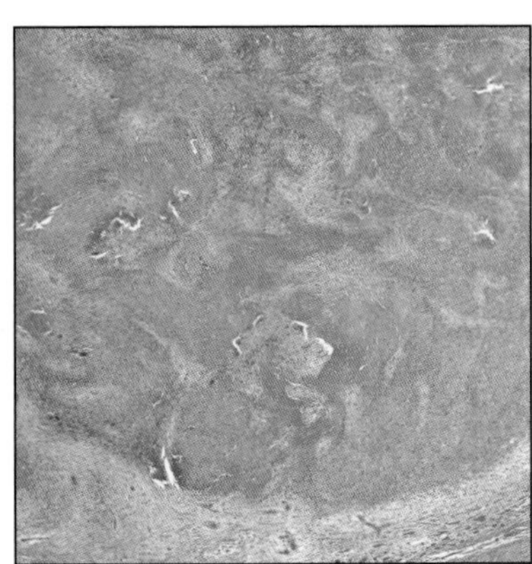

(Left) *Hematoxylin & eosin shows a more subtly calcifying aponeurotic fibroma. Although it demonstrates a classic calcifying focus →, the remainder of the lesion shows features reminiscent of a fibromatosis.* ***(Center)*** *Hematoxylin & eosin shows a predominantly fascicular portion of a calcifying aponeurotic fibroma.* ***(Right)*** *Hematoxylin & eosin shows an adult lesion. It has an overall lobulated appearance. This lesion featured zones of ossification (not shown).*

CALCIFYING FIBROUS TUMOR

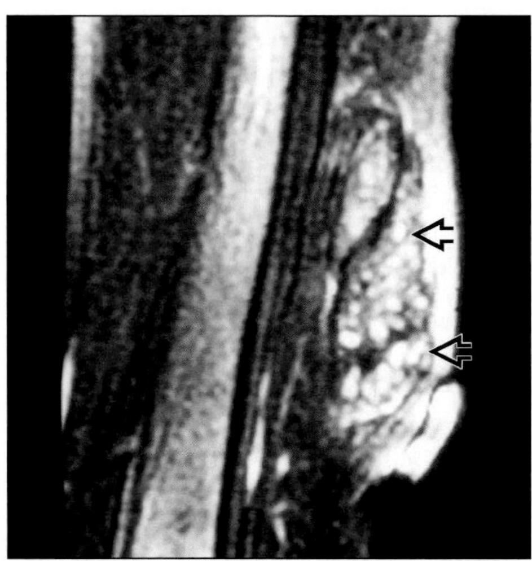

MR shows a soft tissue mass ➢ in the arm of a child. The lesion has its epicenter in the skeletal muscle and subcutaneous soft tissue.

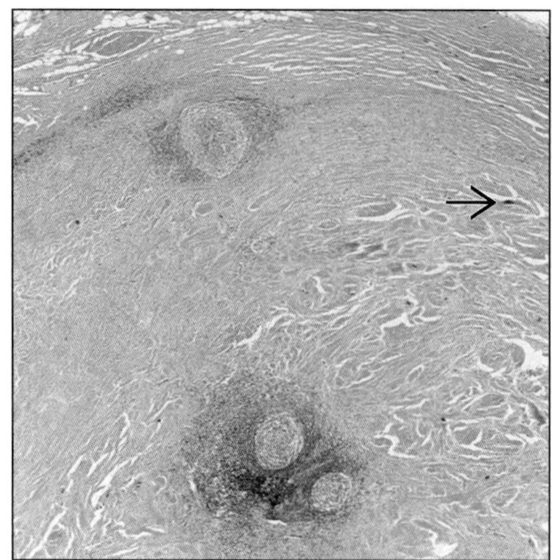

Hematoxylin & eosin shows low magnification of a calcifying fibrous tumor. At this magnification, there are lymphoid aggregates, a hypocellular spindle cell population, and calcifications ➔.

TERMINOLOGY

Abbreviations

- Calcifying fibrous tumor (CFT)

Synonyms

- Calcifying fibrous pseudotumor, childhood fibrous tumor with psammoma bodies

Definitions

- Rare benign hypocellular fibrous lesion composed of fibroblasts, dense collagen deposition, psammomatous and dystrophic calcifications, and lymphoplasmacytic inflammation with lymphoid aggregates
  - May reflect endstage of another lesion, though appears unrelated to inflammatory myofibroblastic tumor based on immunophenotyping

CLINICAL ISSUES

Presentation

- Soft tissue examples
  - Painless soft tissue mass in children and young adults
    - Median age at resection: 18.5 years
    - Lesions often present for many years prior to excision
    - Most in extremities and trunk
    - Usually deep, median size: 5 cm
    - No gender predilection
- Visceral examples
  - Described in pleura, peritoneum, mediastinum, paratesticular, adrenal, heart, lung
    - Most reported in adults with rare pediatric examples
    - Multiplicity not uncommon; reported in both pleura and peritoneum
    - No gender predilection
    - Familial peritoneal example reported (sisters, multifocal lesions)
- Rare cases associated with Castleman disease, inflammatory myofibroblastic tumor, and sclerosing angiomatoid nodular transformation of spleen

Treatment

- Excision

Prognosis

- Excellent

MACROSCOPIC FEATURES

General Features

- Well-marginated, unencapsulated, firm, white masses; sometimes gritty on sectioning

MICROSCOPIC PATHOLOGY

Histologic Features

- Well-marginated, unencapsulated borders
- Hypocellular hyalinized sclerotic tissue with fibroblastic bland nuclei
- Variable inflammatory infiltrate consisting of lymphocytes, plasma cells, and lymphoid aggregates
- Scattered psammomatous and dystrophic calcifications

DIFFERENTIAL DIAGNOSIS

Inflammatory Myofibroblastic Tumor

- Cellular lesions with more abundant inflammation, larger, more atypical myofibroblasts, and ALK expression in subset of cases

Gastrointestinal Stromal Tumor

- Cellular lesions with minimal inflammation, CD117 expression in immunohistochemistry
  - CFT is CD117(-)

CALCIFYING FIBROUS TUMOR

Key Facts

Terminology

- Benign hypocellular fibrous lesion composed of fibroblasts, dense collagen deposition, psammomatous and dystrophic calcifications
  - Lymphoplasmacytic inflammation with lymphoid aggregates
- Possibly endstage of another lesion; appears unrelated to inflammatory myofibroblastic tumor

Clinical Issues

- Painless soft tissue mass in children and young adults
- Visceral examples: Pleura, peritoneum, mediastinum, paratesticular, adrenal, heart, lung
- Multiplicity not uncommon: Pleura and peritoneum
- Rare cases associated with Castleman disease, inflammatory myofibroblastic tumor, and sclerosing angiomatoid nodular transformation of spleen

Immunohistochemistry

Antibody	Reactivity	Staining Pattern	Comment
CD34	Positive	Cytoplasmic	About 2/3 of cases
α1-antichymotrypsin	Positive	Cytoplasmic	Focal (rare cells)
Desmin	Positive	Cytoplasmic	Focal (rare cells)
ALK1	Negative		
S100	Negative		

Fibromatosis

- Cellular lesions without inflammation or calcifications
- Typically CD34(-), display nuclear β-catenin labeling
  - CFT is β-catenin(-)

Fibroma of Tendon Sheath

- Variable cellularity; lacks inflammation and calcifications

Synovial Sarcoma

- Can be calcified
- Cellular sarcomas
- Focal keratin expression, Bcl-2 expression, negative CD34

SELECTED REFERENCES

1. Lee JC et al: Coexisting sclerosing angiomatoid nodular transformation of the spleen with multiple calcifying fibrous pseudotumors in a patient. J Formos Med Assoc. 106(3):234-9, 2007
2. Chen KT: Familial peritoneal multifocal calcifying fibrous tumor. Am J Clin Pathol. 119(6):811-5, 2003
3. Sigel JE et al: Immunohistochemical analysis of anaplastic lymphoma kinase expression in deep soft tissue calcifying fibrous pseudotumor: evidence of a late sclerosing stage of inflammatory myofibroblastic tumor? Ann Diagn Pathol. 5(1):10-4, 2001
4. Pinkard NB et al: Calcifying fibrous pseudotumor of pleura. A report of three cases of a newly described entity involving the pleura. Am J Clin Pathol. 105(2):189-94, 1996
5. Fetsch JF et al: Calcifying fibrous pseudotumor. Am J Surg Pathol. 17(5):502-8, 1993
6. Rosenthal NS et al: Childhood fibrous tumor with psammoma bodies. Clinicopathologic features in two cases. Arch Pathol Lab Med. 112(8):798-800, 1988

IMAGE GALLERY

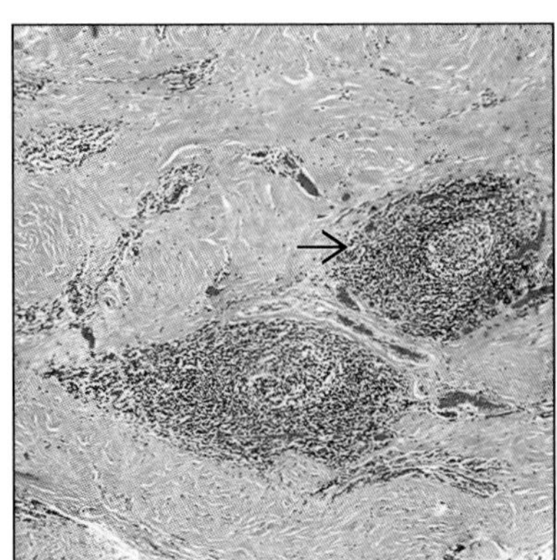

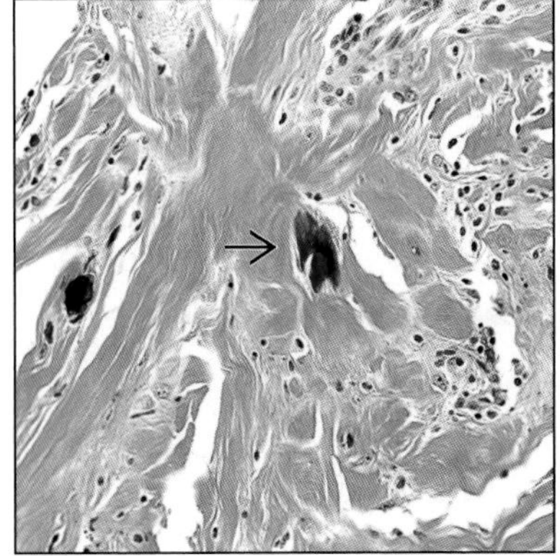

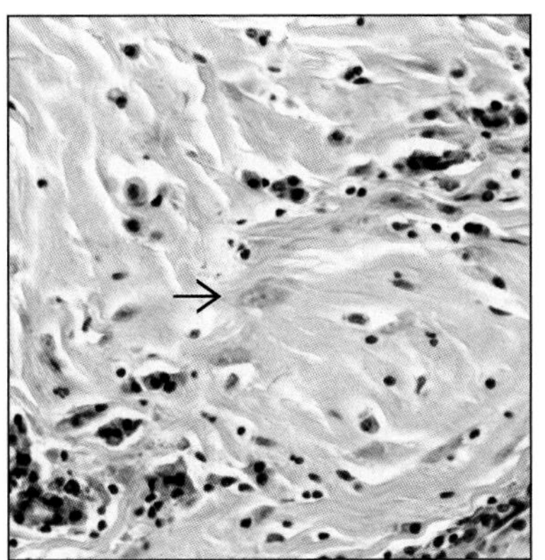

__(Left)__ Hematoxylin & eosin shows higher magnification of a CFT. Note the low cellularity, lymphoid aggregates ⇒, and background lymphocytes and plasma cells. __(Center)__ Hematoxylin & eosin shows calcifications ⇒, scattered chronic inflammatory cells, and fibroblastic nuclei. Calcifications in these lesions can be either dystrophic or psammomatous. __(Right)__ Hematoxylin & eosin shows the bland appearance of the proliferating fibroblasts ⇒ in a calcifying fibrous tumor. Scattered plasma cells, mast cells, and lymphocytes are present in the background.

REACTIVE NODULAR FIBROUS PSEUDOTUMOR OF MESENTERY

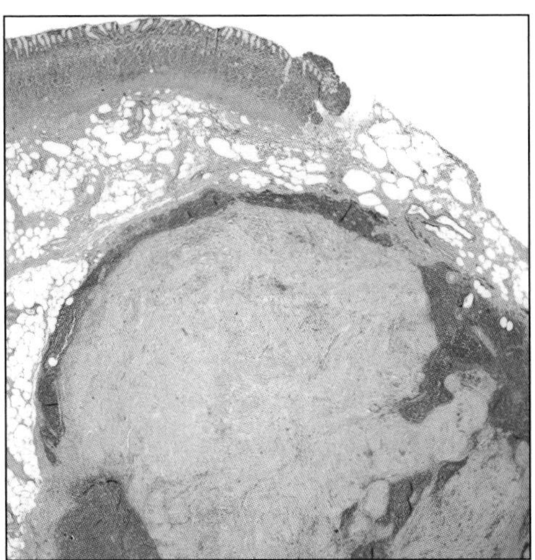

Hematoxylin & eosin shows low magnification of a reactive nodular fibrous pseudotumor involving the mesentery extending up into the deep gastric submucosa.

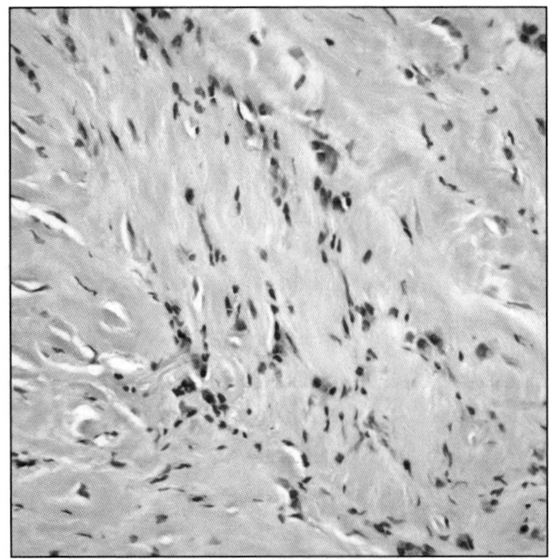

Hematoxylin & eosin shows a higher magnification of the lesion. There are a few plasma cells along with fibroblastic cells and a collagenized background.

TERMINOLOGY

Definitions

- Lesion of mesentery composed of stellate and spindle-shaped cells arranged in collagen-rich stroma with lymphoid aggregates

CLINICAL ISSUES

Epidemiology

- Incidence
  - Rare
- Age
  - Predominantly adults
- Gender
  - No predominance

Presentation

- Obstruction
- Frequent history of prior operations, evidence of prior bowel perforation, or history of pancreatitis
- Some patients have multiple nodules
  - Some lesions associated with foreign bodies
- Most in small bowel (ileal) mesentery
  - Also in colon mesentery and in bed of area of prior pancreatitis

Treatment

- Surgical excision

Prognosis

- Excellent; benign process

MACROSCOPIC FEATURES

Size

- 1.5 cm to > 10 cm

Appearance

- Firm white cut surface

MICROSCOPIC PATHOLOGY

Histologic Features

- Multilobulated appearance
  - Predominantly involving subserosa and extending into submucosa
- Frequent lymphoid aggregates
  - Sparse intralesional mononuclear cells
- Hypocellular spindle cell lesion
  - Bland cytologic features
  - Cells arranged in loose aggregates
  - Stellate and spindle cells
- Abundant collagen
- Most lack calcifications

Predominant Pattern/Injury Type

- Fibrous

Predominant Cell/Compartment Type

- Fibroblast
  - May be multipotential submesothelial/subserosal cells rather than ordinary fibroblasts

ANCILLARY TESTS

PCR

- No *KIT* mutations identified

Electron Microscopy

- Shows myofibroblastic differentiation
  - Prominent rough endoplasmic reticulum, sparse pinocytotic vesicles, subplasmalemmal bundles of microfilaments attached to dense bodies

REACTIVE NODULAR FIBROUS PSEUDOTUMOR OF MESENTERY

Key Facts

Terminology

- Lesion of mesentery composed of stellate and spindle-shaped cells arranged in collagen-rich stroma with lymphoid aggregates

Clinical Issues

- Frequent history of prior operations, evidence of prior bowel perforation, or history of pancreatitis
- Some patients have multiple nodules
- Excellent prognosis; benign process

Microscopic Pathology

- Multilobulated appearance
- Predominantly involving subserosa and extending into submucosa
- Frequent lymphoid aggregates
- Sparse intralesional mononuclear cells
- Hypocellular spindle cell lesion
- Bland cytologic features

Immunohistochemistry

Antibody	Reactivity	Staining Pattern	Comment
AE13	Positive	Cytoplasmic	Usually focal and attributed to submesothelial cell type
CD117	Positive	Cell membrane & cytoplasm	Not associated with *KIT* mutations
Actin-sm	Positive	Cytoplasmic	
CK8/18/CAM5.2	Negative		
S100	Negative		Helpful in excluding GI tract schwannomas, which tend to have lymphoid cuffs
CD34	Negative		
CD68	Negative		
EMA	Negative		
Desmin	Negative		
ALK1	Negative		Unrelated to inflammatory myofibroblastic tumor

DIFFERENTIAL DIAGNOSIS

Calcifying Fibrous Pseudotumor

- In mesentery of adults
- Hypocellular spindle cell lesion
- Prominent psammomatous and dystrophic calcifications
- Lack keratin staining

Gastrointestinal Tract Schwannoma

- Usually centered in muscularis propria of stomach
- Prominent lymphoid cuff around tumor
- Moderate to high cellularity
- Strong S100 expression on immunohistochemistry

SELECTED REFERENCES

1. Saglam EA et al: Reactive nodular fibrous pseudotumor involving the pelvic and abdominal cavity: a case report and review of literature. Virchows Arch. 447(5):879-82, 2005
2. Daum O et al: Reactive nodular fibrous pseudotumors of the gastrointestinal tract: report of 8 cases. Int J Surg Pathol. 12(4):365-74, 2004
3. Yantiss RK et al: Reactive nodular fibrous pseudotumor of the gastrointestinal tract and mesentery: a clinicopathologic study of five cases. Am J Surg Pathol. 27(4):532-40, 2003

IMAGE GALLERY

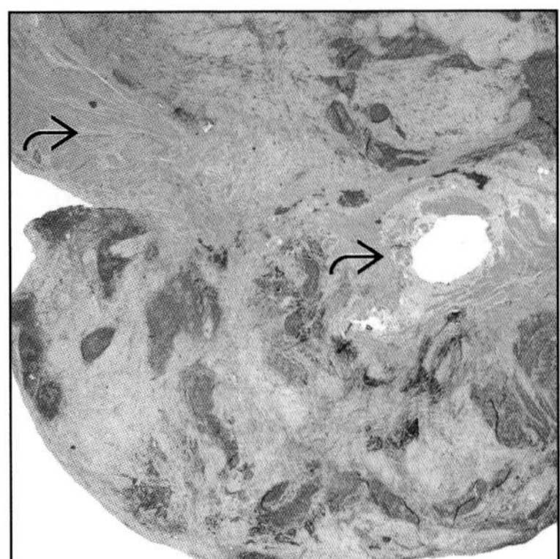

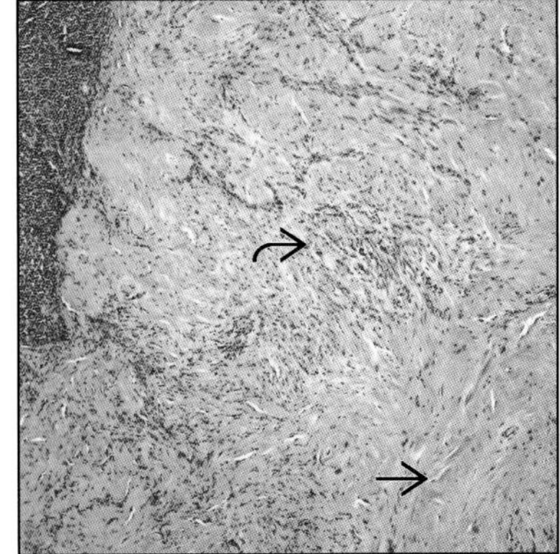

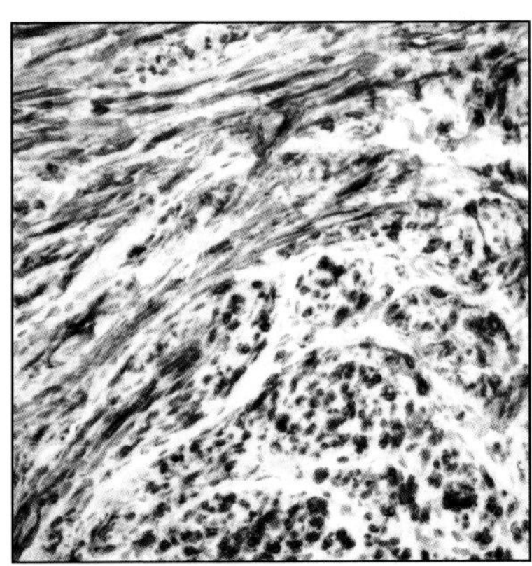

(Left) *Hematoxylin & eosin shows the mesenteric side of a reactive nodular fibrous pseudotumor of the mesentery. The muscularis propria is indicated ⮫. The tumor is lobulated with many lymphoid aggregates but is hypocellular.* ***(Center)*** *Hematoxylin & eosin of a reactive nodular fibrous pseudotumor of mesentery shows essentially acellular zones ⇒ adjacent to hypocellular areas ⮫.* ***(Right)*** *CD117 shows strong immunolabeling of this reactive nodular fibrous pseudotumor of the mesentery (this staining was very focal); this tumor type lacks KIT mutations.*

SCLEROSING FIBROINFLAMMATORY LESIONS

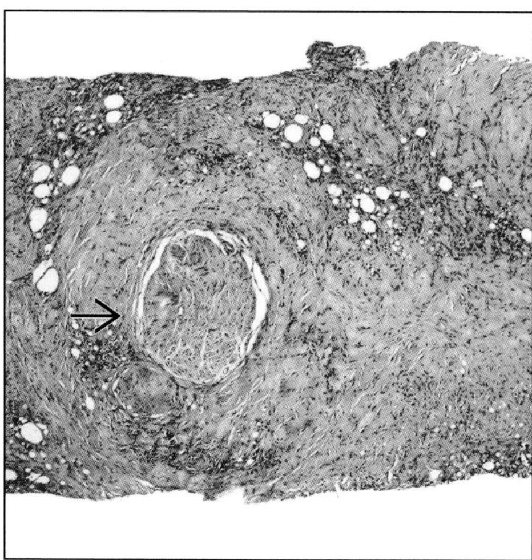

Hematoxylin & eosin shows a needle biopsy specimen from an example of retroperitoneal fibrosis that encased the ureters. The process has surrounded a nerve ➔ *and infiltrates adipose tissue.*

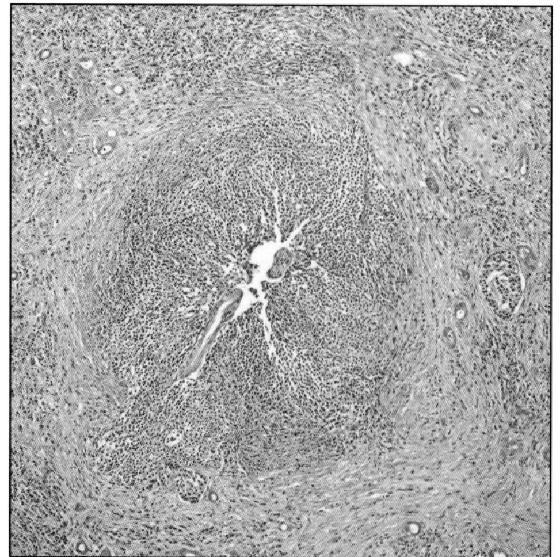

Lymphoplasmacytic sclerosing (autoimmune) pancreatitis is the prototype of the IgG4-related sclerosing disorders. In this field, there is dense lymphoplasmacytic inflammation around a duct.

TERMINOLOGY

Synonyms

- IgG4-related chronic sclerosing disorders

Definitions

- Poorly understood lesions unified by sclerosis, inflammation, variable tumor formation and variable association with elevated serum IgG4/intralesional IgG4-producing plasma cells
  - Lymphoplasmacytic sclerosing pancreatitis (autoimmune pancreatitis)
  - Sclerosing lymphoplasmacytic tubulointerstitial nephritis
  - Reidel struma (thyroiditis)
  - Orbital pseudotumor (chronic sclerosing dacryoadenitis)
  - Chronic sclerosing sialadenitis (Küttner tumor)
  - Retroperitoneal fibrosis (Ormond disease, sometimes called retractile mesenteritis)
    - Associated with various medications, including methysergide, β-blockers, chemotherapeutic agents
  - Aortic inflammatory lesions
  - Some patients manifest several of these lesions simultaneously
- Other lesions less associated with increased IgG4
  - Sclerosing mesenteritis
    - Overlaps with retroperitoneal fibrosis and is thus also sometimes called retractile mesenteritis
  - Plasma cell granuloma (inflammatory myofibroblastic tumor of lung)
    - Subset of such lung lesions is associated with increased serum IgG4 and similar lesions in other sites

ETIOLOGY/PATHOGENESIS

Unknown

- Association with elevated IgG4 in some cases raises possibility of autoimmune or infectious disorder
  - Specific trigger unknown
- No characteristic genetic alteration established

CLINICAL ISSUES

Presentation

- Most present as hard masses in various sites
- Patients with retroperitoneal fibrosis can present with urinary obstructive symptoms
- Most pancreatic examples initially believed to be pancreatic cancer clinically

Treatment

- Surgery for sclerosing mesenteritis
- Steroids for lesions associated with elevated serum IgG4
- For retroperitoneal fibrosis, surgery to reduce ureteral obstruction
  - Added medical therapy includes steroids, methotrexate, cyclophosphamide, and mycophenolate mofetil

Prognosis

- Good overall; most patients respond to treatment
- Occasional examples show progression to lymphomas

MACROSCOPIC FEATURES

General Features

- Hard white tissue with gritty cut surface

SCLEROSING FIBROINFLAMMATORY LESIONS

Key Facts

Terminology

- Group of poorly understood lesions unified by sclerosis and inflammation, with variable tumor formation and variable association with elevated serum IgG4 and intralesional IgG4-producing plasma cells
- IgG4-related chronic sclerosing disorders
  - Lymphoplasmacytic sclerosing pancreatitis (autoimmune pancreatitis)
  - Sclerosing lymphoplasmacytic tubulointerstitial nephritis
  - Reidel struma (thyroiditis)
  - Orbital pseudotumor (chronic sclerosing dacryoadenitis)
  - Chronic sclerosing sialadenitis (Küttner tumor)
  - Retroperitoneal fibrosis (Ormond disease, sometimes called retractile mesenteritis)
- Some patients manifest several of above lesions simultaneously
- Other lesions less associated with increased IgG4
  - Sclerosing mesenteritis
  - Plasma cell granuloma (inflammatory myofibroblastic tumor of lung)

Clinical Issues

- Steroids administered for lesions associated with elevated serum IgG4

Microscopic Pathology

- All lesions feature fibrosis and lymphoplasmacytic inflammation with scattered eosinophils
- IgG4-labeled plasma cells on immunohistochemistry

MICROSCOPIC PATHOLOGY

General Features

- All lesions feature fibrosis and lymphoplasmacytic inflammation with scattered eosinophils; some have additional features
- Lymphoplasmacytic sclerosing pancreatitis (autoimmune pancreatitis)
  - Duct lesions (lymphoplasmacytic inflammation destroying ducts)
  - Obliterative phlebitis
- Sclerosing mesenteritis (a.k.a. retractile mesenteritis)
  - Prominent fat necrosis
  - Calcifications in some cases

DIFFERENTIAL DIAGNOSIS

Inflammatory Myofibroblastic Tumor

- Cellular myofibroblastic proliferation with abundant myofibroblastic spindle cells
- Minimal sclerosis
- Background lymphoplasmacytic inflammation
- Immunohistochemistry: Most cases have few IgG4(+) plasma cells, ALK(+) (~ 60%), keratin(+), actin(+), variable desmin
- *ALK* gene rearrangements in subset of cases

Fibromatosis

- Sweeping fascicles of myofibroblastic cells
- Negligible inflammatory infiltrate
- Immunohistochemistry: Actin(+), variable desmin, β-catenin(+)
- *APC* and β-catenin gene mutations

Lymphoma

- Clonal lymphoid population typically lacking sclerosis
- Most lymphomas lack plasma cell population
- Various well-established translocations, fusion genes

Gastrointestinal Stromal Tumor

- Spindle cell lesion with minimal inflammation
- Immunohistochemistry: CD117(+), CD34(+), variable actin and desmin
- *KIT* mutations

Extranodal Rosai-Dorfman Disease

- Most cases lack sclerosis
- Emperipolesis by lesional histiocytes
- Immunohistochemistry: S100(+), CD1a(-)

SELECTED REFERENCES

1. Inoue D et al: Immunoglobulin G4-related lung disease: CT findings with pathologic correlations. Radiology. 251(1):260-70, 2009
2. Vega J et al: Treatment of idiopathic retroperitoneal fibrosis with colchicine and steroids: a case series. Am J Kidney Dis. 53(4):628-37, 2009
3. Chen TS et al: Are tumefactive lesions classified as sclerosing mesenteritis a subset of IgG4-related sclerosing disorders? J Clin Pathol. 61(10):1093-7, 2008
4. Akram S et al: Sclerosing mesenteritis: clinical features, treatment, and outcome in ninety-two patients. Clin Gastroenterol Hepatol. 5(5):589-96; quiz 523-4, 2007
5. Björnsson E et al: Immunoglobulin G4 associated cholangitis: description of an emerging clinical entity based on review of the literature. Hepatology. 45(6):1547-54, 2007
6. Zhang L et al: IgG4-positive plasma cell infiltration in the diagnosis of autoimmune pancreatitis. Mod Pathol. 20(1):23-8, 2007
7. Kitagawa S et al: Abundant IgG4-positive plasma cell infiltration characterizes chronic sclerosing sialadenitis (Küttner's tumor). Am J Surg Pathol. 29(6):783-91, 2005
8. Zen Y et al: IgG4-positive plasma cells in inflammatory pseudotumor (plasma cell granuloma) of the lung. Hum Pathol. 36(7):710-7, 2005
9. Abraham SC et al: Pancreaticoduodenectomy (Whipple resections) in patients without malignancy: are they all 'chronic pancreatitis'? Am J Surg Pathol. 27(1):110-20, 2003
10. Montgomery E et al: Beta-catenin immunohistochemistry separates mesenteric fibromatosis from gastrointestinal stromal tumor and sclerosing mesenteritis. Am J Surg Pathol. 26(10):1296-301, 2002
11. Emory TS et al: Sclerosing mesenteritis, mesenteric panniculitis and mesenteric lipodystrophy: a single entity? Am J Surg Pathol. 21(4):392-8, 1997

Microscopic and CT Features

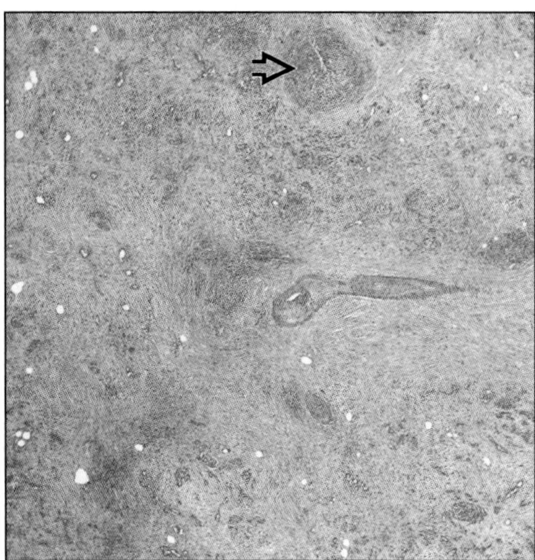

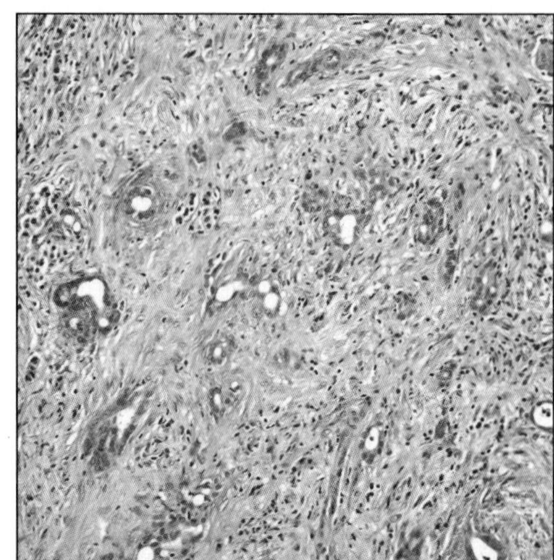

(Left) *Hematoxylin & eosin shows low magnification of lymphoplasmacytic sclerosing (autoimmune) pancreatitis, which usually diffusely enlarges the pancreas. Note the many lymphoid aggregates apparent within an inflamed duct ⮚.* ***(Right)*** *Hematoxylin & eosin shows pancreatic parenchyma in lymphoplasmacytic sclerosing (autoimmune) pancreatitis. The acini are replaced by lymphoplasmacytic cells and sclerosis.*

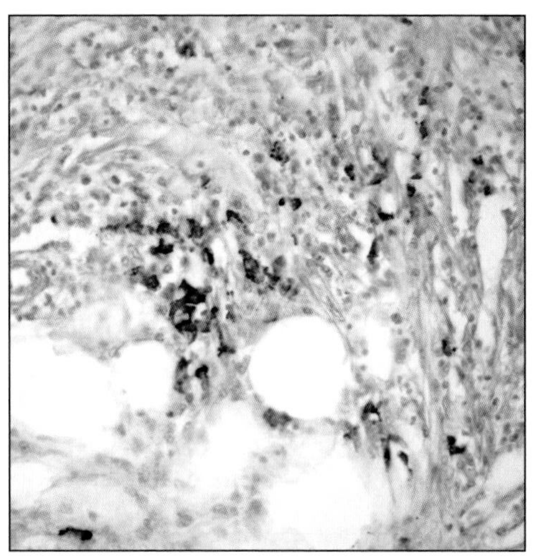

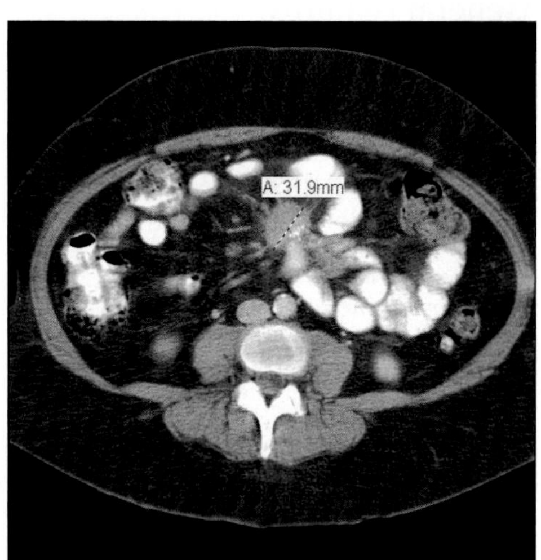

(Left) *IgG4 shows many labeled plasma cells in an example of autoimmune pancreatitis. IgG4 is the least common subclass of IgG. Patients with sclerosing inflammatory disorders, of which lymphoplasmacytic sclerosing pancreatitis is the prototype, often have elevated serum IgG4.* ***(Right)*** *CT shows a fibrotic lesion being measured in the mesentery. Such lesions have been variably termed sclerosing mesenteritis and retractile mesenteritis and are in a spectrum with retroperitoneal fibrosis.*

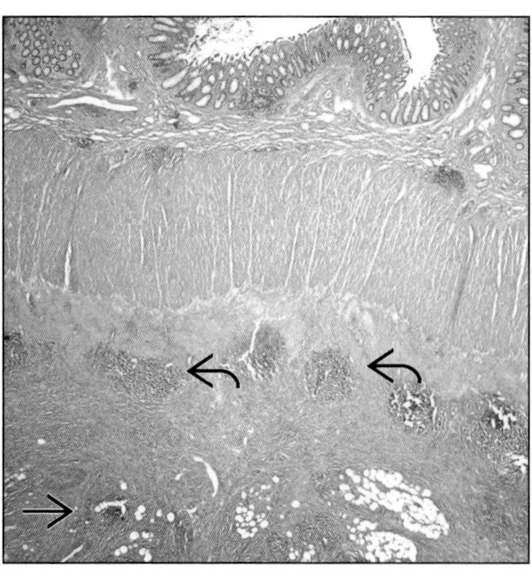

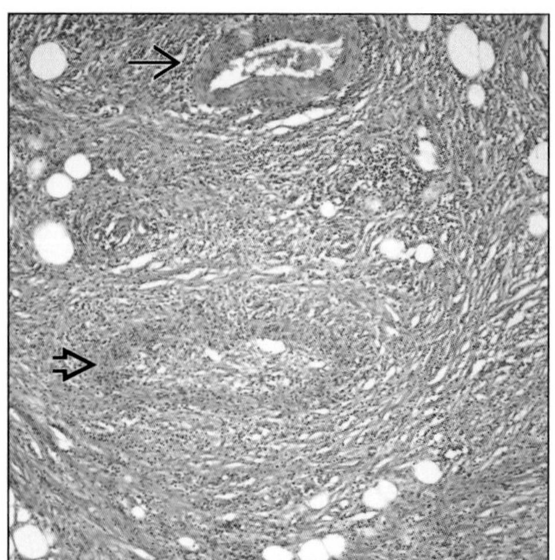

(Left) *Hematoxylin & eosin shows an example of sclerosing mesenteritis. The epicenter of the process is in the colon mesentery ⮕. Note the prominent lymphoid aggregates ⮌. This patient presented with colonic obstruction, and a mass was found on imaging.* ***(Right)*** *Hematoxylin & eosin shows a focus with a lymphocytic phlebitis pattern in an example of sclerosing mesenteritis, which produced a mass. Note the pristine artery ⮕ and compare it to the damaged inflamed vein ⮚.*

Microscopic Features

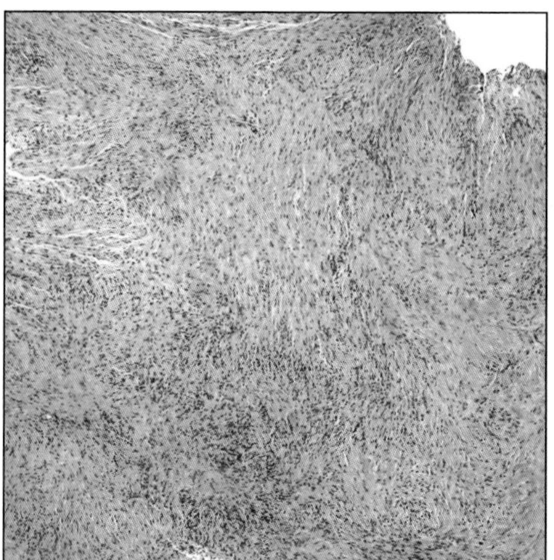

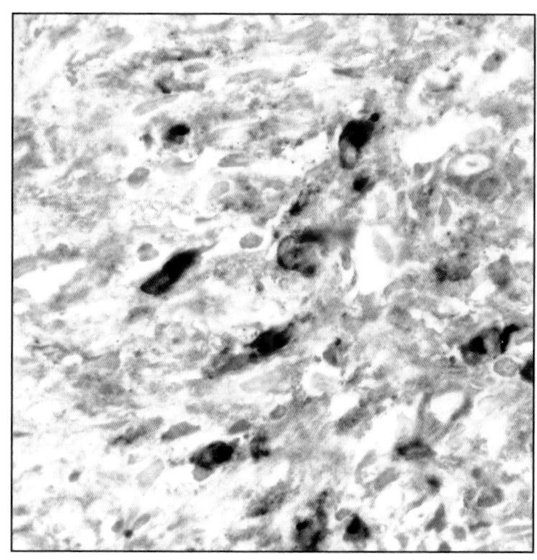

(Left) H&E shows low magnification of an example of orbital pseudotumor (chronic sclerosing dacryoadenitis), which appears similar to other sclerosing fibroinflammatory lesions. This lesion presented as a hard orbital mass in a patient with similar lesions in his lung and abdomen, and elevated serum IgG4. **(Right)** IgG4 shows labeled cells in the orbital pseudotumor (chronic sclerosing dacryoadenitis).

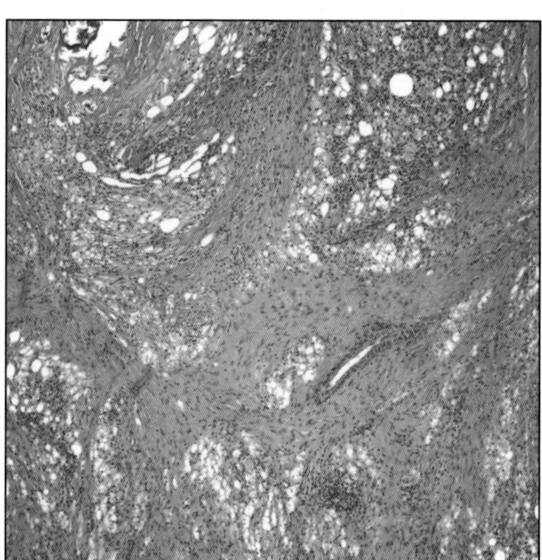

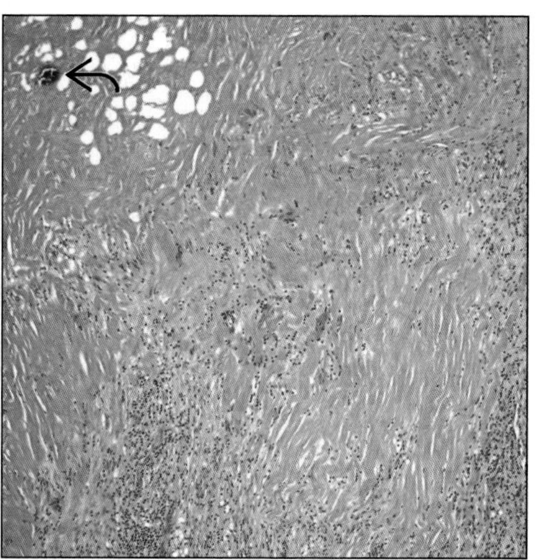

(Left) Hematoxylin & eosin shows an example of sclerosing mesenteritis with fat necrosis, sclerosis, and an inflammatory background rich in lymphocytes and plasma cells. **(Right)** Hematoxylin & eosin shows another example of sclerosing mesenteritis. There is a focus of calcification ⮳ in an area of fat necrosis. The lesion is densely sclerotic with abundant lymphoplasmacytic inflammation, imparting a heterogeneous appearance at low magnification.

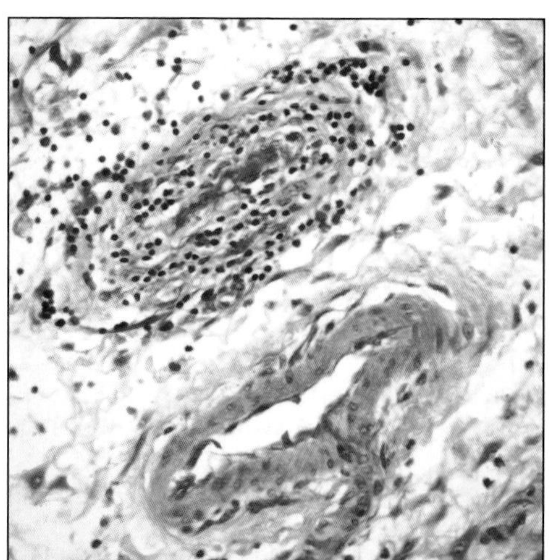

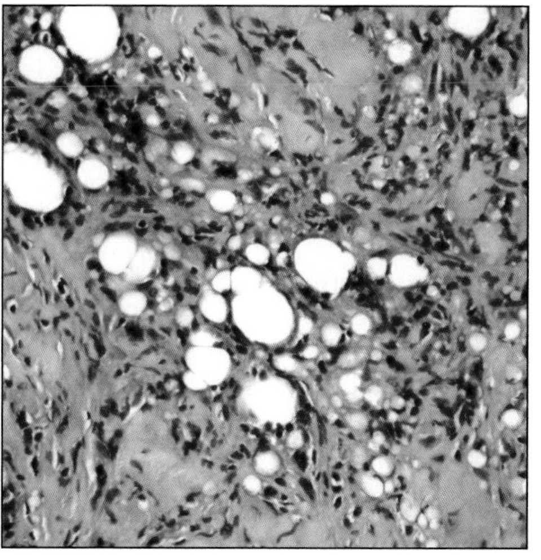

(Left) Hematoxylin & eosin shows a focus of lymphocytic phlebitis in an example of sclerosing mesenteritis. The phlebitis tends to be less destructive than that associated with autoimmune pancreatitis. **(Right)** Hematoxylin & eosin shows an example of retroperitoneal fibrosis, with sclerosis and numerous lymphoplasmacytic cells. Some of these lesions have prominent IgG4-expressing plasma cells. Note that all of the lesions in this category appear similar histologically.

INCLUSION BODY FIBROMATOSIS

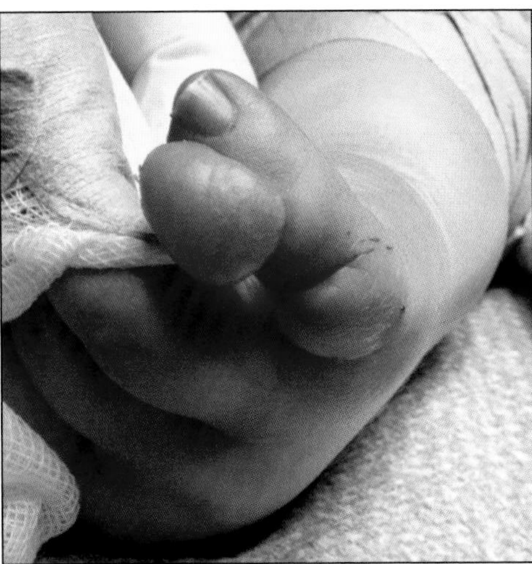

This photograph of a hand shows an exophytic, dome-shaped mass. Patients with inclusion body fibromatosis usually present with clinically evident masses.

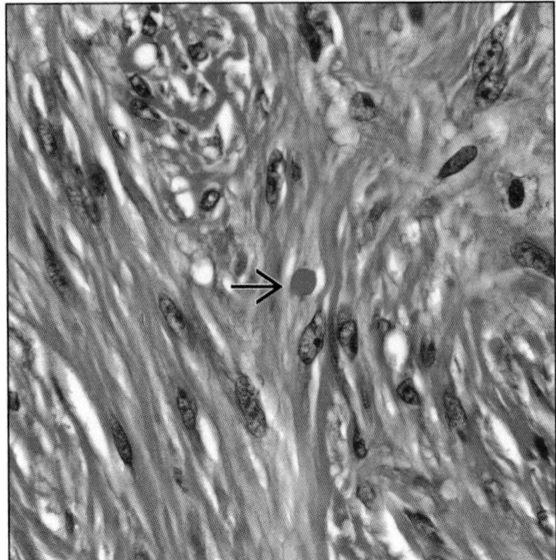

The presence of eosinophilic cytoplasmic inclusions ➔ represents the morphologic hallmark of inclusion body fibromatosis.

TERMINOLOGY

Synonyms

- Infantile digital fibromatosis
- Digital fibrous tumor of childhood
- Reye tumor

Definitions

- Benign proliferation of fibroblasts and myofibroblasts containing scattered eosinophilic spherical inclusions that occur on the digits of young children

CLINICAL ISSUES

Epidemiology

- Incidence
  - Rare fibroblastic/myofibroblastic neoplasm
- Age
  - Occurs usually in 1st year of life
  - Very rare in adult patients
- Gender
  - M = F

Site

- Dorsal aspects of hands or feet
- Rarely synchronous or asynchronous involvement of more than 1 digit
- Thumb or big toe is only very rarely affected
- Extradigital soft tissues (i.e., arm, breast) are extremely rarely affected

Presentation

- Digital enlargement
- Dome-shaped swelling overlying phalanges or interphalangeal joints
- Nontender nodules
- Rarely erosion of bone

Natural History

- May recur locally
- May regress spontaneously
- No progression
- No metastases

Treatment

- Surgical approaches
  - Local excision with preservation of function

Prognosis

- Excellent overall prognosis
- May recur locally
- May show spontaneous regression
- Main prognostic indicator represents adequacy of primary excision

MACROSCOPIC FEATURES

General Features

- Ill-defined neoplasms
- Dermal neoplasms with gray-white, indurated cut surfaces covered by intact skin
- No areas of hemorrhage
- No areas of necrosis

Size

- Nodules of variable size
  - Nodules usually measure < 2 cm

MICROSCOPIC PATHOLOGY

Histologic Features

- Infiltrating fascicles and sheets
- Uniform spindle-shaped fibroblasts and myofibroblasts
- No cytologic atypia
- Elongated spindled nuclei
- Pale eosinophilic fibrillary cytoplasm
- Intracytoplasmic eosinophilic spherical inclusions
  - Often in perinuclear location

INCLUSION BODY FIBROMATOSIS

Key Facts

Terminology
- Benign proliferation of fibroblasts and myofibroblasts containing scattered eosinophilic inclusion bodies that occur on digits of young children

Clinical Issues
- Rare fibroblastic/myofibroblastic neoplasm
- Occurs usually in 1st year of life
- Dorsal aspects of hands or feet
- Digital enlargement
- May recur locally; may show spontaneous regression
- Extradigital soft tissues (i.e., arm, breast) are extremely rarely affected
- Dome-shaped swelling overlying phalanges or interphalangeal joints
- Treatment: Local excision with preservation of function

Macroscopic Features
- Ill-defined neoplasms

Microscopic Pathology
- Infiltrating fascicles
- Uniform spindle-shaped tumor cells
- No cytologic atypia
- Intracytoplasmic eosinophilic spherical inclusions
- Inclusions are trichrome(+)
- Pale eosinophilic fibrillary cytoplasm

Ancillary Tests
- Spindled cells show features of myofibroblasts
- Expression of actins, desmin, calponin, and CD99
- Inclusions show granular &/or filamentous features
- Cytoplasmic filaments extend onto inclusions

  - Lack of refringence helps in distinction from erythrocytes
  - Stain red with Masson trichrome staining
  - PAS(-)
- Rare mitoses
- Variable amount of extracellular collagen

Predominant Pattern/Injury Type
- Fascicular
- Infiltrative

Predominant Cell/Compartment Type
- Myofibroblast

ANCILLARY TESTS

Electron Microscopy
- Spindled cells show features of myofibroblasts
- Tumor cells contain rough endoplasmic reticulum and cytoplasmic aggregates of filaments
- Scattered dense bodies
- Inclusions show granular &/or filamentous features
- Cytoplasmic filaments extend onto inclusions

DIFFERENTIAL DIAGNOSIS

Dermatofibroma
- Hyperplastic, hyperpigmented epidermis
- Stellate appearance
- Storiform growth
- Tumor cells grow around hyalinized collagen bundles
- Admixture of plump spindled and histiocytoid tumor cells
- May contain multinucleated giant cells
- May contain hemosiderin deposits
- Lack of cytoplasmic inclusions

Pilar Leiomyoma
- Nodules and bundles of spindled cells
- Bright eosinophilic fibrillary cytoplasm
- Spindle-shaped, blunt-ended nuclei
- Lack of cytoplasmic inclusions
- HCAD(+)

Neurofibroma
- Elongated spindled tumor cells
- Elongated, wrinkled nuclei
- Lack of cytoplasmic inclusions
- S100(+)
- Muscle markers negative

Extraneural Spindle Cell Perineurioma
- Elongated spindled tumor cells
- May show perivascular accentuation
- Lack of cytoplasmic inclusions
- EMA(+)
- Muscle markers negative

Dermatomyofibroma
- Does not occur in 1st years of life
- Does not occur on fingers and toes
- Plaque-like dermal neoplasms
- Bundles of spindle cells oriented parallel to epidermis
- Tumor cells grow around preexisting adnexal structures
- Lack of cytoplasmic inclusions
- Increased number of fragmented elastic fibers

Superficial Acral Fibromyxoma
- Varying myxoid and collagenous stroma
- Lack of cytoplasmic inclusions
- No/focal expression of actins
- Frequent expression of EMA

Desmoid Fibromatosis
- Occurs usually in deep soft tissues
- Locally aggressive
- High rate of local recurrences
- Nuclear expression of β-catenin
- Numerous vessels
- Perivascular edema

Superficial Solitary Fibrous Tumor
- Usually well-circumscribed, nodular neoplasms
- Varying cellularity
- Numerous hemangiopericytoma-like blood vessels

INCLUSION BODY FIBROMATOSIS

Immunohistochemistry

Antibody	Reactivity	Staining Pattern	Comment
Actin-sm	Positive	Cytoplasmic inclusion	Parallel positivity beneath cell membrane; eosinophilic globules are variably positive
Desmin	Positive	Cytoplasmic	
Calponin	Positive	Cytoplasmic	
CD99	Positive	Cytoplasmic	
Caldesmon	Negative		
S100	Negative		
EMA	Negative		
AE1/AE3	Negative		
β-catenin	Negative		
CD34	Negative		

- No/focal expression of actins
- Usually homogeneous CD34 expression

Myofibroma

- Multinodular growth
- Biphasic growth
  - Small undifferentiated mesenchymal cells associated with hemangiopericytoma-like vessels
  - Mature, spindled, eosinophilic myofibroblasts
- Myxohyaline stroma
- Lack of cytoplasmic inclusions

DIAGNOSTIC CHECKLIST

Clinically Relevant Pathologic Features

- Gross appearance
- Organ distribution
- Age distribution
- Invasive pattern
- Cytoplasmic features

Pathologic Interpretation Pearls

- Ill-defined dermal neoplasms
- Proliferation of fibroblastic/myofibroblastic tumor cells
- Bland cytology of neoplastic cells
- Tumor cells contain characteristic cytoplasmic inclusions
- Expression of actins
- Coexpression of desmin may be present

SELECTED REFERENCES

1. Laskin WB et al: Infantile digital fibroma/fibromatosis: a clinicopathologic and immunohistochemical study of 69 tumors from 57 patients with long-term follow-up. Am J Surg Pathol. 33(1):1-13, 2009
2. Grenier N et al: A range of histologic findings in infantile digital fibromatosis. Pediatr Dermatol. 25(1):72-5, 2008
3. Niamba P et al: Further documentation of spontaneous regression of infantile digital fibromatosis. Pediatr Dermatol. 24(3):280-4, 2007
4. Talbot C et al: Infantile digital fibromatosis. J Pediatr Orthop B. 16(2):110-2, 2007
5. Plusjé LG et al: Infantile-type digital fibromatosis tumour in an adult. Br J Dermatol. 143(5):1107-8, 2000
6. Kawaguchi M et al: A case of infantile digital fibromatosis with spontaneous regression. J Dermatol. 25(8):523-6, 1998
7. Rimareix F et al: Infantile digital fibroma--report on eleven cases. Eur J Pediatr Surg. 7(6):345-8, 1997
8. Falco NA et al: Infantile digital fibromas. J Hand Surg Am. 20(6):1014-20, 1995
9. Hayashi T et al: Infantile digital fibromatosis: a study of the development and regression of cytoplasmic inclusion bodies. Mod Pathol. 8(5):548-52, 1995
10. Pettinato G et al: Inclusion body fibromatosis of the breast. Two cases with immunohistochemical and ultrastructural findings. Am J Clin Pathol. 101(6):714-8, 1994
11. Choi KC et al: Infantile digital fibromatosis. Immunohistochemical and immunoelectron microscopic studies. J Cutan Pathol. 17(4):225-32, 1990
12. Viale G et al: Infantile digital fibromatosis-like tumour (inclusion body fibromatosis) of adulthood: report of two cases with ultrastructural and immunocytochemical findings. Histopathology. 12(4):415-24, 1988
13. Yun K: Infantile digital fibromatosis. Immunohistochemical and ultrastructural observations of cytoplasmic inclusions. Cancer. 61(3):500-7, 1988
14. Fringes B et al: Identification of actin microfilaments in the intracytoplasmic inclusions present in recurring infantile digital fibromatosis (Reye tumor). Pediatr Pathol. 6(2-3):311-24, 1986
15. Mukai M et al: Infantile digital fibromatosis. An electron microscopic and immunohistochemical study. Acta Pathol Jpn. 36(11):1605-15, 1986
16. Purdy LJ et al: Infantile digital fibromatosis occurring outside the digit. Am J Surg Pathol. 8(10):787-90, 1984
17. Faraggiana T et al: Ultrastructural histochemistry of infantile digital fibromatosis. Ultrastruct Pathol. 2(3):241-7, 1981
18. Iwasaki H et al: Infantile digital fibromatosis. Ultrastructural, histochemical, and tissue culture observations. Cancer. 46(10):2238-47, 1980
19. Sarma DP et al: Infantile digital fibroma-like tumor in an adult. Arch Dermatol. 116(5):578-9, 1980
20. Bhawan J et al: A myofibroblastic tumor. Infantile digital fibroma (recurrent digital fibrous tumor of childhood). Am J Pathol. 94(1):19-36, 1979

Microscopic Features

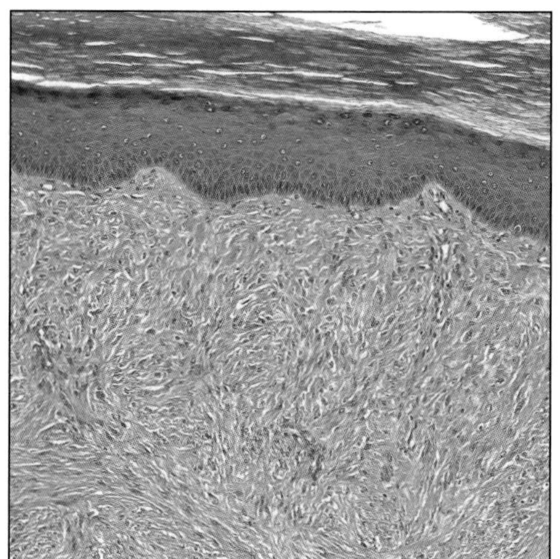

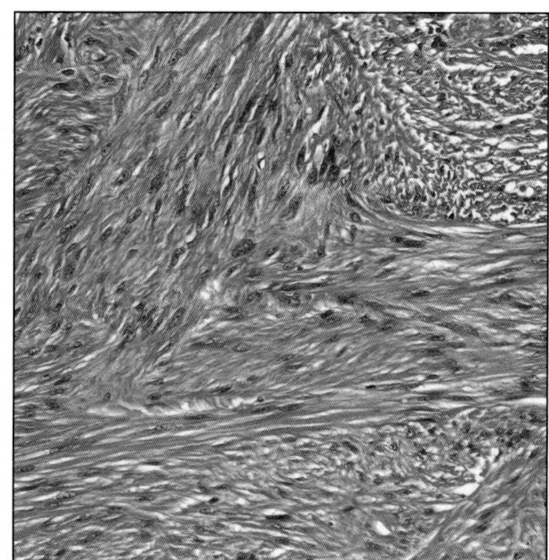

(Left) *Hematoxylin & eosin stains, such as this, show a moderately cellular spindle cell neoplasm of the dermis.* ***(Right)*** *The neoplasm is composed of ill-defined fascicles composed of cytologically bland, spindled fibroblasts and myofibroblasts containing an ill-defined pale eosinophilic cytoplasm and elongated, spindle-shaped nuclei.*

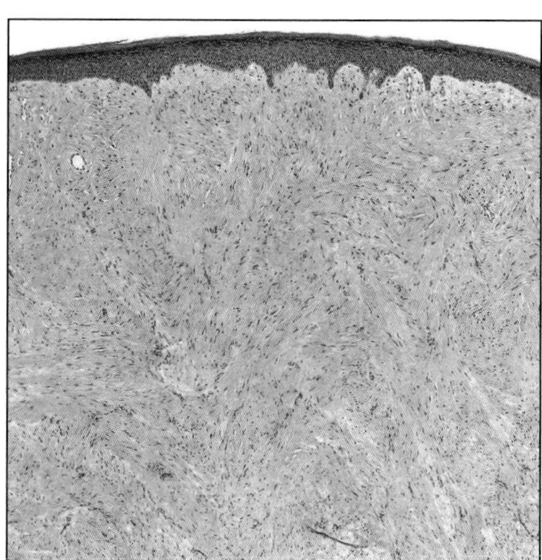

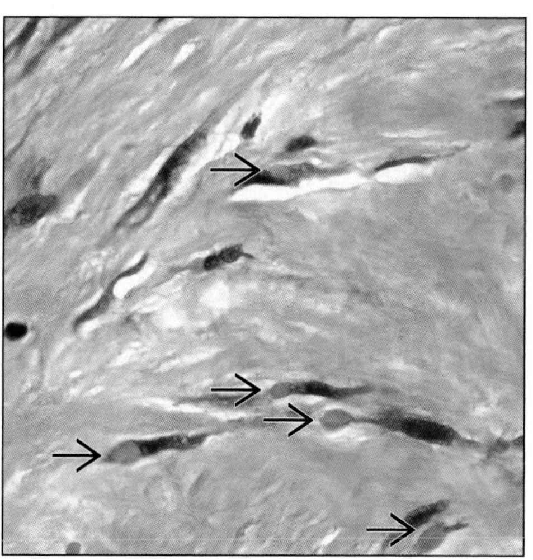

(Left) *A relatively hypocellular spindle cell neoplasm was seen in this case. Note the neoplastic cells set in a collagenous stroma.* ***(Right)*** *Hematoxylin & eosin shows numerous cytoplasmic inclusions ⇒ in this case.*

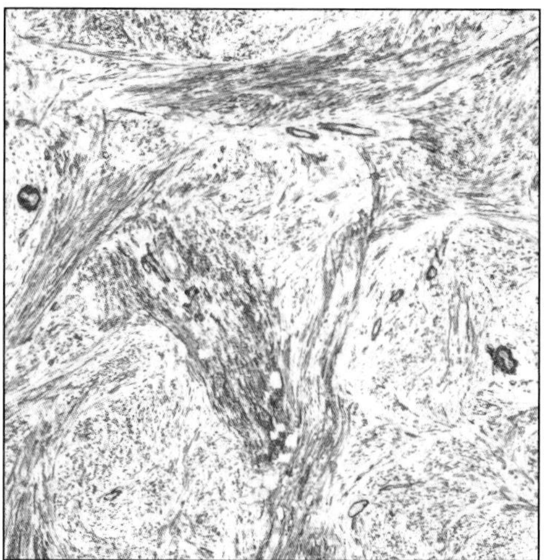

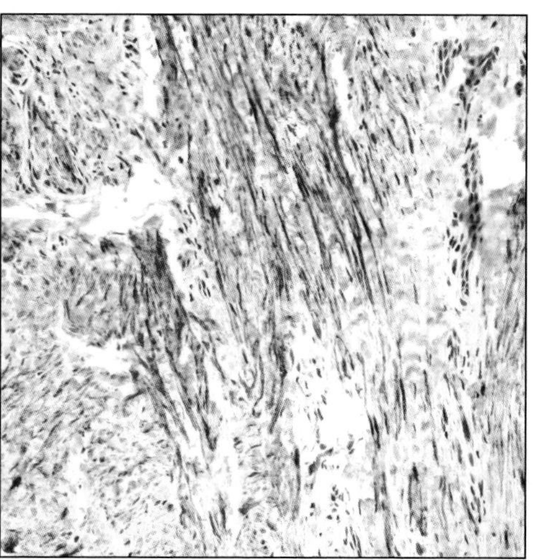

(Left) *Neoplastic cells in inclusion body fibromatosis stain positively for actin-sm in most cases.* ***(Right)*** *In rare cases, a focal coexpression of desmin is noted.*

GINGIVAL FIBROMATOSIS

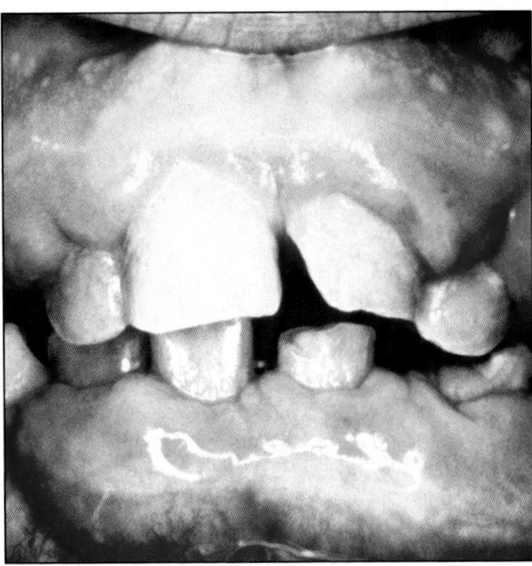

This clinical photograph is from a patient with gingival fibromatosis. The process diffusely involves both the upper and lower gingival tissues. (Courtesy G. Warnock, MD.)

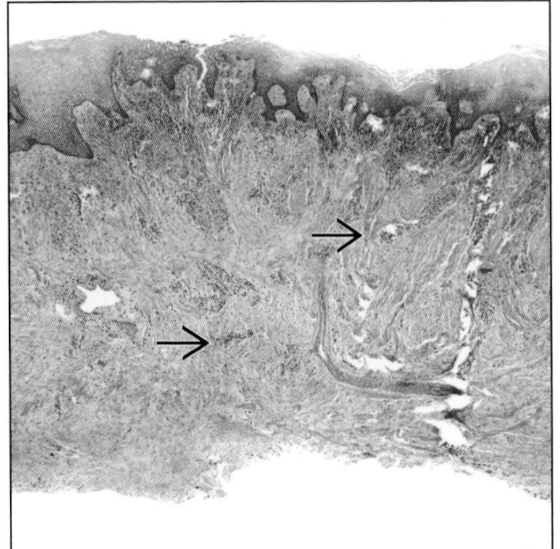

Hematoxylin & eosin of gingival fibromatosis shows a hypocellular fibroblastic lesion with prominent perivascular ⇒ inflammation.

TERMINOLOGY

Synonyms

- Idiopathic gingival fibromatosis, hereditary gingival fibromatosis, hereditary gingival hyperplasia, congenital macrogingivae, generalized hypertrophy of gums, gingival elephantiasis

Definitions

- Rare benign fibroproliferative disorder affecting gums, either idiopathic or familial
  - Isolated familial gingival fibromatosis
  - Isolated idiopathic gingival fibromatosis
  - Gingival fibromatosis associated with hypertrichosis
  - Gingival fibromatosis associated with hypertrichosis, mental retardation, &/or epilepsy
  - Gingival fibromatosis associated with mental retardation, &/or epilepsy
  - Gingival fibromatosis associated with other syndromes
    - Zimmerman-Laband syndrome (autosomal dominant with skeletal anomalies and hepatosplenomegaly)
    - Cherubism (Ramon syndrome)
    - Klippel-Trenaunay-Weber syndrome (vascular malformations)
  - ~ 1/3 of cases are familial
- Virtually identical lesions reported in association with certain medications
  - Phenytoin, cyclosporine A, nifedipine
  - Can be impossible to ascertain etiology of gingival hyperplasia in patients with seizures

ETIOLOGY/PATHOGENESIS

Excess Stimulation of Fibrosis

- Overexpression of connective tissue growth factor in all cases
- Mutation of human *SOS1* (Son of Sevenless-1 gene) responsible for hereditary gingival fibromatosis type 1
  - Stimulates ERK signaling, cell proliferation rate

CLINICAL ISSUES

Presentation

- Slow-growing swelling of gingivae
- Usually extensive and bilateral
- Arises as teeth begin to erupt in childhood
  - Younger age of onset in familial cases
  - Some examples are congenital
- 10% of patients have associated hypertrichosis
  - Present at younger age, female predominance

Treatment

- Excision of hyperplastic tissue
  - Regrowth common
- Removal of teeth seems to reduce regrowth

Prognosis

- Overall good; lesions are benign

MICROSCOPIC PATHOLOGY

Histologic Features

- Hypocellular fibrous proliferation of gingivae
- Calcifications common
- Perivascular lymphoplasmacytic inflammation
- Unremarkable overlying squamous mucosa
  - Some cases with epithelial hyperplasia

Predominant Pattern/Injury Type

- Fibrous

Predominant Cell/Compartment Type

- Fibroblast

GINGIVAL FIBROMATOSIS

Key Facts

Terminology

- Rare benign fibroproliferative disorder affecting gums, either idiopathic or familial
- ~ 1/3 of cases are familial
- Virtually identical lesions reported in association with certain medications
  - Phenytoin, cyclosporine A, nifedipine

Etiology/Pathogenesis

- Mutation of human *SOS1* (Son of Sevenless-1 gene) responsible for hereditary gingival fibromatosis type 1

Microscopic Pathology

- Calcifications common
- Perivascular lymphoplasmacytic inflammation

DIFFERENTIAL DIAGNOSIS

Juvenile Hyaline Fibromatosis

- Patients present with gingival hypertrophy, multiple cutaneous collagenized nodules, joint and skeletal anomalies
- Mutations in *ANTXR2* gene
  - Governs angiogenesis
- Autosomal recessive
- Rare; < 100 cases reported
- Has abundant glassy collagen
  - Chondroid appearance
  - Negligible inflammation

Deep Fibromatosis

- Large soft tissue masses
  - Usually in deep soft tissues of extremities
- Cellular with sweeping fascicles of fibroblasts
- Associated with familial adenomatous polyposis

Medication-associated Gingival Hyperplasia

- Phenytoin (Dilantin)
  - Marked fibrosis
- Cyclosporine A
  - Mild fibrosis
- Nifedipine
  - Intermediate levels of fibrosis
- Histologic appearance of these lesions essentially identical to that in idiopathic and familial forms
  - Fibrosis
  - Calcifications
  - Perivascular inflammation
  - Distinction requires correlation with history

Irritation Fibroma (Focal Fibrous Hyperplasia)

- Typically small lesion rather than diffuse hyperplasia
- Dome-shaped soft tissue mass
  - Usually found on buccal mucosa along line of occlusion
  - Less frequently on lips and tongue
- Submucosal localized fibrous proliferation
- Local removal curative

SELECTED REFERENCES

1. Abo-Dalo B et al: Extensive molecular genetic analysis of the 3p14.3 region in patients with Zimmermann-Laband syndrome. Am J Med Genet A. 143A(22):2668-74, 2007
2. Jang SI et al: Germ line gain of function with SOS1 mutation in hereditary gingival fibromatosis. J Biol Chem. 282(28):20245-55, 2007
3. Coletta RD et al: Hereditary gingival fibromatosis: a systematic review. J Periodontol. 77(5):753-64, 2006
4. Kantarci A et al: Epithelial and connective tissue cell CTGF/CCN2 expression in gingival fibrosis. J Pathol. 210(1):59-66, 2006
5. Takagi M et al: Heterogeneity in the gingival fibromatoses. Cancer. 68(10):2202-12, 1991

IMAGE GALLERY

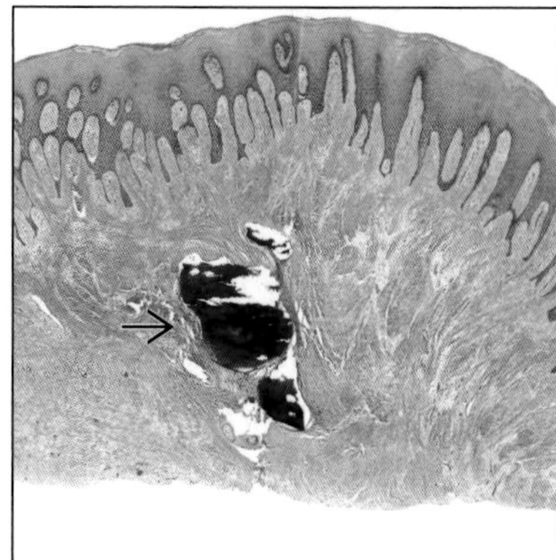

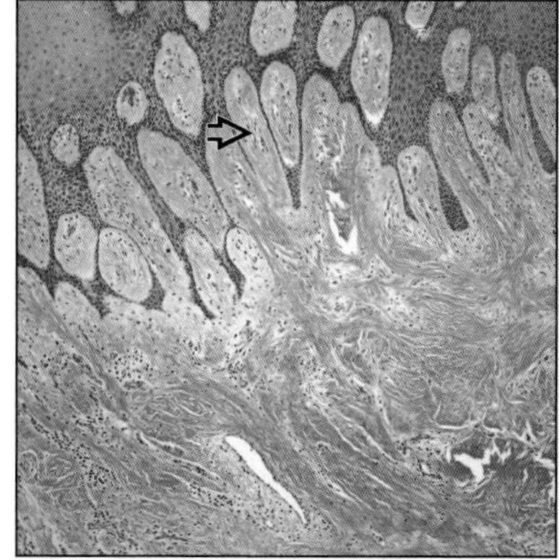

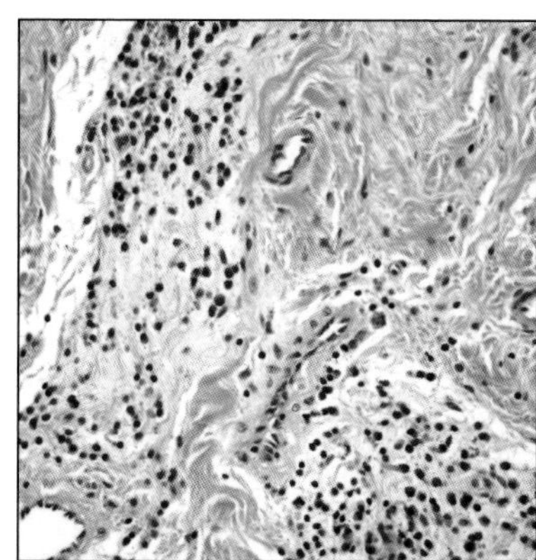

(Left) *Hematoxylin & eosin of gingival fibromatosis shows a longstanding lesion that has become focally calcified* ➔. ***(Center)*** *Hematoxylin & eosin shows prominent collagen deposition in this example of gingival fibromatosis. The overlying squamous mucosa displays pseudoepitheliomatous hyperplasia* ⇨. ***(Right)*** *Hematoxylin & eosin shows focal chronic inflammation in an example of gingival fibromatosis.*

FIBROMATOSIS COLLI

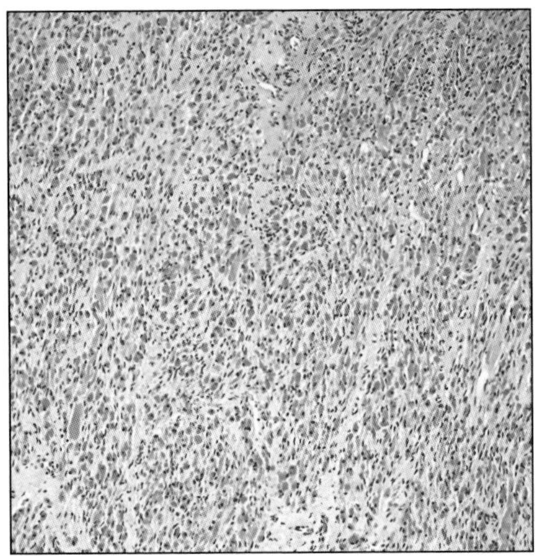

Hematoxylin & eosin shows diffuse fibrosis separating muscle fibers and imparting a fine checkerboard-like pattern in this biopsy specimen from the sternomastoid muscle.

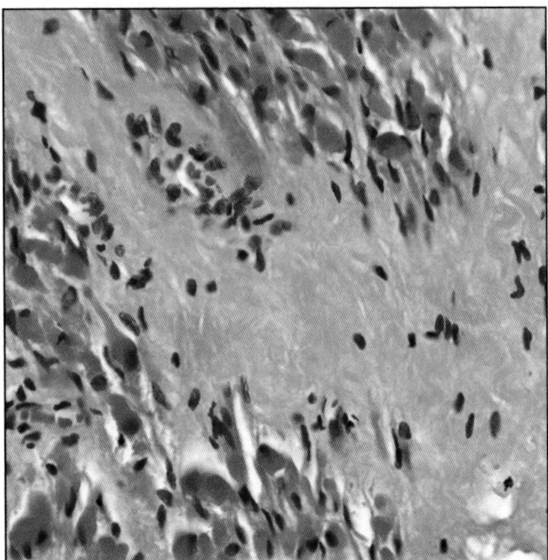

Hematoxylin & eosin shows hypocellular, finely fibrillary collagen forming a focus of confluent fibrosis in this late-stage example of fibromatosis colli.

TERMINOLOGY

Synonyms

- Sternomastoid tumor
- Congenital muscular torticollis
  - Clinical condition with several associated factors
  - Only up to 1/3 have fibromatosis colli

Definitions

- Fibrosing lesion of infants involving muscles of neck

ETIOLOGY/PATHOGENESIS

Developmental Anomaly

- Most cases spontaneous; presumed relation to intrauterine trauma
- Rarely familial

Environmental Exposure

- Obstetric trauma has been proposed as causal factor
  - Breech or forceps delivery
- Associated with muscular torticollis
  - Synchronous or delayed
- Associated with congenital dislocation of hip, anomalies of foot

CLINICAL ISSUES

Epidemiology

- Incidence
  - Rare, < 1% of newborns
- Age
  - Congenital or within 1st 6 months
- Gender
  - Equal incidence

Site

- Lower 1/3 of sternomastoid muscle
- Rarely in trapezius muscle

Presentation

- Painless mass
- Grows rapidly at first, then stops and persists

Natural History

- Most cases eventually regress
- Some persist
  - Can result in torticollis
    - Cervicofacial asymmetry

Treatment

- Options, risks, complications
  - Physiotherapy with stretching in early stages
- Surgical approaches
  - No intervention required in majority of cases
  - Surgery can be required for persistent cases

Prognosis

- Excellent in most cases
- Worse in patients older than 1 year
  - Fibrosis leads to shortening of muscle and deformity

IMAGE FINDINGS

Ultrasonographic Findings

- Isoechoic homogeneous mass
  - Within muscle body

MACROSCOPIC FEATURES

General Features

- Firm white lesion involving part of muscle
- Does not extend into adjacent soft tissue

Size

- Average: 2-3 cm in diameter

FIBROMATOSIS COLLI

Key Facts

Terminology
- Fibrosing lesion of infants involving muscles of head and neck

Etiology/Pathogenesis
- Rarely familial
- Obstetric trauma has been proposed as causal factor
  - Breech or forceps delivery
- Found in up to 1/3 of cases of congenital torticollis

Clinical Issues
- Majority in lower 1/3 of sternomastoid muscle
- Grows rapidly at first then stops and persists
- Most cases eventually regress

Microscopic Pathology
- Variably cellular fibroblastic infiltrate between skeletal muscle bundles
- Early stage more cellular, later scarring
- Muscle fibers swell, then atrophy

MICROSCOPIC PATHOLOGY

Histologic Features
- Variably cellular fibroblastic infiltrate between skeletal muscle bundles
- Early stage proliferative and more cellular
- Fibrosis in later stages
  - Infiltrates between muscle fibers in fine checkerboard-like pattern
  - Eventual confluent scarring
- Muscle fibers swell, then atrophy
  - Occasional fiber regeneration
- Minimal inflammation, no necrosis or atypia

Predominant Pattern/Injury Type
- Fibrous

Predominant Cell/Compartment Type
- Mesenchymal, muscle, skeletal

ANCILLARY TESTS

Immunohistochemistry
- Infiltrating fibroblasts are SMA(+) in early stages
- Lesional cells are β-catenin(-)

DIFFERENTIAL DIAGNOSIS

Nodular Fasciitis
- More circumscribed
- Does not infiltrate between muscle bundles
- Myxoid and storiform areas
- Extravasated red blood cells, lymphocytes

Fibromatosis
- Discrete mass
- Parallel-aligned myofibroblasts
- Mast cells
- β-catenin immunoreactivity in nuclei

DIAGNOSTIC CHECKLIST

Clinically Relevant Pathologic Features
- Age distribution
- Organ distribution

Pathologic Interpretation Pearls
- Typical clinical picture
- Diffusely infiltrative, cellular or hypocellular fibrosis

SELECTED REFERENCES

1. Tatli B et al: Congenital muscular torticollis: evaluation and classification. Pediatr Neurol. 34(1):41-4, 2006
2. Cheng JC et al: The clinical presentation and outcome of treatment of congenital muscular torticollis in infants--a study of 1,086 cases. J Pediatr Surg. 35(7):1091-6, 2000
3. Ho BC et al: Epidemiology, presentation and management of congenital muscular torticollis. Singapore Med J. 40(11):675-9, 1999
4. Lawrence WT et al: Congenital muscular torticollis: a spectrum of pathology. Ann Plast Surg. 23(6):523-30, 1989

IMAGE GALLERY

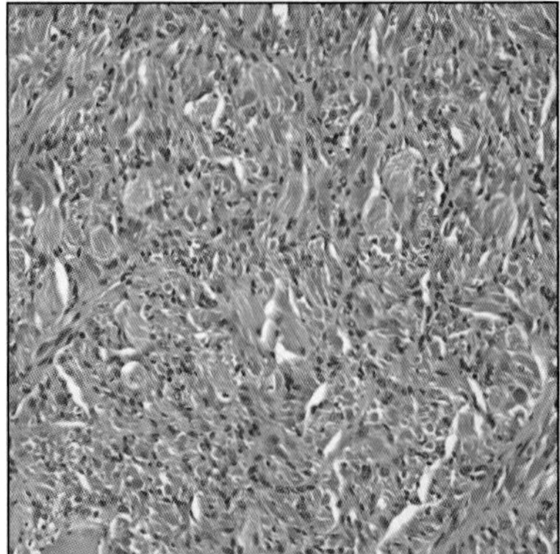

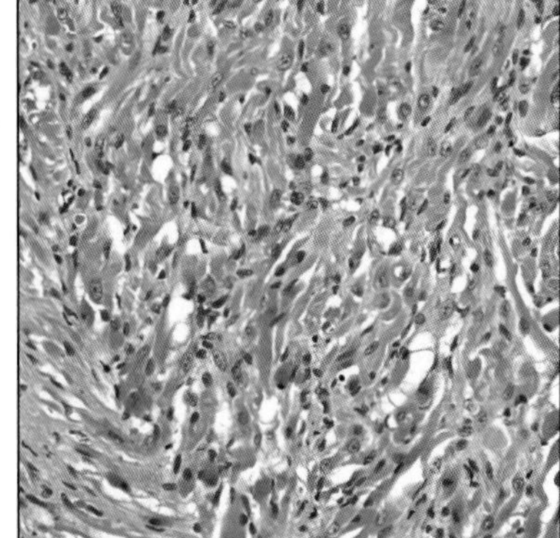

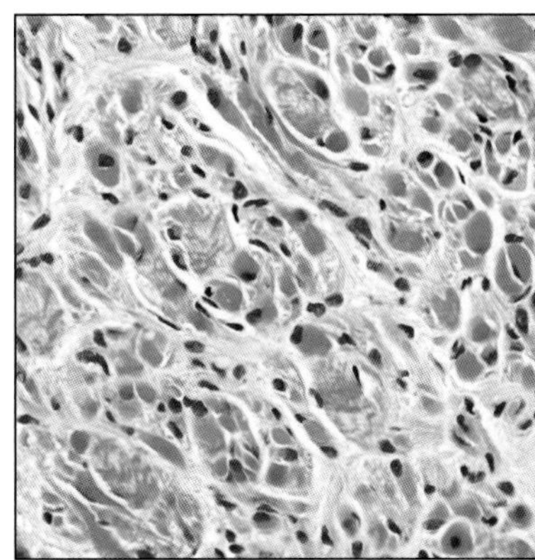

(Left) *Hematoxylin & eosin shows early-stage fibromatosis coli with cellular infiltrate between muscle fibers. The infiltrate includes cellular fibrous tissue and inflammatory cells. The muscle fibers undergo swelling, then atrophy.* ***(Center)*** *Hematoxylin & eosin shows early fibrosis with atrophy of skeletal muscle fibers. Fatty replacement of atrophied muscle is not a feature of this condition.* ***(Right)*** *Hematoxylin & eosin shows late-stage fibrosis with reduction in size of muscle fibers. The skeletal muscle is dissected by the fibrous tissue into small groups of fibers.*

JUVENILE HYALINE FIBROMATOSIS

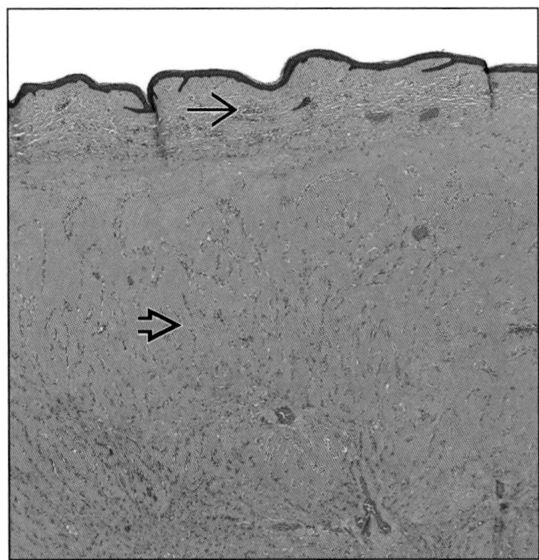

Hematoxylin & eosin shows juvenile hyaline fibromatosis of face in subepithelial tissue ⇨. There is a tumor-free (Grenz) zone → between the epidermis and the lesional tissue.

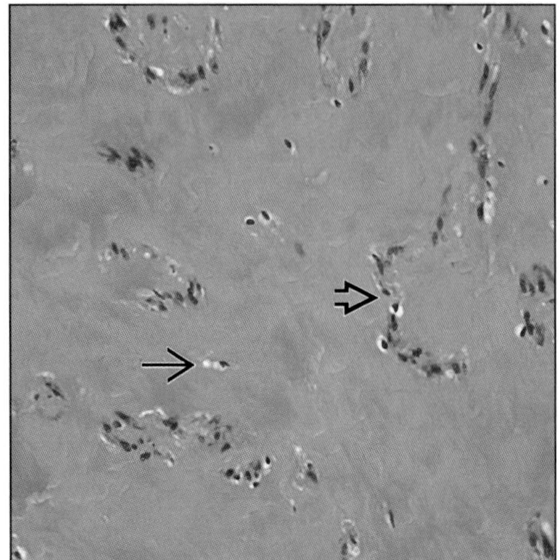

Hematoxylin & eosin shows scattered lesional cells in homogeneous eosinophilic stroma. The cells are small and uniform, arranged in short curved cords ⇨. Some nuclei appear in spaces →.

TERMINOLOGY

Abbreviations

- Juvenile hyaline fibromatosis (JHF)

Synonyms

- Related disorder: Infantile systemic hyalinosis (ISH)
  - Suggested synonym: Hyaline fibromatosis syndrome

Definitions

- Rare autosomal recessive disorder (often found in consanguineous populations) characterized by multiple skin papules and early onset

ETIOLOGY/PATHOGENESIS

Genetic Disorder

- Mutations in *ANTXR2* in both juvenile hyaline fibromatosis and infantile systemic hyalinosis
- Autosomal recessive transmission

CLINICAL ISSUES

Presentation

- Juvenile hyaline fibromatosis
  - Infantile presentation of lesions of scalp, face, neck, retroauricular areas, perineal region, and gingival hypertrophy
  - Joint contractures and motion limitation
  - Osteolytic lesions, mainly in phalanges and distal portions of long bones; cortical defects in subset of patients
- Infantile systemic hyalinosis
  - More severe end of clinical spectrum of mutations in *ANTXR2*
    - Hyaline changes are seen in multiple viscera as well as in skin
    - More prominent than those described in JHF
    - Affected individuals usually die in 1st years of life as result of complications of visceral involvement
  - Infiltration of intestines leads to malabsorption

MACROSCOPIC FEATURES

Skin and Gingival Lesions

- Plaques and papules of skin
- Larger lesions form soft tissue masses
- Gingival hyperplasia

Systemic Lesions

- Infiltration of small bowel and colon forming masses

MICROSCOPIC PATHOLOGY

Histologic Features

- Histologic findings in both JHF and ISH are indistinguishable
  - Round to spindle cell proliferation composed of bland fibroblasts lying in clear spaces simulating chondrocyte lacunae
  - No significant cellular pleomorphism or mitoses
  - Homogeneous, hyalinized, pale, eosinophilic intercellular matrix
  - PAS(+); diastase resistant
  - Displaces normal components of dermis and lamina propria of gingival and intestinal mucosa
  - Early lesions can lack hyaline stroma

DIFFERENTIAL DIAGNOSIS

Fibrodysplasia (Myositis) Ossificans Progressiva

- Rare and autosomal dominant
  - Characterized by soft tissue ossification at multiple sites and skeletal abnormalities of digits and cervical spine

JUVENILE HYALINE FIBROMATOSIS

Key Facts

Terminology
- Related disorder: Infantile systemic hyalinosis (ISH)

Clinical Issues
- Autosomal recessive transmission
- Infantile presentation of lesions of scalp, face, neck, retroauricular areas
  - Gingival hypertrophy
- Cutaneous papules and plaques

Microscopic Pathology
- Uniform round to spindle cells
  - Some in clear spaces
- No significant cellular pleomorphism
- No mitoses or necrosis
- Homogeneous, hyalinized, pale, eosinophilic intercellular matrix
  - PAS(+); diastase resistant
- Blood vessels sparse

- Short great toes
- No gender predominance
- Trauma (accidental or surgical) results in painful soft tissue lesions
  - Progressive ossification of lesions over 2-3 months
- Lesions appear similar to those of myositis ossificans
  - Mitotically active myofibroblasts
  - Variable ossification depending on age of lesions

Infantile Myofibromatosis
- Multiple lesions presenting in infancy
  - Can involve bones, soft tissues, and viscera
    - Pulmonary involvement is poor prognostic feature
- Biphasic lobulated lesions
  - Myoid nodules
  - Hemangiopericytoma-like zones

Desmoid-type Fibromatosis
- Large masses of deep soft tissues, usually solitary
- Cellular fascicular lesions
- Associated with familial adenomatous polyposis (FAP)
- Nuclear immunoreactivity for β-catenin (deep examples)

Calcifying Aponeurotic Fibroma
- Distal extremities of infants and children
- Solitary lesions
- Stippled calcifications and fibrous areas

Nuchal Fibrocartilaginous Tumor
- Solitary lesion of adults
- Associated with prior neck injury
- Posterior aspect of base of neck
  - Junction of nuchal ligament and deep cervical fascia
- Fibrocartilaginous tissue forming mass

SELECTED REFERENCES

1. Nofal A et al: Juvenile hyaline fibromatosis and infantile systemic hyalinosis: A unifying term and a proposed grading system. J Am Acad Dermatol. Epub ahead of print, 2009
2. Tanaka K et al: Abnormal collagen deposition in fibromas from patient with juvenile hyaline fibromatosis. J Dermatol Sci. 55(3):197-200, 2009
3. Al-Malik MI et al: Gingival hyperplasia in hyaline fibromatosis--a report of two cases. J Int Acad Periodontol. 9(2):42-8, 2007
4. Antaya RJ et al: Juvenile hyaline fibromatosis and infantile systemic hyalinosis overlap associated with a novel mutation in capillary morphogenesis protein-2 gene. Am J Dermatopathol. 29(1):99-103, 2007
5. Anadolu RY et al: Juvenile non-hyaline fibromatosis: juvenile hyaline fibromatosis without prominent hyaline changes. J Cutan Pathol. 32(3):235-9, 2005
6. Hanks S et al: Mutations in the gene encoding capillary morphogenesis protein 2 cause juvenile hyaline fibromatosis and infantile systemic hyalinosis. Am J Hum Genet. 73(4):791-800, 2003
7. Rahman N et al: The gene for juvenile hyaline fibromatosis maps to chromosome 4q21. Am J Hum Genet. 71(4):975-80, 2002

IMAGE GALLERY

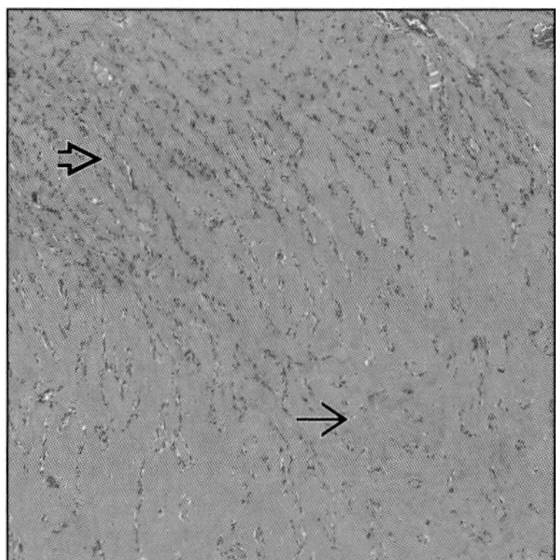

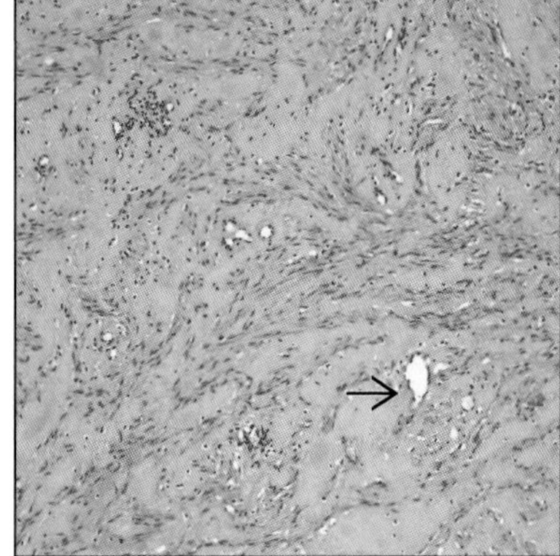

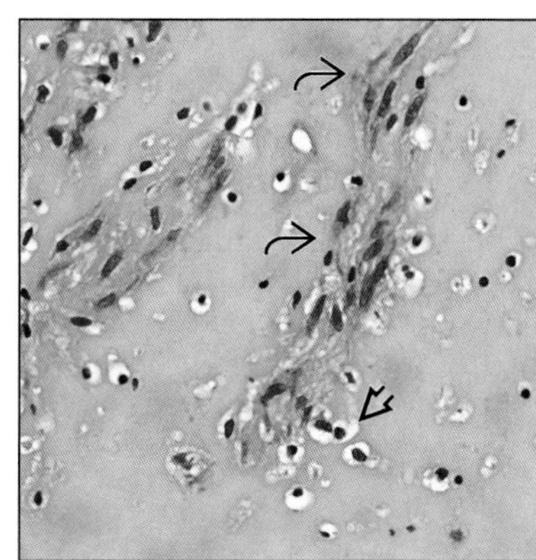

__(Left)__ H&E stain shows cords of cells within characteristic stroma. The cords show a vaguely parallel alignment ⮚. Some parts of the tumor → are less cellular. __(Center)__ H&E stain shows a cellular example with branching cords of spindle cells. Note the occasional thin-walled dilated blood vessels →. __(Right)__ H&E stain shows numerous cells with clear cytoplasm resembling chondrocytes ⮚ and clusters of spindle cells ↗. Note the absence of pleomorphism and mitotic activity. The stroma shows diastase-resistant positivity with PAS staining.

DESMOPLASTIC FIBROBLASTOMA

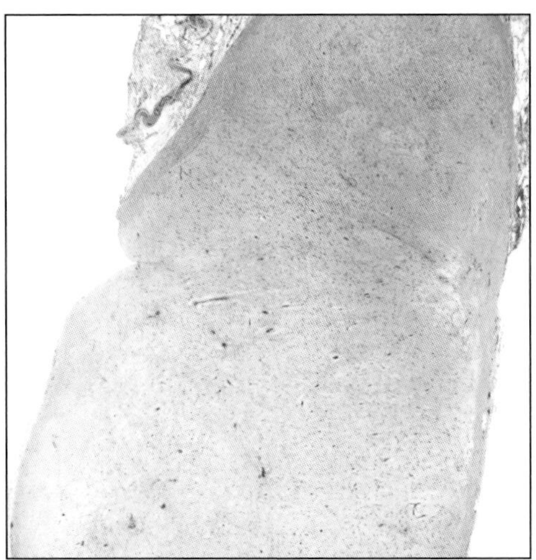

Hematoxylin & eosin shows desmoplastic fibroblastoma. The lesion is a well-circumscribed ovoid or fusiform mass. The hypocellularity is apparent at low power.

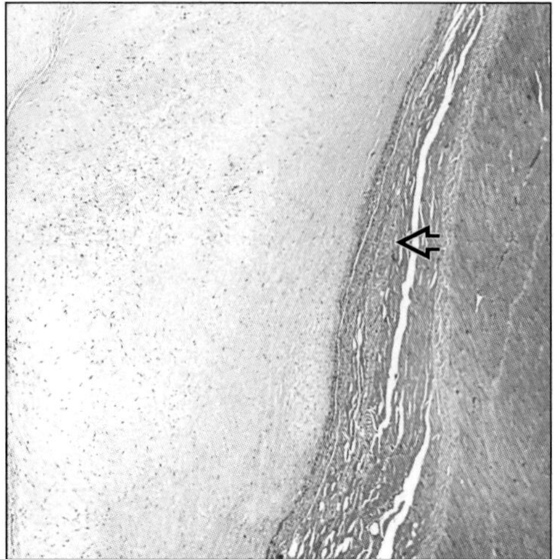

Hematoxylin & eosin shows desmoplastic fibroblastoma. Although most tumors are subcutaneous, some involve skeletal muscle ⇨, which this lesion is seen to abut.

TERMINOLOGY

Abbreviations

- Desmoplastic fibroblastoma (DF)

Synonyms

- Collagenous fibroma

Definitions

- Rare benign fibrous soft tissue neoplasm occurring mainly in adult males and consisting of paucicellular arrays of stellate and spindle fibroblasts
- Reciprocal translocation t(2;11)(q31;q12) found in some cases

ETIOLOGY/PATHOGENESIS

Developmental Anomaly

- Etiology unknown

CLINICAL ISSUES

Epidemiology

- Age
  - All ages, but particularly older adults (5th-6th decades)
- Gender
  - M > F

Site

- Most occur in subcutaneous tissue
- Up to 25% involve skeletal muscle
- Most common in upper extremity (shoulder, upper arm, forearm), followed by lower extremity
- Rare in head and neck

Presentation

- Slow growing
- Painless mass

Treatment

- Surgical approaches
  - Simple complete excision

Prognosis

- Benign; does not recur locally or metastasize

MACROSCOPIC FEATURES

General Features

- Firm, circumscribed, lobulated mass
- White or gray cut surface
- No necrosis or hemorrhage

Size

- Majority of tumors are small (< 4 cm); range: 1.5-20 cm

MICROSCOPIC PATHOLOGY

Histologic Features

- Sparsely cellular
- Patternless distributions of bland spindle or stellate cells
- Hypovascular fibrous or fibromyxoid stroma
- Mitotic figures very rare; no necrosis
- Isolated cases have shown dystrophic calcification and metaplastic bone or small foci of floret-like multinucleated giant cells

Margins

- Generally circumscribed, although many infiltrate adjacent soft tissues

ANCILLARY TESTS

Immunohistochemistry

- Variable positivity for smooth muscle actin

DESMOPLASTIC FIBROBLASTOMA

Key Facts

Terminology
- Rare benign fibrous soft tissue neoplasm occurring mainly in adult males and consisting of paucicellular arrays of stellate and spindle fibroblasts

Clinical Issues
- Usually in older adults (5th to 6th decades)
- Male preponderance
- Most occur in subcutaneous tissue but up to 25% involve skeletal muscle
- Most common in proximal extremity

Microscopic Pathology
- Sparsely cellular patternless distributions of bland spindle or stellate cells
- Hypovascular fibrous or fibromyxoid stroma
- Mitotic figures rare; no necrosis

Ancillary Tests
- Variably SMA(+)

- May show focal weak positivity for S100 protein and rare focal desmin or keratin positivity
- Negative for CD34

Cytogenetics
- Reciprocal translocation t(2;11)(q31;q12) reported in 2 cases; translocation has also been reported in 1 case of fibroma of tendon sheath
- 11q12 breakpoint in 2 further cases

Electron Microscopy
- Tumor cells show features of fibroblasts and myofibroblasts

DIFFERENTIAL DIAGNOSIS

Fibromatosis
- More infiltrative and cellular
- Cells in loose fascicles
- Prominent vascular pattern

Neurofibroma
- Cell nuclei may be buckled or "schwannian"
- Strongly positive for S100 protein

Nodular Fasciitis (Late Stage)
- Foci of increased cellularity
- Chronic inflammation, extravasated red cells

Elastofibroma
- Typically located in subscapular region
- Fragmented elastic fibers

Fibroma of Tendon Sheath
- Peritendinous locations, particularly of hands

Calcifying Fibrous Pseudotumor
- Children and young adults
- Psammomatous calcifications
- Lymphoplasmacytic infiltrate

Low-Grade Fibromyxoid Sarcoma
- More cellular; may show rosette formation
- Characteristic translocations t(7;16) and t(11;16)

SELECTED REFERENCES

1. Sakamoto A et al: Desmoplastic fibroblastoma (collagenous fibroma) with a specific breakpoint of 11q12. Histopathology. 51(6):859-60, 2007
2. Bernal K et al: Translocation (2;11)(q31;q12) is recurrent in collagenous fibroma (desmoplastic fibroblastoma). Cancer Genet Cytogenet. 149(2):161-3, 2004
3. Sciot R et al: Collagenous fibroma (desmoplastic fibroblastoma): genetic link with fibroma of tendon sheath? Mod Pathol. 12(6):565-8, 1999
4. Miettinen M et al: Collagenous fibroma (desmoplastic fibroblastoma): a clinicopathologic analysis of 63 cases of a distinctive soft tissue lesion with stellate-shaped fibroblasts. Hum Pathol. 29(7):676-82, 1998
5. Nielsen GP et al: Collagenous fibroma (desmoplastic fibroblastoma): a report of seven cases. Mod Pathol. 9(7):781-5, 1996
6. Evans HL: Desmoplastic fibroblastoma. A report of seven cases. Am J Surg Pathol. 19(9):1077-81, 1995

IMAGE GALLERY

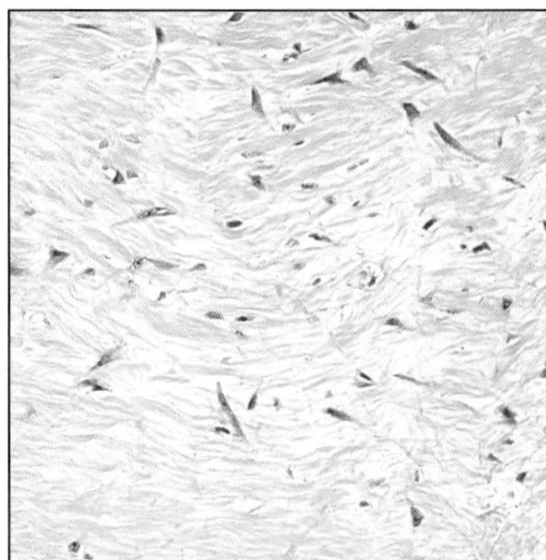

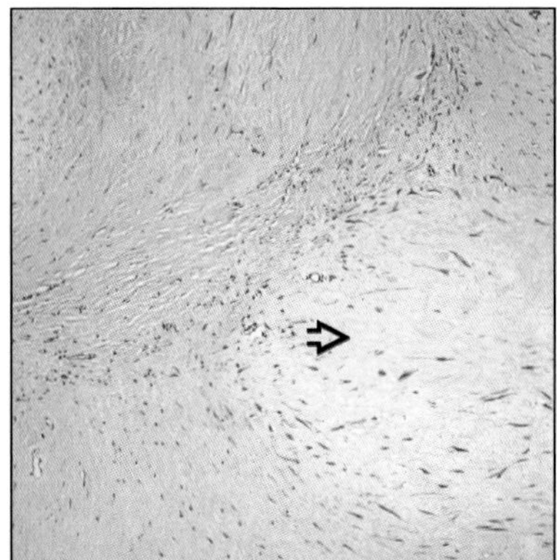

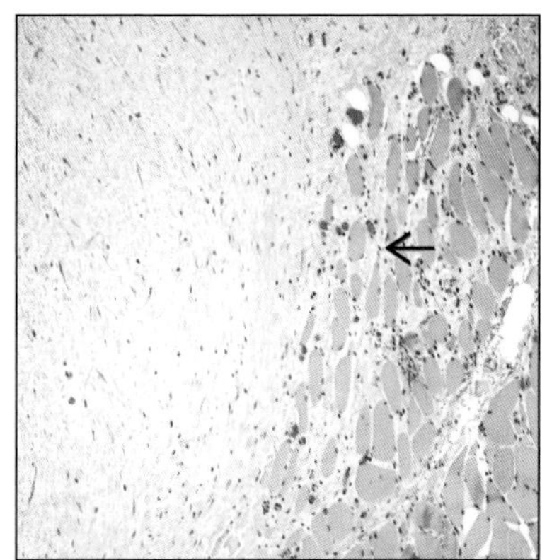

*(**Left**) Hematoxylin & eosin shows stroma that is densely collagenous and contains spindle and stellate fibroblasts in patternless distributions. Vessels are inconspicuous. (**Center**) Hematoxylin & eosin shows the sparsely cellular nature of the lesion. The stroma can be focally myxoid ⇨. Although cells may be plump, no true atypia is seen, and mitotic figures are rare or absent. (**Right**) Hematoxylin & eosin shows desmoplastic fibroblastoma. Although the tumor is largely circumscribed, focal infiltration of surrounding soft tissues may be seen →.*

NODULAR FASCIITIS

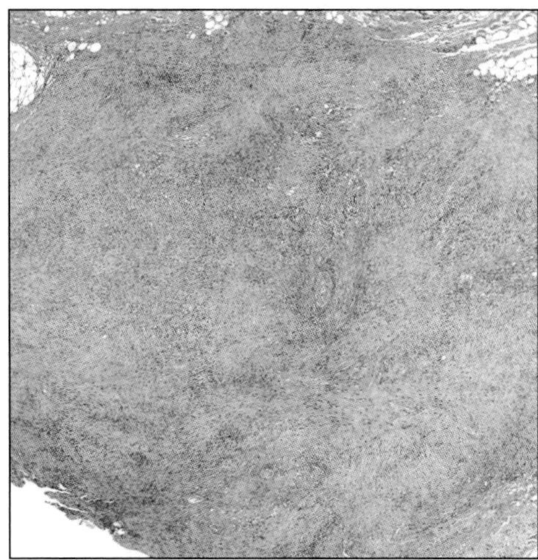

Hematoxylin & eosin shows low magnification of nodular fasciitis. The lesion is nodular and reminiscent of granulation tissue. Note the moderate circumscription.

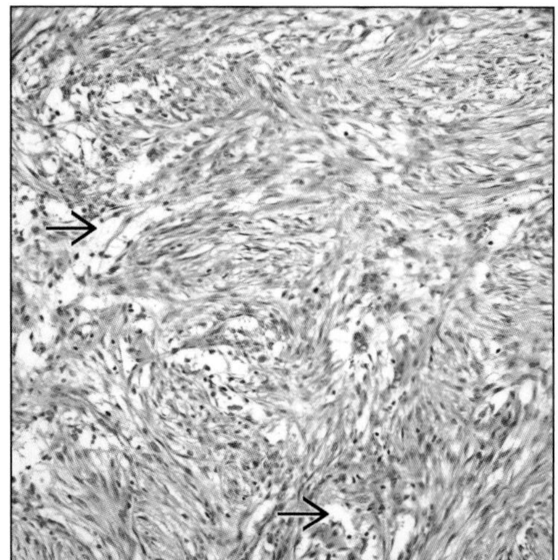

Hematoxylin & eosin shows a loose storiform pattern with cystic spaces ➔ and background lymphocytes and extravasated erythrocytes.

TERMINOLOGY

Abbreviations

- Nodular fasciitis (NF)

Synonyms

- Pseudosarcomatous fasciitis
- Subcutaneous pseudosarcomatous fibromatosis

Definitions

- Rapidly growing myofibroblastic mass-forming proliferation that is often cellular and mitotically active but behaves in benign fashion
  - Typically displays loose storiform pattern, cystic spaces, and strands of keloid-like collagen
- Intravascular fasciitis is rare variant of nodular fasciitis arising from small or medium-sized vessels
  - Presents as soft tissue mass with focal intravascular extension or multinodular predominantly intravascular mass
  - Despite intravascular location, lesion behaves in benign fashion with no tendency to recur or metastasize
- Cranial fasciitis involves soft tissues of scalp and underlying skull of infants
  - Usually erodes bone but may penetrate through bone to involve meninges
  - Fragments of bone may be seen at periphery of lesion
  - Birth trauma presumed inciting stimulus

ETIOLOGY/PATHOGENESIS

Unknown

- History of local trauma in subset

CLINICAL ISSUES

Epidemiology

- Incidence
  - Uncommon but comparatively common among soft tissue lesions
- Age
  - 3rd-4th decades
- Gender
  - M = F

Presentation

- Subcutaneous mass

Treatment

- Simple excision usually curative

Prognosis

- Excellent prognosis
- Seldom recurs, even if incompletely excised

MACROSCOPIC FEATURES

General Features

- Well-marginated but unencapsulated
- Variable mucoid appearance

Sections to Be Submitted

- Usually entire lesion is submitted

Size

- 2-3 cm mass

MICROSCOPIC PATHOLOGY

Histologic Features

- Loose storiform, "feathery" pattern with tissue culture appearance, variable myxoid stroma, cystic spaces, strands of keloid-like collagen
- Mitoses present but no atypical forms

NODULAR FASCIITIS

Key Facts

Clinical Issues

- Age: 3rd-4th decades
- Gender: M = F
- Most lesions are benign and do not recur, even if incompletely excised
- Simple excision is treatment

Microscopic Pathology

- Loose storiform, "feathery" pattern with tissue culture appearance, variable myxoid stroma, cystic spaces, strands of keloid-like collagen
- Mitoses present but no atypical forms
- Osteoclast-like giant cells found in most lesions if sought
- Scattered lymphocytes but essentially no plasma cells
- Extravasated erythrocytes unassociated with hemosiderin
- 3 forms reported: Myxoid, cellular, and fibrous
  - Loose correlation with duration of lesions; myxoid lesion often resected within 10 days after coming to clinical attention; cellular and fibrous forms resected after longer intervals (patterns variable)
- Myofibroblastic differentiation results in expression of some smooth muscle immunohistochemical markers
- Lesions can be mistaken for leiomyosarcomas when mitotically active

- Osteoclast-like giant cells found in most lesions if sought
  - Can be highlighted by CD68
- Scattered lymphocytes but essentially no plasma cells
- Extravasated erythrocytes
  - No associated hemosiderin
- 3 forms reported: Myxoid, cellular, and fibrous
  - Loose correlation with duration of lesions
  - Myxoid lesion often resected within 10 days after coming to clinical attention
  - Cellular and fibrous forms resected after longer intervals
  - Some lesions show several patterns
- Myofibroblastic differentiation results in expression of some smooth muscle immunohistochemical markers
  - Lesions can be mistaken for leiomyosarcomas when mitotically active

Predominant Pattern/Injury Type

- Localized

Predominant Cell/Compartment Type

- Mesenchymal, spindle

Variant Forms

- Nodular myositis
  - Same as nodular fasciitis but intramuscular
  - Debate as to whether such cases are instead early myositis ossificans
- Intravascular fasciitis
  - Typically affects head and neck and distal extremities
  - More solid than classic form
  - Typically displays abundant osteoclast-like giant cells
  - Easily mistaken for leiomyosarcoma based on mitoses
- Cranial fasciitis
  - Lesion of infants sometimes attributed to birth trauma
  - Similar morphology to that of nodular fasciitis but more myxoid background
  - Some reported examples may be fibromatoses
  - Can involve skull itself
- Subsets occur in specific locations
  - Spermatic cord (proliferative funiculitis)
  - Within nerves

ANCILLARY TESTS

Cytology

- Shows myofibroblastic cells
  - Lesions are cellular, which can lead to erroneous impression of sarcoma on aspiration cytology

Frozen Sections

- Seldom requested
- Difficult to distinguish from sarcomas, but lesions lack pleomorphic cells

Flow Cytometry

- Diploid

Cytogenetics

- Rearrangement of 3q21 with group D acrocentric chromosome, t(2;15), t(2;13), marker chromosomes

Electron Microscopy

- Transmission
  - Shows myofibroblastic differentiation

DIFFERENTIAL DIAGNOSIS

Fibrous Histiocytoma

- Typically small superficial lesions
  - Rare deep cellular examples
- Storiform pattern
- Abundant background changes
  - Foamy macrophages, hemosiderin, plasma cells
- Collagen trapping at periphery of lesions
- Superficial lesions have overlying skin changes (epidermal hyperplasia)
- Factor XIII reactive, focal CD68 in background cells
- Variable actin expression
- Tend to recur locally if incompletely excised

NODULAR FASCIITIS

Immunohistochemistry

Antibody	Reactivity	Staining Pattern	Comment
Actin-sm	Positive	Cytoplasmic	Sometimes results in misdiagnosis of leiomyosarcoma
CD68	Positive	Cytoplasmic	Highlights osteoclast-like giant cells
Calponin	Positive	Cytoplasmic	
ALK1	Negative		
Desmin	Negative		Occasional examples show focal staining
S100	Negative		
CK-PAN	Negative		
Myogenin	Negative		
Caldesmon	Negative		

- Rare reports of metastases

Neurofibroma
- Small superficial lesions
  - Subset associated with neurofibromatosis
- Serpentine nuclei
- Shredded-appearing collagen, nuclei "plastered" against collagen
- Background changes
  - Myxoid areas, mast cells
- Immunohistochemistry: S100 protein reactive, variable CD34 supporting cells
- Benign behavior

Fibromatosis
- Large deep infiltrative lesions
  - Shoulder girdle common site
  - Abdominal wall in women in reproductive years
  - Head and neck
- Sweeping fascicles of myofibroblasts
- Uniform collagen deposition
- Prominent vascular pattern
- Highly infiltrative lesions
  - Entrap and destroy skeletal muscle at periphery
- Immunohistochemistry: Actin reactive, nuclear β-catenin
- Prone to local recurrences

Kaposi Sarcoma
- Found in immunocompromised patients (especially AIDS patients)
  - Often involve skin and mucosal surfaces of upper body
  - Rare "classic" cases in distal extremities of elderly men
  - Associated with HHV8 in all settings
- Hyperchromatic spindle cells
- Extravasated erythrocytes, hemosiderin, plasma cells, hyaline globules
- Immunohistochemistry: CD34, CD31, and HHV8 reactive
- Most behave indolently
  - Quasi-neoplastic lesions
    - Often regress if immunosuppression ceases

Leiomyosarcoma
- Wide range of clinical presentation
  - Some involve skin and subcutaneous tissue
- Perpendicularly oriented fascicles
- Brightly eosinophilic cytoplasm
- Hyperchromatic nuclei with blunt ends
- Paranuclear vacuoles
- Immunohistochemistry: Actin, desmin, calponin, and caldesmon reactive
- Outcome related to stage

Malignant Fibrous Histiocytoma (Undifferentiated Pleomorphic Sarcoma)
- Usually large deep lesions
- Storiform pattern
- Pleomorphic nuclei
- Fibroblastic and myofibroblastic differentiation
- Variable expression of smooth muscle markers
- Outcome related to stage
- Overall 5-year survival about 60%

SELECTED REFERENCES

1. Weibolt VM et al: Involvement of 3q21 in nodular fasciitis. Cancer Genet Cytogenet. 106(2):177-9, 1998
2. Birdsall SH et al: Cytogenetic findings in a case of nodular fasciitis of the breast. Cancer Genet Cytogenet. 81(2):166-8, 1995
3. el-Jabbour JN et al: Flow cytometric study of nodular fasciitis, proliferative fasciitis, and proliferative myositis. Hum Pathol. 22(11):1146-9, 1991
4. Montgomery EA et al: Nodular fasciitis. Its morphologic spectrum and immunohistochemical profile. Am J Surg Pathol. 15(10):942-8, 1991
5. Shimizu S et al: Nodular fasciitis: an analysis of 250 patients. Pathology. 16(2):161-6, 1984
6. Daroca PJ Jr et al: Ossifying fasciitis. Arch Pathol Lab Med. 106(13):682-5, 1982
7. Patchefsky AS et al: Intravascular fasciitis: a report of 17 cases. Am J Surg Pathol. 5(1):29-36, 1981
8. Lauer DH et al: Cranial fasciitis of childhood. Cancer. 45(2):401-6, 1980
9. Meister P et al: Nodular fasciitis (analysis of 100 cases and review of the literature). Pathol Res Pract. 162(2):133-65, 1978
10. Allen PW: Nodular fasciitis. Pathology. 4(1):9-26, 1972
11. Konwaler BE et al: Subcutaneous pseudosarcomatous fibromatosis (fasciitis). Am J Clin Pathol. 25(3):241-52, 1955

Microscopic Features

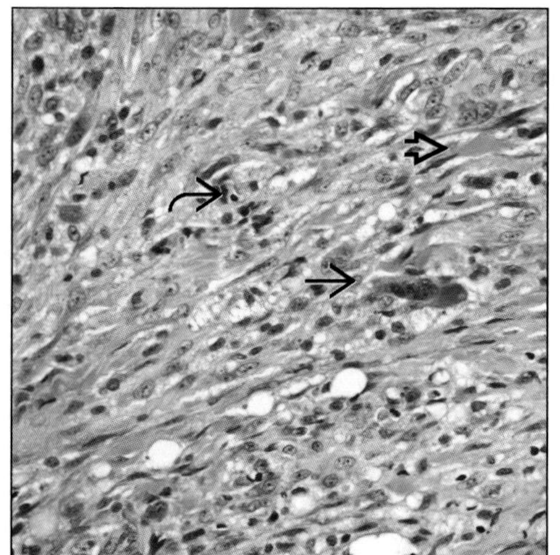

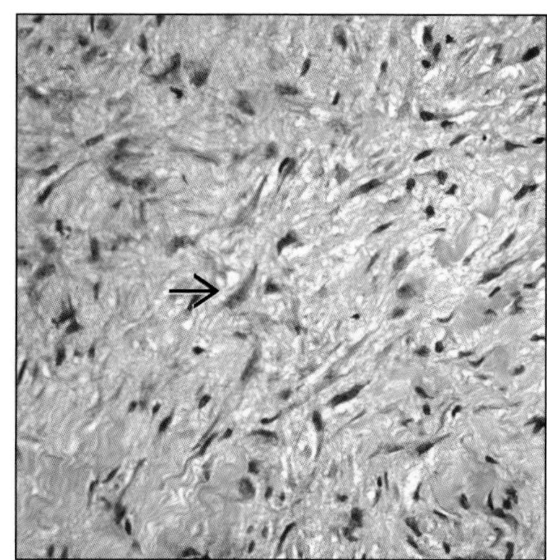

(Left) Hematoxylin & eosin shows the cytologic features of nodular fasciitis. The nuclei are uniform and appear bland. This field shows an osteoclast-like giant cell ➔ and strands of dense collagen ➯. There are scattered background lymphocytes ➚ that appear more hyperchromatic than the proliferating cells. **(Right)** This lesion displays stellate cells and prominent keloid-like collagen. The nuclei are pale with delicate small nucleoli ➔.

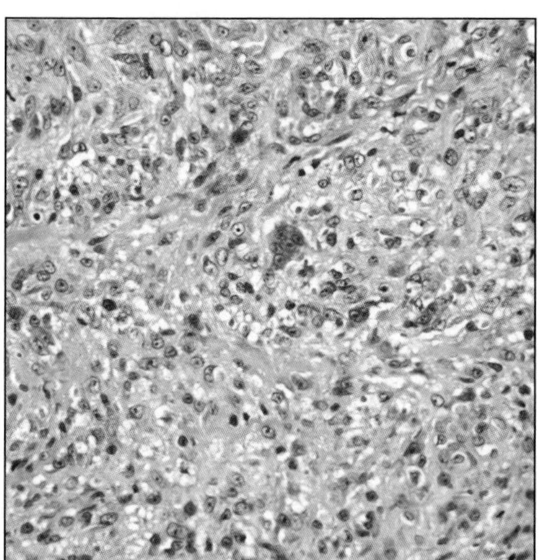

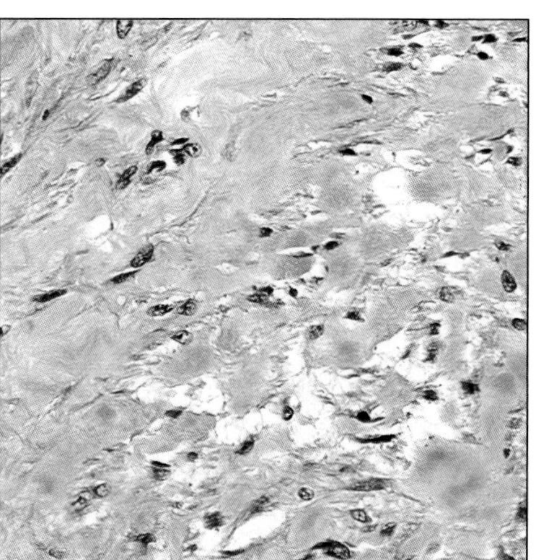

(Left) Hematoxylin & eosin shows delicate nuclear features of nodular fasciitis. Each myofibroblast contains a uniform nucleolus. Scattered extravasated erythrocytes are present without accompanying hemosiderin. **(Right)** Hematoxylin & eosin shows nodular fasciitis with abundant keloid-like collagen. This can be misinterpreted, especially in core biopsy, as fibromatosis (latter has parallel, evenly dispersed, more elongated cells, more uniform collagen, and mast cells).

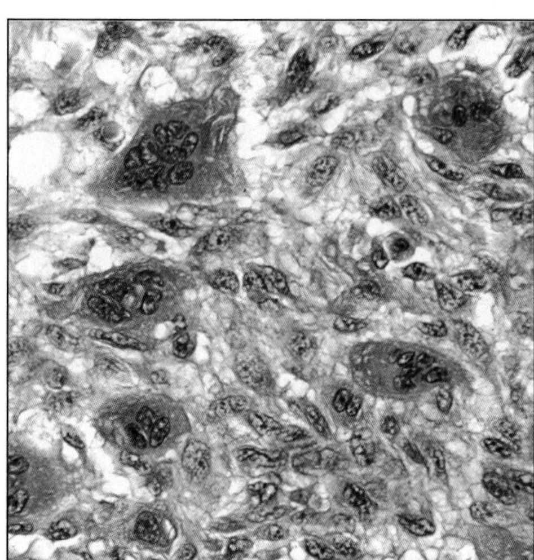

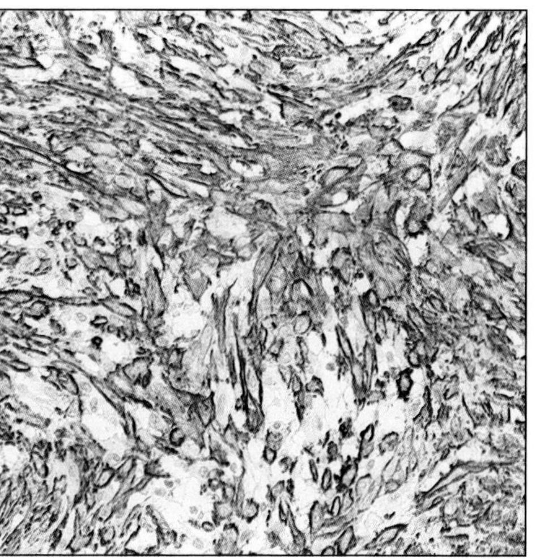

(Left) Hematoxylin & eosin shows an example of nodular fasciitis with prominent multinucleated giant cells. **(Right)** Actin-sm highlights the stellate proliferating myofibroblasts. This feature of nodular fasciitis can lead to a misinterpretation of leiomyosarcoma since mitoses are often found in nodular fasciitis. However, peripheral localization of staining within the cells is characteristic of myofibroblasts. They also lack H-caldesmon unlike smooth muscle cells.

Intravascular and Cranial Fasciitis

(Left) Intraoperative photograph shows an example of intravascular fasciitis that was clinically mistaken for a nerve sheath tumor. **(Right)** Trichrome shows a lesion that nearly occludes the vessel. Despite this, there is no hemosiderin deposition. This does not usually result in any functional impairment, and the lesion presents as a mass. Veins or arteries can be involved, and the lesional tissue sometimes extends through the vessel wall.

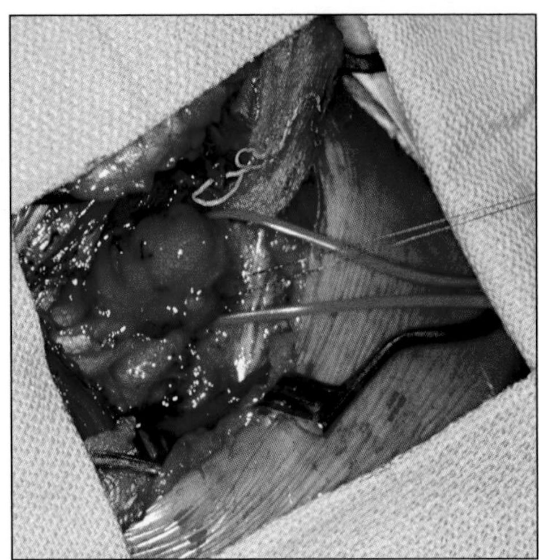

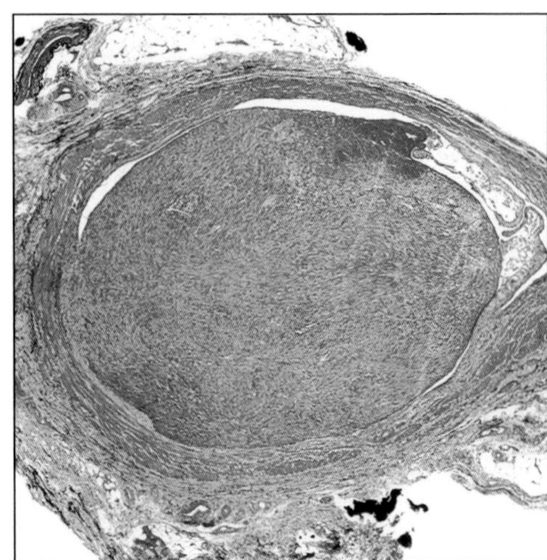

(Left) Hematoxylin & eosin shows the fascicular pattern of intravascular fasciitis, which, like nodular fasciitis, often features giant cells ➙. Note that the lesional cells have much paler nuclei than the lymphocytes and endothelial cells in the field. **(Right)** Hematoxylin & eosin shows intravascular fasciitis that has extended into a small capillary. In this image, the lesional cells ➯ have much paler nuclei than the surrounding endothelial cells ➙.

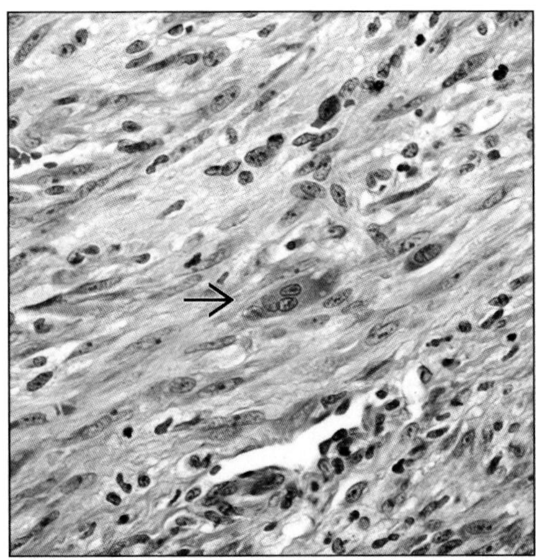

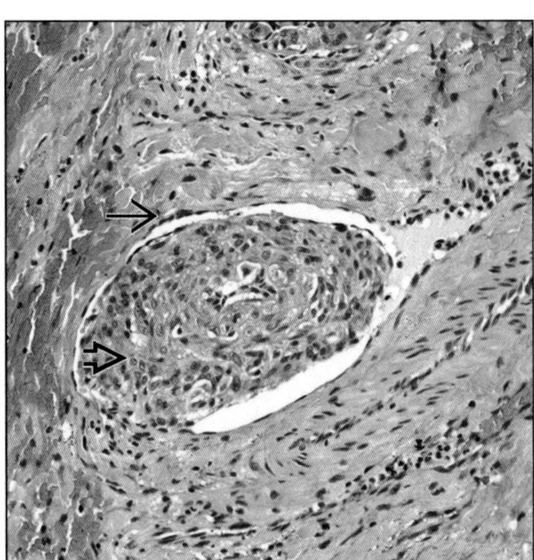

(Left) Hematoxylin & eosin shows an example of cranial fasciitis. At low magnification, the lesion appears loose and myxoid and uniform. It has fewer inflammatory cells and extravasated erythrocytes than typical nodular fasciitis. **(Right)** Hematoxylin & eosin shows cranial fasciitis at high magnification. The proliferating myofibroblasts have similar nuclear features to those of typical nodular fasciitis and intravascular fasciitis.

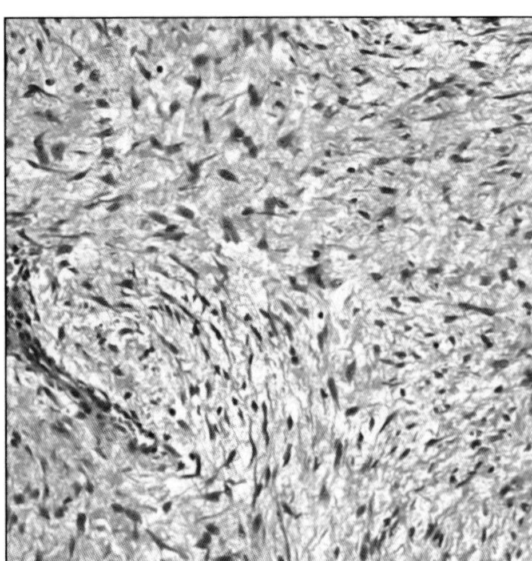

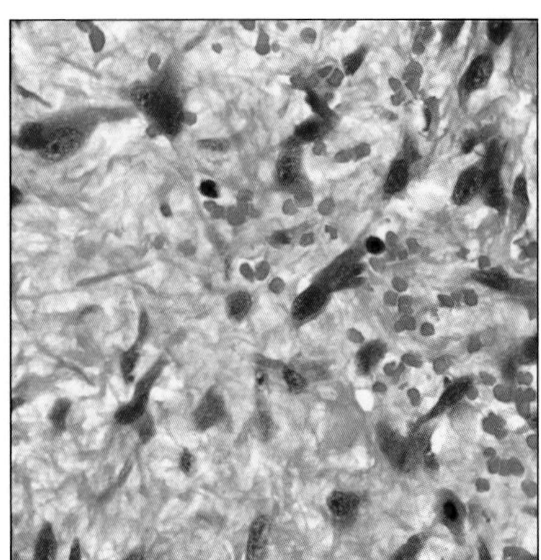

Differential Diagnosis

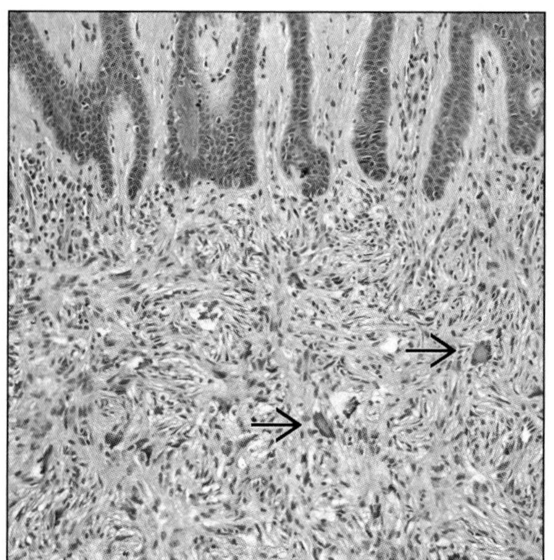

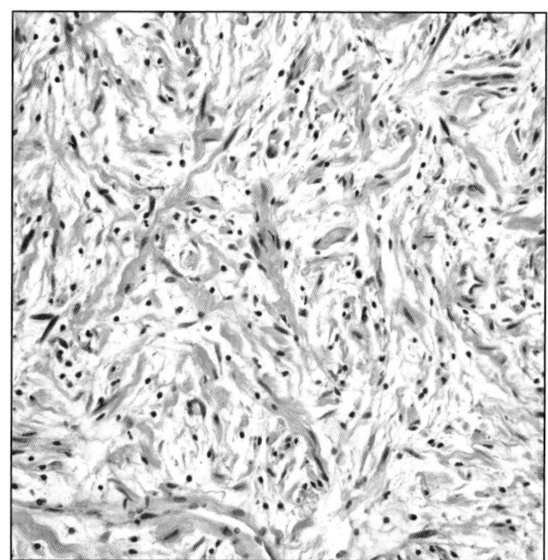

(Left) *Hematoxylin & eosin shows a fibrous histiocytoma (dermatofibroma). The lesion features darker nuclei than those of nodular fasciitis and a background of foam cells, multinucleated cells ⇒, plasma cells, lymphocytes, and hemosiderin. Note the overlying epidermal hyperplasia with increased basal pigmentation.* ***(Right)*** *Hematoxylin & eosin shows a neurofibroma featuring irregularly arranged wiry collagen with dark nuclei closely related to the collagen bundles.*

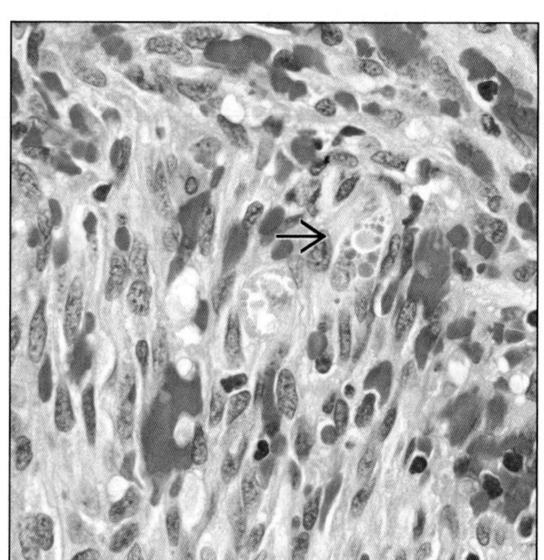

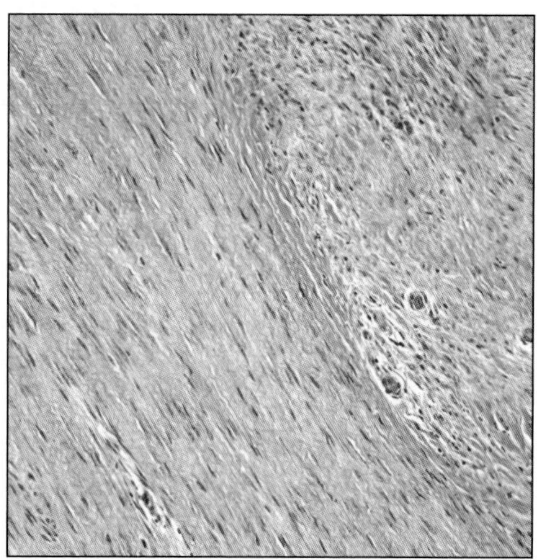

(Left) *Hematoxylin & eosin of Kaposi sarcoma shows hyperchromatic lesional cells and hyaline globules ⇒. The latter are erythrophagolysosomes.* ***(Right)*** *Hematoxylin & eosin shows the sweeping fascicular arrangement of fibromatosis. The collagen is denser than that seen in nodular fasciitis and distributed evenly throughout the lesion. The cells are relatively elongated and slender and aligned in a parallel fashion.*

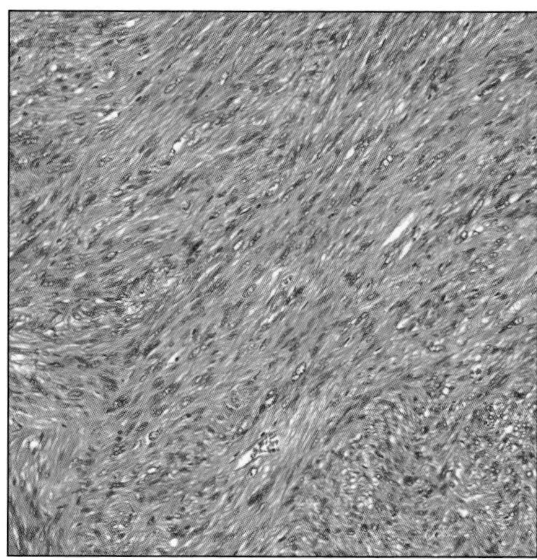

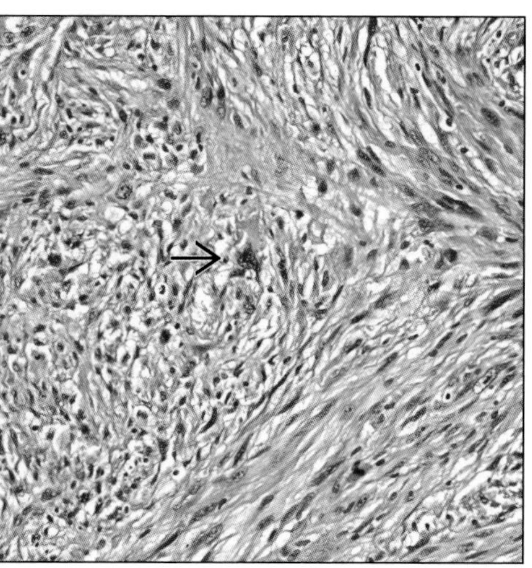

(Left) *Hematoxylin & eosin shows a leiomyosarcoma. The cytoplasm of the proliferating cells is brightly eosinophilic compared to the lesional cells in nodular fasciitis. The nuclei are somewhat hyperchromatic. The fascicles are arranged at right angles to each other, a characteristic feature of leiomyosarcoma.* ***(Right)*** *Hematoxylin & eosin shows a malignant fibrous histiocytoma (pleomorphic undifferentiated sarcoma). Note the storiform pattern and markedly pleomorphic nuclei ⇒.*

PROLIFERATIVE FASCIITIS/MYOSITIS

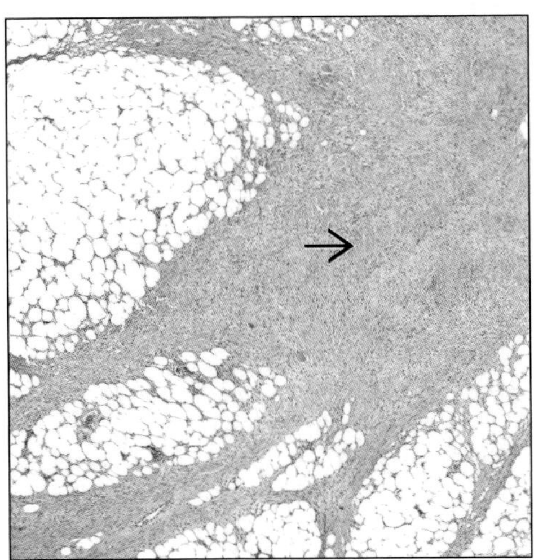

Hematoxylin & eosin shows proliferative fasciitis at low magnification. It tracks along fibrous septa and is somewhat less cellular in the center ⇒, where there is keloid-like collagen.

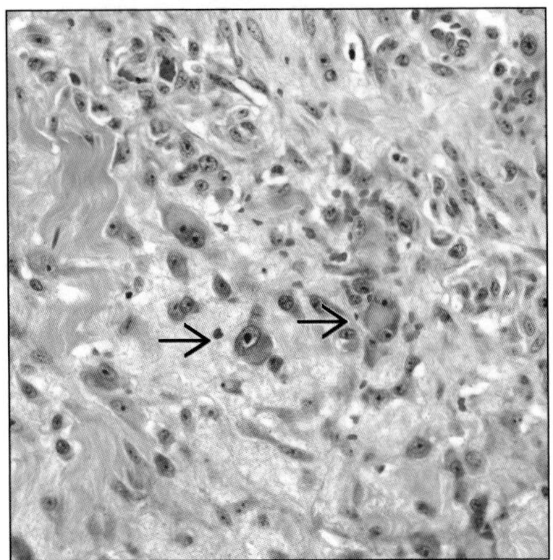

Hematoxylin & eosin shows the so-called ganglion-like cells ⇒ of proliferative fasciitis. These are fibroblasts, but their macronucleoli are reminiscent of those found in ganglion cells.

TERMINOLOGY

Definitions

- Tumefactive subcutaneous (fasciitis) or intramuscular (myositis) proliferation featuring ganglion-like fibroblasts
  - Background of myofibroblasts and fibroblasts similar to those in nodular fasciitis

CLINICAL ISSUES

Epidemiology

- Incidence
  - Rare; less common than nodular fasciitis
- Age
  - Middle-aged and older adults; rare in children
- Gender
  - No predominance

Site

- Proliferative fasciitis: Upper extremity (forearm) > lower extremity > trunk
- Proliferative myositis: Trunk > shoulder girdle > upper arm > thigh

Presentation

- Rapidly growing painless mass; more likely to be painful than nodular fasciitis
- Usually no history of trauma

Treatment

- Simple excision

Prognosis

- Benign lesions
  - Usually no recurrence even with incomplete excision

MACROSCOPIC FEATURES

General Features

- Poorly circumscribed mass extending along connective tissue septa
- Usually 2-3 cm; rare lesions 5 cm

MICROSCOPIC PATHOLOGY

Histologic Features

- Mostly plump stellate to spindled fibroblasts and myofibroblasts
- Extravasated erythrocytes
- Background lymphocytes
- Large ganglion-like fibroblasts
  - Macronucleoli, abundant amphophilic cytoplasm
  - Not true ganglion cells, no Nissl substance
- Mitotic activity common
- Pediatric examples
  - Predominance of ganglion-like cells
  - Exuberant mitotic activity
  - Frequently misinterpreted as sarcomas
- Rare reports of abnormal karyotypes
  - No consistent abnormality reported
  - Diploid on flow cytometry

DIFFERENTIAL DIAGNOSIS

Nodular Fasciitis

- Usually in young adults, 3-5 cm mass
- Loose storiform pattern
- Stellate myofibroblasts, lacks ganglion-like cells
- Background lymphocytes, extravasated erythrocytes
- Benign outcome even if incompletely excised

Dermatofibroma/Fibrous Histiocytoma

- Usually in adults
- Storiform pattern

PROLIFERATIVE FASCIITIS/MYOSITIS

Key Facts

Terminology

- Tumefactive subcutaneous (fasciitis) or intramuscular (myositis) proliferation featuring ganglion-like fibroblasts

Macroscopic Features

- Usually 2-3 cm

Microscopic Pathology

- Mostly plump stellate to spindled fibroblasts and myofibroblasts
- Large ganglion-like fibroblasts
- Macronucleoli, abundant amphophilic cytoplasm
- Mitotic activity common
- Pediatric examples can display exuberant mitotic activity, which can lead to misinterpretation as sarcomas

Immunohistochemistry

Antibody	Reactivity	Staining Pattern	Comment
Vimentin	Positive	Cytoplasmic	Labels both ganglion-like cells and background cells
Actin-sm	Negative		Can label background myofibroblasts
Desmin	Negative		Occasionally labels background myofibroblasts
Myogenin	Negative		Helpful to exclude rhabdomyosarcoma, especially in children
MYOD1	Negative		Helpful to exclude rhabdomyosarcoma, especially in children
Synaptophysin	Negative		
CK-PAN	Negative		
CD34	Negative		

- Background histiocytes, hemosiderin, plasma cells common
- Benign

Embryonal Rhabdomyosarcoma

- Usually involve genital region or head and neck of infants and young children
- Enhanced cellularity beneath mucous membranes (cambium layer)
- Atypical nuclei, usually without prominent nucleoli
- Display skeletal muscle differentiation on immunolabeling
- Responds to chemotherapy; 70-80% 5-year survival

Pleomorphic Rhabdomyosarcoma

- Highly aggressive lesions of adults, often in deep soft tissue of thigh
- Markedly pleomorphic cells
- Skeletal muscle differentiation on immunolabeling
- Poor 5-year survival

High-Grade Undifferentiated Pleomorphic Sarcoma

- Also termed malignant fibrous histiocytoma
- Large mass of deep soft tissues: Buttocks and thighs common
- Pleomorphic spindle cells

SELECTED REFERENCES

1. Meis JM et al: Proliferative fasciitis and myositis of childhood. Am J Surg Pathol. 16(4):364-72, 1992
2. Chung EB et al: Proliferative fasciitis. Cancer. 36(4):1450-8, 1975

IMAGE GALLERY

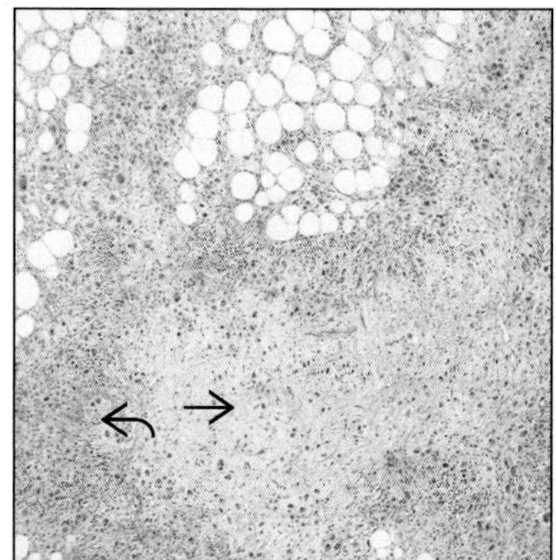

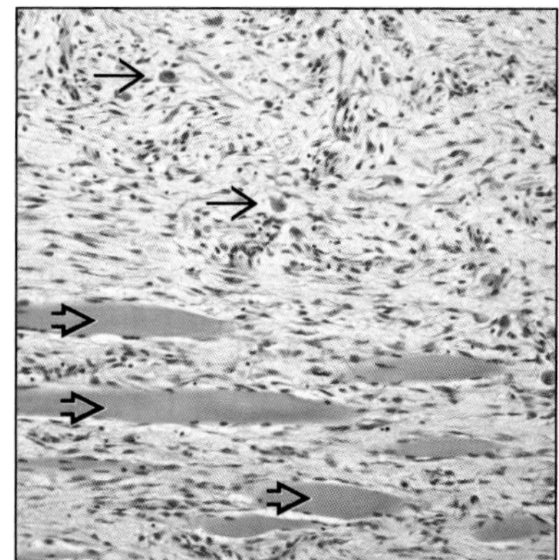

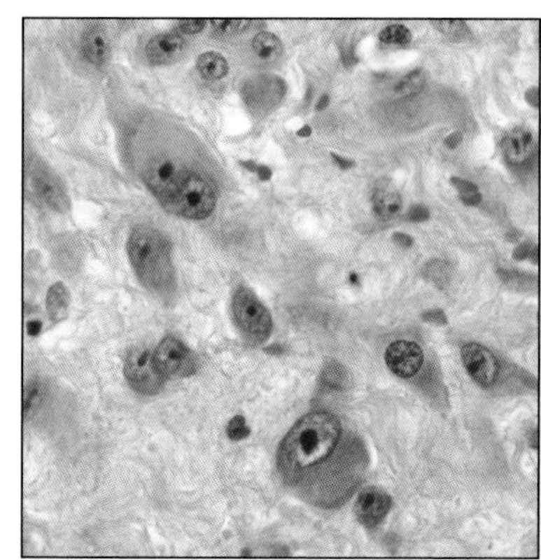

(Left) *Hematoxylin & eosin shows a more tumefactive example of proliferative fasciitis. The central portion ➔ is less cellular than the periphery ↶, which is more like nodular fasciitis.* ***(Center)*** *Hematoxylin & eosin shows proliferative myositis. There are several ganglion-like fibroblasts ➔ and a background that is nodular fasciitis-like. The process separates skeletal myocytes ➲.* ***(Right)*** *Hematoxylin & eosin shows high magnification of ganglion-like cells. This field also shows extravasated erythrocytes, a feature shared with nodular fasciitis.*

ISCHEMIC FASCIITIS

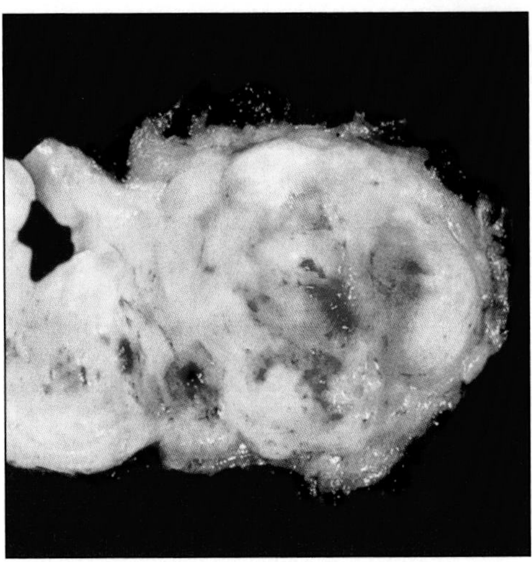

Gross photograph of ischemic fasciitis shows subcutaneous fat with hemorrhage, whitish fibrous tissue, and zonal necrosis.

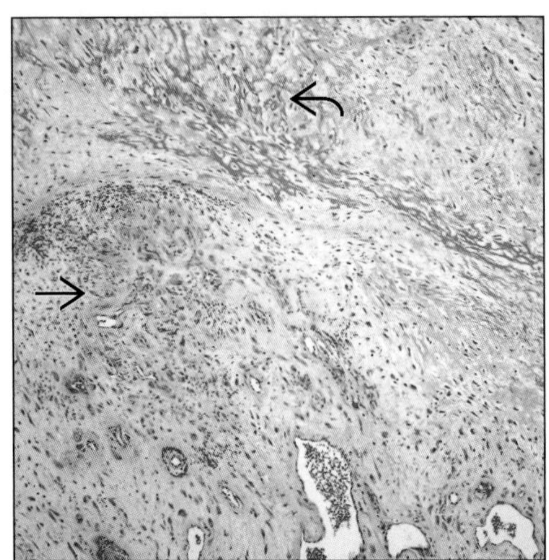

Hematoxylin & eosin shows a zone of fibrinoid necrosis ↩ and an area with vessels and fibroblasts →.

TERMINOLOGY

Synonyms

- Atypical decubital fibroplasia

Definitions

- Pseudosarcomatous proliferation composed of zones of fat and fibrinoid necrosis with ingrowth of capillaries, reactive fibroblasts, and myofibroblasts
  - Initially described as tumefactive pressure sore arising over bony prominences in debilitated patients
  - May also arise in other locations in nondebilitated persons

CLINICAL ISSUES

Epidemiology

- Incidence
  - Rare
- Age
  - Mean: 8th decade
    - Occasionally in younger adult patients
- Gender
  - No predominance

Site

- Usually around limb girdles and sacral region

Presentation

- Painless soft tissue mass
- Patients usually elderly
- Some patients are debilitated/bedridden

Prognosis

- Most cases do not recur following excision
  - Occasional recurrences in debilitated individuals

MACROSCOPIC FEATURES

General Features

- 1-8 cm ill-defined mass with necrosis and hemorrhage on cut surface

MICROSCOPIC PATHOLOGY

Histologic Features

- Ill-defined, focally myxoid masses
  - Lobular configuration
- Most involve deep subcutis
  - A few with extensions into adjacent skeletal muscle or tendon
- Epidermal ulceration typically absent
- Zones of fibrinoid necrosis and prominent myxoid stroma
- Necrotic zones rimmed by ingrowing, ectatic, thin-walled vascular channels
- Atypical enlarged degenerated fibroblasts with abundant basophilic cytoplasm, large hyperchromatic smudged nuclei, and prominent nucleoli
  - Similar to ganglion-like cells in proliferative fasciitis
- Occasional mitoses, including atypical forms

DIFFERENTIAL DIAGNOSIS

Well-Differentiated Liposarcoma

- Large deep soft tissues of proximal extremities and retroperitoneum
- Mature adipose tissue lesion with relatively uniform low-power appearance
- Fat separated by fibrous bands containing atypical hyperchromatic cells, no prominent nucleoli
- Occasional lipoblasts
- Usually no necrosis
- Minimal mitotic activity
- Low-grade sarcoma

ISCHEMIC FASCIITIS

Key Facts

Terminology
- Pseudosarcomatous proliferation

Clinical Issues
- Mean age: 8th decade
- Most cases do not recur following excision

Microscopic Pathology
- Most involve deep subcutis
- Epidermal ulceration typically absent
- Zones of fibrinoid necrosis and prominent myxoid stroma
- Necrotic zones rimmed by ingrowing, ectatic, thin-walled vascular channels
- Atypical enlarged degenerated fibroblasts with abundant basophilic cytoplasm, large hyperchromatic smudged nuclei, and prominent nucleoli

Immunohistochemistry

Antibody	Reactivity	Staining Pattern	Comment
Vimentin	Positive	Cytoplasmic	Strong diffuse pattern
Actin-HHF-35	Positive	Cytoplasmic	Focal in subset of cases, indicating myofibroblastic differentiation
Actin-sm	Positive	Cytoplasmic	Focal in subset of cases, indicating myofibroblastic differentiation
Desmin	Positive	Cytoplasmic	Focal in subset of cases, indicating myofibroblastic differentiation
CD34	Positive	Cell membrane	In atypical cells in some cases
CD68	Positive	Cytoplasmic	Reactive in ~ 2/3
CK-PAN	Negative		
S100	Negative		

Proliferative Fasciitis
- Small distal extremity lesions
- Proliferated along fascial planes in fusiform fashion
- Exuberant myofibroblastic proliferation with delicate vessels, extravasated erythrocytes, scattered lymphocytes
- Reactive fibroblasts with large nucleoli
- Mitoses may be numerous, especially in pediatric cases
- Benign

Nodular Fasciitis
- Small distal extremity lesions
- Exuberant myofibroblastic proliferation with delicate vessels, extravasated erythrocytes, scattered lymphocytes
- Mitoses may be numerous
- Benign

SELECTED REFERENCES

1. Liegl B et al: Ischemic fasciitis: analysis of 44 cases indicating an inconsistent association with immobility or debilitation. Am J Surg Pathol. 32(10):1546-52, 2008
2. Perosio PM et al: Ischemic fasciitis: a juxta-skeletal fibroblastic proliferation with a predilection for elderly patients. Mod Pathol. 6(1):69-72, 1993
3. Montgomery EA et al: Atypical decubital fibroplasia. A distinctive fibroblastic pseudotumor occurring in debilitated patients. Am J Surg Pathol. 16(7):708-15, 1992

IMAGE GALLERY

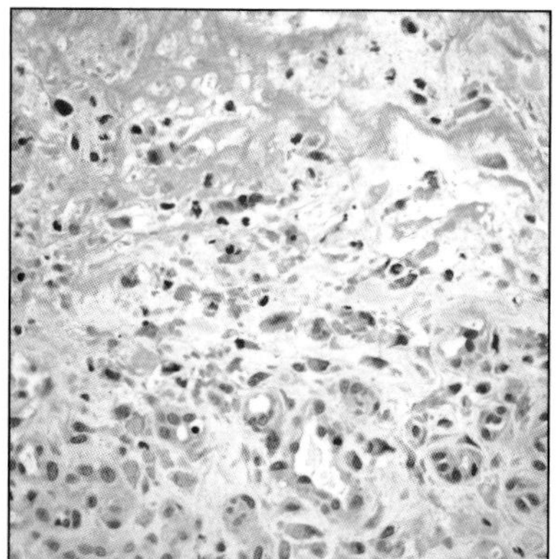

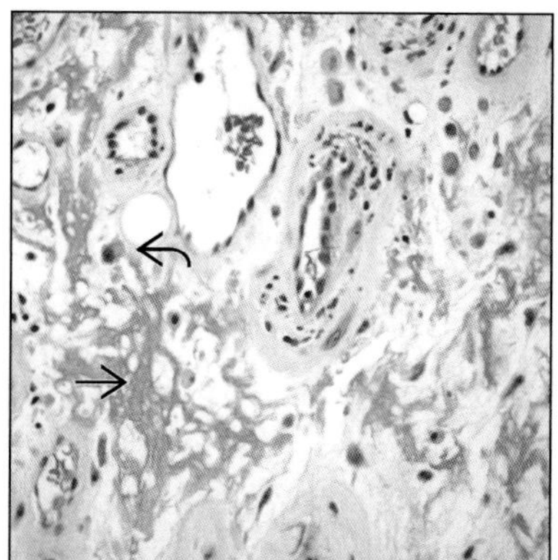

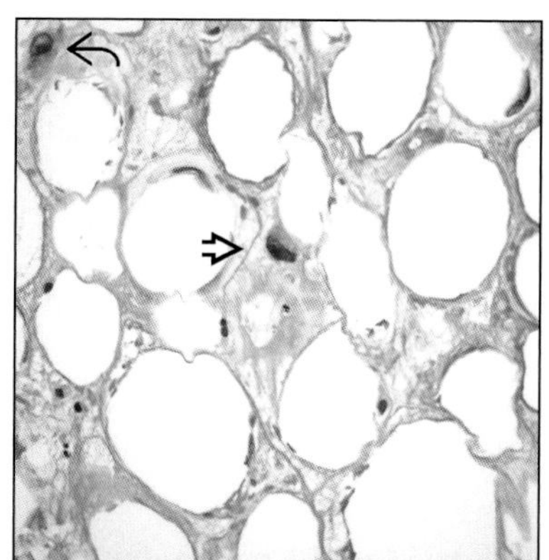

(Left) Hematoxylin & eosin shows the zonation in ischemic fasciitis. The top of the field is necrotic with ingrowth of capillaries and enlarged fibroblasts and myofibroblasts. ***(Center)*** Hematoxylin & eosin shows a few small vessels, fibrinoid necrosis ⇒, and cells with large nucleoli ⇗ reminiscent of those in proliferative fasciitis. ***(Right)*** Hematoxylin & eosin shows cells with large nucleoli ⇗ as well as cells with smudged nuclei ⇨.

FIBROUS HAMARTOMA OF INFANCY

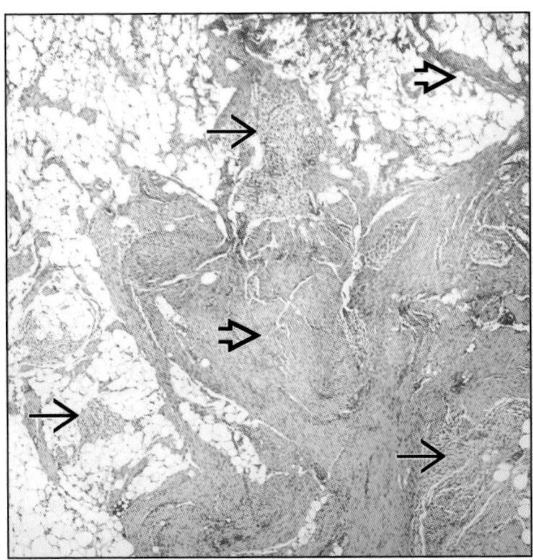

Hematoxylin & eosin shows fibrous hamartoma of infancy. The lesion is poorly defined, with nodules of rounded to ovoid cells ⇨ and fibrous bands of spindle cells ⇨ admixed with mature fat.

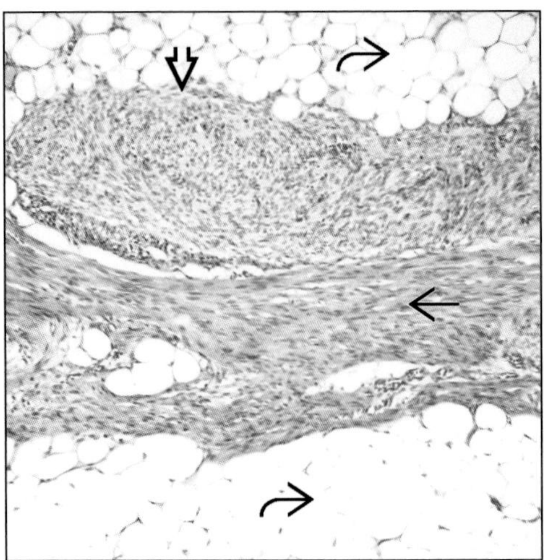

Hematoxylin & eosin shows fibrous hamartoma of infancy. Nodules of immature round to ovoid cells ⇨, situated within mature adipose tissue ⇨, abut the fibrous trabeculae ⇨.

TERMINOLOGY

Abbreviations

- Fibrous hamartoma of infancy (FHI)

Definitions

- Benign superficial fibrous lesion occurring in 1st 2 years of life

ETIOLOGY/PATHOGENESIS

Developmental Anomaly

- No conclusive familial or syndromic associations
  - Rare cases reported in tuberous sclerosis patients

CLINICAL ISSUES

Epidemiology

- Age
  - Infants and children up to 2 years
    - Up to 25% present at birth
  - Rarely in older children
- Gender
  - M > F

Site

- Deep dermis or subcutis
- Most occur in upper body, especially axillary fold
  - Other sites include upper arm, shoulder, forearm, groin, thigh, chest wall, back, neck, and scalp
- Usually solitary
  - Rarely multiple synchronous nodules

Presentation

- Suddenly enlarging mass
- Painless and often freely mobile

Natural History

- Rapid growth, which slows but does not regress

Treatment

- Complete local excision is curative

Prognosis

- Excellent, but can recur if incompletely excised

MACROSCOPIC FEATURES

General Features

- Poorly defined variegated surface
- Admixture of firm white tissue and fat
- Sometimes overlying skin changes (e.g., altered pigmentation)

Size

- Most up to 5 cm, but larger lesions reported

MICROSCOPIC PATHOLOGY

Histologic Features

- "Organoid" growth pattern
- 3 distinct components in varying amounts
  - Intersecting bands and trabeculae of mature fibrous tissue, comprising spindle myofibroblasts and fibroblasts
  - Nests and whorls of immature round, ovoid, or spindle cells
    - In loose myxoid stroma
    - Often arranged around small veins
  - Interspersed mature fat

ANCILLARY TESTS

Immunohistochemistry

- Vimentin in both fibrous and immature areas
- Actin and rarely CD34 or desmin in fibrous areas

Cytogenetics

- Translocations reported in 2 cases

FIBROUS HAMARTOMA OF INFANCY

Key Facts

Terminology

- Benign superficial fibrous lesion occurring during 1st 2 years of life

Clinical Issues

- Congenital in up to 25%
- M > F
- Occur in deep dermis or subcutis
- Typically in upper torso but at variety of sites
- Complete excision is curative
  - Can recur if incompletely excised

Microscopic Pathology

- 3 components in organoid growth pattern
  - Intersecting bands of mature fibrous tissue, comprising spindle myofibroblasts and fibroblasts
  - Nests of immature round, ovoid, or spindle cells in myxoid stroma
  - Interspersed mature fat

  - Reciprocal t(2;3)(q31;q21)
  - Complex t(6;12;8)(q25;q24.3;q13)
  - Raises possibility of FHI being neoplastic rather than hamartomatous

Electron Microscopy

- Transmission
  - Fibroblasts and myofibroblasts in fascicular areas
  - Primitive mesenchymal cells in immature areas
  - Irregular collagen fibers among mature fat

DIFFERENTIAL DIAGNOSIS

Fibromatosis

- No primitive oval cell component
- β-catenin(+) in nuclei

Infantile Fibromatosis/Lipofibromatosis

- Deep-seated
- Predilection for distal extremities
- Can occur in older children (up to early 2nd decade)
- No primitive oval cell component

Lipoblastoma

- Lobulated architecture
- Immature adipocytes

Diffuse Myofibromatosis

- Nodular cell proliferations
- Hemangiopericytoma-like areas

Embryonal Rhabdomyosarcoma

- Occurs in older children
- Cytologic atypia
- Desmin(+)

Infantile Fibrosarcoma

- Cells in sheets
- Lack of organoid pattern

SELECTED REFERENCES

1. Rougemont AL et al: A complex translocation (6;12;8) (q25;q24.3;q13) in a fibrous hamartoma of infancy. Cancer Genet Cytogenet. 171(2):115-8, 2006
2. Lakshminarayanan R et al: Fibrous hamartoma of infancy: a case report with associated cytogenetic findings. Arch Pathol Lab Med. 129(4):520-2, 2005
3. Popek EJ et al: Fibrous hamartoma of infancy in the genital region: findings in 15 cases. J Urol. 152(3):990-3, 1994
4. Sotelo-Avila C et al: Subdermal fibrous hamartoma of infancy: pathology of 40 cases and differential diagnosis. Pediatr Pathol. 14(1):39-52, 1994
5. Efem SE et al: Clinicopathological features of untreated fibrous hamartoma of infancy. J Clin Pathol. 46(6):522-4, 1993
6. Michal M et al: Fibrous hamartoma of infancy. A study of eight cases with immunohistochemical and electron microscopical findings. Pathol Res Pract. 188(8):1049-53, 1992
7. Groisman G et al: Fibrous hamartoma of infancy: an immunohistochemical and ultrastructural study. Hum Pathol. 22(9):914-8, 1991

IMAGE GALLERY

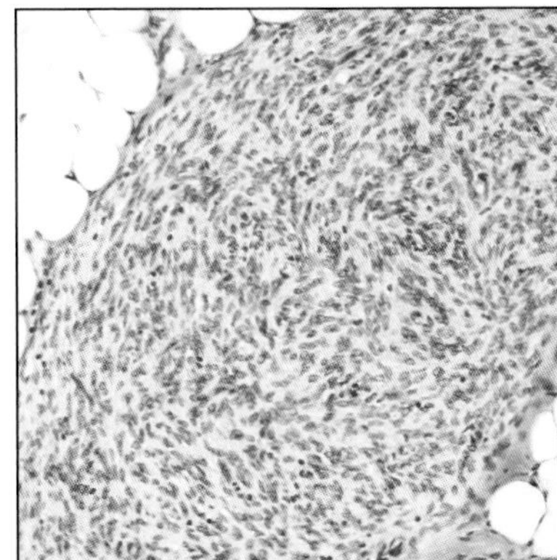

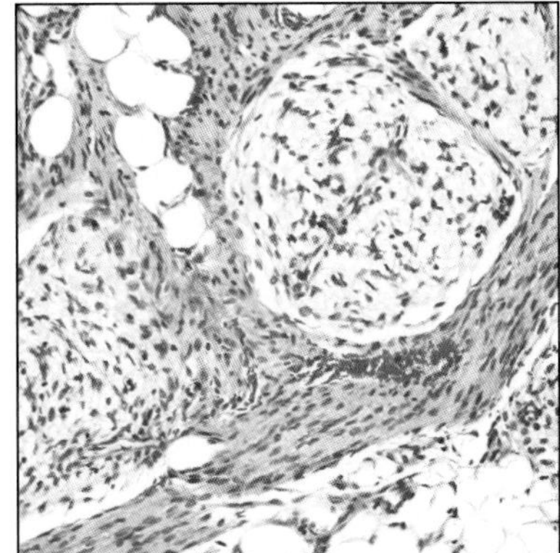

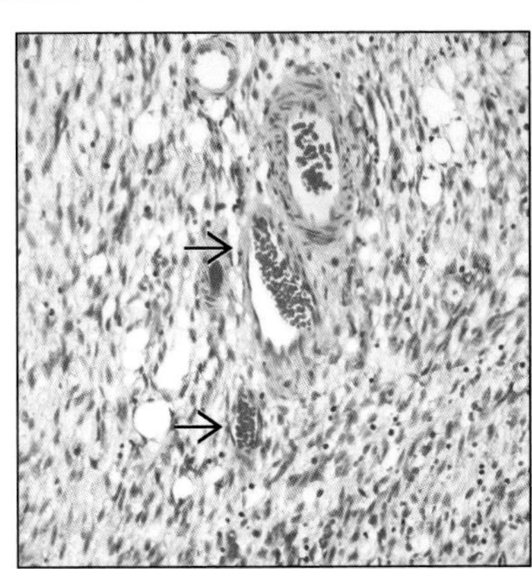

(Left) Hematoxylin & eosin shows fibrous hamartoma of infancy with a nodule composed of sheets of immature cells with bland, ovoid vesicular nuclei. Mitotic figures are absent. (Center) Hematoxylin & eosin shows the 3 components of fibrous hamartoma of infancy. There is prominent myxoid stroma within the nodules. No cellular atypia is seen in any of the elements. (Right) Hematoxylin & eosin shows fibrous hamartoma of infancy. The myxoid zones are often oriented around small veins ⇒.

MYOFIBROMA AND MYOFIBROMATOSIS

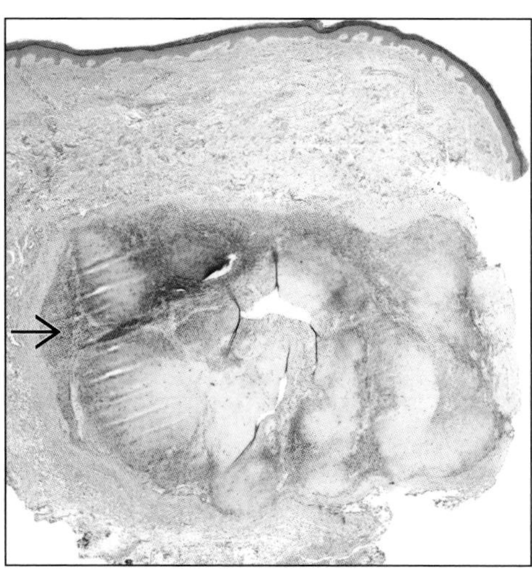

Hematoxylin & eosin shows a cutaneous myofibroma. Note the lobulated appearance at scanning magnification. In this example, the darker hemangiopericytoma-like component is peripheral ➔.

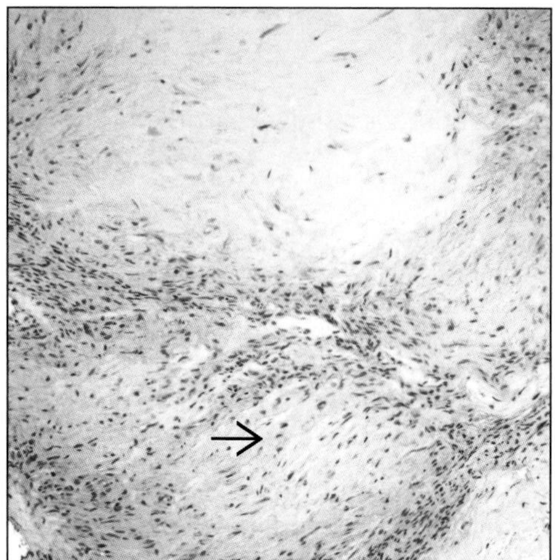

Hematoxylin & eosin shows myoid lobules separated by more cellular areas. The myoid cells have prominent cytoplasmic eosinophilia ➔.

TERMINOLOGY

Synonyms

- Infantile myofibromatosis, congenital generalized fibromatosis
  - Continuum with lesions termed "myopericytoma, infantile hemangiopericytoma"

Definitions

- Benign neoplasms composed of lobules of myoid cells separated by vascularized zones (biphasic pattern)
  - Solitary form (myofibroma)
  - Multicentric form (myofibromatosis)

CLINICAL ISSUES

Epidemiology

- Incidence
  - Solitary form rare but more common than multicentric form
  - Multicentric form extremely rare
  - Rare familial cases
- Age
  - Wide age range (neonates to elderly)
  - Most common in patients from birth to 2 years of age
- Gender
  - Male predominance

Site

- Most solitary examples in subcutaneous tissues of head and neck
  - Trunk, extremities
  - Occasional skeletal example, especially skull
- Multicentric form usually involves soft tissue and bone
  - Usually long bones
  - Visceral sites
    - Gastrointestinal tract
    - Liver, kidney, pancreas

Presentation

- Asymptomatic skin nodules with purplish color (solitary form)
- Visceral lesions with site-specific presentations
- Bone lesions seen as multiple elongated radiolucencies in metaphysis

Treatment

- Simple excision for solitary lesions
- Selective excisions for multicentric form

Prognosis

- Excellent for solitary form
- Outcome for multicentric form is function of involved sites
  - Extensive lung involvement poor prognostic factor

MICROSCOPIC PATHOLOGY

Histologic Features

- Most lesions well marginated
  - Can be locally infiltrative with intravascular and osseous extension and foci of necrosis
- Biphasic pattern
  - Myoid nodules separated by cellular pockets with hemangiopericytoma-like vascular pattern
  - Variable amounts of each component
  - Most cases have minimal mitotic activity
- Spindle cell areas
  - Prominent beneath ulcerated mucosal surfaces
- Myoid nodules
  - Pink cytoplasm and round to tapered nuclei
  - Myxoid change or hyalinization
- Hemangiopericytoma-like areas
  - Cellular but with minimal mitotic activity
  - Round cell similar to glomus cells

MYOFIBROMA AND MYOFIBROMATOSIS

Key Facts

Terminology
- Benign neoplasms composed of lobules of myoid cells separated by vascularized zones (biphasic pattern)
  - Solitary form (myofibroma)
  - Multicentric form (myofibromatosis)
- Synonyms: Infantile myofibromatosis, congenital generalized fibromatosis
  - Continuum with lesions termed "myopericytoma, infantile hemangiopericytoma"

Clinical Issues
- Most common from birth to 2 years of age
- Most solitary examples in subcutaneous tissues of head and neck
- Simple excision for solitary lesions
- Selective excisions for multicentric form
- Extensive lung involvement poor prognostic factor

Microscopic Pathology
- Biphasic pattern
  - Myoid nodules separated by cellular pockets with hemangiopericytoma-like vascular pattern
  - Variable amounts of each component
- Most cases have minimal mitotic activity
- Spindle cell areas
- Prominent beneath ulcerated mucosal surfaces

Ancillary Tests
- Usually label with α-actin and calponin but negative to focal desmin/focal caldesmon
- Negative S100 protein and keratin
- No characteristic alterations or mutation

Immunohistochemistry

Antibody	Reactivity	Staining Pattern	Comment
α1-antichymotrypsin	Positive	Cytoplasmic	Strong labeling in myoid component, minimal in vascular portion
Vimentin	Positive	Cytoplasmic	All components label
S100	Negative		
CD34	Negative		Occasional focal labeling
CK-PAN	Negative		
Desmin	Equivocal	Cytoplasmic	Usually focal and weak (or negative)
Caldesmon	Equivocal	Cytoplasmic	Focal in myofibroma; more labeling in myopericytoma

ANCILLARY TESTS

Immunohistochemistry
- Usually label with α-actin and calponin but not desmin or caldesmon
- Negative S100 protein and keratin

Cytogenetics
- No characteristic alterations or mutation

DIFFERENTIAL DIAGNOSIS

Smooth Muscle Tumors
- Not lobulated
- Perpendicularly oriented fascicles, cigar-shaped nuclei
- Express actins, desmin, caldesmon

Fibromatosis
- Highly infiltrative growth pattern; sweeping fascicles of myofibroblasts
- Express actins, usually not desmin; nuclear β-catenin labeling
- β-catenin and *APC* mutations

Hemangiopericytoma
- No myoid areas
- Infantile form part of continuum with myofibroma

SELECTED REFERENCES

1. Dray MS et al: Myopericytoma: a unifying term for a spectrum of tumours that show overlapping features with myofibroma. A review of 14 cases. J Clin Pathol. 59(1):67-73, 2006
2. Gengler C et al: Solitary fibrous tumour and haemangiopericytoma: evolution of a concept. Histopathology. 48(1):63-74, 2006
3. Mentzel T et al: Myopericytoma of skin and soft tissues: clinicopathologic and immunohistochemical study of 54 cases. Am J Surg Pathol. 30(1):104-13, 2006
4. Montgomery E et al: Myofibromas presenting in the oral cavity: a series of 9 cases. Oral Surg Oral Med Oral Pathol Oral Radiol Endod. 89(3):343-8, 2000
5. Granter SR et al: Myofibromatosis in adults, glomangiopericytoma, and myopericytoma: a spectrum of tumors showing perivascular myoid differentiation. Am J Surg Pathol. 22(5):513-25, 1998
6. Coffin CM et al: Congenital generalized myofibromatosis: a disseminated angiocentric myofibromatosis. Pediatr Pathol Lab Med. 15(4):571-87, 1995
7. Smith KJ et al: Cutaneous myofibroma. Mod Pathol. 2(6):603-9, 1989
8. Jennings TA et al: Infantile myofibromatosis. Evidence for an autosomal-dominant disorder. Am J Surg Pathol. 8(7):529-38, 1984
9. Chung EB et al: Infantile myofibromatosis. Cancer. 48(8):1807-18, 1981

MYOFIBROMA AND MYOFIBROMATOSIS

Microscopic Features

(Left) **Hematoxylin & eosin shows many vessels at the periphery of a myoid nodule in a myofibroma. The stroma has a chondromyxoid appearance. *(Right)* Hematoxylin & eosin shows high magnification of the myoid cells in a myofibroma. Many of the cells have prominent cytoplasmic eosinophilia ⇒, and there are delicate amphophilic cytoplasmic processes ↗.**

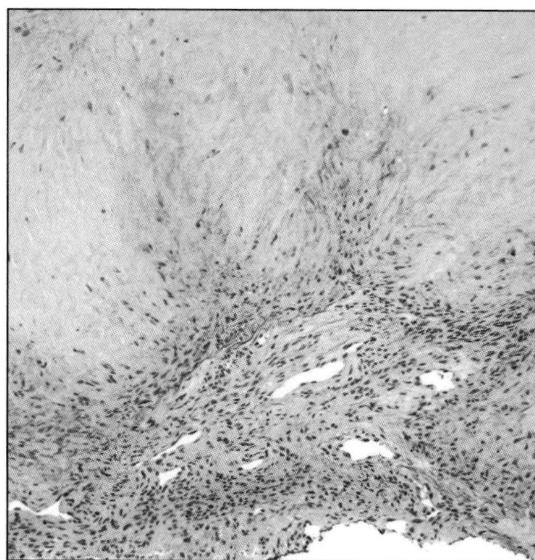

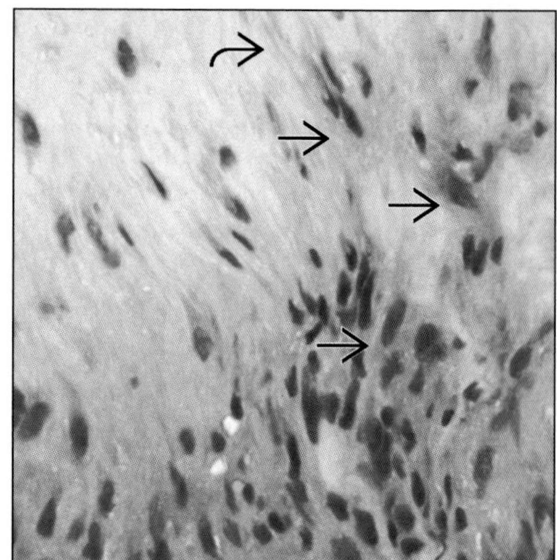

(Left) *Hematoxylin & eosin shows a prominent lobular configuration in a myofibroma. Note the biphasic appearance; the upper portion of the field shows a prominent hemangiopericytomatous vascular pattern ⇨.* ***(Right)*** *Hematoxylin & eosin shows higher magnification of the hemangiopericytoma-like component of a myofibroma.*

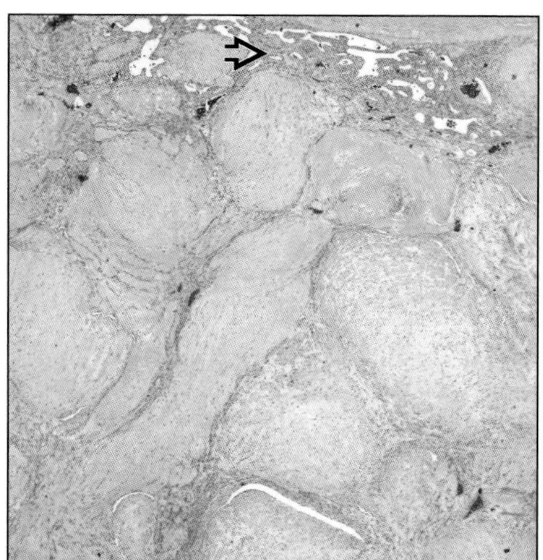

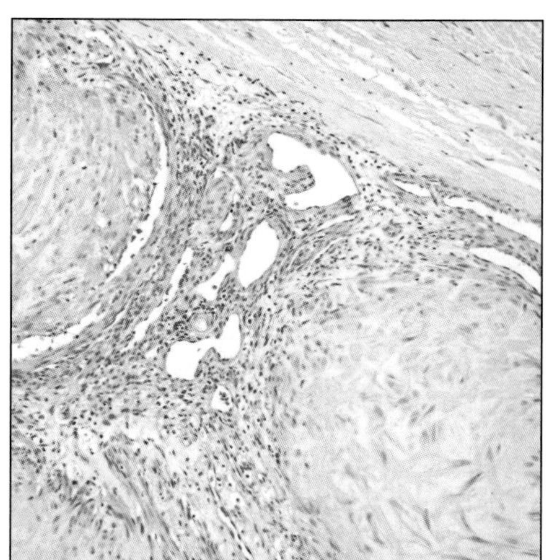

(Left) *Hematoxylin & eosin shows a skeletal myofibroma. There is a vaguely lobulated appearance, and the tumor is infiltrative at the periphery. There is also focal necrosis ⇨.* ***(Right)*** *Hematoxylin & eosin shows a myofibroma of the parotid region of a child. The spindle cells are arranged in nodules.*

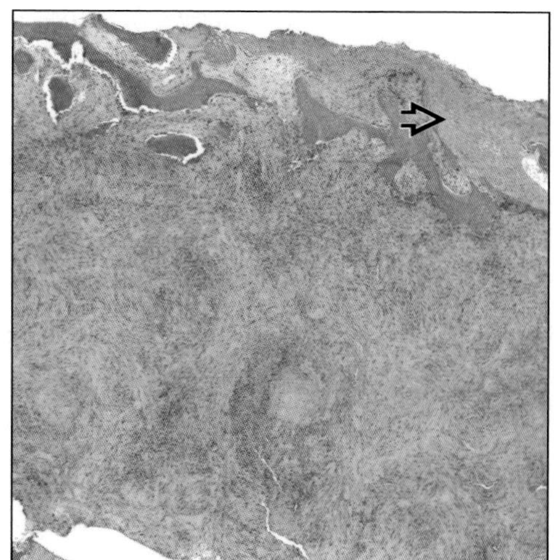

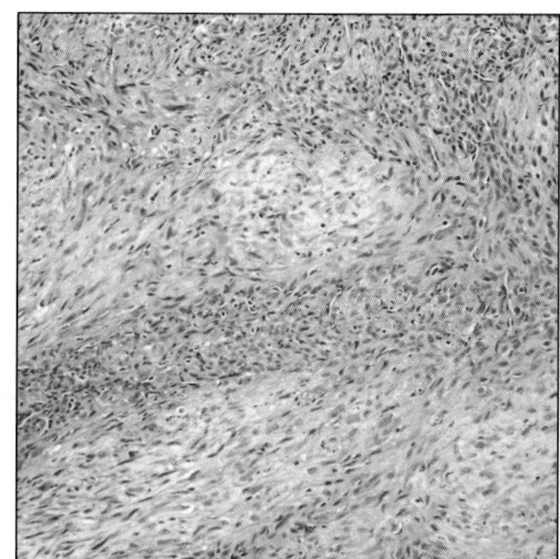

Microscopic Features

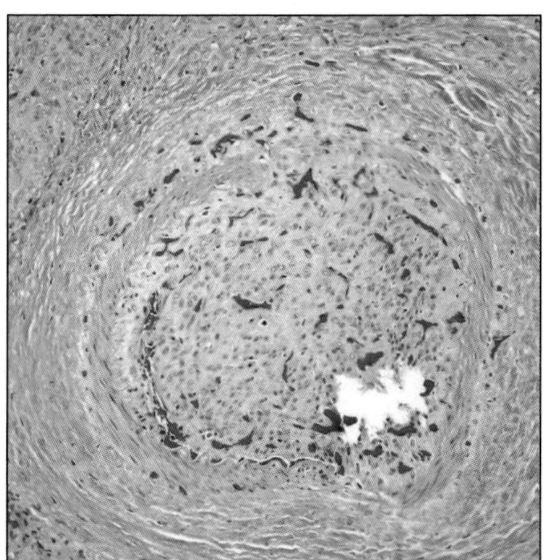

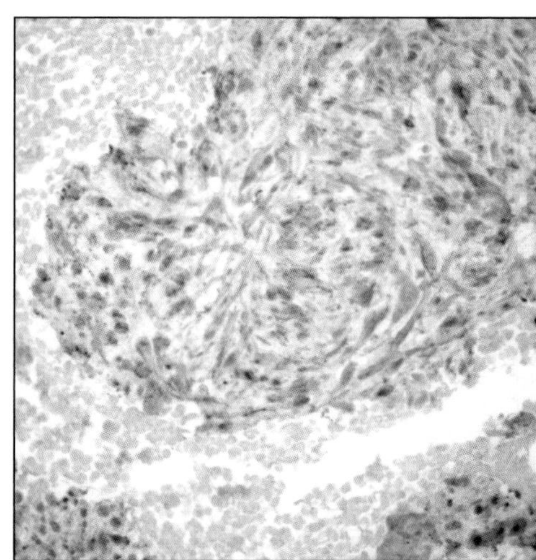

(Left) *Hematoxylin & eosin shows vascular space invasion in a myofibroma. This feature can lead to an erroneous interpretation of malignancy.* ***(Right)*** *Actin-HHF-35 shows cytoplasmic labeling in a myofibroma.*

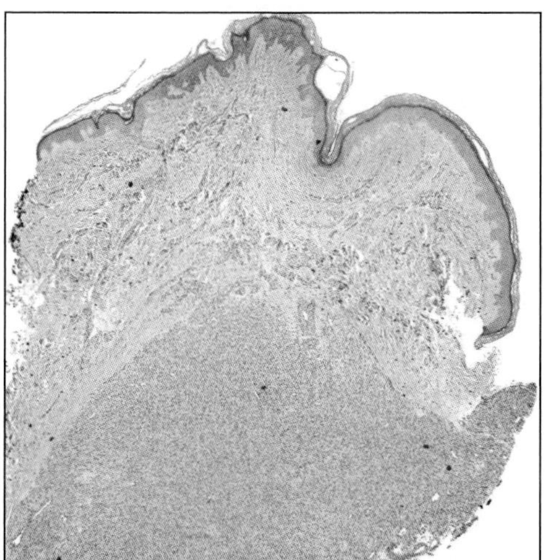

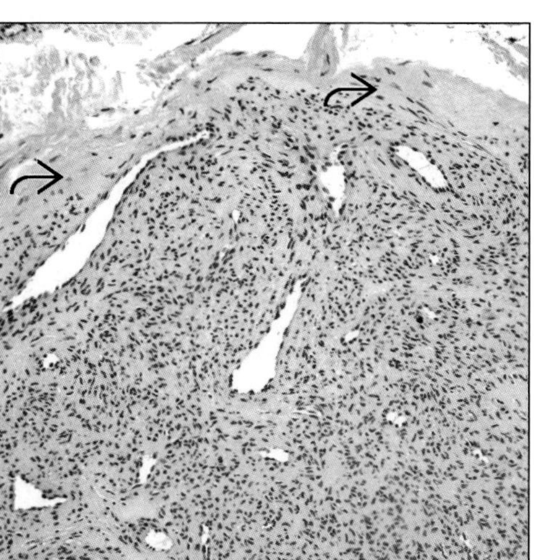

(Left) *Hematoxylin & eosin shows another lesion that has a predominance of hemangiopericytoma-like areas. This lesion would be regarded as "myopericytoma" to underscore this finding.* ***(Right)*** *Hematoxylin & eosin shows higher magnification. Subtle myoid features can be appreciated, particularly at the edge of the nodule ↷.*

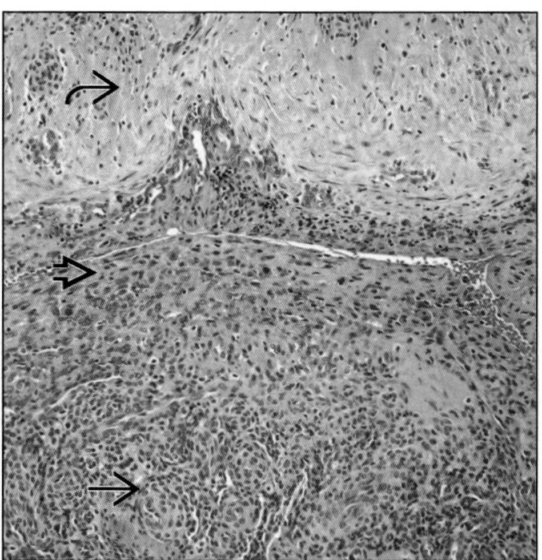

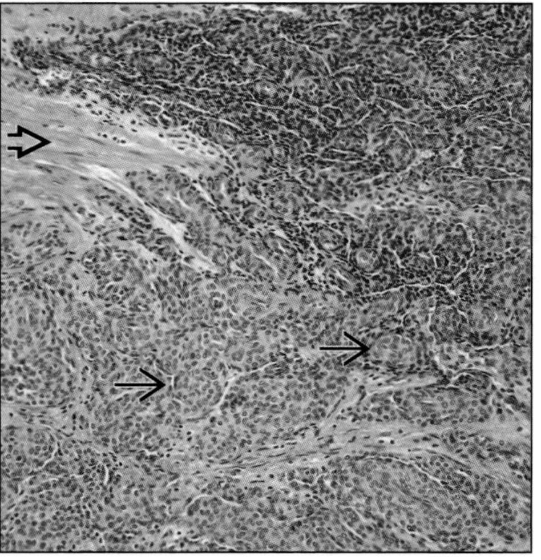

(Left) *Hematoxylin & eosin shows a lesion with myoid ↷, whorled hemangiopericytomatous →, and glomus cell ⇨ areas. Such a lesion would be classified as a myopericytoma, a tumor within a continuum with myofibroma.* ***(Right)*** *Hematoxylin & eosin shows another field from the lesion in the previous image. The cellular areas are alarming but have negligible mitotic activity. Note the myoid area ⇨ and whorled areas →.*

DERMATOMYOFIBROMA

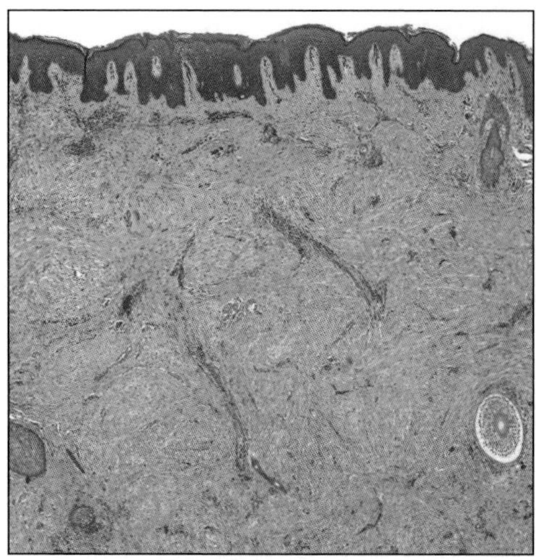

Scanning magnification of a dermatomyofibroma shows a dermal-based, plaque-like spindle proliferation with overlying epidermal hyperplasia, similar to a dermatofibroma.

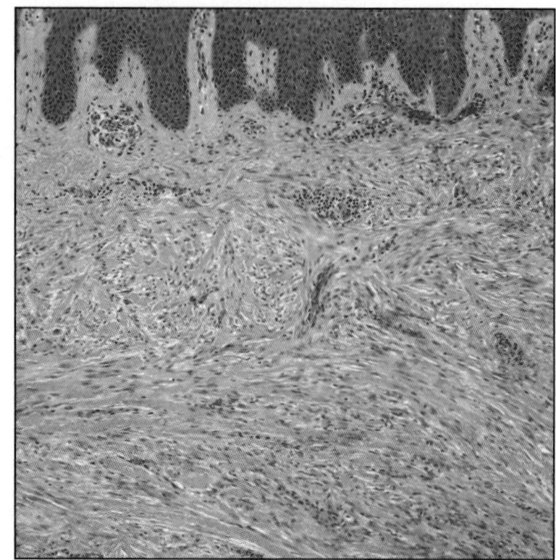

Higher magnification shows a proliferation of bland spindle cells arranged in fascicles, largely running parallel to the epidermis and associated with collagen trapping.

TERMINOLOGY

Synonyms

- Plaque-like dermal fibromatosis

Definitions

- Myofibroblastic tumor with many features similar to dermatofibroma

ETIOLOGY/PATHOGENESIS

Unknown

- May be related to trauma in some cases

CLINICAL ISSUES

Epidemiology

- Incidence
  - Rare tumor
- Age
  - Usually occurs in young adults
- Gender
  - M:F = 1:8

Site

- Typically present in shoulder and axillary regions
  - Also present in trunk, head and neck

Presentation

- Slow-growing indurated plaque or nodule
  - Often red-brown in color
- Rarely may present as multiple lesions

Treatment

- Surgical approaches
  - Complete surgical excision is curative

Prognosis

- Excellent
  - No malignant potential but may continue to enlarge if not completely removed

MACROSCOPIC FEATURES

General Features

- Small, dermal-based nodule

Size

- Usually 1-2 cm in size but occasionally much larger

MICROSCOPIC PATHOLOGY

Histologic Features

- Dermal-based, plaque-like spindle cell proliferation
  - Usually located in reticular dermis but may show involvement of superficial subcutis
  - Adnexal structures are usually preserved
  - Overlying epidermal hyperplasia, similar to dermatofibroma, is often seen
- Tumor is composed of broad fascicles of elongated monomorphous spindle cells
  - Nuclei bland and tapered
  - Uniform chromatin
  - Small nucleoli
  - Cytoplasm eosinophilic, poorly delineated
- Mitotic figures are rare and not atypical
- Elastic fibers are typically increased in numbers and fragmented
  - Highlight with elastic stains

Predominant Pattern/Injury Type

- Fibrous/spindle cell proliferation
- Parallel orientation to epidermis

Predominant Cell/Compartment Type

- Fibroblast, myofibroblast

DERMATOMYOFIBROMA

Key Facts

Terminology

- Myofibroblastic tumor with features overlapping with dermatofibroma

Clinical Issues

- Slow-growing plaque or nodule

Microscopic Pathology

- Dermal-based spindle cell proliferation
- Tumor is composed of broad fascicles of elongated monomorphous spindle cells oriented parallel to surface
- Elastic fibers are typically increased in numbers and fragmented, which may be highlighted with elastic stains

Top Differential Diagnoses

- Dermatofibroma
- Hypertrophic scar

ANCILLARY TESTS

Immunohistochemistry

- Tumor cells variably positive for smooth muscle actin (SMA)
- Cells are negative for muscle specific actin (MSA), desmin, S100, CD34, and FXIIIA

DIFFERENTIAL DIAGNOSIS

Dermatofibroma

- Lacks parallel orientation
- Shows more prominent collagen trapping

Leiomyoma

- Shows more clear-cut smooth muscle differentiation with SMA, MSA, and desmin staining
- Fascicles of spindle cells not typically oriented parallel to epidermis

Hypertrophic Scar

- Dense proliferation of collagen with vertically oriented vessels
- Adnexal structures are lost, as opposed to dermatomyofibroma

Dermatofibrosarcoma Protuberans

- Plaque-like variant can show histologic features similar to dermatomyofibroma
- In dermatofibrosarcoma protuberans, CD34 is typically strongly positive and SMA is negative

DIAGNOSTIC CHECKLIST

Pathologic Interpretation Pearls

- Dermal-based, plaque-like proliferation composed of broad fascicles of elongated monomorphous spindle cells oriented parallel to surface

SELECTED REFERENCES

1. Mentzel T et al: Dermatomyofibroma: clinicopathologic and immunohistochemical analysis of 56 cases and reappraisal of a rare and distinct cutaneous neoplasm. Am J Dermatopathol. 31(1):44-9, 2009
2. Viglizzo G et al: A unique case of multiple dermatomyofibromas. Clin Exp Dermatol. 33(5):622-4, 2008
3. Mortimore RJ et al: Dermatomyofibroma: a report of two cases, one occurring in a child. Australas J Dermatol. 42(1):22-5, 2001
4. Mentzel T et al: Dermatomyofibroma: additional observations on a distinctive cutaneous myofibroblastic tumour with emphasis on differential diagnosis. Br J Dermatol. 129(1):69-73, 1993
5. Cooper PH: Dermatomyofibroma: a case of fibromatosis revisited. J Cutan Pathol. 19(2):81-2, 1992
6. Kamino H et al: Dermatomyofibroma. A benign cutaneous, plaque-like proliferation of fibroblasts and myofibroblasts in young adults. J Cutan Pathol. 19(2):85-93, 1992

IMAGE GALLERY

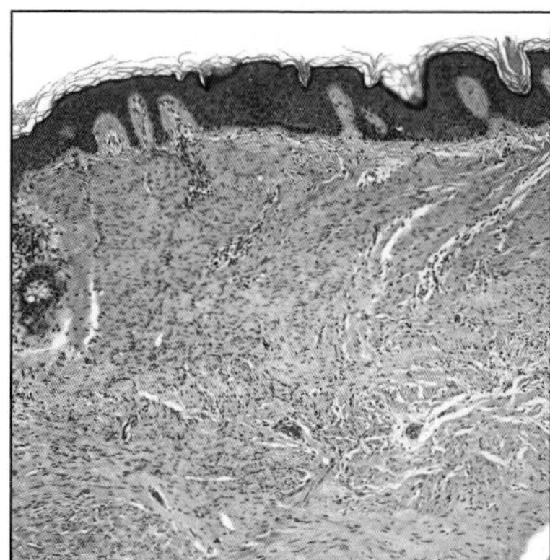

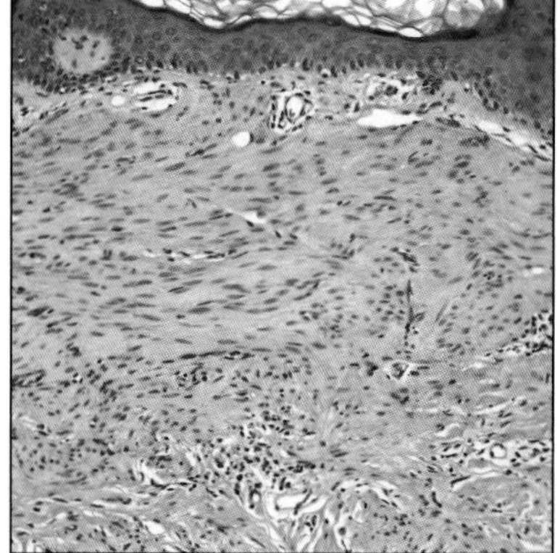

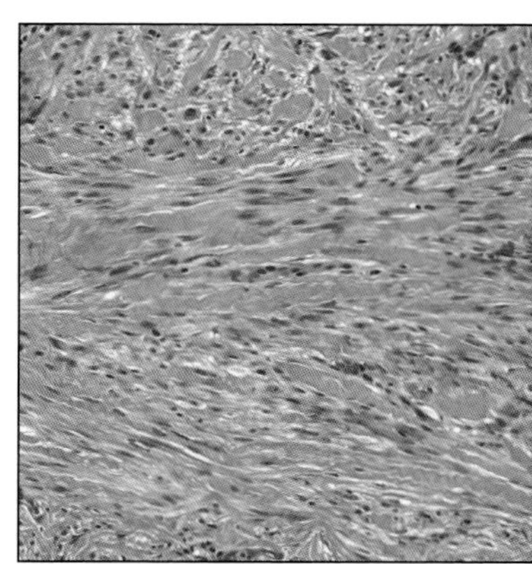

(Left) *Another example of a dermatomyofibroma shows a scar-like plaque of spindle cells in the dermis associated with mild chronic inflammation and increased numbers of small blood vessels.* ***(Center)*** *Higher magnification shows the superficial portion of the lesion closely approaching the epidermis.* ***(Right)*** *High-power examination shows bland cytologic features of the elongated myofibroblastic cells. There is also associated collagen trapping.*

GIANT CELL ANGIOFIBROMA

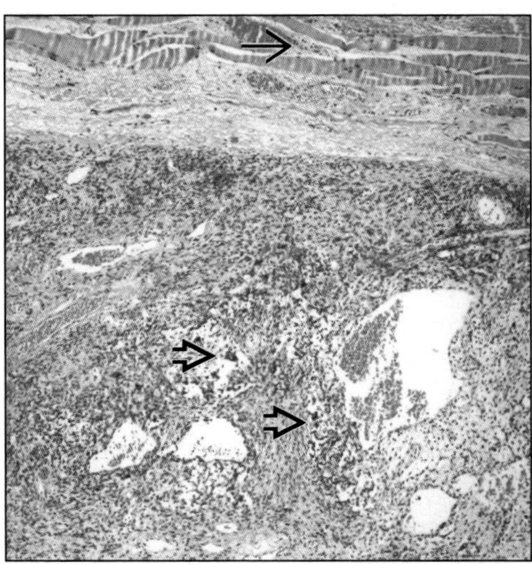

Giant cell angiofibromas are well-circumscribed tumors. The lesion shown here is sharply demarcated from skeletal muscle ➔. Scattered larger nuclei are discernible at low-power examination ➔.

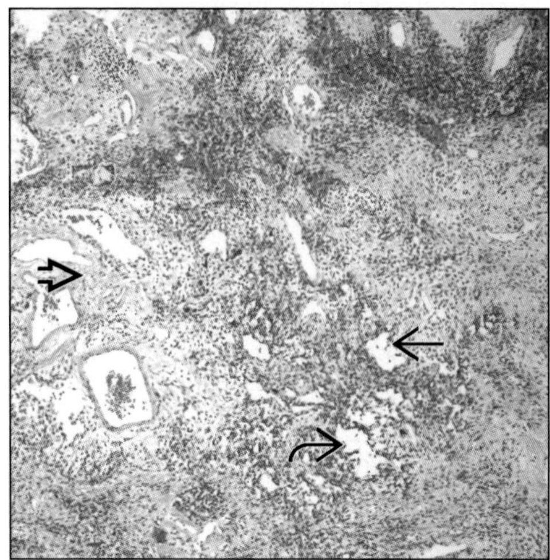

Hypocellular ➔ and hypercellular ➔ areas with ectatic pseudovascular spaces ➔ are present in giant cell angiofibroma.

TERMINOLOGY

Abbreviations

- Giant cell angiofibroma (GCAF)

Definitions

- Benign fibroblastic tumor with multinucleated tumor giant cells and angiectoid spaces
  - May be giant-cell-rich variant of solitary fibrous tumor/hemangiopericytoma (SFT/HP)

CLINICAL ISSUES

Epidemiology

- Age
  - Middle-aged adults
- Gender
  - Orbital lesions predominate in men
  - Extraorbital lesions predominate in women

Site

- Orbital involvement common
- Extraorbital lesions are usually subcutaneous
  - Head and neck
  - Back, axilla, inguinal region
  - Mediastinum and retroperitoneum
  - Vulva

Presentation

- Painful or painless mass
- Typically slow growing

Treatment

- Surgical excision is curative

Prognosis

- Excellent; does not recur following complete surgical excision

MACROSCOPIC FEATURES

General Features

- Well-circumscribed tumor
- Cystic change and hemorrhage common

Size

- Orbital lesions are small in size
- Extraorbital lesions may attain large size

MICROSCOPIC PATHOLOGY

Histologic Features

- Bland round-spindle cell proliferation
- Variable cellularity
- Prominent angiectoid (pseudovascular) spaces
- Multinucleated tumor giant cells
  - Variable number; cluster around angiectoid spaces
  - Nuclei in giant cells resemble those of surrounding round-spindle cells
  - Appear different from osteoclast-type multinucleate giant cells seen in fibrous histiocytoma
- Collagenous or myxoid stroma
- "Hemangiopericytoma-like" or thick-walled blood vessels with perivascular hyalinization
- Single rare example of GCAF with mature fat has been described
  - Supports theory that GCAF is giant-cell-rich variant of SFT/HP

Cytologic Features

- No cytological atypia

ANCILLARY TESTS

Immunohistochemistry

- CD34(+), CD99(+)
  - Both mononuclear and multinucleated cells
- Bcl-2(+) (about 80%); focal EMA or actin-sm positivity

GIANT CELL ANGIOFIBROMA

Key Facts

Terminology

- Benign fibroblastic tumor with multinucleated tumor giant cells and angiectoid spaces
  - May be related to solitary fibrous tumor/ hemangiopericytoma group

Clinical Issues

- Lesion of middle-aged adults; often involves orbit
  - Extraorbital lesions predominate in women
- Does not recur following complete surgical excision

Microscopic Pathology

- Bland spindle to round cell proliferation with variable cellularity
- Prominent angiectoid spaces; cystic change and hemorrhage
- Multinucleated stromal cells around angiectoid spaces
- Tumor cells are CD34(+) and CD99(+)

- Some cases may be hormone receptor positive (ER, PR)

Cytogenetics

- Abnormality of 6q and t(12;17) has been reported in GCAF

DIFFERENTIAL DIAGNOSIS

Giant Cell Fibroblastoma

- a.k.a. **juvenile dermatofibrosarcoma protuberans (DFSP)**
- Also CD34(+); pseudovascular spaces and giant cells present
- Occurs in infants and children; infiltrative margins; more myxoid
- Same cytogenetic abnormality as in DFSP

Schwannoma

- Diffuse strong S100 positivity in tumor cells

Fibrous Histiocytoma

- Polymorphic cell population (spindle cells, histiocytoid cells, macrophages, inflammatory cells)

Monophasic Synovial Sarcoma

- Cellular and fascicular spindle cell tumor
- Lacks pseudovascular spaces and stromal giant cells
- Keratin(+); t(X;18) diagnostic

DIAGNOSTIC CHECKLIST

Clinically Relevant Pathologic Features

- Age distribution
  - Middle-aged adults

Pathologic Interpretation Pearls

- May be giant-cell-rich variant of solitary fibrous tumor/hemangiopericytoma
- Combination of round-spindle cells, pseudovascular spaces, and multinucleated tumor giant cells

SELECTED REFERENCES

1. Guillou L et al: Orbital and extraorbital giant cell angiofibroma: a giant cell-rich variant of solitary fibrous tumor? Clinicopathologic and immunohistochemical analysis of a series in favor of a unifying concept. Am J Surg Pathol. 24(7):971-9, 2000
2. Hayashi N et al: Giant cell angiofibroma of the orbit and eyelid. Ophthalmology. 106(6):1223-9, 1999
3. Fukunaga M et al: Giant cell angiofibroma of the mediastinum. Histopathology. 32(2):187-9, 1998
4. Mikami Y et al: Extraorbital giant cell angiofibromas. Mod Pathol. 10(11):1082-7, 1997
5. Dei Tos AP et al: Giant cell angiofibroma. A distinctive orbital tumor in adults. Am J Surg Pathol. 19(11):1286-93, 1995

IMAGE GALLERY

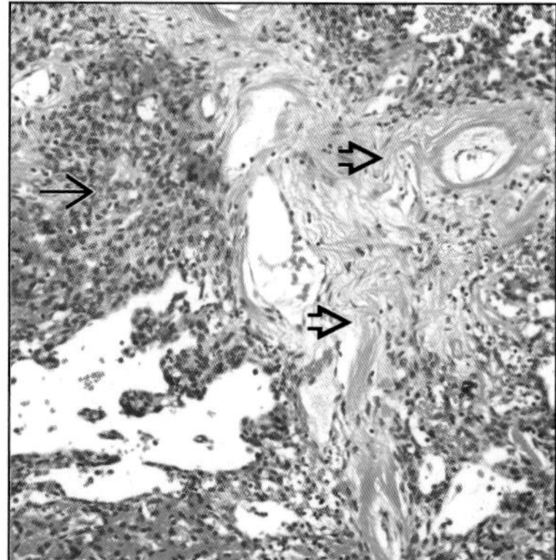

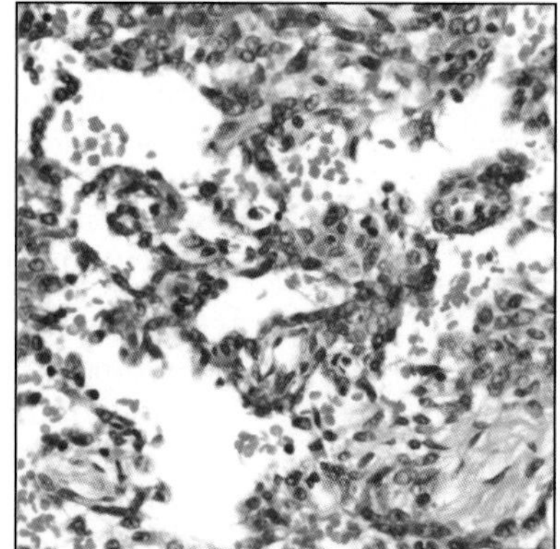

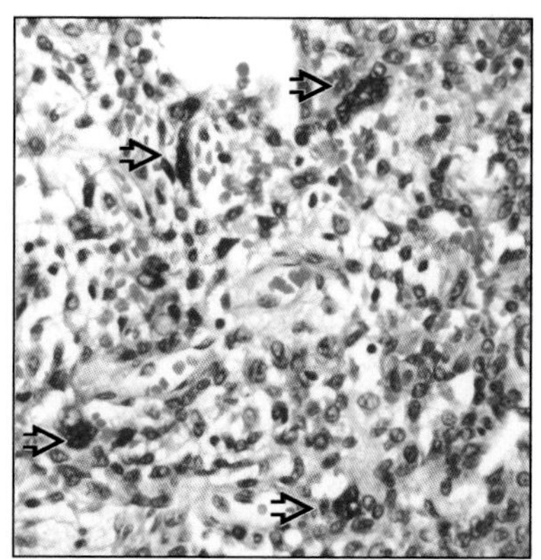

(Left) *Collagenized stroma with perivascular hyalinization ⇒ alternates with more cellular round cell areas on the left →.* ***(Center)*** *The angiectoid pseudovascular spaces are lined by small round cells with high nuclear-to-cytoplasmic ratio.* ***(Right)*** *The nuclei within stromal giant cells ⇒ appear similar to those in the surrounding tumor cells. The multinucleated giant cells tend to cluster around the angiectoid spaces.*

NASOPHARYNGEAL ANGIOFIBROMA

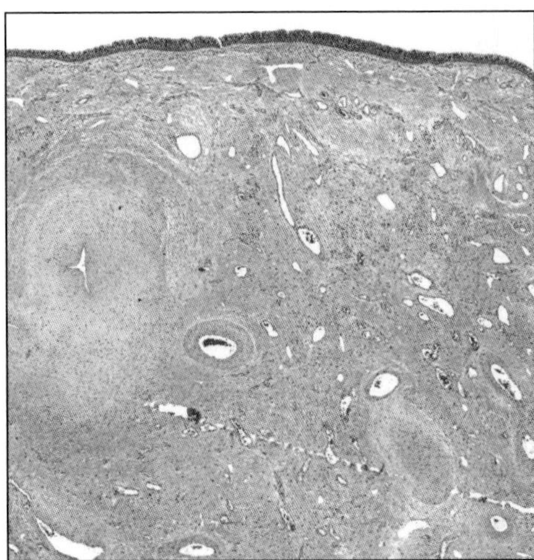

Low magnification shows an intact surface with a wide variety of vessels in a fibrous stroma. Some of the vessels have smooth muscle, and others do not. Patulous and compressed vessels are noted.

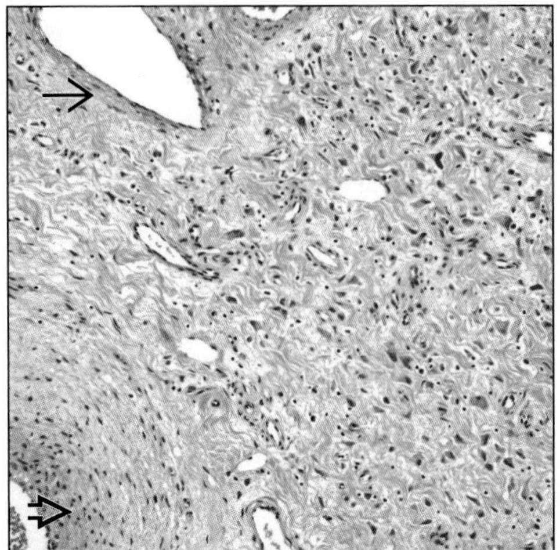

Smooth-muscle-walled vessels ➢ lie close to vessels without smooth muscle ➔. There are also numerous capillaries in the fibrous stroma. The lesion is moderately cellular and lacks atypia.

TERMINOLOGY

Abbreviations

- Juvenile angiofibroma (JNA)
- Angiofibroma (AF)

Synonyms

- Angiomyofibroblastoma-like tumor
- Angiofibroma
- Fibroangioma
- Fibroma

Definitions

- Benign, highly cellular, and richly vascularized mesenchymal neoplasm arising in nasopharynx in males

ETIOLOGY/PATHOGENESIS

Hormonal

- Testosterone-dependent puberty-induced growth can be blocked with estrogen &/or progesterone therapy

Genetic

- Reported association with familial adenomatous polyposis

CLINICAL ISSUES

Epidemiology

- Incidence
  - < 1% of all nasopharyngeal tumors
  - < 0.1% of all head and neck neoplasms
- Age
  - < 20 years old
    - Adolescents to young men
    - Peak in 2nd decade of life
- Gender
  - Males exclusively
  - If diagnosed in female, studies of sex chromosomes required to confirm gender
- Ethnicity
  - Worldwide distribution
  - Higher frequency in Caucasians
    - Favors fair-skinned, red-haired individuals

Site

- Nasopharynx usually affected
- Pterygoid region usually affected
- May expand to involve surrounding structures (30% of cases)
  - Anterior: Nasal cavity and maxillary sinus via roof of nasopharynx
  - Lateral: Temporal and infratemporal fossae via pterygomaxillary fissure, resulting in cheek or intraoral buccal mass
  - Posterior: Middle cranial fossa
  - Superior: Pterygopalatine fossa and orbit via inferior and superior orbital fissures resulting in proptosis
  - Medial: Contralateral side

Presentation

- Nasal obstruction
- Recurrent, spontaneous epistaxis
- Nasal discharge
- Facial deformity (proptosis), exophthalmia, diplopia
- Rhinolalia, sinusitis
- Otitis media, tinnitus, deafness
- Headaches
- Rarely, anosmia or pain
- Symptoms present for 12-24 months (nonspecific presentation)

Treatment

- Options, risks, complications
  - Benign tumor can show aggressive local growth
  - Biopsy is contraindicated due to potential exsanguination
  - Potential for facial deformity if allowed to grow
- Surgical approaches

NASOPHARYNGEAL ANGIOFIBROMA

Key Facts

Terminology

- Benign, highly cellular, and richly vascularized mesenchymal neoplasm arising in nasopharynx in males

Clinical Issues

- Recurrent, spontaneous epistaxis
- Nasopharynx is nearly always affected
- Patients < 20 years old
- Males exclusively
- Recurrences in ~ 20% of patients
- Up to 22 cm in size, mean: 4 cm

Image Findings

- Anterior bowing of posterior wall of maxillary sinus with posterior displacement of pterygoid plates (Holman-Miller sign)
- Angiography identifies feeding vessel(s) and allows for presurgical embolization
- Tumor blush is characteristic

Microscopic Pathology

- Submucosal proliferation of vascular component within fibrous stroma
- Many variably sized disorganized vessels
- Fibrous stroma consists of plump spindle, angular, or stellate-shaped cells
- Variable amounts of fine and coarse collagen fibers
- Elastic tissue is not identified within stroma

Top Differential Diagnoses

- Lobular capillary hemangioma
- Antrochoanal polyp
- Inflammatory polyp

  - Surgery is treatment of choice
  - Definitive resection is frequently associated with significant morbidity
- Drugs
  - Preoperative hormone therapy
    - Not as popular as other modalities
    - Giving estrogens to pubertal males is undesirable
- Radiation
  - Used to manage large, intracranial, or recurrent tumors
- Angiography
  - Selective angiography allows embolization with sclerosing agent or cryotherapy

Prognosis

- Good
- May have fatal exsanguination if incorrectly managed
- Recurrences in ~ 20% of patients
  - Usually develop within 2 years of diagnosis
  - Commonly extend intracranially

IMAGE FINDINGS

General Features

- Best diagnostic clue
  - Anterior bowing of posterior wall of maxillary sinus with posterior displacement of pterygoid plates (Holman-Miller sign)
- Location
  - Nasopharynx with extension into surrounding structures
- Angiography identifies feeding vessel(s) and allows for presurgical embolization
  - Tumor blush is characteristic

CT Findings

- Allows for accurate determination of size and extent
- Enhancement is different from adjacent muscle, accentuated with contrast
- Bony margins may be eroded

MACROSCOPIC FEATURES

General Features

- Polypoid mass with multinodular contour
- Red, gray-tan cut surface

Size

- Mean: 4 cm
- Range: Up to 22 cm

MICROSCOPIC PATHOLOGY

Histologic Features

- Submucosal proliferation of vascular component within fibrous stroma
- Many variably sized disorganized vessels
  - Varying thickness of vessel wall with patchy muscle content
  - Vessels are mostly thin walled, slit-like ("staghorn")
  - Range from capillary size to large, dilated, patulous vessels
- Focal pad-like smooth muscle thickenings within vessel walls
- Endothelial cells may be plump but are usually attenuated
- Fibrous stroma consists of plump spindle, angular, or stellate-shaped cells
- Variable amounts of fine and coarse collagen fibers
- Myxoid degeneration is common (especially in embolized specimens)
  - May see foreign material within vessel walls in embolized cases
- As stroma increases, vascular compression results in virtually nonexistent lumina
- Elastic tissue is not identified within stroma
- Stromal cells may be angulated, multinucleated, and pleomorphic
- Mitotic figures are sparse
- Mast cells may be seen
- Hormone-treated cases show increased collagenization of stroma with fewer but thicker-walled vessels

NASOPHARYNGEAL ANGIOFIBROMA

Immunohistochemistry

Antibody	Reactivity	Staining Pattern	Comment
Vimentin	Positive	Cytoplasmic	All elements of tumor
Actin-sm	Positive	Cytoplasmic	Smooth muscle of vessel walls highlighted
Actin-HHF-35	Positive	Cytoplasmic	Smooth muscle of vessel walls highlighted
Desmin	Positive	Cytoplasmic	Only within larger vessel walls
Androgen receptor	Positive	Nuclear	Stromal cells and endothelial cell nuclei
ER	Positive	Nuclear	Variably reactive, mostly in vascular nuclei
PR	Positive	Nuclear	Variably reactive, mostly in vascular nuclei
FVIIIRAg	Positive	Cytoplasmic	Endothelial cells only
CD34	Positive	Cytoplasmic	Endothelial cells only
CD31	Positive	Cytoplasmic	Endothelial cells only
PDGF-B	Positive	Cytoplasmic	
IGF-2	Positive	Cytoplasmic	
β-catenin-nuclear	Positive	Nuclear	Usually widespread in lesional cells
S100	Negative		Highlights entrapped nerves but not tumor cells

Staging for Nasopharyngeal Angiofibroma

Stage	Radiographic, Clinical, or Pathologic Finding
I	Tumor limited to nasopharynx with no bone destruction
II	Tumor invading nasal cavity, maxillary, ethmoid, and sphenoid sinus with no bone destruction
III	Tumor invading pterygopalatine fossa, infratemporal fossa, orbit, and parasellar region
IV	Tumor with massive invasion of cranial cavity, cavernous sinus, optic chiasm, or pituitary fossa

- Sarcomatous transformation is exceedingly uncommon event
  - Develops following massive doses of radiation

ANCILLARY TESTS

Histochemistry

- Reticulin shows positive black staining around stromal cells and blood vessels
- Elastic van Gieson highlights elastic tissue within vessel walls

Immunohistochemistry

- Vessels are highlighted within myofibroblastic stroma

DIFFERENTIAL DIAGNOSIS

Lobular Capillary Hemangioma

- Lesion is ulcerated; arises from different anatomic site; has granulation-type tissue and lots of inflammation; vessels are more organized

Inflammatory Polyp

- Especially if there are atypical stromal cells; usually more edematous; lacks rich vascular investment

Antrochoanal Polyp

- Arises from different location; heavy stromal fibrosis but usually lacks characteristic vascular pattern of juvenile angiofibroma

SELECTED REFERENCES

1. Bleier BS et al: Current management of juvenile nasopharyngeal angiofibroma: a tertiary center experience 1999-2007. Am J Rhinol Allergy. 23(3):328-30, 2009
2. Carrillo JF et al: Juvenile nasopharyngeal angiofibroma: clinical factors associated with recurrence, and proposal of a staging system. J Surg Oncol. 98(2):75-80, 2008
3. Coutinho-Camillo CM et al: Genetic alterations in juvenile nasopharyngeal angiofibromas. Head Neck. 30(3):390-400, 2008
4. Glad H et al: Juvenile nasopharyngeal angiofibromas in Denmark 1981-2003: diagnosis, incidence, and treatment. Acta Otolaryngol. 127(3):292-9, 2007
5. Tyagi I et al: Staging and surgical approaches in large juvenile angiofibroma--study of 95 cases. Int J Pediatr Otorhinolaryngol. 70(9):1619-27, 2006
6. Thompson LDR et al: Tumours of the Nasopharynx: Nasopharyngeal angiofibroma. Barnes EL et al: Pathology and Genetics of Head and Neck Tumours. World Health Organization Classification of Tumours. Lyon, France: IARC Press. 102-3, 2005
7. Fletcher CD: Distinctive soft tissue tumors of the head and neck. Mod Pathol. 15(3):324-30, 2002
8. Lee JT et al: The role of radiation in the treatment of advanced juvenile angiofibroma. Laryngoscope. 112(7 Pt 1):1213-20, 2002
9. Coffin CM et al: Fibroblastic-myofibroblastic tumors in children and adolescents: a clinicopathologic study of 108 examples in 103 patients. Pediatr Pathol. 11(4):569-88, 1991
10. Makek MS et al: Malignant transformation of a nasopharyngeal angiofibroma. Laryngoscope. 99(10 Pt 1):1088-92, 1989

Microscopic and Immunohistochemical Features

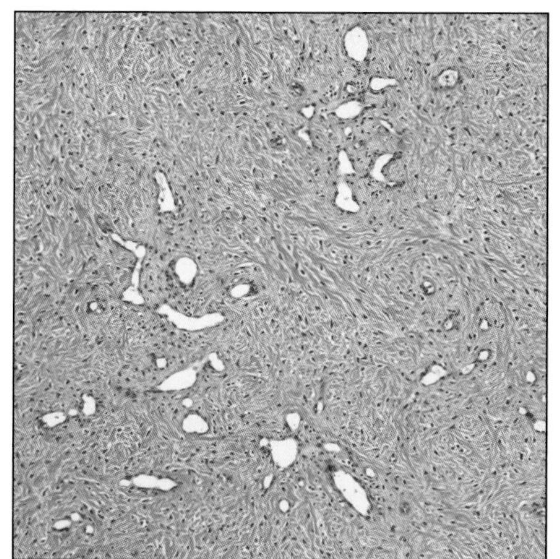

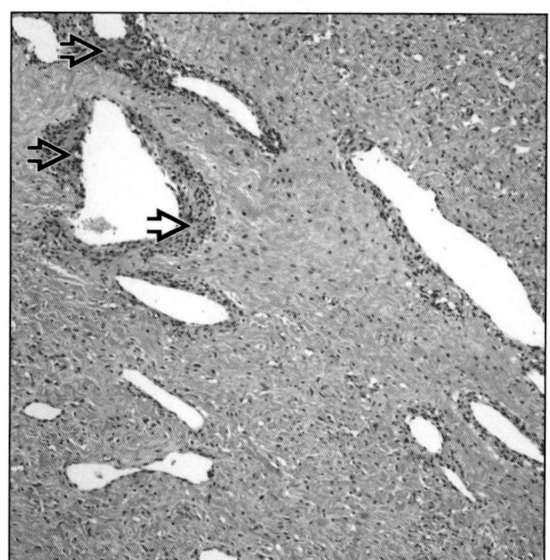

(Left) *Hematoxylin & eosin shows increased collagen deposition often seen in lesions of a long duration. Note how the vessels are compressed and narrowed to a nearly slit-like configuration.* ***(Right)*** *Hematoxylin & eosin shows numerous vessels of various calibers, some with smooth muscle ⇨, set in a heavily collagenized stroma. The stroma shows hypocellularity.*

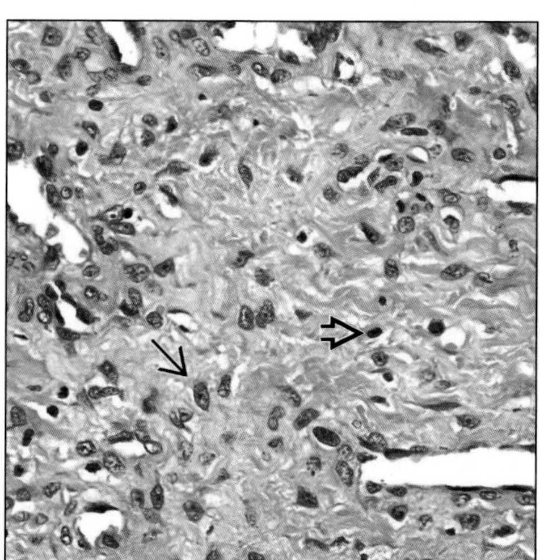

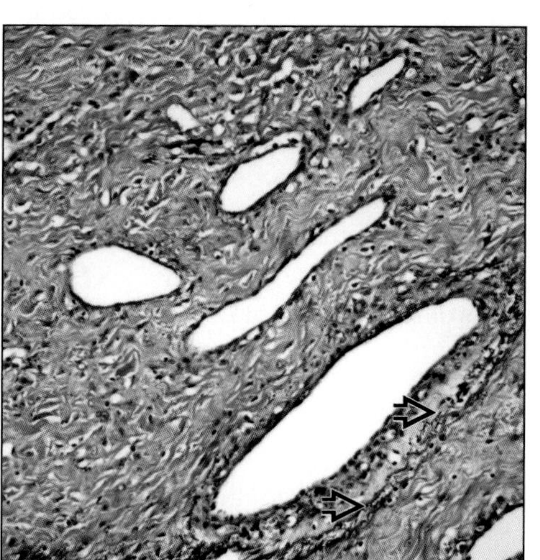

(Left) *The lesional cells have plump ovoid nuclei → and indistinct cell margins. The cells are randomly oriented within fibrous stroma that contains scattered mast cells ⇨ and lymphocytes.* ***(Right)*** *Elastic van Gieson shows elastic tissue (black deposition as short to wavy fragments) in the larger vessel ⇨ but not in the smaller vessels. This results in profuse epistaxis, as the vessels are unable to contract and staunch bleeding.*

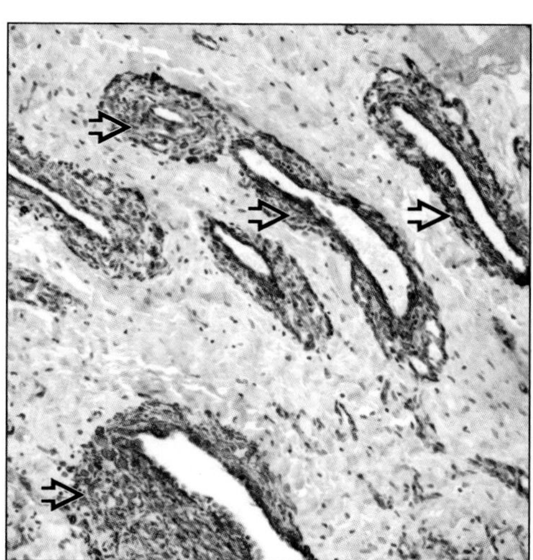

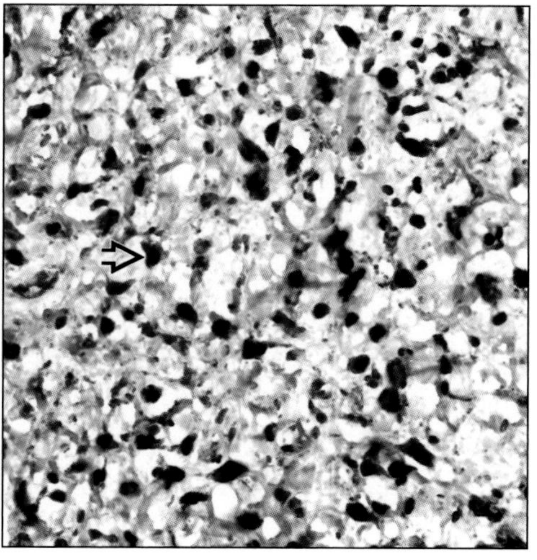

(Left) *Muscle specific actin highlights the muscle walls around vessels ⇨. The variable intensity of the reaction helps to demonstrate the variable amounts of smooth muscle associated with the vessels.* ***(Right)*** *Immunohistochemistry for β-catenin shows strong diffuse positivity in nuclei ⇨ in the majority of the lesional cells. The tumor's architecture, nuclear features, vascular pattern, and absence of SMA in lesional cells allow distinction from fibromatosis.*

FIBROMATOSIS

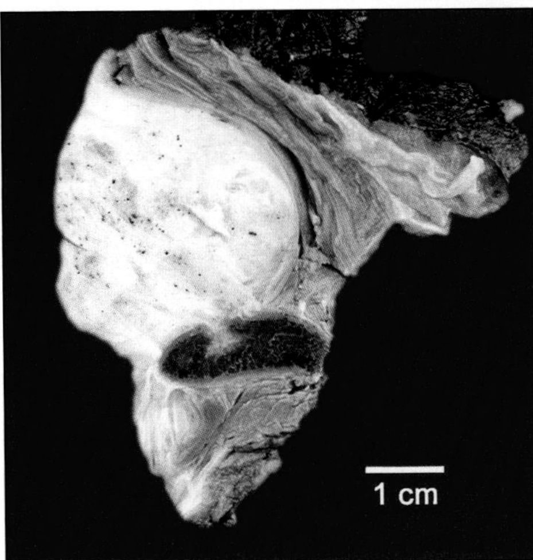

Gross photograph shows a large deep fibromatosis involving the shoulder. This lesion has eroded into the scapula, although typically fibromatoses do not erode bone.

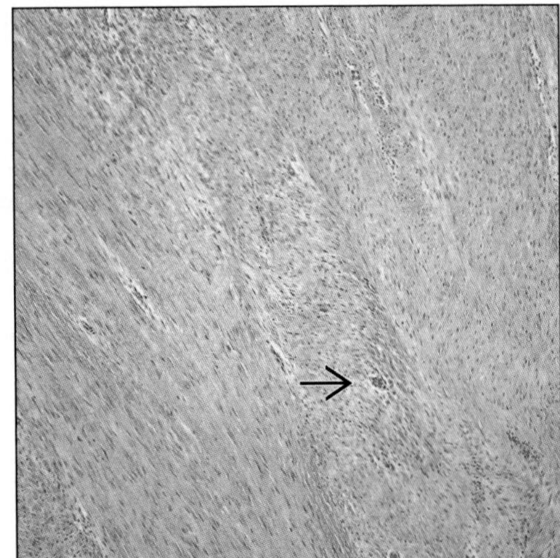

Hematoxylin & eosin shows sweeping fascicles of spindle cells separated by regularly spaced collagen. Even at this magnification, small vessels ➔ are readily apparent.

TERMINOLOGY

Synonyms

- Superficial fibromatoses
  - Palmar fibromatosis: Dupuytren contracture, Dupuytren disease
  - Plantar fibromatosis: Ledderhose disease
  - Penile fibromatosis: Peyronie disease
  - Knuckle pads
- Deep fibromatosis: Aggressive fibromatosis, desmoid tumor

Definitions

- Palmar fibromatosis
  - Nodular myofibroblastic proliferation of volar surface of hand that is prone to local persistence but does not metastasize
- Plantar fibromatosis
  - Nodular myofibroblastic proliferation of plantar surface of foot that is prone to local persistence but does not metastasize
- Peyronie disease
  - Penile fibrous lesion causing various deformities; initially pain with erection, erectile dysfunction
- Knuckle pads
  - Well-circumscribed thickening of skin over metacarpophalangeal and, more commonly, proximal interphalangeal joints
  - Some associated with Dupuytren contractures, most idiopathic
- Deep fibromatosis
  - Myofibroblastic proliferations of deep soft tissues with infiltrative growth pattern
  - Prone to local recurrences but do not metastasize

CLINICAL ISSUES

Epidemiology

- Incidence
  - Palmar fibromatosis
    - 4-6% of Caucasian adults over 50 years of age
    - Reports of up to 75% of Celtic men
    - Uncommon in nonwhites
    - Marked male predominance
  - Plantar fibromatosis
    - 1-2 per 100,000 persons per year (northern Europe)
    - Most patients 30-50 years of age
    - Slight male predominance
  - Penile fibromatosis
    - About 3.5% of white men over 50 years of age
  - Deep fibromatosis
    - 2.4-4.43 new cases per 100,000 persons per year (Scandinavian data)

Presentation

- Superficial fibromatoses present as nodular lesions on palms, soles, knuckles, or penis
  - Most common in older white men
- Deep fibromatoses present as firm large masses
  - Relationship to age and gender
    - In children, no gender predominance: Lesions of shoulders, chest wall, back, thigh, head, and neck
    - In women in childbearing years: Abdominal wall
    - In older adults, no gender predominance: Lesions of shoulders, chest wall, back, thigh, head, and neck
  - Mesenteric fibromatoses
    - Most have asymptomatic abdominal mass
    - Gastrointestinal hemorrhage or perforation
- Lesions associated with familial adenomatous polyposis (FAP)
  - Risk of fibromatoses is 2.56/1,000 person-years
  - Comparative risk is 852x that of general population
- Occasionally associated with scar ("cicatricial fibromatosis")

Treatment

- Superficial fibromatoses treated by excision

Key Facts

Terminology
- Palmar fibromatosis: Dupuytren contracture, Dupuytren disease
- Plantar fibromatosis: Ledderhose disease
- Penile fibromatosis: Peyronie disease
- Deep fibromatosis: Aggressive fibromatosis, desmoid tumor
  - Myofibroblastic proliferations with infiltrative growth pattern that are prone to local recurrences but do not metastasize

Clinical Issues
- Palmar fibromatosis
  - 4-6% of Caucasian adults over 50 years of age
- Deep fibromatosis
  - 2.4-4.43 new cases per 100,000 persons per year (Scandinavian data)
- Recurrences common for both superficial and deep fibromatoses
- Occasional deaths from deep fibromatoses, especially FAP-associated mesenteric fibromatosis

Microscopic Pathology
- Sweeping fascicles of myofibroblasts
- Smooth nuclear membranes
- Delicate nucleoli in most cells
- Occasional cells with stellate cytoplasmic contours
- Occasional foci with storiform pattern similar to nodular fasciitis
- Some cases with keloid-like collagen
- Small but conspicuous vessels
- Open, gaping, thin-walled vessels with perivascular sclerosis often feature of mesenteric fibromatosis

- Nonsurgical treatments for penile lesions
  - Verapamil treatment administered by intraplaque injection
  - Colchicine, aminobenzoate potassium (Potaba), L-carnitine, and liposomal superoxide dismutase
- Deep fibromatoses treated by wide excision
  - For unresectable lesions, radiation, chemotherapy, hormone therapy

Prognosis
- Recurrences common for both superficial and deep fibromatoses
- Occasional deaths from deep fibromatoses
  - FAP-associated mesenteric fibromatosis

MACROSCOPIC FEATURES

General Features
- Superficial fibromatoses
  - Small (1-3 cm), nodular, firm, white lesions; some with gritty cut surface
  - Large, infiltrative, firm, white lesions; some with gritty cut surface

MICROSCOPIC PATHOLOGY

Histologic Features
- Sweeping fascicles of myofibroblasts
  - Smooth nuclear membranes
  - Delicate nucleoli in most cells
  - Occasional cells with stellate cytoplasmic contours
  - Occasional foci with storiform pattern similar to nodular fasciitis
- Uniformly distributed collagen
  - Some cases with keloid-like collagen
- Prominent vascular pattern
  - Small but conspicuous vessels
  - Open, gaping, thin-walled vessels with perivascular sclerosis
- Minimal background inflammation
- Scattered lesional giant cells found in some plantar fibromatoses
  - Rarely found in palmar and deep fibromatoses

DIFFERENTIAL DIAGNOSIS

DDx of Superficial Fibromatoses
- Clear cell sarcoma
  - Most involve hands and feet of young adults
  - Packeted arrangement of spindle cells
  - Scattered giant cells
  - S100 protein, HMB-45, Melan-A positive
  - *EWS-ATF1* gene fusion
- Epithelioid sarcoma
  - Most involve distal upper extremity
  - Epithelioid cells arranged around necrotic zones, reminiscent of granulomatous inflammation
  - Cytokeratin, EMA, CD34 positive
- Tenosynovial giant cell tumor (giant cell tumor of tendon sheath)
  - Usually involves fingers and toes of middle-aged women
  - Rounded cells, giant cells, foamy macrophages, hemosiderin
  - CD68(+), clusterin(+)
- Scar
  - Disorganized myofibroblastic proliferation
  - Lacks nodular configuration
  - Few mast cells
  - β-catenin(-)

DDx of Deep Fibromatoses
- Leiomyoma
  - Multiple anatomic sites, especially female genital tract
  - Perpendicularly oriented fascicles of spindle cells with brightly eosinophilic cytoplasm, blunt-ended nuclei, paranuclear vacuoles, none to few mitoses, bland cytologic features
  - Actin, desmin, calponin, H-caldesmon positive
  - S100 protein, CD34, β-catenin negative

FIBROMATOSIS

Immunohistochemistry

Antibody	Reactivity	Staining Pattern	Comment
β-catenin	Positive	Nuclear	In deep fibromatoses, correlates with β-catenin or *APC* gene mutations (but not in superficial fibromatoses)
Actin-sm	Positive	Cytoplasmic	Reflects myofibroblastic differentiation
Desmin	Negative		
CD34	Negative		
CK-PAN	Negative		
S100	Negative		
CD117	Equivocal	Cell membrane & cytoplasm	Can lead to misinterpretation of mesenteric fibromatosis as gastrointestinal stromal tumor when antigen retrieval is used

- Leiomyosarcoma
  - Multiple anatomic sites, especially female genital tract
  - Perpendicularly oriented fascicles of spindle cells with brightly eosinophilic cytoplasm, blunt-ended nuclei, paranuclear vacuoles, none to few mitoses, atypical cytologic features
  - Actin, desmin, calponin, H-caldesmon positive
  - S100 protein, CD34, β-catenin negative
- Low-grade fibromyxoid sarcoma
  - Deep lesions without gender predilection
  - Disorganized and swirled arrangement of fibroblastic cells with hyperchromatic nuclei, variable myxoid background
  - Cellularity similar to that of fibromatosis
  - Occasionally actin(+)
  - S100 protein, desmin, CD34, β-catenin negative
  - Claudin-1(+), epithelial membrane antigen(+)
  - *FUS-CREB3L2* fusion
- Gastrointestinal stromal tumor
  - Usually involves muscularis propria of stomach
  - Spindled or epithelioid
    - Often with cytoplasmic vacuoles, uniform nuclei
  - CD117, CD34 positive; variable actin, variable desmin
  - S100 protein, β-catenin negative
  - *KIT* mutations
- Sclerosing mesenteritis
  - Usually involves mesentery in adult patients
  - Infiltrative fibroblastic lesion with fat necrosis
    - Prominent inflammation (lymphocytes, plasma cells, foam cells)
  - Actin variable
  - Negative desmin, S100 protein, β-catenin
- Inflammatory myofibroblastic tumor
  - Often involves mesentery in patients with B symptoms
  - Cellular lesions composed of stellate myofibroblasts
    - Abundant inflammation (lymphocytes, plasma cells)
  - Actin(+), desmin variable, ALK(+) (60%), keratin variable (about 75% in mesentery)
  - S100 protein, β-catenin negative
  - Some examples with *ALK* rearrangements

SELECTED REFERENCES

1. Lips DJ et al: The role of APC and beta-catenin in the aetiology of aggressive fibromatosis (desmoid tumors). Eur J Surg Oncol. 35(1):3-10, 2009
2. Lazar AJ et al: Specific mutations in the beta-catenin gene (CTNNB1) correlate with local recurrence in sporadic desmoid tumors. Am J Pathol. 173(5):1518-27, 2008
3. Smith JF et al: Peyronie's disease: a critical appraisal of current diagnosis and treatment. Int J Impot Res. 20(5):445-59, 2008
4. Deyrup AT et al: Estrogen receptor-beta expression in extraabdominal fibromatoses: an analysis of 40 cases. Cancer. 106(1):208-13, 2006
5. Heinrich MC et al: Clinical and molecular studies of the effect of imatinib on advanced aggressive fibromatosis (desmoid tumor). J Clin Oncol. 24(7):1195-203, 2006
6. Ishizuka M et al: Expression profiles of sex steroid receptors in desmoid tumors. Tohoku J Exp Med. 210(3):189-98, 2006
7. Bhattacharya B et al: Nuclear beta-catenin expression distinguishes deep fibromatosis from other benign and malignant fibroblastic and myofibroblastic lesions. Am J Surg Pathol. 29(5):653-9, 2005
8. Fetsch JF et al: Palmar-plantar fibromatosis in children and preadolescents: a clinicopathologic study of 56 cases with newly recognized demographics and extended follow-up information. Am J Surg Pathol. 29(8):1095-105, 2005
9. Evans HL: Multinucleated giant cells in plantar fibromatosis. Am J Surg Pathol. 26(2):244-8, 2002
10. Montgomery E et al: Beta-catenin immunohistochemistry separates mesenteric fibromatosis from gastrointestinal stromal tumor and sclerosing mesenteritis. Am J Surg Pathol. 26(10):1296-301, 2002
11. Montgomery E et al: Superficial fibromatoses are genetically distinct from deep fibromatoses. Mod Pathol. 14(7):695-701, 2001
12. Gurbuz AK et al: Desmoid tumours in familial adenomatous polyposis. Gut. 35(3):377-81, 1994
13. Burke AP et al: Intra-abdominal fibromatosis. A pathologic analysis of 130 tumors with comparison of clinical subgroups. Am J Surg Pathol. 14(4):335-41, 1990
14. Burke AP et al: Mesenteric fibromatosis. A follow-up study. Arch Pathol Lab Med. 114(8):832-5, 1990
15. Häyry P et al: The desmoid tumor. II. Analysis of factors possibly contributing to the etiology and growth behavior. Am J Clin Pathol. 77(6):674-80, 1982
16. Reitamo JJ et al: The desmoid tumor. I. Incidence, sex-, age- and anatomical distribution in the Finnish population. Am J Clin Pathol. 77(6):665-73, 1982

Microscopic, Radiographic, and Gross Features

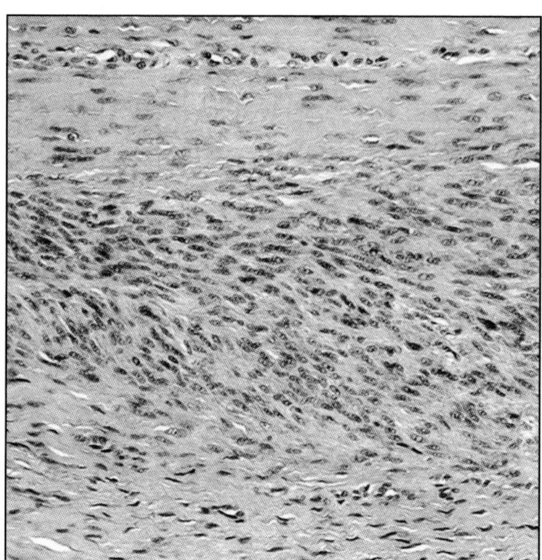

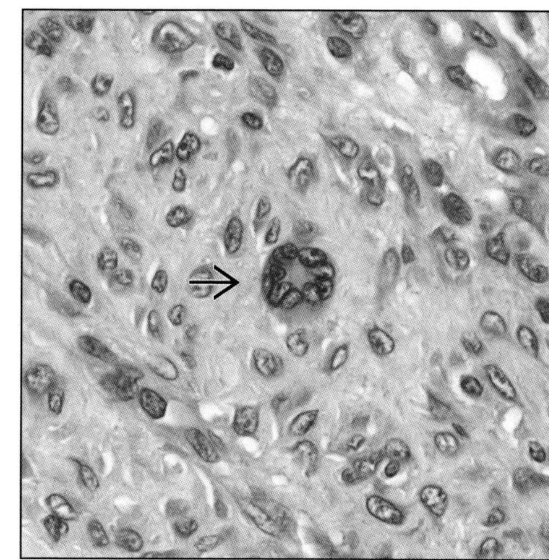

(Left) *Hematoxylin & eosin shows a plantar fibromatosis, which can be fairly large and have pockets of enhanced cellularity that lead to misinterpretations as sarcomas. Superficial fibromatoses can have β-catenin immunolabeling but lack β-catenin and APC gene mutations.* ***(Right)*** *Hematoxylin & eosin shows a giant cell in plantar fibromatosis ⇒. Such cells can also occur in palmar lesions and cause confusion with a tenosynovial giant cell tumor and clear cell sarcoma.*

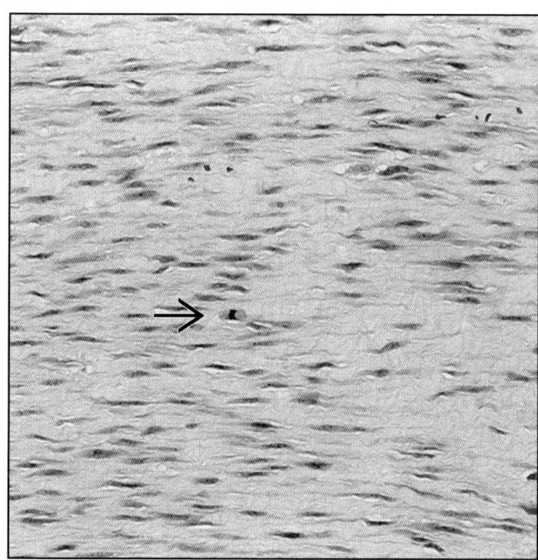

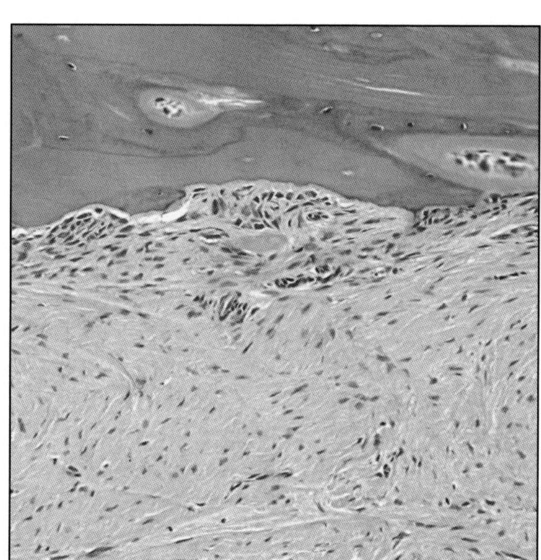

(Left) *Hematoxylin & eosin shows a mitosis in a palmar fibromatosis ⇒. Mitotic activity can be encountered in both palmar and in plantar fibromatoses and should not lead to a concern for malignancy.* ***(Right)*** *Hematoxylin & eosin shows an example of Peyronie disease (penile fibromatosis) that has ossified. Peyronie disease consists of a fibrous proliferation of the tunica albuginea, resulting in a palpable scar and penile curvature, hinging, narrowing, and shortening as well as painful erections.*

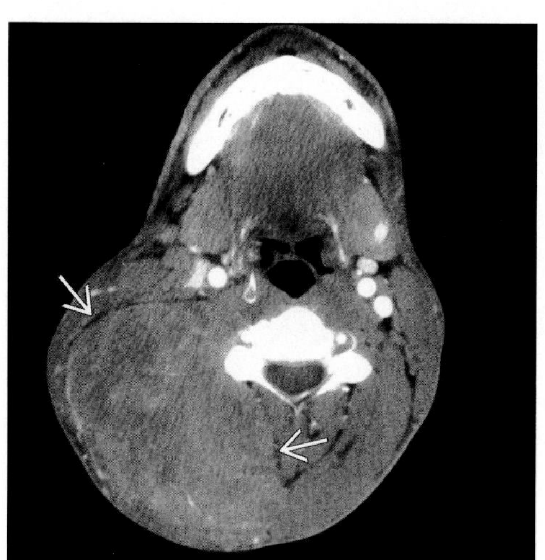

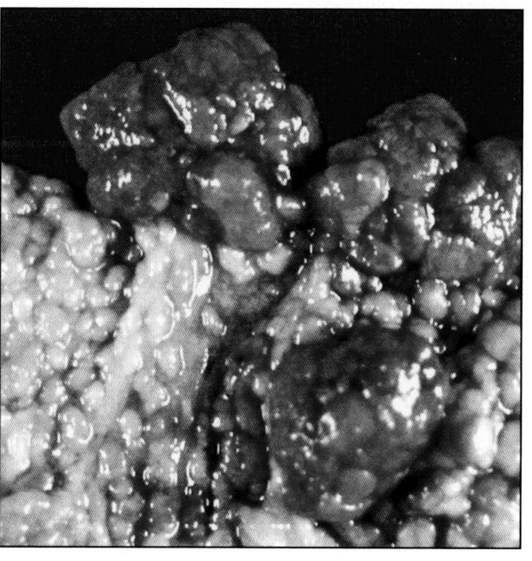

(Left) *Radiologic image shows a large fibromatosis ➡ of the head and neck in an elderly alcoholic man. Although more arise in the shoulder girdles (or in the abdominal wall in young women), the head and neck is a common location for fibromatoses.* ***(Right)*** *Gross photograph shows a colectomy sample from a patient with familial adenomatous polyposis (FAP). FAP patients often have fibromatoses (many times mesenteric) in addition to their colon polyps.*

FIBROMATOSIS

Microscopic Features

*(**Left**) Hematoxylin & eosin shows low magnification of a small intestinal mesenteric fibromatosis. The epicenter of the mass is in the mesentery, but the tumor has infiltrated into the muscularis propria ➙. The lesions are especially prone to recurrences in FAP patients. (**Right**) Hematoxylin & eosin in a mesenteric fibromatosis shows gaping vessels, which appear to be stretched open by the proliferating lesion. This is a characteristic feature of mesenteric fibromatosis.*

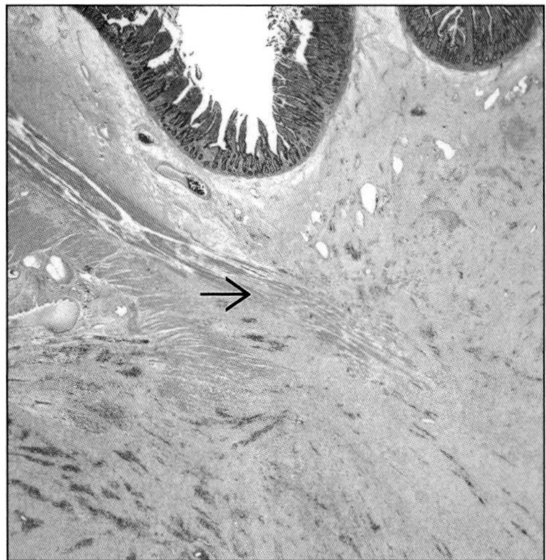

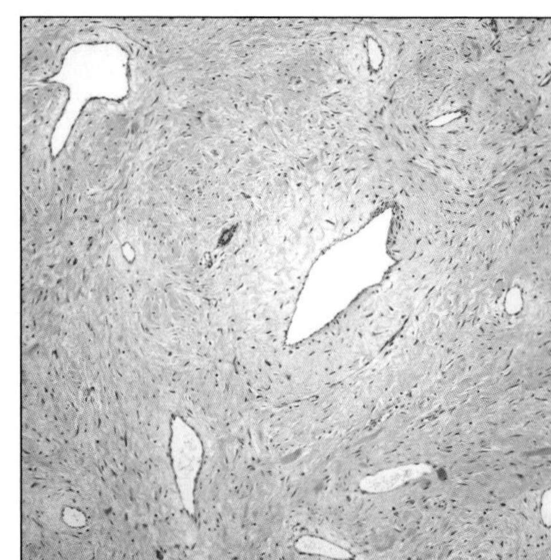

*(**Left**) Hematoxylin & eosin shows a deep fibromatosis proliferating adjacent to a small vessel. The vascular smooth muscle appears more eosinophilic than the myofibroblastic appearance of the lesional cells. (**Right**) Hematoxylin & eosin shows high magnification of a deep fibromatosis. The cells contain nuclei with single delicate nucleoli and bipolar or stellate cytoplasm. Collagen is evenly distributed in most examples but is occasionally keloid-like.*

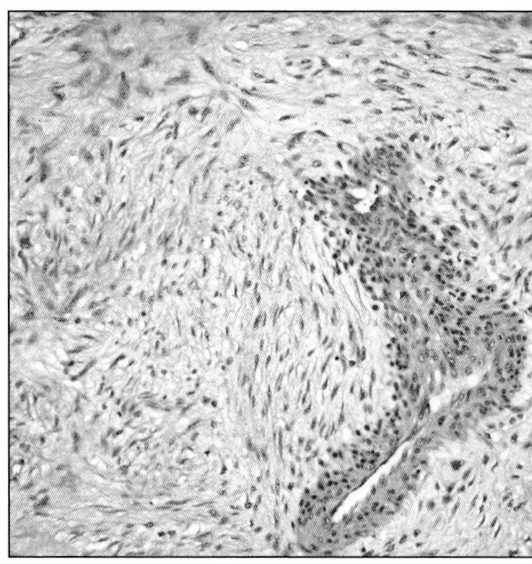

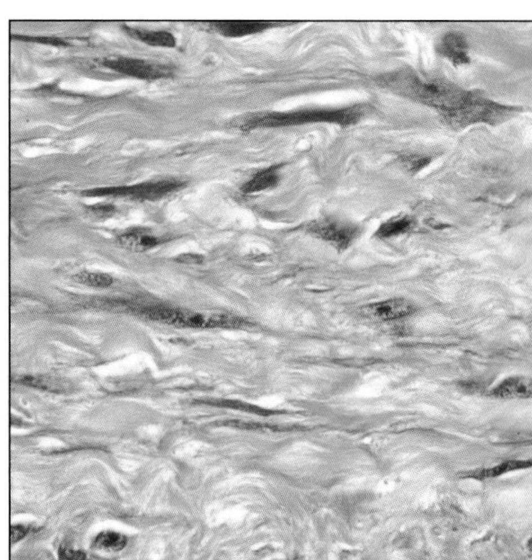

*(**Left**) Hematoxylin & eosin shows a deep fibromatosis infiltrating skeletal muscle. The nuclei of degenerating skeletal myocytes form clusters ➙, imparting an alarming appearance at low magnification. (**Right**) Hematoxylin & eosin shows a collection of degenerating skeletal myocytes in a deep fibromatosis. Compare their dark nuclei ➙ to the pale ones of the fibromatosis ➚. Note that most of the lesional cells have delicate nucleoli, a consistent feature in fibromatoses.*

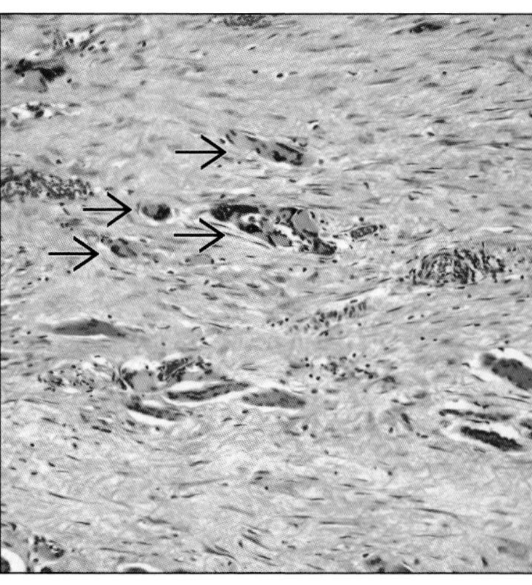

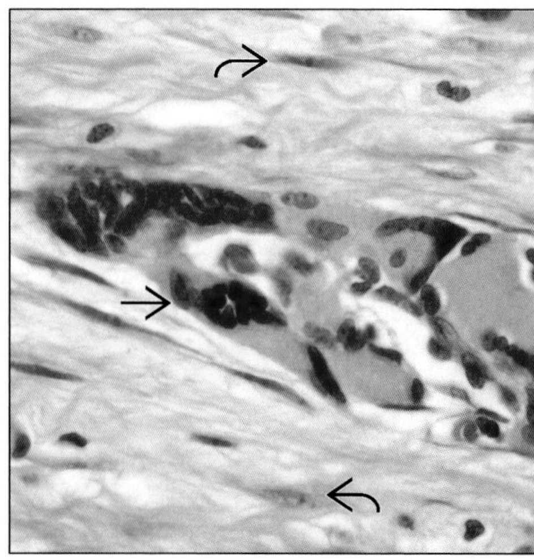

Microscopic Features and Differential Diagnosis

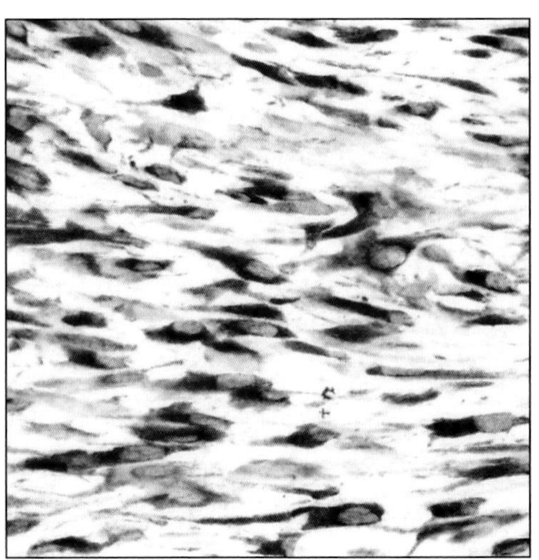

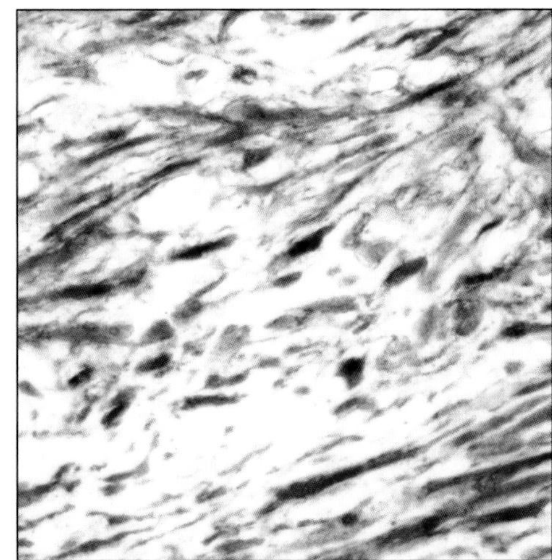

(Left) *CD117 shows strong labeling in a deep fibromatosis. This particular example displays more prominent staining than most fibromatoses, but this feature can result in misdiagnosis as gastrointestinal stromal tumor in mesenteric fibromatoses. Fibromatoses lack KIT mutations and have minimal response to imatinib.* ***(Right)*** *β-catenin shows nuclear staining in a fibromatosis, a reflection of either APC or β-catenin mutations in most fibromatoses.*

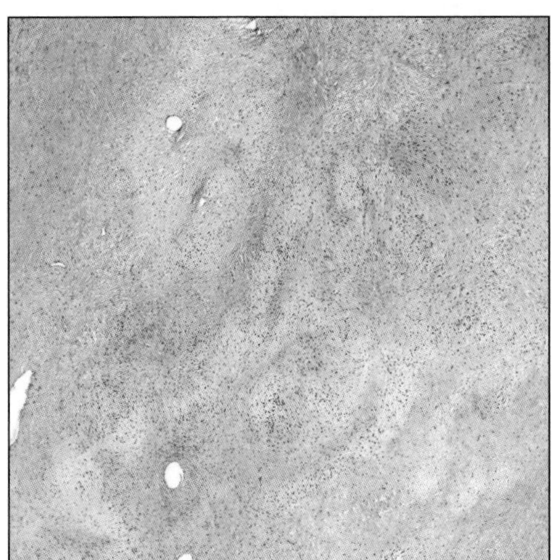

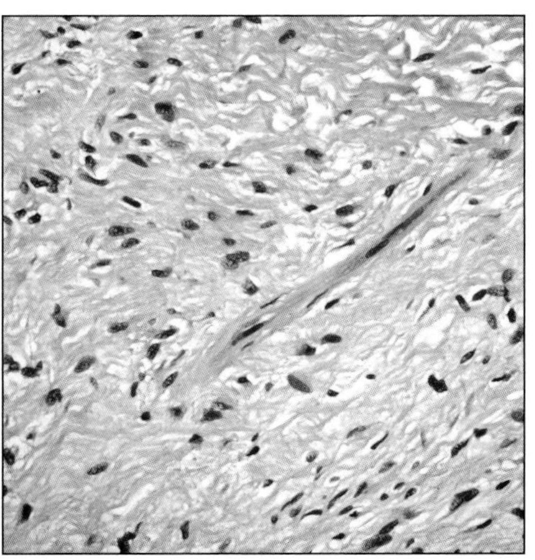

(Left) *Hematoxylin & eosin shows a low-grade fibromyxoid sarcoma. Although the lesion appears similar to a fibromatosis at low magnification, it differs by featuring a less uniformly fascicular low-power appearance.* ***(Right)*** *Hematoxylin & eosin shows a low-grade fibromyxoid sarcoma. The lesional cells are far more hyperchromatic than those of a fibromatosis. These lesions lack nuclear β-catenin and have a characteristic translocation, t(7;16) (q32-34;p11), with a FUS/CREB3L2 fusion gene.*

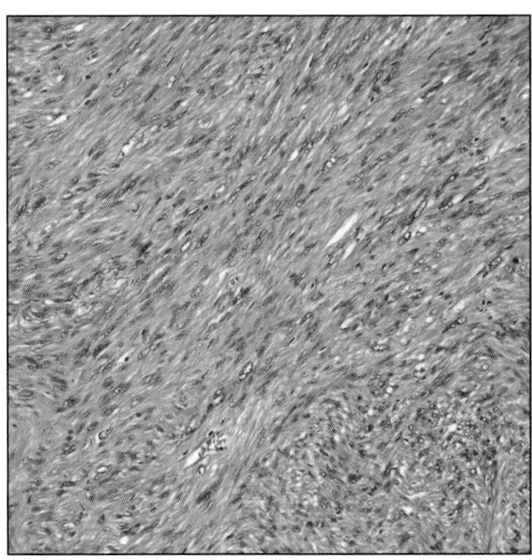

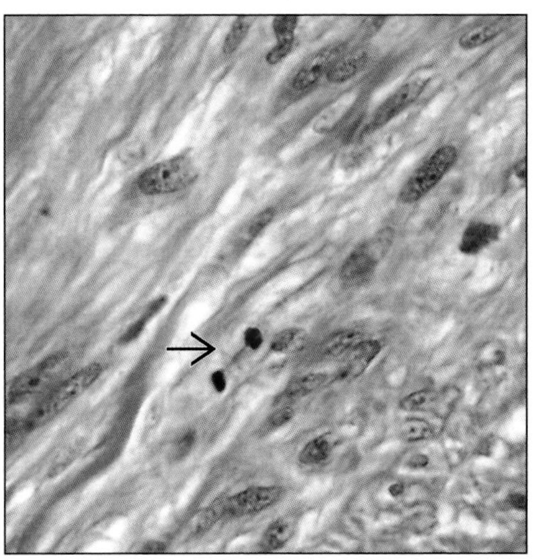

(Left) *Hematoxylin & eosin shows a leiomyosarcoma. The lesional nuclei are larger and more hyperchromatic than those of fibromatoses, and the cytoplasm is strikingly eosinophilic.* ***(Right)*** *Hematoxylin & eosin shows high magnification of a leiomyosarcoma. The nuclear chromatin is coarser than that in fibromatoses. There is an anaphase bridge* ⇒, *a feature of chromosomally unstable tumors (in contrast to the lack of anaphase bridges in tumors with characteristic mutations or translocations).*

LIPOFIBROMATOSIS

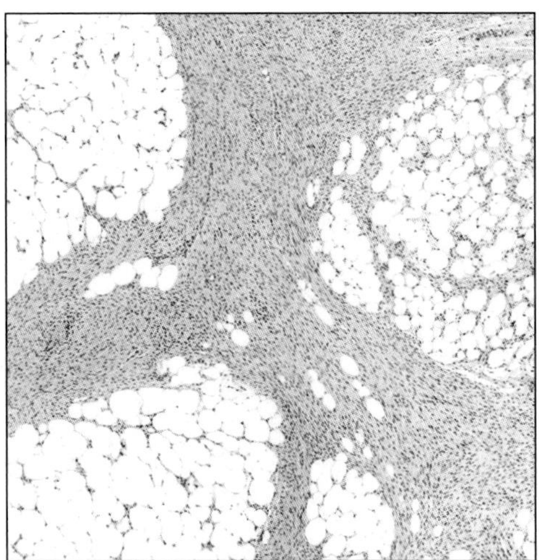

Hematoxylin & eosin shows lipofibromatosis at low magnification. The tumor is fibroblastic, but adipose tissue is an integral part of the lesion. Such tumors usually arise in the hands of children.

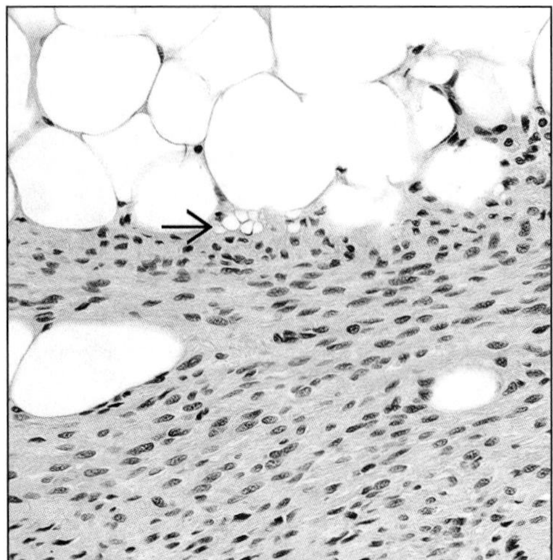

Hematoxylin & eosin shows higher magnification of lipofibromatosis. Cells resembling lipoblasts ⇒ are encountered in the zones where adipose tissue and fibrous components merge.

TERMINOLOGY

Synonyms

- Infantile fibromatosis, nondesmoid type

Definitions

- Fibroadipose tissue tumor of childhood with predilection for distal extremities

ETIOLOGY/PATHOGENESIS

Genetics

- 3-way t(4;9;6) translocation reported in 1 case

CLINICAL ISSUES

Presentation

- Painless mass
- Hands and feet of children
- Median age: 1 year
- Male predominance (M:F = 2:1)

Prognosis

- Local recurrences common
- Risk factors for recurrence
  - Congenital onset, male gender, mitotic activity in fibrous component, incomplete excision
- No metastases reported

MACROSCOPIC FEATURES

General Features

- Yellowish to whitish tan
- Usually has macroscopic fat component

Size

- 1-3 cm, median: 2 cm
- Rare examples > 5 cm

MICROSCOPIC PATHOLOGY

Histologic Features

- Alternating fascicles of fibrous tissue and adipose tissue
- Infiltrative growth pattern
- Overall lobulated arrangement of adipose tissue
- Low mitotic activity
- No nuclear pleomorphism
- Vacuolated (lipoblast-like) cells at areas of interface between adipose and fibrous tissue

DIFFERENTIAL DIAGNOSIS

Lipoblastoma

- Benign; found in infants and children
  - 1st 3 years of life
- Slowly growing masses
- Usually involves extremities
  - Reported in mediastinum, retroperitoneum, trunk, head and neck, various visceral organs
- Admixture of mature and immature adipose tissue
- Lobulated architecture
- Lipoblasts prominent in early lesions in richly vascularized areas
  - Appearances similar to those of myxoid liposarcoma
- Lesions show maturation to mature adipose tissue over time
- Breakpoints in 8q11
- *PLAG1* gene rearrangements

Palmar and Plantar Fibromatosis

- Benign lesions of adults
- Male predominance
- Involve palmar and plantar tendons/aponeuroses
- Fascicular arrangements of myofibroblasts
- Often have β-catenin nuclear labeling but lack mutations

LIPOFIBROMATOSIS

Key Facts

Clinical Issues

- Painless mass
- Hands and feet of children
- Median age: 1 year
- Male predominance (M:F = 2:1)
- Local recurrences common
- No metastases reported

Microscopic Pathology

- Alternating fascicles of fibrous tissue and adipose tissue
- Infiltrative growth pattern
- Overall lobulated arrangement of adipose tissue
- Vacuolated (lipoblast-like) cells
  - Seen at areas of interface between adipose and fibrous tissue

Immunohistochemistry

Antibody	Reactivity	Staining Pattern	Comment
CD34	Positive	Cytoplasmic	Usually focal
Bcl-2	Positive	Cytoplasmic	Usually focal
S100P	Positive	Cytoplasmic	Focal
Actin-sm	Positive	Cytoplasmic	Focal
EMA	Positive	Cytoplasmic	Focal
CD99	Positive	Cytoplasmic	Focal
β-catenin	Negative		

Fibrous Hamartoma of Infancy

- Benign; most present in 1st 2 years of life
- Anterior or posterior axillary fold
- 3 histologic components
  - Adipose tissue
  - Fibrous tissue
  - Primitive cells in myxoid stroma

Fibrolipomatous Hamartoma of Nerve

- a.k.a. lipomatosis of nerve
- Typically affects median nerve
- Benign; infants and children affected
- Associated macrodactyly in 1/3
- Infiltration of perineurium and epineurium by adipose tissue
- Excision necessarily results in nerve damage

Inclusion Body Fibromatosis

- Also called infantile digital fibromatosis
- Benign; presents in 1st year of life
- Dorsal aspect of fingers and toes
- Fascicles of myofibroblasts
- Numerous actin(+) inclusion bodies

SELECTED REFERENCES

1. Thway K et al: Beta-catenin expression in pediatric fibroblastic and myofibroblastic lesions: a study of 100 cases. Pediatr Dev Pathol. 12(4):292-6, 2009
2. Kenney B et al: Chromosomal rearrangements in lipofibromatosis. Cancer Genet Cytogenet. 179(2):136-9, 2007
3. Fetsch JF et al: A clinicopathologic study of 45 pediatric soft tissue tumors with an admixture of adipose tissue and fibroblastic elements, and a proposal for classification as lipofibromatosis. Am J Surg Pathol. 24(11):1491-500, 2000

IMAGE GALLERY

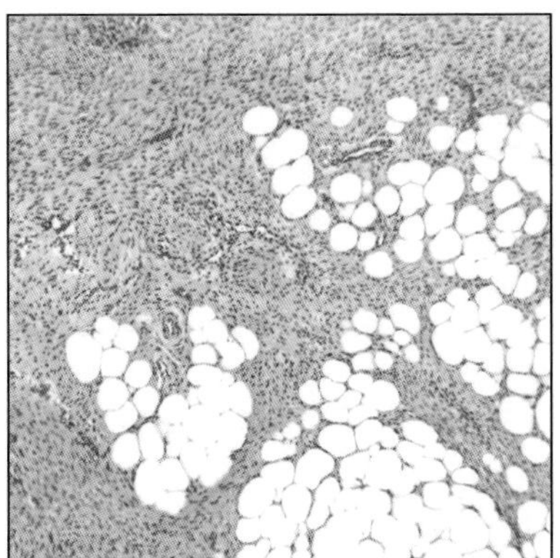

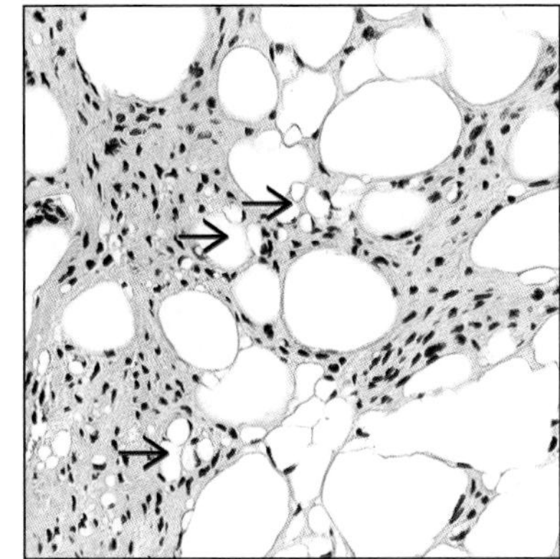

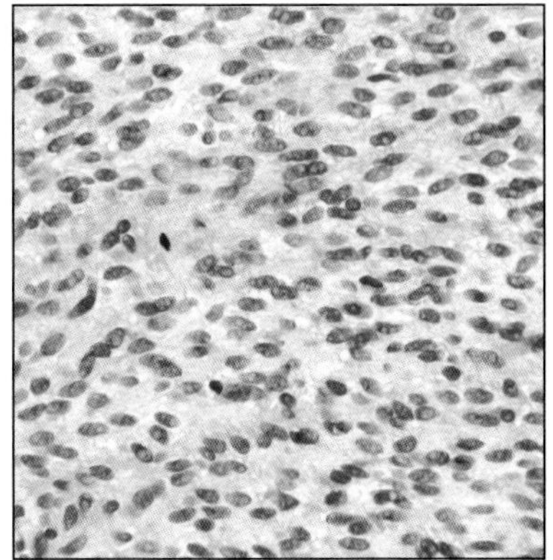

(Left) Hematoxylin & eosin shows the intimate admixture of adipose tissue and fibrous tissue in lipofibromatosis. These lesions are infiltrative and prone to recurrences, although they are benign. (Center) Hematoxylin & eosin shows high magnification of the interface between adipose and fibrous tissue in a lipofibromatosis. There are several cells in this field that resemble lipoblasts ⇒. (Right) Hematoxylin & eosin shows the fibroblastic portion in a cellular pocket from a lipofibromatosis. The area is cellular with uniform nuclei, resembling a plantar fibromatosis.

SOLITARY FIBROUS TUMOR

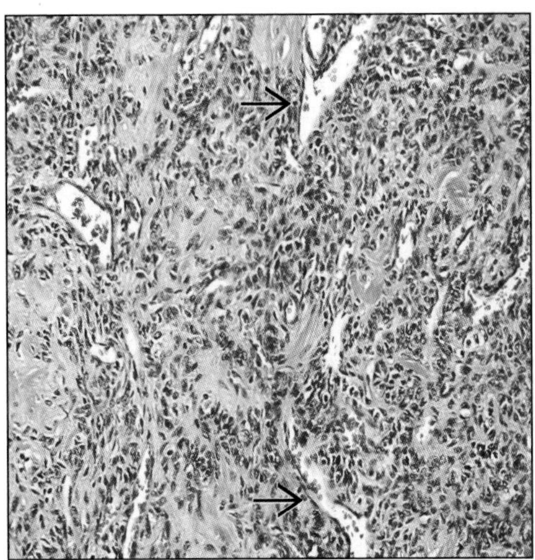

Hematoxylin & eosin shows a solitary fibrous tumor, with spindle to ovoid cells in a collagenous stroma and interspersed hemangiopericytic vessels ➔.

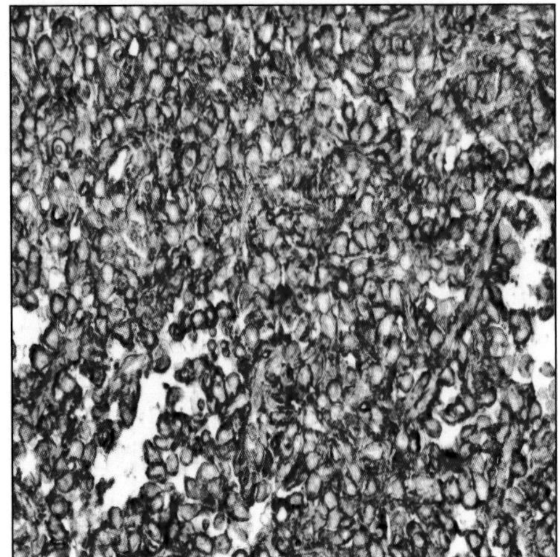

CD34 immunohistochemistry shows characteristic diffuse strong cytoplasmic and membranous positivity throughout the tumor.

TERMINOLOGY

Abbreviations

- Solitary fibrous tumor (SFT)

Synonyms

- Localized fibrous mesothelioma, localized fibrous tumor, submesothelial fibroma, localized fibroma, subpleural fibroma

Definitions

- Fibroblastic mesenchymal tumor with prominent branching (hemangiopericytoma-like) vascular pattern
  - Initially described in pleura but subsequently described in almost any organ or site
  - Many previously diagnosed soft tissue hemangiopericytomas are probably solitary fibrous tumors
- Closely related tumors
  - Lipomatous hemangiopericytoma
  - Giant cell angiofibroma

ETIOLOGY/PATHOGENESIS

Unknown

- Initially considered mesothelial
- Now accepted as mesenchymal tumor

CLINICAL ISSUES

Epidemiology

- Age
  - Adults (range: 20-70 years)
  - Occasionally in children and adolescents
- Gender
  - M = F

Site

- Deep soft tissue
- Viscera
- Subcutaneous tissue and very rarely at cutaneous sites
- Head and neck, including orbit and intracranial sites
- Extrapleural lesions more frequent than pleural

Presentation

- Slow growing
- Painless mass
  - Rarely paraneoplastic syndrome of hypoglycemia due to production of insulin-like growth factor

Treatment

- Surgical approaches
  - Simple surgical resection for benign SFT
  - More extensive surgery for malignant SFT
- Adjuvant therapy
  - Combination of radiation therapy and chemotherapy in malignant SFT

Prognosis

- Long-term follow-up is mandatory due to unpredictable behavior of SFT
- Most are benign
- Up to 15% behave aggressively
- Most tumors with histologically "benign" morphology do not recur or metastasize
- Histologically malignant tumors usually behave aggressively

MACROSCOPIC FEATURES

General Features

- Lobulated, circumscribed mass
  - Malignant tumors may be locally infiltrative
- Firm gray-white or brown cut surface
- Occasional cystic degeneration or hemorrhage

Size

- 1-20 cm (most 5-10 cm)

SOLITARY FIBROUS TUMOR

Key Facts

Terminology

- Fibroblastic mesenchymal tumor with prominent hemangiopericytic branching vascular pattern
- Initially described in pleura
  - Occur in any location
- Closely related tumors
  - Lipomatous hemangiopericytoma
  - Giant cell angiofibroma

Clinical Issues

- Affects adults with equal sex distribution
- Behavior difficult to predict from histological parameters
- Long-term follow-up indicated

Microscopic Pathology

- Fibroblasts with uniform small fusiform, ovoid, or sometimes spindled nuclei, in "patternless" distributions
- Varying proportion of fibrous stroma
- Prominent vascular pattern
- Malignant SFT
  - Hypercellularity, atypia, mitoses > 4/10 HPF, necrosis, and infiltrative margins
- Lipomatous hemangiopericytoma has admixed fat
- Giant cell angiofibroma has spaces lined by multinucleated cells

Ancillary Tests

- Characteristic diffuse immunoreactivity for CD34

MICROSCOPIC PATHOLOGY

Histologic Features

- Classically shows alternating cellularity, with variation between highly cellular and sparsely cellular areas
  - Fibroblasts with uniform small fusiform, ovoid, or sometimes spindled nuclei and scanty cytoplasm
    - Occasional multinucleate giant cells
  - Atypia is unusual
  - "Patternless" pattern of fascicles
  - Varying proportion of fibrous stroma
    - Frequent dense keloid-like hyalinization
    - Stroma may show cracking artifact
    - Amianthoid fibers rarely described
  - Myxoid or cystic change can occur
  - Prominent vascular pattern
    - Frequent perivascular hyalinization
    - Branching or staghorn-shaped large vessels
  - Mitotic figures and necrosis rare
- Malignant solitary fibrous tumor
  - No precise correlation between morphology and behavior, but the following features suggest malignancy
    - Hypercellularity
    - At least focal pleomorphism
    - > 4 mitoses/10 HPF
    - Necrosis
    - Infiltrative margins
    - Can be CD34 positive or negative
  - Rare cases may show abrupt transition from "benign" SFT to high-grade sarcoma
- Lipomatous hemangiopericytoma
  - Areas of typical SFT admixed with variable amount of mature fat
  - Malignant versions rare
- Giant cell angiofibroma
  - Initially described within orbit but occurs in many locations
  - Morphology of typical SFT, with pseudovascular spaces lined by stromal multinucleated giant cells

Predominant Cell/Compartment Type

- Fibroblast

ANCILLARY TESTS

Cytogenetics

- Solitary fibrous tumor
  - Karyotypically diverse
  - Detectable nonconsistent cytogenetic aberrations in most SFTs > 10 cm
- Giant cell angiofibroma
  - No characteristic translocation
  - Abnormality at 6q and t(12;17) in individual cases

Electron Microscopy

- Transmission
  - Ultrastructurally neoplastic cells show fibroblastic differentiation
    - Cells are spindle-shaped with dilated rough endoplasmic reticulum
    - Cells are sometimes more primitive with less fibroblastic differentiation
    - Rare myofibroblastic differentiation

DIFFERENTIAL DIAGNOSIS

Hemangiopericytoma

- More uniformly cellular
- Lack of stromal hyalinization

Benign Fibrous Histiocytoma

- Dermal location
- Poorly demarcated
- Collagen trapping at lesion periphery
- CD34 absent or rarely focal

Spindle Cell Lipoma (for Lipomatous Hemangiopericytoma)

- Usually back, neck, shoulder
- No solid fibroblastic component

SOLITARY FIBROUS TUMOR

Immunohistochemistry

Antibody	Reactivity	Staining Pattern	Comment
CD34	Positive	Cytoplasmic	Diffuse positivity is characteristic for SFT
CD99	Positive	Cell membrane	Diffuse positivity characteristic
Bcl-2	Positive	Nuclear & cytoplasmic	Variable
EMA	Positive	Cell membrane	Variable positivity
Actin-sm	Positive	Cytoplasmic	A few cases
β-catenin	Positive	Nuclear	Present in a subset of cases
CK-PAN	Negative		Helps to exclude synovial sarcoma
Desmin	Negative		
S100	Negative		
CD117	Negative		Helps to exclude gastrointestinal stromal tumor (GIST)

Hemangioma
- No solid fibroblastic component
- Lacks circumscription

Myopericytoma
- Usually in subcutis
- Actin-sm(+)

Dermatofibrosarcoma Protuberans
- Storiform pattern
- Dermal component
- Infiltrative margins
- Hemangiopericytic vascular pattern absent

Synovial Sarcoma
- Biphasic pattern
- Hemangiopericytic pattern but less vascular than SFT
- Focal cytokeratin expression
- Characteristic (X;18) translocations

Ewing Sarcoma
- Small round cell tumor
- Frequently positive for FLI-1
- Usually CD34(-)
- Specific translocations

Gastrointestinal Stromal Tumor
- Fascicular or organoid pattern
- Spindle or epithelioid cells
- CD117(+) and DOG1(+) in most cases
- Can be CD34(+)
- Most show *KIT* or *PDGFRA* oncogenic mutations

Atypical Lipomatous Tumor
- Fibrous septa
- Focal nuclear enlargement and hyperchromasia
- MDM2, CDK4(+)

Dedifferentiated Liposarcoma
- Prominent atypia
- MDM2, CDK4(+)

Fibrosarcoma
- No residual benign SFT component
- No specific markers

SELECTED REFERENCES

1. Erdag G et al: Solitary fibrous tumors of the skin: a clinicopathologic study of 10 cases and review of the literature. J Cutan Pathol. 34(11):844-50, 2007
2. Daigeler A et al: Clinicopathological findings in a case series of extrathoracic solitary fibrous tumors of soft tissues. BMC Surg. 6:10, 2006
3. Qian YW et al: A t(12;17) in an extraorbital giant cell angiofibroma. Cancer Genet Cytogenet. 165(2):157-60, 2006
4. Guillou L et al: Lipomatous hemangiopericytoma: a fat-containing variant of solitary fibrous tumor? Clinicopathologic, immunohistochemical, and ultrastructural analysis of a series in favor of a unifying concept. Hum Pathol. 31(9):1108-15, 2000
5. Guillou L et al: Orbital and extraorbital giant cell angiofibroma: a giant cell-rich variant of solitary fibrous tumor? Clinicopathologic and immunohistochemical analysis of a series in favor of a unifying concept. Am J Surg Pathol. 24(7):971-9, 2000
6. Morimitsu Y et al: Extrapleural solitary fibrous tumor: clinicopathologic study of 17 cases and molecular analysis of the p53 pathway. APMIS. 108(9):617-25, 2000
7. Sigel JE et al: Giant cell angiofibroma of the inguinal region. Ann Diagn Pathol. 4(4):240-4, 2000
8. Dotan ZA et al: Solitary fibrous tumor presenting as perirenal mass associated with hypoglycemia. J Urol. 162(6):2087-8, 1999
9. Hasegawa T et al: Extrathoracic solitary fibrous tumors: their histological variability and potentially aggressive behavior. Hum Pathol. 30(12):1464-73, 1999
10. Chan JK: Solitary fibrous tumour--everywhere, and a diagnosis in vogue. Histopathology. 31(6):568-76, 1997
11. Fukunaga M et al: Extrapleural solitary fibrous tumor: a report of seven cases. Mod Pathol. 10(5):443-50, 1997
12. Khalifa MA et al: Solitary fibrous tumors: a series of lesions, some in unusual sites. South Med J. 90(8):793-9, 1997
13. Miettinen MM et al: Tumor size-related DNA copy number changes occur in solitary fibrous tumors but not in hemangiopericytomas. Mod Pathol. 10(12):1194-200, 1997
14. Nielsen GP et al: Solitary fibrous tumor of soft tissue: a report of 15 cases, including 5 malignant examples with light microscopic, immunohistochemical, and ultrastructural data. Mod Pathol. 10(10):1028-37, 1997
15. Dei Tos AP et al: Giant cell angiofibroma. A distinctive orbital tumor in adults. Am J Surg Pathol. 19(11):1286-93, 1995

Microscopic Features

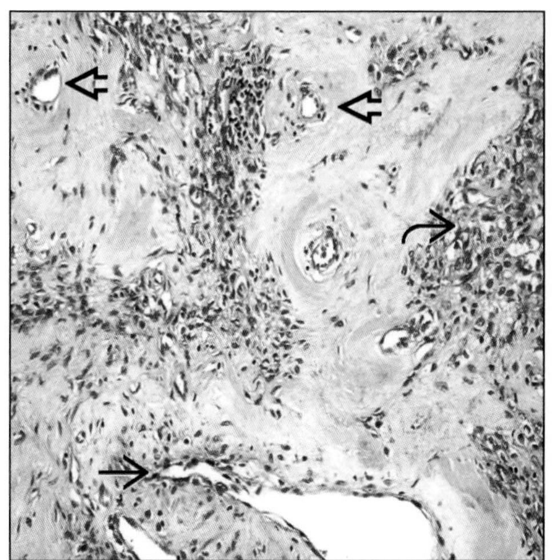

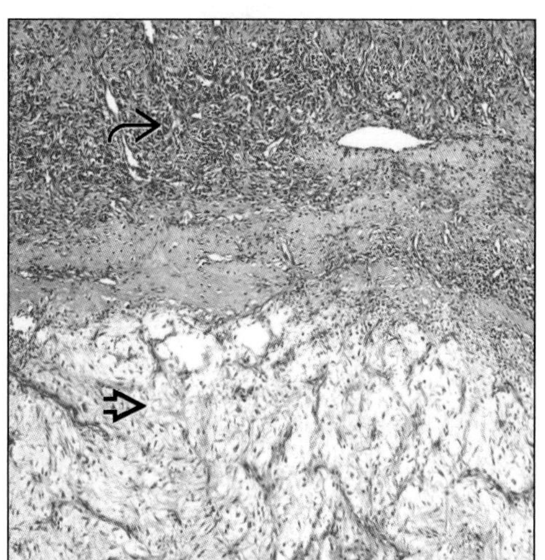

(Left) *Hematoxylin & eosin shows typical transition between cellular areas ⮫ and sparsely cellular collagenous zones. Note the prominent hyalinization of vessel walls ⇨ and the staghorn-shaped vessels →.* ***(Right)*** *Hematoxylin & eosin shows the sharp demarcation between hypercellular ⮫ and hypocellular ⇨ zones. In this case, the hypocellular area is prominently myxoid.*

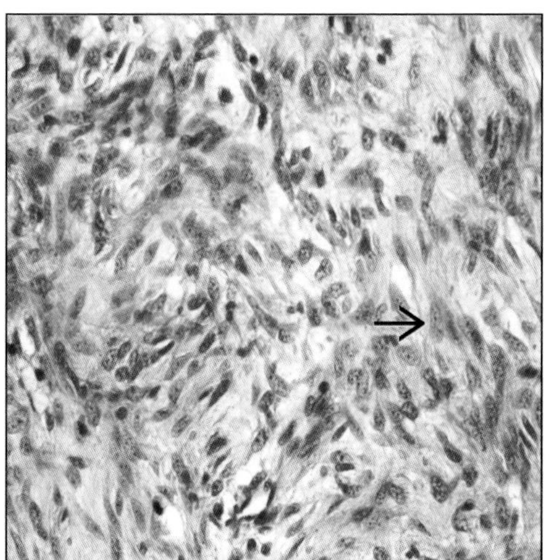

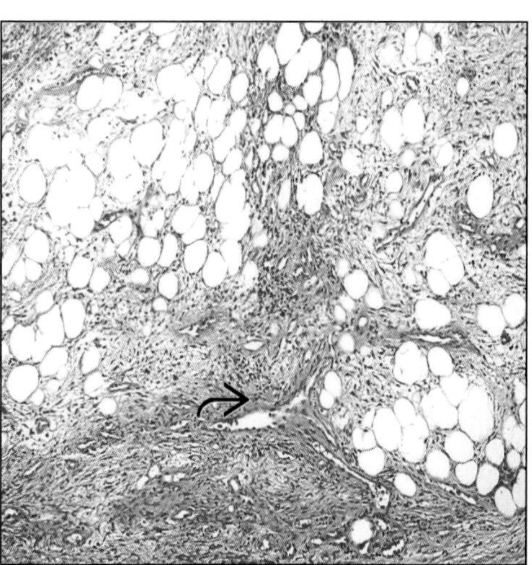

(Left) *Hematoxylin & eosin shows cells with bland, ovoid to spindle nuclei and largely indiscernible cytoplasm. Small nucleoli may be prominent →.* ***(Right)*** *Hematoxylin & eosin shows lipomatous hemangiopericytoma. The lesion shows typical features of solitary fibrous tumor, including branching vessels ⮫, but it is admixed with mature adipose tissue.*

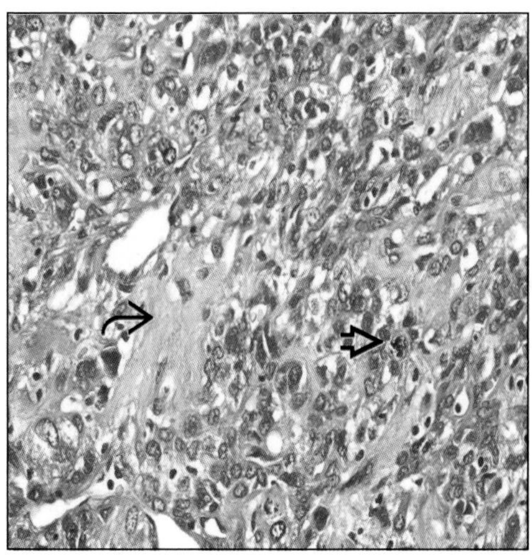

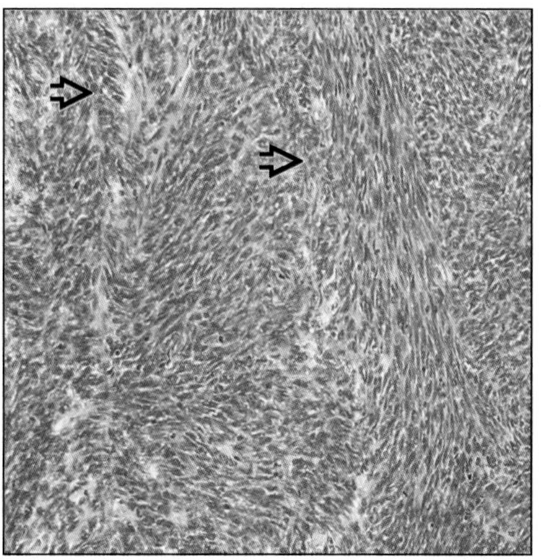

(Left) *Hematoxylin & eosin shows malignant solitary fibrous tumor. Although the tumor shows similar architectural features to usual SFT, such as collagenous stroma ⮫, it is entirely hypercellular. Cellular atypia is prominent, as is an atypical mitotic figure ⇨.* ***(Right)*** *Hematoxylin & eosin shows a malignant solitary fibrous tumor. There is frank sarcomatous change with fascicular or "herringbone," fibrosarcoma-like morphology ⇨ and abundant small mitoses.*

INFLAMMATORY MYOFIBROBLASTIC TUMOR

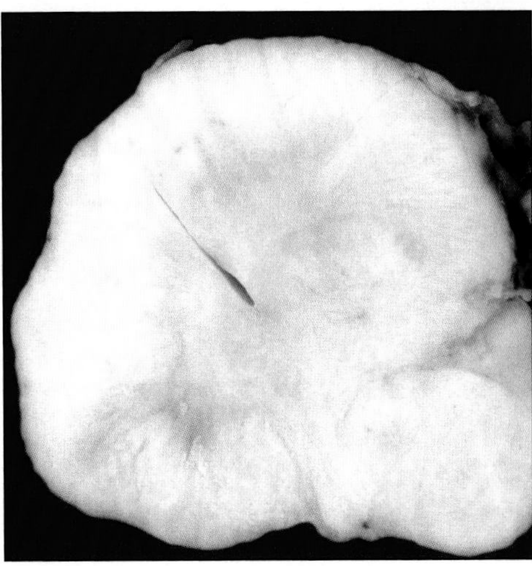

Gross photograph shows a large mesenteric inflammatory myofibroblastic tumor. This lesion formed 1 large mass that compressed one of the kidneys, but many such tumors are multilobulated.

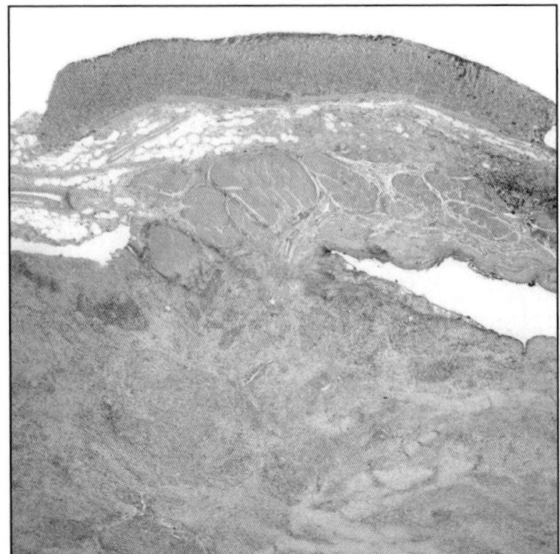

Hematoxylin & eosin shows an inflammatory myofibroblastic tumor involving the gastric mesentery. There are extensions into the outer muscularis propria but not into the mucosa.

TERMINOLOGY

Abbreviations

- Inflammatory myofibroblastic tumor (IMT)

Synonyms

- Inflammatory fibrosarcoma

Definitions

- Myofibroblastic neoplasm of intermediate biologic potential that frequently recurs but rarely metastasizes
- About 1/2 harbor rearrangements of anaplastic lymphoma kinase (*ALK*) gene
  - Alteration activates ALK receptor tyrosine kinase
    - Chromosome 2p23
    - Partners in rearrangements include *ATIC, CARS, TPM3, TPM4, CLTC, RANBP2, SEC31L*

CLINICAL ISSUES

Epidemiology

- Incidence
  - Rare
- Age
  - Often in children and young adults
    - Wide age range overall
- Gender
  - Slight female predominance

Presentation

- Site specific
  - Lung
    - Chest pain, dyspnea
  - Mesentery, omentum, gastrointestinal tract
    - Obstruction
    - B symptoms: Fever, growth retardation, anemia, weight loss
    - Hypergammaglobulinemia, elevated erythrocyte sedimentation rate
  - Soft tissue
    - Painless mass
  - Bladder
    - Hematuria: Controversial since some observers believe bladder lesions are unrelated to IMT in other sites
    - Some regard such lesions in bladder as "pseudosarcomatous myofibroblastic proliferation"
    - Share features (*ALK* alterations, p53 expression, frequent recurrences) with lesions from other sites; 1 reported (post-radiation) case with sarcomatous transformation

Treatment

- Surgery
  - B symptoms relieved by resection of tumor

Prognosis

- 1/4 to 1/3 recur
- Rare metastases (< 5%)

MACROSCOPIC FEATURES

General Features

- Large masses with solid sarcoma-like cut surface
- Often multilobulated

MICROSCOPIC PATHOLOGY

Histologic Features

- Spindled to stellate myofibroblastic cells
  - Some with storiform pattern
  - Some cases fascicular
  - Prominent nucleoli common
  - Highly atypical cells unusual and do not correlate well with outcome
  - Inconspicuous vessels
  - Cells occasionally bulge into vascular spaces
  - Scattered mitotic activity
- Fibroblasts

INFLAMMATORY MYOFIBROBLASTIC TUMOR

Key Facts

Terminology
- Myofibroblastic neoplasm of intermediate biologic potential that frequently recurs but rarely metastasizes
- About 1/2 harbor rearrangements of anaplastic lymphoma kinase (*ALK*) gene

Clinical Issues
- Often in children and young adults
- Wide age range overall
- Mesentery, omentum
- Obstruction
- B symptoms: Fever, growth retardation, anemia, weight loss
- Treatment is surgical
  - B symptoms relieved by resection of tumor
- 1/4 to 1/3 recur
- Rare metastases (< 5%)

Microscopic Pathology
- Spindled to stellate myofibroblastic cells
- Fibroblasts
- Some with storiform pattern
- Some cases fascicular
- Prominent nucleoli common
- Variable fibrosis and keloid-like collagen
- Lymphocytes, plasma cells
- Histiocytes

Ancillary Tests
- Subset is ALK(+), roughly correlating with activation of *ALK* gene rearrangements

---

  - Variable fibrosis and keloid-like collagen
- Inflammatory cells
  - Lymphocytes, plasma cells predominate
  - Histiocytes
  - Variable numbers of neutrophils and eosinophils
- Occasional calcification and ossification

ANCILLARY TESTS

Immunohistochemistry
- Subset is ALK(+), roughly correlating with activation of *ALK* gene rearrangements
- EBV and HHV8 expression reported in some cases, but ALK(+) cases are negative for these viral antigens

DIFFERENTIAL DIAGNOSIS

Inflammatory Fibroid Polyp
- Usually in submucosa of gastric antrum
- Bland spindle cells
- Whorling of proliferating cells around vessels
- Prominent eosinophils
- Scattered lymphocytes
- Immunohistochemistry
  - CD34(+), Cyclin-D1(+), CD117(-), S100 protein(-)
- *PDGFRA* mutations
- Benign

Fibromatosis
- Usually in small bowel mesentery
- Negligible inflammation
- Fascicles of spindle cells with interspersed collagen
- Prominent small caliber vessels
- Immunohistochemistry
  - Actin(+), desmin(-), CD117(±), β-catenin(+)
- *CTNNB1* (β-catenin) or *APC* mutations
- Benign but aggressive
  - Multiple recurrences, no metastases

Gastrointestinal Stromal Tumor (GIST)
- Usually involves muscularis propria of stomach
- Uniform spindle or epithelioid cells
- Usually negligible inflammation
- Immunohistochemistry
  - CD34(+), CD117(+), DOG1(+), S100 protein(-)
- *KIT* or *PDGFRA* mutations
- Most managed with local resection; some treated with imatinib
  - About 20% of patients with gastric GISTs die of disease
  - About 40% of patients with small bowel GISTs die of disease

Inflammatory Liposarcoma
- Retroperitoneum of older adults
- Well-differentiated liposarcoma: Usually mostly T lymphocytes
- Dedifferentiated liposarcoma: Mixed inflammation with many histiocytes and neutrophils
- Background highly atypical hyperchromatic enlarged nuclei
- Often zones of classic well-differentiated lipoma-like liposarcoma
- Immunohistochemistry
  - MDM2(+), CDK4(+)
- Ring chromosomes
- Malignant
  - 5-year survival ~ 75% for well-differentiated liposarcoma
  - 5-year survival ~ 60% for dedifferentiated liposarcoma
  - 10-year survival ~ 5-10% for dedifferentiated liposarcoma

Inflammatory Leiomyosarcoma
- Deep soft tissues of older adults
- Similar to IMT in inflamed areas but with more nuclear atypia
- Often have areas of classic leiomyosarcoma
- Immunohistochemistry
  - Actin(+), desmin (+), ALK(-)
- No characteristic molecular alterations
- Behaves as high-grade sarcoma

INFLAMMATORY MYOFIBROBLASTIC TUMOR

Immunohistochemistry

Antibody	Reactivity	Staining Pattern	Comment
Actin-sm	Positive	Cytoplasmic	Often focal
Desmin	Positive	Cytoplasmic	Often focal or negative
MDM2	Positive	Nuclear	Can lead to confusion with inflammatory well-differentiated liposarcoma
p53	Positive	Nuclear	~ 80% of cases
CK-PAN	Positive	Cytoplasmic	1/4 to 1/3 of cases (depending on series)
Cyclin-D1	Positive	Nuclear	
ALK1	Positive	Cytoplasmic	More commonly reactive in pediatric cases (~ 2/3) than in older adult cases (~ 1/3)
Myogenin	Negative		Occasional false-positives
S100P	Negative		

Sclerosing Mesenteritis

- Mesenteric masses
- Infiltrative borders
- Prominent sclerosis with infiltration between fat septa
- Fat necrosis, foamy macrophages
- Immunohistochemistry
  - Actin (variable), desmin (usually negative), ALK(-), β-catenin(-)
  - Some examples have prominent IgG4 immunolabeling
- Benign; small percentage of recurrence
  - Poor response to steroids; treatment usually surgical excision

Calcifying Fibrous (Pseudo)Tumor (CFT)

- Soft tissues in children, mesenteric in adults
  - Sometimes multiple small nodules
- Hypocellular lesions
- Bland fibroblasts
- Plasma cells and lymphocytes
- Psammomatous and dystrophic calcifications
- Immunohistochemistry
  - Actin (variable), desmin(-), ALK(-)
  - Many studies report negative ALK in all cases, which argues against theory that CFT is "burned out" IMT
- Benign

Lymphoma

- Many subtypes
- Monotonous clonal proliferation of various types lymphoid cells
- Seldom spindled
- Evaluated with wide panel of lymphoid markers depending on appearance
- Malignant; outcome depends on subtype

Extranodal Rosai-Dorfman Disease

- Spindled histiocytes with lymphoplasmacytic backdrop
- Emperipolesis
- Immunohistochemistry
  - S100 protein(+), CD68(+), ALK(-), CD1a(-)
- Most cases behave indolently with occasional aggressive behavior
- Often treated with steroids
  - Possibly autoimmune with unknown immunologic trigger

SELECTED REFERENCES

1. Coffin CM et al: Inflammatory myofibroblastic tumor: comparison of clinicopathologic, histologic, and immunohistochemical features including ALK expression in atypical and aggressive cases. Am J Surg Pathol. 31(4):509-20, 2007
2. Patel AS et al: RANBP2 and CLTC are involved in ALK rearrangements in inflammatory myofibroblastic tumors. Cancer Genet Cytogenet. 176(2):107-14, 2007
3. Harik LR et al: Pseudosarcomatous myofibroblastic proliferations of the bladder: a clinicopathologic study of 42 cases. Am J Surg Pathol. 30(7):787-94, 2006
4. Montgomery EA et al: Inflammatory myofibroblastic tumors of the urinary tract: a clinicopathologic study of 46 cases, including a malignant example inflammatory fibrosarcoma and a subset associated with high-grade urothelial carcinoma. Am J Surg Pathol. 30(12):1502-12, 2006
5. Yamamoto H et al: Absence of human herpesvirus-8 and Epstein-Barr virus in inflammatory myofibroblastic tumor with anaplastic large cell lymphoma kinase fusion gene. Pathol Int. 56(10):584-90, 2006
6. Sirvent N et al: ALK probe rearrangement in a t(2;11;2)(p23;p15;q31) translocation found in a prenatal myofibroblastic fibrous lesion: toward a molecular definition of an inflammatory myofibroblastic tumor family? Genes Chromosomes Cancer. 31(1):85-90, 2001
7. Lawrence B et al: TPM3-ALK and TPM4-ALK oncogenes in inflammatory myofibroblastic tumors. Am J Pathol. 157(2):377-84, 2000
8. Griffin CA et al: Recurrent involvement of 2p23 in inflammatory myofibroblastic tumors. Cancer Res. 59(12):2776-80, 1999
9. Coffin CM et al: Inflammatory myofibroblastic tumor, inflammatory fibrosarcoma, and related lesions: an historical review with differential diagnostic considerations. Semin Diagn Pathol. 15(2):102-10, 1998
10. Coffin CM et al: Extrapulmonary inflammatory myofibroblastic tumor (inflammatory pseudotumor). A clinicopathologic and immunohistochemical study of 84 cases. Am J Surg Pathol. 19(8):859-72, 1995
11. Meis JM et al: Inflammatory fibrosarcoma of the mesentery and retroperitoneum. A tumor closely simulating inflammatory pseudotumor. Am J Surg Pathol. 15(12):1146-56, 1991

Microscopic Features

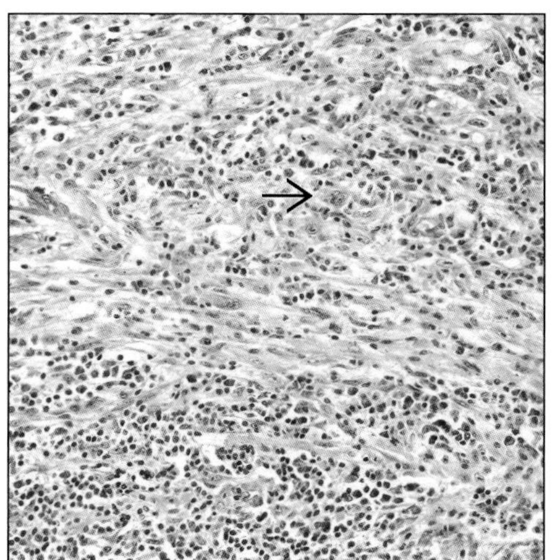

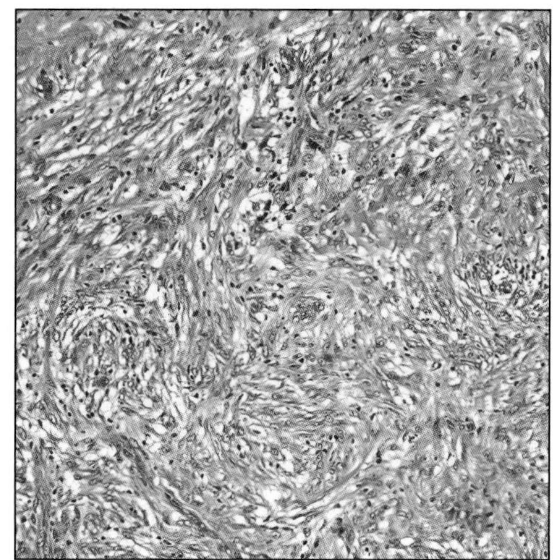

(Left) *Hematoxylin & eosin shows a mesenteric inflammatory myofibroblastic tumor with a prominent lymphoplasmacytic backdrop and a fascicular arrangement. The proliferating myofibroblastic cells often feature large nucleoli* ⇒. *Because of the atypia, they were initially described as "inflammatory fibrosarcoma."* ***(Right)*** *Hematoxylin & eosin shows an inflammatory myofibroblastic tumor that is less inflamed than the previous example. Note the storiform pattern.*

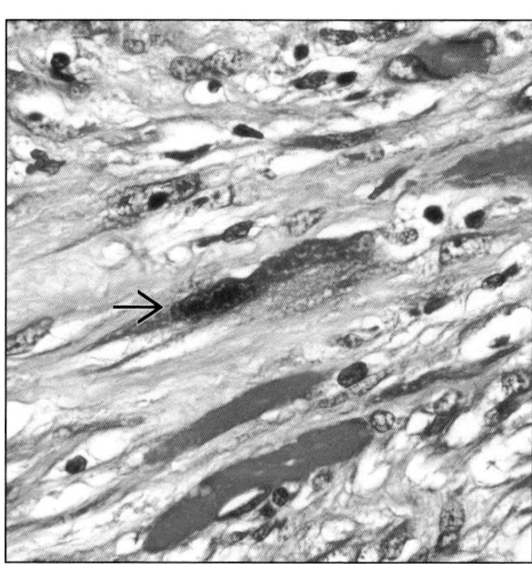

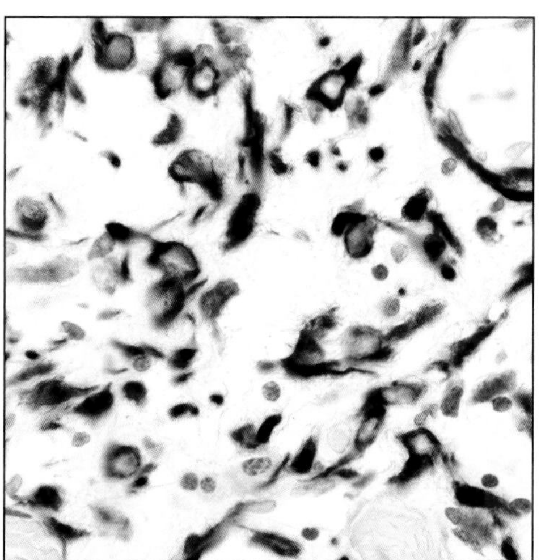

(Left) *Hematoxylin & eosin shows high magnification of a myofibroblastic nuclei in an inflammatory myofibroblastic tumor. Note the prominent nucleoli* ⇒. *The cells have stellate to spindled, eosinophilic to amphophilic cytoplasm.* ***(Right)*** *CK-PAN shows strong cytoplasmic staining in an inflammatory myofibroblastic tumor. Keratin staining is common in these tumors, and its presence should not lead to a diagnosis of sarcomatoid carcinoma.*

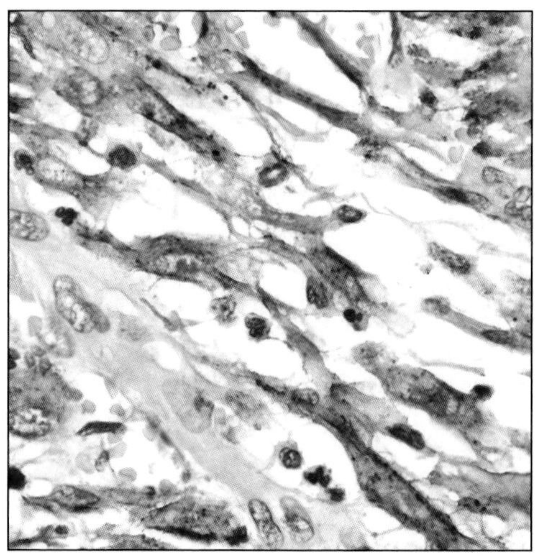

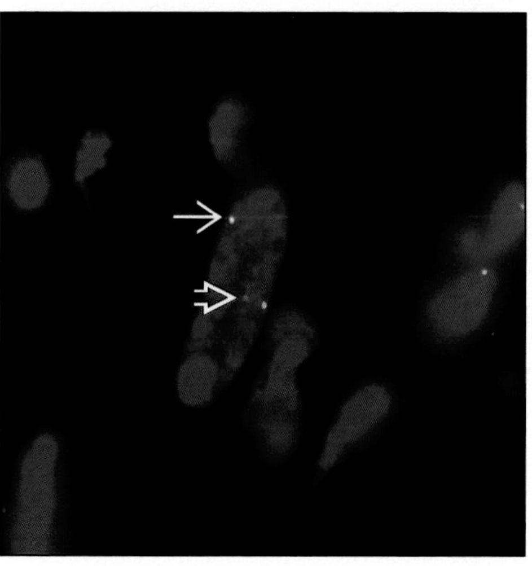

(Left) *ALK1 shows cytoplasmic labeling.* ***(Right)*** *In situ hybridization shows a rearrangement of the ALK gene. When the 2p23 breakpoint on chromosome 2 is rearranged (involved in a translocation), the orange and green signals are separated and visualized as distinct signals more than 1 signal width apart* ➡. *The abnormal specimen thus has 1 fusion for the normal chromosome 2* ➡, *and 1 orange and 1 green signal for the rearranged chromosome 2 (1O1G1F).*

LOW-GRADE MYOFIBROBLASTIC SARCOMA

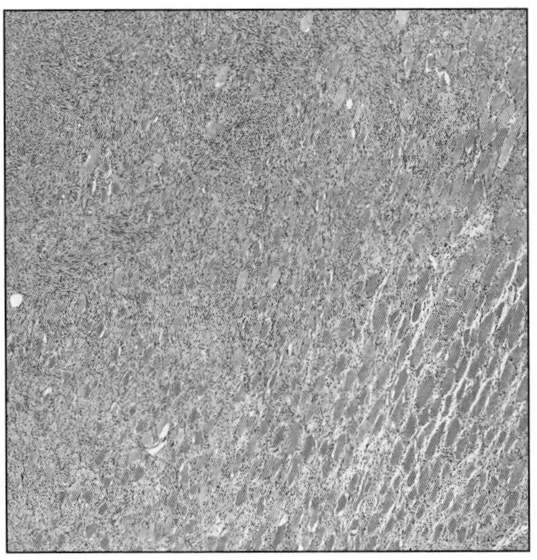

Low-grade myofibroblastic sarcoma is characterized by a diffuse infiltration of preexisting structures, as in this case, in which a diffuse infiltration of preexisting skeletal muscle is seen.

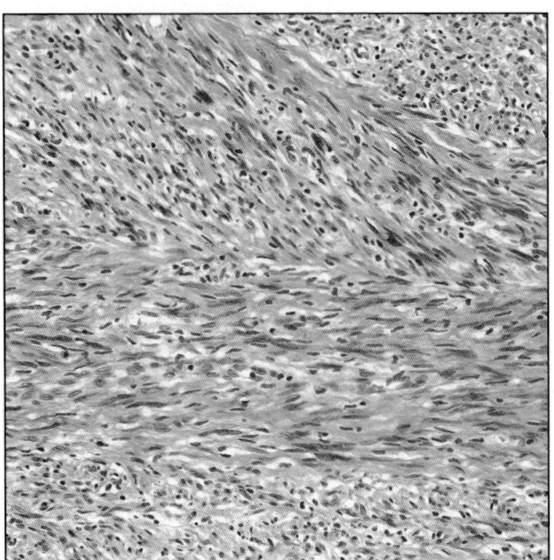

Low-grade myofibroblastic sarcoma composed of spindled cells shows myofibroblastic features. Tumor cells contain an ill-defined, pale eosinophilic cytoplasm and fusiform, slightly atypical nuclei.

TERMINOLOGY

Abbreviations

- Low-grade myofibroblastic sarcoma (LGMFS)

Synonyms

- Myofibrosarcoma

Definitions

- Distinct atypical myofibroblastic neoplasm with fibromatosis-like morphologic features

CLINICAL ISSUES

Epidemiology

- Incidence
  - Rare low-grade sarcoma
- Age
  - Occurs predominantly in adult patients
  - Children are rarely affected
- Gender
  - Slight male predominance

Site

- Wide anatomic distribution
- Occurs frequently in head and neck region
  - Tongue and oral cavity are preferred locations
- Occurs frequently in extremities
- Subcutaneous and deep soft tissue
- Very rare in dermal location

Presentation

- Deep mass
- Painless mass

Treatment

- Surgical approaches
  - Complete excision

Prognosis

- Locally aggressive behavior
- Increased rate of local recurrences
- Often repeated local recurrences
- Metastases occur only rarely and often after prolonged time interval

IMAGE FINDINGS

Radiographic Findings

- Destructive growth pattern

MACROSCOPIC FEATURES

General Features

- Firm tumor mass
- Infiltrative, ill-defined neoplasms
- Pale gray-white, fibrous cut surfaces

Size

- May reach considerable size

MICROSCOPIC PATHOLOGY

Histologic Features

- Diffusely infiltrative growth
- Tumor cells may grow diffusely between individual preexisting cells and structures
- Cellular spindle cell fascicles
- May show storiform growth
- Hypocellular neoplasms are rare
- Collagenous stroma
- Focal stromal hyalinizations may be seen
- Stroma may contain increased number of thin-walled capillaries
- Low to moderate degree of cytologic atypia
- Mitoses may be seen
- Usually no tumor necrosis
- May progress to higher grade malignant neoplasm

LOW-GRADE MYOFIBROBLASTIC SARCOMA

Key Facts

Terminology
- Low-grade myofibroblastic sarcoma represents distinct atypical myofibroblastic neoplasm with fibromatosis-like morphologic features

Clinical Issues
- Occurs frequently in head and neck region
- Occurs frequently in extremities
- Occurs only rarely in dermis
- Increased rate of local recurrences
- Metastases occur only rarely and often after prolonged time interval
- Occurs predominantly in adult patients
- Occurs only rarely in children

Microscopic Pathology
- Diffusely infiltrative growth
- Cellular spindle cell fascicles
- Low to moderate degree of cytologic atypia
- Usually no tumor necrosis
- Spindle-shaped tumor cells
- Ill-defined, pale eosinophilic cytoplasm
- Nuclei are elongated with evenly distributed chromatin
- Nuclei are vesicular with indentations and small nucleoli
- Variable expression of actin &/or desmin
- No expression of HCAD, β-catenin, and myogenin
- Tumor cells show ultrastructural features of myofibroblasts
- May progress to higher grade malignant neoplasm

Cytologic Features
- Spindle-shaped tumor cells
- Ill-defined, pale eosinophilic cytoplasm
- Fusiform nuclei
- Nuclei are elongated with evenly distributed chromatin
- Nuclei are vesicular with indentations and small nucleoli
- Moderate nuclear atypia with enlarged, hyperchromatic, and irregular nuclei

ANCILLARY TESTS

Electron Microscopy
- Tumor cells show myofibroblastic features
  - Indented, clefted nuclei
  - Variable amount of rough endoplasmic reticulum
  - Subplasmalemmal myofilaments (stress fibers) with focal densities
  - Paucity of subplasmalemmal attachment plaques
  - Absent basal lamina and pinocytotic vesicles
- Abundant extracellular collagen

DIFFERENTIAL DIAGNOSIS

Desmoid Fibromatosis
- Infiltrative growth but no diffuse "growing through preexisting structures"
- No cytologic atypia
- Perivascular edema
- β-catenin(+)
- Desmin usually negative
- Focal and weak expression of actins

Leiomyosarcoma
- Often pushing margins
- Spindled tumor cells with deep eosinophilic, fibrillary cytoplasm
- Spindled, cigar-shaped nuclei
- Paranuclear vacuoles
- HCAD(+)

Fibrosarcoma
- Extremely rare
- Herringbone growth pattern
- Small rim of cytoplasm and enlarged spindled nuclei
- No expression of myogenic immunohistochemical markers

Spindle Cell Rhabdomyosarcoma
- Very rare
- Scattered rhabdomyoblasts
- Focal nuclear expression of myogenin

Inflammatory Myofibroblastic Tumor
- Prominent inflammatory infiltrate (lymphocytes, plasma cells)
- Spindled and histiocytoid tumor cells
- ALK expression especially in cases arising in children and adolescents

Infantile Fibrosarcoma
- Children and adolescents are affected
- Plump, spindled, round tumor cells with enlarged nuclei
- Numerous mitoses
- Often tumor necrosis

Myofibroma/Myofibromatosis
- Biphasic growth
  - Primitive mesenchymal tumor cells associated with hemangiopericytoma-like growing capillaries
  - Mature myofibroblastic tumor cells set in collagenous/myxohyaline stroma
- No prominent atypia
- No desmin expression

Solitary Fibrous Tumor
- Well-circumscribed nodular neoplasms
- No strong expression of myogenic markers
- CD34(+)

Extraneural Spindle Cell Perineurioma
- Well-circumscribed nodular neoplasms
- Elongated spindled tumor cells

LOW-GRADE MYOFIBROBLASTIC SARCOMA

Immunohistochemistry

Antibody	Reactivity	Staining Pattern	Comment
Actin-sm	Positive	Cytoplasmic	Variably positive
Desmin	Positive	Cytoplasmic	Variably positive
CD34	Positive	Cytoplasmic	Focal positivity
Calponin	Positive	Cytoplasmic	Nonspecific
FN1	Positive	Cytoplasmic	Nonspecific
Caldesmon	Negative		
β-catenin	Negative		
S100	Negative		
CK-PAN	Negative		
Myogenin	Negative		

- Elongated, thin cytoplasmic processes
- EMA(+)
- Myogenic markers are usually negative

Low-Grade Fibromyxoid Sarcoma

- Bland, elongated, spindled tumor cells
- Whorling and swirling of neoplastic cells
- Arcades of blood vessels
- EMA expression in many cases

DIAGNOSTIC CHECKLIST

Clinically Relevant Pathologic Features

- Organ distribution
- Invasive pattern
- Nuclear features

Pathologic Interpretation Pearls

- Ill-defined, diffusely infiltrative neoplasm
- Cellular spindle cell fascicles
- Tumor cells contain ill-defined, pale eosinophilic cytoplasm and elongated fusiform nuclei
- Low to moderate degree of cytologic atypia

SELECTED REFERENCES

1. Demarosi F et al: Low-grade myofibroblastic sarcoma of the oral cavity. Oral Surg Oral Med Oral Pathol Oral Radiol Endod. 108(2):248-54, 2009
2. Agaimy A et al: Low-grade abdominopelvic sarcoma with myofibroblastic features (low-grade myofibroblastic sarcoma): clinicopathological, immunohistochemical, molecular genetic and ultrastructural study of two cases with literature review. J Clin Pathol. 61(3):301-6, 2008
3. Qiu X et al: Inflammatory myofibroblastic tumor and low-grade myofibroblastic sarcoma: a comparative study of clinicopathologic features and further observations on the immunohistochemical profile of myofibroblasts. Hum Pathol. 39(6):846-56, 2008
4. Watanabe K et al: Fibronexus in low-grade myofibrosarcoma: a case report. Ultrastruct Pathol. 32(3):97-100, 2008
5. Carlson JW et al: Immunohistochemistry for beta-catenin in the differential diagnosis of spindle cell lesions: analysis of a series and review of the literature. Histopathology. 51(4):509-14, 2007
6. Coyne JD: Low-grade myofibroblastic sarcoma of the piriform fossa: a case report with a literature review of a tumour with a predilection for the head and neck. Br J Oral Maxillofac Surg. 45(4):335-7, 2007
7. Jay A et al: Low-grade myofibroblastic sarcoma of the tongue. Oral Surg Oral Med Oral Pathol Oral Radiol Endod. 104(5):e52-8, 2007
8. Perez-Montiel MD et al: Differential expression of smooth muscle myosin, smooth muscle actin, h-caldesmon, and calponin in the diagnosis of myofibroblastic and smooth muscle lesions of skin and soft tissue. Am J Dermatopathol. 28(2):105-11, 2006
9. Bhattacharya B et al: Nuclear beta-catenin expression distinguishes deep fibromatosis from other benign and malignant fibroblastic and myofibroblastic lesions. Am J Surg Pathol. 29(5):653-9, 2005
10. Fisher C: Low-grade sarcomas with CD34-positive fibroblasts and low-grade myofibroblastic sarcomas. Ultrastruct Pathol. 28(5-6):291-305, 2004
11. Fisher C: Myofibroblastic malignancies. Adv Anat Pathol. 11(4):190-201, 2004
12. Roth TM et al: Low-grade myofibroblastic sarcoma of the vulva. Gynecol Oncol. 92(1):361-4, 2004
13. González-Cámpora R et al: Myofibrosarcoma (low-grade myofibroblastic sarcoma) with intracytoplasmic hyaline (fibroma-like) inclusion bodies. Ultrastruct Pathol. 27(1):7-11, 2003
14. Kuhnen C et al: [Myofibroblastic sarcoma of the thoracic wall. Change in appearance in tumour recurrence.] Pathologe. 24(2):128-35, 2003
15. Bisceglia M et al: Myofibrosarcoma of the upper jawbones: a clinicopathologic and ultrastructural study of two cases. Ultrastruct Pathol. 25(5):385-97, 2001
16. Chang SE et al: A case of cutaneous low-grade myofibroblastic sarcoma. J Dermatol. 28(7):383-7, 2001
17. Bisceglia M et al: Low-grade myofibroblastic sarcoma of the salivary gland. Am J Surg Pathol. 23(11):1435-6, 1999
18. Mentzel T et al: Low-grade myofibroblastic sarcoma: analysis of 18 cases in the spectrum of myofibroblastic tumors. Am J Surg Pathol. 22(10):1228-38, 1998
19. Smith DM et al: Myofibrosarcoma of the head and neck in children. Pediatr Pathol Lab Med. 15(3):403-18, 1995
20. Eyden BP et al: Myofibrosarcoma of subcutaneous soft tissue of the cheek. J Submicrosc Cytol Pathol. 24(3):307-13, 1992

LOW-GRADE MYOFIBROBLASTIC SARCOMA

Gross and Microscopic Features

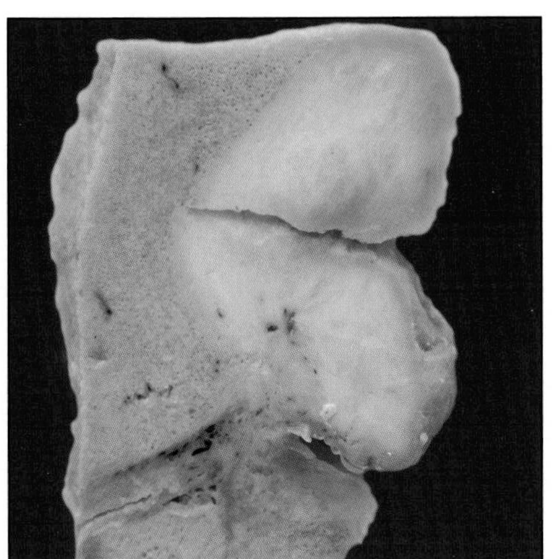
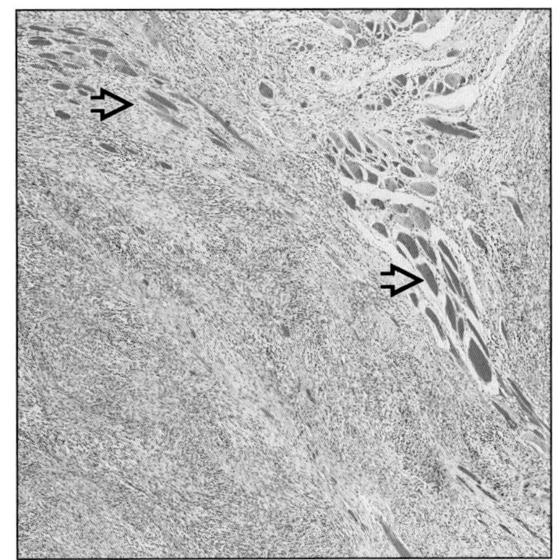

(Left) *Gross photograph shows a low-grade myofibroblastic sarcoma arising in the testis. White and indurated cut surfaces are seen.* ***(Right)*** *This low-grade myofibroblastic sarcoma arose on the lower lip of a 46-year-old man. A diffuse infiltration of preexisting skeletal muscle fibers is seen on this low-power view* ➪.

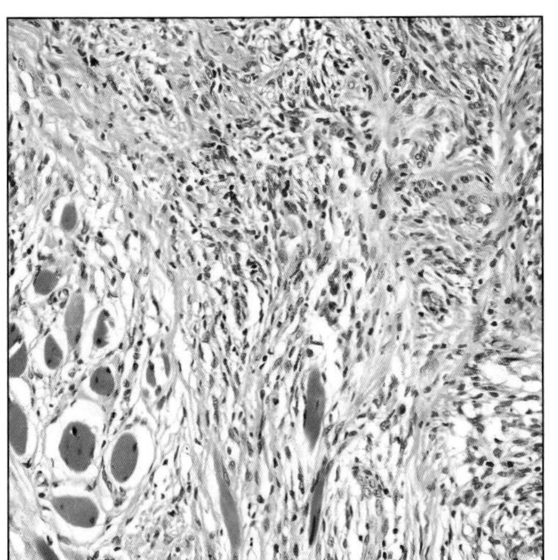
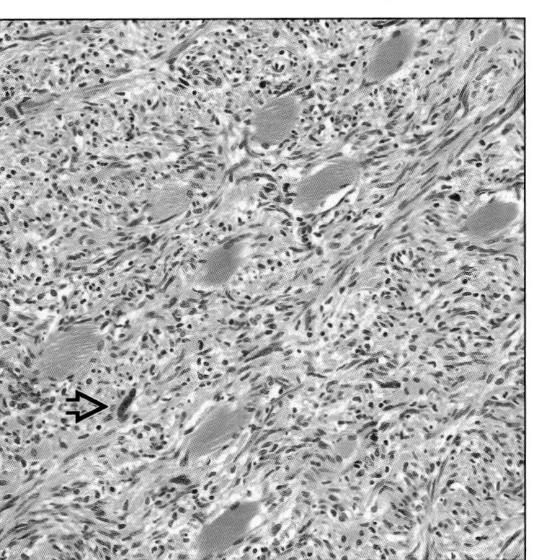

(Left) *This infiltrating neoplasm is composed of spindled tumor cells that are set in a collagenous stroma with scattered inflammatory cells.* ***(Right)*** *Preexisting skeletal muscle fibers are diffusely infiltrated by neoplastic cells in a characteristic fashion. Neoplastic cells contain enlarged nuclei with irregular borders* ➪.

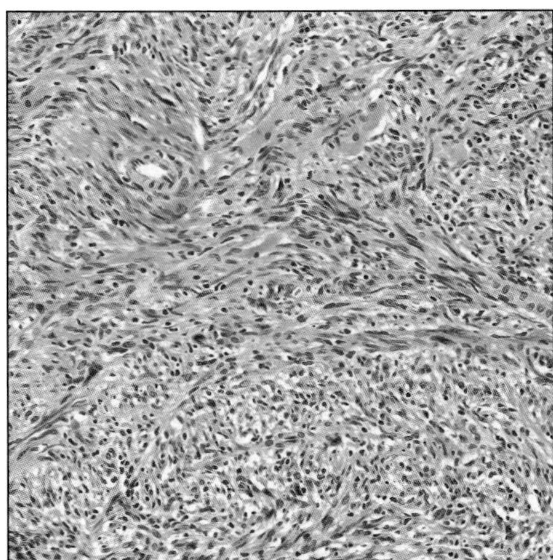
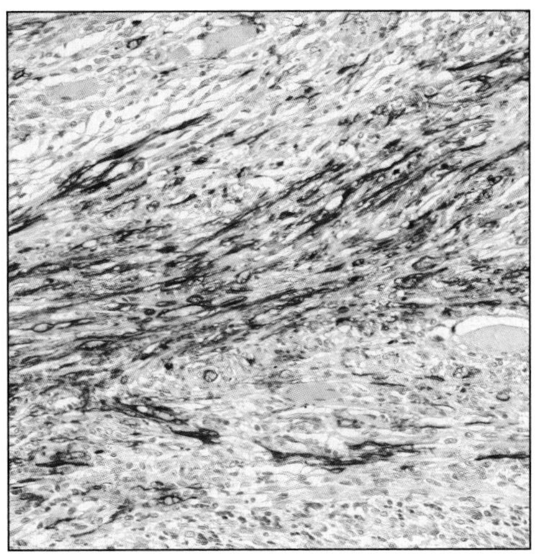

(Left) *Neoplastic spindled cells in low-grade myofibroblastic sarcoma are arranged in ill-defined bands and fascicles. The neoplastic cells contain an ill-defined, pale eosinophilic cytoplasm and enlarged nuclei that are either hyperchromatic or vesicular with small nucleoli and indentations.* ***(Right)*** *Neoplastic cells in this low-grade myofibroblastic sarcoma show a cytoplasmic expression of actin-sm.*

LOW-GRADE MYOFIBROBLASTIC SARCOMA

Microscopic Features and Electron Microscopy

*(**Left**) This example of a low-grade myofibroblastic sarcoma arose on the thigh of a young male patient. Note the diffuse infiltration of skeletal muscle fibers. (**Right**) Neoplastic cells are arranged in ill-defined bands and diffusely infiltrate preexisting muscle fibers.*

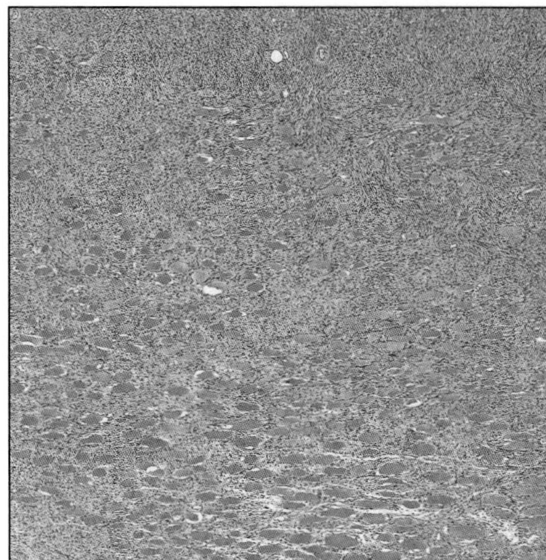

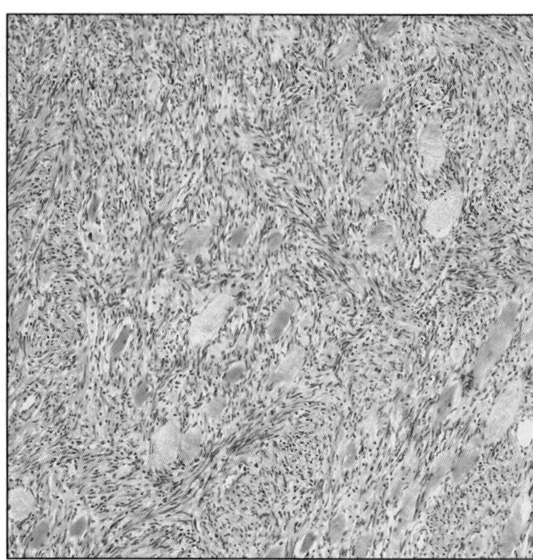

*(**Left**) Neoplastic cells contain elongated, wavy nuclei showing often irregular borders. The collagenous stroma contains narrow vessels. (**Right**) Hematoxylin & eosin shows diffuse infiltration of preexisting muscle fibers in a chessboard fashion. Spindled tumor cells contain enlarged and irregularly configurated nuclei ⇨.*

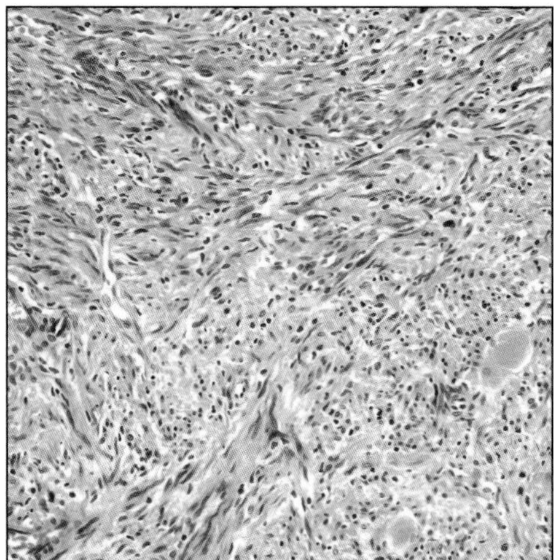

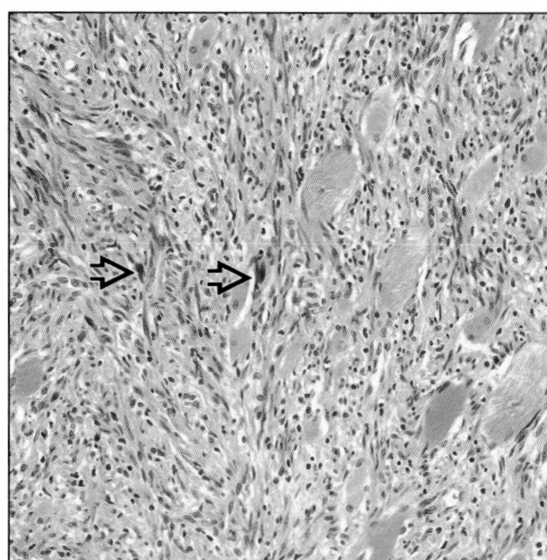

*(**Left**) Electron micrograph of neoplastic myofibroblast shows subplasmalemmal myofilaments (stress fibers) ➡ with focal densities ↪. This extends through the cell membrane as a fibronexus fibril (not shown). Note the rough endoplasmic reticulum ⇨. (**Right**) Ultrastructurally, neoplastic cells contain spindled nuclei with small nucleoli and irregular borders. Abundant rough endoplasmic reticulum is seen in the cytoplasm ⇨. Collagen fibers surround neoplastic cells ➡.*

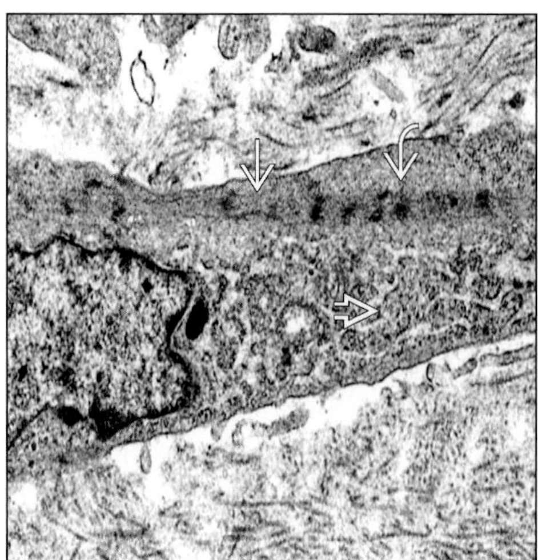

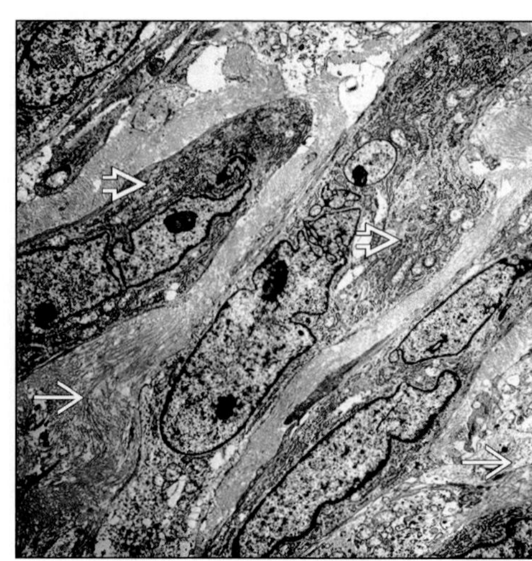

Microscopic Features

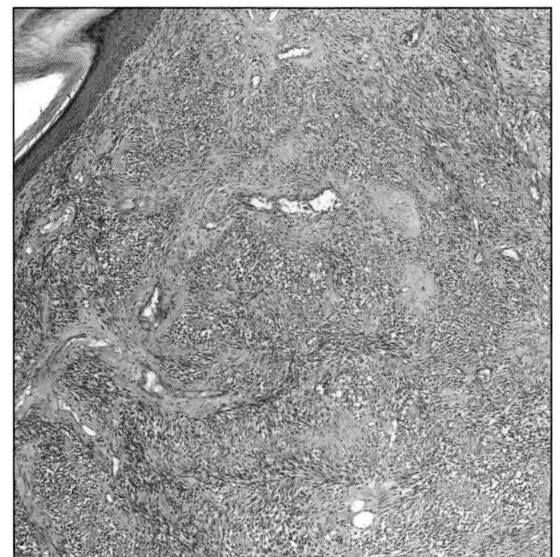

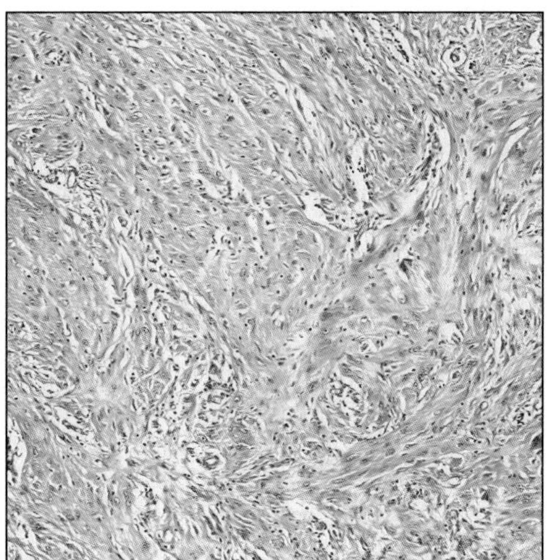

(Left) *Hematoxylin & eosin shows a rare case of a superficially located, dermal low-grade myofibroblastic sarcoma composed of atypical, plump spindled tumor cells set in a collagenous stroma.* ***(Right)*** *A 39-year-old female patient developed an ill-defined soft tissue neoplasm on the left shoulder, initially diagnosed as desmoid fibromatosis, that recurred multiple times. The hypocellular neoplasm is composed of plump spindled tumor cells set in a prominent collagenous stroma.*

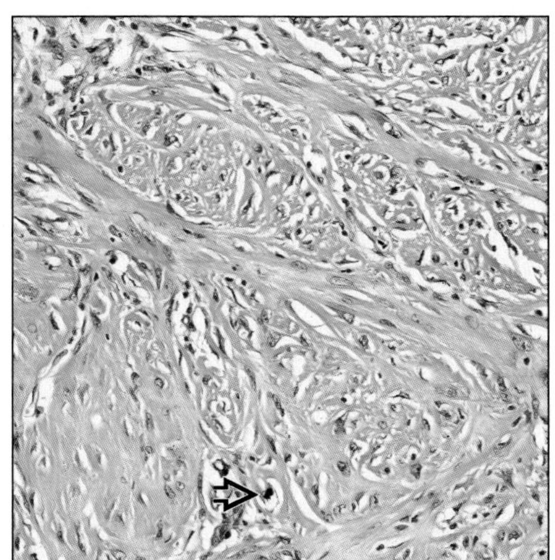

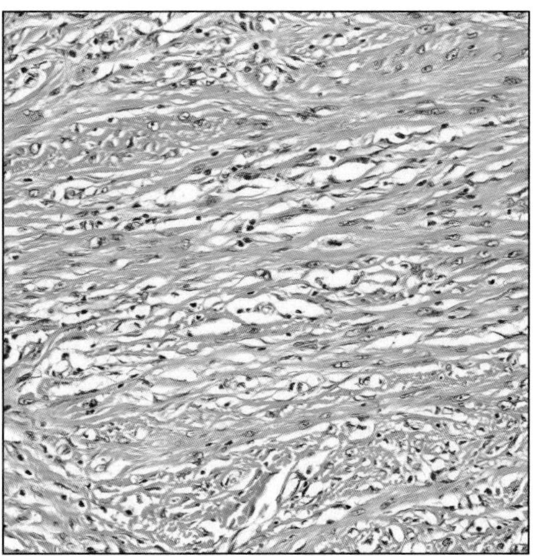

(Left) *Tumor cells are arranged in ill-defined bands and contain enlarged vesicular nuclei. Note the scattered mitoses ⇨, unusual in desmoid fibromatosis.* ***(Right)*** *Hematoxylin & eosin shows tumor cells containing an ill-defined, pale eosinophilic cytoplasm and enlarged vesicular nuclei with small nucleoli and irregular indentations.*

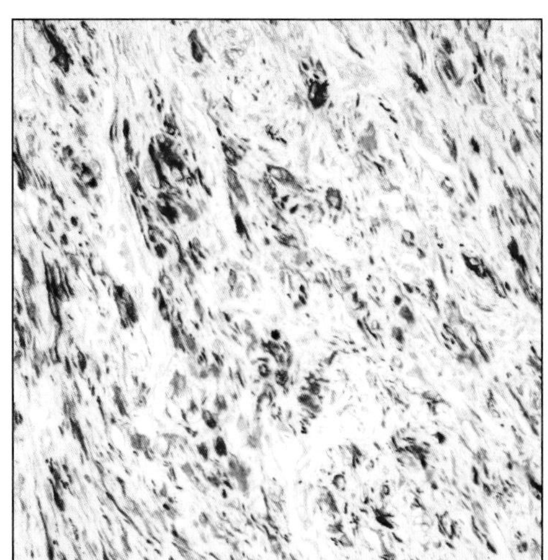

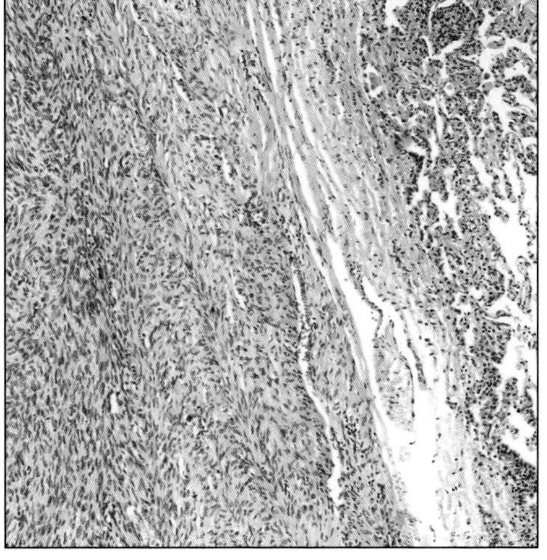

(Left) *Neoplastic cells stain positively for desmin (which would be unusual in cases of desmoid fibromatosis).* ***(Right)*** *Hematoxylin & eosin in this 39-year-old woman shows lung metastases that developed 17 years after the primary low-grade myofibroblastic sarcoma had been excised.*

INFANTILE FIBROSARCOMA

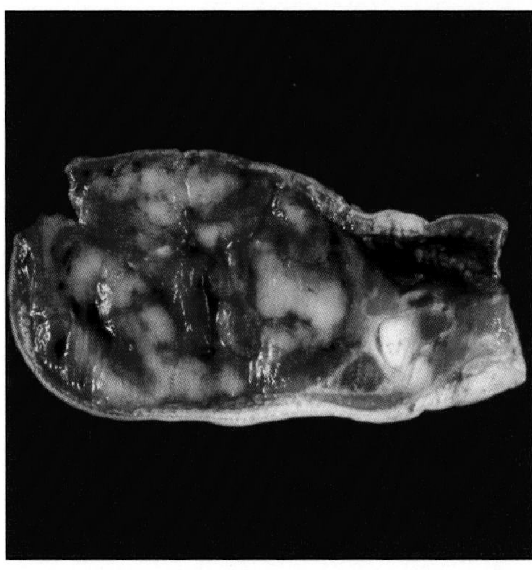

Gross photograph shows a large, hemorrhagic, congenital soft tissue neoplasm arising on the arm of a 13-day-old female baby.

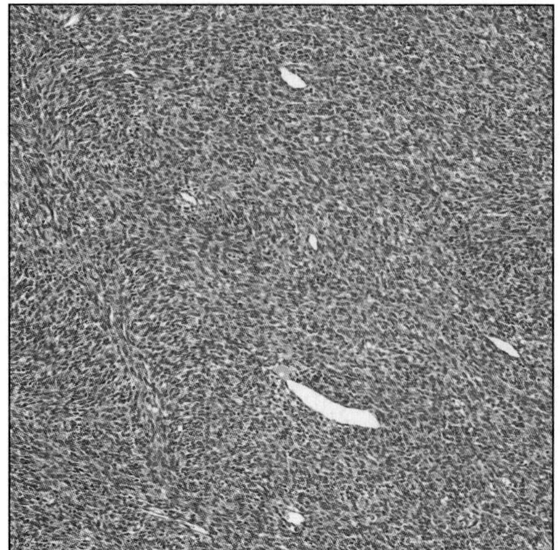

Hematoxylin & eosin shows a cellular neoplasm containing numerous thin-walled blood vessels. The neoplasm is composed of plump spindled, immature-appearing fibroblastic tumor cells.

TERMINOLOGY

Synonyms

- Congenital fibrosarcoma
- Juvenile fibrosarcoma
- Aggressive infantile fibromatosis

Definitions

- Occurs in infants and young children and represents a low-grade fibrosarcoma that carries favorable prognosis

CLINICAL ISSUES

Epidemiology

- Incidence
  - Accounts for ~ 12% of mesenchymal malignancies in infants
- Age
  - Congenital or in 1st 2 years of life
  - Rare in children older than 2 years
- Gender
  - Slight male predominance

Site

- Superficial and deep soft tissues of extremities are most common sites
- More rarely seen on trunk and in head and neck region
- Very rare in retroperitoneum and in mesentery

Presentation

- Limb enlargement
- Painless mass
  - Solitary neoplasms
  - Usually very large neoplasms
  - Overlying skin may be ulcerated
- Suddenly enlarging mass

Natural History

- Often short preoperative duration

Treatment

- Surgical approaches
  - Complete excision with tumor-free margins
- Adjuvant therapy
  - Chemotherapy has been proven effective

Prognosis

- Recurrence rate varies (5-50%)
- Metastases are very rare
- Mortality ranges from 5-25%
- Spontaneous regression has been reported
- Favorable prognosis

IMAGE FINDINGS

General Features

- Usually large soft tissue mass
- Shows heterogeneous enhancement pattern
- May show osseous erosion

MACROSCOPIC FEATURES

General Features

- Poorly circumscribed, lobulated soft tissue tumor
- Infiltration of adjacent tissues
- Firm gray-white cut surfaces
- Variable myxoid changes
- Areas of hemorrhage and necrosis are sometimes present

MICROSCOPIC PATHOLOGY

Histologic Features

- Cellular neoplasms

INFANTILE FIBROSARCOMA

Key Facts

Terminology

- Occurs in infants and young children; represents low-grade fibrosarcoma that carries favorable prognosis

Clinical Issues

- Congenital or arises in 1st two years of life
- Superficial and deep soft tissues of extremities are most common sites
- Solitary neoplasms
- Usually very large neoplasms
- Recurrence rate varies (5-50%)
- Metastases very rare
- Favorable prognosis
- Complete excision with tumor-free margins

Microscopic Pathology

- Cellular neoplasms
- Composed of intersecting fascicles of primitive, immature tumor cells
- Usually little cellular pleomorphism
- Numerous mitoses
- Areas of tumor necrosis &/or hemorrhages are frequent
- Often prominent vessels with hemangiopericytoma-like pattern
- Primitive ovoid and spindled tumor cells

Ancillary Tests

- Most cases contain chromosomal translocation t(12;15)(p13;q26)
- *NTRK3-ETV6* fusion

- Composed of intersecting fascicles of primitive, immature tumor cells
- Often sheets of solidly packed, immature, spindled tumor cells
- Primitive ovoid and spindled tumor cells
- Usually little cellular pleomorphism
- Numerous mitoses
- Areas of tumor necrosis &/or hemorrhage frequent
- Variable collagen formation
- Scattered inflammatory cells often noted
- Often prominent vessels with hemangiopericytoma-like pattern

Predominant Pattern/Injury Type

- Fascicular

Predominant Cell/Compartment Type

- Fibroblast
- Myofibroblast

ANCILLARY TESTS

Cytogenetics

- Most cases contain chromosomal translocation t(12;15)(p13;q26)
- *NTRK3-ETV6* fusion
- Oncogenic activation of *NTRK3* receptor tyrosine kinase gene
- In addition trisomies for chromosomes 8, 11, 17, and 20 are characteristic
- Similar genetic profile is seen in cellular congenital mesoblastic nephroma

Electron Microscopy

- Cellular features of fibroblasts and myofibroblasts seen
- Large tumor cell nuclei
- Dilated rough endoplasmic reticulum
- Abundant lysosomes
- Cytoplasmic filaments

DIFFERENTIAL DIAGNOSIS

Cellular Infantile Fibromatosis

- No metastatic potential
- Diffuse infiltration
- Often myxoid stromal changes
- Lower proliferative activity
- Usually no tumor necrosis
- No t(12;15)(p13;q26)

Desmoid Fibromatosis

- No metastatic potential
- More mature, bland spindled tumor cells
- Low proliferative activity
- Perivascular edema
- Nuclear expression of β-catenin
- No t(12;15)(p13;q26)

Infantile Myofibroma/Myofibromatosis

- Biphasic growth
  - Mature spindled myogenic tumor cells
  - Immature ovoid tumor cells with numerous vessels showing hemangiopericytoma-like pattern
- Homogeneous expression of actins
- No t(12;15)(p13;q26)

Spindle Cell Rhabdomyosarcoma

- Arise predominantly in paratesticular location
- Scattered rhabdomyoblasts
- Expression of desmin and myogenin
- No t(12;15)(p13;q26)

Infantile Rhabdomyofibrosarcoma

- Extremely rare
- Poor clinical outcome
- Combination of fibrosarcomatous tumor areas and scattered rhabdomyoblasts
- Focal expression of desmin and myogenin
- No t(12;15)(p13;q26)

Leiomyosarcoma

- Rare in young children
- Smooth muscle cytomorphology

INFANTILE FIBROSARCOMA

Immunohistochemistry

Antibody	Reactivity	Staining Pattern	Comment
Vimentin	Positive	Cytoplasmic	
Actin-HHF-35	Positive	Cytoplasmic	Variable expression
Actin-sm	Positive	Cytoplasmic	Variable expression
Desmin	Positive	Cytoplasmic	Variable expression
NSE	Positive	Cytoplasmic	Variable expression
Myogenin	Negative		
S100	Negative		
AE1/AE3	Negative		

  - Dense eosinophilic fibrillary cytoplasm
  - Cigar-shaped nuclei
  - Perinuclear vacuoles
- Expression of H-caldesmon
- No t(12;15)(p13;q26)

Inflammatory Myofibroblastic Tumor
- Occurs often in viscera and in deep soft tissues
- Sometimes systemic symptoms
- Multinodular, lobular neoplasms
- More mature myofibroblastic tumor cells
- Often myxoid stromal changes
- Prominent inflammatory infiltrate
- No t(12;15)(p13;q26)

Low-Grade Myofibroblastic Sarcoma
- Tends to occur in adults
- Diffuse infiltration of preexisting structures
- More mature myofibroblastic tumor cells
- Lower proliferative activity
- Usually no tumor necrosis
- No t(12;15)(p13;q26)

DIAGNOSTIC CHECKLIST

Clinically Relevant Pathologic Features
- Gross appearance
- Organ distribution

Pathologic Interpretation Pearls
- Immature-appearing plump spindled tumor cells
- Fibroblastic/myofibroblastic neoplasm
- Low degree of cytologic atypia
- Numerous mitoses
- Often areas of tumor necrosis
- Characteristic genetic changes

SELECTED REFERENCES

1. Russell H et al: Infantile fibrosarcoma: clinical and histologic responses to cytotoxic chemotherapy. Pediatr Blood Cancer. 53(1):23-7, 2009
2. Alaggio R et al: Morphologic Overlap between Infantile Myofibromatosis and Infantile Fibrosarcoma: A Pitfall in Diagnosis. Pediatr Dev Pathol. 11(5):355-62, 2008
3. Ferguson WS: Advances in the adjuvant treatment of infantile fibrosarcoma. Expert Rev Anticancer Ther. 3(2):185-91, 2003
4. McCahon E et al: Non-resectable congenital tumors with the ETV6-NTRK3 gene fusion are highly responsive to chemotherapy. Med Pediatr Oncol. 40(5):288-92, 2003
5. Loh ML et al: Treatment of infantile fibrosarcoma with chemotherapy and surgery: results from the Dana-Farber Cancer Institute and Children's Hospital, Boston. J Pediatr Hematol Oncol. 24(9):722-6, 2002
6. Sandberg AA et al: Updates on the cytogenetics and molecular genetics of bone and soft tissue tumors: congenital (infantile) fibrosarcoma and mesoblastic nephroma. Cancer Genet Cytogenet. 132(1):1-13, 2002
7. Adem C et al: ETV6 rearrangements in patients with infantile fibrosarcomas and congenital mesoblastic nephromas by fluorescence in situ hybridization. Mod Pathol. 14(12):1246-51, 2001
8. Cecchetto G et al: Fibrosarcoma in pediatric patients: results of the Italian Cooperative Group studies (1979-1995). J Surg Oncol. 78(4):225-31, 2001
9. Dubus P et al: The detection of Tel-TrkC chimeric transcripts is more specific than TrkC immunoreactivity for the diagnosis of congenital fibrosarcoma. J Pathol. 193(1):88-94, 2001
10. Mrad K et al: [Infantile fibrosarcoma: a clinicopathological and molecular study of five cases.] Ann Pathol. 21(5):387-92, 2001
11. Sheng WQ et al: Congenital-infantile fibrosarcoma. A clinicopathologic study of 10 cases and molecular detection of the ETV6-NTRK3 fusion transcripts using paraffin-embedded tissues. Am J Clin Pathol. 115(3):348-55, 2001
12. Argani P et al: Detection of the ETV6-NTRK3 chimeric RNA of infantile fibrosarcoma/cellular congenital mesoblastic nephroma in paraffin-embedded tissue: application to challenging pediatric renal stromal tumors. Mod Pathol. 13(1):29-36, 2000
13. Bourgeois JM et al: Molecular detection of the ETV6-NTRK3 gene fusion differentiates congenital fibrosarcoma from other childhood spindle cell tumors. Am J Surg Pathol. 24(7):937-46, 2000
14. Knezevich SR et al: A novel ETV6-NTRK3 gene fusion in congenital fibrosarcoma. Nat Genet. 18(2):184-7, 1998
15. Knezevich SR et al: ETV6-NTRK3 gene fusions and trisomy 11 establish a histogenetic link between mesoblastic nephroma and congenital fibrosarcoma. Cancer Res. 58(22):5046-8, 1998
16. Rubin BP et al: Congenital mesoblastic nephroma t(12;15) is associated with ETV6-NTRK3 gene fusion: cytogenetic and molecular relationship to congenital (infantile) fibrosarcoma. Am J Pathol. 153(5):1451-8, 1998
17. Variend S et al: Are infantile myofibromatosis, congenital fibrosarcoma and congenital haemangiopericytoma histogenetically related? Histopathology. 26(1):57-62, 1995
18. Chung EB et al: Infantile fibrosarcoma. Cancer. 38(2):729-39, 1976

Microscopic Features

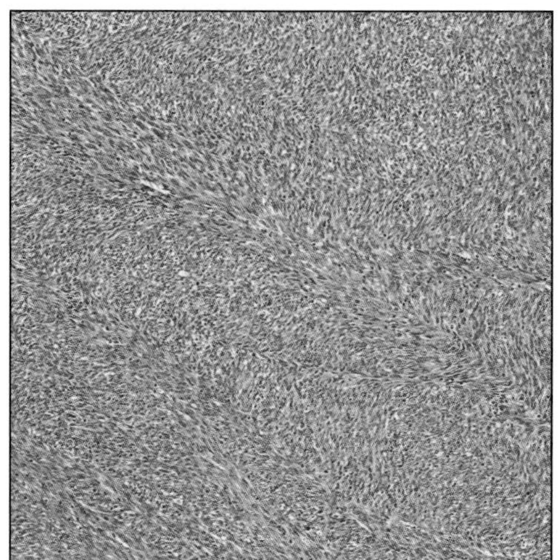

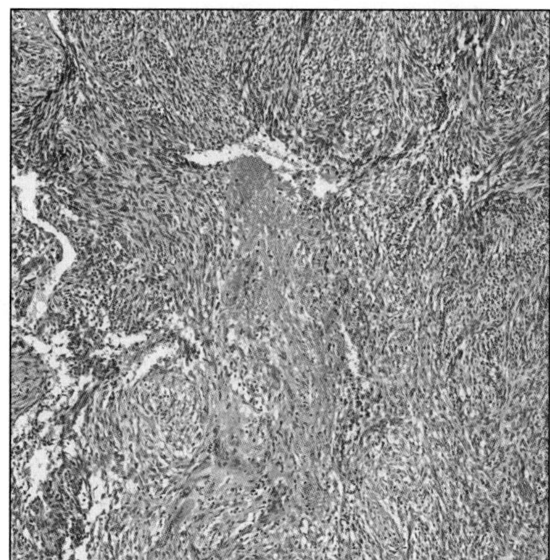

(Left) *This example of an infantile fibrosarcoma arose on the abdominal wall of a 2-month-old male baby. The neoplasm is composed of plump spindled tumor cells arranged in ill-defined fascicles.* ***(Right)*** *As in this case, areas of hemorrhage and tumor necrosis are often present in infantile fibrosarcoma.*

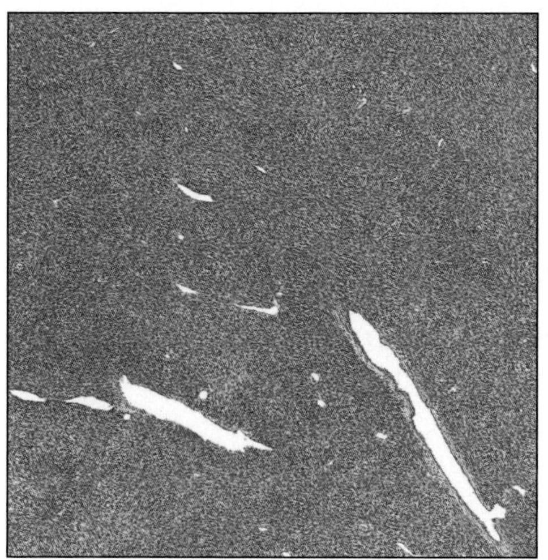

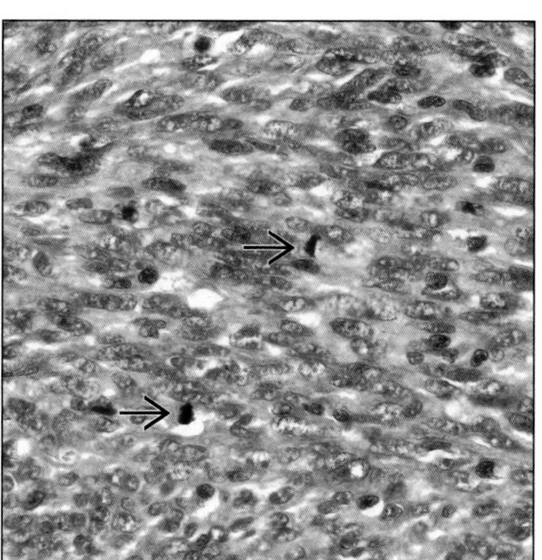

(Left) *The cellular tumor tissue contains numerous thin-walled blood vessels, which may show a hemangiopericytoma-like growth.* ***(Right)*** *High-power view shows immature-appearing plump spindled tumor cells containing enlarged nuclei. Note the numerous mitotic figures ⇾.*

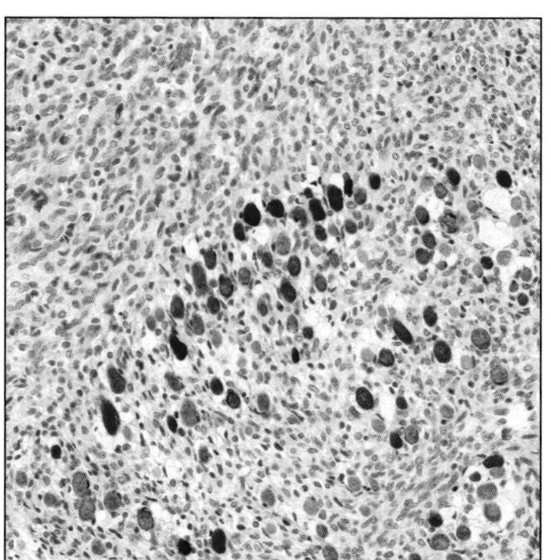

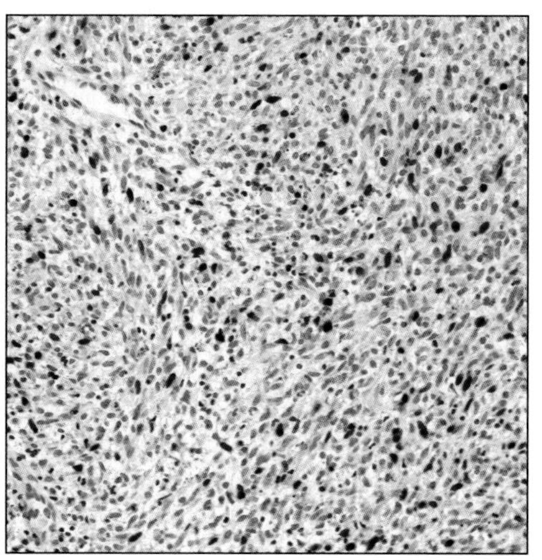

(Left) *Desmin shows preexisting skeletal muscle fibers in this case of a diffusely infiltrating infantile fibrosarcoma.* ***(Right)*** *Ki-67 antibodies reveal an increased proliferative activity of neoplastic cells in infantile fibrosarcoma.*

MYXOINFLAMMATORY FIBROBLASTIC SARCOMA

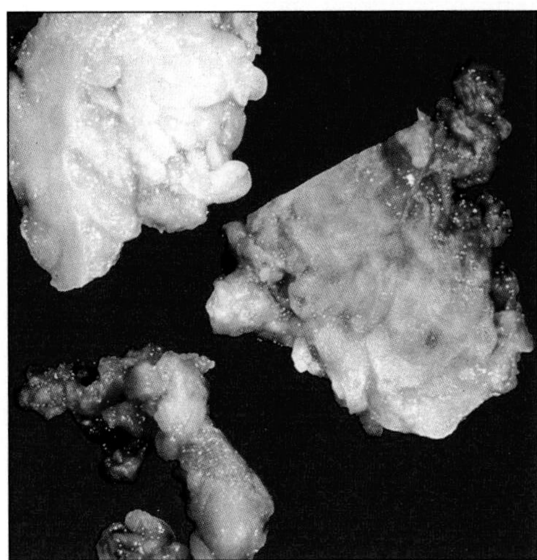

This is a gross specimen of a myxoinflammatory fibroblastic sarcoma. This particular lesion was highly infiltrative and clinically mistaken for pigmented villonodular tenosynovitis.

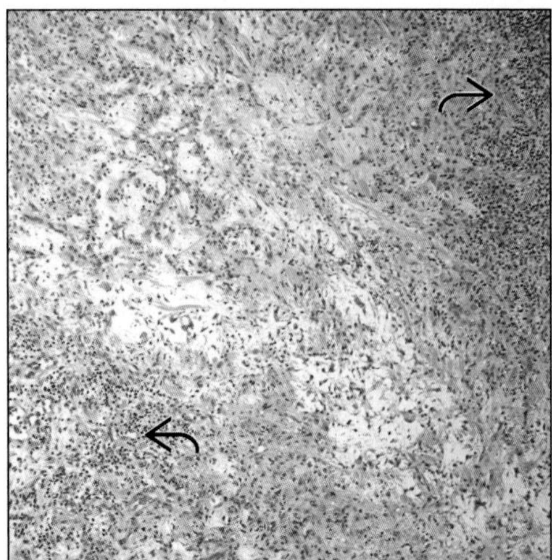

At scanning magnification, myxoinflammatory fibroblastic sarcoma displays a generous inflammatory background and scattered myxoid zones. Lymphoid cells are prominent at the edges of the field ⮫.

TERMINOLOGY

Synonyms

- Acral myxoinflammatory fibroblastic sarcoma, inflammatory myxohyaline tumor

Definitions

- Low-grade fibroblastic sarcoma characterized by typical acral presentation and inflammatory background often rich in eosinophils

CLINICAL ISSUES

Presentation

- Slow-growing infiltrative mass usually affecting distal extremities (hands and feet) of adults

Prognosis

- Recurrences are common, but metastases are rare

MACROSCOPIC FEATURES

General Features

- Infiltrative masses

Size

- 1-10 cm, usually 3-4 cm

MICROSCOPIC PATHOLOGY

Histologic Features

- Poorly marginated tumor with fibrosis, hyalinization, myxoid stroma, and inflammatory components
  - Various lesions have different proportions of each component
- Inflammatory component shows variable mixtures of lymphoplasmacytic cells, eosinophils, neutrophils, histiocytes
- Lesional cells are fibroblasts ultrastructurally
- Scattered enlarged atypical fibroblasts, some with macronucleoli
- Areas with prominent myxoid change
  - Fibroblasts often vacuolated as "pseudolipoblasts"
- Low mitotic rate
  - Low proliferative index using Ki-67

ANCILLARY TESTS

Immunohistochemistry

- Variable expression of CD34, CD68, EGFR, CD163, CD117, EMA
- Negative CD15, CD30, CD45 in cells with macronucleoli
- No demonstration of various viral agents

Cytogenetics

- t(1;10) and amplification of 3p11-12, which myxoinflammatory fibroblastic sarcoma shares with hemosiderotic fibrolipomatous tumor
- t(2;6)(q31;p21.3) reported

DIFFERENTIAL DIAGNOSIS

Extranodal Hodgkin Disease

- Patients usually have history of nodal disease
- Usually no myxoid areas
- Background mostly lymphoid cells, neutrophils not common
- Reed-Sternberg cells label with CD15, CD30, and are lymphoid rather than fibroblastic

Myxofibrosarcoma

- Usually in proximal extremities of older persons
- Typically superficial and lobulated rather than infiltrative
- Abundance of myxoid stroma
- Richly vascular

MYXOINFLAMMATORY FIBROBLASTIC SARCOMA

Key Facts

Clinical Issues

- Slow-growing infiltrative mass usually affecting distal extremities (hands and feet) of adults
- Recurrences are common, but metastases are rare

Microscopic Pathology

- Poorly marginated tumor with fibrosis, hyalinization, myxoid stroma, and inflammatory components
- Inflammatory component shows variable mixtures of lymphoplasmacytic cells, eosinophils, neutrophils, histiocytes
- Scattered enlarged atypical fibroblasts, some with macronucleoli
- Areas with prominent myxoid change
- Low mitotic rate
- Lesional cells are fibroblasts ultrastructurally

Ancillary Tests

- Variable expression of CD34, CD68, EGFR, CD163, CD117, EMA
- t(1;10) and amplification of 3p11-12, which it shares with hemosiderotic fibrolipomatous tumour
- Negative CD15, CD30, CD45 in cells with macronucleoli

Top Differential Diagnoses

- Extranodal Hodgkin disease
- Myxofibrosarcoma
- Pigmented villonodular tenosynovitis
- Hemosiderotic fibrohistiocytic lipomatous lesion
- Viral infection
- Epithelioid sarcoma

- Inflammatory cells a minor component
- No hyalinized zones

Pigmented Villonodular Tenosynovitis

- Also termed tenosynovial giant cell tumor, diffuse type
- Often presents in knee joint area of young women
- Proliferated around joint space
- Proliferation of uniform rounded cells
- Background of hemosiderin, histiocytes, lymphoplasmacytic cells
- Eosinophils and neutrophils not a feature
- Not myxoid
- No enlarged atypical cells

Hemosiderotic Fibrohistiocytic Lipomatous Lesion

- Classically involves the feet
- May form spectrum with both myxoinflammatory fibroblastic sarcoma and with pleomorphic hyalinizing angiectatic tumor
    - However, no metastases have been recorded for either hemosiderotic fibrohistiocytic lipomatous lesion or pleomorphic hyalinizing angiectatic tumor
    - Shares t(1;10) and amplification of 3p11-12
- Tracks along connective tissue septa
- Spindle cells, abundant hemosiderin, histiocytes
- Neutrophils and eosinophils not features
- Strongly CD34(+)

Viral Infection

- Usually involves organs and lymph nodes
- Infectious agents can be demonstrated by immunohistochemistry or molecular testing
- Viral cytopathic effect consists of nuclear (Cytomegalovirus and herpes simplex virus) or cytoplasmic (Cytomegalovirus) inclusions
- Cytomegalovirus effect best seen in stromal cells
- Herpes simplex viral effect often seen in epithelial cells

Epithelioid Sarcoma

- Distal extremities of adults
- Neoplastic cells surround zones of necrosis
    - Appearance mimics granulomatous process
- Minimal inflammation
- CD34(+), pankeratin(+), CK5/6(-), loss of nuclear INI1
- Malignant
    - Metastases to regional nodes as well as systemic metastases and death

Clear Cell Sarcoma

- Also termed "melanoma of soft parts"
- Distal extremities of adults
- Often centered in tendons or aponeuroses
    - "Packeted" growth pattern
- Uniform cells with uniform macronucleoli
- S100 protein(+), HMB-45(+), Melan-A(+), MITF1(+)
- Characteristic translocation and gene fusion
    - t(12;22)(q13;q12) that results in fusion of *EWS* and *ATF1* genes

SELECTED REFERENCES

1. Hallor KH et al: Two genetic pathways, t(1;10) and amplification of 3p11-12, in myxoinflammatory fibroblastic sarcoma, haemosiderotic fibrolipomatous tumour, and morphologically similar lesions. J Pathol. 217(5):716-27, 2009
2. Baumhoer D et al: Myxoinflammatory fibroblastic sarcoma: investigations by comparative genomic hybridization of two cases and review of the literature. Virchows Arch. 451(5):923-8, 2007
3. Ida CM et al: Myxoinflammatory fibroblastic sarcoma showing t(2;6)(q31;p21.3) as a sole cytogenetic abnormality. Cancer Genet Cytogenet. 177(2):139-42, 2007
4. Jurcić V et al: Myxoinflammatory fibroblastic sarcoma: a tumor not restricted to acral sites. Ann Diagn Pathol. 6(5):272-80, 2002
5. Lambert I et al: Acral myxoinflammatory fibroblastic sarcoma with unique clonal chromosomal changes. Virchows Arch. 438(5):509-12, 2001
6. Meis-Kindblom JM et al: Acral myxoinflammatory fibroblastic sarcoma: a low-grade tumor of the hands and feet. Am J Surg Pathol. 22(8):911-24, 1998
7. Montgomery EA et al: Inflammatory myxohyaline tumor of distal extremities with virocyte or Reed-Sternberg-like cells: a distinctive lesion with features simulating inflammatory conditions, Hodgkin's disease, and various sarcomas. Mod Pathol. 11(4):384-91, 1998

MYXOINFLAMMATORY FIBROBLASTIC SARCOMA

Microscopic Features

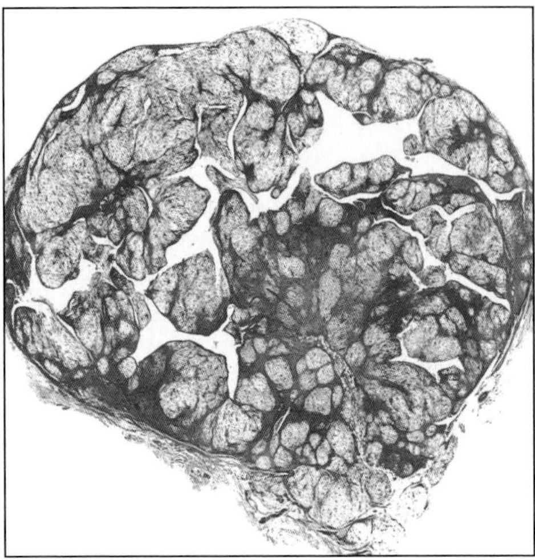
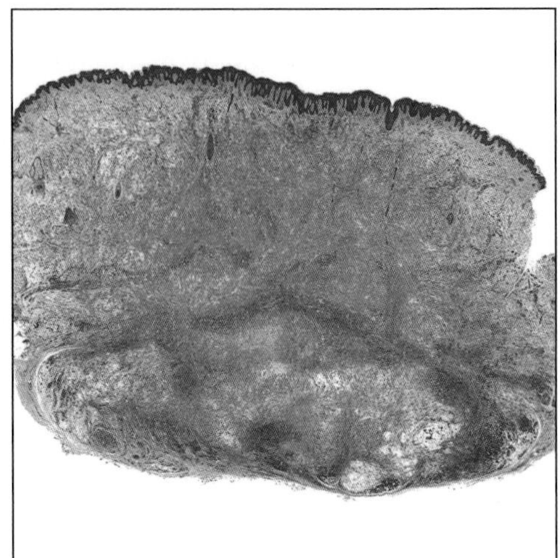

(Left) *This image shows a myxoinflammatory fibroblastic sarcoma at low magnification. This lesion is characterized by myxoid areas. This example also has prominent cleft-like spaces.* ***(Right)*** *This myxoinflammatory fibroblastic sarcoma is superficial and shows a myxoinflammatory expansion of the subcutaneous fat. Such neoplasms can also be associated with tendons and have an infiltrative appearance. A prominent lymphoid infiltrate is present throughout the neoplasm.*

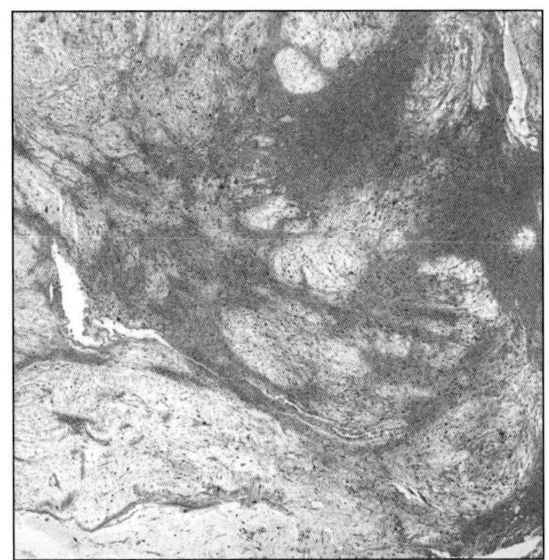
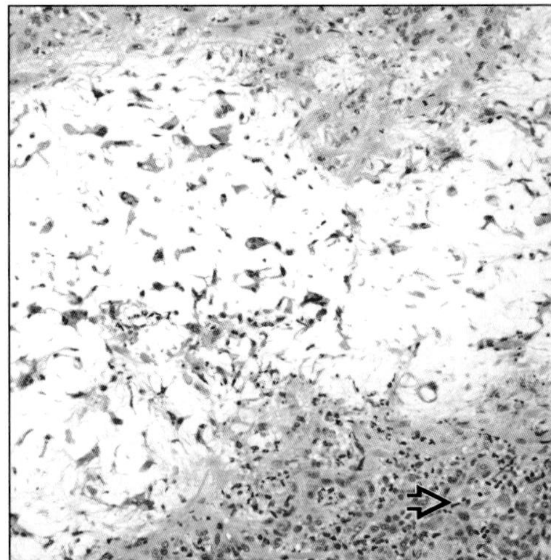

(Left) *This myxoinflammatory fibroblastic sarcoma has pockets of myxoid matrix interspersed with more solid fibroinflammatory zones.* ***(Right)*** *This myxoinflammatory fibroblastic sarcoma shows the junction of a myxoid area with an inflammatory area. The cells suspended in the myxoid matrix are enlarged and hyperchromatic. Note the lymphocytes in the lower right portion of the image ⇨.*

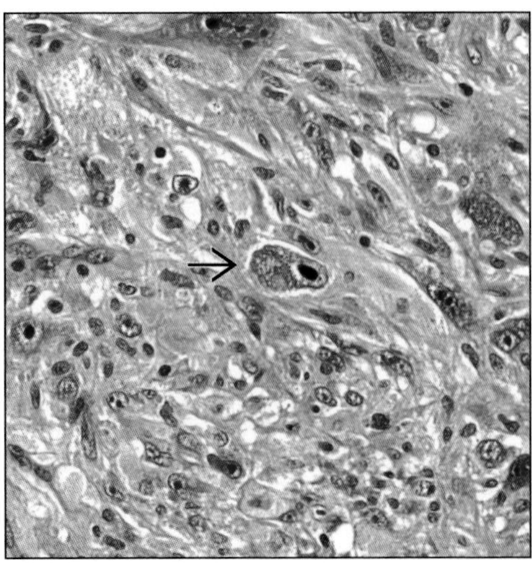
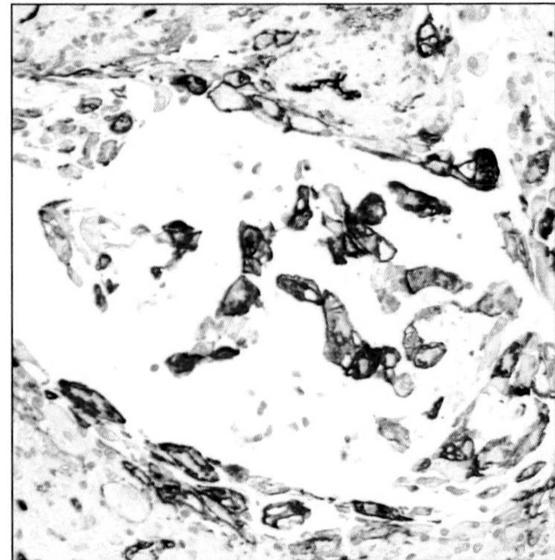

(Left) *There are markedly epithelioid cells within this myxoinflammatory fibroblastic sarcoma. In this field, the cells also display a granular cytoplasmic appearance. The cell in the center has a striking macronucleolus →.* ***(Right)*** *CD34 expression is commonly found in myxoinflammatory fibroblastic sarcoma. Focal keratin expression in myxoinflammatory fibroblastic sarcoma can suggest epithelioid sarcoma as well, but there is retention of INI1 in myxoinflammatory fibroblastic sarcoma.*

Microscopic Features

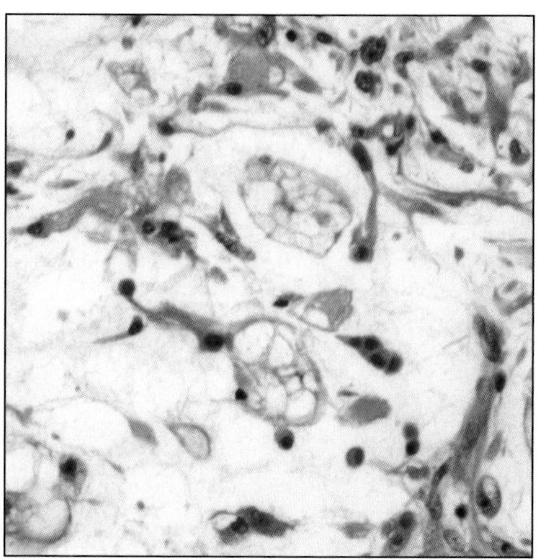

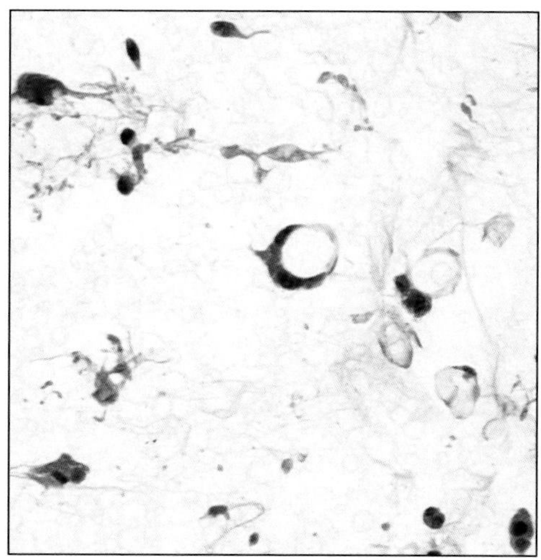

(Left) *This myxoinflammatory fibroblastic sarcoma shows abundant myxoid matrix. In this field, the neoplasm appears similar to myxofibrosarcoma (myxoid malignant fibrous histiocytoma) but lacks the rich vascular pattern of myxofibrosarcoma and has inflammatory features.* ***(Right)*** *This myxoinflammatory fibroblastic sarcoma is characterized by hyperchromatic nuclei embedded in myxoid mucopolysaccharide matrix.*

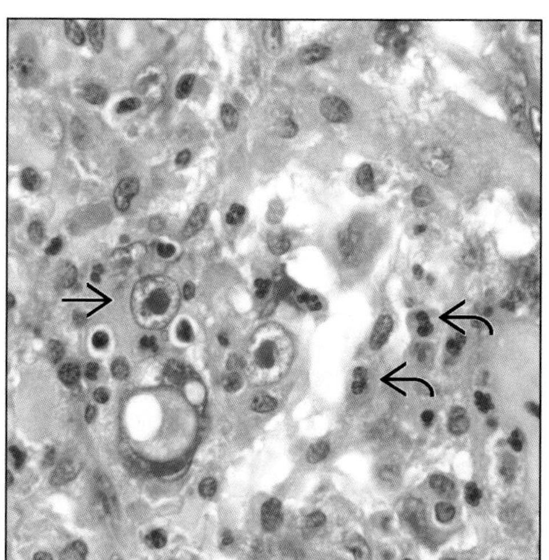

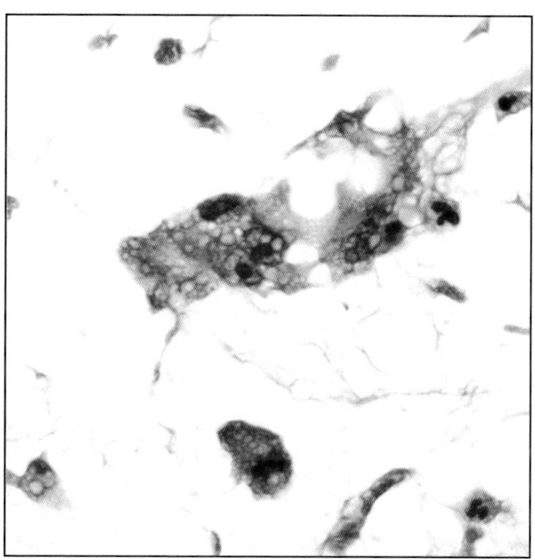

(Left) *The fibroblasts in myxoinflammatory fibroblastic sarcoma often have macronucleoli ⇒. Paired with the frequent eosinophils in many examples ↷, the presence of the prominent nucleoli in many cells can lead to a misinterpretation of Hodgkin disease.* ***(Right)*** *A myxoid focus in a myxoinflammatory fibroblastic sarcoma is shown. The cell in the center, with a pair of nuclei with macronucleoli, is reminiscent of a Reed-Sternberg cell.*

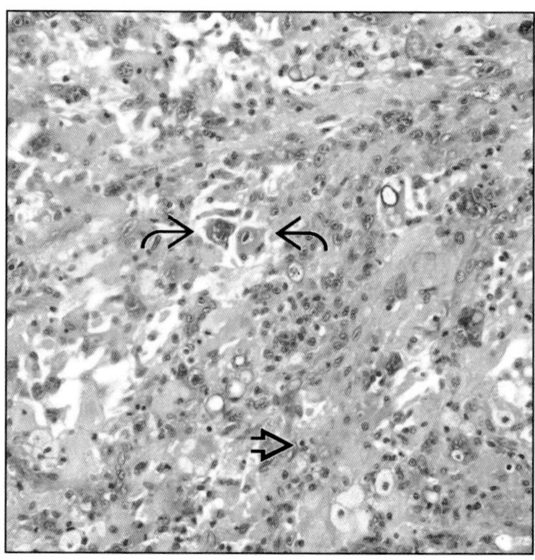

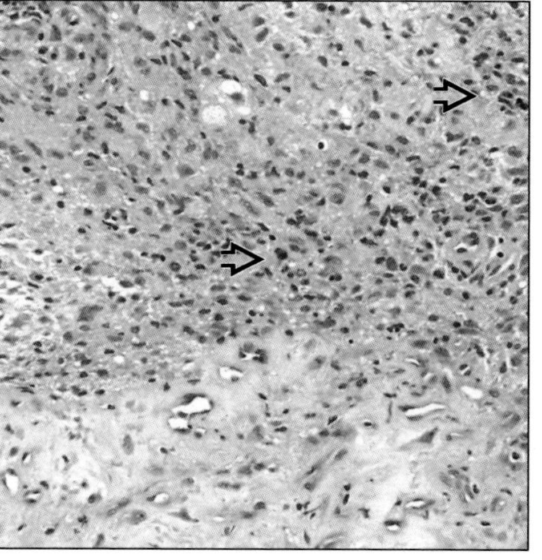

(Left) *This is a hyalinized portion of a myxoinflammatory fibroblastic sarcoma. Based on areas such as this, these neoplasms were 1st described as "inflammatory myxohyaline tumors." Note the cells with macronucleoli ↷ and the scattered lymphoid cells in the background ⇨.* ***(Right)*** *This particular example of myxoinflammatory fibroblastic sarcoma has fairly abundant hemosiderin deposition ⇨. The lower portion of the field has a hyalinized appearance.*

Differential Diagnosis

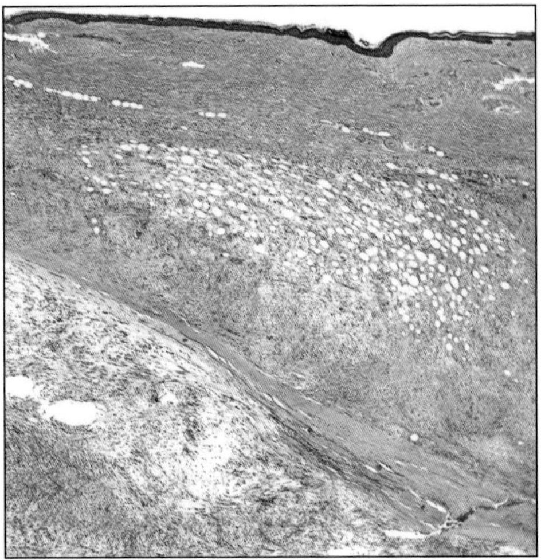

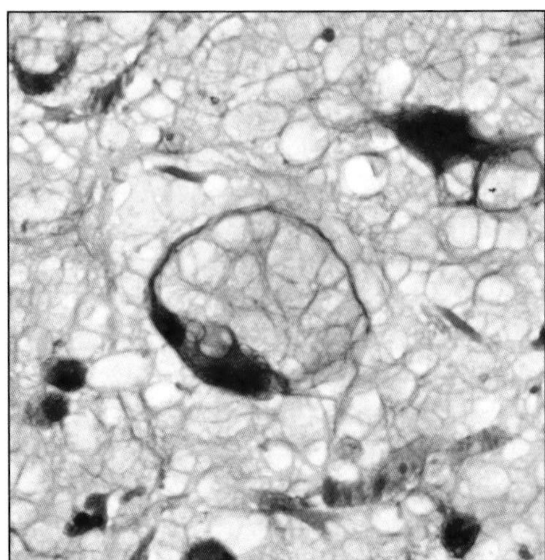

(Left) *This is a myxofibrosarcoma (myxoid malignant fibrous histiocytoma). This superficial lesion arose in the thigh. It appears similar to myxoinflammatory fibroblastic sarcoma but differs by being richly vascular and by lacking prominent inflammation.* ***(Right)*** *This atypical fibroblast from a myxofibrosarcoma appears similar to the cells in myxoinflammatory fibroblastic sarcoma and contains abundant mucopolysaccharide matrix, which is also present in the stroma surrounding the cell.*

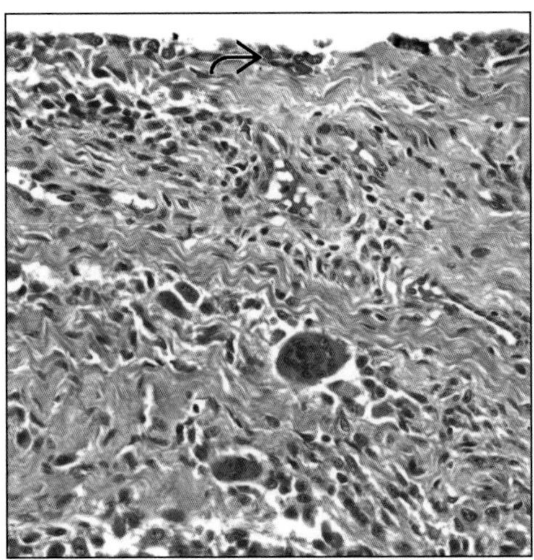

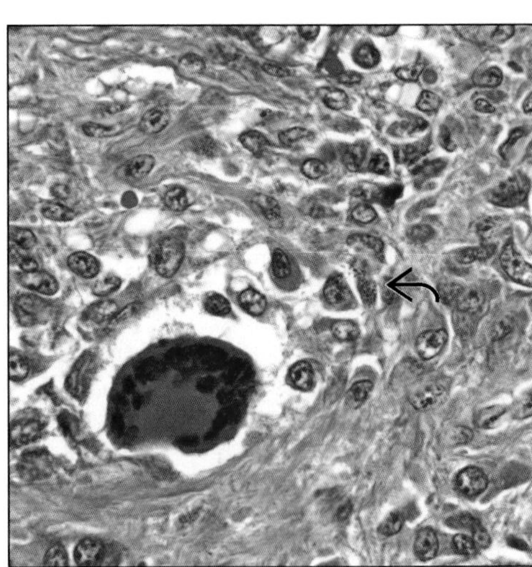

(Left) *Pigmented villonodular tenosynovitis appears similar to myxoinflammatory fibroblastic sarcoma clinically but differs histologically, consisting of giant cells and uniform uninucleate cells. Note the layer of pigmented synovium on the surface ➚.* ***(Right)*** *At high magnification, pigmented villonodular tenosynovitis features multinucleated giant cells, uniform cells with single nuclei, and hemosiderin ➚. These lesions often affect the knee joint.*

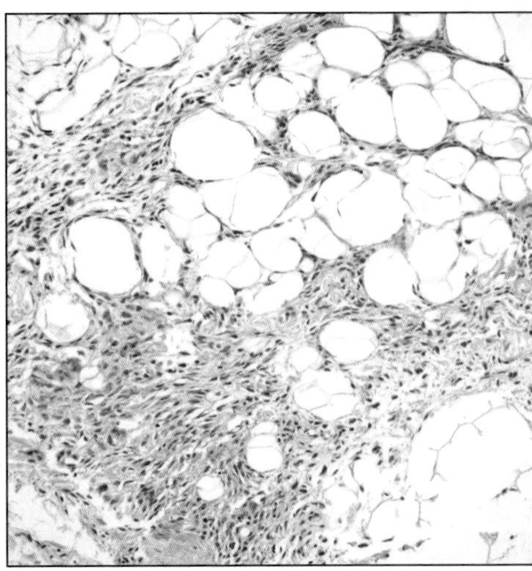

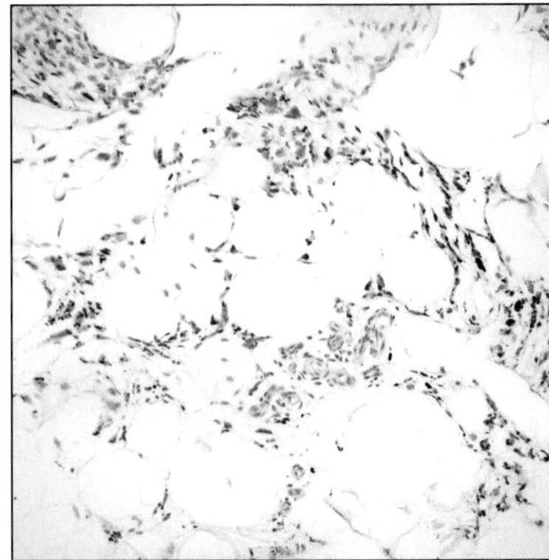

(Left) *Hemosiderotic fibrohistiocytic lipomatous lesion, which is shown here, may form a spectrum with both myxoinflammatory fibroblastic sarcoma and with pleomorphic hyalinizing angiectatic tumor. It typically arises on the foot and consists of CD34-reactive spindle cells, fat, and abundant hemosiderin, which is often inconspicuous on routine H&E stains but readily apparent on iron staining.* ***(Right)*** *Hemosiderotic fibrohistiocytic lipomatous lesion often shows abundant iron on iron stains.*

Differential Diagnosis

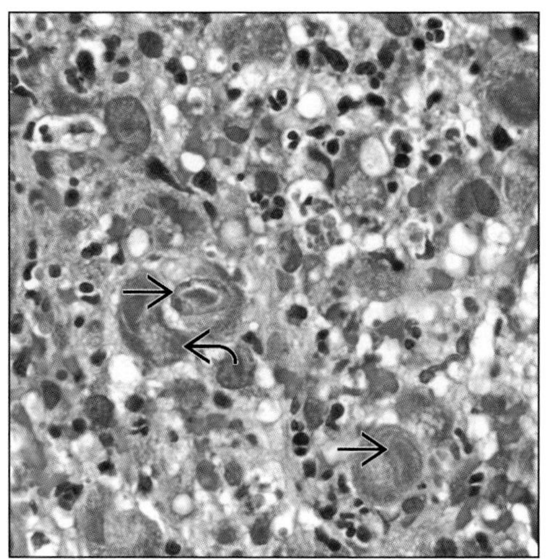

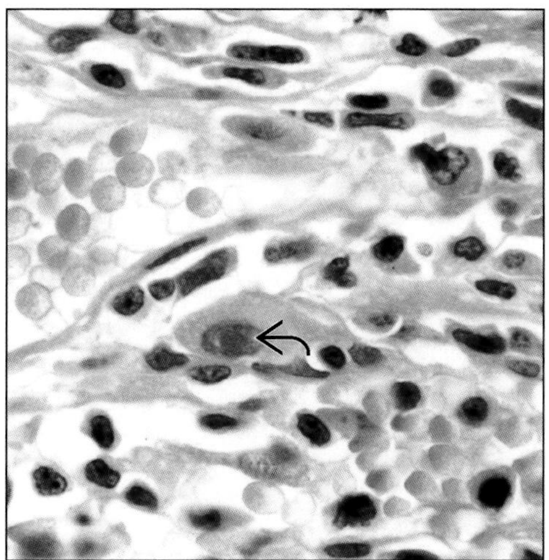

(Left) *This example of Cytomegalovirus infection is from a colon biopsy specimen, although stromal rather than epithelial cells show the classic viral cytopathic effect. The nuclei contain inclusions rather than macronucleoli ➔. There are also cytoplasmic inclusions ➚.* ***(Right)*** *This image shows a cytomegalovirus nuclear inclusion in an endothelial cell ➚, a typical pattern for cytomegalovirus viral cytopathic effect.*

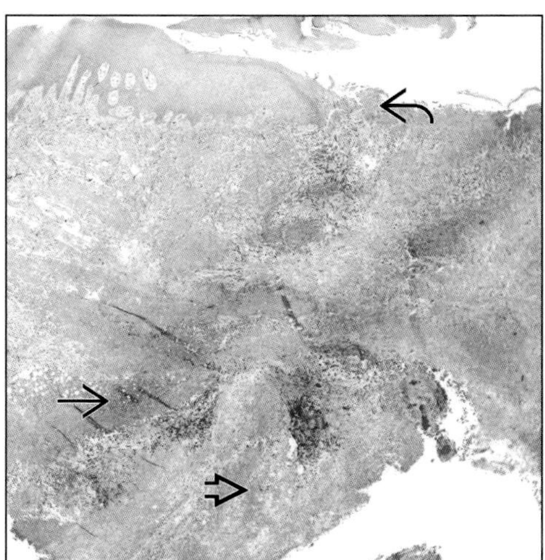

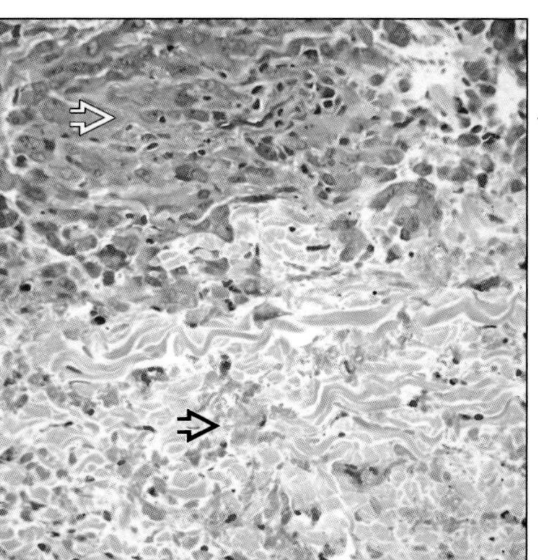

(Left) *This image is from an epithelioid sarcoma that affected the distal forearm of a young adult. The lesion affected an aponeurosis, but the overlying skin is ulcerated ➚. A rim of lesional cells ➔ surrounds a zone of necrosis ⇨, an overall pattern reminiscent of granulomatous inflammation.* ***(Right)*** *High magnification of an epithelioid sarcoma shows the lesional cells ⇨ adjacent to a confluent area of necrosis ⇨. There is essentially no inflammation.*

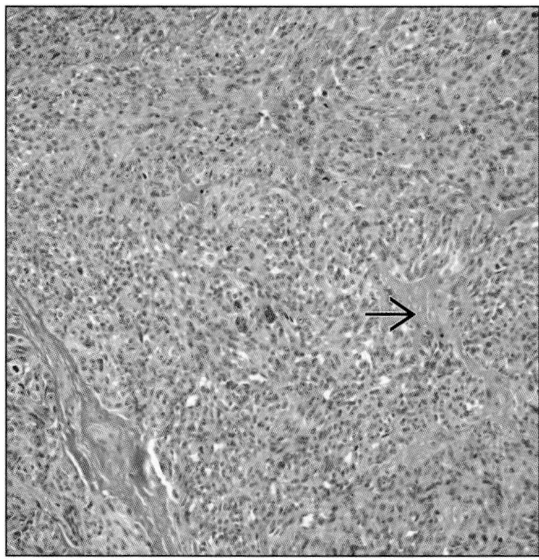

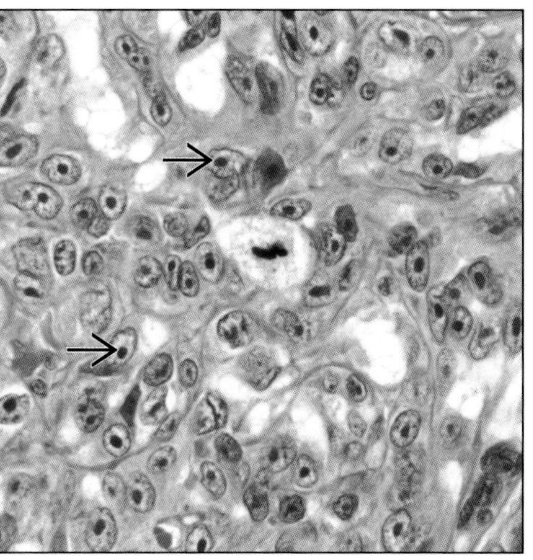

(Left) *This is a clear cell sarcoma that arose in the foot of a young adult. The lesion infiltrated a tendon ➔. At this magnification, there is no myxoid change and no inflammation.* ***(Right)*** *Clear cell sarcomas have very uniform cells (a feature of sarcomas associated with characteristic translocations) and normal mitoses. Each cell has a uniform large nucleolus ➔. These tumors typically harbor an EWS-ATF1 fusion gene (or an alternate EWS-CREB1 fusion gene).*

ADULT-TYPE FIBROSARCOMA

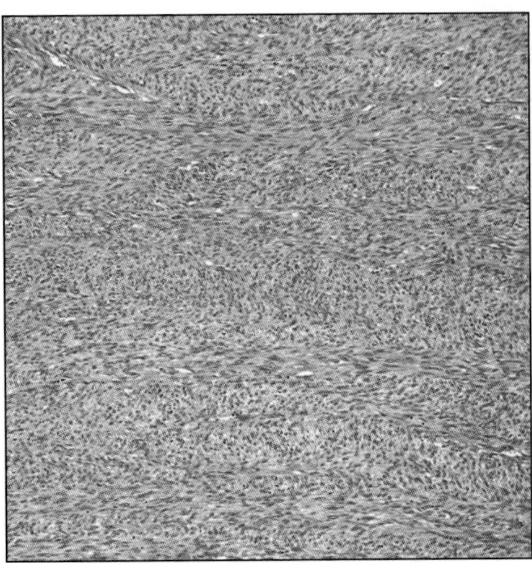

This shows a typically cellular low-grade fibrosarcoma with uniform spindle cells arranged in long intersecting fascicles in a so-called herringbone pattern. No necrosis is seen.

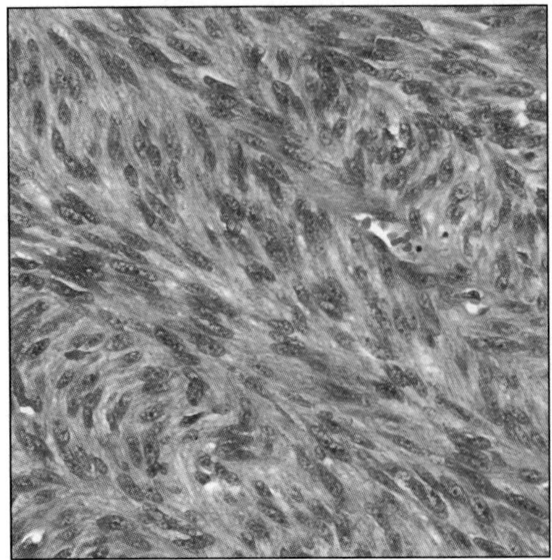

This well-differentiated fibrosarcoma shows uniform tapered spindle cells. The nuclei are elongated, and some have a small nucleolus.

TERMINOLOGY

Definitions

- Soft tissue sarcoma composed of fibroblasts
- Lacks features of named fibrosarcoma subtypes
- Now very rare; mostly a diagnosis of exclusion
- Pleomorphic variants are currently classified as undifferentiated sarcoma/malignant fibrous histiocytoma
- Conclusive diagnosis can require electron microscopy

ETIOLOGY/PATHOGENESIS

De Novo

- Exceptionally rare if strictly defined

Arising in Course of Other Tumor

- Fibrosarcoma in dermatofibrosarcoma
  - Probable origin of many superficial adult fibrosarcomas
- Malignant solitary fibrous tumor
- Component of other fibrosarcoma subtypes, e.g., sclerosing epithelioid fibrosarcoma

Post Irradiation

- Usually therapeutic
- Long time interval before sarcoma develops

CLINICAL ISSUES

Site

- Proximal limbs, head and neck

Presentation

- Painful or painless mass

Treatment

- Surgical approaches
  - Adequate local excision
  - Pulmonary metastasectomy in selected cases

Prognosis

- Few modern studies
  - Older series represent a mixture of sarcoma types
- Relates to grade
- Local recurrence in 12-79%
- Metastasis in 9-63%
  - To lungs, bone, and rarely lymph node

MACROSCOPIC FEATURES

General Features

- Circumscribed, pseudoencapsulated
- Some subcutaneous, most deep (intramuscular)
- Firm, white, focal necrosis in some

Size

- Variable, can exceed 20 cm

MICROSCOPIC PATHOLOGY

Histologic Features

- Fascicular architecture
  - Characteristic "herringbone" or "chevron" pattern
- Elongated spindle cells
  - Slender, tapered, sometimes wavy nuclei
  - Variable hyperchromasia and pleomorphism
  - Variable mitotic activity, can include abnormal forms
- Scanty cytoplasm
- Variable stromal collagen
  - Delicate intercellular network
  - Focal sclerosis or hyalinization
- Rare focal myxoid change
- Rare multinucleated tumor cells

Predominant Pattern/Injury Type

- Fascicular

ADULT-TYPE FIBROSARCOMA

Key Facts

Terminology
- Soft tissue sarcoma composed of fibroblasts
- Lacks features of named fibrosarcoma subtypes

Etiology/Pathogenesis
- Exceptionally rare if strictly defined

Microscopic Pathology
- Fascicular architecture
- Characteristic "herringbone" or "chevron" pattern
- Elongated spindle cells, slender, tapered, sometimes wavy nuclei
- Scanty cytoplasm

Ancillary Tests
- Most cases negative for all immunohistochemical markers except vimentin
- Some express CD34 focally or diffusely
- Some superficial examples have *COL1A1-PDGFB* fusion transcripts like dermatofibrosarcoma

Predominant Cell/Compartment Type
- Fibroblast

ANCILLARY TESTS

Immunohistochemistry
- Most cases negative except for very focal SMA
- Some express CD34 focally or diffusely

Cytogenetics
- Some superficial examples have *COL1A1-PDGFB* fusion transcripts like dermatofibrosarcoma

Electron Microscopy
- Abundant rough endoplasmic reticulum
- No external lamina, junctions, or organized filaments

DIFFERENTIAL DIAGNOSIS

Low-Grade Fibromyxoid Sarcoma
- Less cellular
- Myxoid and fibrous areas with whorling
- Pleomorphism usually absent at 1st occurrence
- Nuclei less elongated, more squarely shaped
- Specific translocation t(7;16)(q34;p11)

Low-Grade Myofibrosarcoma
- Cells have more cytoplasm
- Multifocal positivity for SMA

Synovial Sarcoma
- Younger age, any location, most common around knee
- Biphasic pattern with gland formation in 1/3
- Shorter, ovoid uniform cells, overlapping nuclei
- Mast cells frequent
- EMA(+) or CK(+) in 95%, CD34(-) in 95%
- Specific translocation t(X;18)(p11;q11)

Malignant Peripheral Nerve Sheath Tumor
- Association with neurofibromatosis type 1
- Often originates in neurofibroma or large nerve
- Alternating myxoid and cellular areas
- Spindle cells with wavy or bullet-shaped nuclei
- S100 protein(+) in 2/3 of cases

Fibromatosis
- Less cellular, cells evenly dispersed in mature collagen
- Myofibroblasts, punctate nucleoli
- Nuclear immunoreactivity for β-catenin

SELECTED REFERENCES

1. Sheng WQ et al: Expression of COL1A1-PDGFB fusion transcripts in superficial adult fibrosarcoma suggests a close relationship to dermatofibrosarcoma protuberans. J Pathol. 194(1):88-94, 2001
2. Scott SM et al: Soft tissue fibrosarcoma. A clinicopathologic study of 132 cases. Cancer. 64(4):925-31, 1989
3. Pritchard DJ et al: Fibrosarcoma of bone and soft tissues of the trunk and extremities. Orthop Clin North Am. 8(4):869-81, 1977

IMAGE GALLERY

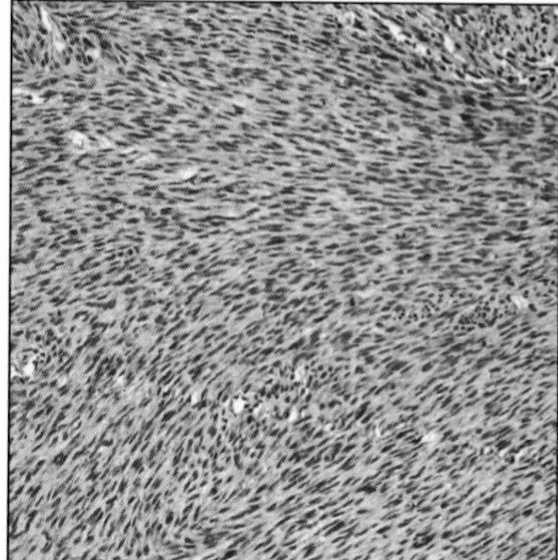

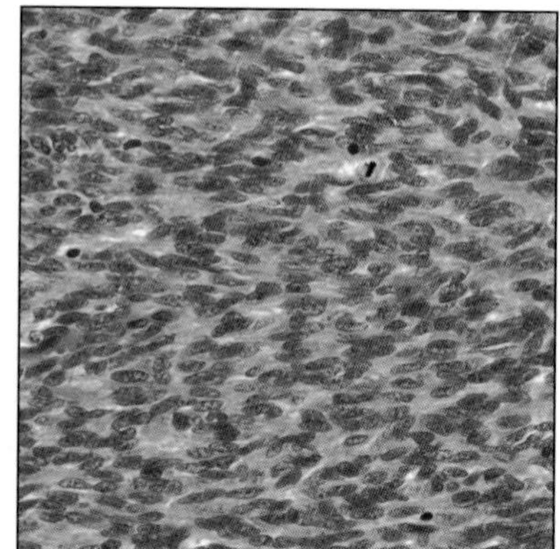

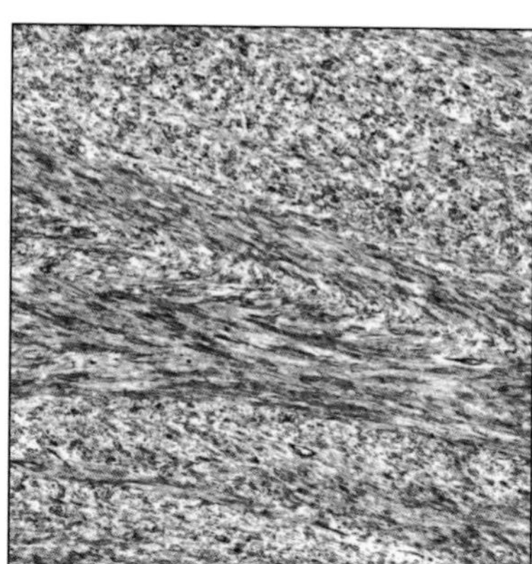

*(**Left**) This higher grade fibrosarcoma displays nuclear hyperchromasia and focal pleomorphism. The fascicular architecture is retained. (**Center**) Moderately differentiated fibrosarcoma is shown with marked cellularity, nuclear variation, and mitotic activity. (**Right**) Positivity for CD34 can be seen in fibrosarcoma arising in dermatofibrosarcoma or solitary fibrous tumor and in fibrosarcoma without antecedent tumor. Other markers are negative except very focal SMA in some cases.*

MYXOFIBROSARCOMA

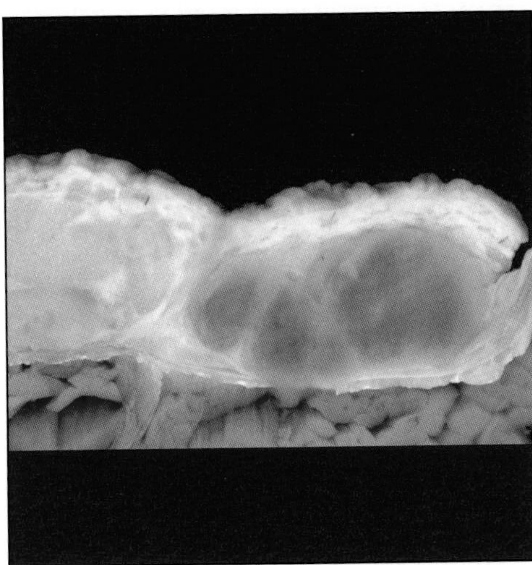

Grossly, cases of myxofibrosarcoma often show a multinodular growth with myxoid cut surfaces, as shown here.

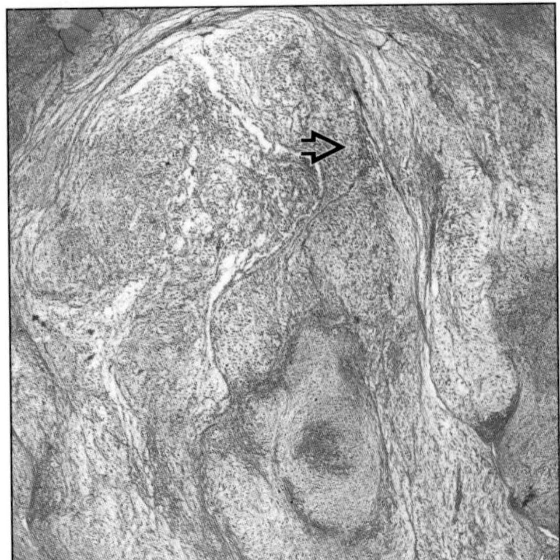

Myxofibrosarcoma is characterized by a variable cellularity and is composed of atypical fibroblastic cells that are set in a prominent myxoid stroma with numerous elongated curvilinear vessels ⇨.

TERMINOLOGY

Abbreviations

- Myxofibrosarcoma (MFS)

Synonyms

- Myxoid malignant fibrous histiocytoma

Definitions

- Myxofibrosarcoma represents a spectrum of malignant fibroblastic neoplasms with variably myxoid stroma and characteristic elongated curvilinear vessels

CLINICAL ISSUES

Epidemiology

- Incidence
  - One of the most common sarcomas in elderly patients
- Age
  - Affects mainly patients in 6th-8th decade
  - Exceptionally rare in patients < 20 years old
- Gender
  - Slight male predominance

Site

- Majority arise in limbs, including limb girdles (lower > upper extremities)
- More rarely on trunk, head and neck region
- Very rarely on hands and feet
- Extremely rare in retroperitoneum and in abdominal cavity
- 2/3 of cases arise in dermal/subcutaneous tissues

Presentation

- Painless mass
- Slow growing

Treatment

- Surgical approaches
  - Complete wide excision

Prognosis

- Local, often repeated recurrences in up to 50-60% of cases unrelated to histologic grade
- Low-grade malignant neoplasms usually do not metastasize
  - May show tumor progression in subsequent recurrences and may acquire metastatic potential
- Intermediate- and high-grade malignant neoplasms may develop metastases in 30-35% of cases
- Overall 5-year survival is 60-70%
- Depth of lesions and grade of malignancy do not influence recurrence rate
- Percentage of metastases and tumor-associated mortality are higher in deep-seated neoplasms & high-grade malignant neoplasms
- Local recurrences within < 12 months increase tumor associated mortality
- Proliferative activity, percentage of aneuploid cells, and tumor vascularity are associated with histologic tumor grade

MACROSCOPIC FEATURES

General Features

- Superficially located neoplasms consist of multiple, variably gelatinous or firmer nodules
- Deep-seated neoplasms often present as single mass with myxoid cut surfaces
- Areas of tumor necrosis may be seen in high-grade neoplasms

MICROSCOPIC PATHOLOGY

Histologic Features

- Broad spectrum of cellularity, cytologic atypia, and proliferative activity reflected by 3 grades of malignancy

MYXOFIBROSARCOMA

Key Facts

Terminology
- Myxofibrosarcoma represents a spectrum of malignant fibroblastic neoplasms with variably myxoid stroma and characteristic elongated curvilinear vessels

Clinical Issues
- One of the most common sarcomas in elderly patients
- Majority arises in limb, including limb girdles (lower > upper extremities)
- 2/3 of cases arise in dermal/subcutaneous tissues
- Local, often repeated recurrences in up to 50-60% of cases unrelated to histologic grade
- Intermediate- and high-grade malignant neoplasms may develop metastases in 30-35% of cases

Macroscopic Features
- Superficially located neoplasms consist of multiple, variably gelatinous or firmer nodules
- Deep-seated neoplasms often present as single mass with myxoid cut surfaces

Microscopic Pathology
- Broad spectrum of cellularity, cytologic atypia, and proliferative activity reflected by 3 grades of malignancy
- Multinodular growth, spindled and stellate atypical fibroblastic cells
- Myxoid stroma with elongated, curvilinear, thin-walled vessels
- Often pseudolipoblasts are present

- Low-grade malignant myxofibrosarcoma
  - Hypocellular neoplasms
  - Few noncohesive tumor cells
  - Ill-defined eosinophilic cytoplasm
  - Enlarged hyperchromatic nuclei
- Intermediate-grade malignant myxofibrosarcoma
  - More cellular and pleomorphic than low-grade neoplasms
  - No solid areas
  - No tumor necrosis
- High-grade malignant myxofibrosarcoma
  - Large parts are composed of solid sheets and cellular fascicles
  - Spindled and pleomorphic tumor cells
  - Bizarre, multinucleated tumor giant cells
  - Numerous, often atypical mitoses
  - Areas of tumor necrosis may be present
  - At least focally, areas of lower grade neoplasm with prominent myxoid stroma and numerous curvilinear vessels
- Multinodular growth with incomplete fibrous septa
- Myxoid stroma
- Prominent elongated, curvilinear, thin-walled blood vessels
- Foci of inflammatory cells may be present

Cytologic Features
- Spindled and stellate atypical fibroblastic cells
- Often pseudolipoblasts are present
  - Pseudolipoblasts are vacuolated neoplastic fibroblastic cells

ANCILLARY TESTS

Cytogenetics
- Complex karyotypes
- Often triploid and tetraploid chromosome numbers
- No activating mutations of *GNAS1*

Electron Microscopy
- Majority of cells shows features of fibroblastic differentiation
  - Oval tumor cells with clefted nuclei
  - Prominent rough endoplasmic reticulum

DIFFERENTIAL DIAGNOSIS

Superficial Angiomyxoma
- Lobular growth
- No prominent cytologic atypia
- Often dilated vessels with slightly fibrosed vessel walls
- Perivascular neutrophils

Superficial Acral Fibromyxoma
- Arises in hands and feet and is often seen in nail bed region
- Fascicles of spindled tumor cells
- No prominent cytologic atypia
- Varying collagenous and myxoid stroma

Intramuscular Myxoma
- No multinodular growth
- Usually hypocellular neoplasm
- Usually only few capillaries
- No prominent cytologic atypia

Juxtaarticular Myxoma
- Arises usually around large joints
- Cystic changes may be seen
- No prominent cytologic atypia

Myxoid Neurofibroma
- Nodular or diffuse growth
- No nuclear atypia
- S100(+)

Myxoid Dermatofibrosarcoma Protuberans
- Often diffuse infiltration of dermis and subcutis
- No prominent cytologic atypia
- Homogeneous expression of CD34

Myxoid Liposarcoma
- Frequently in deep soft tissues of lower extremity
- Small undifferentiated mesenchymal tumor cells and vacuolated lipoblasts

MYXOFIBROSARCOMA

Immunohistochemistry

Antibody	Reactivity	Staining Pattern	Comment
Vimentin	Positive	Cytoplasmic	
CD68	Negative		
Desmin	Negative		
S100	Negative		
CK-PAN	Negative		
CD34	Equivocal	Cytoplasmic	Reflects fibroblastic differentiation
Actin-sm	Equivocal	Cytoplasmic	Reflects focal myofibroblastic differentiation

- No prominent cytologic atypia
- Delicate plexiform vascular pattern

Low-Grade Fibromyxoid Sarcoma

- Mainly in deep soft tissues
- Bland spindled tumor cells
- Alternating myxoid and fibrous stroma
- Whorling and swirling growth pattern of tumor cells
- Arcades of blood vessels
- Frequent expression of EMA
- *FUS* translocation

Myxoinflammatory Fibroblastic Sarcoma

- Frequently arises in subcutaneous tissues of hands, wrists, feet, and ankles
- Spindled, polygonal, and bizarre ganglion-like tumor cells with huge inclusion-like nucleoli
- Prominent mixed inflammatory infiltrate

Myxoid Leiomyosarcoma

- No multinodular growth
- Spindled eosinophilic tumor cells
- Expression of myogenic markers (actin-sm, desmin, HCAD)

Myxoid Malignant Peripheral Nerve Sheath Tumor

- Fascicular arrangement of spindle-shaped tumor cells
- Often perivascular whorling of tumor cells
- In about 1/2 of cases, focal expression of S100

Dedifferentiated Liposarcoma

- Often in retroperitoneal &/or intraabdominal location
- Rim of atypical lipomatous tumor
- Nuclear expression of MDM2 &/or CDK4

Pleomorphic Liposarcoma

- Contains pleomorphic lipoblasts

DIAGNOSTIC CHECKLIST

Clinically Relevant Pathologic Features

- Organ distribution
- Age distribution
- Gross appearance

Pathologic Interpretation Pearls

- Frequently in elderly patients
- Frequently superficial dermal/subcutaneous tissues of lower extremities
- Multinodular neoplasms
- Spectrum of variably cellular atypical fibroblastic neoplasms
- Myxoid stromal changes with characteristic elongated curvilinear blood vessels

SELECTED REFERENCES

1. Willems SM et al: Cellular/intramuscular myxoma and grade I myxofibrosarcoma are characterized by distinct genetic alterations and specific composition of their extracellular matrix. J Cell Mol Med. 13(7):1291-301, 2009
2. Nascimento AF et al: Epithelioid variant of myxofibrosarcoma: expanding the clinicomorphologic spectrum of myxofibrosarcoma in a series of 17 cases. Am J Surg Pathol. 31(1):99-105, 2007
3. Willems SM et al: Local recurrence of myxofibrosarcoma is associated with increase in tumour grade and cytogenetic aberrations, suggesting a multistep tumour progression model. Mod Pathol. 19(3):407-16, 2006
4. Mansoor A et al: Myxofibrosarcoma presenting in the skin: clinicopathological features and differential diagnosis with cutaneous myxoid neoplasms. Am J Dermatopathol. 25(4):281-6, 2003
5. Mentzel T et al: The association between tumour progression and vascularity in myxofibrosarcoma and myxoid/round cell liposarcoma. Virchows Arch. 438(1):13-22, 2001
6. Mentzel T et al: Myxofibrosarcoma. Clinicopathologic analysis of 75 cases with emphasis on the low-grade variant. Am J Surg Pathol. 20(4):391-405, 1996
7. Merck C et al: Myxofibrosarcoma. A malignant soft tissue tumor of fibroblastic-histiocytic origin. A clinicopathologic and prognostic study of 110 cases using multivariate analysis. Acta Pathol Microbiol Immunol Scand Suppl. 282:1-40, 1983
8. Angervall L et al: Myxofibrosarcoma. A study of 30 cases. Acta Pathol Microbiol Scand A. 85A(2):127-40, 1977
9. Weiss SW et al: Myxoid variant of malignant fibrous histiocytoma. Cancer. 39(4):1672-85, 1977

Gross and Microscopic Features

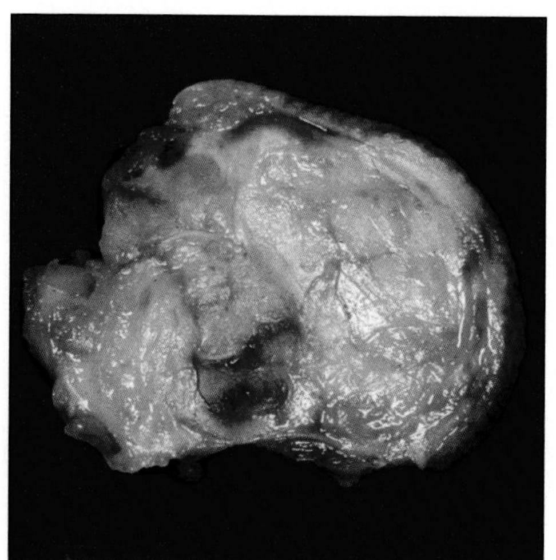

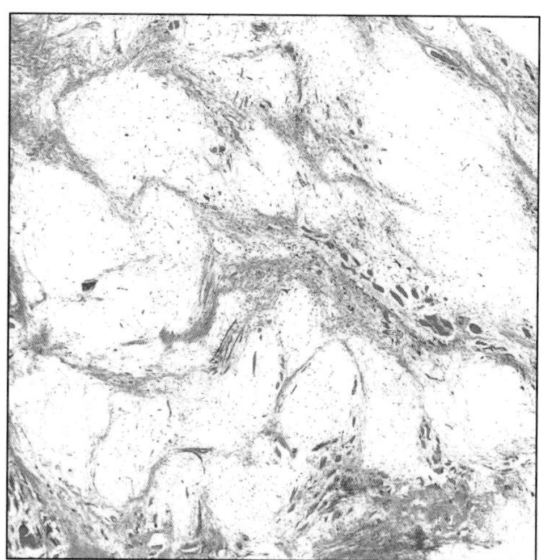

*(**Left**) A case of low-grade myxofibrosarcoma is shown with myxoid, gelatinous cut surfaces. (**Right**) Low-power view shows a deep-seated, intramuscular, low-grade myxofibrosarcoma. Note the characteristic multinodular growth and the presence of thin fibrous septa.*

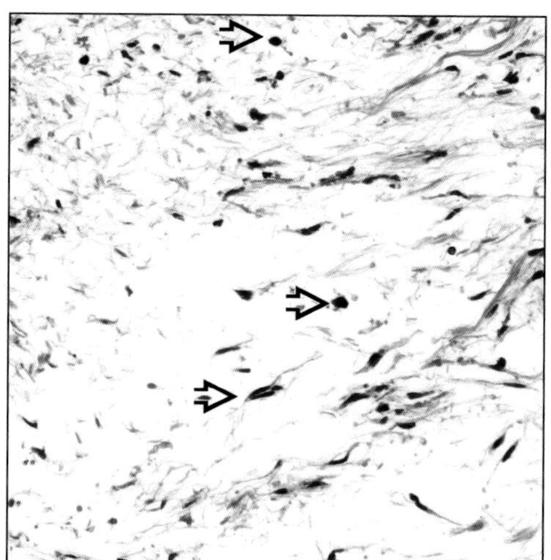

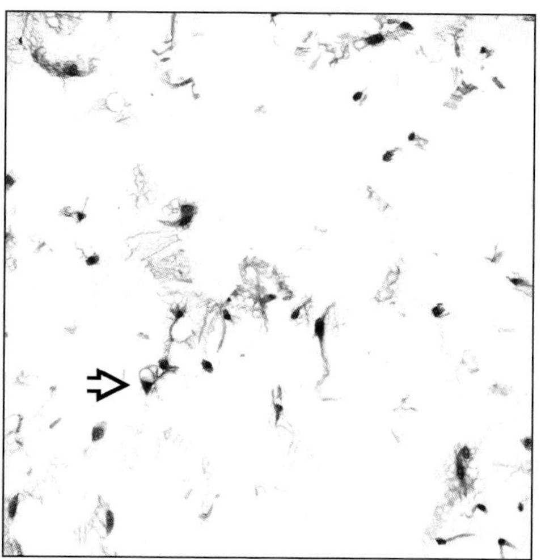

*(**Left**) Despite a low cellularity, cases of low-grade myxofibrosarcoma are composed of atypical fibroblastic tumor cells containing enlarged and hyperchromatic nuclei ➩. (**Right**) Scattered vacuolated tumor cells containing cytoplasmic mucin (so-called pseudolipoblasts) ➩ are often seen mimicking myxoid liposarcoma.*

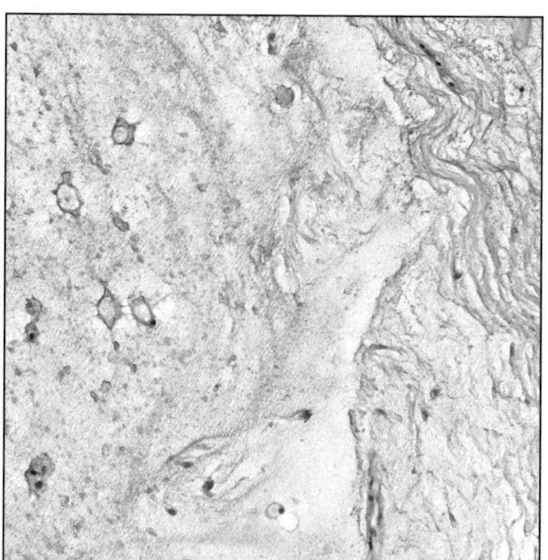

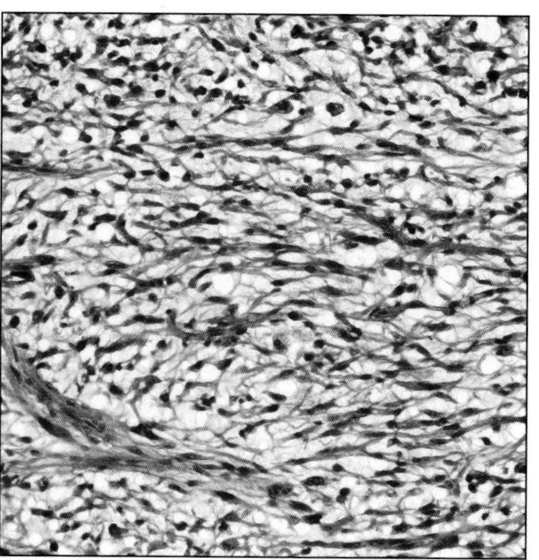

*(**Left**) Alcian blue staining reveals the presence of abundant mucin in the cytoplasm of neoplastic cells. (**Right**) Cases of intermediate-grade malignant myxofibrosarcoma show an increased cellularity of atypical fibroblastic tumor cells.*

MYXOFIBROSARCOMA

Microscopic and Gross Features

*(**Left**) Higher power view of an intermediate-grade malignant myxofibrosarcoma shows atypical tumor cells with enlarged hyperchromatic nuclei. Note the scattered multivacuolated pseudolipoblasts ⇨. (**Right**) A high-grade, deep-seated myxofibrosarcoma is shown with firm gray-white cut surfaces. Myxoid changes are seen only focally.*

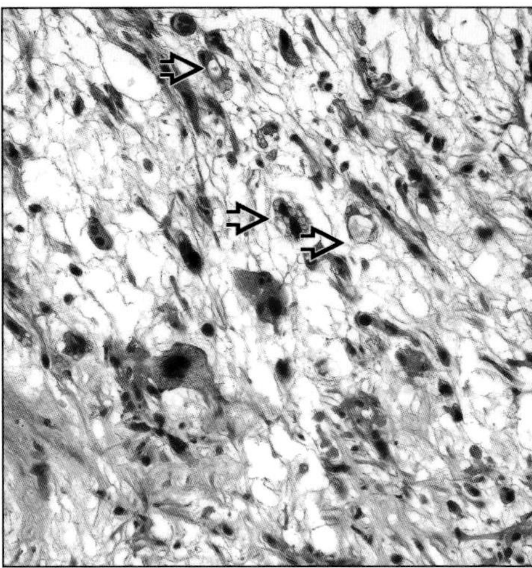

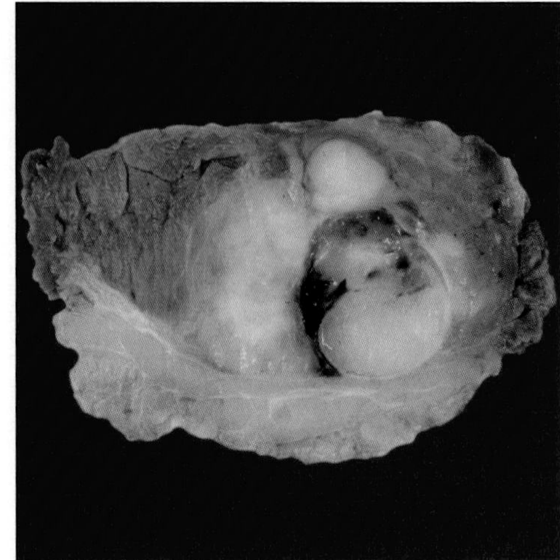

*(**Left**) Cases of high-grade myxofibrosarcoma show features of a high-grade, pleomorphic sarcoma with increased proliferative activity and areas of tumor necrosis ⇨. (**Right**) Often multinucleated tumor giant cells ↩ containing abundant eosinophilic cytoplasm mimicking a myogenic neoplasm are seen in high-grade malignant myxofibrosarcoma.*

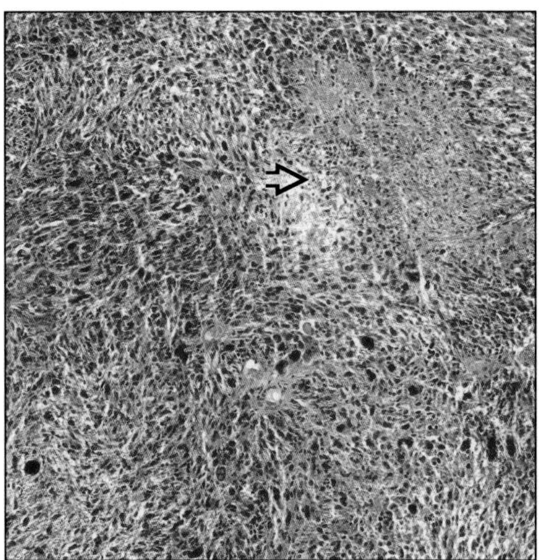

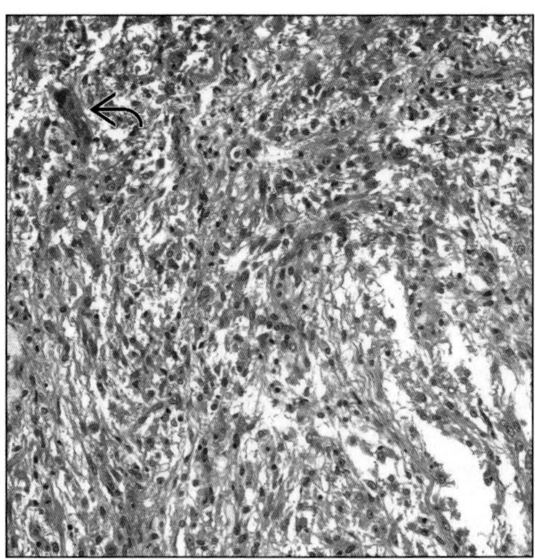

*(**Left**) At least focally, areas of lower cellularity containing abundant myxoid stroma are seen in cases of high-grade malignant myxofibrosarcoma. (**Right**) In this high-grade malignant myxofibrosarcoma, foci with features of an intermediate-grade malignant neoplasm with abundant myxoid stroma and characteristic elongated blood vessels are seen.*

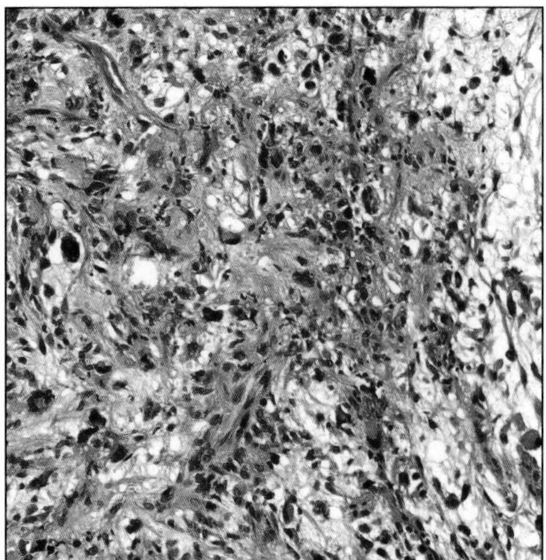

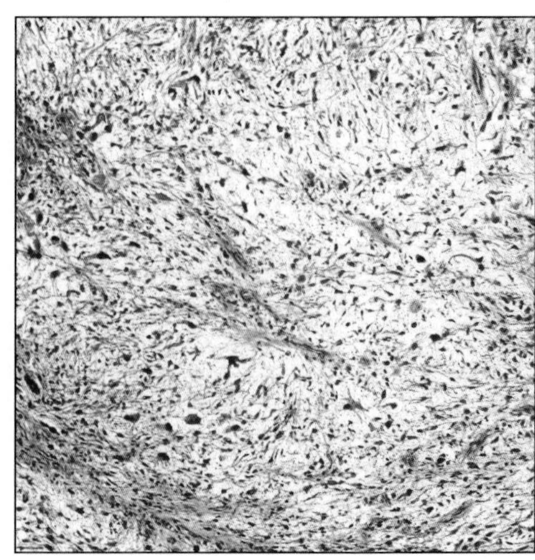

Variant Microscopic and Gross Features

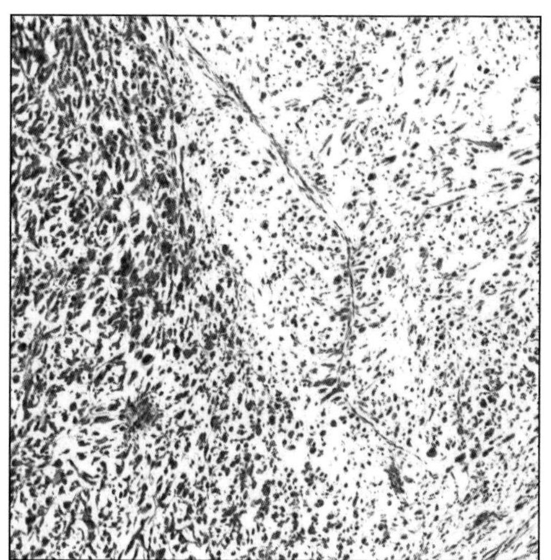

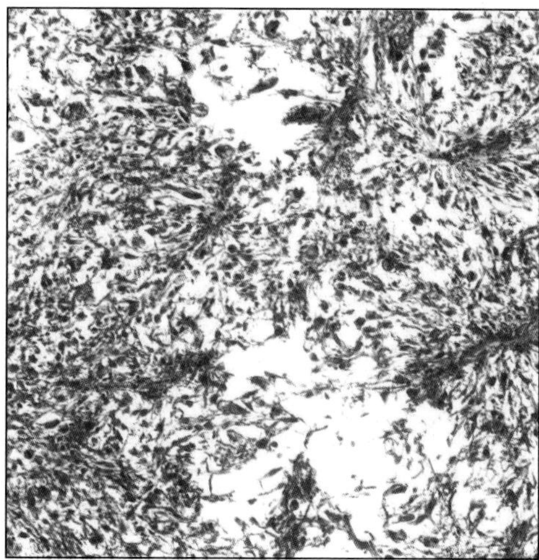

(Left) *Tumor cells in this intermediate-grade malignant myxofibrosarcoma stained focally positive for α-smooth muscle actin.* ***(Right)*** *The expression of CD34 in a number of cases of myxofibrosarcoma confirms the fibroblastic line of differentiation in these neoplasms.*

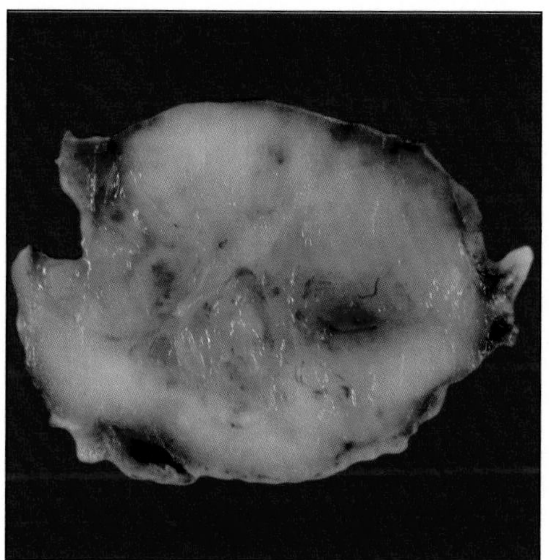

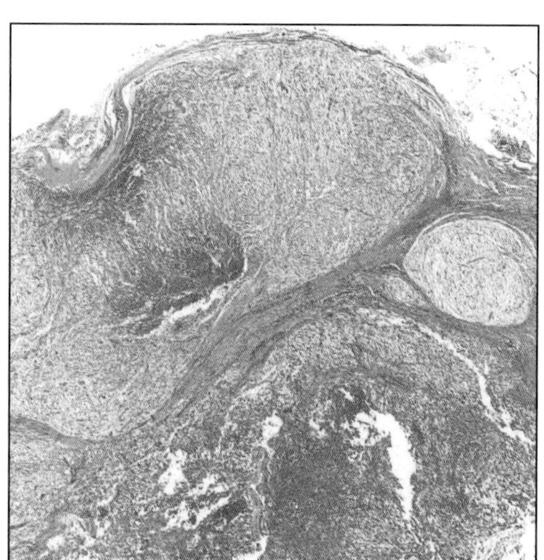

(Left) *This myxofibrosarcoma arose on the lateral aspect of the neck in a middle-aged female patient. Grossly, myxoid cut surfaces are present.* ***(Right)*** *Low-power view shows a multinodular neoplasm with fibrous septa and prominent myxoid stromal changes.*

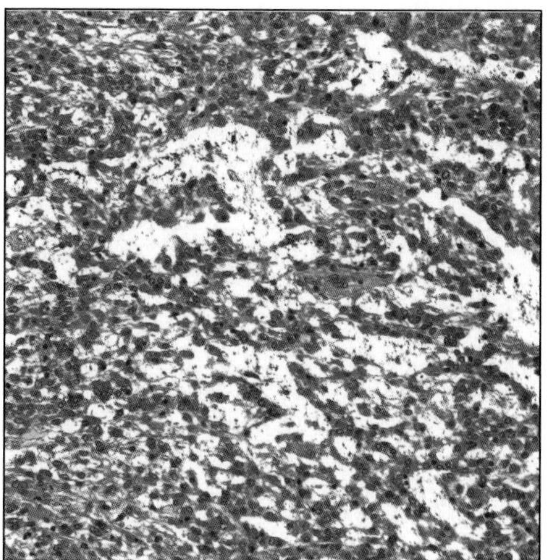

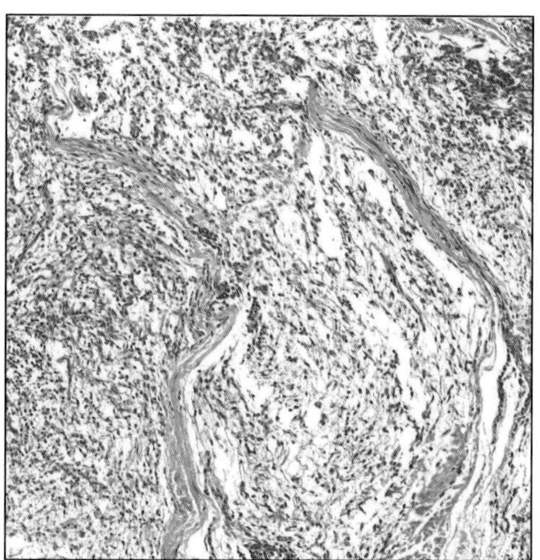

(Left) *The neoplasm is composed of atypical epithelioid tumor cells with abundant eosinophilic cytoplasm and round, vesicular nuclei. This case represents a rare epithelioid cell variant of myxofibrosarcoma.* ***(Right)*** *At least focally, atypical spindled and stellate tumor cells were present.*

LOW-GRADE FIBROMYXOID SARCOMA

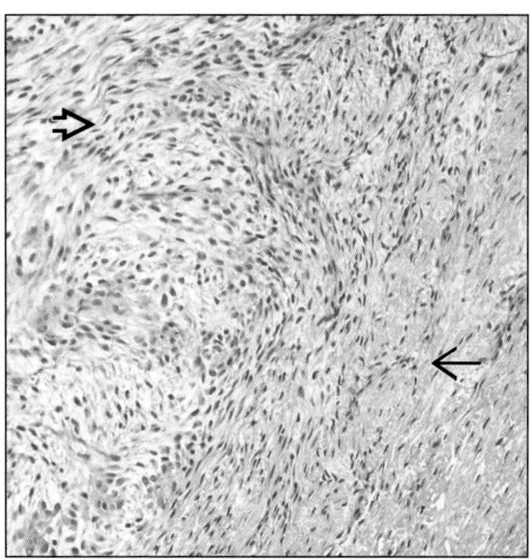

Hematoxylin & eosin shows low-grade fibromyxoid sarcoma, as well as the interface between the myxoid areas ⇨ and the collagenous areas → of the tumor.

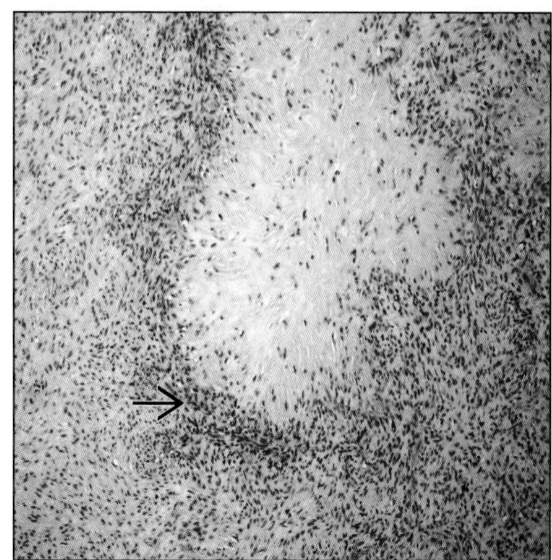

Hematoxylin & eosin shows low-grade fibromyxoid sarcoma with a giant rosette, composed of sparsely cellular collagenous tissue cuffed by a cellular distribution of tumor cells →.

TERMINOLOGY

Abbreviations

- Low-grade fibromyxoid sarcoma (LGFMS)

Synonyms

- Fibrosarcoma, fibromyxoid type; hyalinizing spindle cell tumor with giant rosettes

Definitions

- Malignant fibroblastic neoplasm composed of bland spindle cells in collagenous and myxoid matrix, often with prominent collagenous nodules
- Characterized by specific translocations producing fusion oncogenes
- Despite histologically low-grade morphology, up to 30% can metastasize

ETIOLOGY/PATHOGENESIS

Characteristic Translocations

- Produce chimeric fusion genes
- Cellular origin still unknown but mesenchymal neoplasm with cells of fibroblastic type

CLINICAL ISSUES

Epidemiology

- Incidence
  - True incidence unknown
  - Tumor probably underreported in literature due to its morphologic resemblance to other benign and malignant tumors
- Age
  - Adults (typically in 4th decade), but wide age distribution
    - Significant proportion occur in patients < 18 years old
- Gender
  - M > F

Site

- Mainly deep-seated but can also occur in dermis and subcutis
- Proximal extremities (especially lower limbs) and trunk
- Rarely other locations, including viscera
- Superficial lesions have higher incidence in childhood

Presentation

- Painless mass
  - Many are of long duration

Treatment

- Surgical approaches
  - Wide excision
  - Long-term follow-up is mandatory, in view of potential for late metastases

Prognosis

- Recurrence rates of up to 21%
  - Recurrence is lower in superficial cases
- Metastatic rate of approximately 30% in genetically confirmed cases
  - > 80% of metastases appeared after 9 years
  - No reported metastases in superficial tumors

MACROSCOPIC FEATURES

General Features

- Well-defined mass
- White cut surface, often with glistening myxoid areas
- Sometimes cystic foci, but necrosis rare

MICROSCOPIC PATHOLOGY

Histologic Features

- Lobulated and partially circumscribed, but frequent microscopic infiltration into adjacent soft tissue

LOW-GRADE FIBROMYXOID SARCOMA

Key Facts

Terminology
- Malignant fibroblastic neoplasm composed of bland spindles in collagenous matrix, often with prominent collagenous nodules
- Characterized by specific translocations producing fusion oncogenes

Clinical Issues
- Adults (typically in 4th decade)
- More common in males
- Mainly deep-seated but can also occur superficially
- Proximal extremities (especially lower limbs) and trunk
- Rarely other locations, including viscera
- Recurrence rates of up to 21%
- Recurrence is lower in superficial cases
- Metastatic rate of approximately 30% in genetically confirmed cases

Microscopic Pathology
- Whorled distributions of bland fibroblasts
- Collagenous or myxoid matrix, often in distinct zones
- Owing to bland morphology, tumors often mistaken for variety of benign or low-grade neoplasms

Ancillary Tests
- CD34 positivity in some cases
- Occasional EMA and claudin-1 positivity, which can make distinction from perineurioma difficult
- Balanced translocations
- t(7;16)(q32-34;p11) *FUS, CREB3L2*
- t(11;16)(p11;p11) *FUS, CREB3L1*

- Sparsely to moderately cellular arrays of bland fibroblasts
- Whorled or loosely fascicular distributions
- Collagenous or myxoid matrix, often in distinct zones
  - Abrupt transition to myxoid foci is characteristic
- Cells display angulated, slightly squared nuclei with pale, even chromatin and indistinct fibrillary cytoplasm
- Pleomorphism is unusual
- Mitoses rare
- Approximately 10% show greater cellularity and atypia, more similar to usual intermediate-grade fibrosarcomas
- Hyalinizing spindle cell tumor with giant rosettes
  - Morphologic variant of LGFMS, though term is now used infrequently
  - Prominent paucicellular hyalinized rosette-like nodules, bordered by more rounded tumor cells
  - Similar to typical LGFMS in cytogenetic abnormalities and behavior
- Recurrences of LGFMS frequently show increased cellularity, pleomorphism, and mitotic activity
  - May show transition to frank high-grade spindle cell sarcoma
  - Foci of higher grade sarcoma at presentation, however, not thought to be prognostically adverse
- Relationship between LGFMS and sclerosing epithelioid fibrosarcoma is also suggested

ANCILLARY TESTS

Immunohistochemistry
- Almost always negative for desmin, actin-sm, S100 protein, and pancytokeratin
- Occasional CD34, EMA, and claudin-1 positivity make distinction from perineurioma more difficult

Cytogenetics
- Balanced translocations
- t(7;16)(q32-34;p11) *FUS, CREB3L2*
- t(11;16)(p11;p11) *FUS, CREB3L1*
- Relationship between genetic and histologic findings not yet established
- No relationship between genetic findings and clinical outcome

Electron Microscopy
- Transmission
  - Cells show features of primitive fibroblasts, with paucity of organelles but abundant vimentin-type intermediate filaments

DIFFERENTIAL DIAGNOSIS

Fibromatosis
- Sweeping fascicular pattern
- Myofibroblasts with elongated nuclei and small nucleoli
- Characteristic vascular pattern
- Nuclear β-catenin positivity

Neurofibroma (Especially Myxoid Neurofibroma)
- Variable degree of S100 protein positivity
- Cells with elongated buckled nuclei

Cellular Myxoma
- Lack of pronounced fibrous zones

Nodular Fasciitis
- Superficial location
- Spindle and stellate fibroblasts with tissue culture appearance
- Related phenomena (e.g., extravasated erythrocytes, giant cells)
- Mitoses may be frequent
- Smooth muscle actin positivity

Perineurioma
- Superficial location
- Elongated spindle cells with bipolar processes
- Perivascular whorls
- CD34, EMA, GLUT1, and claudin-1 positivity

LOW-GRADE FIBROMYXOID SARCOMA

Immunohistochemistry

Antibody	Reactivity	Staining Pattern	Comment
Vimentin	Positive	Cytoplasmic	
CD34	Positive	Cytoplasmic	Occasional
EMA	Positive	Cell membrane	Occasional
Claudin-1	Positive	Cell membrane & cytoplasm	Occasional
Desmin	Negative		
Actin-sm	Negative		
AE1/AE3	Negative		
S100	Negative		
β-catenin	Negative		Helps distinguish from fibromatosis

Myxofibrosarcoma

- Subcutaneous locations, in elderly patients
- Atypical hyperchromatic nuclei
- More prominent myxoid stroma
- Stromal vascularity

Myxoid Dermatofibrosarcoma Protuberans

- Superficial location
- Tight storiform fascicular pattern
- Diffuse CD34 positivity

Myxoid Liposarcoma

- Superficial location
- Absence of fibrous zones
- Often contains lipoblasts
- Prominent curvilinear vascular pattern
- Characteristic t(12;16) translocation

Malignant Peripheral Nerve Sheath Tumor

- Elongated cells with buckled nuclei
- Nuclear atypia
- Variable focal S100 protein expression
- Loosely fascicular growth pattern

SELECTED REFERENCES

1. Fisher C: Soft tissue sarcomas with non-EWS translocations: molecular genetic features and pathologic and clinical correlations. Virchows Arch. 456(2):153-66, 2010
2. Thway K et al: Claudin-1 is expressed in perineurioma-like low-grade fibromyxoid sarcoma. Hum Pathol. 40(11):1586-90, 2009
3. Jakowski JD et al: Primary intrathoracic low-grade fibromyxoid sarcoma. Hum Pathol. 39(4):623-8, 2008
4. Matsuyama A et al: DNA-based polymerase chain reaction for detecting FUS-CREB3L2 in low-grade fibromyxoid sarcoma using formalin-fixed, paraffin-embedded tissue specimens. Diagn Mol Pathol. 17(4):237-40, 2008
5. Saito R et al: Low-grade fibromyxoid sarcoma of intracranial origin. J Neurosurg. 108(4):798-802, 2008
6. Guillou L et al: Translocation-positive low-grade fibromyxoid sarcoma: clinicopathologic and molecular analysis of a series expanding the morphologic spectrum and suggesting potential relationship to sclerosing epithelioid fibrosarcoma: a study from the French Sarcoma Group. Am J Surg Pathol. 31(9):1387-402, 2007
7. Panagopoulos I et al: Characterization of the native CREB3L2 transcription factor and the FUS/CREB3L2 chimera. Genes Chromosomes Cancer. 46(2):181-91, 2007
8. Matsuyama A et al: Molecular detection of FUS-CREB3L2 fusion transcripts in low-grade fibromyxoid sarcoma using formalin-fixed, paraffin-embedded tissue specimens. Am J Surg Pathol. 30(9):1077-84, 2006
9. Billings SD et al: Superficial low-grade fibromyxoid sarcoma (Evans tumor): a clinicopathologic analysis of 19 cases with a unique observation in the pediatric population. Am J Surg Pathol. 29(2):204-10, 2005
10. Mertens F et al: Clinicopathologic and molecular genetic characterization of low-grade fibromyxoid sarcoma, and cloning of a novel FUS/CREB3L1 fusion gene. Lab Invest. 85(3):408-15, 2005
11. Panagopoulos I et al: The chimeric FUS/CREB3l2 gene is specific for low-grade fibromyxoid sarcoma. Genes Chromosomes Cancer. 40(3):218-28, 2004
12. Reid R et al: Low-grade fibromyxoid sarcoma and hyalinizing spindle cell tumor with giant rosettes share a common t(7;16)(q34;p11) translocation. Am J Surg Pathol. 27(9):1229-36, 2003
13. Storlazzi CT et al: Fusion of the FUS and BBF2H7 genes in low grade fibromyxoid sarcoma. Hum Mol Genet. 12(18):2349-58, 2003
14. Bejarano PA et al: Hyalinizing spindle cell tumor with giant rosettes--a soft tissue tumor with mesenchymal and neuroendocrine features. An immunohistochemical, ultrastructural, and cytogenetic analysis. Arch Pathol Lab Med. 124(8):1179-84, 2000
15. Folpe AL et al: Low-grade fibromyxoid sarcoma and hyalinizing spindle cell tumor with giant rosettes: a clinicopathologic study of 73 cases supporting their identity and assessing the impact of high-grade areas. Am J Surg Pathol. 24(10):1353-60, 2000
16. Lane KL et al: Hyalinizing spindle cell tumor with giant rosettes: a distinctive tumor closely resembling low-grade fibromyxoid sarcoma. Am J Surg Pathol. 21(12):1481-8, 1997
17. Evans HL: Low-grade fibromyxoid sarcoma. A report of 12 cases. Am J Surg Pathol. 17(6):595-600, 1993

Microscopic Features

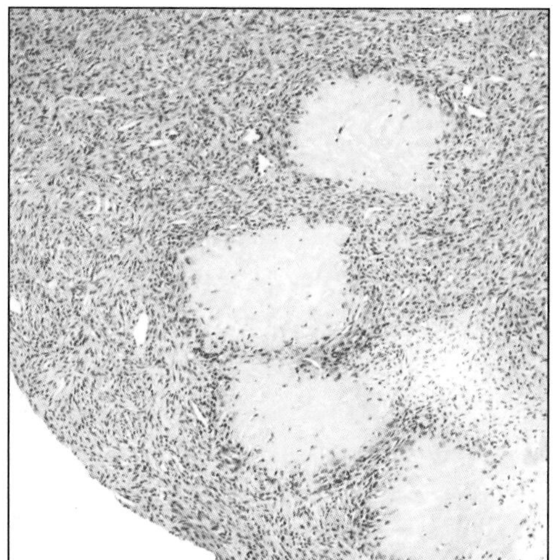

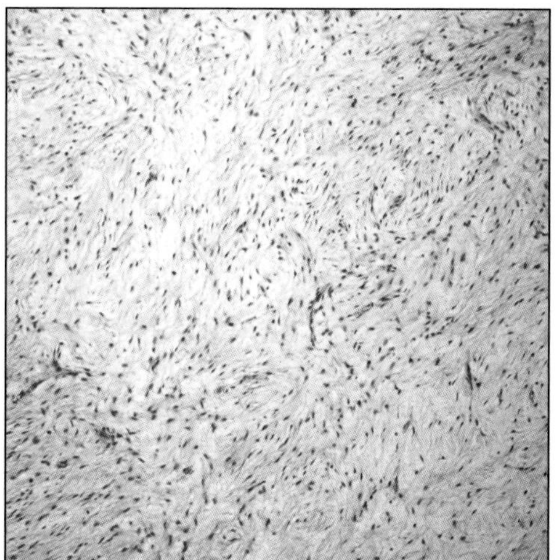

(Left) *Hematoxylin & eosin shows needle core biopsy specimen of LGFMS, with prominent collagenous rosette formation. Rosettes, if present, often vary in distribution and may not be sampled, making the diagnosis difficult.* ***(Right)*** *Hematoxylin & eosin shows LGFMS at low power, with loosely fascicular distributions of spindle cells. Cellularity is frequently only sparse to moderate, and the morphology can be reminiscent of benign spindle cell lesions.*

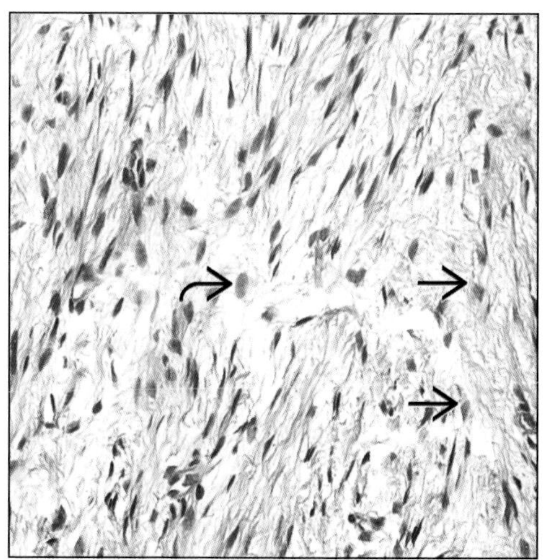

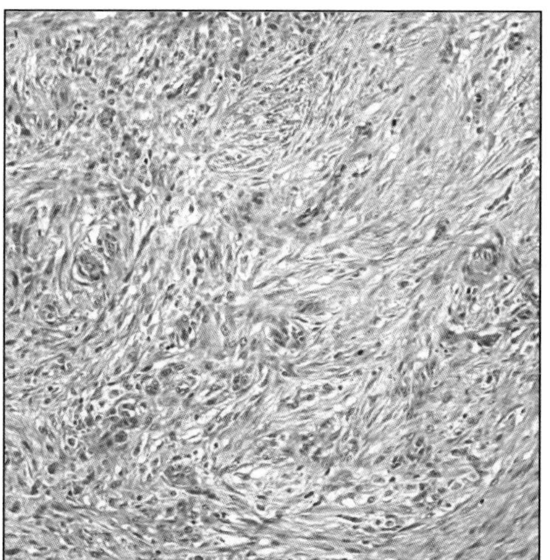

(Left) *Hematoxylin & eosin shows LGFMS. The cells have ovoid ↪, or slightly angulated and squared nuclei →, with delicate, even chromatin and inconspicuous nucleoli. Note the lack of atypia. The stroma is myxoid and delicately collagenous.* ***(Right)*** *Hematoxylin & eosin shows LGFMS with prominent collagenous stroma with a loosely fascicular pattern. This can be mistaken for fibromatosis.*

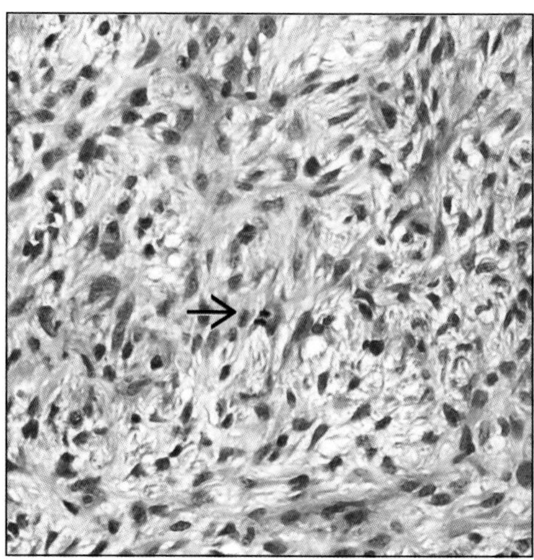

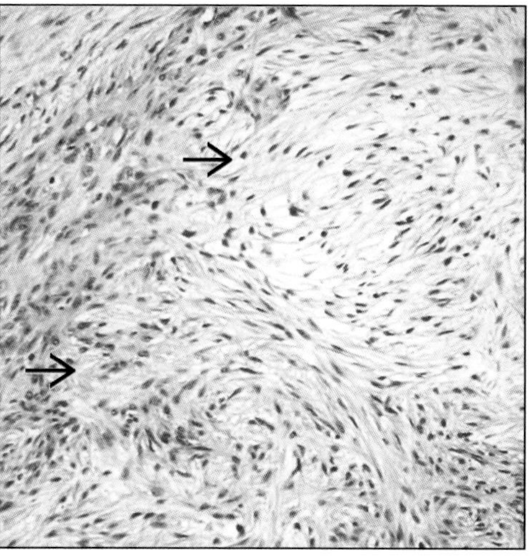

(Left) *Hematoxylin & eosin shows recurrent low-grade fibromyxoid sarcoma. The tumor in this example shows high cellularity with occasional mitoses →.* ***(Right)*** *Hematoxylin & eosin shows LGFMS with nodular formations of cells in a myxoid stroma →. The appearances are reminiscent of myxofibrosarcoma, but no cellular atypia is apparent.*

SCLEROSING EPITHELIOID FIBROSARCOMA

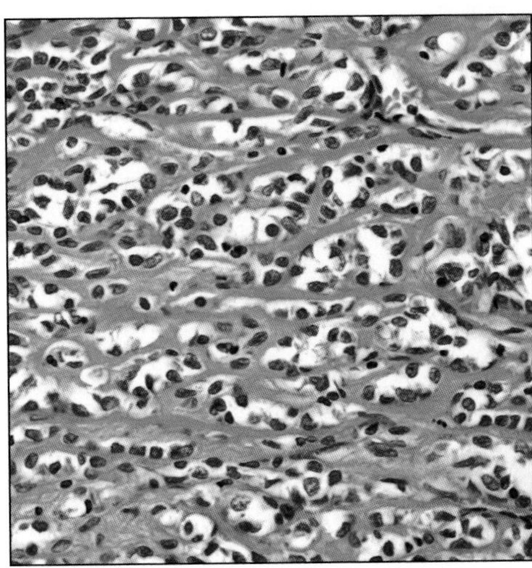

Hematoxylin & eosin shows nests of cells with clear cytoplasm and ovoid, occasionally folded nuclei in a fibrous stroma. Ultrastructurally, these cells show features of fibroblasts.

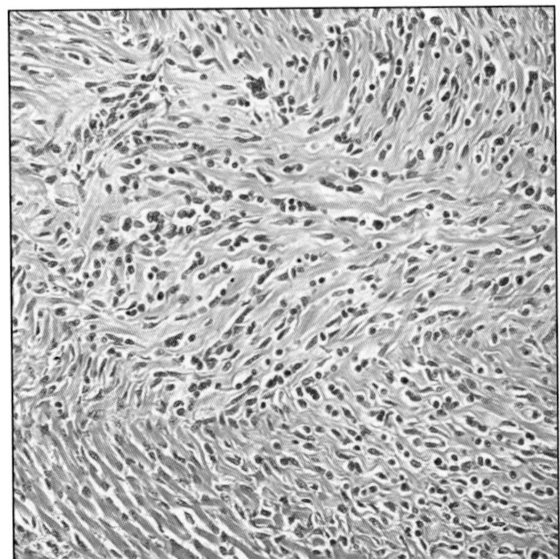

Hematoxylin & eosin shows cords or files of polygonal cells, some with eosinophilic cytoplasm, infiltrating dense fibrous stroma. This can mimic carcinoma, notably lobular carcinoma of the breast.

TERMINOLOGY

Definitions

- Fibrosarcoma variant characterized by at least focal epithelioid cytomorphology and areas of dense fibrosis

ETIOLOGY/PATHOGENESIS

Environmental Exposure

- Occasional example attributed to therapeutic irradiation

CLINICAL ISSUES

Epidemiology

- Incidence
  - Rare: ~ 60 examples reported
- Age
  - Adults, peak in 5th decade
- Gender
  - Slightly more common in females

Site

- Limbs and limb girdles, trunk, shoulder, neck
  - Rarely in visceral sites, e.g., large intestine, ovary, base of penis, pituitary
- Deep muscle
  - Around periosteum or fascia
- Can involve or arise in bone including skull, rib, sacrum

Presentation

- Deep mass
- Painful or painless mass

Treatment

- Surgical approaches
  - Adequate local excision
    - Can require amputation especially when bone involved
- Adjuvant therapy
  - Chemotherapy or radiation therapy can be tried to control recurrence and metastasis

Prognosis

- Histologically of variable grade but clinically aggressive, especially in long term
  - Local recurrence in > 50%
  - Metastasis in 43-86%
  - 5-year survival is 43-75%

MACROSCOPIC FEATURES

General Features

- In deep soft tissue
- Multinodular
- Circumscribed or infiltrative
- Very hard, can show calcification or ossification
- Occasionally cystic

Sections to Be Submitted

- Lesion should be extensively sampled to detect cellular areas

Size

- Variable
  - 2 to > 20 cm in maximum dimension

MICROSCOPIC PATHOLOGY

Histologic Features

- Dense fibrosis divides tumor into cellular islands
  - Nests and cords of polygonal cells
  - Cells can lose cohesion, imparting alveolar appearance
  - Ovoid, sometimes angulated nuclei, occasional pleomorphism

SCLEROSING EPITHELIOID FIBROSARCOMA

Key Facts

Terminology
- Fibrosarcoma variant characterized by at least focal epithelioid cytomorphology and areas of dense fibrosis

Clinical Issues
- Around periosteum or fascia
- Histologically of variable grade but clinically aggressive, especially in long term

Macroscopic Features
- Multinodular

Microscopic Pathology
- Dense fibrosis divides tumor into cellular islands
- Nests and cords of polygonal cells
- Ovoid, sometimes angulated nuclei, occasional pleomorphism
- Can form files of epithelial-like cells
- Other patterns of fibrosarcoma can coexist
  - Adult-type fibrosarcoma
  - Low-grade fibromyxoid sarcoma
- Stroma can show myxohyaline change, calcification, or osteochondroid metaplasia
- Focal hemangiopericytic pattern in some cases

Ancillary Tests
- Epithelioid and spindle cells show features of fibroblasts

Diagnostic Checklist
- Can resemble carcinoma
  - Epithelial markers usually absent
- Can resemble lymphoma
  - Lymphoid markers absent

  - Low mitotic index
  - Clear or eosinophilic cytoplasm
- Cells can form files that simulate scirrhous breast carcinoma or sclerosing lymphoma
- Stroma has range of features
  - Myxohyaline change
  - Pericellular collagen strands can resemble osteoid
  - Calcification
  - Osteochondroid metaplasia
- Focal hemangiopericytic pattern in some cases
- Occasional focal necrosis
- Other patterns of fibrosarcoma can coexist
  - Spindle cell fascicular areas often present, resembling adult-type fibrosarcoma
  - Foci resembling low-grade fibromyxoid sarcoma occasionally seen

Predominant Pattern/Injury Type
- Fibrous

Predominant Cell/Compartment Type
- Fibroblast

ANCILLARY TESTS

Cytogenetics
- Amplification of 12q13 and 12q15 sequences
- Rearrangements of 10p11

Electron Microscopy
- Transmission
  - Epithelioid and spindle cells show features of fibroblasts
    - Abundant rough endoplasmic reticulum
    - Whorls of cytoplasmic filaments
    - Intracytoplasmic collagen
  - Some cases have primitive cell junctions
  - Tonofilaments in occasional example
  - Sarcomere formation in occasional example
    - Immunoreactivity for desmin always negative

DIFFERENTIAL DIAGNOSIS

Metastatic Carcinoma
- Clinical evidence of primary carcinoma
- Absence of fibrosarcoma-like non-pleomorphic spindle component
- Absence of dense acellular hyaline areas
- Widespread positivity for epithelial immunohistochemical markers

Sclerosing Lymphoma
- Relatively uniform cytology
- Presence of lymphoid immunohistochemical markers

Low-Grade Fibromyxoid Sarcoma
- Fibrous and myxoid areas juxtaposed
- Absence of epithelioid cell morphology
- Absence of pleomorphism
- Specific translocation t(7;16)(q33;p11)

Fibromatosis
- Uniform distribution of cells within collagen
- Absence of nests of epithelioid cells
- Absence of pleomorphism
- Immunoreactivity for SMA
- Nuclear positivity for β-catenin in > 80% of cases

Alveolar Soft Part Sarcoma
- Alveolar pattern throughout
- Cells larger than in sclerosing epithelioid fibrosarcoma
  - Rounded nuclei
  - More abundant cytoplasm
- Characteristic crystals on PAS staining and electron microscopy
- Nuclear immunoreactivity for TFE3
- Specific translocation t(X;17(p11;q25)

Alveolar Rhabdomyosarcoma
- Nests of cells in dense fibrous stroma
- Rhabdomyoblasts with eosinophilic cytoplasm
- Multinucleated wreath-like cells
- Immunoreactive for desmin and myogenin (in nuclei)

SCLEROSING EPITHELIOID FIBROSARCOMA

Immunohistochemistry

Antibody	Reactivity	Staining Pattern	Comment
Vimentin	Positive	Cytoplasmic	100%, nonspecific
β-catenin-cytoplasm	Positive	Cytoplasmic	100%, nonspecific
Bcl-2	Positive	Cytoplasmic	90%, nonspecific
EMA/MUC1	Positive	Cell membrane & cytoplasm	~ 45%, focal
MDM2	Positive	Nuclear	Reported in 1 case, 70% of cells
Actin-sm	Negative		
Desmin	Negative		
AE1/AE3	Equivocal	Cytoplasmic	Occasional case, focal
CK8/18/CAM5.2	Equivocal	Cytoplasmic	Occasional case, focal
S100P	Equivocal	Nuclear & cytoplasmic	Occasional case, focal
Ki-67	Equivocal	Nuclear	< 5% of cells, in all cases

Sclerosing (Pseudovascular) Rhabdomyosarcoma

- Spindle and primitive round cells
- Occasional rhabdomyoblasts
- Pseudovascular pattern
- Hyaline or chondroid stroma
- Desmin (dot-like) positivity in cytoplasm
- MYOD1 and focal myogenin positivity in nuclei

DIAGNOSTIC CHECKLIST

Pathologic Interpretation Pearls

- Look for foci of typical adult fibrosarcoma
  - Herringbone fascicles of long tapered spindle cells
- Can resemble carcinoma
  - Epithelial markers rarely positive in sclerosing epithelioid fibrosarcoma
- Can resemble lymphoma
  - Lymphoid markers negative in sclerosing epithelioid fibrosarcoma

SELECTED REFERENCES

1. Ossendorf C et al: Sclerosing epithelioid fibrosarcoma: case presentation and a systematic review. Clin Orthop Relat Res. 466(6):1485-91, 2008
2. Frattini JC et al: Sclerosing epithelioid fibrosarcoma of the cecum: a radiation-associated tumor in a previously unreported site. Arch Pathol Lab Med. 131(12):1825-8, 2007
3. Guillou L et al: Translocation-positive low-grade fibromyxoid sarcoma: clinicopathologic and molecular analysis of a series expanding the morphologic spectrum and suggesting potential relationship to sclerosing epithelioid fibrosarcoma: a study from the French Sarcoma Group. Am J Surg Pathol. 31(9):1387-402, 2007
4. Massier A et al: Sclerosing epithelioid fibrosarcoma of the pituitary. Endocr Pathol. 18(4):233-8, 2007
5. Battiata AP et al: Sclerosing epithelioid fibrosarcoma: a case report. Ann Otol Rhinol Laryngol. 114(2):87-9, 2005
6. Bhattacharya B et al: Nuclear beta-catenin expression distinguishes deep fibromatosis from other benign and malignant fibroblastic and myofibroblastic lesions. Am J Surg Pathol. 29(5):653-9, 2005
7. Chow LT et al: Primary sclerosing epithelioid fibrosarcoma of the sacrum: a case report and review of the literature. J Clin Pathol. 57(1):90-4, 2004
8. Hu WW et al: [Sclerosing epithelioid fibrosarcoma: a clinicopathologic study of eight cases] Zhonghua Bing Li Xue Za Zhi. 33(4):337-41, 2004
9. Ogose A et al: Sclerosing epithelioid fibrosarcoma with der(10)t(10;17)(p11;q11). Cancer Genet Cytogenet. 152(2):136-40, 2004
10. Watanabe K et al: Epithelioid fibrosarcoma of the ovary. Virchows Arch. 445(4):410-3, 2004
11. Genevay M et al: [Recent entities in soft tissue tumor pathology. Part 2] Ann Pathol. 23(2):135-48, 2003
12. Hindermann W et al: [Sclerosing epithelioid fibrosarcoma] Pathologe. 24(2):103-8, 2003
13. Abdulkader I et al: Sclerosing epithelioid fibrosarcoma primary of the bone. Int J Surg Pathol. 10(3):227-30, 2002
14. Jiao YF et al: Overexpression of MDM2 in a sclerosing epithelioid fibrosarcoma: genetic, immunohistochemical and ultrastructural study of a case. Pathol Int. 52(2):135-40, 2002
15. Antonescu CR et al: Sclerosing epithelioid fibrosarcoma: a study of 16 cases and confirmation of a clinicopathologically distinct tumor. Am J Surg Pathol. 25(6):699-709, 2001
16. Arya M et al: A rare tumour in the pelvis presenting with lower urinary symptoms: 'sclerosing epithelioid fibrosarcoma'. Eur J Surg Oncol. 27(1):121-2, 2001
17. Hanson IM et al: Evidence of nerve sheath differentiation and high grade morphology in sclerosing epithelioid fibrosarcoma. J Clin Pathol. 54(9):721-3, 2001
18. Bilsky MH et al: Sclerosing epithelioid fibrosarcomas involving the neuraxis: report of three cases. Neurosurgery. 47(4):956-9; discussion 959-60, 2000
19. Donner LR et al: Sclerosing epithelioid fibrosarcoma: a cytogenetic, immunohistochemical, and ultrastructural study of an unusual histological variant. Cancer Genet Cytogenet. 119(2):127-31, 2000
20. Eyden BP et al: Sclerosing epithelioid fibrosarcoma: a study of five cases emphasizing diagnostic criteria. Histopathology. 33(4):354-60, 1998
21. Gisselsson D et al: Amplification of 12q13 and 12q15 sequences in a sclerosing epithelioid fibrosarcoma. Cancer Genet Cytogenet. 107(2):102-6, 1998
22. Reid R et al: Sclerosing epithelioid fibrosarcoma. Histopathology. 28(5):451-5, 1996
23. Meis-Kindblom JM et al: Sclerosing epithelioid fibrosarcoma. A variant of fibrosarcoma simulating carcinoma. Am J Surg Pathol. 19(9):979-93, 1995

Microscopic Features

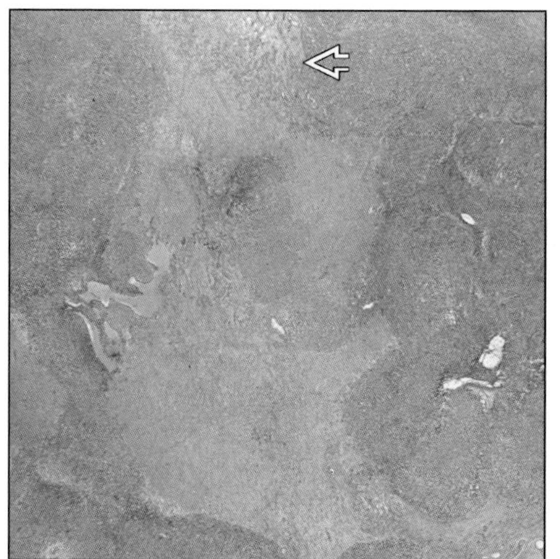

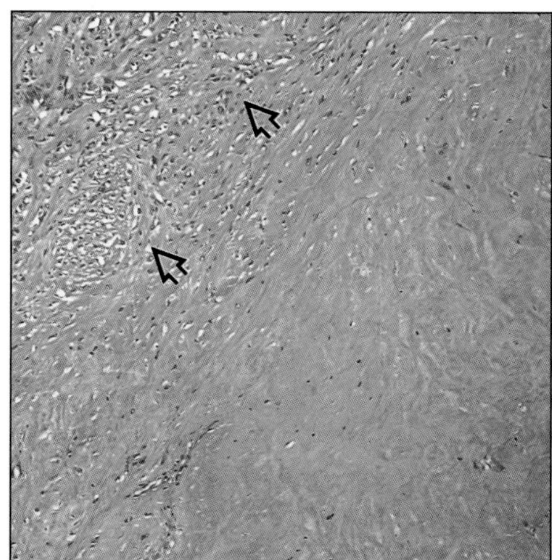

(Left) *Hematoxylin & eosin shows multiple nodules and islands of cells in dense fibrous stroma. Note cords and nests of cells ➡. Focal calcification or ossification can be seen within the stroma in some cases.* ***(Right)*** *Hematoxylin & eosin shows area of dense sclerosis with marked hypocellularity. Note the transition to more cellular focus with nests of cells displaying epithelioid and clear cell morphology ⇨.*

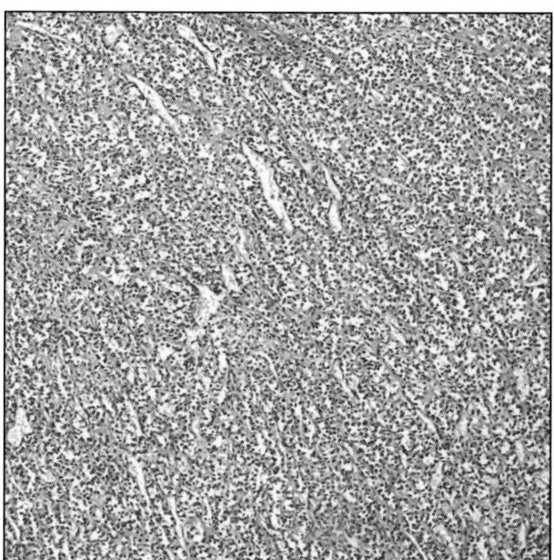

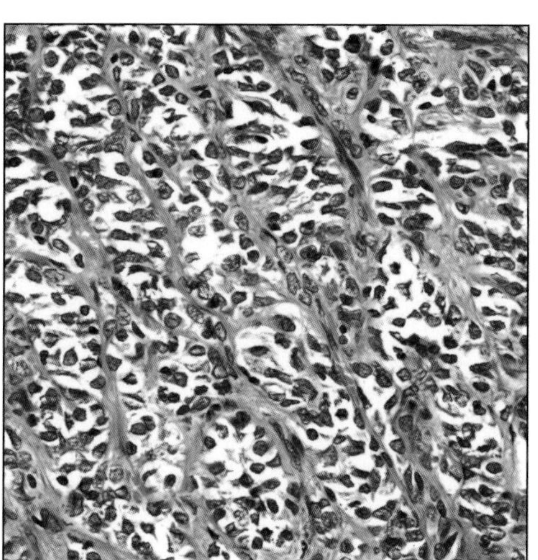

(Left) *Hematoxylin & eosin shows sheet-like architecture of nests of polygonal cells with clear cytoplasm. The nests are separated by thin fibrous bands. This is a characteristic appearance, but it can be confused with alveolar soft part sarcoma or renal cell carcinoma.* ***(Right)*** *Hematoxylin & eosin higher magnification shows elongated cell nests within slender fibrous bands. The cells have ovoid angulated nuclei, sometimes with grooves. The cytoplasm is focally clear.*

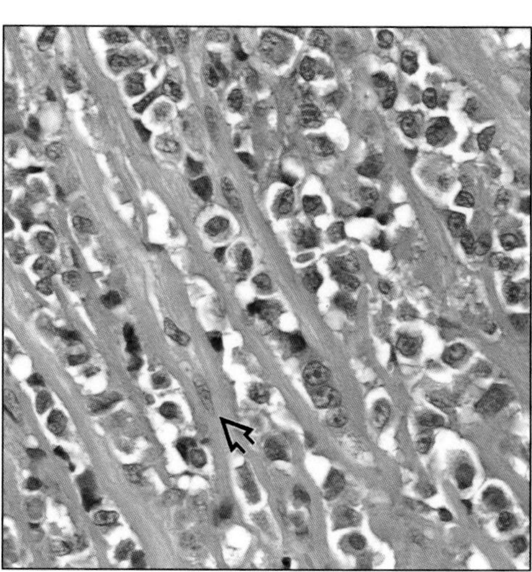

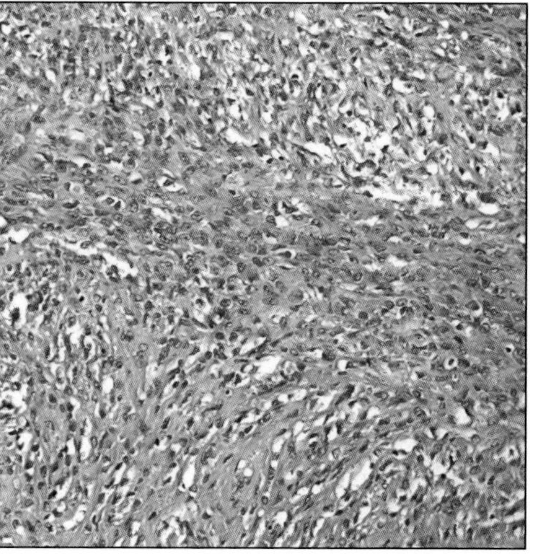

(Left) *Hematoxylin & eosin shows files of rounded cells separated by thick bands of collagen with an occasional fibroblast ⇨. This appearance can be indistinguishable from sclerosing lymphoma or carcinoma without immunohistochemistry, especially in a small biopsy specimen.* ***(Right)*** *A fascicular pattern of spindle cells resembles typical or adult fibrosarcoma. This pattern is often present focally within the tumor, which should therefore be thoroughly sampled.*

Fibrohistiocytic Lesions

Benign

Intermediate

Malignant

DERMATOFIBROMA (BENIGN FIBROUS HISTIOCYTOMA)

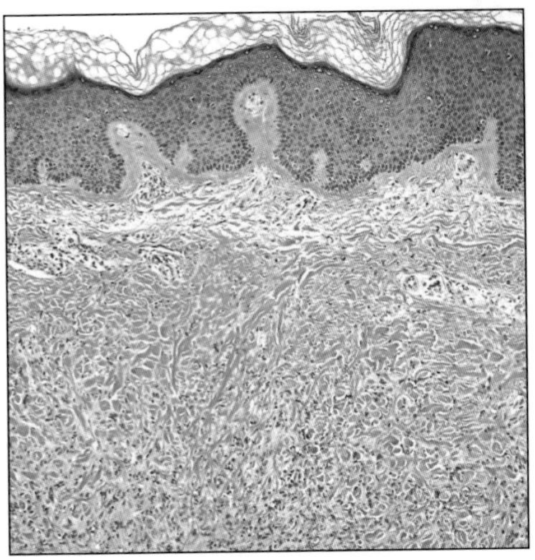

Classic dermatofibroma shows a dermal-based proliferation of bland spindled to histiocytic-appearing cells, associated with a Grenz zone and overlying epidermal hyperplasia and basilar pigmentation.

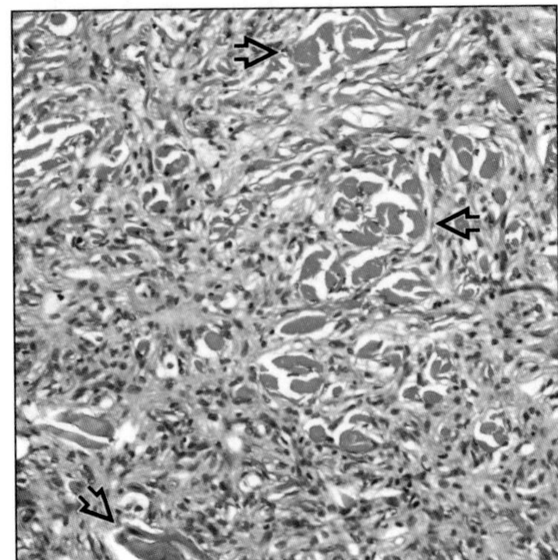

Higher power examination of a classic dermatofibroma shows a proliferation of bland spindled to histiocytoid cells entrapping numerous hyalinized balls of collagen ➯.

TERMINOLOGY

Abbreviations

- Dermatofibroma (DF)
- Fibrous histiocytoma (FH)

Synonyms

- Cutaneous fibrous histiocytoma
- Sclerosing hemangioma
- Histiocytoma
- Epithelioid cell histiocytoma

Definitions

- Common, benign, limited proliferation of mesenchymal cells in dermis
- Lineage not well defined, although commonly referred to as "fibrohistiocytic"

ETIOLOGY/PATHOGENESIS

Unknown

- Evidence supports both reactive and neoplastic pathogenesis
  - Histiocytic population may be clonal; fibroblast/myofibroblastic population may be polyclonal (reactive)
- Tumor may be preceded by local trauma, including insect bite in some cases
  - However, often no inciting event identified

CLINICAL ISSUES

Epidemiology

- Incidence
  - Common tumors in most populations
- Age
  - All ages, but most common in 4th and 5th decades
- Gender
  - Affects males and females equally

Site

- Typically occur on distal extremities but may present at any cutaneous site

Presentation

- Firm, isolated, flesh-colored subcutaneous papule or nodule
  - New DFs are typically pink (vascular); older DFs are brown (overlying melanocyte hyperplasia)
- Multiple DFs occur in immunosuppressed populations
- "Dimpling" sign when in vivo DF is pinched by fingers

Treatment

- Excision usually curative

Prognosis

- Excellent in vast majority of cases
  - Local recurrence potential significant (up to 30%) with cellular variant
  - Metastasis and death from some cellular and atypical tumors reported
    - Usually large and deep lesions

MACROSCOPIC FEATURES

General Features

- Firm, circumscribed but nonencapsulated, dermal-based tumor
- White to yellow cut surface
- Can have cystic changes and hemorrhage

MICROSCOPIC PATHOLOGY

Histologic Features

- Dermal-based proliferation of typically bland spindled to histiocytic-appearing cells
  - Either spindled (fibroblastic) or histiocytoid cells may predominate

DERMATOFIBROMA (BENIGN FIBROUS HISTIOCYTOMA)

Key Facts

Terminology
- Benign limited proliferation of histiocytic and fibroblastic cells in dermis

Etiology/Pathogenesis
- Evidence supports both neoplastic and reactive pathogenesis

Clinical Issues
- Affects all ages and both sexes but most common in young adults
- Excellent prognosis in vast majority of cases
- Metastasis and death in rare cases of cellular and atypical tumors

Microscopic Pathology
- Dermal-based proliferation of typically bland spindled to histiocytic-appearing cells
- Collagen trapping at periphery
- Overlying epithelial basilar induction with hyperpigmentation
- Adjacent adnexal hyperplasia

Ancillary Tests
- FXIIIA(+), CD163(+), CD68(+), CD34(-)

Top Differential Diagnoses
- Basal cell carcinoma
  - CD20(+) Merkel cells overlying DF
- Angiosarcoma and Kaposi sarcoma
  - CD31 and HHV8 are negative in aneurysmal DF
- Dermatofibrosarcoma protuberans
  - Deep subcutaneous extension and fat entrapment
  - CD34, CD163, and FXIIIA usually allow for distinction

- Early lesions typically show more histiocytes and lymphocytes
- Established lesions show greater cellularity and spindled cells
- Older lesions show more fibrosis
- Spindled cells show elongated eosinophilic cytoplasmic processes
- "Histiocytic" type cells are larger, epithelioid-shaped, and have abundant pale vacuolated cytoplasm
- Cytologic atypia and pleomorphism are usually minimal

- Tumors are grossly circumscribed but microscopically have irregular, often jagged borders
- Collagen trapping at periphery
  - Spheres of intensely eosinophilic collagen (so-called "collagen balls") separated by bands of pale fibrohistiocytic cells
- Grenz zone
  - Tumor often spares band of superficial dermis
- Folliculosebaceous induction and basilar epidermal hyperplasia overlying DF
  - Can mimic basal cell carcinoma if basilar induction is marked
- Adjacent adnexal hyperplasia
- Overlying melanocyte hyperplasia occasionally seen
  - So-called "dirty sock" sign

Predominant Pattern/Injury Type
- Ill-defined borders
- Nodular proliferation
- Fibrous
- Histiocytic

Predominant Cell/Compartment Type
- "Fibrohistiocytic"

Histologic Subtypes
- **Aneurysmal (hemosiderotic/sclerosing hemangioma variant)**
  - Pseudovascular spaces, hemosiderin, reactive spindle and epithelioid cells
    - May mimic vascular tumor, including Kaposi sarcoma and angiosarcoma
  - Aneurysmal DF can show some cytologic atypia but lacks high-grade atypia and shows only a few mitoses
- **Cellular**
  - Uncommon, often large, deeply penetrating tumors
    - May show overlap with atypical dermatofibroma
    - Occasional mitoses and multinucleated cells are seen
    - Up to 12% of cases may show focal central necrosis
  - Most likely subtype to recur
    - Complete conservative excision should be recommended
- **Epithelioid cell histiocytoma**
  - Nodular to sheet-like, well-circumscribed proliferation in papillary dermis
    - Often has associated epidermal collarette
  - Clinical and histologic mimic of intradermal Spitz nevus but negative for melanocytic markers
- **Atypical/pseudosarcomatous/"DF with monster cells"**
  - Shows population of atypical cells with nuclear hyperchromasia and prominent nucleoli, often with abundant cytoplasm
    - Mitotic figures are sparse, usually not atypical in appearance
  - Some cases have been reported to metastasize
    - Complete excision should be recommended
- **Lipidized**
  - Often large tumors, typically present in ankle region
  - Numerous large foamy cells are present, with a few hemosiderin-containing cells
  - Stromal hyalinization is typically present, which may be "wiry" or "keloidal" in appearance
- Many other rare variants described, including granular cell, clear cell, histiocytic/xanthomatous, osteoclastic, myxoid, keloidal/scar-like, palisading, deep penetrating (may mimic dermatofibrosarcoma protuberans [DFSP]), and lichenoid

DERMATOFIBROMA (BENIGN FIBROUS HISTIOCYTOMA)

ANCILLARY TESTS

Immunohistochemistry

- FXIIIA(+), CD163(+), HMGA1/HMGA2(+), MMP-11(+)
  - CD68 often positive; highlights histiocytic-appearing cells
  - Actin-sm often positive; may indicate myofibroblastic differentiation
- CD34 typically negative but may show focal staining, especially at periphery of lesion
- Nestin(-), S100(-), desmin(-)

DIFFERENTIAL DIAGNOSIS

Dermatofibrosarcoma Protuberans (DFSP)

- Shows monotonous proliferation of spindled cells
- Typically extends deeply along septa of subcutaneous fat
  - Typically CD34(+), nestin(+), CD163(-), HMGA1/HMGA2(-), FXIIIA(±)

Basal Cell Carcinoma (BCC)

- In superficial biopsies, BCC can be difficult to distinguish from benign follicular induction overlying DF
  - CK20 highlights Merkel cells in basal layer overlying DF; these cells are absent in BCC

Angiosarcoma

- Aneurysmal variant of DF can have atypical cells, pseudovascular spaces, and mitoses
  - Aneurysmal DF is negative for vascular markers, including CD31, CD34, and HHV8

Kaposi Sarcoma

- Nodular/tumor stage Kaposi sarcoma shows cellular spindle cell proliferation
- Slit-like vascular spaces and extravasated red blood cells are often present
  - Immunohistochemistry shows CD31 and HHV8 positivity

Atypical Fibroxanthoma (AFX)

- Dermal nodule composed of highly atypical spindled and pleomorphic epithelioid cells
- Typically occurs in heavily sun-damaged skin (especially head and neck area) of elderly patients
  - Both AFX and DF are positive for nonspecific markers, including CD68, CD10, and vimentin
  - FXIIIA may show greater positivity in DF

DIAGNOSTIC CHECKLIST

Clinically Relevant Pathologic Features

- Cellularity and atypia
- Tumor size (more aggressive cases typically large and deep)

Pathologic Interpretation Pearls

- "Collagen balls"
- Basilar epidermal induction with hyperpigmentation
- Adnexal and melanocytic hyperplasia

SELECTED REFERENCES

1. Fernandez-Flores A et al: Mitosis in dermatofibroma: a worrisome histopathologic sign that does not necessarily equal recurrence. J Cutan Pathol. 35(9):839-42, 2008
2. Gleason BC et al: Deep "benign" fibrous histiocytoma: clinicopathologic analysis of 69 cases of a rare tumor indicating occasional metastatic potential. Am J Surg Pathol. 32(3):354-62, 2008
3. Mori T et al: Expression of nestin in dermatofibrosarcoma protuberans in comparison to dermatofibroma. J Dermatol. 35(7):419-25, 2008
4. Kim HJ et al: Stromelysin-3 expression in the differential diagnosis of dermatofibroma and dermatofibrosarcoma protuberans: comparison with factor XIIIa and CD34. Br J Dermatol. 157(2):319-24, 2007
5. Fletcher CD: The evolving classification of soft tissue tumours: an update based on the new WHO classification. Histopathology. 48(1):3-12, 2006
6. Sachdev R et al: Expression of CD163 in dermatofibroma, cellular fibrous histiocytoma, and dermatofibrosarcoma protuberans: comparison with CD68, CD34, and Factor XIIIa. J Cutan Pathol. 33(5):353-60, 2006
7. Mahmoodi M et al: Anti-cytokeratin 20 staining of Merkel cells helps differentiate basaloid proliferations overlying dermatofibromas from basal cell carcinoma. J Cutan Pathol. 32(7):491-5, 2005
8. Li N et al: Differential expression of HMGA1 and HMGA2 in dermatofibroma and dermatofibrosarcoma protuberans: potential diagnostic applications, and comparison with histologic findings, CD34, and factor XIIIa immunoreactivity. Am J Dermatopathol. 26(4):267-72, 2004
9. Hui P et al: Clonal analysis of cutaneous fibrous histiocytoma (dermatofibroma). J Cutan Pathol. 29(7):385-9, 2002
10. Kaddu S et al: Atypical fibrous histiocytoma of the skin: clinicopathologic analysis of 59 cases with evidence of infrequent metastasis. Am J Surg Pathol. 26(1):35-46, 2002
11. Massone C et al: Multiple eruptive dermatofibromas in patients with systemic lupus erythematosus treated with prednisone. Int J Dermatol. 41(5):279-81, 2002
12. Nuovo M et al: Utility of HHV8 RNA detection for differentiating Kaposi's sarcoma from its mimics. J Cutan Pathol. 28(5):248-55, 2001
13. Chen TC et al: Dermatofibroma is a clonal proliferative disease. J Cutan Pathol. 27(1):36-9, 2000
14. Vanni R et al: Cytogenetic evidence of clonality in cutaneous benign fibrous histiocytomas: a report of the CHAMP study group. Histopathology. 37(3):212-7, 2000
15. Ammirati CT et al: Multiple eruptive dermatofibromas in three men with HIV infection. Dermatology. 195(4):344-8, 1997
16. Li DF et al: Dermatofibroma: superficial fibrous proliferation with reactive histiocytes. A multiple immunostaining analysis. Cancer. 74(1):66-73, 1994
17. Altman DA et al: Differential expression of factor XIIIa and CD34 in cutaneous mesenchymal tumors. J Cutan Pathol. 20(2):154-8, 1993
18. Santa Cruz DJ et al: Aneurysmal ("angiomatoid") fibrous histiocytoma of the skin. Cancer. 47(8):2053-61, 1981

Microscopic Features

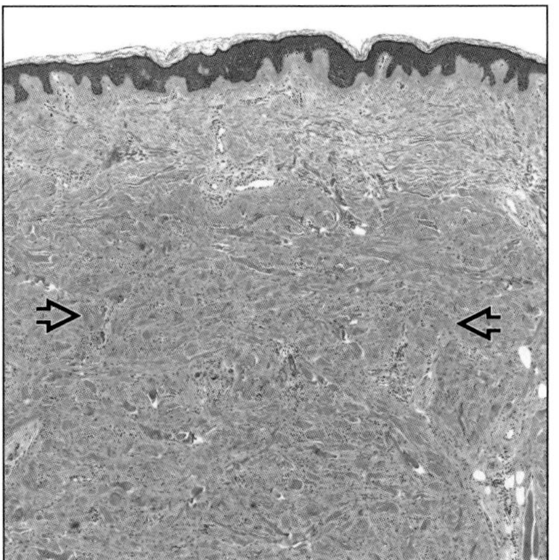

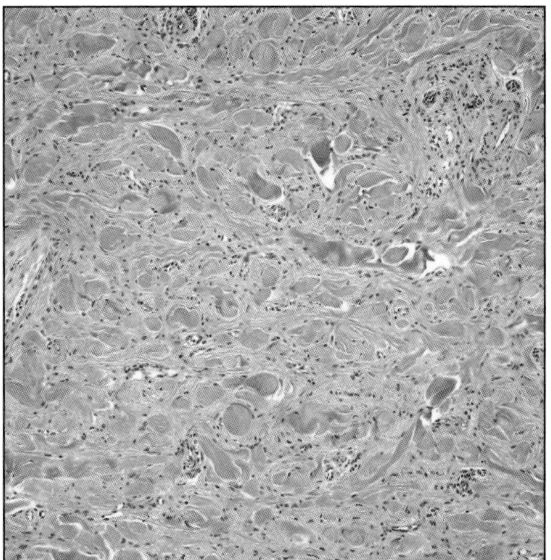

(Left) *Scanning magnification of a scar-like dermatofibroma with thickened, keloidal collagen bundles ⇨ is shown.* ***(Right)*** *Higher power view of scar-like dermatofibroma shows dense and glassy-appearing bundles of keloidal collagen.*

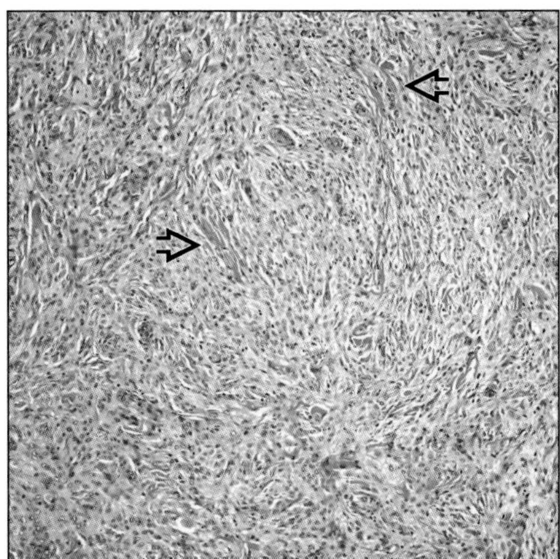

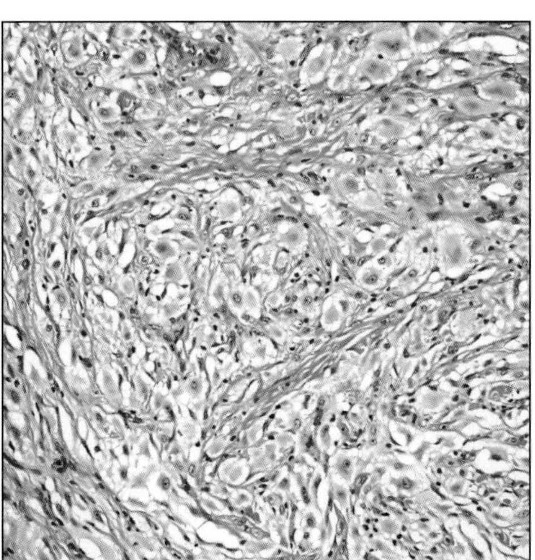

(Left) *Histiocytic-predominant dermatofibroma shows a proliferation of large, epithelioid-appearing cells with abundant pale/vacuolated cytoplasm and scattered entrapped collagen bundles ⇨.* ***(Right)*** *Higher power examination of histiocytic dermatofibroma shows the large cells with abundant pale to vacuolated cytoplasm and bland-appearing nuclei.*

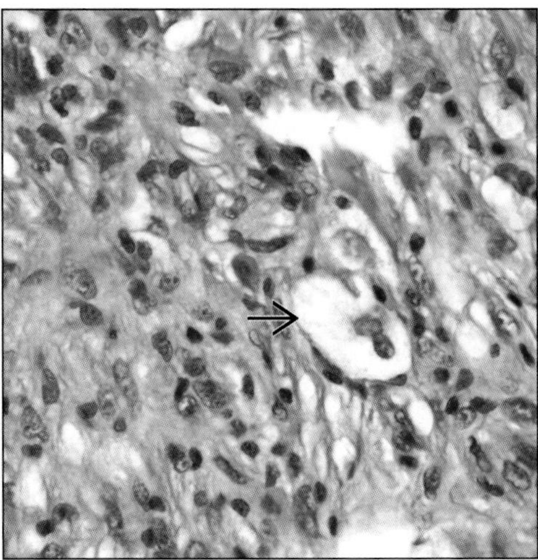

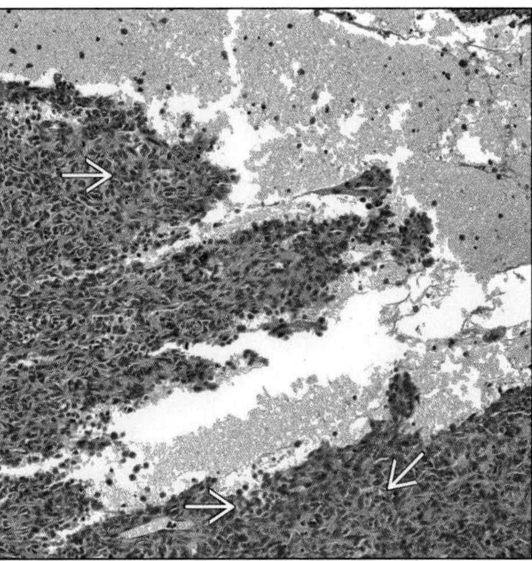

(Left) *Lipidized dermatofibroma shows proliferation of bland histiocytoid cells and scattered multivacuolated cells with nuclear indentation, simulating lipoblasts →.* ***(Right)*** *An example of aneurysmal fibrous histiocytoma shows large, irregular, blood-filled spaces and prominent hemosiderin deposition ➔.*

DERMATOFIBROMA (BENIGN FIBROUS HISTIOCYTOMA)

Microscopic Features

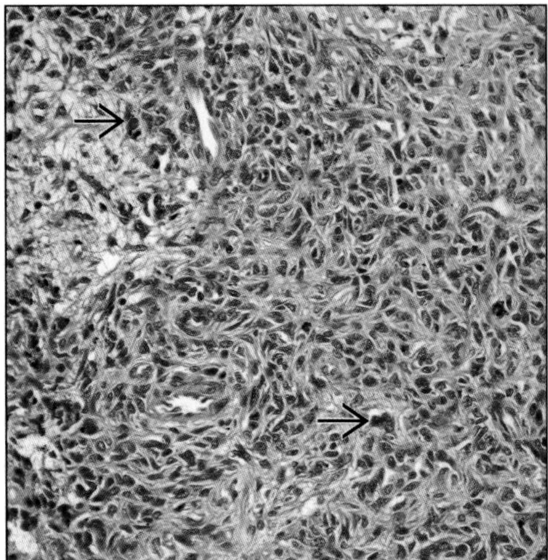

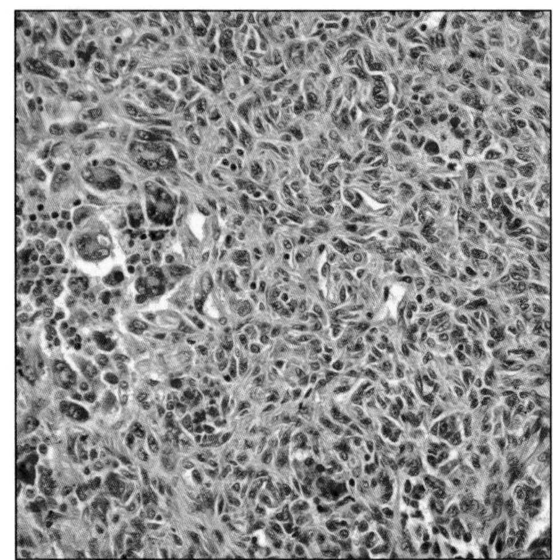

(Left) *Higher magnification of an aneurysmal fibrous histiocytoma shows bland spindled cells and scattered hemosiderin-laden macrophages* →. ***(Right)*** *Another area of aneurysmal fibrous histiocytoma shows numerous hemosiderin-laden macrophages.*

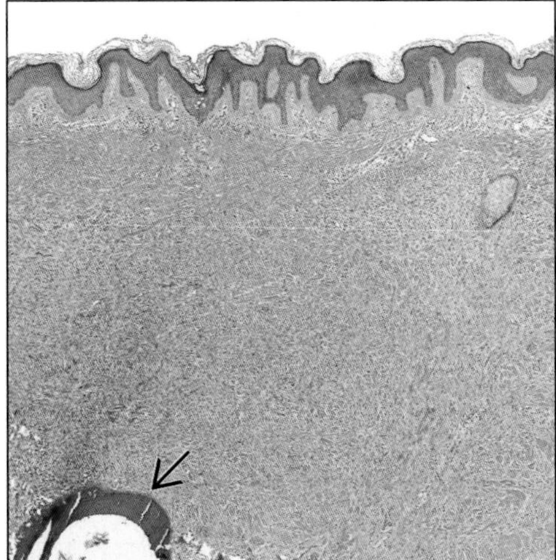

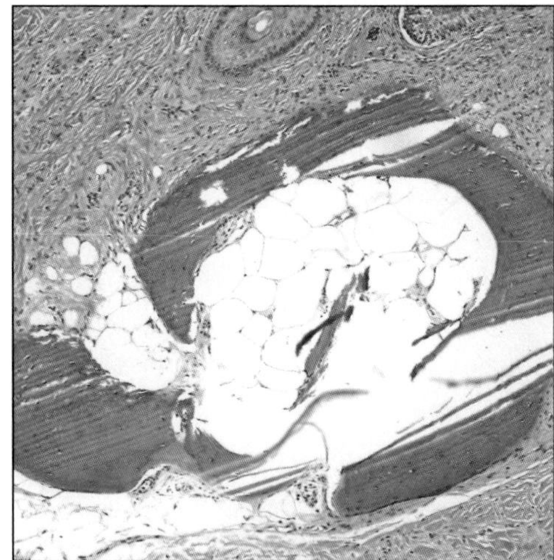

(Left) *Scanning magnification shows an otherwise typical dermatofibroma with a small associated osteoma cutis* →. ***(Right)*** *Higher magnification shows the osteoma cutis surrounded by an otherwise typical-appearing dermatofibroma.*

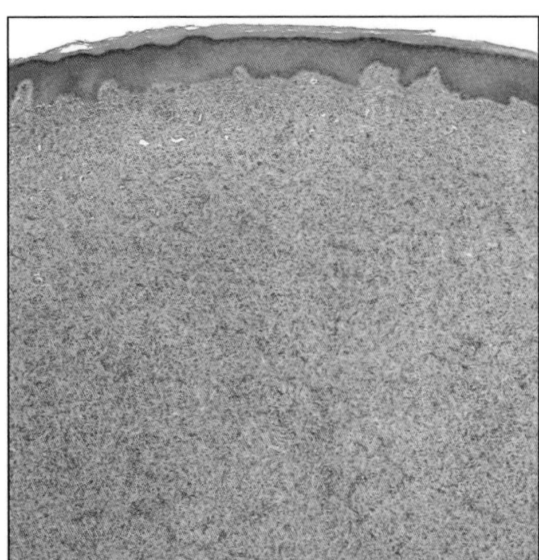

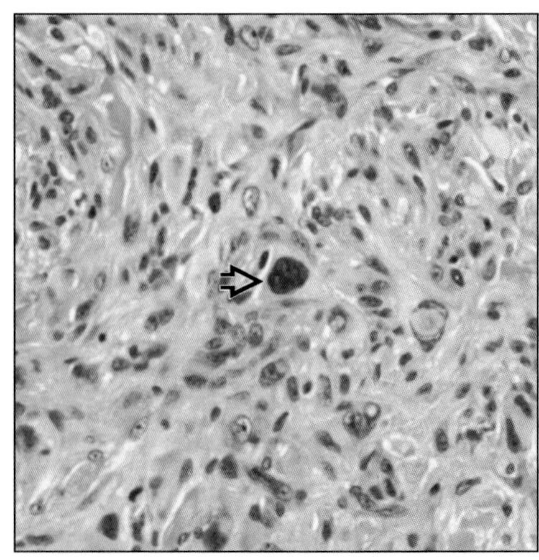

(Left) *Low-power view of a cellular dermatofibroma shows a dense proliferation of spindled and histiocytic-appearing cells with mild atypia.* ***(Right)*** *Higher power view of a cellular dermatofibroma with focal atypia shows scattered bizarre-appearing cells with enlarged, irregular, hyperchromatic nuclei* ⇨.

Microscopic and Immunohistochemical Features

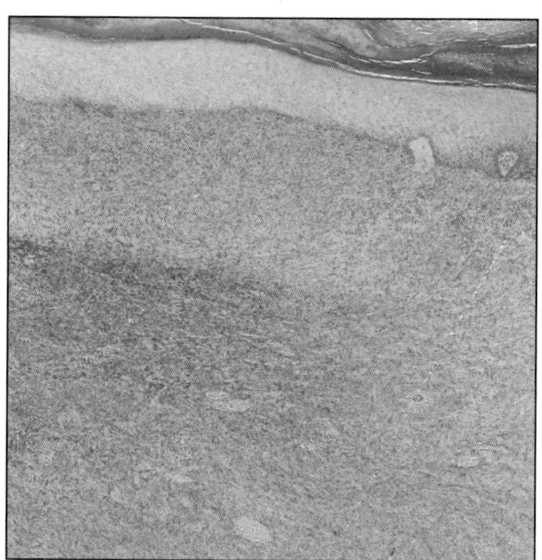

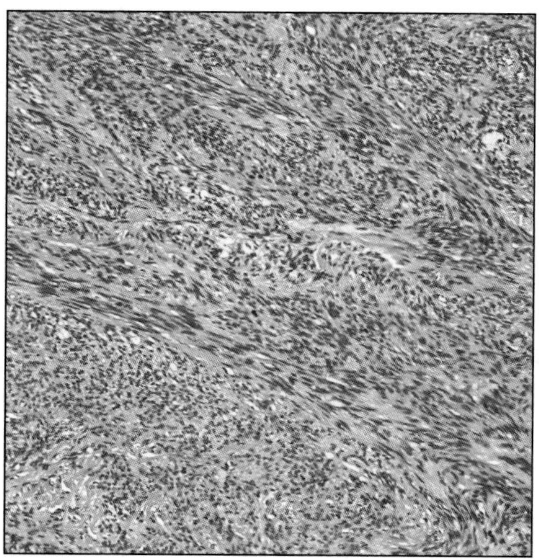

(Left) *Low-power view of a large and highly cellular dermatofibroma with atypia is shown. The tumor fills the dermis and presses directly against the epidermis (loss of the normal Grenz zone).* ***(Right)*** *Higher power view shows quite marked atypia and a focal fascicular growth pattern, raising the possibility of a low-grade sarcoma (fibrosarcoma-like) arising in a cellular fibrous histiocytoma.*

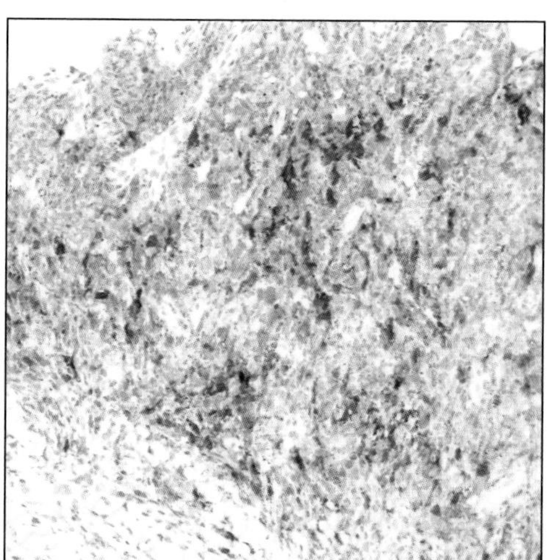

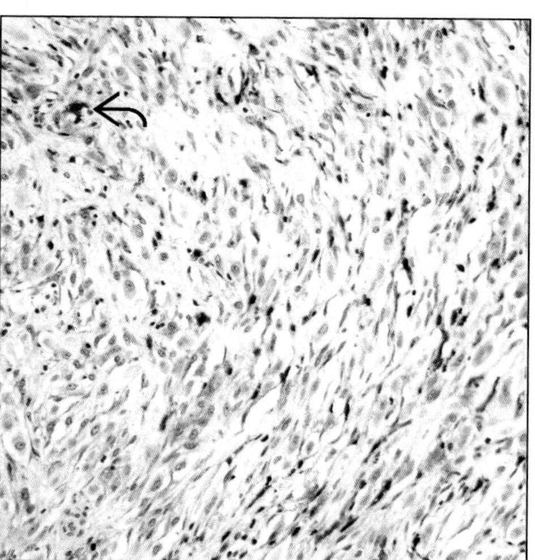

(Left) *Positive FXIIIA shows strong staining of many of the spindled and dendritic-appearing tumor cells.* ***(Right)*** *Weakly positive FXIIIA stain in another case shows weak staining of the tumoral spindled cells and stronger staining of scattered dermal dendritic cells ⮫.*

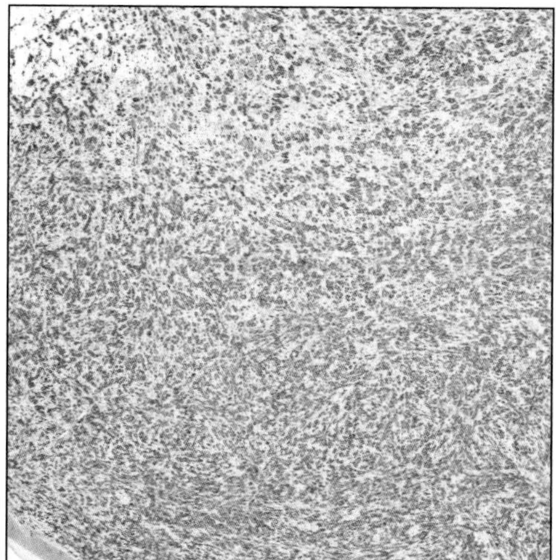

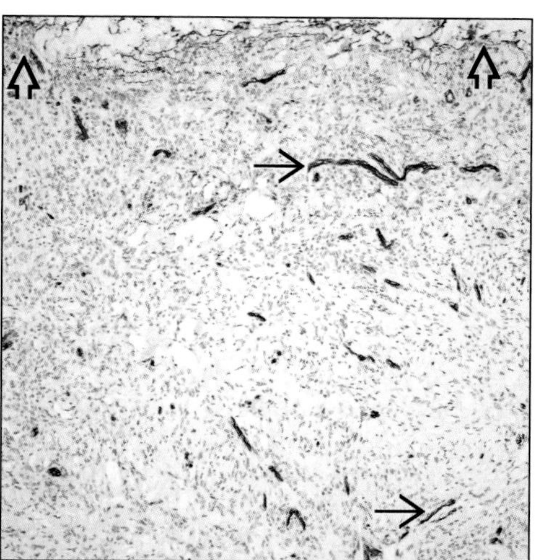

(Left) *Positive CD163 shows strong and diffuse staining in a histiocytic-type dermatofibroma.* ***(Right)*** *CD34 strongly highlights vessels → and shows background staining of peripheral stroma ⇨ but is negative within the tumoral cells.*

DEEP BENIGN FIBROUS HISTIOCYTOMA

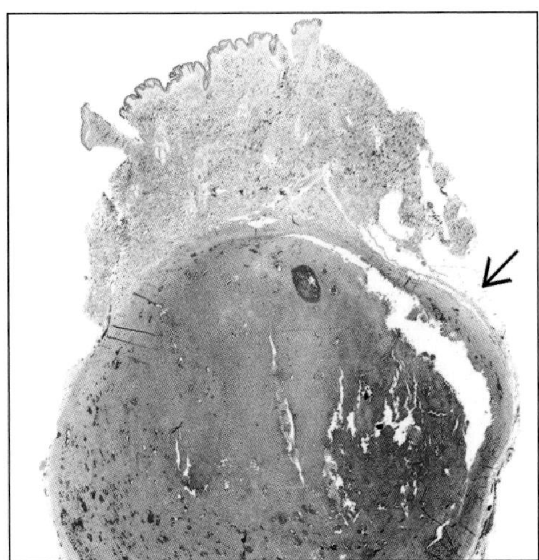

Low magnification shows a deep benign fibrous histiocytoma (BFH). The lesion is in subcutaneous fat ⇒ and has a pseudocapsule (in contrast to cutaneous BFH), with a slightly infiltrative border.

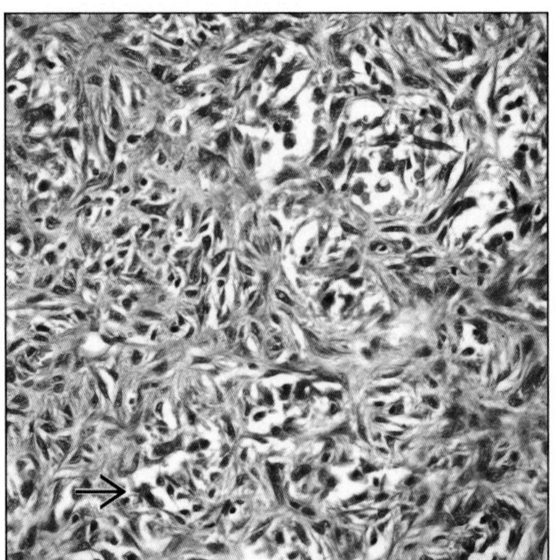

This deep fibrous histiocytoma displays a prominent storiform pattern and hemosiderin deposition ⇒. The individual cells are plump with round nuclei.

TERMINOLOGY

Abbreviations

- Deep benign fibrous histiocytoma (BFH)

Synonyms

- Deep dermatofibroma

CLINICAL ISSUES

Epidemiology

- Incidence
  - Rare
- Age
  - Median: ≈ 40 years
- Gender
  - Slight male predominance

Presentation

- Painless mass of subcutaneous tissue
  - Most common location is lower extremity
  - Followed by upper extremity, trunk, and head and neck
- Rare visceral lesions involving retroperitoneum, mediastinum, pelvis reported

Treatment

- Excision

Prognosis

- Local recurrences common (about 20%)
- Rare metastases and rarer tumor-associated deaths
  - Still regarded as benign overall since metastases vanishingly rare
  - No reliable features to predict aggressive behavior: Necrosis and prior recurrence may be factors
  - Cutaneous BFH also rarely associated with metastases, but usually with indolent course

MACROSCOPIC FEATURES

General Features

- Well marginated with yellow-tan firm cut surface, frequently encapsulated

Size

- Usually 2-3 cm (subcutaneous lesions)
- Visceral lesions can be very large (up to 25 cm reported)

MICROSCOPIC PATHOLOGY

Histologic Features

- Well marginated, often with pseudocapsule (except where tumor extends into cutis; collagen trapping)
- Storiform pattern
- Plump ovoid to spindle cells
- Indistinct pale cytoplasm
- Bland nuclei, vesicular chromatin, delicate nucleoli
- Variable lymphocytes, plasma cells, foam cells, osteoclast-like giant cells
- Staghorn, branching vessels in some cases
- Variable hyalinization
- Variable hemorrhage and hemosiderin (aneurysmal change)
- Rare cases with atypical nuclei
- Occasional cases with prominent mitotic activity

DIFFERENTIAL DIAGNOSIS

Dermatofibrosarcoma Protuberans

- Superficial, abutting on epidermis
- Common in shoulder girdle region
- Highly infiltrative growth pattern with entrapped skin appendages
- Monotonous repetitive storiform pattern
- Uniform cells

DEEP BENIGN FIBROUS HISTIOCYTOMA

Key Facts

Clinical Issues

- Painless mass of subcutaneous tissue
- Most common location is lower extremity
- Local recurrences common (about 20%)
- Rare metastases and rarer tumor-associated deaths

Macroscopic Features

- Well marginated with yellow-tan firm cut surface

Microscopic Pathology

- Well marginated, sometimes with pseudocapsule (except where tumor extends into cutis; collagen trapping)
- Storiform pattern
- Bland nuclei, vesicular chromatin, delicate nucleoli
- Variable lymphocytes, plasma cells, foam cells, osteoclast-like giant cells

Immunohistochemistry

Antibody	Reactivity	Staining Pattern	Comment
CD68	Positive	Cytoplasmic	Highlights lesional histiocytes and some lesional cells
CD34	Negative	Cytoplasmic	May be positive in ~ 40%, though usually focal
Actin-HHF-35	Negative	Cytoplasmic	May be positive in ~ 1/3 of cases, though usually focal
Desmin	Negative	Cytoplasmic	Occasional focal staining
S100	Negative		
AE1/AE3	Negative		
CK-PAN	Negative		

- Negligible inflammatory component, no giant cells
- Consistently CD34(+)

Solitary Fibrous Tumor

- Deep soft tissues (usually not subcutaneous)
- Wiry collagen and monotonous angulated cells
- Prominent hemangiopericytoma-like vascular pattern
- Negligible inflammatory background
- Consistently CD34(+) and Bcl-2(+)

High-Grade Pleomorphic Undifferentiated Sarcoma

- Malignant fibrous histiocytoma
- Deep extremities of older patients (7th decade)
  - Often intramuscular, involving thigh
- Striking nuclear pleomorphism, necrosis, numerous mitoses common
- Most cases have scant inflammatory component

SELECTED REFERENCES

1. Gleason BC et al: Deep "benign" fibrous histiocytoma: clinicopathologic analysis of 69 cases of a rare tumor indicating occasional metastatic potential. Am J Surg Pathol. 32(3):354-62, 2008
2. Guillou L et al: Metastasizing fibrous histiocytoma of the skin: a clinicopathologic and immunohistochemical analysis of three cases. Mod Pathol. 13(6):654-60, 2000
3. Colome-Grimmer MI et al: Metastasizing cellular dermatofibroma. A report of two cases. Am J Surg Pathol. 20(11):1361-7, 1996
4. Zelger B et al: Deep penetrating dermatofibroma versus dermatofibrosarcoma protuberans. A clinicopathologic comparison. Am J Surg Pathol. 18(7):677-86, 1994
5. Fletcher CD: Benign fibrous histiocytoma of subcutaneous and deep soft tissue: a clinicopathologic analysis of 21 cases. Am J Surg Pathol. 14(9):801-9, 1990

IMAGE GALLERY

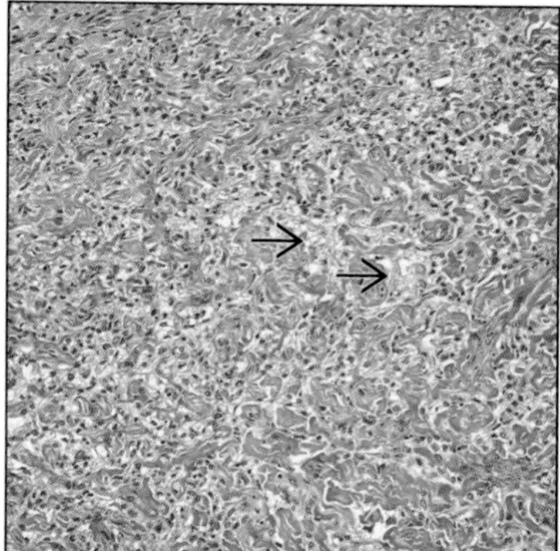

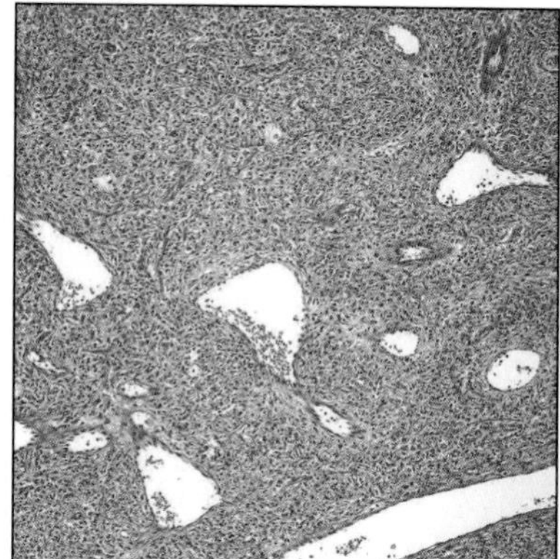

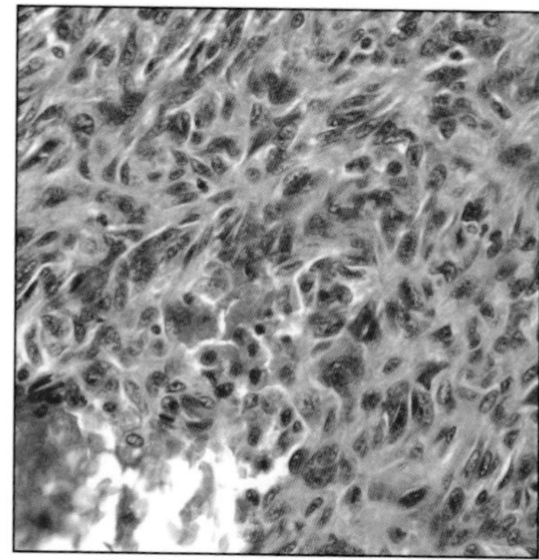

*(**Left**) Numerous foamy histiocytes ⮕ abound in this deep fibrous histiocytoma, which displays a loose storiform pattern. (**Center**) A prominent hemangiopericytoma-like vascular pattern is a common feature of deep benign fibrous histiocytoma. (**Right**) This deep fibrous histiocytoma is composed of plump cells with delicate nucleoli. A few of the nuclei are mildly atypical. Note the hemorrhage in this focus.*

GIANT CELL TUMOR OF TENDON SHEATH

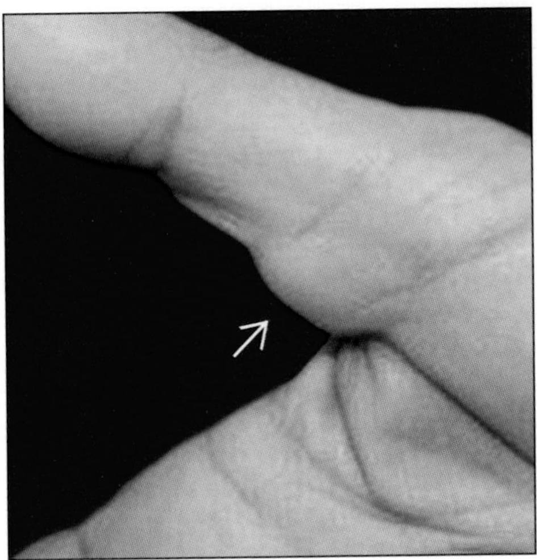

Giant cell tumor of tendon sheath (GCTTS) typically presents as a painless, slow-growing mass that arises from a tendon sheath, most often on the volar aspect of a finger, such as this thumb mass ➔.

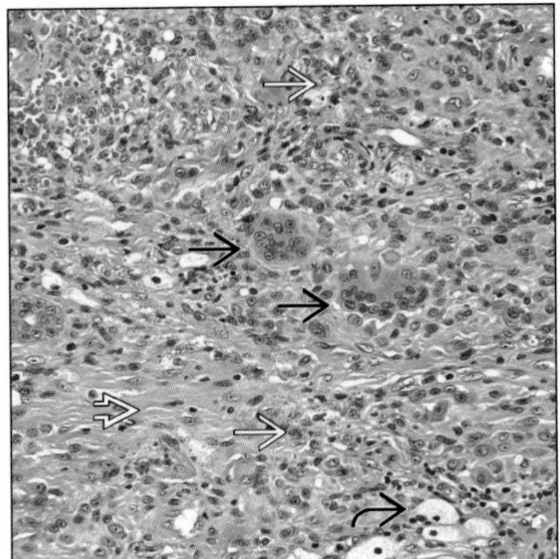

GCTTS has a mixture of mononuclear stromal cells, multinucleated giant cells ➔, and macrophages, including xanthoma cells ➔. Stromal fibrosis ➔ and hemosiderin deposits ➔ are very common.

TERMINOLOGY

Abbreviations

- Giant cell tumor of tendon sheath (GCTTS)

Synonyms

- Localized tenosynovial giant cell tumor, localized pigmented villonodular synovitis (PVNS), nodular tenosynovitis

Definitions

- Benign soft tissue tumor of synovial origin
  - Polymorphous population of neoplastic stromal cells, macrophages, and osteoclast-like giant cells
  - Well circumscribed, noninvasive

ETIOLOGY/PATHOGENESIS

Histogenesis

- Neoplastic growth
  - Balanced translocation involving 1p13 (*CSF1* gene) in many tumors
    - *CSF1* overexpression by neoplastic stromal cells
    - Recruitment and activation of intratumoral macrophages by CSF1R activation

CLINICAL ISSUES

Epidemiology

- Incidence
  - 2nd most common tumor of hand
- Age
  - Any age, peak 3rd-4th decade
- Gender
  - Women outnumber men 2:1

Site

- Digits (85%)
  - Especially fingers (75%)
  - Tendon sheath (usually volar) or interphalangeal joint
- Large joints (10%)
  - Ankle, knee, wrist, elbow
  - Bursa
  - Intraarticular tumors called localized PVNS

Presentation

- Painless mass
- Slow growing
- Uncommon findings: Triggering, carpal and ulnar tunnel syndromes

Treatment

- Surgical approaches
  - Complete local excision

Prognosis

- Benign but recurs locally (around 20%)
- Risk factors for recurrence: Degenerative joint disease, distal phalanx, interphalangeal joint of thumb, osseous erosion

IMAGE FINDINGS

Radiographic Findings

- Soft tissue mass
- Cortical bony erosion (10%)
  - Rarely invades bone to mimic primary bone tumor

MR Findings

- Lobulated mass with low T1 and T2 signal

MACROSCOPIC FEATURES

General Features

- Well circumscribed
- Partially encapsulated
- Lobular configuration with surface clefting
  - Sometimes grooved along tendon interface

GIANT CELL TUMOR OF TENDON SHEATH

Key Facts

Terminology

- Localized tenosynovial giant cell tumor, localized pigmented villonodular synovitis (PVNS), nodular tenosynovitis
- Benign soft tissue tumor of synovial origin
- Polymorphous population of stromal cells, macrophages, and osteoclast-like giant cells
- Arises from tendon sheath, intraarticular site, or bursa

Etiology/Pathogenesis

- Neoplastic growth
- Balanced translocation involving 1p13 (*CSF1* gene) in many tumors

Clinical Issues

- Most common tumor of hand
- Any age, peak 3rd-4th decade
- Digits (85%)
- Large joints (10)%
- Intraarticular tumors called localized PVNS
- Benign but recurs locally (around 20%)

Macroscopic Features

- Average size: 1.1 cm (range: 0.5-6 cm)

Microscopic Pathology

- Well demarcated
- Multinodular with fibrous septa
- Stromal fibrosis
- Mitotic rate 1-20 per 10 high-power fields (average: 5/10)

Top Differential Diagnoses

- Diffuse-type tenosynovial giant cell tumor/PVNS
- Giant cell tumor of soft tissue

- Variegated cut surface: Tan, red-brown, yellow

Size

- Average size: 1.1 cm (range: 0.5-6 cm)
    - Large joint tumors bigger than digital tumors (average: 2 cm)

MICROSCOPIC PATHOLOGY

Histologic Features

- Well demarcated
- Multinodular with fibrous septa
- Stromal fibrosis
    - Can mimic osteoid
    - Can be extensive
- Hemosiderin deposits
- Discohesive areas render pseudoglandular histology
- Cleft-like spaces lined by synoviocytes
- Distal tumors can invade dermis

Cytologic Features

- Polymorphous population
    - Stromal cells with pale cytoplasm and round, spindle, or reniform nuclei
    - Large epithelioid macrophages with eosinophilic cytoplasm and vesicular nuclei
    - Osteoclast-like giant cells
        - Giant cells can be sparse in some tumors
    - Xanthoma cells and siderophages
- Mitotic rate 1-20 per 10 high-power fields (average: 5/10)

ANCILLARY TESTS

Immunohistochemistry

- Stromal cells: CD68, few cells SMA, desmin in 50% of tumors
- Giant cells: CD68, CD45, TRAP

DIFFERENTIAL DIAGNOSIS

Diffuse-type Tenosynovial Giant Cell Tumor/ PVNS

- Similar microscopically to GCTTS
- Diffuse intraarticular tumors form villonodular masses (PVNS)
    - Large joints, knee most common site
- Diffuse extraarticular tumors invade adjacent tissues
    - Often have fewer giant cells and less lobular architecture

Giant Cell Tumor of Soft Tissue

- More uniform, less polymorphous mononuclear stromal cell population
- Less stromal fibrosis
- Often encased by shell of bone

Giant Cell Tumor of Bone

- Identical histology to giant cell tumor of soft tissue
- Primary osseous tumor but can invade soft tissue

SELECTED REFERENCES

1. Darwish FM et al: Giant cell tumour of tendon sheath: experience with 52 cases. Singapore Med J. 49(11):879-82, 2008
2. Cupp JS et al: Translocation and expression of CSF1 in pigmented villonodular synovitis, tenosynovial giant cell tumor, rheumatoid arthritis and other reactive synovitides. Am J Surg Pathol. 31(6):970-6, 2007
3. Nilsson M et al: Molecular cytogenetic mapping of recurrent chromosomal breakpoints in tenosynovial giant cell tumors. Virchows Arch. 441(5):475-80, 2002
4. Reilly KE et al: Recurrent giant cell tumors of the tendon sheath. J Hand Surg Am. 24(6):1298-302, 1999
5. Ushijima M et al: Giant cell tumor of the tendon sheath (nodular tenosynovitis). A study of 207 cases to compare the large joint group with the common digit group. Cancer. 57(4):875-84, 1986

GIANT CELL TUMOR OF TENDON SHEATH

Radiographic, Gross, and Microscopic Features

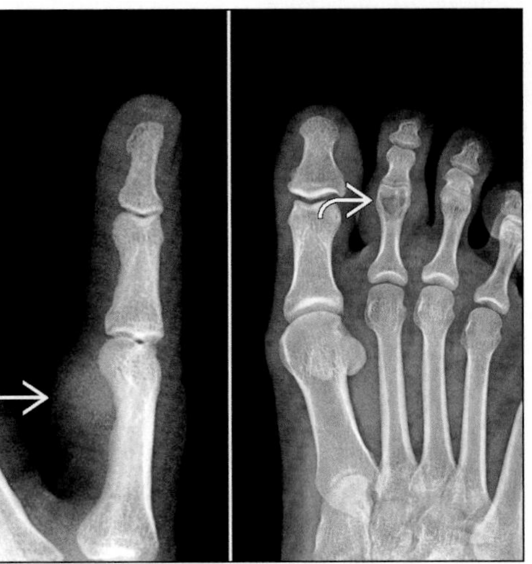

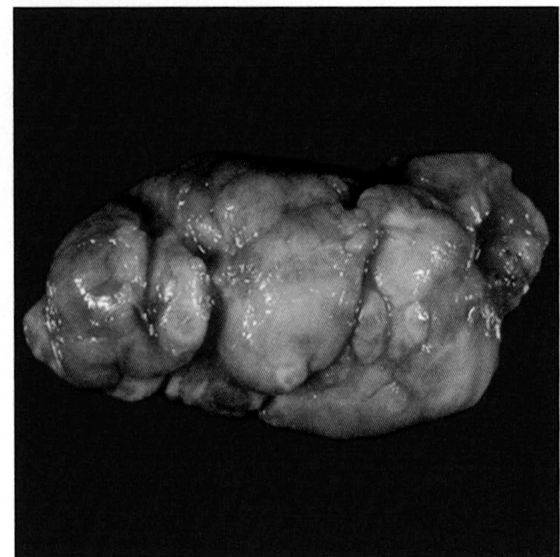

(Left) *Radiographically, GCTTS presents as a soft tissue mass, most frequently located on the palmar side of a finger ➔. Around 10% erode the cortex as seen here. Rare tumors invade into medullary bone mimicking a primary bone tumor ➔, such as this proximal interphalangeal tumor of the 2nd toe.* ***(Right)*** *Grossly, GCTTS is well demarcated, yellow to red-brown, and typically has a lobular configuration with surface clefting as depicted. Average size is 1.1 cm, ranging from 0.5 to 6 cm.*

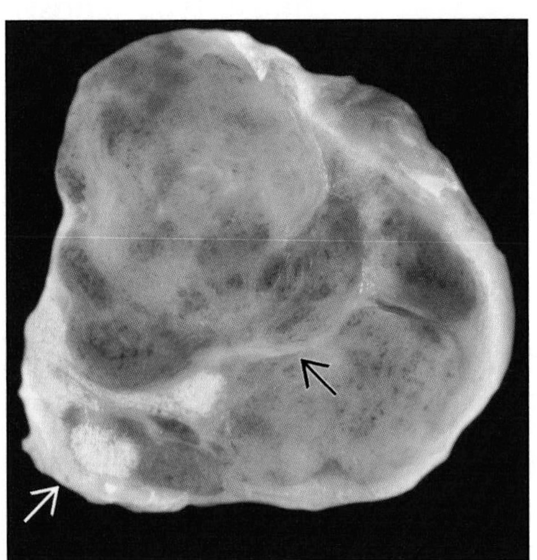

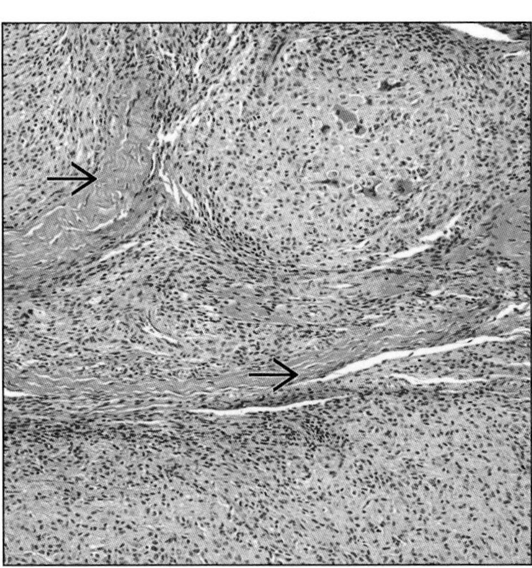

(Left) *GCTTS is well circumscribed, partially encapsulated, and has a multinodular, variegated appearance on cut surface. In this example, fibrous septa ➔ divide and surround tumor nodules. Mottled areas of tan, gold, red-brown, and yellow are present. The bright yellow areas ➔ represent xanthoma cells.* ***(Right)*** *GCTTSs lobular/multinodular architecture is highlighted by this low-power micrograph. Note the long, thick fibrous septa ➔ that divide the tumor into nodules.*

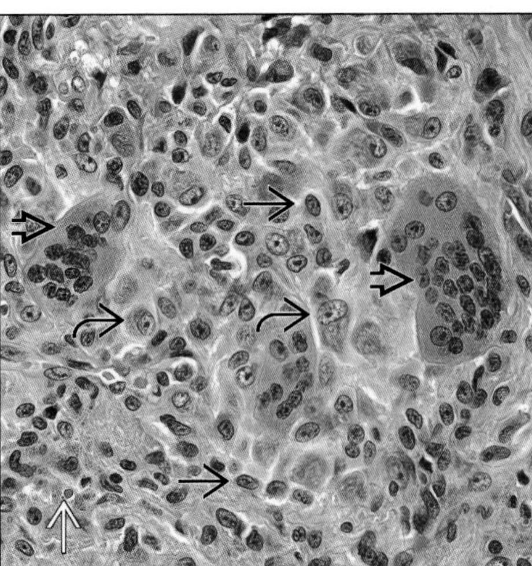

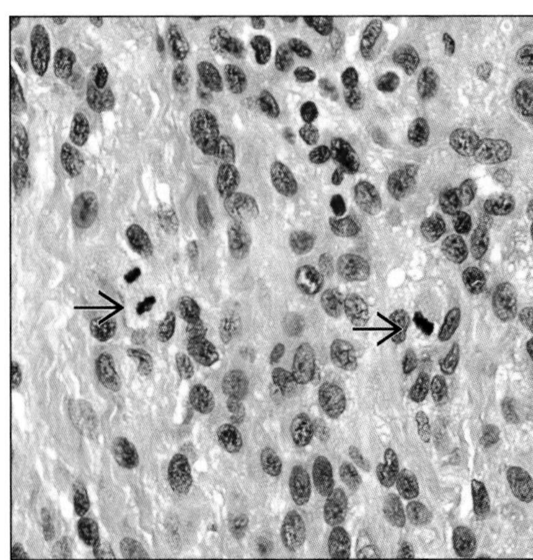

(Left) *GCTTS is composed of a polymorphous population of mononuclear stromal cells with small round, spindle, or reniform nuclei ➔, epithelioid macrophages with abundant eosinophilic cytoplasm and larger vesicular nuclei ➔, and osteoclast-like giant cells ➔. Note the hemosiderin deposits ➔.* ***(Right)*** *Mitotic activity ranges from 1 to 20 mitoses per 10 HPF (average 5/10). Brisk mitotic activity therefore is not uncommon, as shown by 2 mitotic figures in a single field ➔.*

Microscopic Features

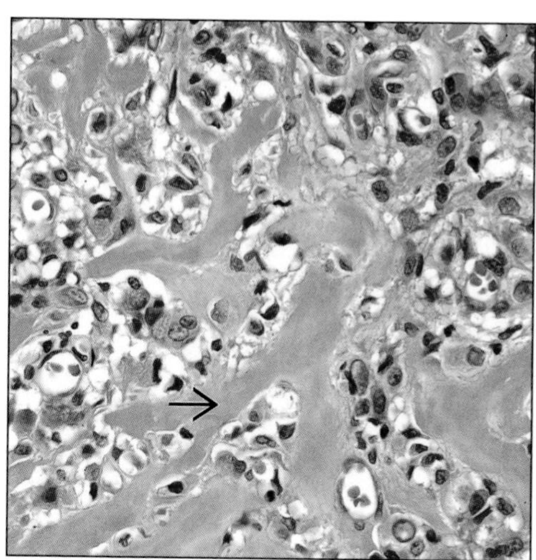

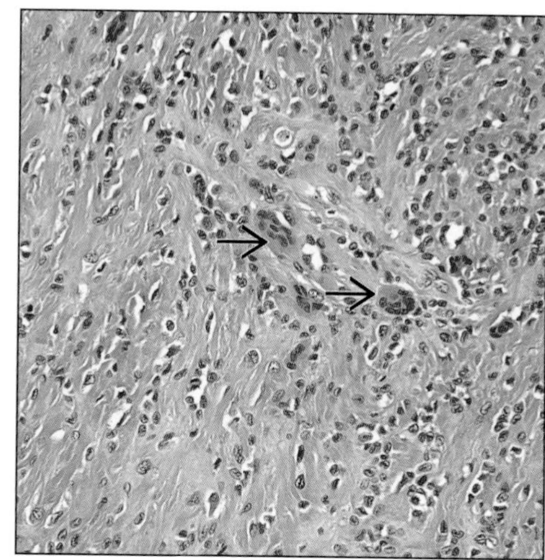

(Left) *Stromal fibrosis is invariably present in GCTTS but highly variable in its extent. In some instances, fibrosis consists of lace-like, hyalinized collagen that resembles osteoid* ➔. ***(Right)*** *Occasionally, fibrosis can be very extensive, affecting large areas of a tumor. This low-power micrograph shows diffuse stromal fibrosis that entraps mononuclear cells and multinucleated giant cells* ➔.

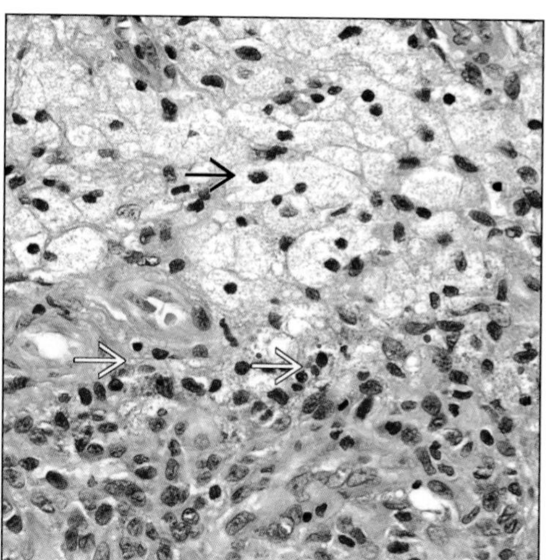

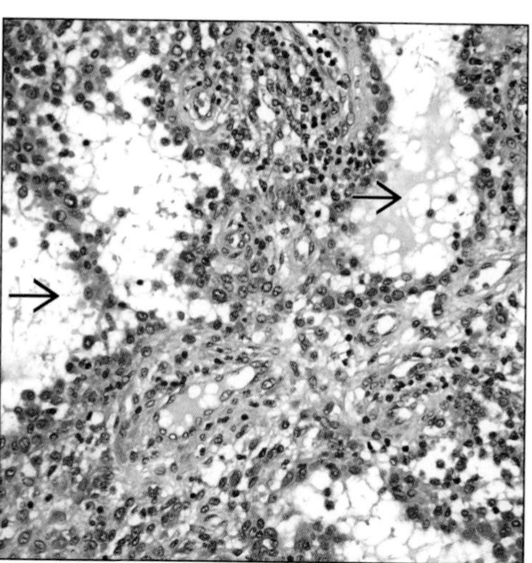

(Left) *Sheets and clusters of xanthoma cells are very frequent in GCTTS. Xanthoma cells (foamy macrophages) have copious, finely vacuolated cytoplasm and small central nuclei as depicted* ➔. *Siderophages (hemosiderin-laden macrophages)* ➔ *are also common.* ***(Right)*** *Areas of cellular discohesion are not uncommon in GCTTS. In some tumors, it can be so pronounced as to form cystic spaces* ➔, *creating a pseudoglandular pattern.*

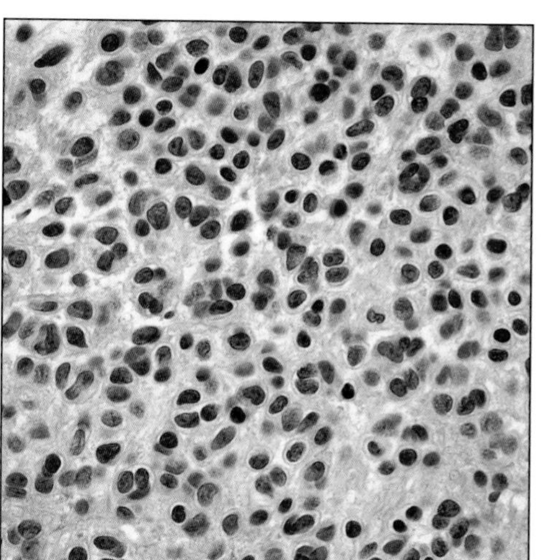

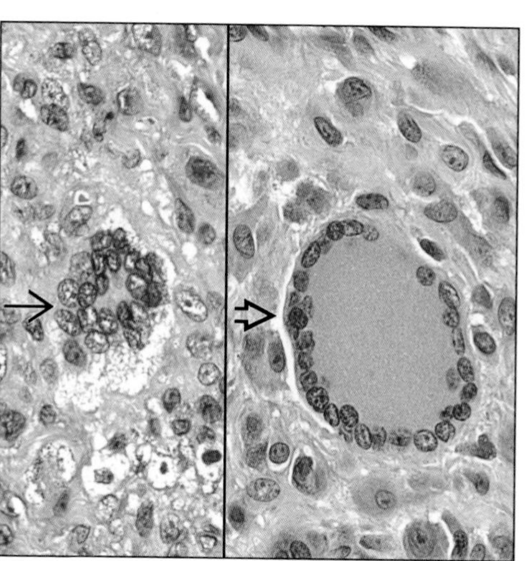

(Left) *Occasionally GCTTS can have very few giant cells as in this example, which is consists of a rather uniform population of mononuclear stromal cells with round nuclei.* ***(Right)*** *Although the multinucleated giant cells are usually osteoclast-like, occasional tumors can have Touton-type* ➔ *or Langhans-type* ➔ *giant cells.*

DIFFUSE-TYPE GIANT CELL TUMOR

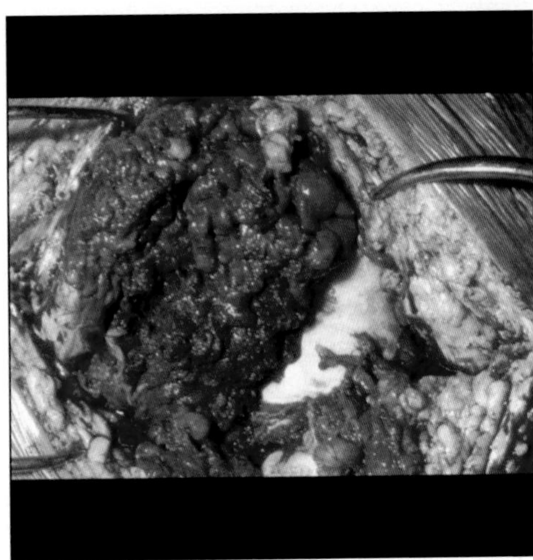

Diffuse-type giant cell tumor (or PVNS) typically presents as an intraarticular tumor, 75-80% occurring in the knee. It covers most of the synovial surface and has a villonodular pattern and brown color.

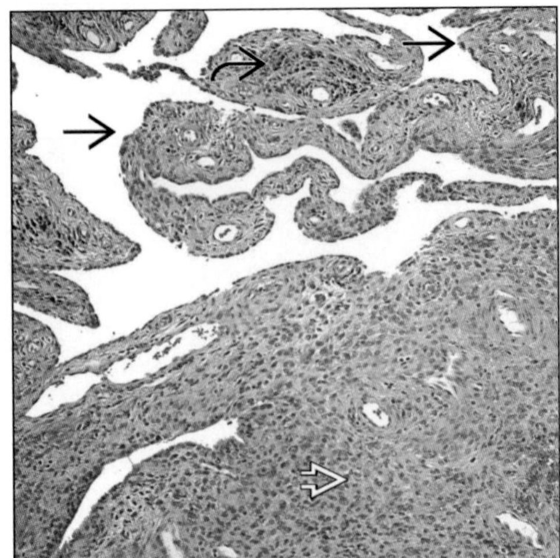

Microscopically, DTGCT has a villonodular architecture composed of elongated villi ⇨, solid cellular areas containing stromal cells and giant cells ➡, and hemosiderin deposits ⇗.

TERMINOLOGY

Abbreviations

- Diffuse-type giant cell tumor (DTGCT)

Synonyms

- Pigmented villonodular synovitis (PVNS), diffuse-type tenosynovial giant cell tumor

Definitions

- Benign, locally aggressive neoplastic proliferation of synovial origin
  - Intraarticular tumors within large joints
  - Extraarticular invasive tumors of tendon sheath or bursal origin

ETIOLOGY/PATHOGENESIS

Neoplastic Proliferation

- Balanced translocation involving 1p13 (*CSF1*) in most tumors
  - Most often fused with 2q35 (*COL6A3*)
- Trisomy 5 or 7 in some tumors

CLINICAL ISSUES

Epidemiology

- Incidence
  - Rare, annual incidence 1.8 patients/million
- Age
  - Average age 35 years, wide range (1st-7th decades)
- Gender
  - Women slightly outnumber men

Site

- Intraarticular
  - Knee (75-80%)
  - Hip (15%)
  - Ankle, elbow, shoulder, temporal mandibular joint, spine
- Extraarticular
  - Knee region most common
  - Foot, wrist, groin, elbow, digits

Presentation

- Painful mass
- Hemorrhagic effusion
- Decreased range of motion
- Long duration of symptoms (years)

Treatment

- Surgical approaches
  - Wide local excision
  - Total synovectomy
  - Prosthetic joint replacement in advanced cases
- Drugs
  - Response to imatinib in relapsing tumors reported
- Radiation
  - May improve local control

Prognosis

- Locally aggressive
  - High recurrence rate (20-50%)
  - Multiple relapses common

IMAGE FINDINGS

General Features

- Ill-defined periarticular soft tissue mass
- Cortical erosions and subchondral cysts

MR Findings

- Low signal on T1 and T2
- Enhancement with contrast
- MR signal voids secondary to hemosiderin ("blooming")

DIFFUSE-TYPE GIANT CELL TUMOR

Key Facts

Terminology
- Pigmented villonodular synovitis (PVNS)
- Benign, locally aggressive neoplastic proliferation of synovial origin
- Intra- or extraarticular

Etiology/Pathogenesis
- Balanced translocation involving 1p13 (*CSF1*)

Clinical Issues
- Average age: 35 years, range: 1st-7th decades
- Knee (75-80%)
- High recurrence rate (20-50%)

Image Findings
- Low signal on T1 and T2, enhancement with contrast
- MR signal voids secondary to hemosiderin

Macroscopic Features
- Most of synovial surface affected
- Villous, nodular, or villonodular
- Extraarticular tumors form multinodular masses
- Large, usually > 5 cm

Microscopic Pathology
- Thin delicate villi and broad papillary structures
- Solid cellular areas with multinodular architecture
- Mononuclear stromal cells
- Osteoclastic giant cells
- Xanthoma cells, hemosiderin, fibrosis

Top Differential Diagnoses
- Localized tenosynovial giant cell tumor
- Hemarthrosis
- Giant cell tumor of soft tissue

MACROSCOPIC FEATURES

General Features
- Most of synovial surface affected
- Villous, nodular, or villonodular
  - Heterogeneous synovial projections (thin villi, thick papillae, nodules)
- Firm to sponge-like
- Variegated cut surface (brown, tan, yellow)
- Poorly demarcated from adjacent soft tissue
- Extraarticular tumors form multinodular masses

Size
- Large, usually > 5 cm

MICROSCOPIC PATHOLOGY

Histologic Features
- Elongated villi
  - Vary from thin delicate villi to broad papillary structures
  - Lined by 1 to a few layers of synoviocytes
- Solid cellular areas with multinodular architecture
  - Fibrous septa surround nodules
  - Minimal to marked stromal fibrosis
    - Irregular hyalinized collagen mimics osteoid
  - Hemosiderin deposits usually abundant

Cytologic Features
- Mononuclear stromal cells with round to oval or reniform nuclei and abundant cytoplasm
- Synoviocytes line villi and cleft-like spaces
- Osteoclastic giant cells
- Macrophages
  - Xanthoma cells
  - Siderophages

DIFFERENTIAL DIAGNOSIS

Localized Tenosynovial Giant Cell Tumor
- Well circumscribed and encapsulated
- Lacks villi
- Otherwise identical microscopic features
- Localized to digits (85%)

Hemarthrosis
- Villiform synovial hyperplasia with hemosiderosis
- Lacks solid cellular areas
- History of repetitive hemarthrosis (e.g., trauma or hemophilia)

Giant Cell Tumor of Soft Tissue
- Identical histology to giant cell tumor of bone
  - Uniform mononuclear stromal cells and numerous osteoclastic giant cells
  - Metaplastic bone may be present
- Less heterogeneous population of cells
- Less stromal fibrosis

Malignant PVNS
- Malignant cytoarchitectural features
  - Pleomorphic spindle cells
  - High mitotic rate and necrosis
  - May be history of radiation therapy

SELECTED REFERENCES

1. Blay JY et al: Complete response to imatinib in relapsing pigmented villonodular synovitis/tenosynovial giant cell tumor (PVNS/TGCT). Ann Oncol. 19(4):821-2, 2008
2. Murphey MD et al: Pigmented villonodular synovitis: radiologic-pathologic correlation. Radiographics. 28(5):1493-518, 2008
3. Nilsson M et al: Molecular cytogenetic mapping of recurrent chromosomal breakpoints in tenosynovial giant cell tumors. Virchows Arch. 441(5):475-80, 2002
4. Fletcher JA et al: Trisomy 5 and trisomy 7 are nonrandom aberrations in pigmented villonodular synovitis: confirmation of trisomy 7 in uncultured cells. Genes Chromosomes Cancer. 4(3):264-6, 1992
5. Dorwart RH et al: Pigmented villonodular synovitis of synovial joints: clinical, pathologic, and radiologic features. AJR Am J Roentgenol. 143(4):877-85, 1984

DIFFUSE-TYPE GIANT CELL TUMOR

Radiographic, Gross, and Microscopic Features

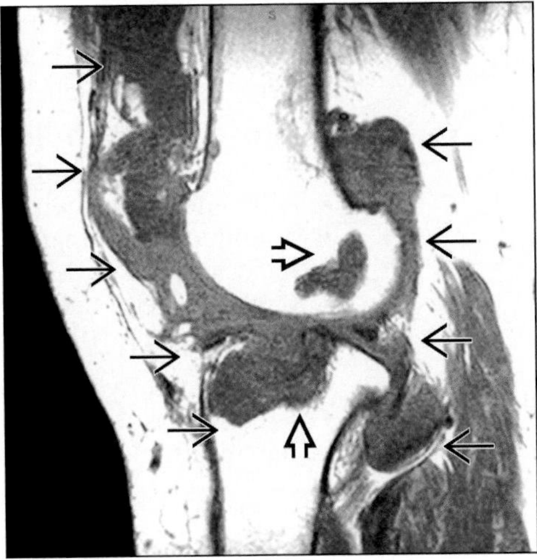

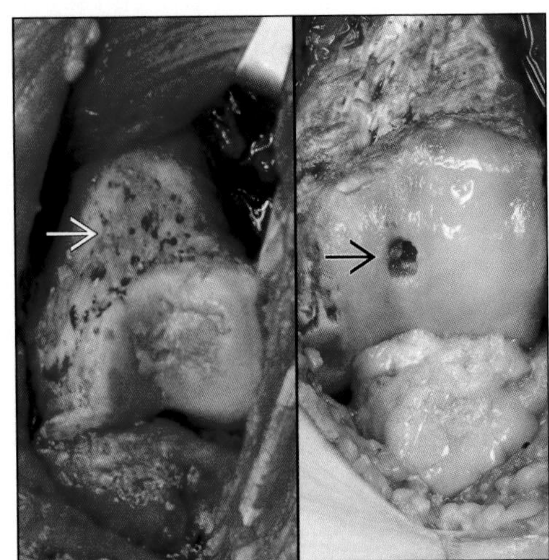

(Left) Sagittal T1-weighted MR of knee highlights an advanced, locally destructive case of DTGCT (PVNS). Tumor forms a large mass involving both anterior and posterior synovium →, which erodes into distal femur and proximal tibia ⇨. On MR, DTGCT shows low signal on T1 and T2 and enhances with contrast. **(Right)** Intraoperative post-synovectomy images from 2 patients with DTGCT of the knee illustrate multiple surface bone erosions ➡ and penetration of the articular cartilage →.

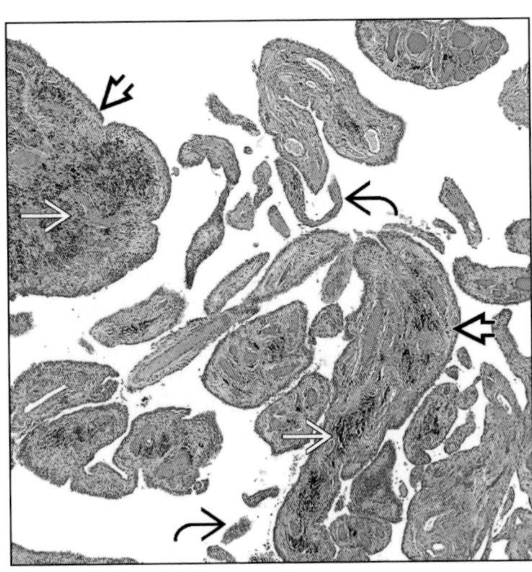

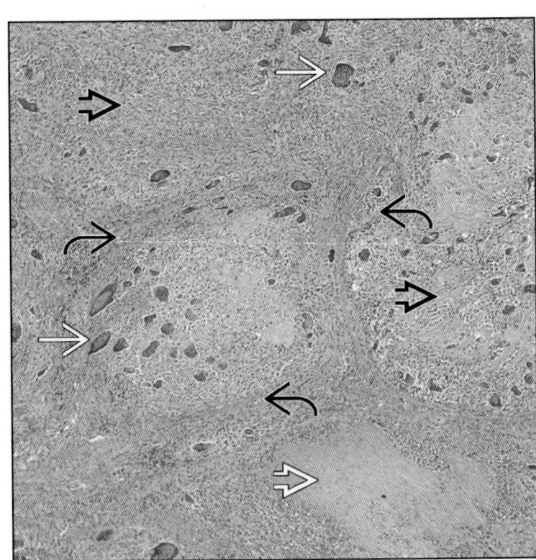

(Left) Intraarticular DTGCT (PVNS) forms long villous processes that extend into the synovial space. They vary from thin and delicate ↪ to broad ⇨ and are lined by synoviocytes. Hemosiderin is often abundant in the villi ➡. **(Right)** In the solid areas, DTGCT has a multinodular architecture composed of cellular areas ⇨ separated by fibrous septa ↪. Giant cells ➡ and zones of stromal fibrosis ➡ are also seen.

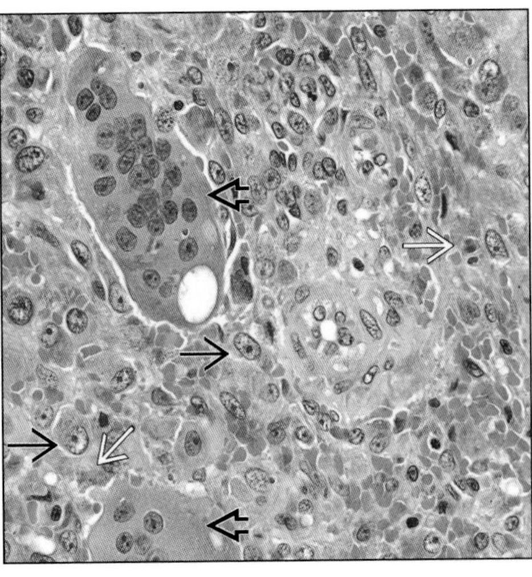

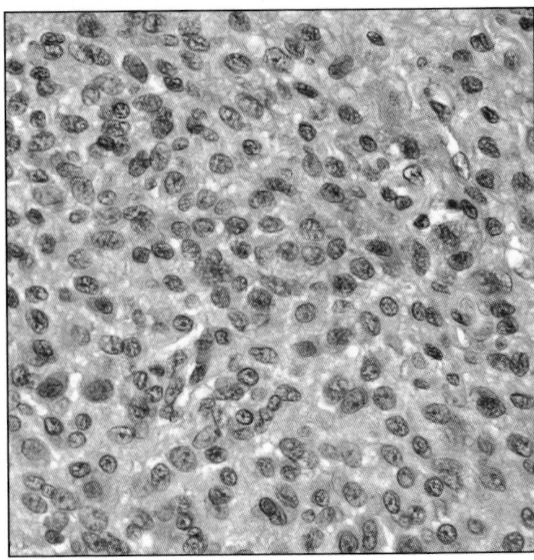

(Left) DTGCT typically has a mix of histiocytic stromal cells with ovoid to reniform nuclei and eosinophilic cytoplasm → and osteoclastic giant cells ⇨. Note the presence of stromal hemorrhage and hemosiderin deposits ➡. **(Right)** Zones of mononuclear cells with few or no giant cells are common. This image depicts a monotonous population of histiocytoid stromal cells with uniform round to oval nuclei, ill-defined eosinophilic cytoplasm, and benign cytological features.

Microscopic and Radiographic Features

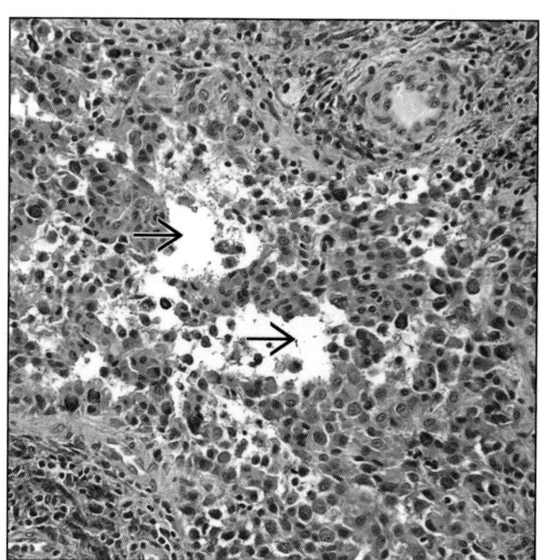

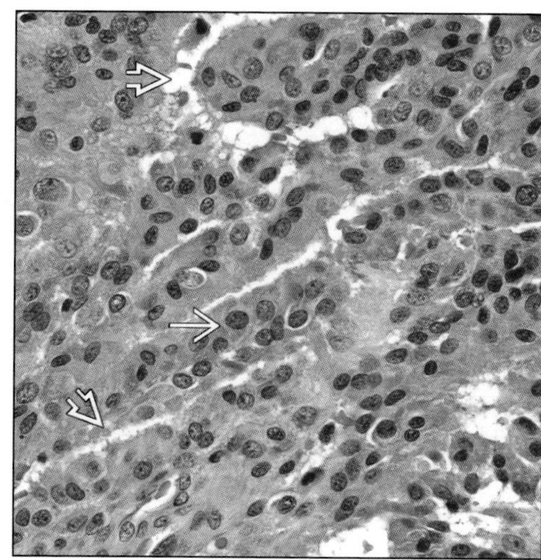

(Left) *In areas, the cells become discohesive and form irregular cystic spaces* ➔. ***(Right)*** *Slit-like clefted areas lined by synoviocytes can be present within DTGCT. This micrograph depicts linear clear spaces* ➔ *rimmed by plump synoviocytes with abundant eosinophilic cytoplasm and rounded nuclei* ➔.

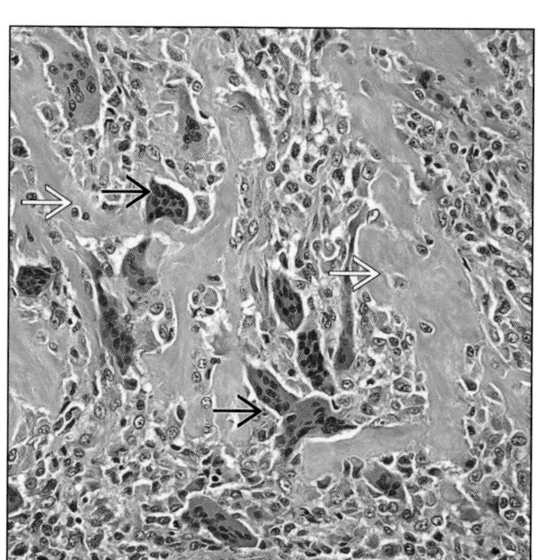

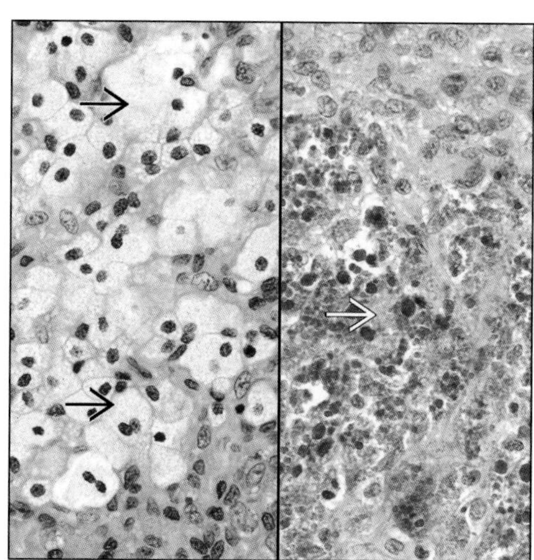

(Left) *Stromal fibrosis and hyalinization are common in DTGCT. Hyalinized collagen can form irregular branching structures that mimic osteoid* ➔. *Numerous osteoclastic giant cells are present* ➔. ***(Right)*** *Clusters of xanthoma cells (foamy macrophages)* ➔ *are common. They have abundant vacuolated lipid-filled cytoplasm, which imparts a yellow color to the gross tissue. Hemosiderin deposits secondary to remote hemorrhage are common and can be abundant, as illustrated* ➔.

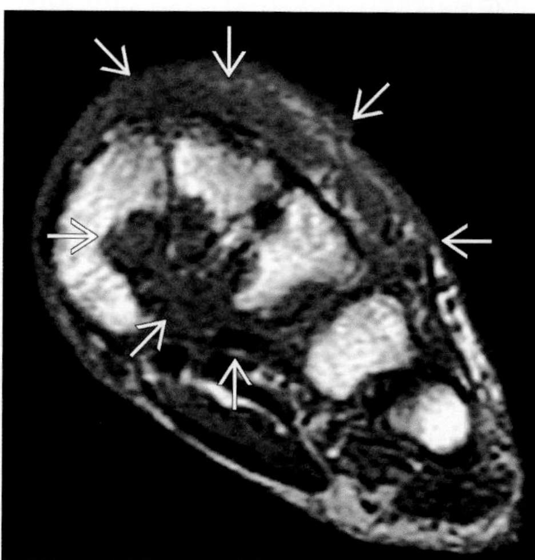

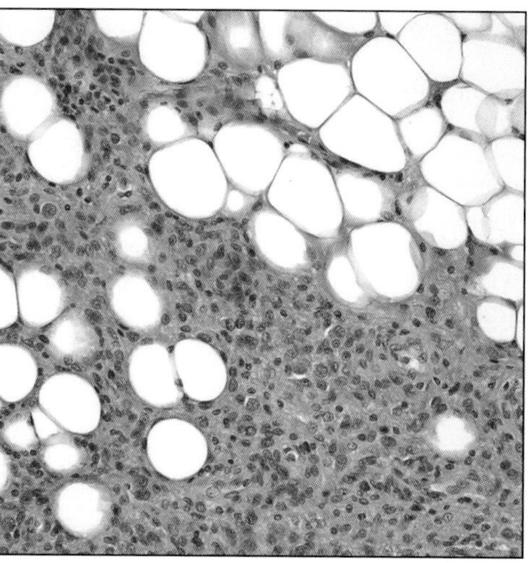

(Left) *Extraarticular DTGCT present as an invasive soft tumor tumor associated with tendon sheath or bursa. This T1-weighted MR depicts a low signal mass that diffusely infiltrates between metatarsals to involve both deep and superficial compartments of the foot* ➔. ***(Right)*** *Unlike localized giant cell tumor of tendon sheath, which is usually encased by a pseudocapsule, DTGCT invades adjacent tissues as illustrated by infiltration and entrapment of adipose tissue.*

JUVENILE XANTHOGRANULOMA

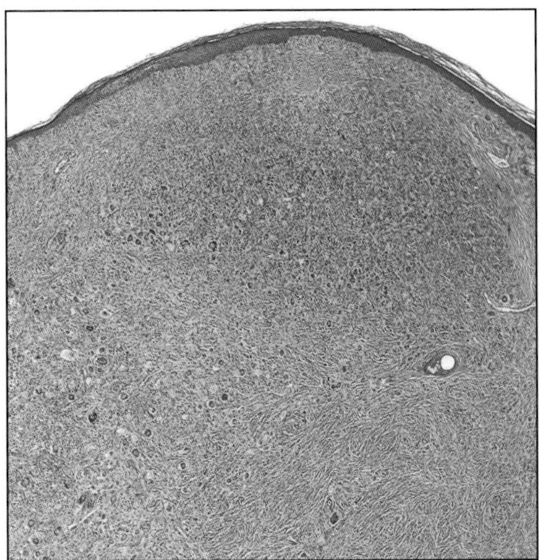

This is a typical appearance of a juvenile xanthogranuloma removed from the face of a small boy. The lesion is uniform and cellular and proliferates under the skin with no Grenz zone.

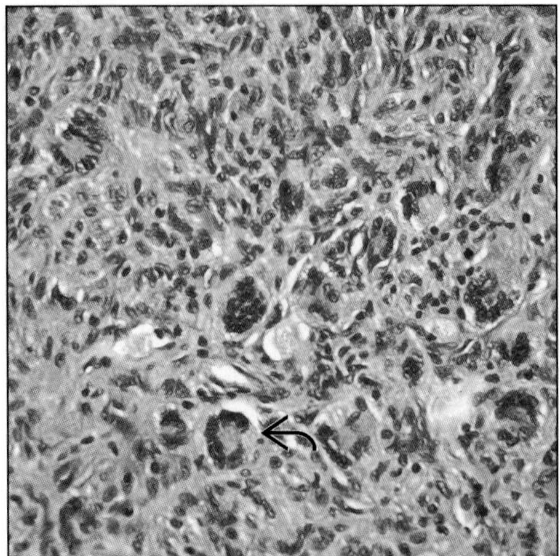

Many Touton giant cells ⇾ can be seen in this juvenile xanthogranuloma. The background cells are spindled to ovoid with eosinophilic cytoplasm, which shows only minimal lipid in this case.

TERMINOLOGY

Abbreviations

- Juvenile xanthogranuloma (JXG)

Synonyms

- Nevoxanthoendothelioma

Definitions

- Stable or regressing histiocytic lesion that usually occurs in childhood
  - Form of non-Langerhans histiocytosis

CLINICAL ISSUES

Epidemiology

- Incidence
  - Rare
- Age
  - Majority under 3 years
    - Visceral examples almost exclusively in infants and children
  - 13-30% in older children and adults
- Gender
  - Slight male predominance

Presentation

- Solitary cutaneous lesion in majority of cases
  - Head and neck > trunk > extremities
- Up to 10% of patients with multiple cutaneous lesions
- Up to 5% of patients with visceral-systemic disease

Treatment

- Excision
- Chemotherapy administered to rare patients with systemic disease

Prognosis

- Usually excellent
  - Most lesions regress or stabilize (including large visceral ones)
  - Rare deaths associated with multiorgan disease

MICROSCOPIC PATHOLOGY

Histologic Features

- Mononuclear cells
- Multinucleated cells ± Touton features
- Spindle cells
  - Variable finely vacuolated cytoplasm
  - Often lightly eosinophilic
- Variable lipid and foamy histiocytes
  - Minimal lipid in early lesion
- Inflammatory cell background
  - Chronic inflammatory cells
    - Eosinophils, consistent finding
  - Neutrophils uncommon
- Negligible nuclear atypia
- Minimal mitotic activity

DIFFERENTIAL DIAGNOSIS

Langerhans Cell Histiocytosis

- Usually presents as skeletal disease
- Atypical histiocytic cells
- Background eosinophils
- S100(+), CD1a(+)

Xanthoma

- Foamy histiocytes
- No Touton giant cells
- No background inflammation
- Can be associated with hyperlipidemia
  - Usually lesions of adults
- Benign

Fibrous Histiocytoma/Dermatofibroma

- Usually in adults

JUVENILE XANTHOGRANULOMA

Key Facts

Terminology

- Stable or regressing histiocytic lesion that usually occurs in childhood
  - Form of non-Langerhans histiocytosis

Clinical Issues

- Majority in individuals under 3 years
- Visceral examples almost exclusively in infants and children
- Solitary cutaneous lesion in majority of cases
- Head and neck > trunk > extremities

Microscopic Pathology

- Mononuclear cells
- Multinucleated cells ± Touton features
- Spindle cells
- Inflammatory cell background
- Eosinophils, consistent finding
- Variable lipid and foamy histiocytes

Immunohistochemistry

Antibody	Reactivity	Staining Pattern	Comment
CD68	Positive	Cytoplasmic	Essentially all cases reactive
FXIIIA	Positive	Nuclear	Essentially all cases reactive
S100	Positive	Nuclear & cytoplasmic	Most cases are negative; usually staining is weak
CD1a	Negative		

- Prominent storiform pattern
- Eosinophils usually inconspicuous
- Peripheral collagen trapping in cutaneous examples
- Overlying epidermal hyperplasia in skin lesions
- Intralesional hemorrhage, hemosiderin
- Benign
  - Rare metastases but no deaths associated with skin lesion

Rosai-Dorfman Disease

- Also called sinus histiocytosis with massive lymphadenopathy
- Usually involves lymph nodes but may present in skin and soft tissues
- Also form of non-Langerhans histiocytosis
- Histiocytes and lymphoid aggregates
- Emperipolesis, key diagnostic feature
- Histiocytes are S100(+), CD1a(-)
- Most patients have good outcome

Reticulohistiocytoma

- Lesions of adults
- Brown-yellow papules at any site
- Nodules of brightly eosinophilic histiocytes, some multinucleated
- Nuclear atypia
- CD68(+), S100(-), CD1a(-)
- Benign

SELECTED REFERENCES

1. Janssen D et al: Clonality in juvenile xanthogranuloma. Am J Surg Pathol. 31(5):812-3, 2007
2. Janssen D et al: Juvenile xanthogranuloma in childhood and adolescence: a clinicopathologic study of 129 patients from the kiel pediatric tumor registry. Am J Surg Pathol. 29(1):21-8, 2005
3. Dehner LP: Juvenile xanthogranulomas in the first two decades of life: a clinicopathologic study of 174 cases with cutaneous and extracutaneous manifestations. Am J Surg Pathol. 27(5):579-93, 2003
4. Zelger B et al: Juvenile and adult xanthogranuloma. A histological and immunohistochemical comparison. Am J Surg Pathol. 18(2):126-35, 1994

IMAGE GALLERY

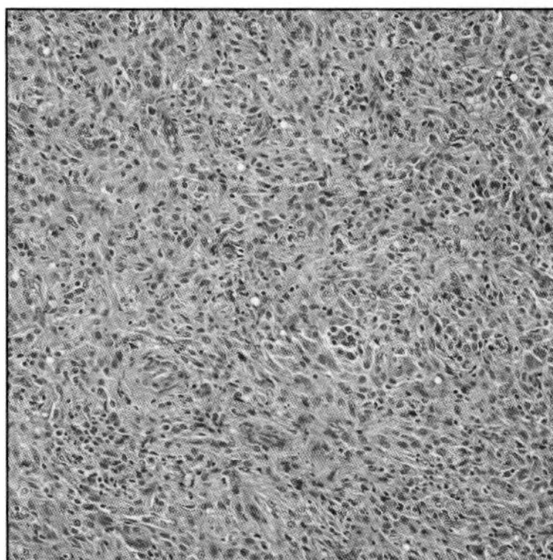

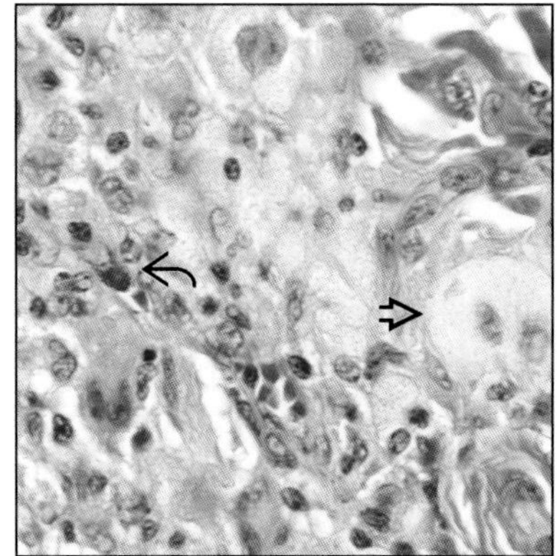

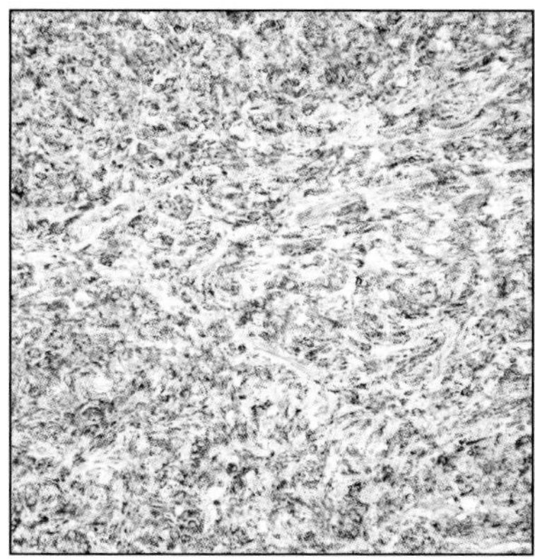

(Left) *This cellular example of juvenile xanthogranuloma features an inflammatory background composed mostly of mononuclear cells.* ***(Center)*** *Eosinophils ⇗ and foamy histiocytes ⇨ are commonly encountered in juvenile xanthogranuloma.* ***(Right)*** *Essentially all examples of juvenile xanthogranuloma are reactive with CD68 (shown) and factor XIIIA antibodies on immunohistochemistry but negative for S100 and CD1a.*

RETICULOHISTIOCYTOMA

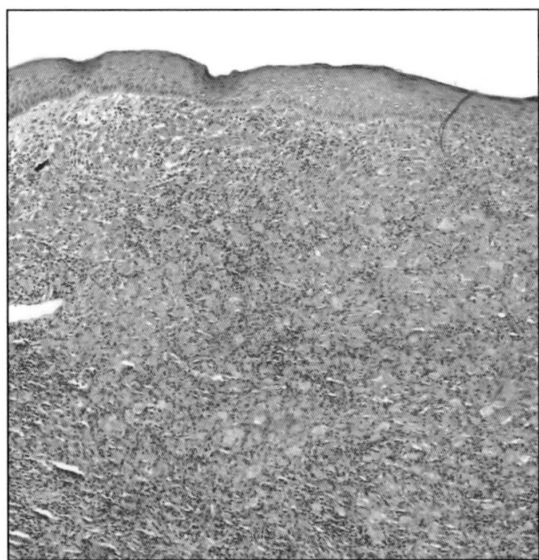

Low-power examination shows a dense nodular to sheet-like collection of large histiocytic cells in the dermis.

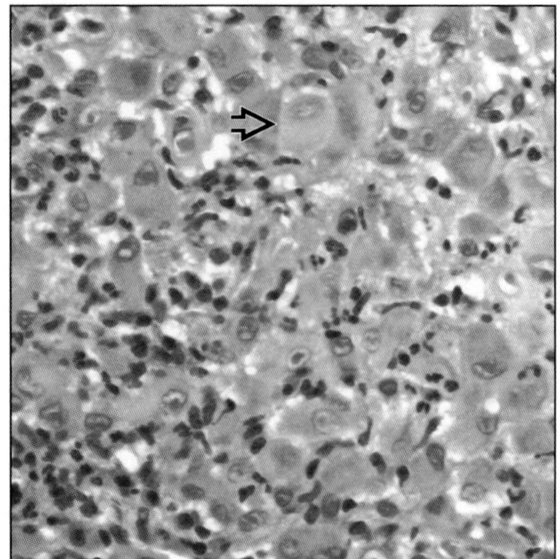

High-power view shows large histiocytic cells with abundant dense, glassy-appearing cytoplasm ➡ and a background inflammatory infiltrate containing neutrophils and eosinophils.

TERMINOLOGY

Synonyms

- Solitary cutaneous reticulohistiocytoma (SCR)
- Reticulohistiocytic granuloma
- Giant cell reticulohistiocytoma

Definitions

- Proliferation of histiocytes with abundant dense, glassy-appearing, eosinophilic cytoplasm

ETIOLOGY/PATHOGENESIS

Environmental Exposure

- May be related to stimuli, such as insect bites, infection, trauma, or ruptured folliculitis or cyst

CLINICAL ISSUES

Epidemiology

- Incidence
  - Rare tumor
- Age
  - Usually occurs in adults > 40 years old
    - However, some cases have been reported in adolescents
- Gender
  - Equal male and female incidence
- Ethnicity
  - Most cases occur in Caucasians

Site

- Usually head and neck region, including mucosal sites
  - However, may present at any cutaneous site

Presentation

- Skin papule or nodule
  - Usually single lesion, but several may be present in some cases
- Firm, rapidly growing lesion
- Usually appear as red-brown or yellow-brown
- May be preceded by trauma in some cases
- Lack of systemic symptoms, including fever, weight loss, or weakness (which may be seen in multicentric reticulohistiocytosis)

Treatment

- Surgical approaches
  - Complete conservative excision is curative
    - Usually not required unless lesion is very large or fails to resolve

Prognosis

- Excellent; lesions often involute spontaneously
- No definite relationship with more aggressive multicentric reticulohistiocytosis
  - However, multiple skin lesions should suggest possibility of generalized cutaneous reticulohistiocytosis

MACROSCOPIC FEATURES

General Features

- Dermal-based, nodular, well-circumscribed but unencapsulated lesion

Size

- Lesions typically range in size from 0.5-2 cm

MICROSCOPIC PATHOLOGY

Histologic Features

- Dermal-based nodular proliferation of large mononuclear and multinucleated histiocytes
  - Cells show characteristic abundant glassy/hyalinized-appearing eosinophilic cytoplasm
  - Some cells may show finely granular cytoplasm

RETICULOHISTIOCYTOMA

Key Facts

Terminology
- Proliferation of histiocytes with abundant dense, glassy-appearing eosinophilic cytoplasm

Clinical Issues
- Usually occurs in adults > 40 years old, but cases have been reported in adolescents
- Usually head and neck region, including mucosal sites, but may present at any cutaneous site
- Usually red-brown or yellow-brown appearing

Microscopic Pathology
- Dermal-based nodular proliferation of large mononuclear and multinucleated histiocytes
- Cells show characteristic abundant glassy/hyalinized-appearing eosinophilic cytoplasm
- Occasional Touton-type giant cells containing lipid may be present
- Early lesions characterized by more mononuclear cells with lymphocytes

Ancillary Tests
- Cells typically are typically positive for CD68 (KP1), CD163, and lysozyme

Top Differential Diagnoses
- Multicentric reticulohistiocytosis and generalized cutaneous reticulohistiocytosis
- Juvenile xanthogranuloma (JXG)
- Langerhans cell histocytosis (LCH)
- Rosai-Dorfman disease (sinus histiocytosis with massive lymphadenopathy)

  - Occasional Touton-type giant cells containing lipid may be present but not prominent
  - Cytologic atypia is usually minimal, and mitoses are few and nonatypical
  - No infiltrative features are present
- Overlying epidermis may show atrophy/thinning
  - Often Grenz zone separating infiltrate from epidermis
- Early lesions characterized by background inflammatory infiltrate with many small mononuclear cells and lymphocytes
- Later lesions show greater numbers of large mononuclear and multinucleated cells with background infiltrate, including neutrophils and eosinophils
- Phagocytosis of inflammatory cells and collagen may be present
- Occasional bizarre-appearing cells may be present but do not indicate malignancy
- Rare cases may show deep subcutaneous, and even lymph node, involvement

Predominant Pattern/Injury Type
- Inflammatory, granulomatous

Predominant Cell/Compartment Type
- Histiocyte

ANCILLARY TESTS

Histochemistry
- Periodic acid-Schiff with diastase digestion and Sudan black
  - Reactivity: Positive
  - Staining pattern
    - Cytoplasmic; highlights granules

Immunohistochemistry
- Cells are typically positive for CD68 (KP1), CD163, and lysozyme
- Variable positivity reported for FXIIIA, CD64, and α-1-antitrypsin
- S100(-) in most cases but has been reported to be rarely positive (usually focal)
- Cells negative for CD1a, CD3, CD20, CD34, actin, desmin, HMB-45, Melan-A

Electron Microscopy
- Large cells showing abundant granular cytoplasm containing numerous mitochondria, phagolysosomes, dense bodies, and myelin figures
    - Also contain so-called "pleomorphic cytoplasmic inclusions"
    - Highly complex structures consisting mainly of unit membranes, which may surround vesicles
- Birbeck granules are absent

DIFFERENTIAL DIAGNOSIS

Multicentric and Generalized Cutaneous Reticulohistiocytosis
- These entities show different clinical features
  - Multicentric cutaneous reticulohistiocytosis (MCR) presents with multiple lesions involving skin, mucosal sites, joints, and occasionally internal organs
    - MCR may show aggressive course with destructive arthropathy and constitutional symptoms
  - Generalized cutaneous reticulohistiocytosis (GCR) is characterized by eruption of multiple small cutaneous lesions
    - Some cases may progress to MCR
- Histologically, there is considerable overlap with solitary reticulohistiocytoma, but some differences have been described
  - Solitary lesions may be better circumscribed and show more multinucleated giants cells
  - Neutrophils and xanthomatized cells have been reported to be more common in solitary reticulohistiocytoma
  - FXIIIA expression may be lower in systemic cases

RETICULOHISTIOCYTOMA

Juvenile Xanthogranuloma (JXG)

- Typically occurs in children, but some cases occur in adults ("adult-type xanthogranuloma")
- Multiple papules are common, and dozens of lesions have been reported in some cases
- Histologically, typically show more foamy histiocytes and Touton-type giant cells with peripheral wreath-like arrangement of nuclei
  - Cells lack dense glassy eosinophilic cytoplasm of reticulohistiocytoma
- Cells positive by immunohistochemistry for CD68 and CD163, but negative for S100 and CD1a

Langerhans Cell Histocytosis (LCH)

- LCH includes Letterer-Siwe, Hand-Schüller-Christian, eosinophilic granuloma, and congenital self-healing reticulohistiocytosis variants
- Predominantly occur in children
  - Also 2nd peak in elderly adults (usually eosinophilic granuloma variant)
- Typically characterized by multiple skin lesions and systemic involvement (especially bone)
- Histologic examination shows proliferation of mononuclear cells in dermis and occasionally in epidermis
  - Cells show large folded or reniform vesicular nuclei and abundant eosinophilic cytoplasm
  - Cells lack dense eosinophilic cytoplasm of reticulohistiocytoma
  - Background infiltrate often contains numerous eosinophils and variable numbers of lymphocytes
- CD1a and S100 should be positive in vast majority of cases (both are negative in reticulohistiocytoma)

Rosai-Dorfman Disease

- Also known as sinus histiocytosis with massive lymphadenopathy (SHML)
- Often show concomitant lymphadenopathy and constitutional symptoms
- Lesions may be solitary or multiple
- Histologic examination shows proliferation of large pale-staining histiocytes with emperipolesis of lymphocytes, plasma cells, and erythrocytes
  - Cells lack dense glassy cytoplasm of reticulohistiocytoma
- S100(+) (negative in reticulohistiocytoma), CD1a(-)

DIAGNOSTIC CHECKLIST

Pathologic Interpretation Pearls

- Nodular proliferation of large mononuclear and multinucleated histiocytes
  - Cells show characteristic abundant glassy/ hyalinized-appearing eosinophilic cytoplasm
  - Occasional Touton-type giant cells containing lipid may be present but not prominent (as in juvenile xanthogranuloma)
- Cells typically positive for CD68, CD163, and lysozyme
- Cells typically negative for S100, CD1a, CD3, CD20, and CD34

SELECTED REFERENCES

1. Caputo R et al: Unusual variants of non-Langerhans cell histiocytoses. J Am Acad Dermatol. 57(6):1031-45, 2007
2. Chen CH et al: Multicentric reticulohistiocytosis presenting with destructive polyarthritis, laryngopharyngeal dysfunction, and a huge reticulohistiocytoma. J Clin Rheumatol. 12(5):252-4, 2006
3. Miettinen M et al: Reticulohistiocytoma (solitary epithelioid histiocytoma): a clinicopathologic and immunohistochemical study of 44 cases. Am J Surg Pathol. 30(4):521-8, 2006
4. Wang KH et al: Cutaneous Rosai-Dorfman disease: clinicopathological profiles, spectrum and evolution of 21 lesions in six patients. Br J Dermatol. 154(2):277-86, 2006
5. Nguyen TT et al: Expression of CD163 (hemoglobin scavenger receptor) in normal tissues, lymphomas, carcinomas, and sarcomas is largely restricted to the monocyte/macrophage lineage. Am J Surg Pathol. 29(5):617-24, 2005
6. Bakri SJ et al: Recurrent solitary reticulohistiocytoma of the eyelid. Ophthal Plast Reconstr Surg. 19(2):162-4, 2003
7. Ka MM et al: [Multicentric reticulohistiocytosis with a 20-year follow-up .] Rev Med Interne. 23(9):779-83, 2002
8. Busam KJ et al: Immunohistochemical distinction of epithelioid histiocytic proliferations from epithelioid melanocytic nevi. Am J Dermatopathol. 22(3):237-41, 2000
9. Burgdorf WH et al: The non-Langerhans' cell histiocytoses in childhood. Cutis. 58(3):201-7, 1996
10. Shy SW et al: A solitary congenital self-healing histiocytosis. Report of a case and review of the literature. Pathol Res Pract. 192(8):869-74; discussion 875-6, 1996
11. Suwabe H et al: Reticulohistiocytoma involving the skin, subcutaneous tissue and a regional lymph node. Pathol Int. 46(7):531-7, 1996
12. Hunt SJ et al: Solitary reticulohistiocytoma in pregnancy: immunohistochemical and ultrastructural study of a case with unusual immunophenotype. J Cutan Pathol. 22(2):177-81, 1995
13. Zelger B et al: Reticulohistiocytoma and multicentric reticulohistiocytosis. Histopathologic and immunophenotypic distinct entities. Am J Dermatopathol. 16(6):577-84, 1994
14. Caputo R et al: Solitary reticulohistiocytosis (reticulohistiocytoma) of the skin in children: report of two cases. Arch Dermatol. 128(5):698-9, 1992
15. Chun SI et al: Congenital self-healing reticulohistiocytosis--report of a case of the solitary type and review of the literature. Yonsei Med J. 33(2):194-8, 1992
16. Anaguchi S et al: [Solitary reticulohistiocytic granuloma--a report of three cases and a review of literature.] Nippon Hifuka Gakkai Zasshi. 101(7):735-42, 1991
17. Coode PE et al: Multicentric reticulohistiocytosis: report of two cases with ultrastructure, tissue culture and immunology studies. Clin Exp Dermatol. 5(3):281-93, 1980
18. Davies BT et al: The so-called reticulohistiocytoma of the skin; a comparison of two distinct types. Br J Dermatol. 67(6):205-11, 1955

Microscopic and Immunohistochemical Features

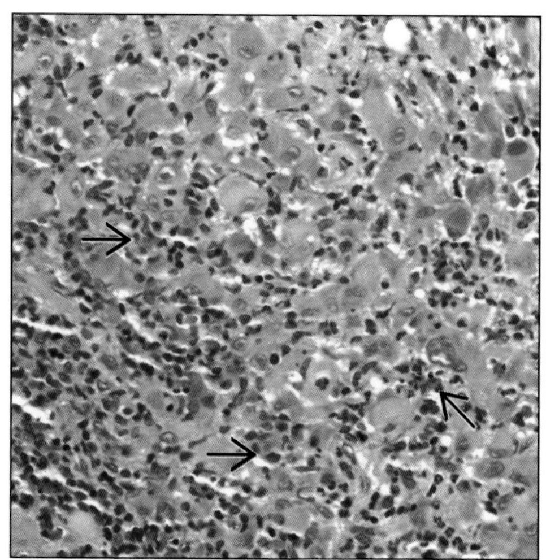

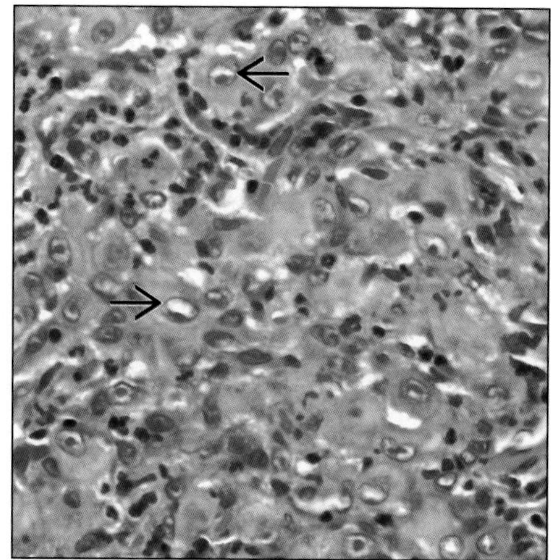

(Left) *Intermediate-power view shows sheets of eosinophilic cells associated with an inflammatory infiltrate containing lymphocytes, neutrophils, and eosinophils* ➔. ***(Right)*** *Higher power examination shows the cytologic features of the cells, with abundant dense eosinophilic to glassy-appearing cytoplasm and vesicular nuclei* ➔ *with prominent nucleoli.*

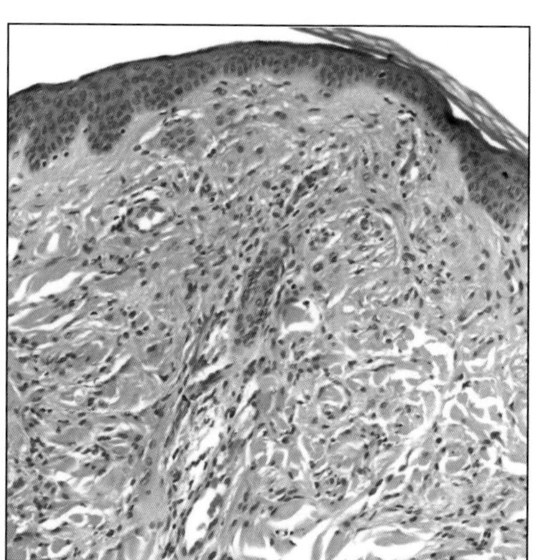

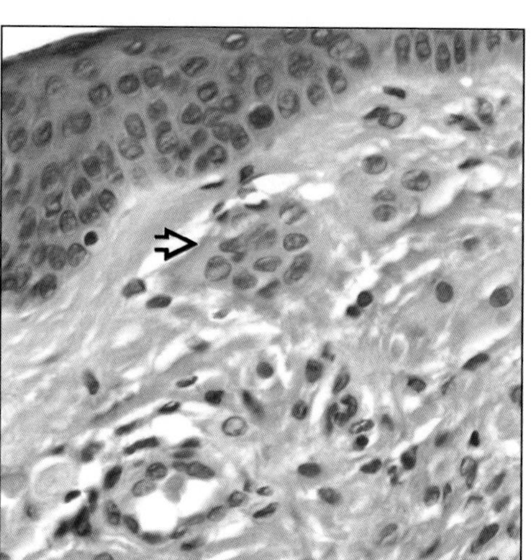

(Left) *Low-power view of a hypocellular lesion shows only scattered large histiocytes in the superficial dermis.* ***(Right)*** *Higher power examination of the cells shows typical histologic features of reticulohistiocytoma, with enlarged mononuclear and multinucleated* ⇨ *cells with abundant eosinophilic cytoplasm.*

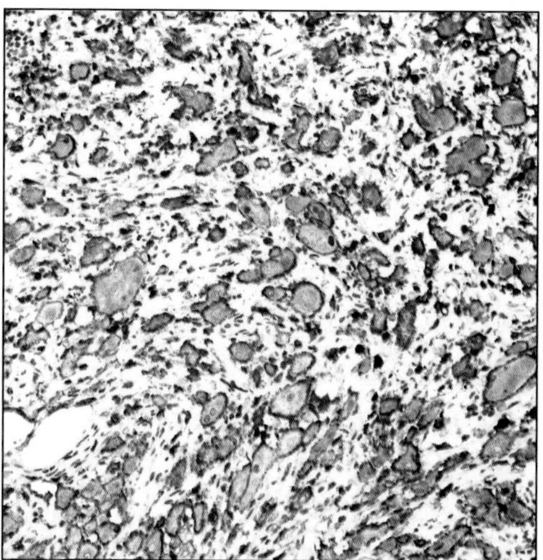

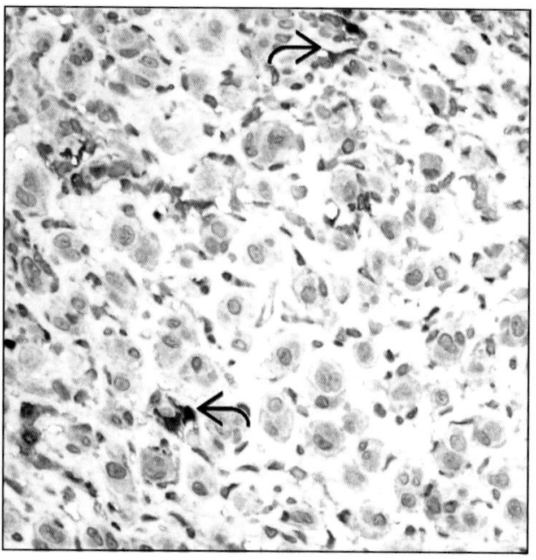

(Left) *CD163 immunohistochemical stain is strongly and diffusely positive, highlighting the tumoral cell cytoplasm and membranes.* ***(Right)*** *S100 is essentially negative, with only very weak cytoplasmic, and no nuclear, staining. A few background dendritic cells are strongly positive* ↷.

MULTICENTRIC RETICULOHISTIOCYTOSIS

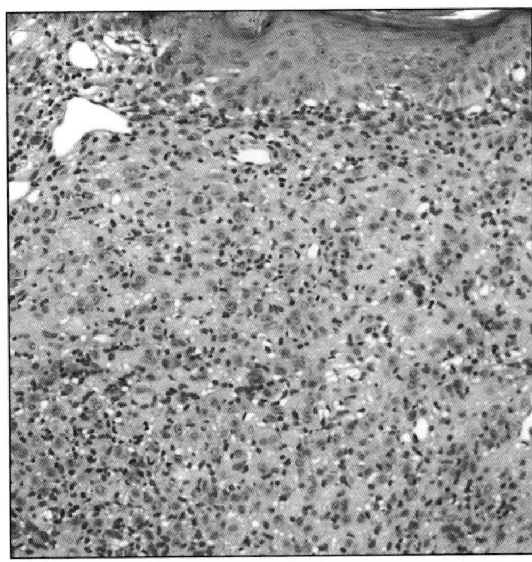

Low-power examination shows a dermal-based proliferation containing numerous enlarged histiocytic-appearing cells associated with a background mixed inflammatory infiltrate.

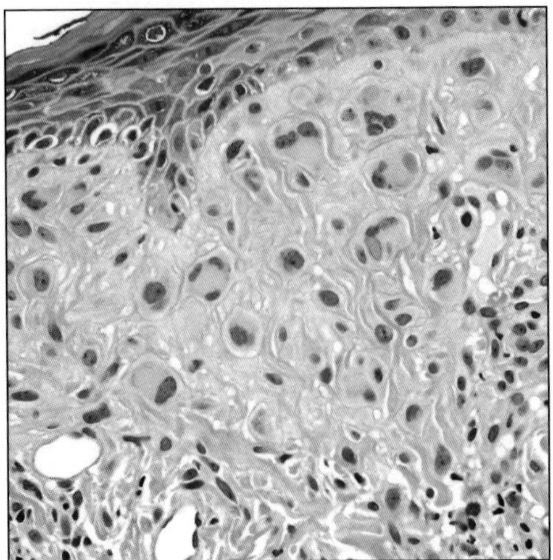

Higher magnification shows a population of enlarged histiocytic cells with abundant dense eosinophilic cytoplasm and 1 to several oval to reniform nuclei.

TERMINOLOGY

Abbreviations

- Multicentric reticulohistiocytosis (MCR)

Synonyms

- Giant cell reticulohistiocytosis
- Reticulohistiocytosis of skin and synovia

Definitions

- Proliferation of large histiocytes with dense eosinophilic cytoplasm involving multiple organs

ETIOLOGY/PATHOGENESIS

Associated Conditions

- Association with autoimmune disorders and internal malignancies

CLINICAL ISSUES

Epidemiology

- Age
  - Most cases occur in adults > 40 years old

Presentation

- Multiple nodules and arthropathy
  - Most patients present with multiple cutaneous/ mucocutaneous papulonodules as well as severe arthropathy and other visceral symptoms

Treatment

- Drugs
  - Immunosuppressive medications typically used
  - Underlying autoimmune disease or malignancy should be treated

Prognosis

- Variable; some cutaneous lesions may regress
- Osteoarticular involvement shows progressive course in approximately 50% of cases

MACROSCOPIC FEATURES

General Features

- Dermal-based, nodular, nonencapsulated lesion

Size

- Typically range from 2 mm to 2 cm in diameter

MICROSCOPIC PATHOLOGY

Histologic Features

- Dermal-based nodular proliferation of large mononuclear and multinucleated histiocytes
  - Cells show characteristic abundant glassy/ hyalinized-appearing eosinophilic cytoplasm
  - Some cells may show finely granular cytoplasm
  - Cytologic atypia is minimal; only few mitoses
  - Less well circumscribed than solitary reticulohistiocytoma but no infiltrative features
- Overlying epidermis may show atrophy/thinning
- Early lesions characterized by background inflammatory infiltrate with many small mononuclear cells and lymphocytes
- Later lesions show greater numbers of large cells and neutrophils and eosinophils

ANCILLARY TESTS

Immunohistochemistry

- Cells are typically positive for histiocytic markers, including CD68, lysozyme, and CD45
  - Variable reactivity reported for FXIIIA; may be greater than in solitary reticulohistiocytoma
- Cells are negative for S100, CD1a, and MAC387

MULTICENTRIC RETICULOHISTIOCYTOSIS

Key Facts

Terminology
- Giant cell reticulohistiocytosis

Clinical Issues
- Most cases occur in adults > 40 years old
- Multiple nodules and arthropathy
- Prognosis is variable; some cutaneous lesions may regress
- Osteoarticular involvement shows progressive course in 1/2 of cases

Microscopic Pathology
- Dermal-based nodular proliferation of large mononuclear and multinucleated histiocytes
- Cells show characteristic abundant glassy/hyalinized-appearing eosinophilic cytoplasm
- Occasional Touton-type giant cells containing lipid may be present but not prominent
- There is often overlying epidermal atrophy

DIFFERENTIAL DIAGNOSIS

Solitary Reticulohistiocytoma and Generalized Cutaneous Reticulohistiocytosis
- Solitary reticulohistiocytoma (SR) is characterized by single papular or nodular lesion
  - Histologically, there is considerable overlap with MCR, but some differences have been described
    - Solitary lesions may be better circumscribed and show more multinucleated giants cells and neutrophils
- Generalized cutaneous reticulohistiocytosis (GCR) is characterized by eruption of multiple small cutaneous lesions
  - Some cases may progress to MCR

Juvenile Xanthogranuloma (JXG)
- Typically single lesion occurring in children, but some cases occur in adults
- Histologically, typically shows more foamy histiocytes and Touton-type giant cells with peripheral wreath-like arrangement of nuclei

Langerhans Cell Histocytosis (LCH)
- Predominantly occur in children, but 2nd peak in elderly adults (usually eosinophilic granuloma variant)
- Typically characterized by multiple skin lesions and systemic involvement (especially bone)
- Cells show large, folded, or reniform vesicular nuclei and abundant eosinophilic cytoplasm
- CD1a and S100 are positive

DIAGNOSTIC CHECKLIST

Pathologic Interpretation Pearls
- Nodular proliferation of large mononuclear and multinucleated histiocytes
  - Cells show characteristic abundant glassy/hyalinized-appearing eosinophilic cytoplasm

SELECTED REFERENCES

1. Luz FB et al: Multicentric reticulohistiocytosis: a proliferation of macrophages with tropism for skin and joints, part I. Skinmed. 6(4):172-8, 2007
2. Chen CH et al: Multicentric reticulohistiocytosis presenting with destructive polyarthritis, laryngopharyngeal dysfunction, and a huge reticulohistiocytoma. J Clin Rheumatol. 12(5):252-4, 2006
3. Baghestani S et al: Multicentric reticulohistiocytosis presenting with papulonodular skin eruption and polyarthritis. Eur J Dermatol. 15(3):196-200, 2005
4. Snow JL et al: Malignancy-associated multicentric reticulohistiocytosis: a clinical, histological and immunophenotypic study. Br J Dermatol. 133(1):71-6, 1995
5. Coode PE et al: Multicentric reticulohistiocytosis: report of two cases with ultrastructure, tissue culture and immunology studies. Clin Exp Dermatol. 5(3):281-93, 1980

IMAGE GALLERY

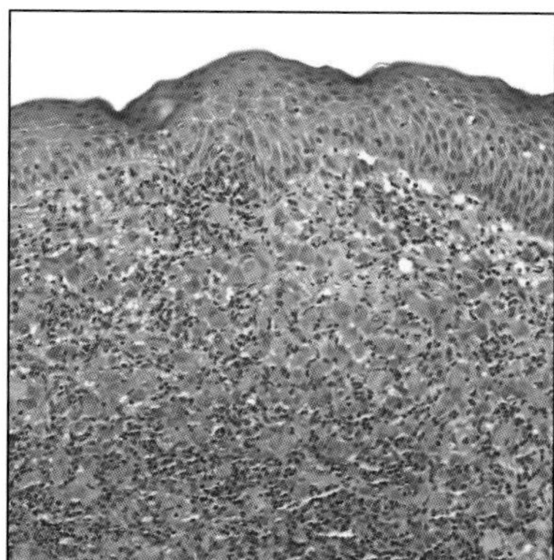

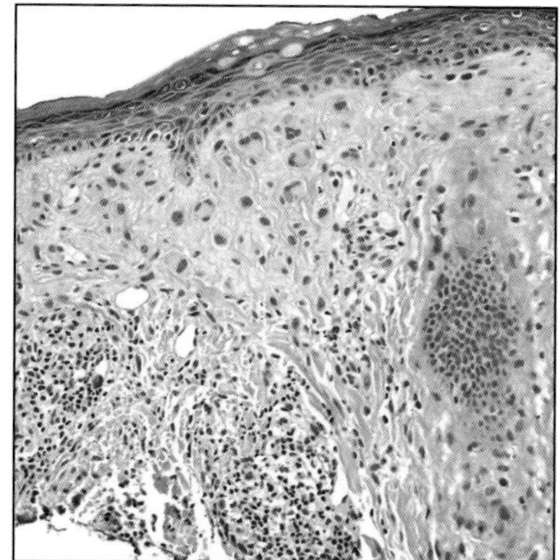

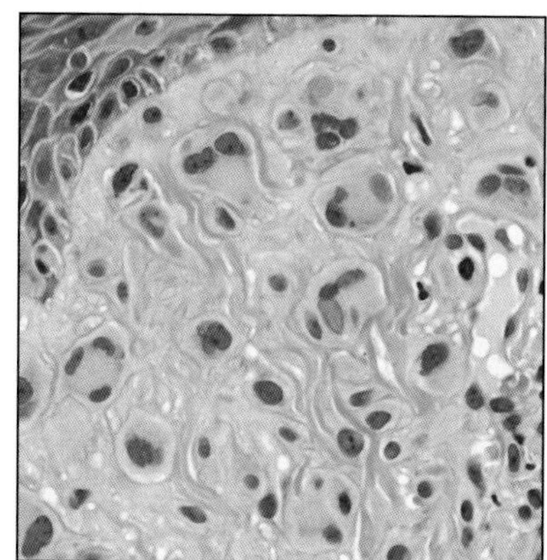

(Left) *Low-power examination of multicentric reticulohistiocytosis shows a dermal infiltrate of large histiocytic cells with abundant dense eosinophilic cytoplasm.* ***(Center)*** *Another example of multicentric reticulohistiocytosis shows a dermal-based proliferation of large epithelioid histiocytes and a mild associated chronic inflammatory infiltrate.* ***(Right)*** *High-power view shows the cytologic features of the large histiocytic cells with abundant dense eosinophilic cytoplasm and bland, oval to reniform nuclei with small nucleoli.*

MISCELLANEOUS XANTHOMAS

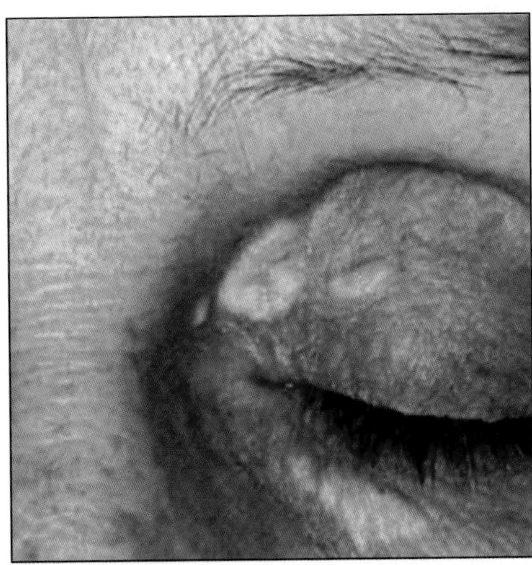

Xanthelasmas typically symmetrically involve bilateral upper and lower eyelids and periorbital skin. Sharply demarcated soft yellow papules and plaques with a yellow color are characteristic.

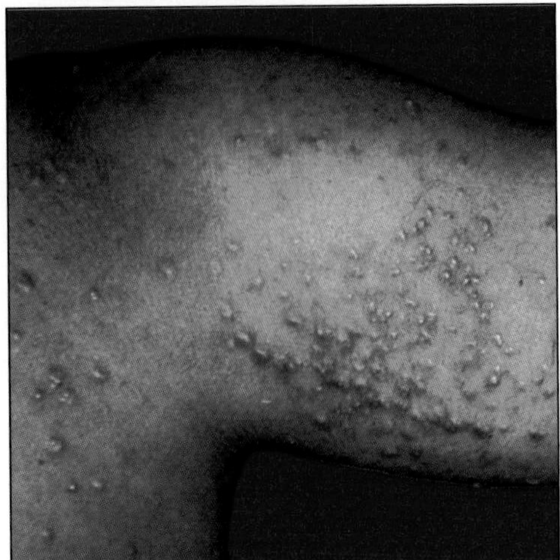

Eruptive xanthomas are characterized by the sudden appearance of crops of small yellow papules with an erythematous base. Eruptive xanthomas typically occur in the buttock, thigh, and shoulder regions.

TERMINOLOGY

Definitions

- Mass-forming collection of lipidized macrophages
- Reactive process usually resulting from altered serum lipid levels

ETIOLOGY/PATHOGENESIS

Hereditary or Nonhereditary

- Associated with hereditary lipoproteinemias and occasionally secondary lipoproteinemias (e.g., diabetes, hypothyroidism, primary biliary cirrhosis)
- May also occur in normolipemic patients

CLINICAL ISSUES

Presentation

- Usually occur in skin and subcutaneous tissue
- Occasionally arise in deep soft tissues (tendon, synovium, bone)
- Classified based on clinical features
  - **Xanthelasma**
    - Soft yellow plaques; predilection for eyelids and periorbital skin; often bilateral
  - **Eruptive xanthoma**
    - Sudden onset of small yellow papules with erythematous halo; predilection for gluteal region, thigh, and shoulders
  - **Tuberous xanthoma**
    - Firm yellow subcutaneous nodules and plaques; predilection for elbow, knee, gluteal region, and fingers
  - **Tendinous xanthoma**
    - Soft tissue mass associated with tendons, ligaments, &/or fascia; predilection for hands, feet, and Achilles tendon
    - May impair joint function but often asymptomatic
  - **Plane xanthoma**
    - Variably sized yellow macules; predilection for palmar creases
    - In normolipemic patients, consider underlying reticuloendothelial malignancy
  - **Cerebrotendinous xanthomatosis**
    - Rare autosomal recessive disease; sterol 27-hydroxylase gene (*CYP27A*) mutation
    - Enzyme involved in bile acid synthesis; defect results in accumulation of cholestanol, which is deposited systemically
    - Bilateral Achilles tendon xanthomas and cataracts; CNS symptoms include ataxia, dementia, dysarthria, psychiatric disturbances, and seizures

Treatment

- May regress with medical therapy for hyperlipidemia or underlying cause if secondary
- Conservative excision can be employed for large or symptomatic lesions

Prognosis

- Excellent prognosis; surgically treated lesions may recur

MACROSCOPIC FEATURES

General Features

- Diffuse or circumscribed with variegated yellow, tan, and white appearance

Size

- Generally a few millimeters to centimeters depending on type
- Tendinous xanthomas can be quite large (up to 20 cm)

MISCELLANEOUS XANTHOMAS

Key Facts

Terminology
- Mass-forming collection of lipidized macrophages
- Reactive process usually resulting from altered serum lipid levels

Etiology/Pathogenesis
- Associated with hereditary lipoproteinemias and occasionally secondary lipoproteinemias
- May also occur in normolipemic patients

Clinical Issues
- Usually occur in skin and subcutaneous tissue
- Occasionally arise in deep soft tissues (tendon, synovium, bone)
- Classified based on clinical features and gross appearance
- Excellent prognosis

Microscopic Pathology
- Specific classification requires clinicopathologic correlation
- Generally consist of mixtures of foamy and nonfoamy macrophages with secondary changes including inflammation, fibrosis and cholesterol cleft formation

Top Differential Diagnoses
- Giant cell tumor of tendon sheath
- Juvenile xanthogranuloma
- Plexiform xanthoma
- Lipidized benign fibrous histiocytoma (dermatofibroma)
- Verruciform xanthoma

Clinical Forms of Xanthoma

Feature	Xanthelasma	Eruptive	Tuberous	Tendinous	Plane
Lipoprotein association	None or IIa, III	I, III, V, secondary	IIa, III, secondary	IIa, secondary	None, III, secondary
Characteristic location	Eyelids	Buttock	Elbow, knee, buttock, finger	Hand, foot, ankle (Achilles)	Palm creases
Characteristic histopathology	Foamy macrophages	Foamy and nonfoamy macrophages	Foamy macrophages, cholesterol clefts, inflammation, fibrosis	Foamy macrophages, cholesterol clefts, inflammation, fibrosis	Foamy macrophages

Hyperlipoproteinemia (Fredrickson) Classification

	I	IIa	IIb	III	IV	V
Elevated lipoprotein	Chylomicrons	LDL	LDL, VLDL	Chylomicrons, VLDL remnants	VLDL	Chylomicrons, VLDL
Molecular defect	Lipoprotein lipase, apoC-II	LDL receptor, apoB-100	Unknown	ApoE	Unknown	Unknown

MICROSCOPIC PATHOLOGY

Histologic Features
- Specific classification requires clinicopathologic correlation
- Consist of mixtures of foamy and nonfoamy macrophages with variable inflammation, fibrosis, and cholesterol cleft formation
- Xanthelasmas and plane xanthomas consist of sheets of foamy macrophages
- Eruptive xanthomas consist mostly of nonfoamy macrophages with some foamy macrophages
- Tuberous and tendinous xanthomas consist of sheets of foamy macrophages with chronic inflammation, fibrosis, and cholesterol clefts with giant cells

DIFFERENTIAL DIAGNOSIS

Giant Cell Tumor of Tendon Sheath
- Usually solitary; resembles tendinous xanthoma but contains multinucleated giant cells and hemosiderin

Juvenile Xanthogranuloma
- Usually young children; more heterogeneous with Touton giant cells and acute inflammation

Plexiform Xanthoma
- Usually normolipemic; plexiform growth pattern

Lipidized Benign Fibrous Histiocytoma
- Usually lower leg (ankle predominant); demonstrates dermal collagen entrapment

Verruciform Xanthoma
- Most are intraoral or anogenital; verrucous epithelium with parakeratin plugs and stromal foam cells

SELECTED REFERENCES

1. Moghadasian MH: Cerebrotendinous xanthomatosis: clinical course, genotypes and metabolic backgrounds. Clin Invest Med. 27(1):42-50, 2004
2. Cruz PD Jr et al: Dermal, subcutaneous, and tendon xanthomas: diagnostic markers for specific lipoprotein disorders. J Am Acad Dermatol. 19(1 Pt 1):95-111, 1988
3. Parker F: Xanthomas and hyperlipidemias. J Am Acad Dermatol. 13(1):1-30, 1985

MISCELLANEOUS XANTHOMAS

Microscopic and Clinical Features

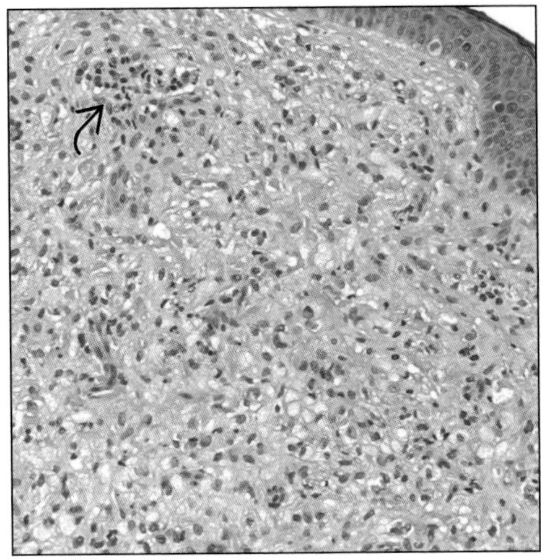

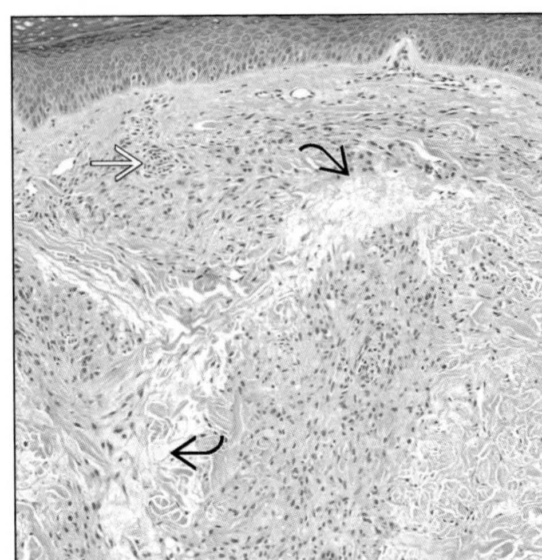

*(**Left**) Xanthelasmas (and plane xanthomas) consist of a sheet-like infiltrate of foamy macrophages involving the dermis and surrounding adnexal structures. Small areas of chronic inflammation ⇗ may be present, but fibrosis & cholesterol clefts are not typical. (**Right**) Eruptive xanthoma is characterized by sheets of macrophages within the dermis. Extravascular lipid deposits with a blue-gray amorphous appearance are often seen ⇗ between dermal collagen bundles. Sparse perivascular inflammatory infiltrate ➡ can also be seen.*

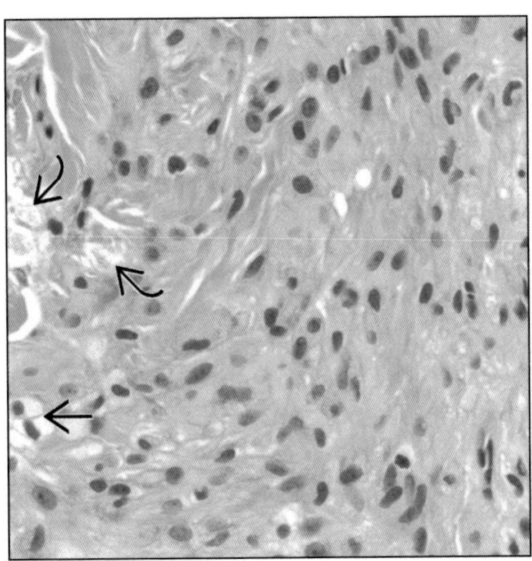

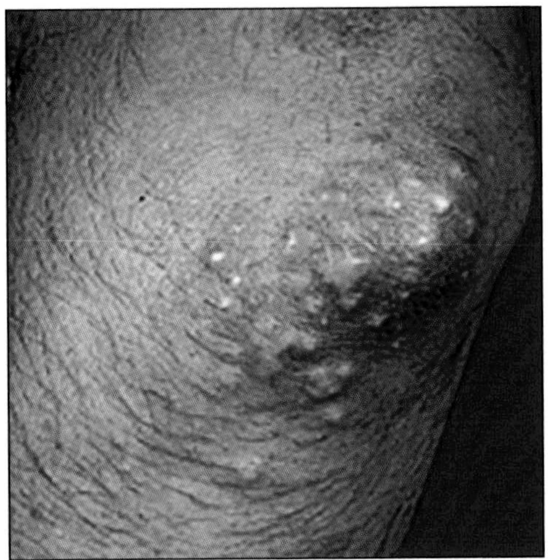

*(**Left**) In contrast to other forms of xanthoma, the cells in eruptive xanthoma are nonfoamy in early lesions. Note rare foamy macrophages → and extravascular lipid ⇗. (**Right**) Tuberous xanthoma is shown involving the knee. Tuberous xanthomas appear as firm yellow-red subcutaneous nodules and occur at pressure areas such as the buttock and extensor surfaces of the knee and elbow. Smaller nodules often coalesce to form larger nodules or plaques.*

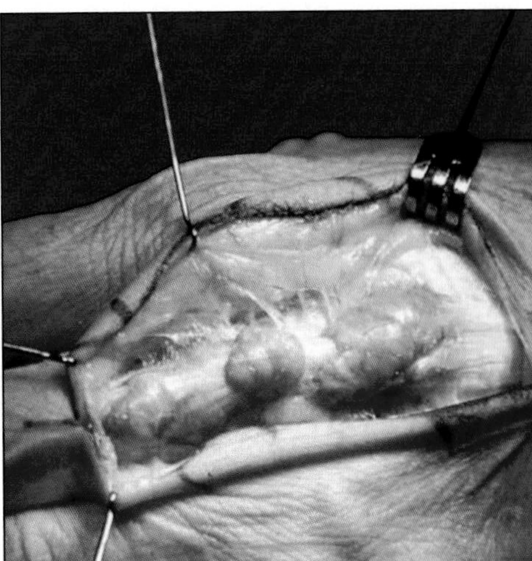

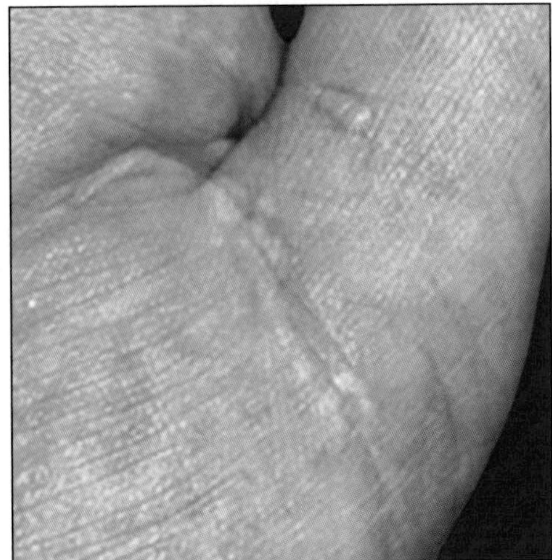

*(**Left**) Intraoperative photo shows tendinous xanthomas involving a hand extensor tendon. Tendinous xanthomas typically present as skin-colored soft tissue nodules and may be attached to tendons or ligaments. (**Right**) Plane xanthomas appear as small yellow macules that often involve skin creases, especially palmar creases, but can occur at any site.*

Microscopic Features

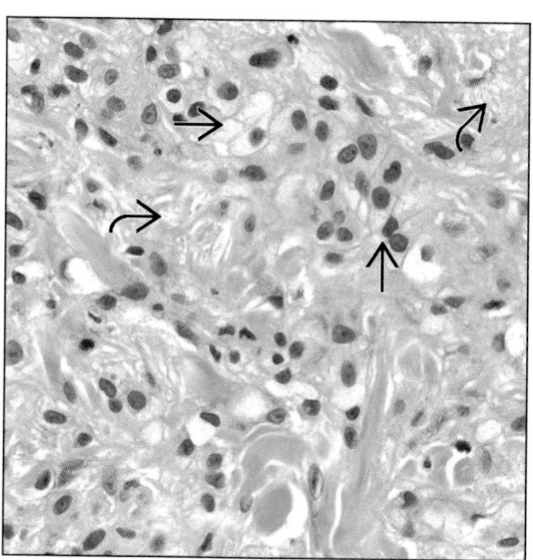

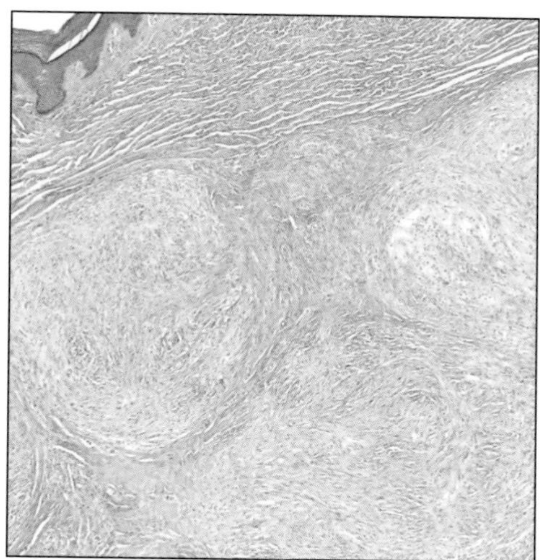

(Left) *Older eruptive xanthomas accumulate more foamy macrophages ➔ and consist of a mixture of foamy and nonfoamy cells. Again, note areas of lace-like blue-gray extravascular lipid between dermal collagen bundles ➔.* ***(Right)*** *Tuberous xanthomas consist of a nodular infiltrate of foamy macrophages involving the dermis and may be uninodular or multinodular, as in this example.*

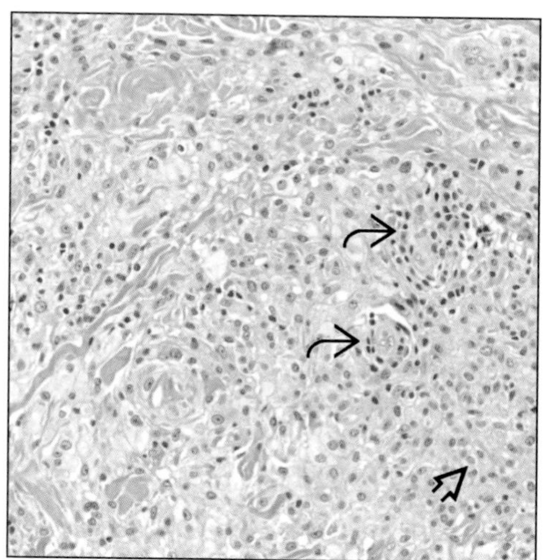

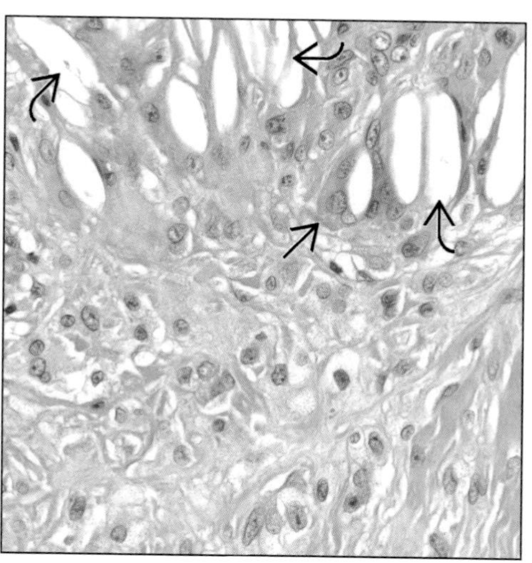

(Left) *Large aggregates of foam cells growing in sheets is typical of tuberous xanthoma. Some early lesions will have nonfoamy cells ➔ as well. Patchy nonspecific inflammation ➔ is often present and frequently is perivascular in early stage lesions.* ***(Right)*** *Unlike the other forms of xanthoma, tuberous (and tendinous) xanthomas usually have secondary changes including collections of extracellular cholesterol with cholesterol cleft formation ➔ and associated giant cells ➔.*

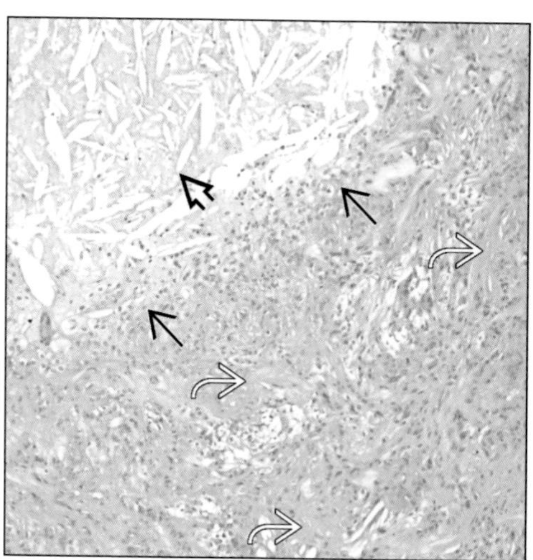

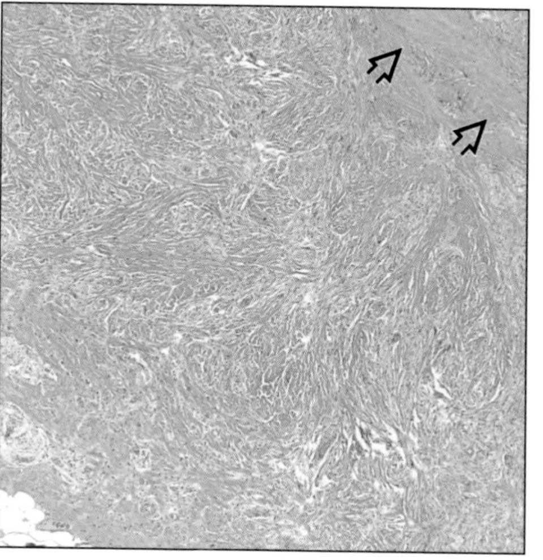

(Left) *Other secondary changes in tuberous (and tendinous) xanthomas include varying degrees of fibrosis ➔ and foci of necrosis ➔ containing amorphous eosinophilic debris with cholesterol clefts and a surrounding rim of foamy macrophages ➔.* ***(Right)*** *Tendinous xanthomas are histologically identical to tuberous xanthomas except that they involve deeper structures, such as tendons ➔ and ligaments.*

PLEXIFORM XANTHOMA

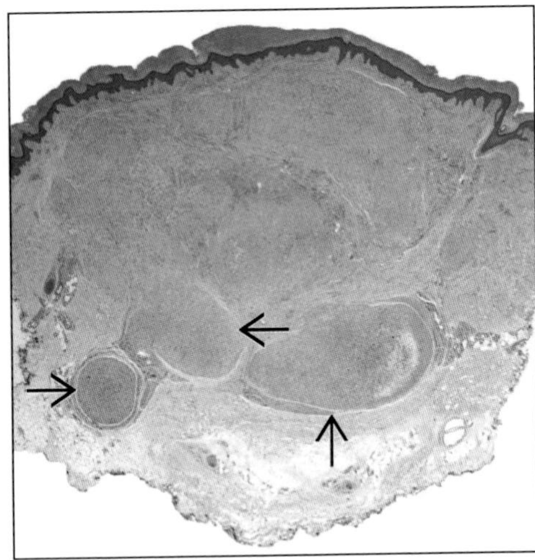

A multinodular proliferation with a plexiform architecture filling the dermis is typical of plexiform xanthoma. The deep nodules ⇒ tend to be more well developed than the superficial ones.

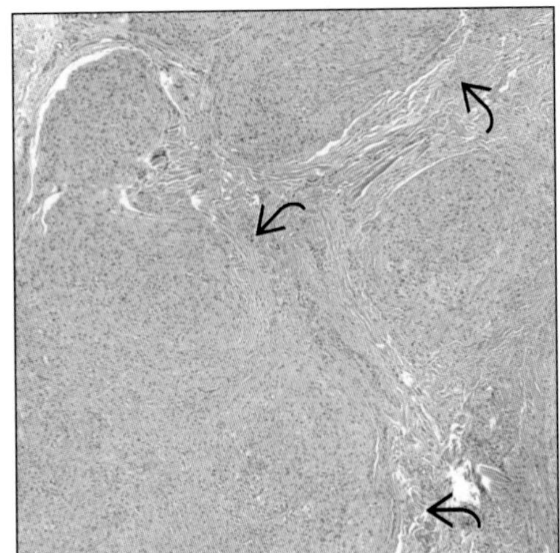

Medium-power view shows the typical appearance of plexiform xanthoma, with variably sized nodules arranged in a plexiform configuration and with associated fibrosis ⇒.

TERMINOLOGY

Definitions

- Superficial (dermis/subcutis) nodular proliferation of lipid-laden macrophages with plexiform arrangement

CLINICAL ISSUES

Epidemiology

- Incidence
  - Rare
    - Only single case reports and small series in the literature
- Age
  - Tend to occur in young adults (4th decade)
- Gender
  - Men affected more frequently than women

Site

- Most often occur in extremities
  - Tend to occur on extensor surfaces
  - Elbow and knee region most frequent subsites

Presentation

- Dermal-based cutaneous nodule
- ± hyperlipidemia

Treatment

- Surgical approaches
  - Conservative excision

Prognosis

- Nonprogressive
- Local recurrences do occur with inadequate excision

MACROSCOPIC FEATURES

General Features

- Yellow to orange dermal nodule
- Plexiform arrangement may be observed macroscopically
- May be multifocal

Size

- 1-5 cm (mean: 2.7 cm)

MICROSCOPIC PATHOLOGY

Histologic Features

- Nodular proliferation located within dermis with plexiform arrangement
  - May have superficial subcutaneous extension
- Nodules composed of sheets of monomorphic foamy macrophages
- Sparse lymphocytic inflammatory infiltrate
- Variable numbers of multinucleated giant cells
- Cholesterol clefts and necrosis absent to focal
- Stromal sclerosis often present around nodules

Immunohistochemistry

- Foamy cells are positive for macrophage markers (CD68, CD163)
- Foamy cells are negative for S100 protein

DIFFERENTIAL DIAGNOSIS

Plexiform Xanthomatous Tumor

- Almost exclusively occur in young adult men (mean: 45 years)
  - Most occur in upper and lower extremities (knees and elbows most frequent)
- Rarely have dyslipidemia or family history of dyslipidemia
- Neoplastic proliferation with overlapping histology of plexiform xanthoma
  - Relationship to plexiform xanthoma uncertain (may be the same entity)

PLEXIFORM XANTHOMA

Key Facts

Clinical Issues

- Rare
- Tend to occur in young adults (4th decade)
- Most often occur in extremities
  - Elbow and knee regions most frequent
- Dermal-based cutaneous nodule
- May or may not have dyslipidemia
- Local recurrences do occur with inadequate excision

Microscopic Pathology

- Nodular and plexiform proliferation of foamy macrophages located within dermis

Top Differential Diagnoses

- Plexiform xanthomatous tumor
- Schwannoma (plexiform)
- Lipidized benign fibrous histiocytoma
- Plexiform fibrohistiocytic tumor
- Tuberous and tendinous xanthoma

- Plexiform arrangement of nodules composed of foamy macrophages
- Tend to have more subcutaneous extension than plexiform xanthoma
- Compared to plexiform xanthoma, plexiform architecture and fibrosis more well developed

Schwannoma (Plexiform)

- Spindle cell proliferation with variable cellularity (Antoni A and B areas) and neural phenotype
  - May rarely have plexiform arrangement (plexiform schwannoma)
- May have foamy cells, but these do not predominate
- Strongly S100 protein positive

Plexiform Fibrohistiocytic Tumor

- Typically occurs in children and adolescents, and both men and women affected
- Biphasic: Fascicles of spindle cells with fibromatosis-like appearance and small nodules of epithelioid cells
- Rare cases have xanthomatous change but limited in extent compared to plexiform xanthoma

Tuberous and Tendinous Xanthoma

- Similar histology but lack plexiform arrangement
- Men and women both affected
- Personal/family history of dyslipidemia is often present

Ancient Hematoma

- Typically trauma related
- Tend to be much larger than plexiform xanthoma (up to 20 cm)
- Located within deep soft tissue and with a central cavity
- Mixture of cell types including epithelioid macrophages, foamy macrophages, hemosiderin-laden macrophages, and multinucleated giant cells
- May have striking plexiform arrangement

Lipidized Benign Fibrous Histiocytoma

- No distinct male predilection
- Lack plexiform architecture of plexiform xanthoma

SELECTED REFERENCES

1. Michal M et al: Plexiform xanthomatous tumor: a report of 20 cases in 12 patients. Am J Surg Pathol. 26(10):1302-11, 2002
2. Mentzel T et al: Ancient hematoma: a unifying concept for a post-traumatic lesion mimicking an aggressive soft tissue neoplasm. Mod Pathol. 10(4):334-40, 1997
3. Michal M: Plexiform xanthomatous tumor. A report of three cases. Am J Dermatopathol. 16(5):532-6, 1994
4. Beham A et al: Plexiform xanthoma: an unusual variant. Histopathology. 19(6):565-7, 1991

IMAGE GALLERY

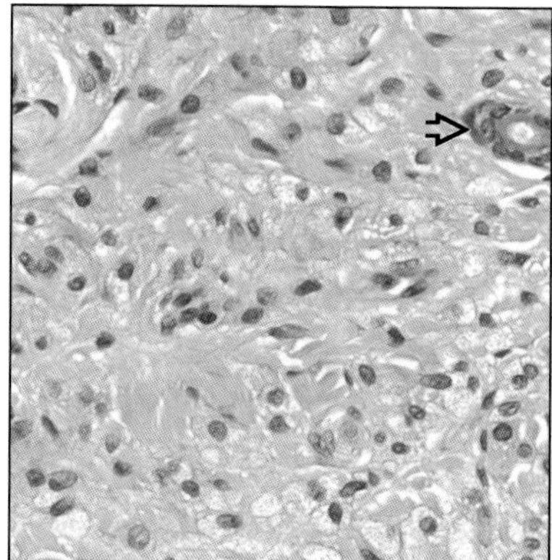

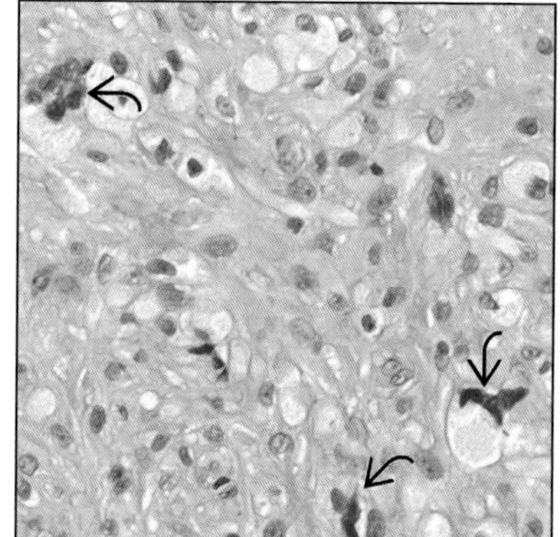

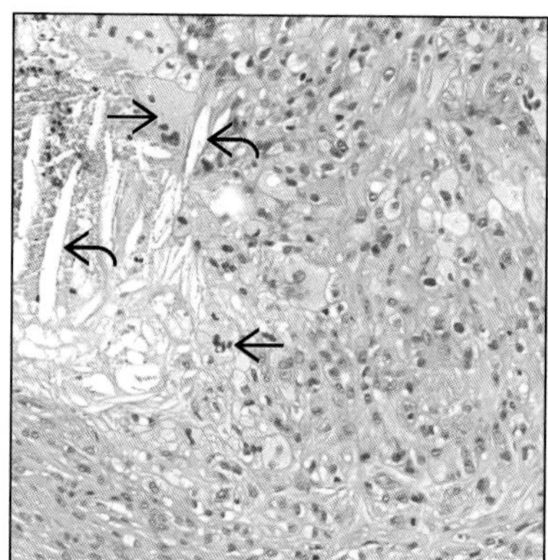

(Left) *Similar to xanthomas, the nodules consist of monomorphic round macrophages with foamy cytoplasm and associated stromal collagen. The proliferation can displace or surround ⇨ (eccrine sweat gland) cutaneous adnexal structures.* ***(Center)*** *Multinucleated giant cells →, often with foamy cytoplasm, are often present in variable numbers.* ***(Right)*** *Focal areas of necrosis with cholesterol crystals → and associated giant cells → may be present in some lesions.*

CELLULAR NEUROTHEKEOMA

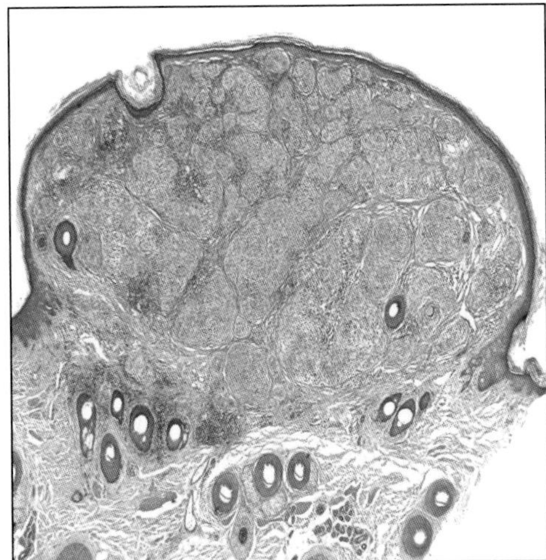

Hematoxylin & eosin of a transverse section of whole tumor shows the smooth, dome-shaped outline. The lesion is confined to the dermis. The epidermis is thinned except at the lateral margins.

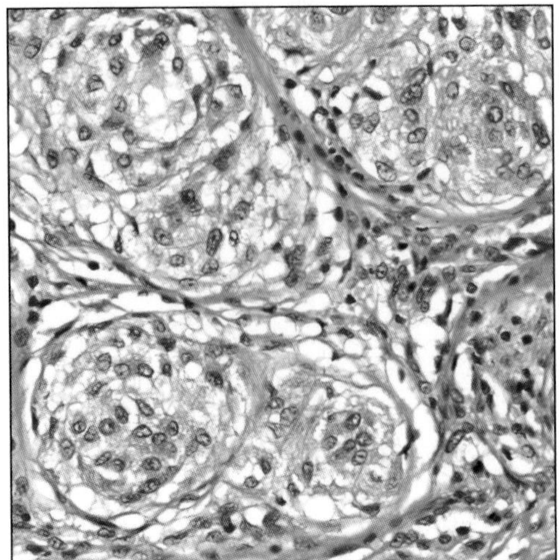

Hematoxylin & eosin shows rounded nests of cells separated by thin fibrous septa with some lymphocytes. The cells have uniform nuclei, a moderate amount of cytoplasm, and variably distinct cell margins.

TERMINOLOGY

Definitions

- Multinodular dermal tumor composed of nests of rounded cells separated by delicate fibrous septa
- Differs from dermal nerve sheath myxoma (a.k.a. neurothekeoma)
- Cell type unknown; considered fibrohistiocytic

CLINICAL ISSUES

Epidemiology

- Incidence
  - Rare
- Age
  - Young adults, most 15-25 years
- Gender
  - M = F
- Ethnicity
  - No predilection

Site

- Head and neck and upper extremity most common

Presentation

- Slow growing
  - Elevated dermal nodule
  - Painless

Treatment

- Surgical approaches
  - Simple excision

Prognosis

- Reported cases have behaved in benign fashion
- Occasional recurrence, especially if incompletely excised
- Atypical histologic features have no prognostic significance

MACROSCOPIC FEATURES

General Features

- Rounded or dome-shaped skin lesion
- Pale or tan

Size

- ≤ 2 cm diameter

MICROSCOPIC PATHOLOGY

Histologic Features

- ~ 50% confined to dermis; 48% involve superficial subcutis
- Nests of rounded cells
  - Uniform nuclei, scanty cytoplasm
  - Occasional spindling of cells, especially in myxoid areas
- Nests separated by thin fibrous septa
- Myxoid change in 20%
  - 30% are mixed cellular and myxoid lesions
- Nuclear atypia in 25%
- Mitoses occasionally seen up to 3 per 10 HPF
- Multinucleated cells in 40%
- Osteoclast-like cells in 30%
- Occasional plexiform pattern

Predominant Pattern/Injury Type

- Nested

Predominant Cell/Compartment Type

- Mesenchymal, fibrohistiocytic

DIFFERENTIAL DIAGNOSIS

Dermal Nerve Sheath Myxoma

- Circumscribed
- Delicate internal septa between myxoid lobules
- Vacuolated Schwann cells

CELLULAR NEUROTHEKEOMA

Key Facts

Terminology
- Multinodular dermal tumor composed of nests of rounded cells separated by delicate fibrous septa
- Differs from dermal nerve sheath myxoma (a.k.a. neurothekeoma)

Clinical Issues
- Young adults, most 15-25 years
- Head and neck and upper extremity most common sites
- Elevated dermal nodule
- Reported cases have behaved in benign fashion

Microscopic Pathology
- ~ 50% confined to dermis
- 48% involve superficial subcutis
- Nests of rounded cells
- Occasional spindling of cells, especially in myxoid areas
- Myxoid change in 20%
- Nuclear atypia in 25%
- Mitoses: ≤ 3 per 10 high-power fields
- Osteoclast-like cells in 30%
- Occasional plexiform pattern

Top Differential Diagnoses
- Dermal nerve sheath myxoma
  - Circumscribed, S100 positive
- Plexiform fibrohistiocytic tumor
  - Based at dermal-subcutaneous junction
  - Also has multinucleated cells and fibroblasts
  - Fibroblastic variant with fascicles in subcutis
- Melanocytic nevus
  - S100 protein positive

Immunohistochemistry

Antibody	Reactivity	Staining Pattern	Comment
Actin-sm	Positive	Cytoplasmic	30-60% of cases
CD63	Positive	Cytoplasmic	Same as NKI-C3; in 90% but not specific
MITF	Positive	Nuclear	80% of cases
CD68	Positive	Cytoplasmic	Nonspecific finding
Podoplanin	Positive	Cell membrane	100%; not in plexiform fibrohistiocytic tumor
S100	Negative		Contrast with dermal nerve sheath myxoma
HMB-45	Negative		Helps to exclude melanoma
melan-A103	Negative		Helps to exclude melanoma

- S100 protein positive
- EMA(+) perineurial cells peripherally

Plexiform Fibrohistiocytic Tumor
- Based at dermal-subcutaneous junction
- Extends into dermis and subcutaneous fat
- Fibrohistiocytic nodules consist of histiocyte-like cells, multinucleated cells, fibroblasts
- Fibroblastic pattern in 17%
  - Plexiform bundles of spindle cells within collagen
- Mixed fibroblastic and fibrohistiocytic pattern in 40%
- Podoplanin(-)

Melanocytic Nevus
- Junctional activity in many
- S100(+)

Melanoma
- Nuclear atypia with prominent nucleoli
- Abnormal mitoses
- S100(+); HMB-45(+), Melan-A(+) in some

Epithelioid Cutaneous Fibrous Histiocytoma
- Overlying epidermal hyperplasia
- Cells not organized in nests
- NKI-C3 (CD63)(-) and MITF(-)

SELECTED REFERENCES

1. Jaffer S et al: Neurothekeoma and plexiform fibrohistiocytic tumor: mere histologic resemblance or histogenetic relationship? Am J Surg Pathol. 33(6):905-13, 2009
2. Kaddu S et al: Podoplanin expression in fibrous histiocytomas and cellular neurothekeomas. Am J Dermatopathol. 31(2):137-9, 2009
3. Alkhalidi H et al: Cellular neurothekeoma with a plexiform morphology: a case report with a discussion of the plexiform lesions of the skin. J Cutan Pathol. 34(3):264-9, 2007
4. Fetsch JF et al: Neurothekeoma: an analysis of 178 tumors with detailed immunohistochemical data and long-term patient follow-up information. Am J Surg Pathol. 31(7):1103-14, 2007
5. Hornick JL et al: Cellular neurothekeoma: detailed characterization in a series of 133 cases. Am J Surg Pathol. 31(3):329-40, 2007
6. Sachdev R et al: Frequent positive staining with NKI/C3 in normal and neoplastic tissues limits its usefulness in the diagnosis of cellular neurothekeoma. Am J Clin Pathol. 126(4):554-63, 2006
7. Page RN et al: Microphthalmia transcription factor and NKI/C3 expression in cellular neurothekeoma. Mod Pathol. 17(2):230-4, 2004
8. Busam KJ et al: Atypical or worrisome features in cellular neurothekeoma: a study of 10 cases. Am J Surg Pathol. 22(9):1067-72, 1998

CELLULAR NEUROTHEKEOMA

Microscopic Features

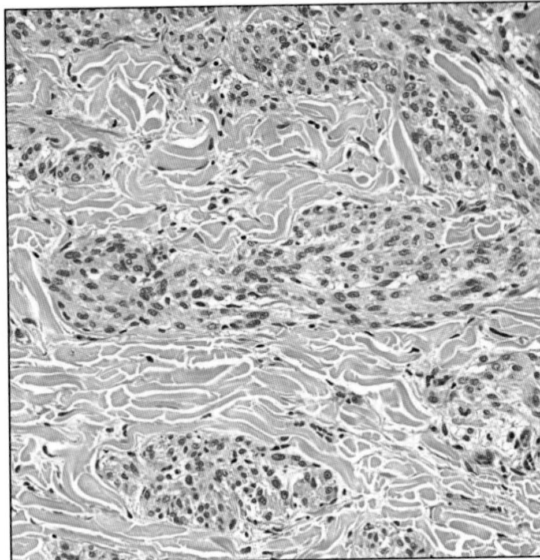

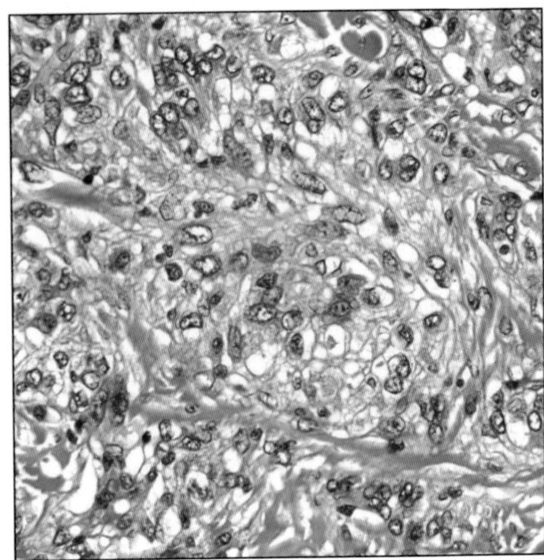

(Left) *Hematoxylin & eosin shows cellular neurothekeoma with confluent dermal nests forming irregularly shaped cellular aggregates. This variant can be misdiagnosed as a nerve sheath tumor or melanocytic lesion.* ***(Right)*** *Hematoxylin & eosin shows cellular features. The nuclei are uniform, rounded, and mostly vesicular, and some have inconspicuous nuclei. The cytoplasm is darkly eosinophilic, finely granular, or focally clear.*

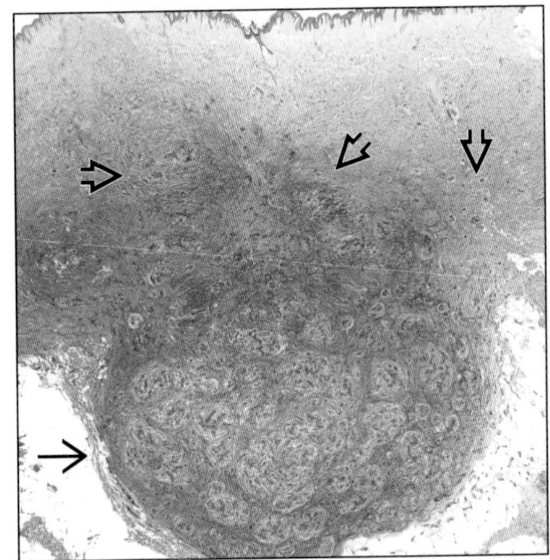

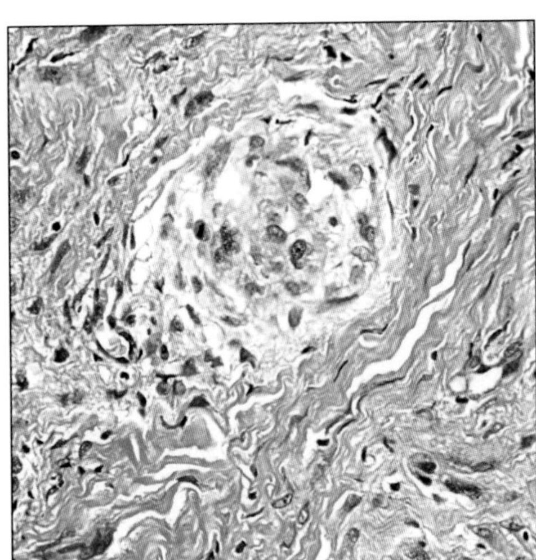

(Left) *Hematoxylin & eosin shows a tumor forming a nodular cluster of cell nests at the dermal-subcutaneous junction →, protruding into fat. Numerous single nests of lesional cells are dispersed throughout the overlying dermis ⇨.* ***(Right)*** *Hematoxylin & eosin of the dermal nests at higher magnification shows small numbers of rounded cells arranged in an ill-defined whorl, with myxoid stroma around the margin. About 20% of cellular neurothekeomas show prominent myxoid change.*

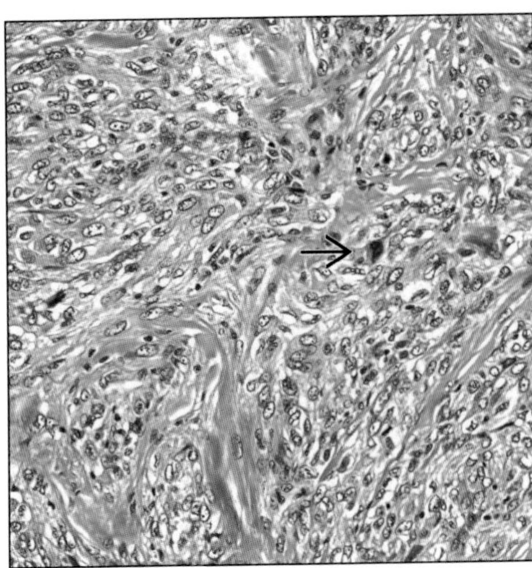

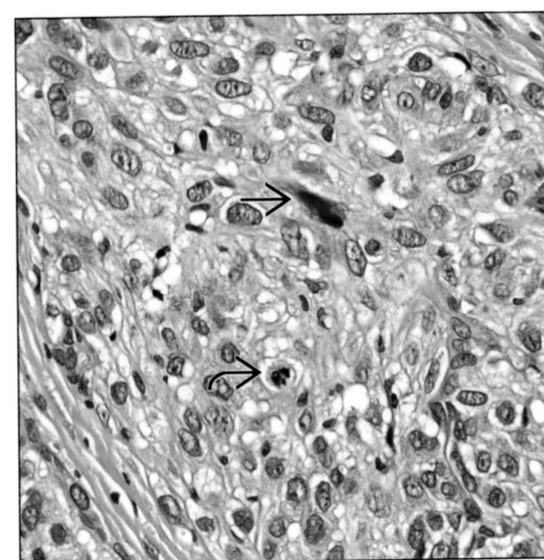

(Left) *Hematoxylin & eosin shows atypical cellular neurothekeoma. The cell nests are larger and more irregularly shaped than usual. Note the scattered hyperchromatic nuclei →.* ***(Right)*** *Hematoxylin & eosin shows atypical cellular neurothekeoma at higher magnification. Note the mild variation in nuclear shape and size, focal hyperchromasia →, and a mitotic figure ↪. Up to 3 mitoses per 10 high-power fields can be seen, but this does not indicate malignant potential.*

Microscopic Features

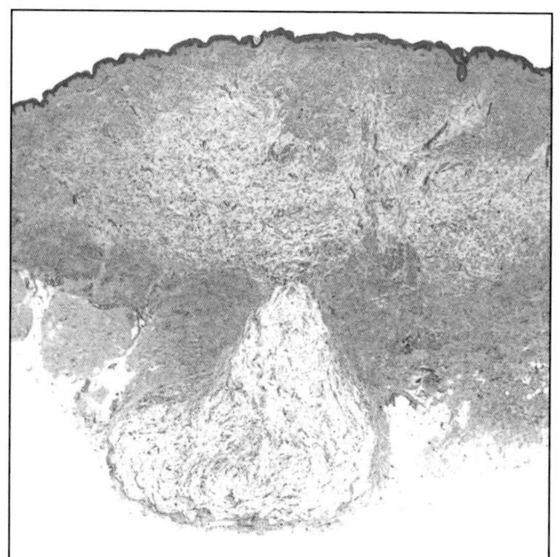

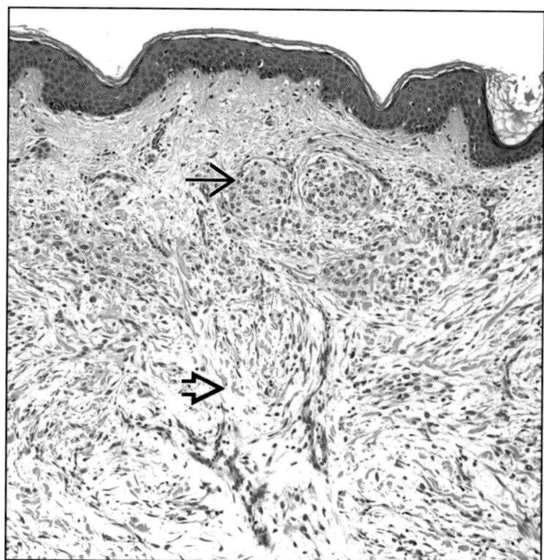

(Left) *Low-power view shows an example of cellular neurothekeoma with myxoid change and a nodule extending, unusually, into subcutis. The cellular composition differs from that of plexiform fibrohistiocytic tumor, which additionally has multinucleated and spindle cells and rarely shows myxoid change.* ***(Right)*** *This hematoxylin & eosin of cellular neurothekeoma shows focal myxoid change ➯ with gradual transition from more typical areas → in the superficial dermis.*

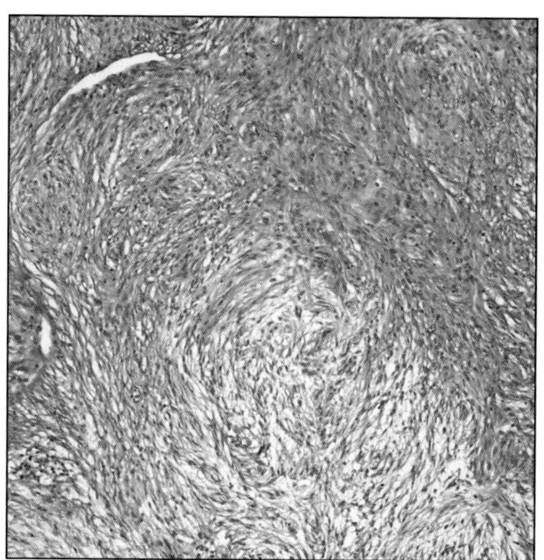

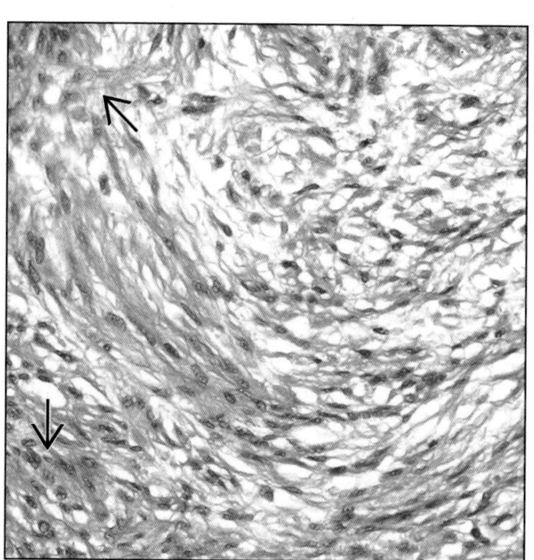

(Left) *Hematoxylin & eosin shows a myxoid variant of cellular neurothekeoma. Note that the myxoid and cellular areas merge. The cells assume a spindled shape in the latter.* ***(Right)*** *Hematoxylin & eosin shows a myxoid variant of cellular neurothekeoma. There is a vaguely whorled pattern of spindle cells that retain the typical nuclear and cytoplasmic features. Note the residual foci of the more typical rounded cells at the corners of the field →.*

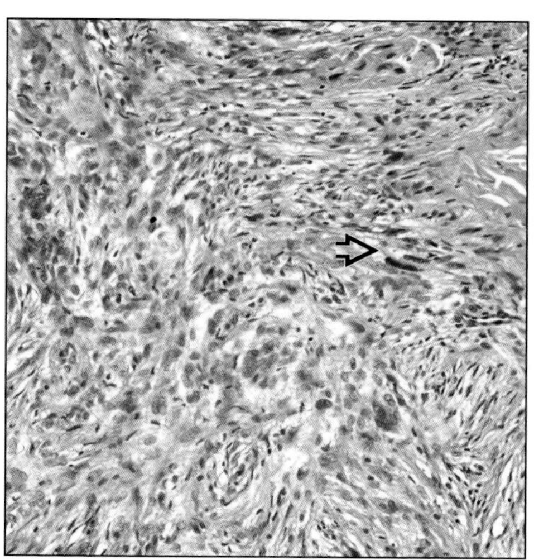

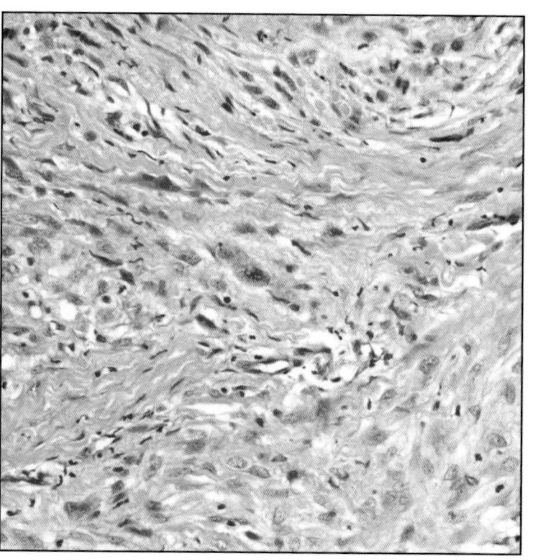

(Left) *This hematoxylin & eosin of a cellular neurothekeoma shows the usual pattern of nests of cells with uniform cytologic features in the lower half of the field and transition to spindle cells in the upper half, where there is also focal nuclear atypia ➯.* ***(Right)*** *Hematoxylin & eosin at higher magnification shows spindled cells lying within fibrous rather than myxoid stroma. The cell margins are indistinct. This is a difficult diagnosis in the absence of typical areas.*

MULTINUCLEATE CELL ANGIOHISTIOCYTOMA

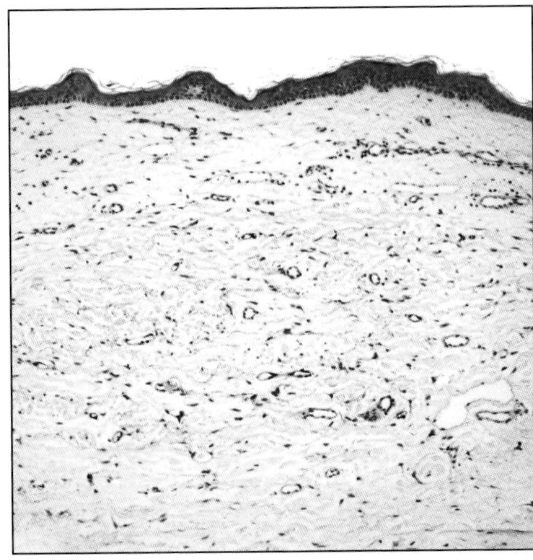

Low-power examination of hematoxylin & eosin stained section shows a dermal-based proliferation of small vessels with focal telangiectasia and increased numbers of stromal cells.

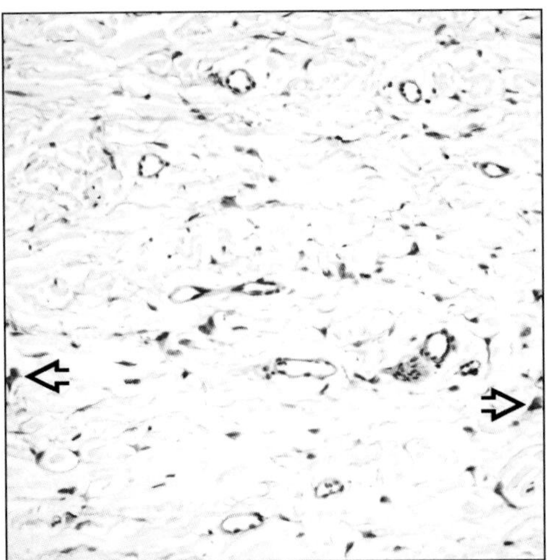

Higher power view shows a proliferation of numerous small blood vessels and scattered enlarged, angulated mononuclear and multinucleated ➲ stromal cells.

TERMINOLOGY

Abbreviations

- Multinucleate cell angiohistiocytoma (MCAH)

Definitions

- Proliferation of vessels and multinucleated stromal cells

ETIOLOGY/PATHOGENESIS

Unknown

- May be nonneoplastic reactive process

CLINICAL ISSUES

Epidemiology

- Age
  - Usually presents in patients > 40 years old
- Gender
  - Typically occurs in females

Site

- Most cases have been reported on legs (calves and thighs) or hands
  - Others sites rarely described, including oral mucosa

Presentation

- Multiple grouped round to oval papules
  - Usually described as red to violet lesions
  - May rarely be generalized
  - Rarely, may coalesce into 1 large annular lesion
- May be asymptomatic or pruritic

Prognosis

- Excellent; no malignant potential described
- Treatment not necessary; some lesions may regress spontaneously

MACROSCOPIC FEATURES

General Features

- Well-circumscribed, nonencapsulated, dermal-based lesion

MICROSCOPIC PATHOLOGY

Histologic Features

- Increased numbers of superficial small to telangiectatic vessels in reticular dermis
  - Endothelial cells show hyperchromatic nuclei
  - Do not show slit-like spaces suggestive of Kaposi sarcoma
- Proliferation of enlarged, angulated multinucleated cells
  - Cells show 3-10 nuclei, which may be arranged in ring or aggregated together
  - Nuclear hyperchromasia and mild atypia present
    - However, no frank atypia or pleomorphism
  - No/rare mitotic figures identified
- No infiltrative features identified
- Surrounding stroma may show inflammatory infiltrate
  - Consists of lymphocytes, plasma cells, mast cells, and neutrophils

Predominant Pattern/Injury Type

- Vascular and fibrohistiocytic

ANCILLARY TESTS

Immunohistochemistry

- Multinucleated cells are typically positive for FXIIIA and vimentin
  - CD68 staining is variably positive
- Stromal cells are positive for FXIIIA, vimentin, and lysozyme

MULTINUCLEATE CELL ANGIOHISTIOCYTOMA

Key Facts

Terminology
- Proliferation of vessels and multinucleated stromal cells

Etiology/Pathogenesis
- May be nonneoplastic reactive process

Clinical Issues
- Usually occur in patients > 40 years old
- Multiple grouped papules
- Typically in females

Microscopic Pathology
- Increased numbers of superficial small to telangiectatic vessels
- Proliferation of enlarged, angulated multinucleated cells
- No infiltrative features identified
- Nuclear hyperchromasia and mild atypia present

- Vessels are positive for CD31, CD34, and FVIIIRAg; HHV8 is negative

DIFFERENTIAL DIAGNOSIS

Kaposi Sarcoma
- Proliferation of atypical spindle cells and slit-like blood vessels; plasma cells usually present
- Multinucleate cells not identified
- Immunoreactive for HHV8 (in nuclei)

Giant Cell Angioblastoma
- Exceptionally rare tumor; present at birth or shortly thereafter
- Concentric arrays of spindle cells around small vessels

Pleomorphic Fibroma
- Polypoid lesion, likely related to fibroepithelial polyp
- Large, atypical-appearing, multinucleated pleomorphic fibroblasts present
- Proliferation of small vessels not prominent, as in MCAH

DIAGNOSTIC CHECKLIST

Pathologic Interpretation Pearls
- Proliferation of enlarged, angulated multinucleated cells associated with numerous small vessels
  - Cells show 3-10 nuclei, which may be arranged in ring or clumped together

SELECTED REFERENCES

1. Jaconelli L et al: Multinucleate cell angiohistiocytoma: report of three new cases and literature review. Dermatol Online J. 15(2):4, 2009
2. Rawal YB et al: Multinucleate cell angiohistiocytoma: an uncommon mucosal tumour. Clin Exp Dermatol. 34(3):333-6, 2009
3. Pérez LP et al: Multinucleate cell angiohistiocytoma. Report of five cases. J Cutan Pathol. 33(5):349-52, 2006
4. Puig L et al: Multinucleate cell angiohistiocytoma: a fibrohistiocytic proliferation with increased mast cell numbers and vascular hyperplasia. J Cutan Pathol. 29(4):232-7, 2002
5. Sass U et al: Multinucleate cell angiohistiocytoma: report of two cases with no evidence of human herpesvirus-8 infection. J Cutan Pathol. 27(5):258-61, 2000
6. Chang SN et al: Generalized multinucleate cell angiohistiocytoma. J Am Acad Dermatol. 35(2 Pt 2):320-2, 1996
7. Cribier B et al: Multinucleate cell angiohistiocytoma. A review and report of four cases. Acta Derm Venereol. 75(5):337-9, 1995
8. Shapiro PE et al: Multinucleate cell angiohistiocytoma: a distinct entity diagnosable by clinical and histologic features. J Am Acad Dermatol. 30(3):417-22, 1994
9. Jones WE et al: Multinucleate cell angiohistiocytoma: an acquired vascular anomaly to be distinguished from Kaposi's sarcoma. Br J Dermatol. 122(5):651-63, 1990
10. Smolle J et al: Multinucleate cell angiohistiocytoma: a clinicopathological, immunohistochemical and ultrastructural study. Br J Dermatol. 121(1):113-21, 1989

IMAGE GALLERY

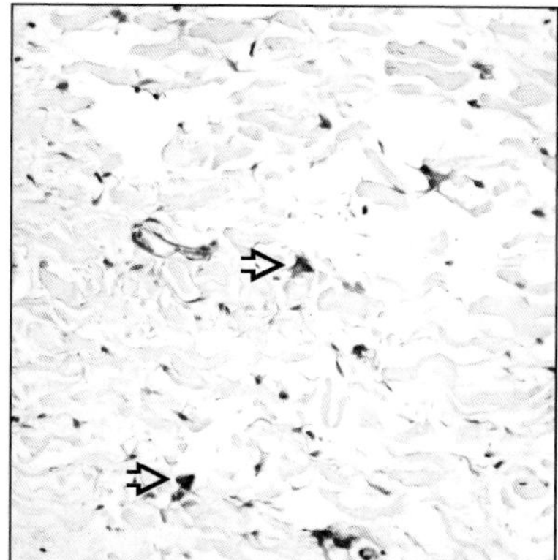
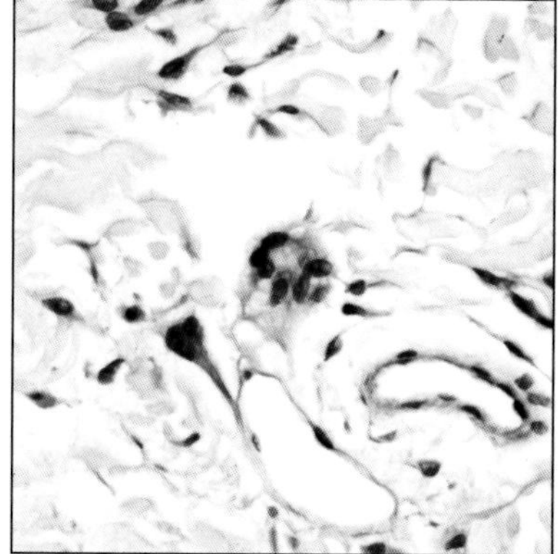
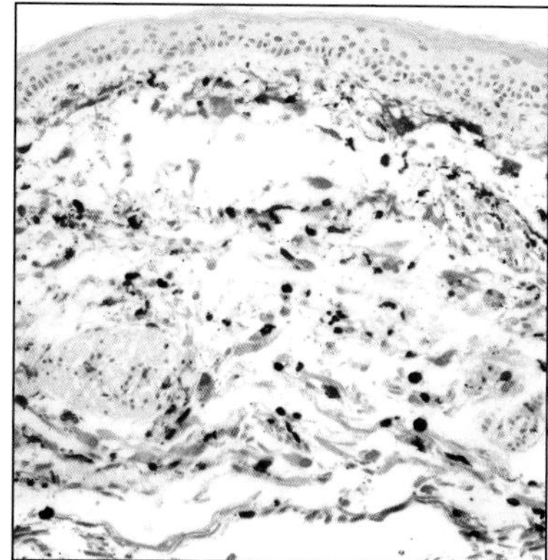

*(**Left**) Histologic section shows scattered enlarged multinucleated cells ➡ with nuclear hyperchromasia. (**Center**) High-power examination of the multinucleated cells shows clumping or a wreath-like arrangement of the nuclei. (**Right**) FXIIIA immunohistochemistry shows strong cytoplasmic staining of many of the lesional cells.*

DERMATOFIBROSARCOMA PROTUBERANS

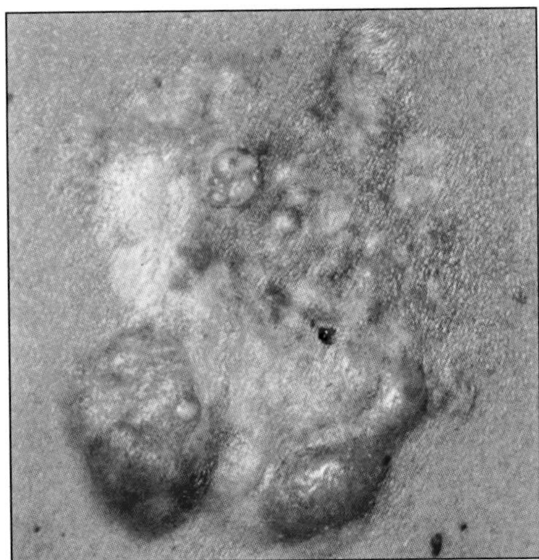

Dermatofibrosarcoma protuberans is characterized clinically by an exophytic, multinodular growth in most cases.

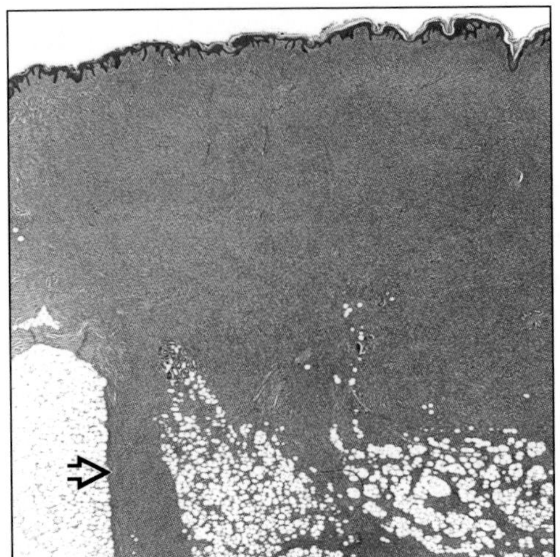

Low-power view of a dermatofibrosarcoma protuberans shows the characteristic diffuse infiltration of subcutaneous fat by neoplastic cells that grow along fibrous septa ➡.

TERMINOLOGY

Abbreviations

- Dermatofibrosarcoma protuberans (DFSP)

Definitions

- Superficially located low-grade fibroblastic sarcoma
- Can progress to fibrosarcomatous dermatofibrosarcoma protuberans

CLINICAL ISSUES

Epidemiology

- Incidence
  - Rare neoplasm
  - One of most frequent superficially located sarcomas
- Age
  - Young adults
  - Rare in childhood or older age
- Gender
  - Slight male predominance

Site

- Trunk (chest, back, shoulder, abdominal wall)
- Proximal extremities > distal extremities
- Head and neck region
- Rare in genital areas

Presentation

- Slowly growing nodular dermal neoplasm
- Often history of slow but persistent growth
- Can show rapid enlargement due to tumor progression
- Can show rapid enlargement in pregnancy
- Rarely plaque-like growth

Treatment

- Surgical approaches
  - Wide excision (2-3 cm)
- Adjuvant therapy
  - Imatinib treatment in advanced and metastatic cases

Prognosis

- Locally aggressive growth
- Increased number of often repeated local recurrences
- Metastases extremely rare (< 0.5%)
- May progress to fibrosarcomatous DFSP

MACROSCOPIC FEATURES

General Features

- Indurated dermal plaques
- 1 or more tumor nodules
  - Multiple protuberant tumors are often seen in recurrent cases
- Firm gray-white cut surface
- Usually no tumor necrosis
- Rarely subcutaneous

Sections to Be Submitted

- Numerous sections have to be submitted
- Resection margins have to be carefully assessed

Size

- May reach considerable size

MICROSCOPIC PATHOLOGY

Histologic Features

- Diffuse infiltration of dermis and subcutis
- Infiltration along fibrous septa of subcutaneous fat
  - Characteristic honeycomb pattern
  - Tumor cells encase skin appendages
- Storiform growth pattern
- Uniform spindled tumor cells
  - Plump spindled or elongated wavy nuclei
  - Only mild cytologic atypia, < 5 mitoses per 10 high-power fields
- Collagenous stroma with small vessels
- May contain pigmented melanocytic cells (pigmented DFSP, so-called Bednar tumor)

DERMATOFIBROSARCOMA PROTUBERANS

Key Facts

Terminology
- Dermatofibrosarcoma represents superficially located low-grade fibroblastic sarcoma that may show progression to fibrosarcomatous dermatofibrosarcoma protuberans

Clinical Issues
- Young adults
- Rare in childhood
- Trunk (chest, back, shoulder, abdominal wall)
- Proximal > distal extremities > head/neck region
- Slowly growing nodular dermal neoplasm
- Wide excision is necessary
- Imatinib treatment in advanced and metastatic cases
- Increased number of often repeated local recurrences
- Metastases are extremely rare (< 0.5%)
- May show progression to fibrosarcomatous DFSP

Microscopic Pathology
- Diffuse infiltration of dermis and subcutis
- Infiltration along fibrous septa of subcutaneous fat
- Characteristic honeycomb infiltration of subcutaneous fat
- Storiform growth
- Uniform spindled tumor cells
- Homogeneous expression of CD34
- Giant cell fibroblastoma
  - Hypocellular neoplasms with angiectoid spaces and multinucleated giant cells
- Fibrosarcomatous DFSP
  - Abrupt or gradual transition
  - Cellular spindle cell fascicles with increased atypia and proliferative activity

- May show prominent myxoid changes (myxoid DFSP)
- May contain bundles and nests of myofibroblastic cells (DFSP with myoid differentiation)
- May rarely show flat, plaque-like growth (plaque-like DFSP, atrophic DFSP)
- May rarely show granular cell changes (granular DFSP)

Margins
- Ill defined, infiltrative

Predominant Pattern/Injury Type
- Diffuse

Predominant Cell/Compartment Type
- Spindle
- Fibroblast

Giant Cell Fibroblastoma
- Primarily affects children in 1st decade of life, rarely adults
- Strong male predilection
- Locally aggressive neoplasm, frequent local recurrence
- Metastases have not been reported yet
- Hypocellular, with myxoid to collagenous stroma
- Spindled tumor cells and scattered mono- &/or multinucleated giant cells
- Irregular branching angiectoid spaces

Fibrosarcomatous DFSP
- Represents morphologic form of progression (grade 2 malignancy)
  - 10-15% metastasize, and sometimes cause death
- Occurs de novo or more rarely in local recurrence
- Abrupt or gradual fibrosarcomatous transformation
- Often nodular, rather well-circumscribed growth
- Cells arranged in cellular "herringbone" fascicles
- Increased atypia and mitotic index
- Increased p53 expression

ANCILLARY TESTS

Immunohistochemistry
- CD34 diffusely positive
  - Can be lost in fibrosarcomatous transformation
- CD99 can be weakly positive
- Apoprotein D(+)
- SMA(-) except in myoid nodules
- S100 protein(-) except in pigmented cells (Bednar)
- EMA sometimes positive in cytoplasm
- Cytokeratin(-)
- Desmin(-)

Molecular Genetics
- Characteristic translocation t(17;22)(q22;q13)
  - *COL1A1-PDGFB* fusion product
- Ring chromosomes in some cases
- Neoplastic cells have also PDGFB receptors on cell surface
  - Autocrine stimulation of tumor cell growth

Electron Microscopy
- No specific features
- "Satellite" nuclei
- Fragments of external lamina

DIFFERENTIAL DIAGNOSIS

(Cellular) Dermatofibroma (Fibrous Histiocytoma)
- Very common lesion
- Most lesions occur on distal extremities
- Single papules, nodules
- Epidermal hyperplasia, hyperpigmentation
- Stellate appearance
- Polymorphous cellular infiltrate
- Focal (radial) infiltration of subcutis
- CD34(-) (focal peripheral positivity in cellular examples)

Dermatomyofibroma
- Superficial, plaque-like dermal neoplasms
- Elongated spindled cells with myofibroblastic features
- Cells oriented parallel to surface
- Tumor cells grow around adnexal structures
- Increased number of small elastic fibers

DERMATOFIBROSARCOMA PROTUBERANS

Diffuse Neurofibroma

- Short spindle cells without storiform pattern
- Presence of Meissner-like corpuscles is common
- S100 protein diffusely positive
- CD34 focally positive

Extraneural Spindle Cell Perineurioma

- Elongated tumor cells with thin, elongated cytoplasmic processes
- Often perivascular whorls
- EMA(+) and claudin-1(+)
- CD34(+) in some cases
- Electron microscopy is diagnostic
  - Continuous externa lamina
  - Pinocytotic vesicles

Collagenous Fibroma

- Well-circumscribed, nodular dermal neoplasm
- Low cellularity
- Characteristic stromal sclerosis
  - Laminated "plywood" pattern

Pilar Leiomyoma

- Bundles and nests of eosinophilic spindled cells
- Deep eosinophilic, often fibrillary cytoplasm
- Cigar-shaped nuclei
  - Rectangular rather than tapered outline
- Expression of actin and desmin
- CD34(-)

Plaque-like CD34(+) Dermal Fibroma

- Benign superficial plaque-like proliferation
- Tumor cells spare adnexal structures
- Does not show molecular changes of DFSP
- Benign clinical behavior

Pleomorphic Dermal Sarcoma NOS (So-called "MFH")

- Pleomorphic tumor cells
- Numerous multinucleated tumor giant cells
- Diffuse nuclear atypia and atypical mitoses
- Areas of tumor necrosis

Malignant Peripheral Nerve Sheath Tumor

- Rare in superficial location
- Associated neurofibroma may be present
- Wavy spindle cells
- Variable nuclear pleomorphism
- Focal expression of S100 in half of cases
- Only focal CD34 expression

Spindle Cell (Desmoplastic) Malignant Melanoma

- Often in actinically damaged skin in elderly patients
- Often associated with lentigo maligna
- Homogeneous expression of S100

DIAGNOSTIC CHECKLIST

Pathologic Interpretation Pearls

- Storiform growth of relatively bland spindled tumor cells
- Characteristic diffuse infiltration of subcutis
- Homogeneous expression of CD34
- Characteristic molecular changes
- Fibrosarcomatous change identified by
  - Fascicular instead of storiform architecture
  - Increased mitoses, often > 10 per 10 high-power fields

SELECTED REFERENCES

1. Llombart B et al: Dermatofibrosarcoma protuberans: clinical, pathological, and genetic (COL1A1-PDGFB) study with therapeutic implications. Histopathology. 54(7):860-72, 2009
2. Bague S et al: Dermatofibrosarcoma protuberans presenting as a subcutaneous mass: a clinicopathological study of 15 cases with exclusive or near-exclusive subcutaneous involvement. Am J Dermatopathol. 30(4):327-32, 2008
3. Handolias D et al: Imatinib as effective therapy for dermatofibrosarcoma protuberans: proof of concept of the autocrine hypothesis for cancer. Future Oncol. 4(2):211-7, 2008
4. Jha P et al: Giant cell fibroblastoma: an update and addition of 86 new cases from the Armed Forces Institute of Pathology, in honor of Dr. Franz M. Enzinger. Ann Diagn Pathol. 11(2):81-8, 2007
5. Reimann JD et al: Myxoid dermatofibrosarcoma protuberans: a rare variant analyzed in a series of 23 cases. Am J Surg Pathol. 31(9):1371-7, 2007
6. Linn SC et al: Gene expression patterns and gene copy number changes in dermatofibrosarcoma protuberans. Am J Pathol. 163(6):2383-95, 2003
7. Terrier-Lacombe MJ et al: Dermatofibrosarcoma protuberans, giant cell fibroblastoma, and hybrid lesions in children: clinicopathologic comparative analysis of 28 cases with molecular data--a study from the French Federation of Cancer Centers Sarcoma Group. Am J Surg Pathol. 27(1):27-39, 2003
8. Bowne WB et al: Dermatofibrosarcoma protuberans: A clinicopathologic analysis of patients treated and followed at a single institution. Cancer. 88(12):2711-20, 2000
9. Goldblum JR et al: Sarcomas arising in dermatofibrosarcoma protuberans: a reappraisal of biologic behavior in eighteen cases treated by wide local excision with extended clinical follow up. Am J Surg Pathol. 24(8):1125-30, 2000
10. Davis DA et al: Atrophic and plaquelike dermatofibrosarcoma protuberans. Am J Dermatopathol. 20(5):498-501, 1998
11. Mentzel T et al: Fibrosarcomatous ("high-grade") dermatofibrosarcoma protuberans: clinicopathologic and immunohistochemical study of a series of 41 cases with emphasis on prognostic significance. Am J Surg Pathol. 22(5):576-87, 1998
12. Calonje E et al: Myoid differentiation in dermatofibrosarcoma protuberans and its fibrosarcomatous variant: clinicopathologic analysis of 5 cases. J Cutan Pathol. 23(1):30-6, 1996

Microscopic Features and Ancillary Techniques

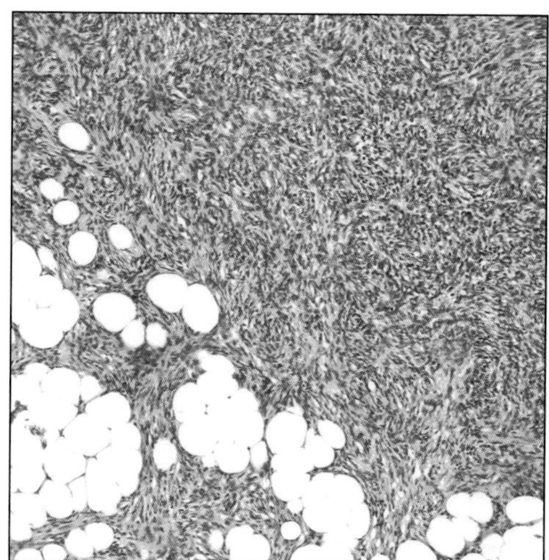

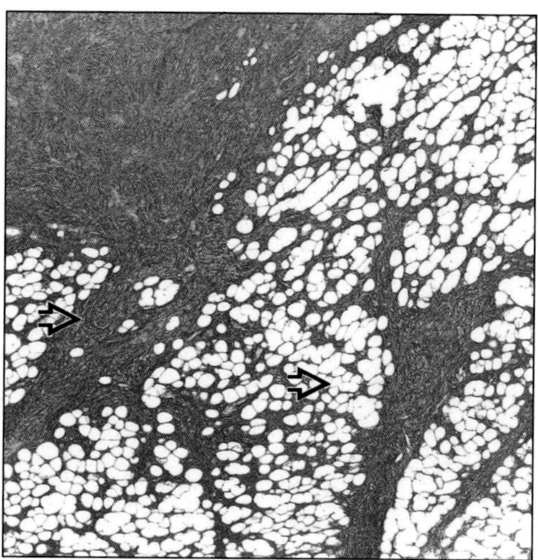

(Left) *The neoplastic spindled tumor cells are arranged in a storiform growth pattern and contain an ill-defined, pale eosinophilic cytoplasm and elongated fusiform nuclei.* ***(Right)*** *Neoplastic cells in DFSP stain homogeneously positive for CD34. Note the tumor cell growth along preexisting fibrous septa* ⇨.

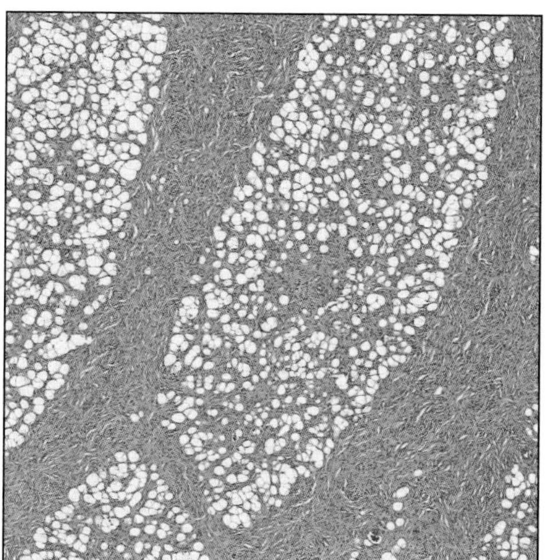

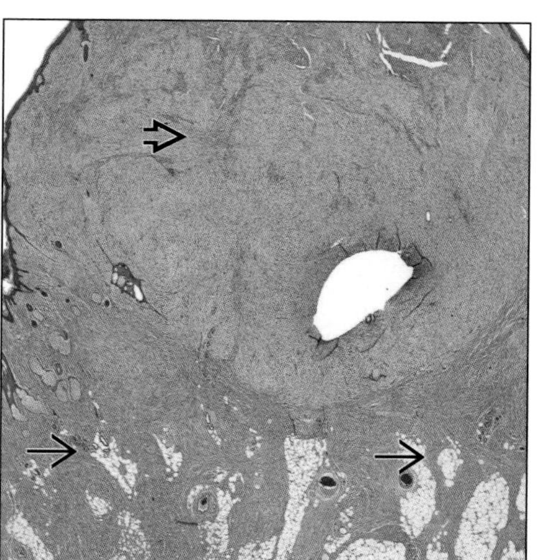

(Left) *A characteristic diffuse infiltration of subcutaneous fat is seen in the DFSP areas at the base of the neoplasm. This honeycombing pattern is much more extensive than in dermatofibroma, in which there are typically short radial extensions into fat.* ***(Right)*** *A case of DFSP with superficially located myofibroblastic differentiation is seen. On top, spindled myofibroblastic cells are noted* ⇨*, whereas diffuse infiltration by DFSP-like areas is seen in deeper parts of the neoplasm* →.

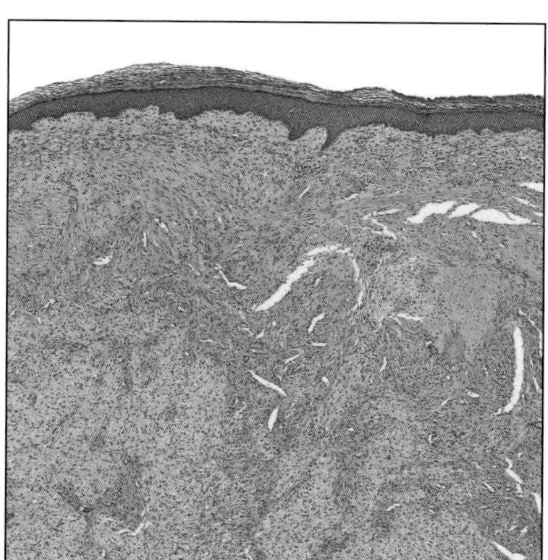

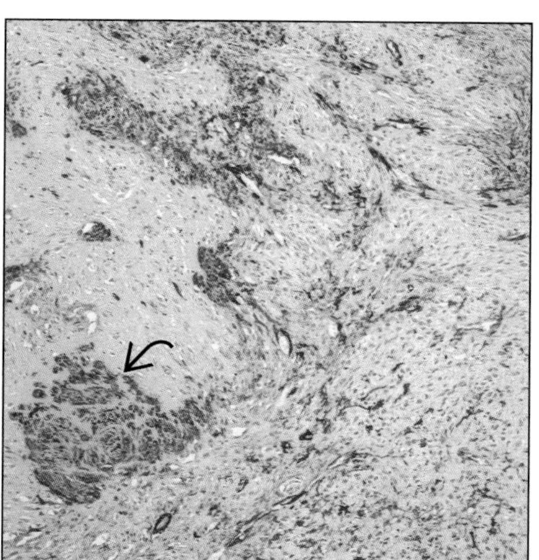

(Left) *DFSP with myofibroblastic differentiation is shown. The myofibroblastic cells are arranged in ill-defined bundles and nodules and set in a myxohyaline stroma.* ***(Right)*** *The myofibroblastic component* ↶ *stains positively for smooth muscle actin. It is negative for CD34, which is demonstrable in the adjacent dermatofibrosarcomatous component.*

DERMATOFIBROSARCOMA PROTUBERANS

Clinical and Microscopic Features

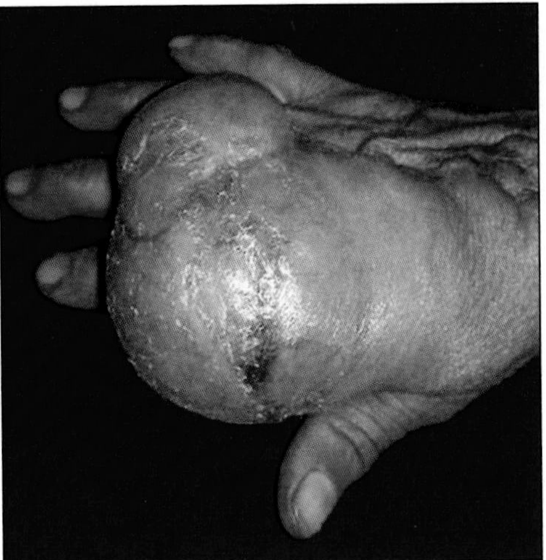

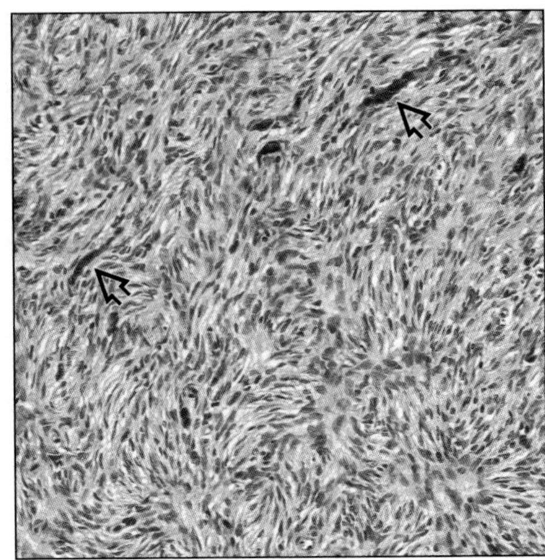

(Left) *Clinical photograph shows a case of a recurrent DFSP with associated pigmented melanocytic cells (pigmented DFSP).* ***(Right)*** *In addition to spindled fibroblastic tumor cells, scattered elongated pigmented melanocytic cells are seen ⊳. This is known as Bednar tumor. The finding is of no prognostic significance. Similar cells can be found in fibrosarcomatous DFSP and in giant cell fibroblastoma.*

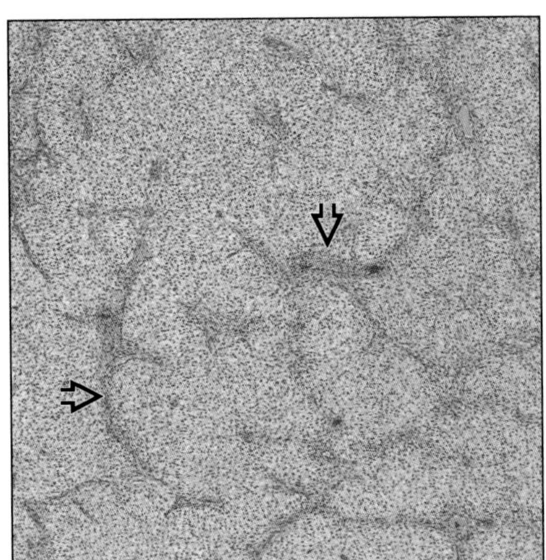

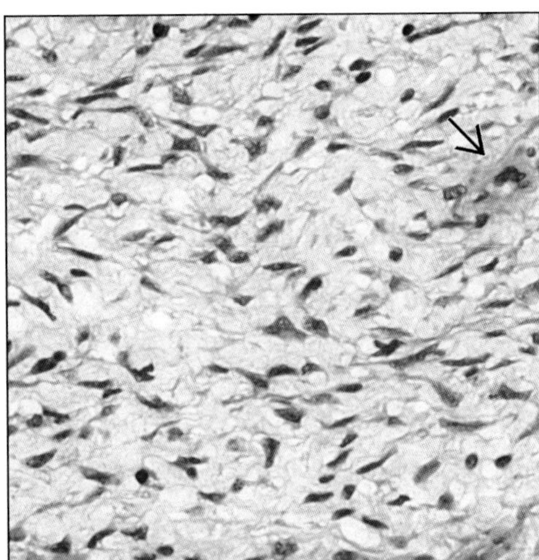

(Left) *Myxoid DFSP is a rare variant characterized by prominent myxoid stromal changes. Note the numerous blood vessels with slightly fibrosed walls ⊳. A more typical nonmyxoid pattern is sometimes seen focally.* ***(Right)*** *Myxoid dermatofibrosarcoma shows stellate or spindle cells in a myxoid stroma. There is a residual storiform pattern, although the cells are widely separated by the stroma material. A blood vessel is seen with a thickened wall →.*

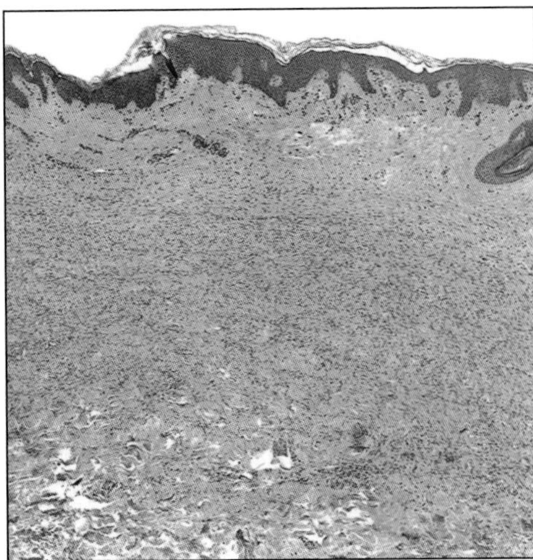

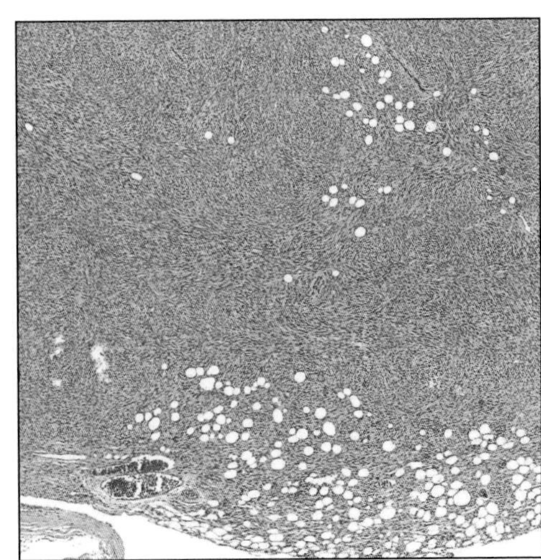

(Left) *Rare cases of plaque-like DFSP show a plaque-like growth of bland spindled tumor cells. These neoplasms are easily misdiagnosed as benign mesenchymal neoplasms.* ***(Right)*** *Fibrosarcomatous DFSP shows tumor areas with at least focally increased cellularity, increased nuclear atypia, and increased proliferative activity. This change can be abrupt or gradual.*

Microscopic Features and Ancillary Techniques

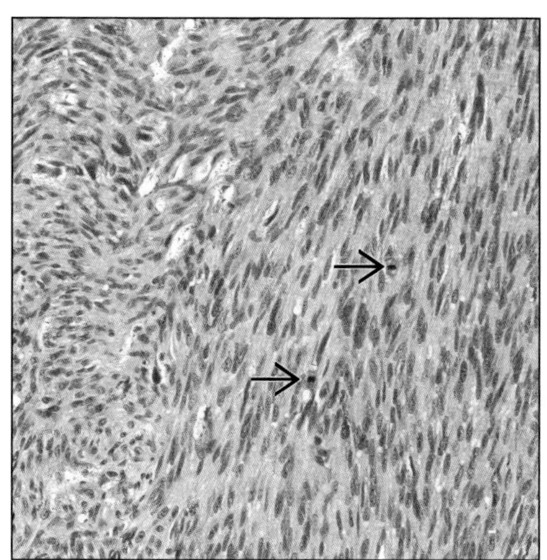

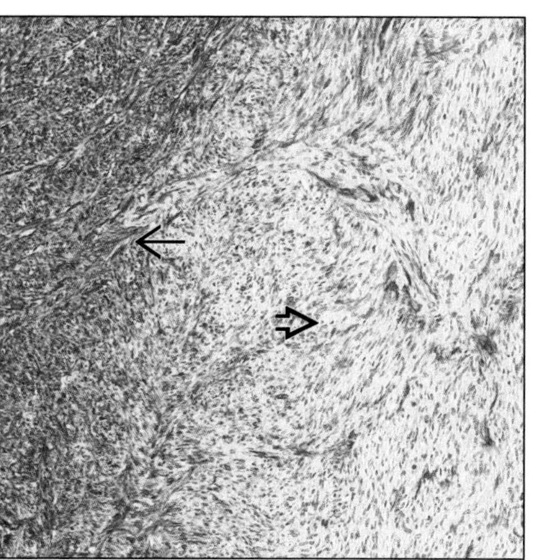

(Left) *Tumor cells in fibrosarcomatous areas contain enlarged nuclei. An increased number of mitotic figures is usually seen ⇒, but necrosis is rare.* ***(Right)*** *Focal loss of CD34 expression ⇨ is seen in a number of cases of fibrosarcomatous DFSP, compared with the residual adjacent dermatofibrosarcoma ⇒. However, some cases retain diffuse CD34 immunoreactivity.*

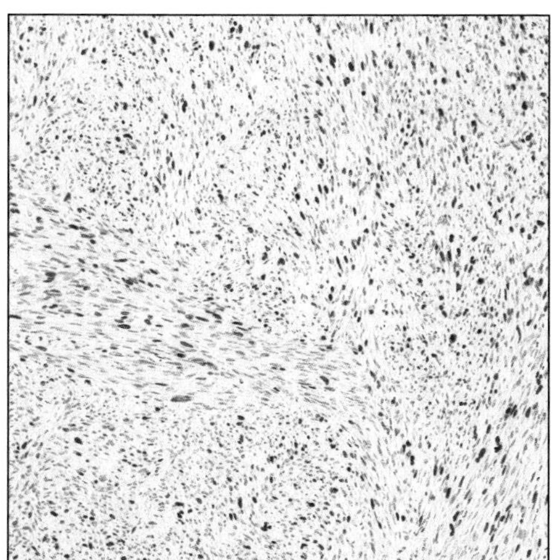

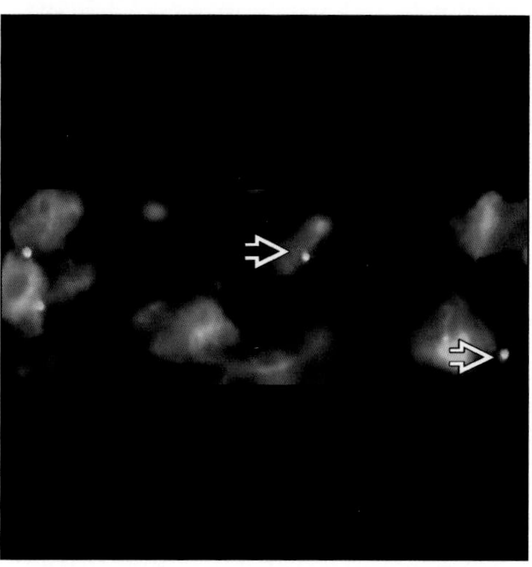

(Left) *Ki-67 antibodies highlight the increased proliferative activity in fibrosarcomatous areas.* ***(Right)*** *FISH analysis of DFSP shows the characteristic 17;22 translocation. Green BACs labeling the region on chromosome 22 are fused with red BACs labeling the region on chromosome 17 ⇨.*

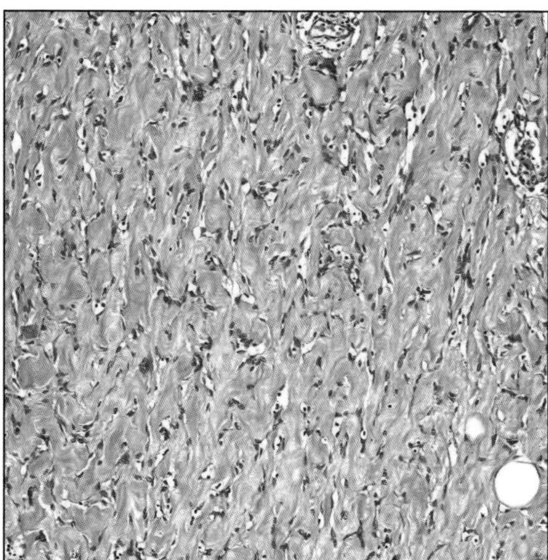

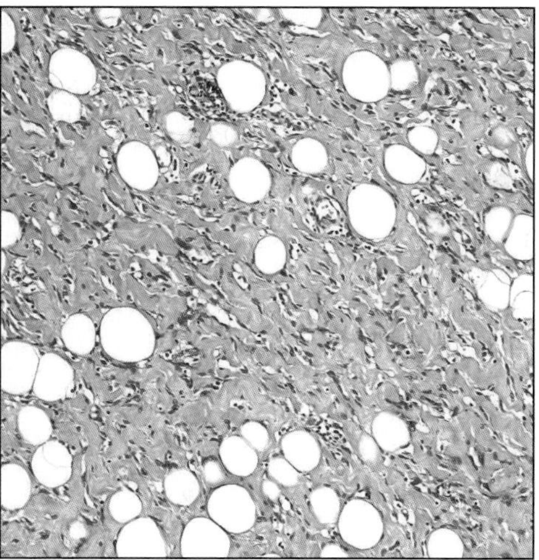

(Left) *Giant cell fibroblastoma is composed of spindled and multinucleated giant cells set in a collagenous stroma. Note the numerous narrow pseudovascular spaces lined by neoplastic (not endothelial) cells.* ***(Right)*** *Diffuse infiltration of subcutaneous tissue is seen in many examples of giant cell fibroblastoma, such as this case.*

PLEXIFORM FIBROHISTIOCYTIC TUMOR

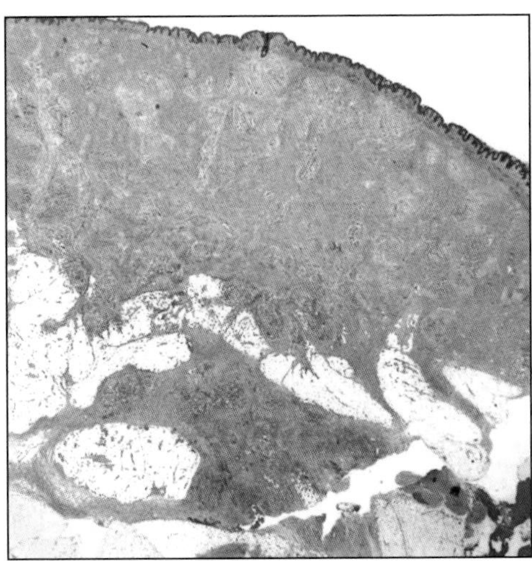

Hematoxylin & eosin shows plexiform fibrohistiocytic tumor (PFHT) at the dermal subcutaneous interface with a plexiform appearance. Note the extensions into the dermis and subcutis.

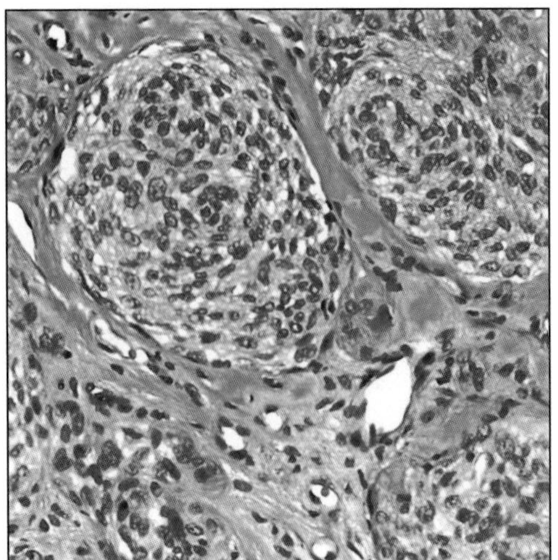

Hematoxylin & eosin shows a dermal ball-like growth pattern of histiocytoid cells (plexiform) as part of a histiocytic-type of PFHT.

TERMINOLOGY

Abbreviations

- Plexiform fibrohistiocytic tumor (PFT/PFHT)

Synonyms

- Debatably deep form of cellular neurothekeoma

Definitions

- Borderline tumor of fibrohistiocytic phenotype involving dermis and subcutis in infiltrative growth pattern, sparing adnexa

CLINICAL ISSUES

Epidemiology

- Incidence
  - Rare
- Age
  - Children and young adults
  - Range: 1-77 years; median: 20 years
- Gender
  - Slight male predominance

Site

- Upper extremity is most common site
- Followed by lower extremities and trunk
- Rare in head and neck

Presentation

- Subcutaneous mass

Treatment

- Wide excision with careful patient follow-up
  - Examination of regional lymph nodes, possibly chest imaging

Prognosis

- Low metastatic potential, usually only to regional lymph nodes
- Usually no systemic metastases, except in 1 case to lung

MACROSCOPIC FEATURES

General Features

- Often nodular protuberant lesions, involving dermis and subcutis

MICROSCOPIC PATHOLOGY

Histologic Features

- Dermal-subcutaneous interface
- Infiltrative growth pattern
- Morphologically divided into 3 groups
  - Fibroblastic
  - Histiocytic with osteoclast-type giant cells
  - Mixed
- Cannonball-like or plexiform arrangement of cells
- Occasional metaplastic bone formation
- Absence of cellular pleomorphism
- Low mitotic activity, occasional pleomorphism
- Dense hyalinization, occasional myxoid change
- Hemorrhage and chronic inflammation observed

Predominant Pattern/Injury Type

- Infiltrative

Predominant Cell/Compartment Type

- Mesenchymal, fibrohistiocytic

Immunohistochemistry

- Positive for SMA in fibroblasts and CD68 (and CD163) in histiocytes
- S100 protein, CD34, desmin, cytokeratin, FVIIIRAg, and lysozyme negative
- Nonspecific markers of cellular neurothekeoma, PGP-9.5, S100-A6, MITF, NK1C3 (CD57) may be positive

PLEXIFORM FIBROHISTIOCYTIC TUMOR

Key Facts

Terminology

- Borderline tumor of fibrohistiocytic phenotype with histiocytic and osteoclast-type giant cells rich; cannonball-like pattern &/or spindled fibroblastic pattern, involving dermis and subcutis in infiltrative growth pattern and sparing adnexa

Microscopic Pathology

- Dermal subcutaneous border
- Infiltrative growth pattern
- Cannonball growth pattern
- Histiocytic with osteoclast type giant cells
- Fibroblastic, spindled
- SMA(+) fibroblastic
- CD68(+) histiocytic

Top Differential Diagnoses

- May be on spectrum with cellular neurothekeoma
  - PFHT involves subcutis rather than just dermis
  - PFHT on extremities and trunk rather than face

DIFFERENTIAL DIAGNOSIS

Giant Cell Tumor of Soft Parts

- Multinodular
- Bland
- Osteoclast-type giant cells
- Not infiltrative
- Lacks spindled pattern

Nodular Fasciitis

- Nodular
- Fascial based
- Myxoid degeneration and extravasation of erythrocytes
- Not plexiform

Fibromatosis

- Infiltrative
- Deep, into skeletal muscle
- Elongate vessels
- β-catenin(+)

Myofibromatosis

- Smooth muscle and hemangiopericytoma-like areas
- Usually face or deep
- Lacks giant cells and plexiform pattern

Fibrous Hamartoma of Infancy

- Spindled component infiltrates fat
- Also has immature mesenchymal and collagenous components
- Axillary in newborns

Cutaneous Pilar Leiomyoma

- Plexiform pattern
- Intersecting fascicles
- Desmin(+)

Cellular Neurothekeoma

- Related or identical lesion to PFHT
- Usually younger children
- Usually face
- Usually dermal only

SELECTED REFERENCES

1. Moosavi C et al: An update on plexiform fibrohistiocytic tumor and addition of 66 new cases from the Armed Forces Institute of Pathology, in honor of Franz M. Enzinger, MD. Ann Diagn Pathol. 11(5):313-9, 2007
2. Remstein ED et al: Plexiform fibrohistiocytic tumor: clinicopathologic analysis of 22 cases. Am J Surg Pathol. 23(6):662-70, 1999
3. Fisher C: Atypical plexiform fibrohistiocytic tumour. Histopathology. 30(3):271-3, 1997
4. Hollowood K et al: Plexiform fibrohistiocytic tumour: clinicopathological, immunohistochemical and ultrastructural analysis in favour of a myofibroblastic lesion. Histopathology. 19(6):503-13, 1991
5. Enzinger FM et al: Plexiform fibrohistiocytic tumor presenting in children and young adults. An analysis of 65 cases. Am J Surg Pathol. 12(11):818-26, 1988

IMAGE GALLERY

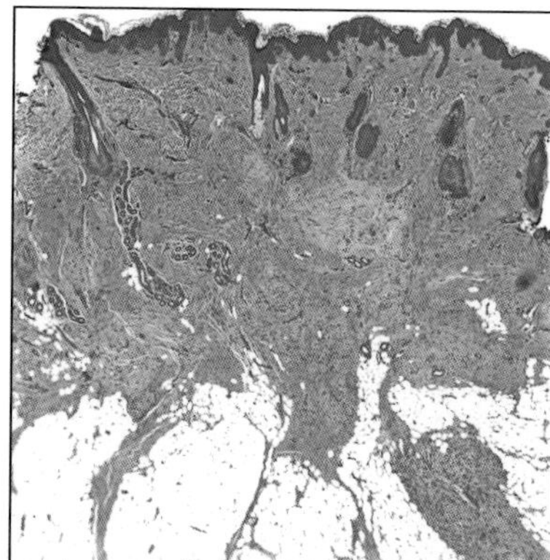
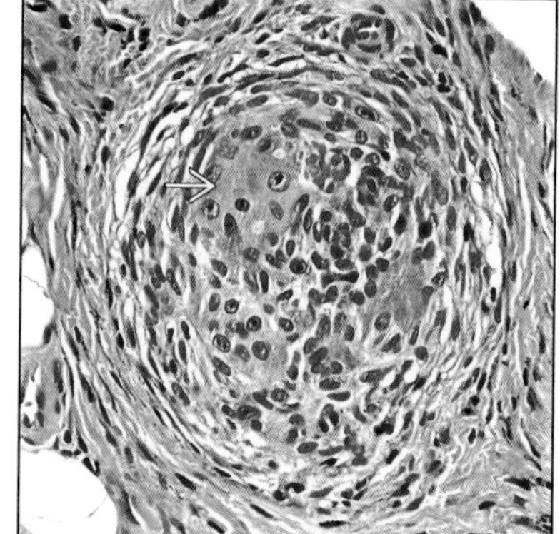
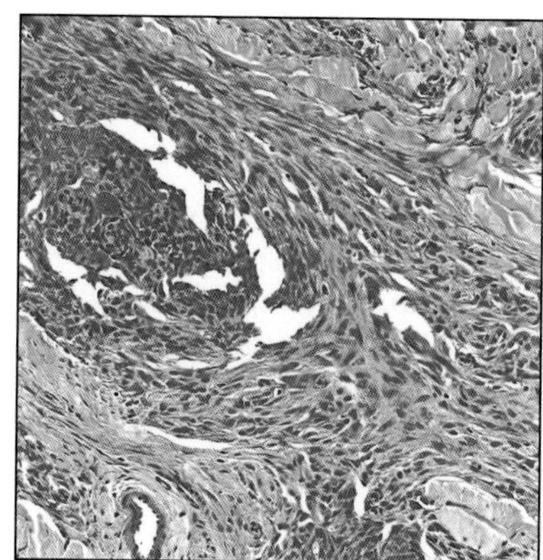

*(**Left**) Hematoxylin & eosin shows that the lesion is present at the dermal subcutaneous interface, with a ball-like and infiltrative growth pattern. The balls are usually histiocytic, and the infiltrative component is fibroblastic. (**Center**) Hematoxylin & eosin shows balls of histiocytoid cells with osteoclast-type giant cells ➡. Giant cell tumor of soft parts is similar but has fewer giant cells and is less infiltrative. (**Right**) Hematoxylin & eosin shows a mixed-type of PFHT that has both balls (histiocytic) and sheets (fibroblastic) of plexiform and infiltrative tumor cells.*

GIANT CELL TUMOR OF SOFT TISSUE

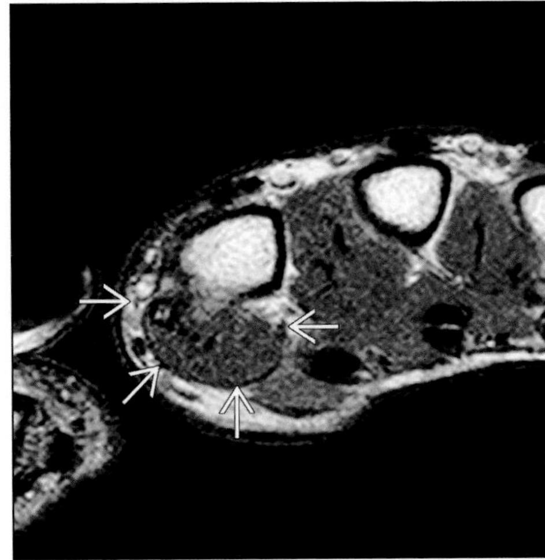

Giant cell tumor of soft tissue presents as an extraskeletal soft tissue tumor, depicted in this MR image by a well-circumscribed mass arising in the index finger ➡ of a 21-year-old man.

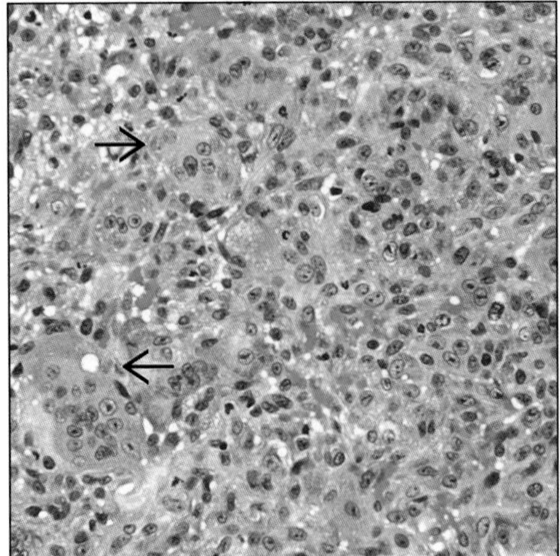

Microscopically, giant cell tumor of soft tissue is identical to giant cell tumor of bone composed of mononuclear stromal cells and multinuclear osteoclastic giant cells ➡ that are uniformly distributed throughout the tumor.

TERMINOLOGY

Abbreviations

- Giant cell tumor of soft tissue (GCTST)

Synonyms

- Soft tissue giant cell tumor of low malignant potential
- Extraskeletal giant cell tumor
- Osteoclastoma of soft tissue

Definitions

- Benign soft tissue neoplasm composed of mononuclear stromal cells, osteoclastic giant cells, and metaplastic bone
  - Microscopically identical to giant cell tumor of bone

CLINICAL ISSUES

Epidemiology

- Incidence
  - Rare, exact incidence unknown
  - Associated with Paget disease of bone
    - Can be multifocal
- Age
  - Average: Around 40 years
    - Wide range: 1-86 years
- Gender
  - Women = men

Site

- Arm, thigh, and calf most common sites
  - Others: Hand, finger, shoulder, foot, buttock, groin, hip, head and neck, abdominal wall, chest wall, flank, back, ischiorectal fossa, presacral, peripancreatic
- Superficial (subcutaneous) in 2/3
- Deep (subfascial) in 1/3

Presentation

- Painless mass

Natural History

- Benign
- Local recurrence in around 10%
- No established reports of metastasis

Treatment

- Surgical approaches
  - Complete local excision

Prognosis

- Very good

IMAGE FINDINGS

Radiographic Findings

- Soft tissue mass
- Peripheral mineralization in some
- Deep-seated tumors can saucerize underlying bone

MACROSCOPIC FEATURES

General Features

- Most tumors well circumscribed
- Multinodular
- Red-brown
- Peripheral rim of ossification in 1/2
- Hemorrhagic cystic spaces

Size

- Average size: 3.5 cm
  - Range: 0.7-10 cm

MICROSCOPIC PATHOLOGY

Histologic Features

- Well circumscribed
- Multinodular with fibrous septa
- Peripheral rim of metaplastic ossification
  - Can extend into center of tumor

GIANT CELL TUMOR OF SOFT TISSUE

Key Facts

Terminology
- Benign soft tissue neoplasm composed of mononuclear stromal cells, osteoclastic giant cells, and metaplastic bone
- Microscopically identical to giant cell tumor of bone

Clinical Issues
- Average age: Around 40 years; wide range: 1-86 years
- Arm, thigh, and calf most common sites
- Superficial (subcutaneous) in 2/3
- Local recurrence in around 10%
- No established reports of metastasis

Macroscopic Features
- Average size: 3.5 cm

Microscopic Pathology
- Well circumscribed
- Multinodular with fibrous septa
- Peripheral rim of metaplastic ossification
- Hemorrhage and cystic hemorrhage
- Mononuclear stromal cells
  - Oval to spindle-shaped nuclei
  - No significant cytological atypia
- Osteoclastic giant cells
  - Evenly distributed throughout tumor

Top Differential Diagnoses
- Giant cell tumor of tendon sheath/diffuse-type giant cell tumor
- Undifferentiated pleomorphic sarcoma with giant cells
- Extraskeletal recurrence of giant cell tumor of bone

- Hemorrhage and cystic hemorrhage
  - Aneurysmal bone cyst-like changes
  - Hemosiderin
- Variable amount of stromal fibrosis
- Vascular invasion in 1/3

Cytologic Features
- Mononuclear stromal cells
  - Oval to spindle-shaped nuclei
  - Ill-defined cytoplasm and cytoplasmic boundaries
  - No significant cytological atypia
  - Mitoses readily identified
    - Average: Around 2-5/10 HPF
    - Rare cases with > 30/10 HPF
    - No atypical mitotic figures
- Osteoclastic giant cells
  - Evenly distributed throughout tumor
- Xanthoma cell (foamy macrophages) in some

ANCILLARY TESTS

Immunohistochemistry
- Stromal cells positive for CD68 and SMA
- Giant cells positive for CD68 and TRAP

DIFFERENTIAL DIAGNOSIS

Giant Cell Tumor of Tendon Sheath/Diffuse-type Giant Cell Tumor
- Synovial-based or intraarticular tumor
- More heterogeneous population of cells
  - Macrophages
    - Xanthoma cells and siderophages
  - Synoviocytes
    - Line villous extensions or intralesional clefts

Undifferentiated Pleomorphic Sarcoma with Giant Cells
- High-grade sarcoma with numerous osteoclastic giant cells
- Pleomorphic stromal cells, atypical mitotic figures, necrosis

Extraskeletal Recurrence of Giant Cell Tumor of Bone
- Grossly and microscopically indistinguishable from giant cell tumor of soft tissue
- Clinical history of giant cell tumor of bone

DIAGNOSTIC CHECKLIST

Clinically Relevant Pathologic Features
- Tissue distribution

Pathologic Interpretation Pearls
- Microscopically identical to giant cell tumor of bone
- Essential to distinguish GCTST from soft tissue sarcoma

SELECTED REFERENCES

1. O'Connell JX et al: Giant cell tumors of soft tissue: a clinicopathologic study of 18 benign and malignant tumors. Am J Surg Pathol. 24(3):386-95, 2000
2. Oliveira AM et al: Primary giant cell tumor of soft tissues: a study of 22 cases. Am J Surg Pathol. 24(2):248-56, 2000
3. Folpe AL et al: Soft tissue giant cell tumor of low malignant potential: a proposal for the reclassification of malignant giant cell tumor of soft parts. Mod Pathol. 12(9):894-902, 1999
4. Galed-Placed I et al: Giant-cell tumor in soft parts in a patient with osseous Paget's disease: diagnosis by fine-needle aspiration. Diagn Cytopathol. 19(5):352-4, 1998
5. Guccion JG et al: Malignant giant cell tumor of soft parts. An analysis of 32 cases. Cancer. 29(6):1518-29, 1972
6. Salm R et al: Giant-cell tumours of soft tissues. J Pathol. 107(1):27-39, 1972

GIANT CELL TUMOR OF SOFT TISSUE

Radiographic and Microscopic Features

(Left) Radiographically, GCTST presents as a soft tissue mass ➔. Although most occur in the subcutis, 1/3 involve the deep soft tissue, such as this tumor that saucerizes the clavicle ⇨. GCTST can be associated with Paget disease of bone, as in this 64-year-old man. **(Right)** Most often GCTST presents as a well-circumscribed mass. This low-power micrograph illustrates sharp demarcation of tumor ⇨ from overlying fibroadipose tissue by a thick fibrous pseudocapsule →.

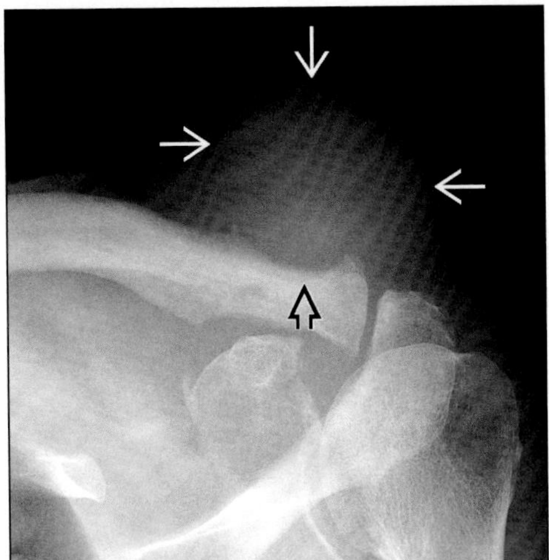

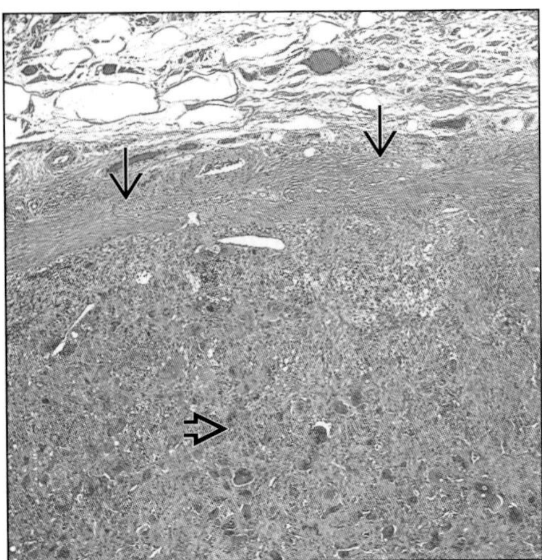

(Left) Most tumors have a multinodular architecture defined by fibrous septa → that divide it into cellular nodules ⇨. Giant cells ↩ are easily identified even at low power. **(Right)** Metaplastic ossification is present in approximately 1/2 of GCTST. It typically forms a peripheral rind of woven bone →. However, ossification can also extend into the center of the mass.

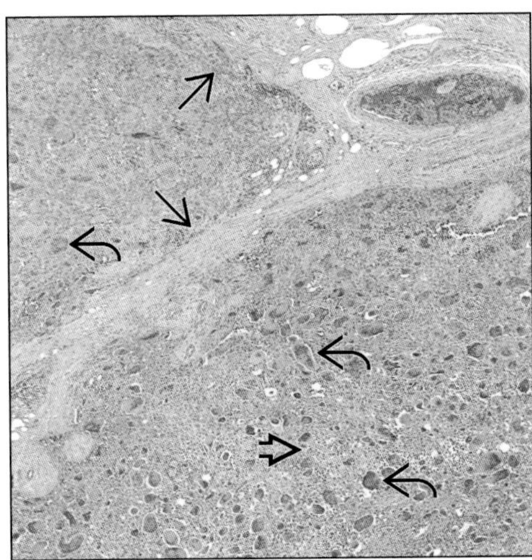

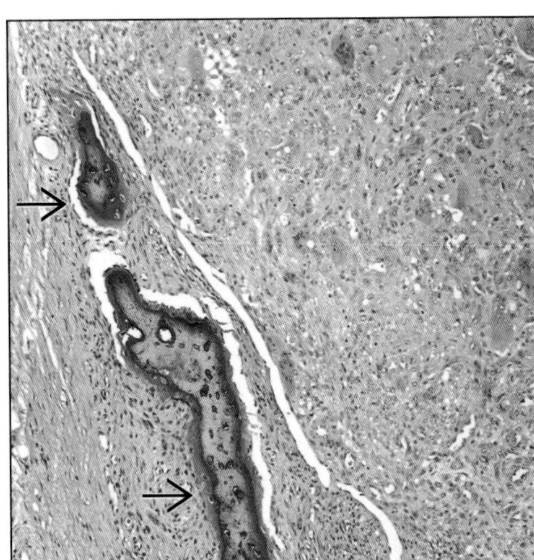

(Left) GCTST is composed of uniform mononuclear stromal cells with round to oval nuclei and ill-defined cytoplasmic borders →. Osteoclastic giant cells ⇨ are abundant and evenly distributed throughout the tumor. Although mitoses are readily identified in most tumors, none is atypical. **(Right)** Like giant cell tumor of bone, GCTST can have a storiform pattern depicted by short curvilinear fascicles of plump spindle cells that intersect within the center of the field.

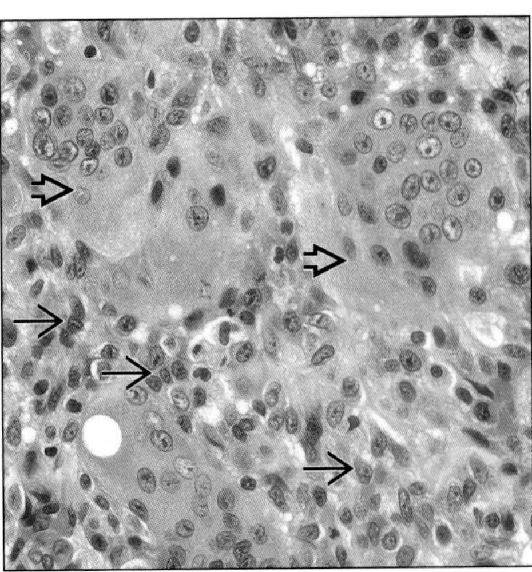

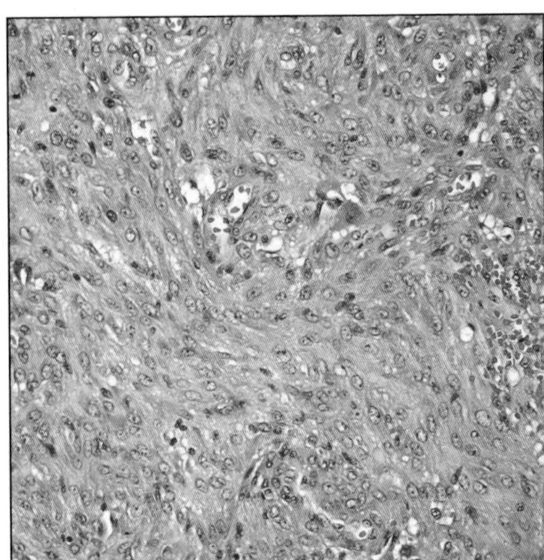

GIANT CELL TUMOR OF SOFT TISSUE

Microscopic Features

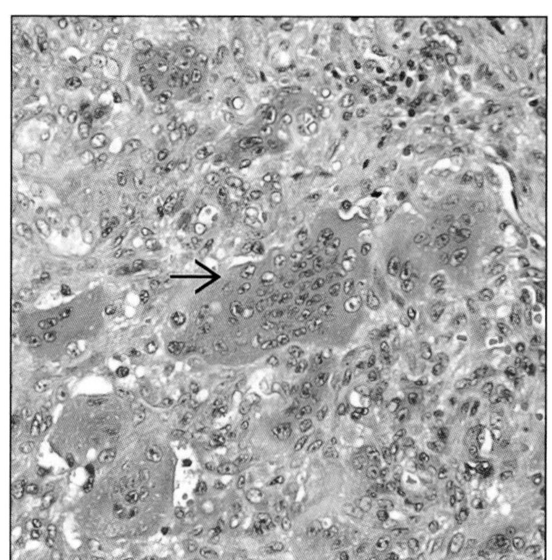

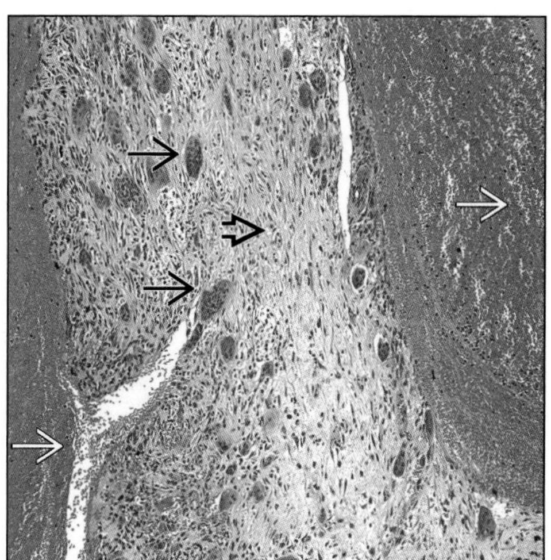

(Left) *As in giant cell tumor of bone, the osteoclastic giant cells in GCTST can be huge and harbor high numbers of nuclei* →. ***(Right)*** *Stromal hemorrhage is very common and presents as extravasated red blood cells, blood-filled cystic areas, or aneurysmal bone cyst-like change. This micrograph depicts aneurysmal bone cyst-like change in a giant cell tumor characterized by blood pools* ➡ *separated by an edematous fibrous trabecula* ⇨ *that contains giant cells* →.

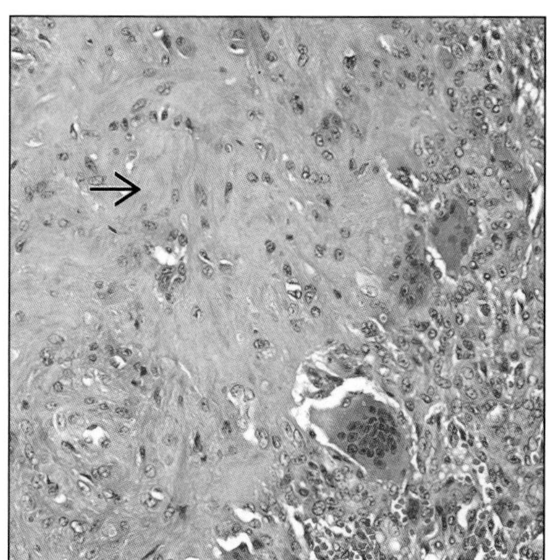

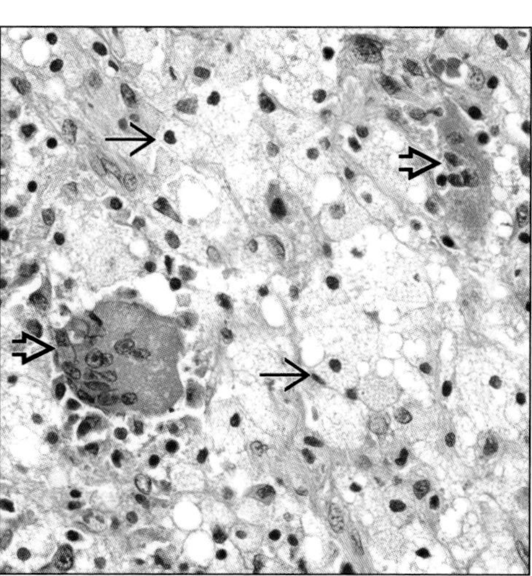

(Left) *Stromal fibrosis is common in GCTST. It can sometimes form large sheets of hyalinized collagenous matrix* →. ***(Right)*** *Areas containing sheets of xanthoma cells (foamy macrophages) can be seen in GCTST. These cells contain abundant phagocytized lipid material, which imparts a microvacuolar cytoplasm* →. *Here they are admixed with osteoclastic giant cells* ⇨.

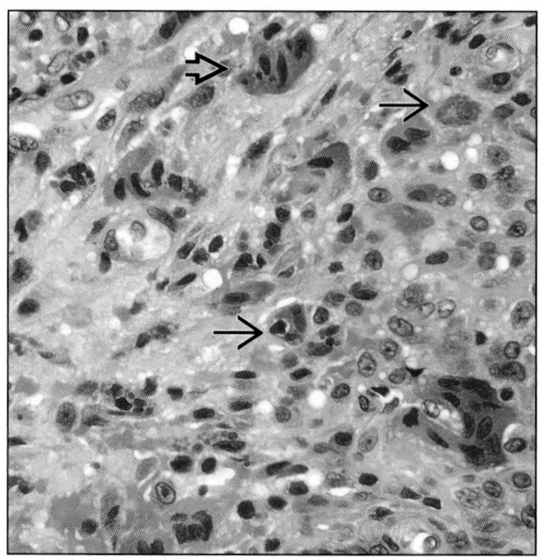

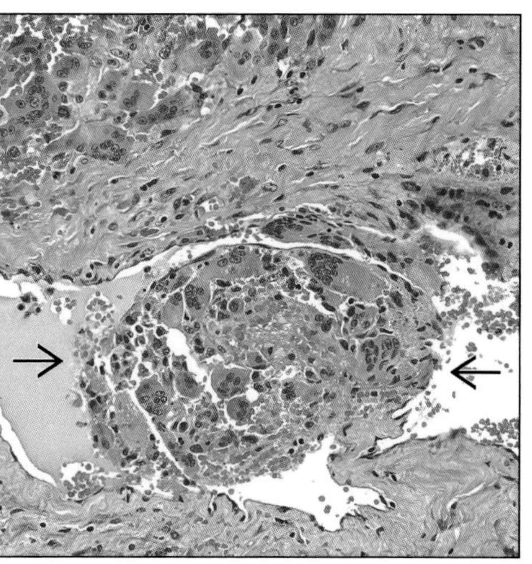

(Left) *Stromal hemorrhage is common in GCTST, as is hemosiderin deposition. This micrograph illustrates hemosiderin pigment within macrophages* → *as well as in osteoclastic giant cells* ⇨. ***(Right)*** *Vascular invasion* → *can be seen in approximately 1/3 of GCTST. As in giant cell tumor of bone, vascular invasion does not have prognostic value nor does it indicate an increased risk of metastasis.*

ATYPICAL FIBROXANTHOMA

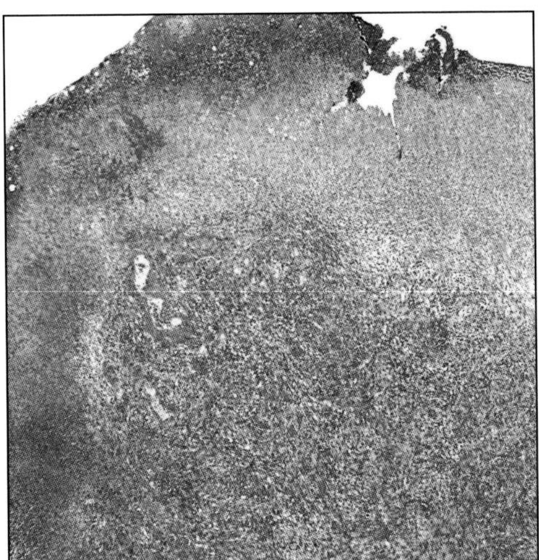

Histologic section at low magnification shows a large, dermal-based nodular tumor with overlying ulceration and serum crusting.

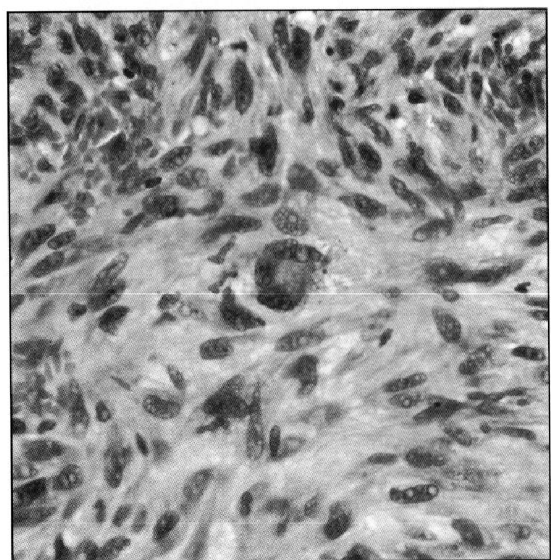

Histologic section at high magnification shows a proliferation of highly pleomorphic spindled and multinucleated tumor cells.

TERMINOLOGY

Abbreviations

- Atypical fibroxanthoma (AFX)

Synonyms

- Superficial malignant fibrous histiocytoma (MFH)/ pleomorphic sarcoma

Definitions

- Dermal-based, low-grade mesenchymal neoplasm showing no specific lineage of differentiation

ETIOLOGY/PATHOGENESIS

Environmental Exposure

- Likely related to UV exposure, as most cases occur in sun-damaged skin

CLINICAL ISSUES

Epidemiology

- Age
  - Typically occurs in elderly patients
- Gender
  - May have slight male predominance

Site

- Head and neck in general is most commonly affected area
  - Scalp is most common location
  - Pinna is most common site on ear

Presentation

- Skin nodule, asymptomatic in most cases
  - Dermal-based lesion
  - May show overlying ulceration or bleeding/crusting
- Regional lymph node metastases may be found in small number of cases

Treatment

- Surgical approaches
  - Complete and wide surgical excision
    - Mohs surgery is also effective
  - Unresectable or metastatic cases may be treated with chemoradiation

Prognosis

- Good
- Rate of local recurrence is low
  - < 10%
- Majority of cases do not metastasize
  - Cases with subcutaneous involvement are considered MFH and can metastasize

MACROSCOPIC FEATURES

General Features

- Large, nodular, unencapsulated, dermal-based tumors

MICROSCOPIC PATHOLOGY

Histologic Features

- Proliferation of markedly atypical and pleomorphic spindled and epithelioid-appearing cells
  - Variants include spindle cell, clear cell, granular, chondroid, and osteoid
  - Cytoplasm of tumor cells is abundant, eosinophilic, and sometimes foamy
- Scattered large, bizarre-appearing multinucleated giant cells
- Numerous mitoses, including highly atypical forms

Predominant Pattern/Injury Type

- Spindled

Predominant Cell/Compartment Type

- Mesenchymal

ATYPICAL FIBROXANTHOMA

Key Facts

Terminology
- Atypical fibroxanthoma (AFX)
- Dermal-based, low-grade mesenchymal neoplasm showing no specific lineage of differentiation

Clinical Issues
- Mass lesion, may be ulcerated or bleeding

Microscopic Pathology
- Highly atypical and pleomorphic proliferation of spindled to epithelioid-appearing cells
- Scattered large, bizarre-appearing multinucleated cells

Ancillary Tests
- Immunohistochemistry is key in confirming diagnosis
  - Essentially excluding specific diagnoses
- Negative for melanocytic markers, cytokeratins (especially HMWCKs), p63, muscle and vascular markers
- Positive for nonspecific markers including CD68, CD10, CD99, and vimentin

Top Differential Diagnoses
- Sarcomatoid carcinoma (typically SCC)
  - Metastatic carcinoma should be considered
- Spindle cell melanoma
- Leiomyosarcoma

Diagnostic Checklist
- Depth of involvement: Subcutaneous extension implies more aggressive behavior
- Poorly differentiated malignancies often showing bizarre tumor cells and nonspecific IHC findings

ANCILLARY TESTS

Immunohistochemistry
- IHC is key in confirming diagnosis
  - Essentially excluding specific diagnoses
- Positive for nonspecific markers, including CD68, CD10, CD99, and vimentin

Electron Microscopy
- Transitional forms from fibroblasts to large giant cells, with intermediate forms exhibiting features of both

DIFFERENTIAL DIAGNOSIS

Sarcomatoid Carcinoma
- Typically SCC, but metastatic poorly differentiated carcinoma should be considered
- Positive: High molecular weight cytokeratins (CK5/6, CK903) and p63 (especially primary cutaneous)
  - May or may not show staining for AE1/AE3, EMA, and CAM5.2

Spindle Cell and Desmoplastic Melanoma
- Junctional component may be present in some cases
- Positive: S100, ± Mart-1/Melan-A, HMB-45, tyrosinase, MITF

Leiomyosarcoma
- Positive: SMA, actin-sm, desmin (most cases)
  - Focal actin-sm in some AFXs, likely indicating myofibroblastic differentiation

Other Sarcomas
- Much less likely, including metastatic sarcoma
- Angiosarcoma: CD31(+), CD34(+)
  - Other vascular neoplasms are less likely
- Malignant peripheral nerve sheath tumor
  - Usually deep-seated lesions
  - Focal to weak S100(+) in 50-70% of cases

DIAGNOSTIC CHECKLIST

Clinically Relevant Pathologic Features
- Depth of involvement (subcutaneous extension implies more aggressive behavior)

Pathologic Interpretation Pearls
- Poorly differentiated malignancy often shows bizarre tumor cells and nonspecific IHC findings

SELECTED REFERENCES

1. Ang GC et al: More than 2 decades of treating atypical fibroxanthoma at mayo clinic: what have we learned from 91 patients? Dermatol Surg. 35(5):765-72, 2009
2. Gleason BC et al: Utility of p63 in the differential diagnosis of atypical fibroxanthoma and spindle cell squamous cell carcinoma. J Cutan Pathol. 36(5):543-7, 2009
3. Ferri E et al: Atypical fibroxanthoma of the external ear in a cardiac transplant recipient: case report and the causal role of the immunosuppressive therapy. Auris Nasus Larynx. 35(2):260-3, 2008
4. González-García R et al: Atypical fibroxanthoma of the head and neck: report of 5 cases. J Oral Maxillofac Surg. 65(3):526-31, 2007
5. Hultgren TL et al: Immunohistochemical staining of CD10 in atypical fibroxanthomas. J Cutan Pathol. 34(5):415-9, 2007
6. Ríos-Martín JJ et al: Granular cell atypical fibroxanthoma: report of two cases. Am J Dermatopathol. 29(1):84-7, 2007
7. Farley R et al: Diagnosis and management of atypical fibroxanthoma. Skinmed. 5(2):83-6, 2006
8. Hartel PH et al: CD99 immunoreactivity in atypical fibroxanthoma and pleomorphic malignant fibrous histiocytoma: a useful diagnostic marker. J Cutan Pathol. 33 Suppl 2:24-8, 2006
9. Murali R et al: Clear cell atypical fibroxanthoma - report of a case with review of the literature. J Cutan Pathol. 33(5):343-8, 2006
10. Seavolt M et al: Atypical fibroxanthoma: review of the literature and summary of 13 patients treated with mohs micrographic surgery. Dermatol Surg. 32(3):435-41; discussion 439-41, 2006

ATYPICAL FIBROXANTHOMA

Microscopic Features

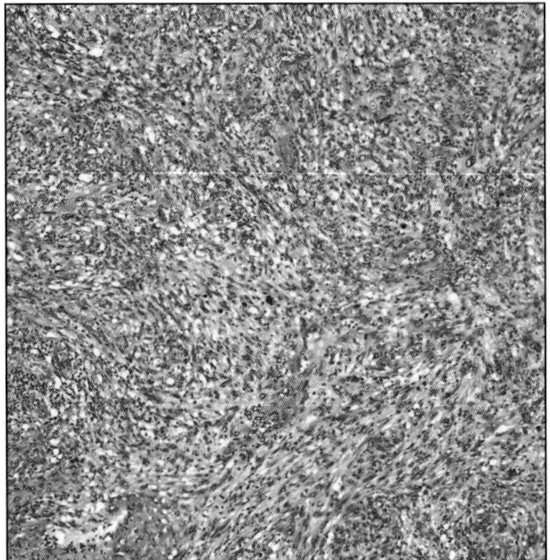
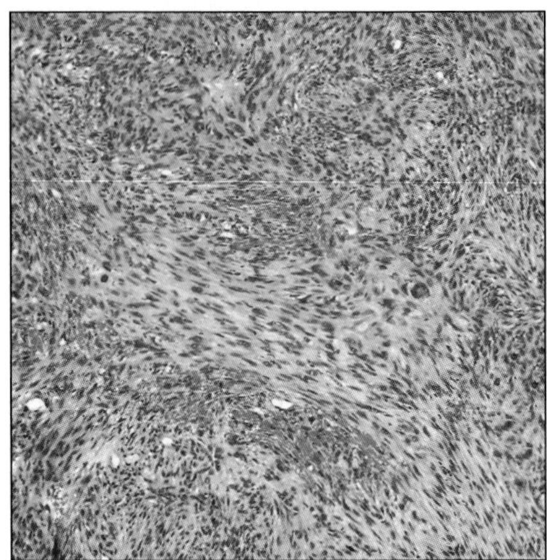

(Left) *Histiologic examination shows a cellular proliferation composed of sheet-like and haphazard fascicles of tumor cells associated with an inflamed and edematous stroma.* ***(Right)*** *Higher power histologic examination shows areas of spindle cells forming dense, short fascicles.*

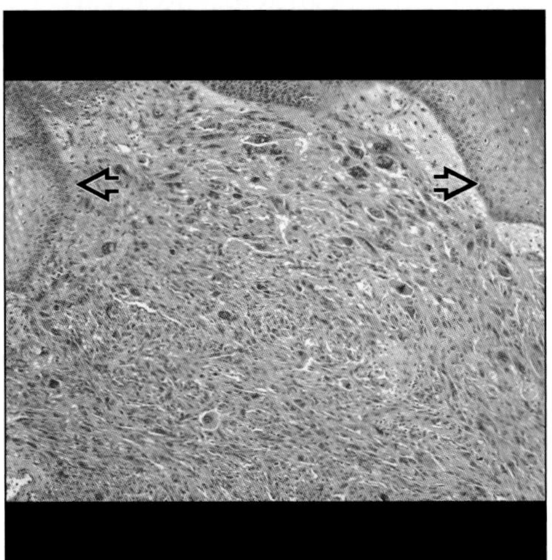
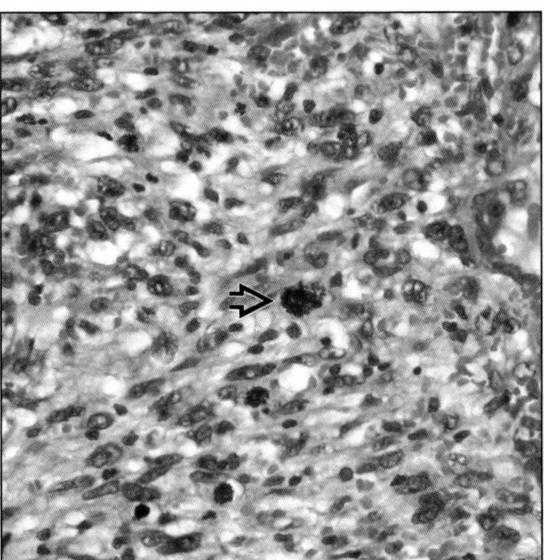

(Left) *Histologic examination shows a superficial portion of the tumor with a proliferation of markedly atypical spindled cells, epithelioid cells, and many multinucleated tumor cells. The tumor closely abuts, but does not involve, the overlying epidermis ⇨.* ***(Right)*** *This slide shows highly atypical cells with numerous mitoses, including atypical forms ⇨.*

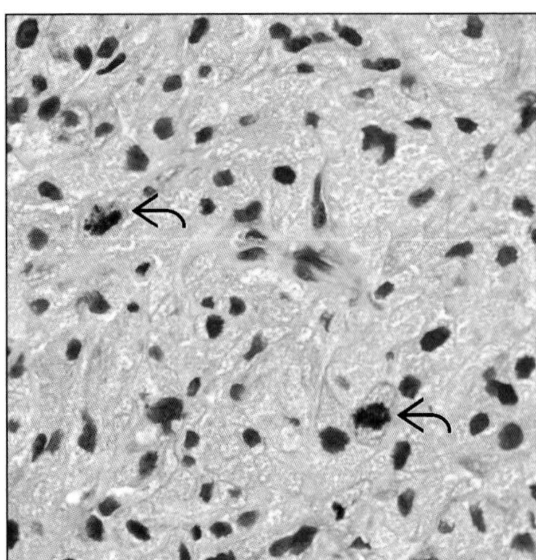
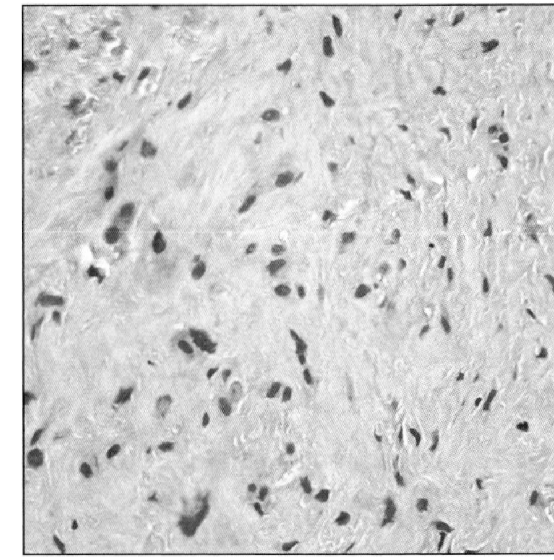

(Left) *An example of the granular cell variant of AFX shows large, bizarre-appearing histiocytoid cells containing abundant granular cytoplasm, similar to a malignant granular cell tumor. Mitoses are easily found ↶.* ***(Right)*** *Histologic section shows an example of an unusual hypocellular AFX case with a chondromyxoid-appearing stroma (chondroid AFX).*

Ancillary Techniques

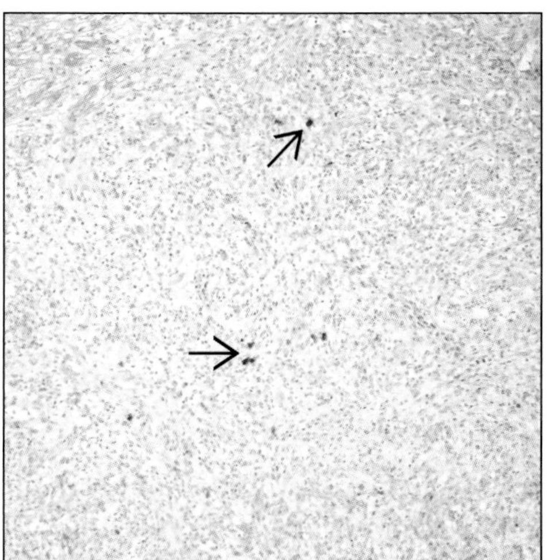

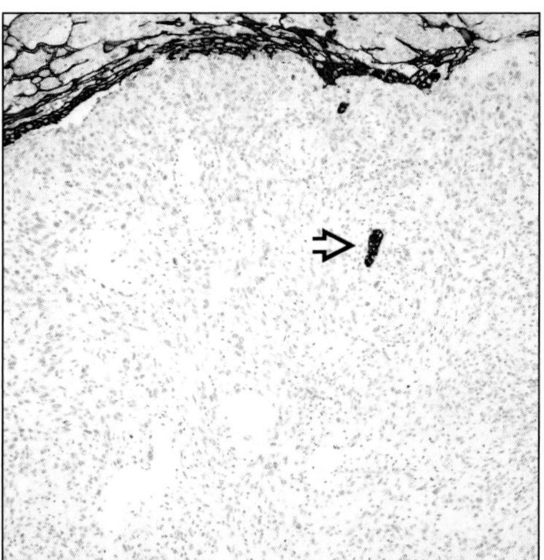

*(**Left**) S100 stained section shows no staining of the tumor cells but highlights a few intradermal dendritic cells ➔. (**Right**) High molecular weight cytokeratin stain shows positivity within the epidermis and a few adnexal ducts ➔ but is negative within the tumor cells.*

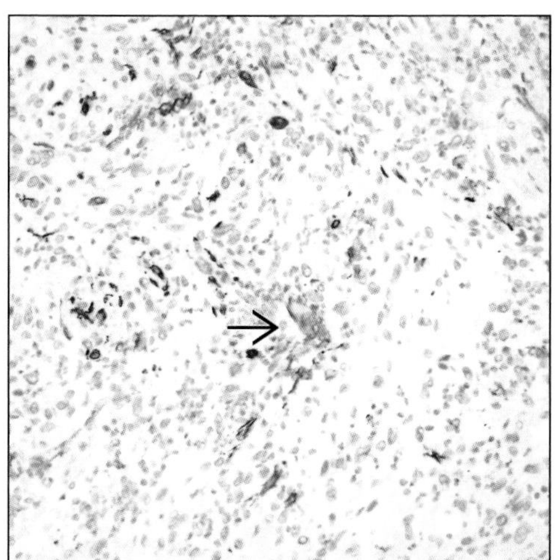

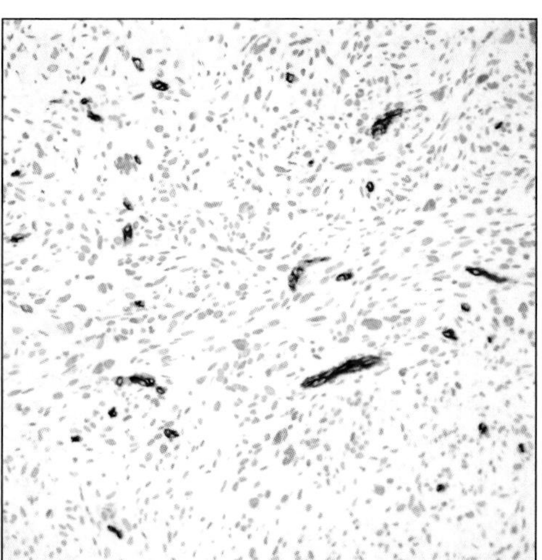

*(**Left**) Smooth muscle actin stain shows scattered weakly positive cells ➔, likely indicating myofibroblastic differentiation. (**Right**) CD34 immunohistochemical stain shows strong positive staining of vessels but is negative within the tumor cells.*

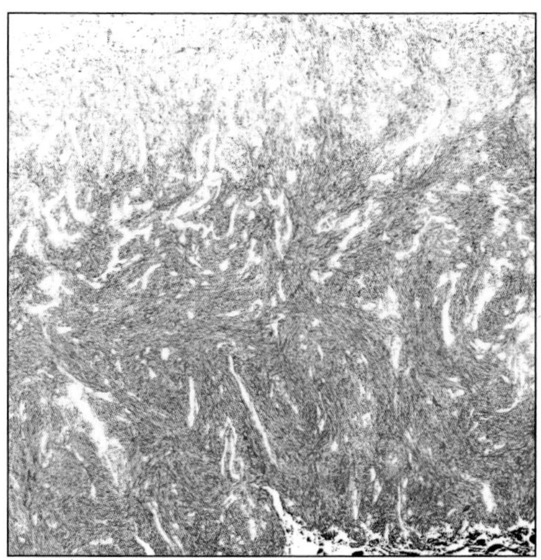

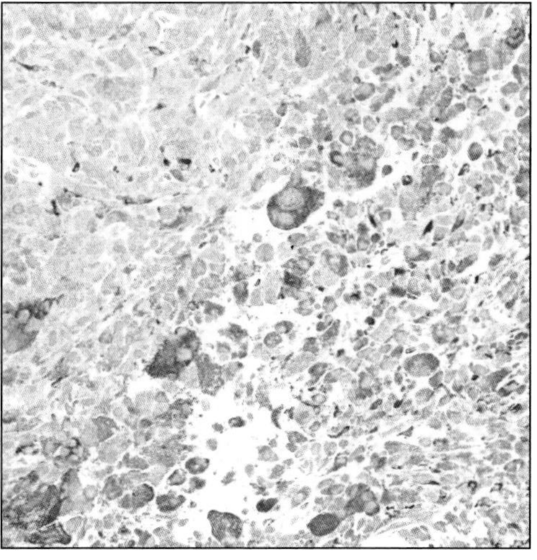

*(**Left**) CD10 stain shows strong and diffuse staining of the tumor cells, a finding that is not specific but is helpful, as it is typically seen in AFX. (**Right**) CD68 stain shows moderate to strong cytoplasmic staining of most of the tumor cells, especially the large multinucleated tumor giant cells.*

UNDIFFERENTIATED PLEOMORPHIC SARCOMA

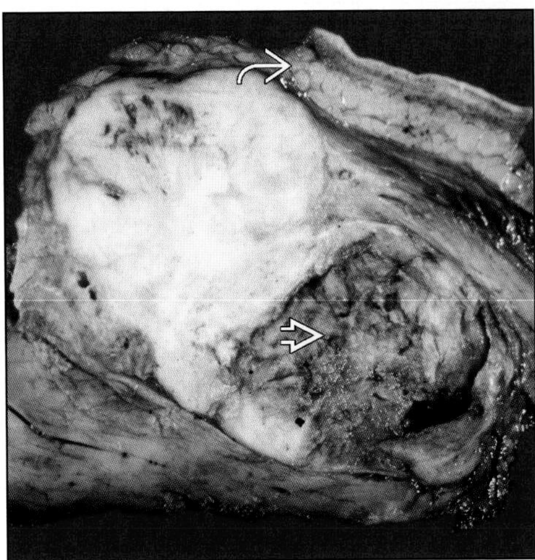

Gross photograph of pleomorphic undifferentiated sarcoma shows lobulated tumor within skeletal muscle and focally abutting the subcutis ➦. Necrosis is a prominent feature ➪.

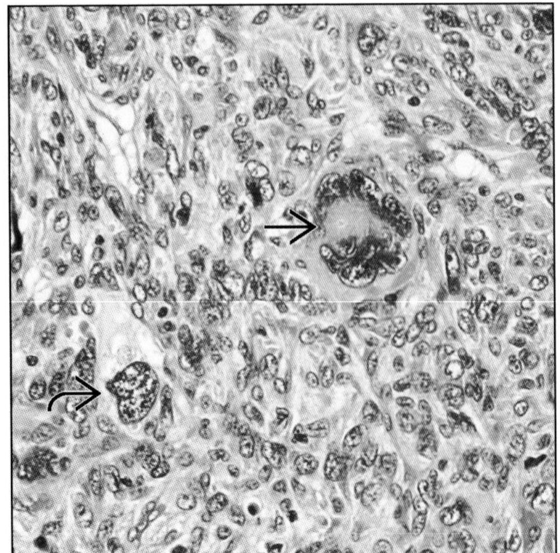

Microscopically, pleomorphic undifferentiated sarcoma is hypercellular with sheets of markedly anaplastic spindle and epithelioid cells, including bizarre ➦ and multinucleated ➔ forms.

TERMINOLOGY

Synonyms

- Pleomorphic sarcoma
- Undifferentiated high-grade sarcoma
- Malignant fibrous histiocytoma (MFH)

Definitions

- Anaplastic sarcoma composed of pleomorphic spindle and polygonal cells
- No other definable differentiation, other than fibroblastic or myofibroblastic
- Morphologic pattern shared by poorly differentiated or anaplastic tumors of different lineages
  - Diagnosis of pleomorphic sarcoma is therefore one of exclusion

ETIOLOGY/PATHOGENESIS

Environmental Exposure

- Can occur at site of previous irradiation
- Rarely secondary to chronic ulceration or scarring

CLINICAL ISSUES

Epidemiology

- Incidence
  - Most common adult soft tissue sarcoma
  - Incidence increases with age
- Age
  - Older adults
  - Very rare in adolescents and young adults
- Gender
  - Slight male predominance

Site

- Deep soft tissue
- Most in extremities
  - Lower limb > upper limb
- May also arise on trunk
- Most intraabdominal examples represent dedifferentiated liposarcoma
- Smaller numbers occur superficially

Presentation

- Enlarging mass
  - Painful or painless
- Small proportion of patients have metastases at presentation

Prognosis

- Usually high-grade tumors
- Local recurrence in up to 1/3 of cases
- Pulmonary metastases in up to 1/2 of cases
- Superficial tumors have better prognosis than deep ones
- Myoid differentiation is prognostically adverse, with earlier metastasis
  - Applies whether differentiation is morphologic (leiomyosarcoma, myofibrosarcoma, rhabdomyosarcoma) or only immunohistochemical (actin, desmin)
- Dedifferentiated liposarcoma has comparatively low metastatic rate

MACROSCOPIC FEATURES

General Features

- Lobulated
- Generally circumscribed
- Heterogeneous cut surface
  - Firm, solid, and softer myxoid areas
- Necrosis
- Hemorrhage

Sections to Be Submitted

- Thorough sampling required to demonstrate any possible lines of differentiation
  - e.g., lipoblastic, epithelial

UNDIFFERENTIATED PLEOMORPHIC SARCOMA

Key Facts

Terminology
- Anaplastic sarcoma composed of pleomorphic spindle and polygonal cells
- No other definable differentiation, other than fibroblastic or myofibroblastic

Etiology/Pathogenesis
- Small proportion of cases occur post irradiation or secondary to chronic ulceration/scarring

Clinical Issues
- Most common adult soft tissue sarcoma
- Most frequent in deep soft tissue of extremities
- Usually high-grade tumors
- Pulmonary metastases in up to 1/2 of cases
- Older adults

Macroscopic Features
- Thorough sampling required to demonstrate any possible lines of differentiation
- Heterogeneous cut surface
- Necrosis and hemorrhage

Microscopic Pathology
- Diagnosis of exclusion
- Morphology shared by many tumors of different lineages
- Storiform pattern, loose fascicles or sheets
- Markedly atypical cells
- Abundant mitoses and necrosis
- No discernible microscopic features of differentiation
- Immunohistochemical panel required to exclude tumors with specific differentiation

Size
- Often large at presentation

MICROSCOPIC PATHOLOGY

Histologic Features
- Storiform or loose fascicles and sheets
- Markedly atypical cells
  - Spindle or polygonal
  - Bizarre and multinucleate forms frequent
  - Can have abundant foamy cytoplasm
- Abundant and atypical mitoses
- Necrosis
- Stroma ranges from fibrous to focally myxoid
- Chronic inflammation, including macrophages
- No discernible microscopic differentiation

ANCILLARY TESTS

Immunohistochemistry
- Use panel to exclude tumors with specific differentiation
- Focal smooth muscle actin
  - Often in subplasmalemmal distribution
    - Indicates myofibroblastic differentiation
- May express CD34
- No evidence of histiocytic differentiation

Cytogenetics
- Complex nonspecific cytogenetic abnormalities

DIFFERENTIAL DIAGNOSIS

Melanoma
- Cells often have nested architecture
- Overlying skin may show junctional activity
- Expresses S100 protein, melanocytic markers

Anaplastic Carcinoma
- At least focal expression of epithelial antigens
- Epithelium may show dysplastic or in situ changes

Anaplastic Large Cell Lymphoma
- Variably positive for CD45, CD30, ALK1

Atypical Fibroxanthoma
- Histologically identical
- Dermal location, typically sun-damaged skin

Myxofibrosarcoma
- Subcutis or deep soft tissue
- Lobulated architecture, myxoid stroma
- Higher grades resemble pleomorphic sarcoma

Pleomorphic Leiomyosarcoma
- Focal fascicular architecture
- Focal smooth muscle cytology, e.g., blunt-ended nuclei
- Immunoreactive for desmin, SMA, and H-caldesmon

Pleomorphic Rhabdomyosarcoma
- Pleomorphic rhabdomyoblasts
- Expresses desmin and myogenin

Pleomorphic Liposarcoma
- Pleomorphic, multivacuolated lipoblasts

Dedifferentiated Liposarcoma
- Most frequent in internal trunk
- Can have adjacent well-differentiated liposarcoma
- Amplification of MDM2, CDK4 (by IHC or FISH)

SELECTED REFERENCES

1. Deyrup AT et al: Myoid differentiation and prognosis in adult pleomorphic sarcomas of the extremity: an analysis of 92 cases. Cancer. 98(4):805-13, 2003
2. Fletcher CD et al: Clinicopathologic re-evaluation of 100 malignant fibrous histiocytomas: prognostic relevance of subclassification. J Clin Oncol. 19(12):3045-50, 2001
3. Le Doussal V et al: Prognostic factors for patients with localized primary malignant fibrous histiocytoma: a multicenter study of 216 patients with multivariate analysis. Cancer. 77(9):1823-30, 1996
4. Weiss SW et al: Malignant fibrous histiocytoma: an analysis of 200 cases. Cancer. 41(6):2250-66, 1978

UNDIFFERENTIATED PLEOMORPHIC SARCOMA

Gross and Microscopic Features

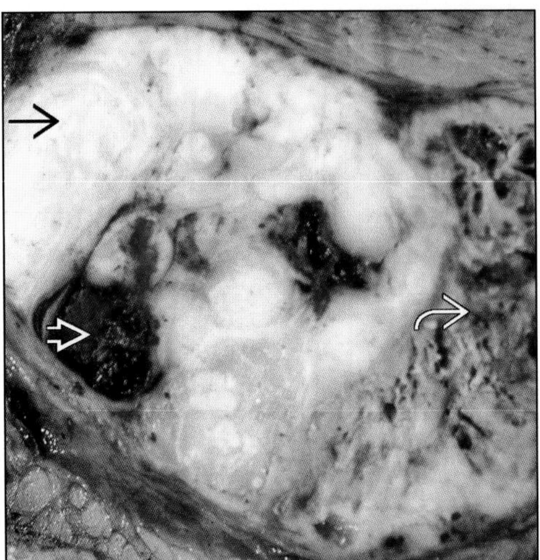

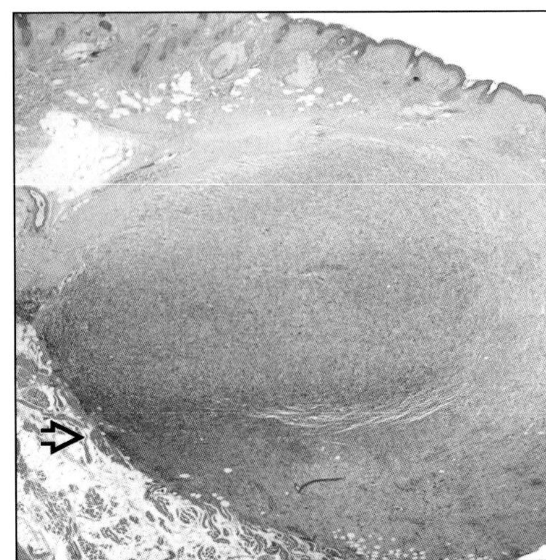

*(**Left**) Gross photograph of pleomorphic undifferentiated sarcoma shows viable intramuscular tumor with solid, white to tan colored cut surface, as well as foci of hemorrhage and extensive necrosis that accounts for almost half of the tumor volume. (**Right**) Tumors can be superficially located. This example is fairly well demarcated and located in the deep dermis and subcutis, although focally abutting skeletal muscle.*

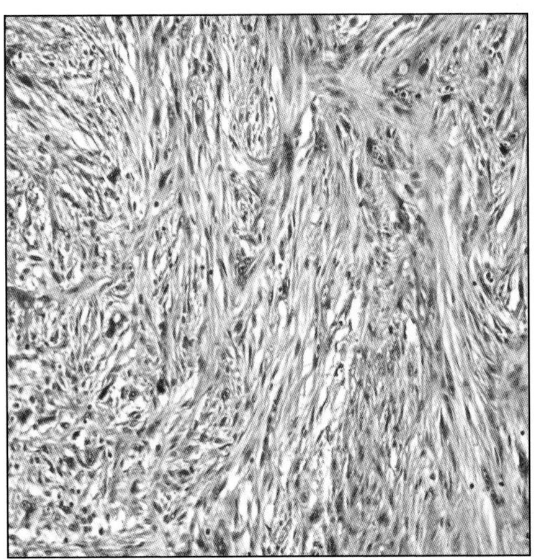

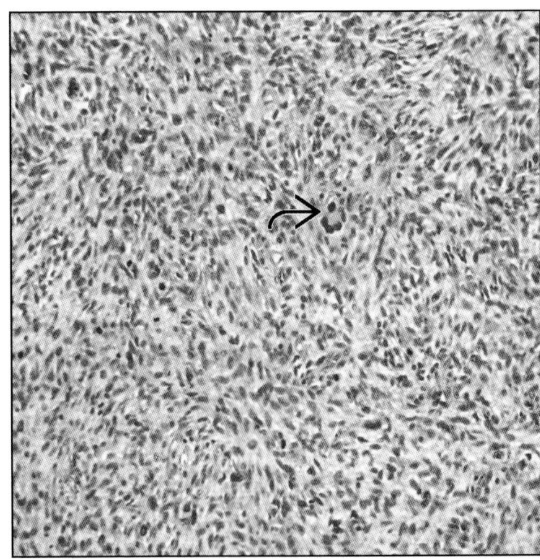

*(**Left**) The cells are spindled in this field and are arranged in loosely fascicular distributions within collagenous stroma. Nuclear pleomorphism and cellular hyperchromasia are discernible even at low power. (**Right**) The cellularity is high, and the architecture can vary from loosely fascicular to storiform to sheet-like. This case shows a more storiform or short fascicular pattern. Tumor giant cells are interspersed and can be a prominent feature.*

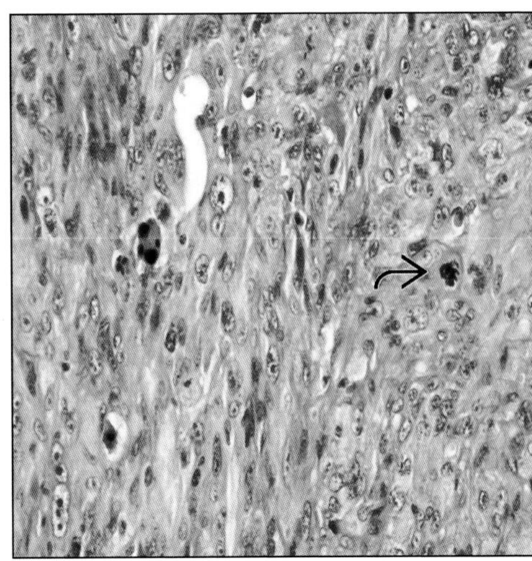

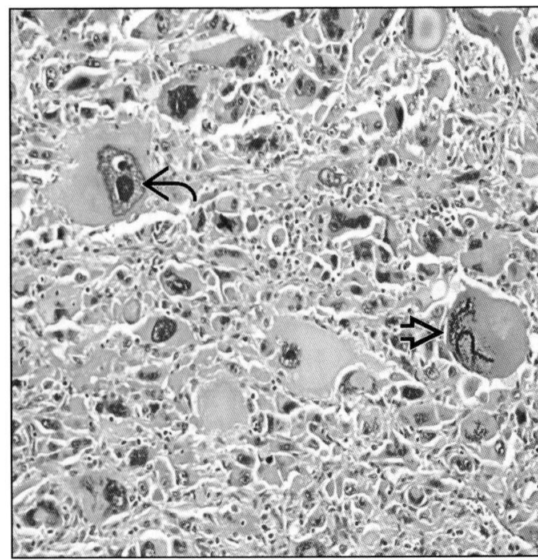

*(**Left**) This pleomorphic undifferentiated sarcoma is composed of streams and fascicles of cells, many of which are epithelioid, with vesicular nuclei and prominent large nucleoli. Mitotic figures are readily identified. (**Right**) The anaplasia in this example is striking, with polygonal cells that vary greatly in size. Note the huge, often bizarre nuclei, prominent nucleoli, and abundant amphophilic cytoplasm. There is also a markedly atypical mitotic figure.*

Microscopic Features and Ancillary Techniques

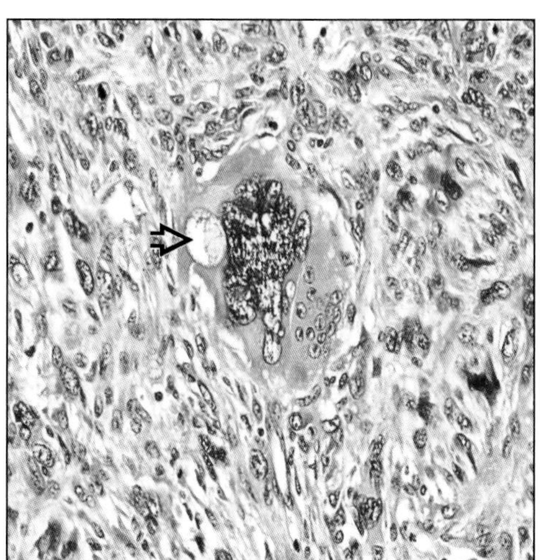
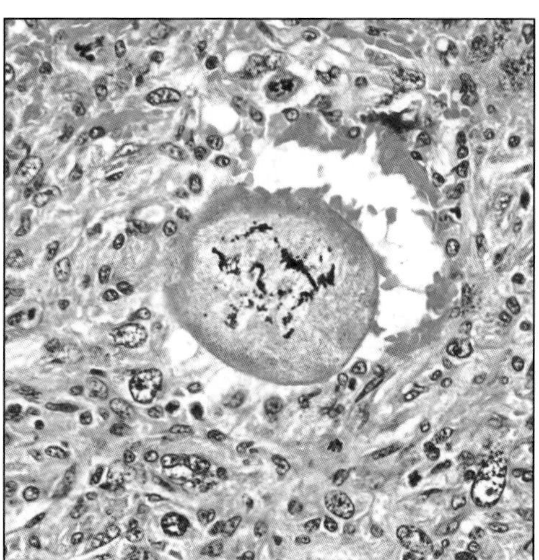

*(**Left**) This cell is both bizarre and multinucleate and is several times the size of its neighbors, which are themselves enlarged. A cytoplasmic inclusion ⇨ is also seen within the large cell, and its nuclear chromatin is coarse and irregular. These differ from osteoclast-like giant cells, which have multiple uniform nuclei. (**Right**) A similarly enlarged neoplastic cell shows a large, fragmented atypical mitotic figure. Stromal hemorrhage and inflammation may also be features.*

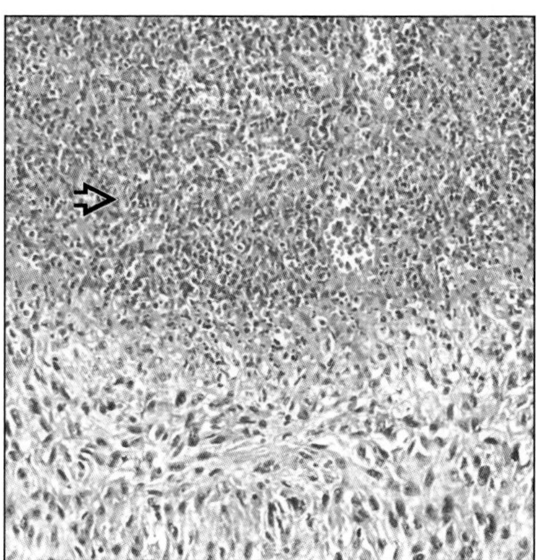
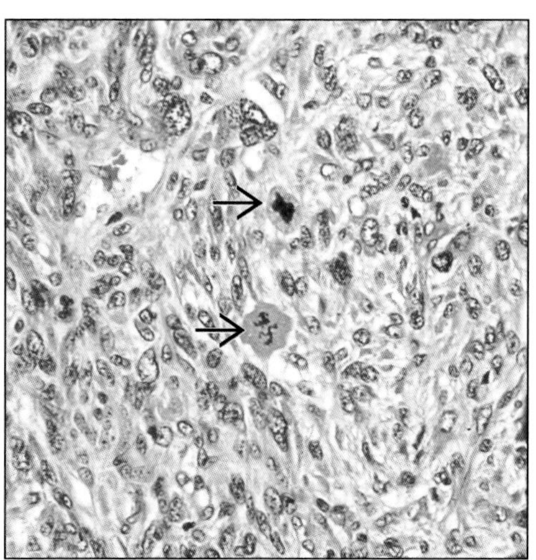

*(**Left**) Necrosis ⇨ is a common finding in pleomorphic undifferentiated sarcoma and is often seen on gross examination. It can sometimes account for most of the tumor. (**Right**) This example is hypercellular, and atypical mitoses are easily discernible →. This tumor shows no morphologically identifiable line of differentiation. A wide immunohistochemical panel is therefore required to exclude any specific mesenchymal lineage, carcinoma, or melanoma.*

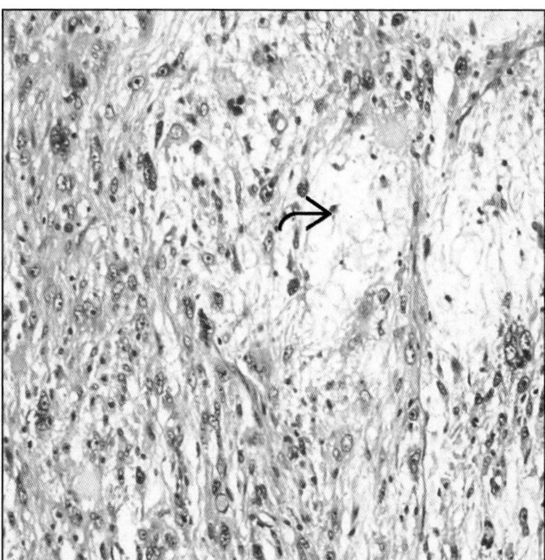
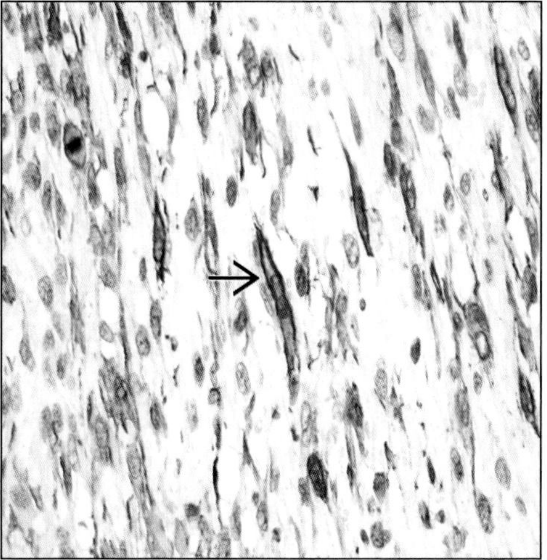

*(**Left**) This pleomorphic undifferentiated sarcoma developed as recurrence of previous myxofibrosarcoma. Residual myxofibrosarcomatous zones are apparent ↪, which are less cellular, with prominent myxoid stroma and a lobulated architecture. (**Right**) With immunohistochemistry, polygonal and spindled tumor cells show focal expression of SMA, with subplasmalemmal linear distribution →, typical of myofibroblastic differentiation.*

UNDIFFERENTIATED PLEOMORPHIC SARCOMA WITH GIANT CELLS

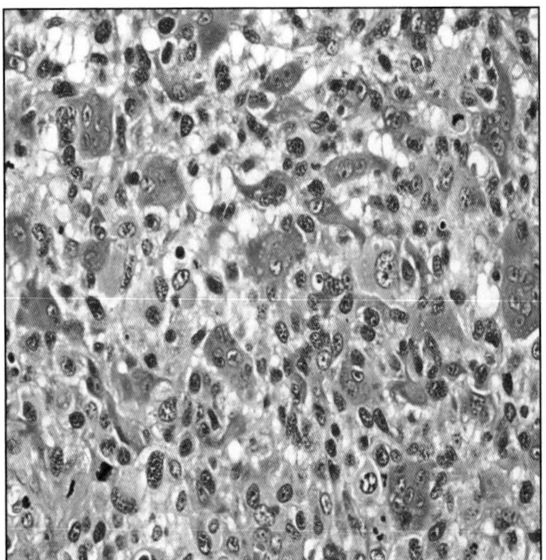

Osteoclast-like giant cells are admixed with tumor cells in this example of giant cell MFH. The giant cells show plump nuclei with prominent nucleoli but lack the pleomorphism and marked atypia of the tumor cells.

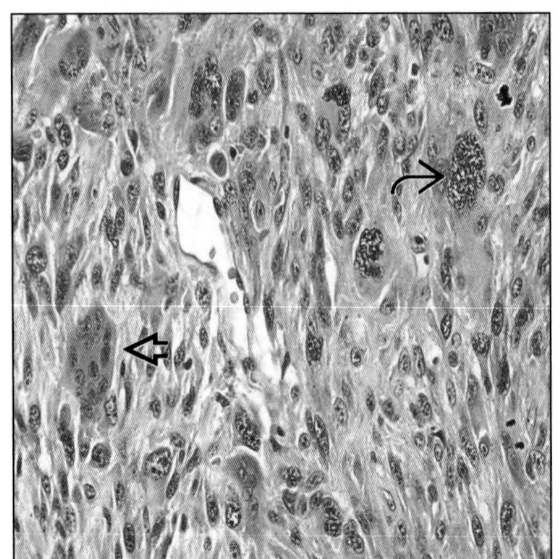

Osteoclast-like giant cells ⇨ and tumor giant cells ↪ are often intermingled. Note the much larger size of tumor nuclei compared to those of the giant cells.

TERMINOLOGY

Abbreviations

- Giant cell malignant fibrous histiocytoma (MFH)

Synonyms

- Malignant giant cell tumor of soft parts
- Giant cell sarcoma
- Malignant osteoclastoma
- Pleomorphic undifferentiated sarcoma with giant cells

Definitions

- Malignant pleomorphic spindle and polygonal cell sarcoma with osteoclast-type giant cells
- Morphology shared with several other pleomorphic malignant tumors of other lineages

CLINICAL ISSUES

Epidemiology

- Age
  - Older adults
    - Rare cases in children and adolescents
- Gender
  - M = F

Site

- Mostly in deep soft tissue
  - Extremity or trunk
- Can also occur superficially

Presentation

- Painless mass
  - Usually nonspecific symptoms

Prognosis

- Similar to that of other pleomorphic sarcomas
- Superficial tumors have better prognosis than deep ones

MACROSCOPIC FEATURES

General Features

- Hemorrhage
- Necrosis

Size

- Usually large
- Deep tumors larger than superficial ones

MICROSCOPIC PATHOLOGY

Histologic Features

- Sheets of markedly atypical spindle and polygonal cells
- Prominent intermixed osteoclast-type giant cells
  - Usually lack atypia
  - Giant cells often contain ingested material
- Hemorrhage
  - Formation of large cystic hemorrhagic spaces
- Necrosis
- Mitotic figures prominent
  - Often atypical forms
- Focal osteoid or mature bone may be present
  - Malignant osteoid absent

Predominant Pattern/Injury Type

- Neoplastic

Predominant Cell/Compartment Type

- Undifferentiated, pleomorphic

ANCILLARY TESTS

Immunohistochemistry

- Morphology shared by other tumors of different lineages

UNDIFFERENTIATED PLEOMORPHIC SARCOMA WITH GIANT CELLS

Key Facts

Terminology

- Malignant pleomorphic spindle and polygonal cell sarcoma with osteoclast-type giant cells
- Tumor morphology shared with several other pleomorphic malignant tumors of different lineages

Clinical Issues

- Older adults
- Mostly in deep soft tissue
- Extremity or trunk

Microscopic Pathology

- Sheets of markedly atypical spindle and polygonal cells
- Prominent intermixed osteoclast-type giant cells that lack atypia

Ancillary Tests

- As morphology is shared by other tumors of different lineages, features of specific differentiation need exclusion

  - Features of specific differentiation therefore need exclusion by broad panel of immunohistochemical markers

DIFFERENTIAL DIAGNOSIS

Giant Cell Tumor of Soft Tissues

- Ovoid and polygonal cells
- Atypia absent or minimal
- Usually in subcutaneous tissue
- Multinodular growth pattern

Giant Cell Tumor of Bone with Soft Tissue Extension

- Bony destruction
- Atypia absent or minimal

Extraskeletal Osteosarcoma

- Malignant tumoral osteoid laid down by cytologically atypical cells

Leiomyosarcoma with Giant Cells

- At least focal fascicular architecture
- Areas of more typical morphology of leiomyosarcoma also present
- Focal expression of desmin and smooth muscle markers
  - Expression more pronounced than sometimes seen in MFH

Anaplastic Carcinoma

- At least focal expression of cytokeratin or EMA
- Foci of better differentiated carcinoma may be present
- Patient may have history of primary carcinoma
  - Typical sites
    - Thyroid
    - Pancreas
    - Breast
    - Kidney
- Dysplastic changes or carcinoma in situ may be present in overlying epithelium

SELECTED REFERENCES

1. O'Connell JX et al: Giant cell tumors of soft tissue: a clinicopathologic study of 18 benign and malignant tumors. Am J Surg Pathol. 24(3):386-95, 2000
2. Folpe AL et al: Soft tissue giant cell tumor of low malignant potential: a proposal for the reclassification of malignant giant cell tumor of soft parts. Mod Pathol. 12(9):894-902, 1999
3. Hollowood K et al: Malignant fibrous histiocytoma: morphologic pattern or pathologic entity? Semin Diagn Pathol. 12(3):210-20, 1995
4. Angervall L et al: Malignant giant cell tumor of soft tissues: a clinicopathologic, cytologic, ultrastructural, angiographic, and microangiographic study. Cancer. 47(4):736-47, 1981
5. Guccion JG et al: Malignant giant cell tumor of soft parts. An analysis of 32 cases. Cancer. 29(6):1518-29, 1972

IMAGE GALLERY

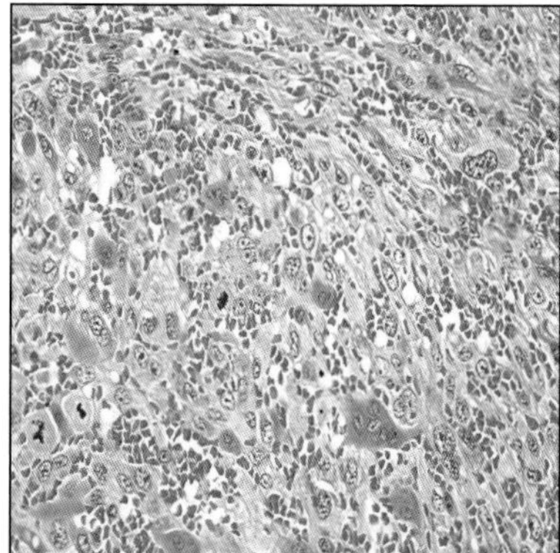

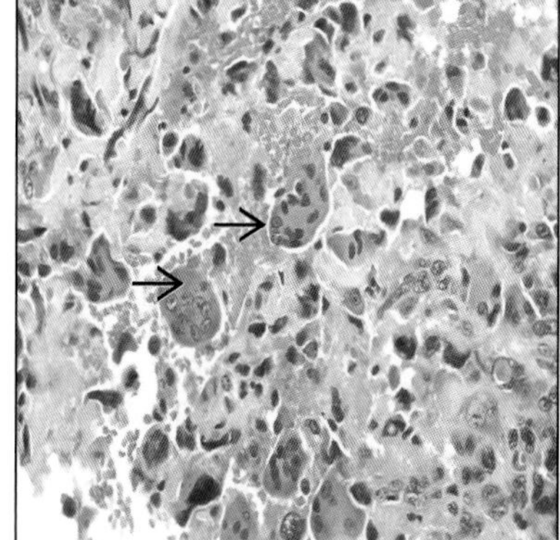

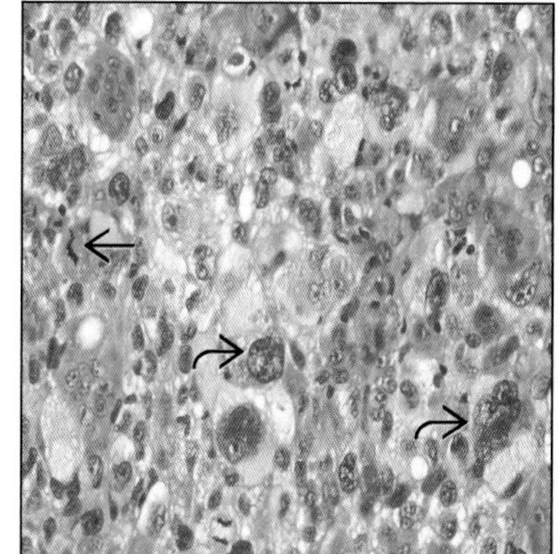

(Left) *Hemorrhage is a frequent feature, and there is often formation of large hemorrhagic cystic spaces, as in this example of giant cell malignant fibrous histiocytoma.* ***(Center)*** *The osteoclast-like giant cells often contain ingested material, in this case hemosiderin* ➔. ***(Right)*** *This tumor shares features of typical MFH, including the presence of bizarre pleomorphic cells* ➔ *and numerous atypical mitotic figures* ➔.

UNDIFFERENTIATED PLEOMORPHIC SARCOMA WITH PROMINENT INFLAMMATION

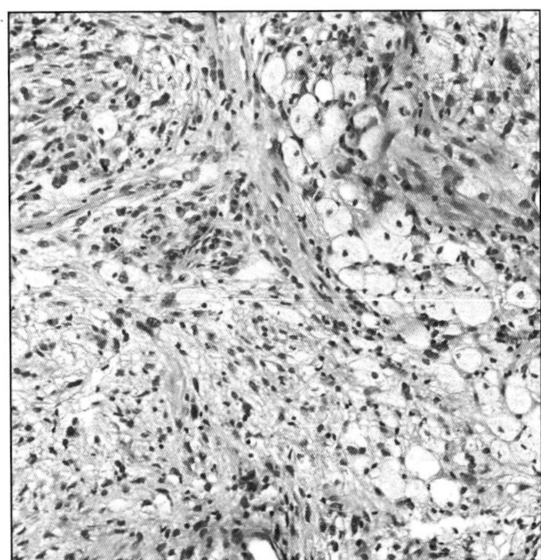

Inflammatory malignant fibrous histiocytoma is shown with sheets of large cells with abundant foamy cytoplasm. The inflammatory background is apparent even at low power.

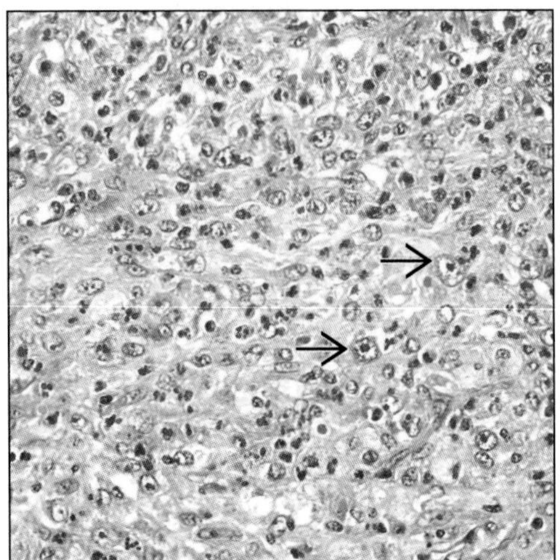

Inflammatory malignant fibrous histiocytoma contains a prominent infiltrate of neutrophils. Large atypical cells with vesicular nuclei and prominent nucleoli are also easily identifiable ⇒.

TERMINOLOGY

Abbreviations

- Inflammatory malignant fibrous histiocytoma (MFH)

Synonyms

- Undifferentiated pleomorphic sarcoma with prominent inflammation

Definitions

- Pleomorphic undifferentiated malignant neoplasm with large, variably atypical xanthomatous cells admixed with atypical spindle cells and prominent acute and chronic inflammatory cell infiltrate
- Although designated as specific subtype of MFH, many of these are now thought to represent dedifferentiated liposarcomas

ETIOLOGY/PATHOGENESIS

Environmental Exposure

- Etiology unknown for most cases
- A few cases have occurred post radiation

CLINICAL ISSUES

Epidemiology

- Incidence
  - Rarest form of MFH
- Age
  - Middle-aged and elderly adults
- Gender
  - M = F

Site

- Predilection for retroperitoneum
- Other soft tissue sites
- Can occur in visceral organs

Presentation

- Deep mass
  - May present with systemic symptoms
    - e.g., fever, leukocytosis, or eosinophilia

Prognosis

- Aggressive tumors
  - Recurrence common
  - Eventual metastases in many patients

MACROSCOPIC FEATURES

General Features

- Often large
- Cut surface may have yellow color due to large number of xanthomatous cells

MICROSCOPIC PATHOLOGY

Histologic Features

- Sheets of large xanthomatous cells
  - Variably atypical nuclei
    - Anaplastic as well as bland forms
  - Foamy cytoplasm
- Prominent acute and chronic inflammatory cell infiltrate
  - Numerous interspersed neutrophils
    - Neutrophils unassociated with necrosis
  - Other cells include histiocytes, lymphocytes, plasma cells, and eosinophils
- Admixed atypical cells
  - Vesicular or hyperchromatic nuclei
  - Often large nucleoli
  - Multinucleate or Reed-Sternberg-like forms may be present
- Phagocytosis of neutrophils or red cells may be seen
- Often focal storiform architecture
- Variably collagenous background

UNDIFFERENTIATED PLEOMORPHIC SARCOMA WITH PROMINENT INFLAMMATION

Key Facts

Terminology
- Pleomorphic undifferentiated malignant neoplasm with histiocytic and inflammatory cell infiltrate

Microscopic Pathology
- Sheets of variably atypical xanthomatous cells
- Prominent inflammatory cell infiltrate, particularly neutrophils
- Admixed atypical cells with large nucleoli
  - May include Reed-Sternberg-like forms
- Phagocytosis of cells
- Can have focal storiform architecture

Ancillary Tests
- Cytogenetic and molecular studies show that inflammatory MFHs share similar structural and genetic abnormalities to dedifferentiated liposarcoma
  - Suggests that most inflammatory MFHs are dedifferentiated liposarcomas
- No other specific lines of differentiation identifiable

ANCILLARY TESTS

Immunohistochemistry
- Occasional CD68 expression within tumor cells
- CDK4 and MDM2 positivity shown in both inflammatory MFH and dedifferentiated liposarcoma (DDL)
- No other specific lines of differentiation identifiable
  - Useful in excluding poorly differentiated neoplasms of other lineages
- Tumor negative for hematolymphoid markers, such as CD45, CD15, and CD30

In Situ Hybridization
- Amplifications of MDM2 and CDK4 previously shown

Array CGH
- 12q13-15 amplification or gain shown
  - Cytogenetic and molecular studies show that inflammatory MFH shares similar structural and genetic abnormalities to DDL
    - Suggests that most inflammatory MFHs are dedifferentiated liposarcomas

DIFFERENTIAL DIAGNOSIS

Anaplastic Carcinoma
- Cytokeratin(+)
- Primary site may be found

Lymphoma
- Patient may have lymphadenopathy
- Expression of hematolymphoid markers
- Neutrophil phagocytosis not seen

Inflammatory Myofibroblastic Tumor
- Lymphocytes are predominant inflammatory component
- Actin-sm expression
- ALK1 expression or *ALK* gene rearrangement in proportion of patients

SELECTED REFERENCES

1. Coindre JM et al: Inflammatory malignant fibrous histiocytomas and dedifferentiated liposarcomas: histological review, genomic profile, and MDM2 and CDK4 status favour a single entity. J Pathol. 203(3):822-30, 2004
2. Fukunaga M et al: Radiation-induced inflammatory malignant fibrous histiocytoma of the ileum. APMIS. 107(9):837-42, 1999
3. Khalidi HS et al: Inflammatory malignant fibrous histiocytoma: distinction from Hodgkin's disease and non-Hodgkin's lymphoma by a panel of leukocyte markers. Mod Pathol. 10(5):438-42, 1997
4. Roques AW et al: Inflammatory fibrous histiocytoma in the left upper abdomen with a leukemoid blood picture. Cancer. 43(5):1800-4, 1979
5. Kyriakos M et al: Inflammatory fibrous histiocytoma. An aggressive and lethal lesion. Cancer. 37(3):1584-1606, 1976

IMAGE GALLERY

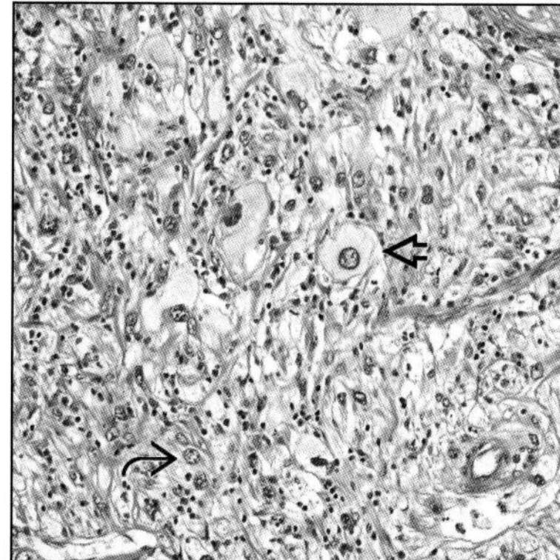

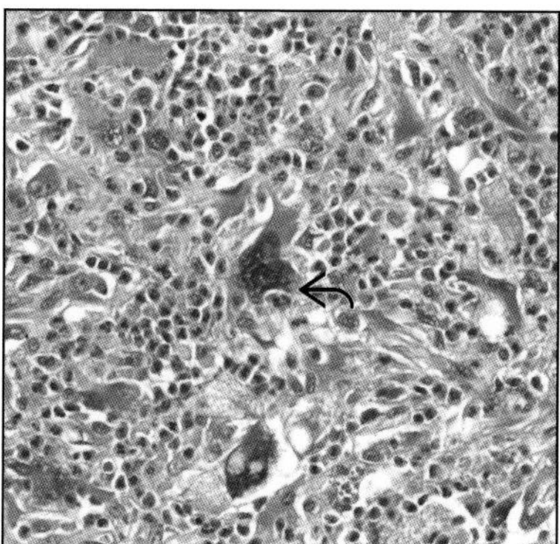

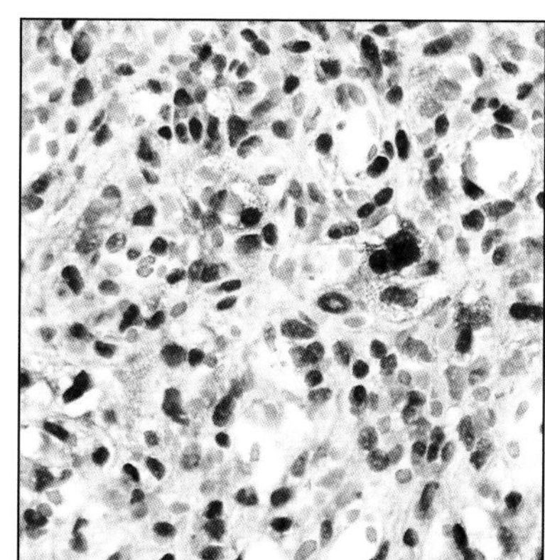

(Left) *The foamy cells are of varying size and pleomorphism. There are small forms ➚, as well as much larger, atypical foamy cells ➪.* ***(Center)*** *Pleomorphic spindle cells are interspersed. The large multinucleate tumor cell in the center is seen phagocytosing a neutrophil ➚.* ***(Right)*** *Tumor nuclei show strong positivity for CDK4, supporting evidence that some inflammatory malignant fibrous histiocytomas represent dedifferentiated liposarcomas.*

Genital Stromal Tumors

Benign

FIBROEPITHELIAL STROMAL POLYP

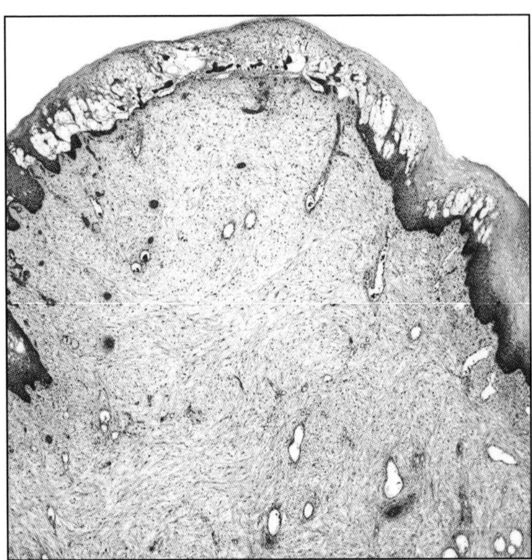

Fibroepithelial stromal polyps are typically edematous at low magnification, with overlying reactive epithelial changes. Note that the lesion abuts the overlying epithelium without a Grenz zone.

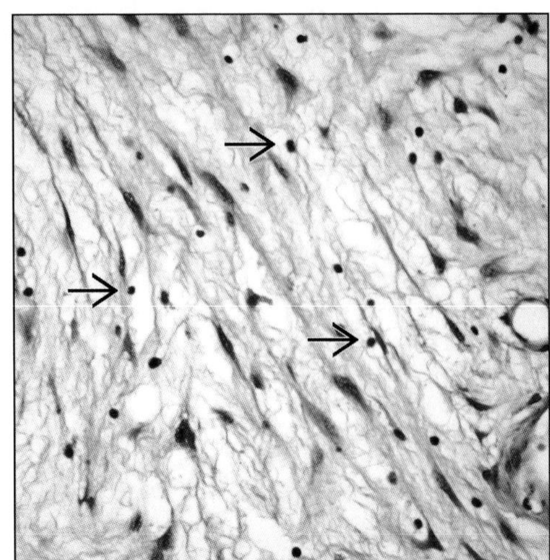

At high magnification, most fibroepithelial stromal polyps consist of bland-appearing stellate to spindle cells in an edematous background with scattered inflammatory cells →.

TERMINOLOGY

Abbreviations

- Fibroepithelial stromal polyp (FSP)

Synonyms

- Cellular pseudosarcomatous fibroepithelial stromal polyp, pseudosarcoma botryoides

Definitions

- Benign polyps, usually involving vagina of women of reproductive age, composed of fibroblastic cells in edematous stroma

CLINICAL ISSUES

Epidemiology

- Incidence
  - Relatively common
- Age
  - Reproductive years
- Gender
  - Women

Presentation

- Polypoid lesions presenting in vagina or vulva
- Possible relationship to hormonal factors
  - Discovered in antenatal examinations
  - Some regress in puerperium
  - Association with hormone usage

Treatment

- Simple excision

Prognosis

- Occasional recurrences, especially with subsequent pregnancies
- Benign

MACROSCOPIC FEATURES

General Features

- Round to villiform polypoid lesions closely apposed to overlying mucosa/skin

Size

- 1-3 cm

MICROSCOPIC PATHOLOGY

Histologic Features

- Coating of unremarkable or hyperplastic squamous mucosa
  - No Grenz zone between lesion and overlying mucosa/skin
- Spindle to stellate cells
  - Tapering cytoplasmic processes
  - Multinucleation and nuclear enlargement common
    - Multinucleate cell with wreath-like appearance
- Fibrous, edematous, or myxoid stroma
- Thick- or thin-walled vessels more prominent in center of lesion
- Larger lesions can undergo torsion
  - Imparts striking edema/myxoid change
- Can be highly cellular, mimicking sarcomas (often in pregnancy)

DIFFERENTIAL DIAGNOSIS

Aggressive Angiomyxoma

- Poorly circumscribed large masses, nonpolypoid
- Multinucleated cells uncommon
- Same immunolabeling pattern as FSP

Angiomyofibroblastoma

- Well-circumscribed masses rather than polyps
- Grenz zone between lesion and overlying mucosa/skin
- Plump plasmacytoid cells proliferating around vessels

FIBROEPITHELIAL STROMAL POLYP

Key Facts

Clinical Issues

- Polypoid lesions presenting in vagina or vulva
- Possible relationship to hormonal factors
- Simple excision; occasional recurrences, especially with subsequent pregnancies

Microscopic Pathology

- Coating of unremarkable or hyperplastic squamous mucosa
- No Grenz zone between lesion and overlying mucosa/skin
- Spindle to stellate cells
- Tapering cytoplasmic processes
- Multinucleation and nuclear enlargement common
- Multinucleate cell with wreath-like appearance
- Fibrous, edematous, or myxoid stroma
- Can be highly cellular, mimicking sarcomas (often in pregnancy)

Immunohistochemistry

Antibody	Reactivity	Staining Pattern	Comment
Vimentin	Positive	Cytoplasmic	
Desmin	Positive	Cytoplasmic	Most cases reactive
ERP	Positive	Nuclear	
PRP	Positive	Nuclear	
MYOD1	Negative	Nuclear	Helps exclude botryoid rhabdomyosarcoma in cellular examples
Myogenin	Negative	Nuclear	Helps exclude botryoid rhabdomyosarcoma in cellular examples
S100	Negative		
CK-PAN	Negative		

- Same immunolabeling pattern as FSP

Cellular Angiofibroma

- Well-circumscribed masses rather than polyps
- Grenz zone between lesion and overlying mucosa/skin
- Spindle cells and abundant collagen
- Thick-walled hyalinized vessels
- Same immunolabeling pattern as FSP

Superficial Cervicovaginal Myofibroblastoma

- Well-circumscribed masses rather than polyps
- Grenz zone between lesion and overlying mucosa/skin
- Ovoid to spindle-shaped vessels
- No clustering around vessels and no thick-walled vessels
- Same immunolabeling pattern as FSP

Botryoid Rhabdomyosarcoma

- Young patients, polypoid masses
- Cells proliferate under mucosa ("cambium layer")
- Cytologically malignant cells
- Desmin, myogenin, MYOD1 immunoreactivity

SELECTED REFERENCES

1. Nucci MR et al: Cellular pseudosarcomatous fibroepithelial stromal polyps of the lower female genital tract: an underrecognized lesion often misdiagnosed as sarcoma. Am J Surg Pathol. 24(2):231-40, 2000
2. Miettinen M et al: Vaginal polyps with pseudosarcomatous features. A clinicopathologic study of seven cases. Cancer. 51(6):1148-51, 1983
3. Norris HJ et al: Polyps of the vagina. A benign lesion resembling sarcoma botryoides. Cancer. 19(2):227-32, 1966

IMAGE GALLERY

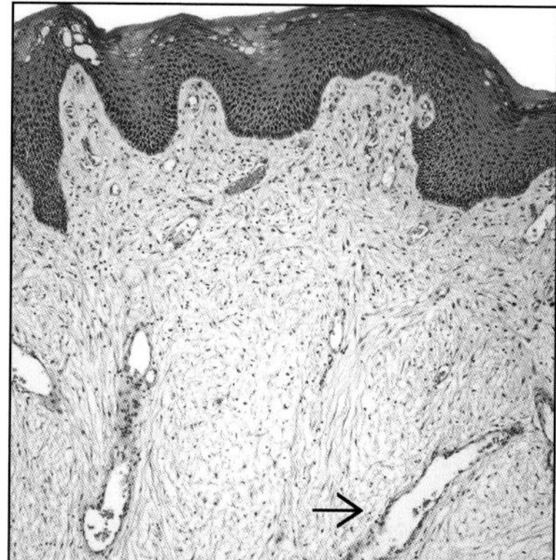

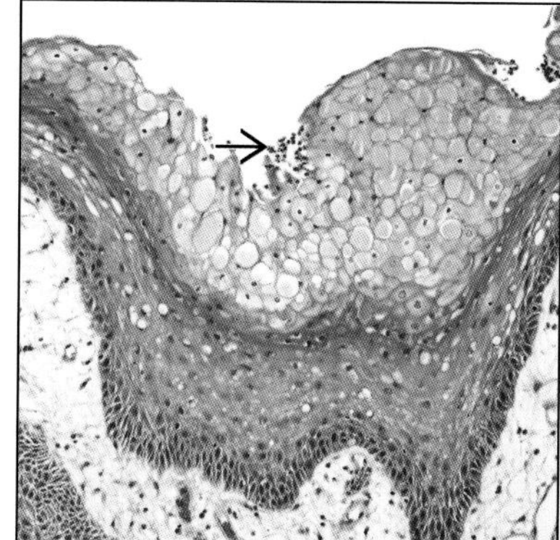

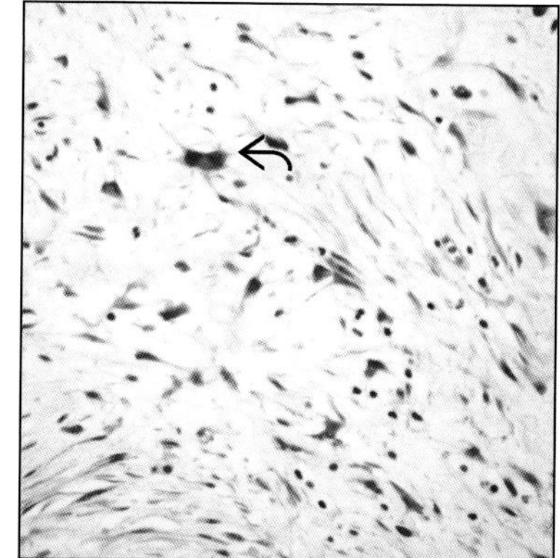

(Left) *In addition to abutting the epithelium, the fibroblastic cells of fibroepithelial stromal polyps proliferate adjacent to the vascular endothelial cells ⇒.* ***(Center)*** *Since fibroepithelial stromal polyps prolapse into the vaginal lumen, they often display overlying reactive epithelial changes. In this example the surface shows acute inflammation ⇒.* ***(Right)*** *Enlarged multinucleated "pseudosarcomatous" cells ↶ are common in fibroepithelial stromal polyps.*

DEEP (AGGRESSIVE) ANGIOMYXOMA

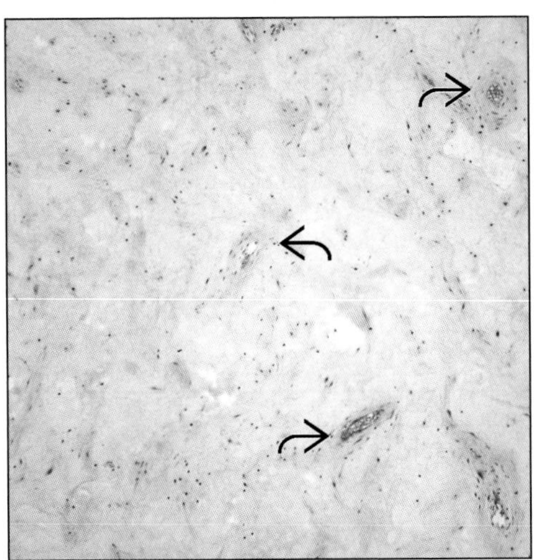

This is the typical loose myxoid hypocellular appearance of aggressive angiomyxoma. The vessels have somewhat thick walls ➚, and overall cellularity is low.

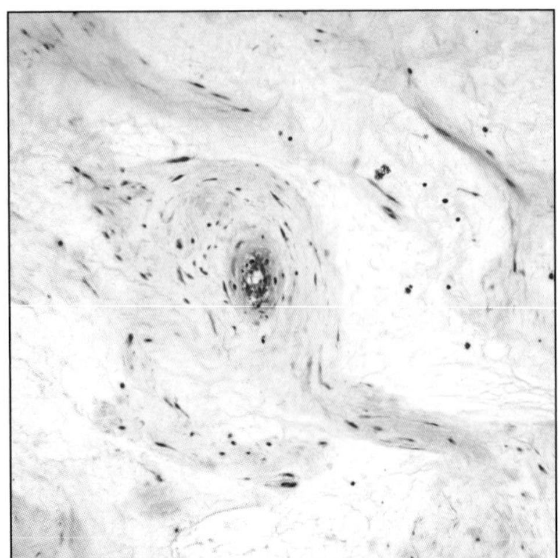

A characteristic feature of aggressive angiomyxoma is the appearance of lesional cells spinning off a vessel that they encircle. This example has mildly atypical nuclei but is devoid of mitoses.

TERMINOLOGY

Synonyms

- Aggressive angiomyxoma of female pelvis and perineum
  - Also known to arise in men

Definitions

- Hypocellular myxoid neoplasm with prominent vessels, typically of deep pelvic tissues
  - Can be locally aggressive but does not metastasize

CLINICAL ISSUES

Presentation

- Deep soft tissue mass in genital region
  - Vulvovaginal (women)
    - Typicall in women of reproductive age
  - Inguinoscrotal (men)

Treatment

- Surgical excision
- Reports of responses to gonadotrophin-releasing hormone agonists and antiestrogens

Prognosis

- Benign, but recurrences common

IMAGE FINDINGS

MR Findings

- Well-defined mass displacing adjacent structures
- Isointense relative to muscle on T1-weighted images, hyperintense on T2-weighted images
- Enhances avidly after gadolinium contrast with characteristic "swirled" internal pattern

CT Findings

- Well-defined mass displacing adjacent structures
- Low attenuation relative to muscle

MACROSCOPIC FEATURES

General Features

- Poorly circumscribed gelatinous mass
- Most examples > 10 cm

MICROSCOPIC PATHOLOGY

Histologic Features

- Hypocellular lesion
  - Infiltrative growth pattern
- Small bland ovoid and spindled cells
- Abundant myxoid stroma
- No mitotic activity
- Negligible nuclear atypia
- Stromal mast cells and erythrocytes
- Numerous vessels with sizes ranging from capillaries to thick-walled larger vessels
- Perivascular lesional cells radiate around vessels

DIFFERENTIAL DIAGNOSIS

Angiomyofibroblastoma

- Grossly well marginated
- Usually < 5 cm
- Alternating hypercellular and hypocellular zones
- Cells with plump epithelioid cytoplasm
- Delicate capillary sized vessels
- ER(+), PR(+), variable desmin and CD34

Cellular Angiofibroma

- Well-circumscribed lesions
- Most common in vulva
- Rim of fat
- Spindle cells and wispy collagen
- Numerous small vessels

DEEP (AGGRESSIVE) ANGIOMYXOMA

Key Facts

Clinical Issues

- Deep soft tissues of vulvovaginal region
  - Typically in women in reproductive age group
- Benign, but recurrences common

Macroscopic Features

- Poorly circumscribed gelatinous mass
- Most examples > 10 cm

Microscopic Pathology

- Infiltrative growth pattern
- Small bland ovoid and spindled cells
- Abundant myxoid stroma
- No mitotic activity
- Numerous vessels with sizes ranging from capillaries to thick-walled larger vessels
- Perivascular lesional cells radiate from around vessels

Immunohistochemistry

Antibody	Reactivity	Staining Pattern	Comment
ERP	Positive	Nuclear	Nearly all cases
PRP	Positive	Nuclear	Nearly all cases
Desmin	Positive	Cytoplasmic	Most cases
Actin-sm	Positive	Cytoplasmic	Variable
CD34	Positive	Cytoplasmic	Variable
HMGA2	Positive	Nuclear	Reported in about 1/2 of cases

  - Some with thick hyalinized walls with fibrinoid change
- ER(+), PR(+), variable desmin and CD34

Superficial Myofibroblastoma of Lower Female Genital Tract

- a.k.a. superficial cervicovaginal myofibroblastoma
- Polypoid cervical or vaginal masses
- Well marginated/polypoid
- Grenz zone
- Cells with bland ovoid, spindle, or stellate nuclei, often with wavy appearance, embedded in finely collagenous stroma
- Sometimes thick collagen bundles
- ER(+), PR(+), variable desmin and CD34
- Probably forms spectrum with "fibroepithelial stromal polyp"

SELECTED REFERENCES

1. McCluggage WG: Recent developments in vulvovaginal pathology. Histopathology. 54(2):156-73, 2009
2. McCluggage WG et al: Aggressive angiomyxoma of the vulva: Dramatic response to gonadotropin-releasing hormone agonist therapy. Gynecol Oncol. 100(3):623-5, 2006
3. Jeyadevan NN et al: Imaging features of aggressive angiomyxoma. Clin Radiol. 58(2):157-62, 2003
4. Fetsch JF et al: Aggressive angiomyxoma: a clinicopathologic study of 29 female patients. Cancer. 78(1):79-90, 1996
5. Steeper TA et al: Aggressive angiomyxoma of the female pelvis and perineum. Report of nine cases of a distinctive type of gynecologic soft-tissue neoplasm. Am J Surg Pathol. 7(5):463-75, 1983

IMAGE GALLERY

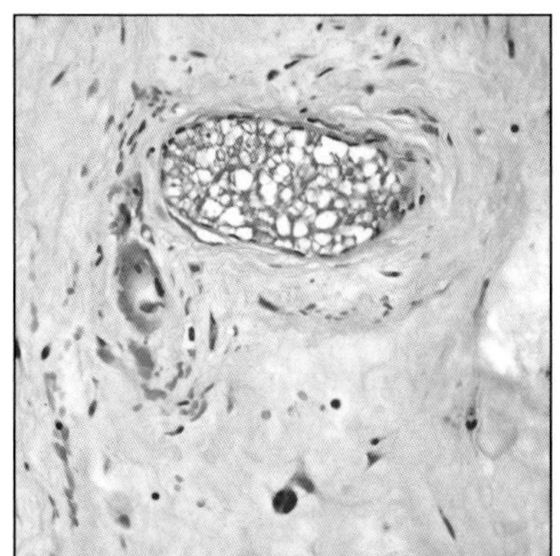

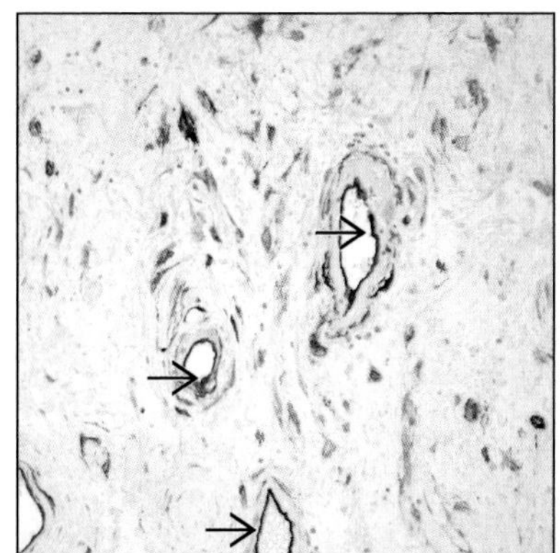

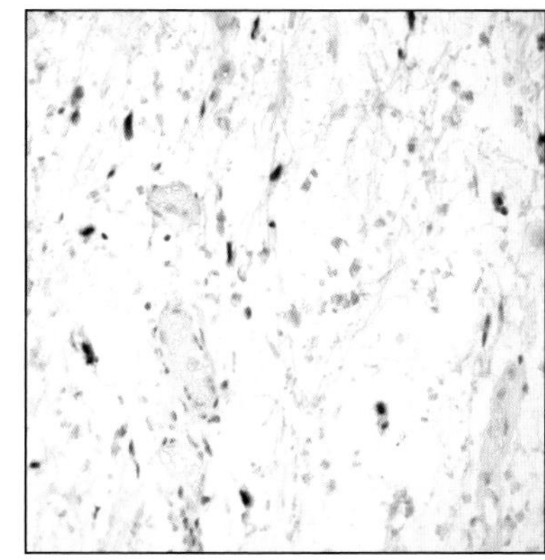

(Left) *A hyperchromatic cell in an aggressive angiomyxoma is shown. The background shows abundant myxoid matrix without wiry collagen.* ***(Center)*** *Aggressive angiomyxomas have a variable immunolabeling pattern. This example shows fairly strong CD34 labeling. Note the internal control endothelial cells ⇒ that strongly express CD34.* ***(Right)*** *Estrogen receptor is often expressed by the lesional cells in aggressive angiomyxomas, even those that arise in men.*

ANGIOMYOFIBROBLASTOMA

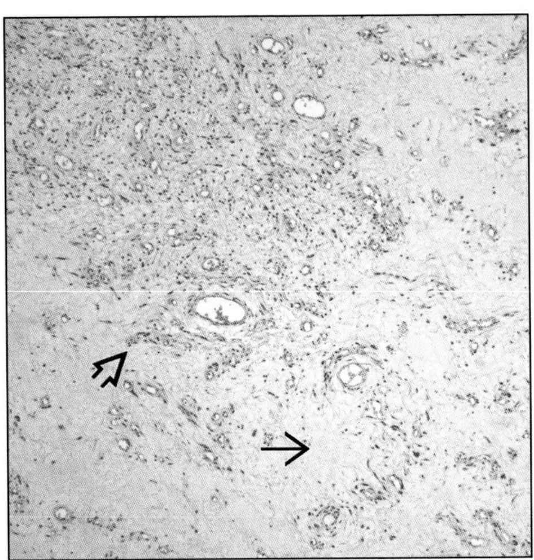

Angiomyofibroblastoma is characterized by numerous capillary-sized vessels ➢, alternating zones of cellularity and more fibrous areas →, without necrosis.

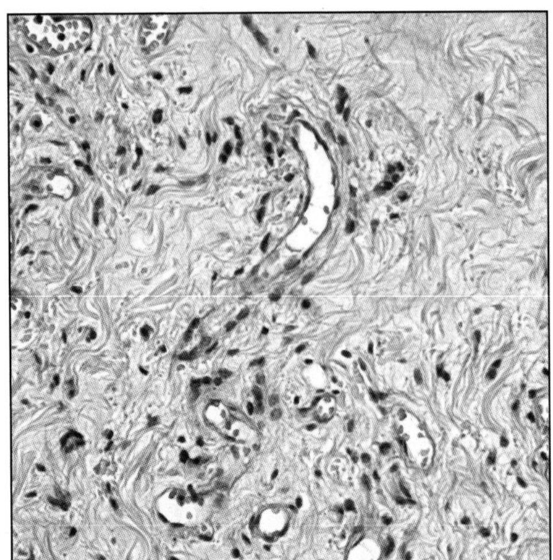

The stromal cells tend to cluster around the prominent yet delicate vascular component. The intervening tissue is sparsely cellular and contains slender collagen fibrils. The cells lack nuclear atypia.

TERMINOLOGY

Abbreviations

- Angiomyofibroblastoma (AMF)

Definitions

- Benign stromal tumor composed of numerous capillaries and myofibroblasts

ETIOLOGY/PATHOGENESIS

Cell of Origin

- Subepithelial mesenchyme of distal female genital tract

CLINICAL ISSUES

Epidemiology

- Age
  - Typically women of reproductive age

Site

- Vulva
- Vagina

Presentation

- Most common signs/symptoms
  - Painless mass
    - Often thought to represent cyst

Treatment

- Local excision

Prognosis

- Excellent
- No recurrent potential

MACROSCOPIC FEATURES

General Features

- Well circumscribed
- Tan-white
- Rubbery cut surface

Size

- Usually < 5 cm

MICROSCOPIC PATHOLOGY

Histologic Features

- Nonencapsulated
- Well demarcated
- Rich vascular component
  - Numerous thin-walled capillaries
- Alternating zones of cellularity
- Variably edematous to collagenous matrix
- Plump, ovoid (plasmacytoid) to spindle-shaped cells
  - Cells cluster around capillaries
- Less commonly, may have lipomatous component
- Rarely, associated with malignant transformation

Margins

- Well circumscribed

ANCILLARY TESTS

Immunohistochemistry

- Typically desmin(+)
- ER and PR usually positive
- S100 and CD34 variably positive
- Smooth muscle actin usually negative

ANGIOMYOFIBROBLASTOMA

Key Facts

Terminology

- Benign stromal tumor composed of numerous capillaries and myofibroblasts

Clinical Issues

- Often thought to represent a cyst
- Local excision
- No recurrent potential

Microscopic Pathology

- Well demarcated
- Numerous thin-walled capillaries
- Alternating zones of cellularity
- Variably edematous to collagenous matrix
- Plump, ovoid (plasmacytoid) to spindle-shaped cells
- Cells cluster around capillaries

Ancillary Tests

- Typically desmin positive

DIFFERENTIAL DIAGNOSIS

Deep Angiomyxoma

- Infiltrative, not circumscribed, margins
- Uniformly cellular (lacks alternating zones of cellularity seen in AMF)
- Less vascular; contains medium to large-sized vessels

Cellular Angiofibroma

- More uniformly cellular
- Less vascular; contains medium-sized vessels, often with hyalinized walls
- Typically positive for CD34

Fibroepithelial Stromal Polyp

- Typically polypoid
  - Overlying squamous epithelium
  - May have thin connecting stalk
- Vascular component tends to be central (vascular core)
  - Medium to large-sized vessels
- Does not have distinct margin
- Stellate and multinucleate cells are characteristic
  - Often located beneath epithelial surface at epithelial-stromal interface
  - May be present around central vasculature

DIAGNOSTIC CHECKLIST

Pathologic Interpretation Pearls

- Stromal cells tend to be spindled in tumors from postmenopausal women

SELECTED REFERENCES

1. Cao D et al: Lipomatous variant of angiomyofibroblastoma: report of two cases and review of the literature. Int J Gynecol Pathol. 24(2):196-200, 2005
2. McCluggage WG et al: Angiomyofibroblastoma of the vagina. J Clin Pathol. 53(10):803, 2000
3. Nucci MR et al: Vulvovaginal soft tissue tumours: update and review. Histopathology. 36(2):97-108, 2000
4. Fukunaga M et al: Vulval angiomyofibroblastoma. Clinicopathologic analysis of six cases. Am J Clin Pathol. 107(1):45-51, 1997
5. Laskin WB et al: Angiomyofibroblastoma of the female genital tract: analysis of 17 cases including a lipomatous variant. Hum Pathol. 28(9):1046-55, 1997
6. Nielsen GP et al: Angiomyofibroblastoma of the vulva and vagina. Mod Pathol. 9(3):284-91, 1996
7. Hisaoka M et al: Angiomyofibroblastoma of the vulva: a clinicopathologic study of seven cases. Pathol Int. 45(7):487-92, 1995
8. Fletcher CD et al: Angiomyofibroblastoma of the vulva. A benign neoplasm distinct from aggressive angiomyxoma. Am J Surg Pathol. 16(4):373-82, 1992

IMAGE GALLERY

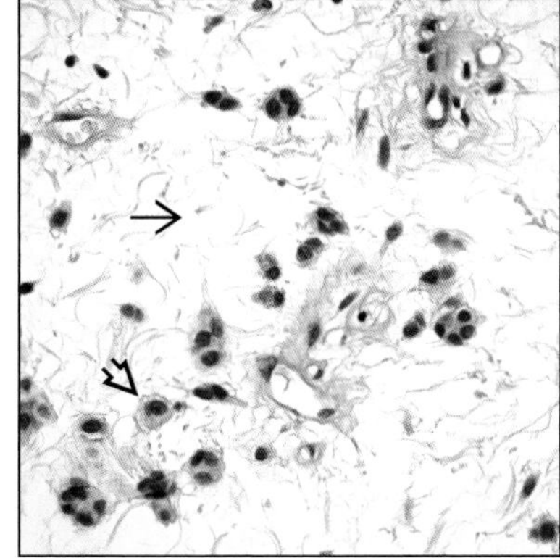

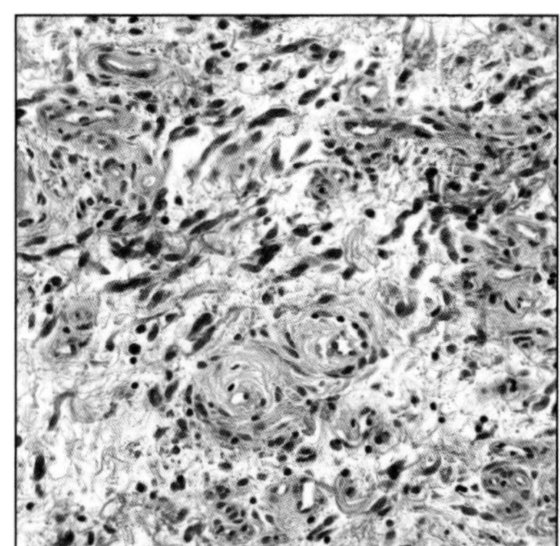

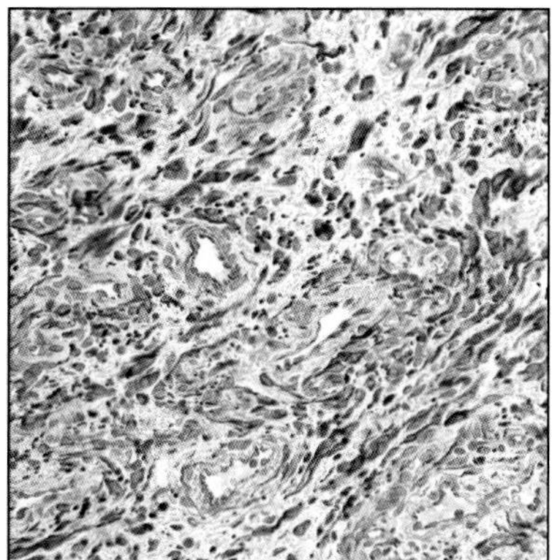

(Left) *The plump plasmacytoid stromal cells ⇨ surround thin-walled capillaries. Note edematous matrix →.* ***(Center)*** *The stromal cells are spindled in this tumor from a postmenopausal patient; however, the cells maintain their relationship to the vasculature.* ***(Right)*** *The tumor cells typically are diffusely immunoreactive for desmin, as seen here.*

CELLULAR ANGIOFIBROMA

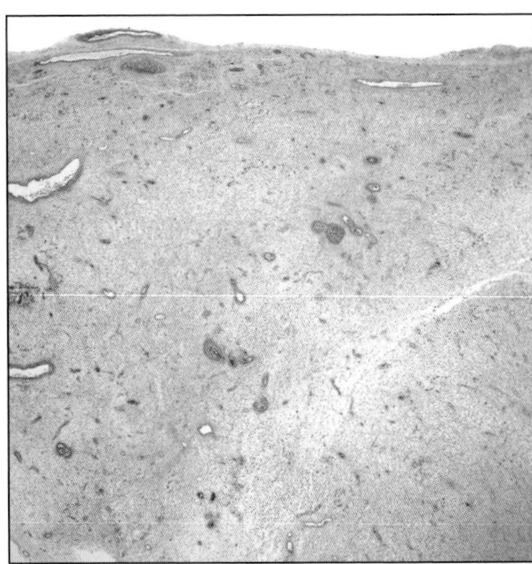

At low magnification, this cellular angiofibroma is well marginated but unencapsulated. Note the prominent vessels, readily apparent even at scanning magnification.

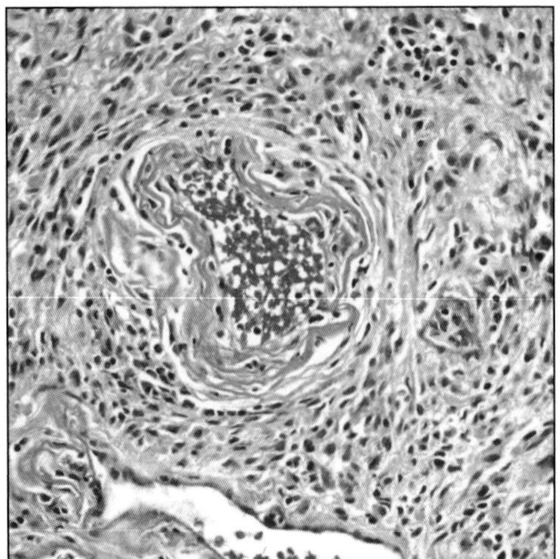

Thick hyalinized vessels are characteristic of cellular angiofibroma. The lesion is moderately cellular and consists of a uniform population of spindle cells and background collagen fibrils.

TERMINOLOGY

Synonyms

- Angiomyofibroblastoma-like tumor of male genital tract

Definitions

- Well-marginated tumor of genital stroma composed of uniform population of bland spindle-shaped cells, wispy collagen, and thick-walled hyalinized vessels
- Resembles spindle cell lipoma with 13q- and RB/13q14 allelic loss in some cases

CLINICAL ISSUES

Epidemiology

- Incidence
  - Rare
- Age
  - Middle-aged patients
- Gender
  - More common in women

Presentation

- Females
  - Usually in vulva, occasionally in vagina
- Males
  - Inguinoscrotal region

Prognosis

- Benign lesions
  - Recurrences rare
  - Examples with sarcomatous features have exhibited benign behavior

MACROSCOPIC FEATURES

General Features

- Subcutaneous
- Well circumscribed ("shelled out")
- Firm to rubbery gray-white cut surface
- Necrosis rare

Size

- Median: 2-3 cm in females
- Median: 6-7 cm in males

MICROSCOPIC PATHOLOGY

Histologic Features

- Well marginated, surrounded by entrapped fat at periphery
- Moderately cellular
- Uniform spindle cells
  - Occasional palisading
  - Rare examples with atypical nuclei/"sarcomatous" transformation
    - Benign clinical outcomes reported for such cases
- Fibrous stroma with wispy collagen
- Mitoses not numerous
- Highly vascular
  - Small to medium-sized
  - Hyalinized vessels common and characteristic
- About 10% contain abundant mature fat

DIFFERENTIAL DIAGNOSIS

Aggressive Angiomyxoma

- Large masses
- Deep soft tissue of genital region of women in reproductive years
- Poorly marginated gelatinous mass
- Paucicellular myxoid lesion
- Spindled to stellate cells
- Prominent stromal vessels
- Smooth muscle and lesional cells radiate from around vessels
- Variable CD34, desmin, smooth muscle actin, ER, PR

CELLULAR ANGIOFIBROMA

Key Facts

Terminology
- Synonym: Angiomyofibroblastoma-like tumor of male genital tract

Clinical Issues
- Middle-aged patients
- More common in women
- Subcutaneous; usually in vulva or inguinoscrotal region
- Benign lesions
- Recurrences rare
- Examples with sarcomatous features have exhibited benign behavior

Microscopic Pathology
- Uniform spindle cells
- Fibrous stroma with wispy collagen
- Highly vascular
- Hyalinized vessels common and characteristic
- About 10% contain abundant fat

Immunohistochemistry

Antibody	Reactivity	Staining Pattern	Comment
CD34	Positive	Cytoplasmic	About 60%
Desmin	Positive	Cytoplasmic	About 10%
Actin-sm	Positive	Cytoplasmic	About 20%
ERP	Positive	Nuclear	About 50% in women; about 20% in men
PRP	Positive	Nuclear	About 90% in women; about 20% in men
S100	Negative		

Angiomyofibroblastoma
- Vulvar lesions of reproductive-age and early postmenopausal women
- Well marginated
- Alternating high and low cellularity
- Epithelioid cells with ample eosinophilic cytoplasm
- Spindle cells
- Prominent vascularity
- Tumor cells aggregate around vessels
- Variable CD34, desmin, smooth muscle actin, ER, PR

Superficial Cervicovaginal Myofibroblastoma
- Also termed superficial myofibroblastoma of lower female genital tract
- Superficial lamina propria of cervix, vagina, vulva
- Well circumscribed
- Uninvolved skin/mucosal Grenz zone
- Moderate cellularity
- Bland cells with ovoid nuclei
- Delicately collagenous stroma
- Variable CD34, desmin, smooth muscle actin, ER, PR

SELECTED REFERENCES

1. Chen E et al: Cellular angiofibroma with atypia or sarcomatous transformation: clinicopathologic analysis of 13 cases. Am J Surg Pathol. 34(5):707-14, 2010
2. Iwasa Y et al: Cellular angiofibroma: clinicopathologic and immunohistochemical analysis of 51 cases. Am J Surg Pathol. 28(11):1426-35, 2004
3. Laskin WB et al: Angiomyofibroblastoma-like tumor of the male genital tract: analysis of 11 cases with comparison to female angiomyofibroblastoma and spindle cell lipoma. Am J Surg Pathol. 22(1):6-16, 1998
4. Nucci MR et al: Cellular angiofibroma: a benign neoplasm distinct from angiomyofibroblastoma and spindle cell lipoma. Am J Surg Pathol. 21(6):636-44, 1997

IMAGE GALLERY

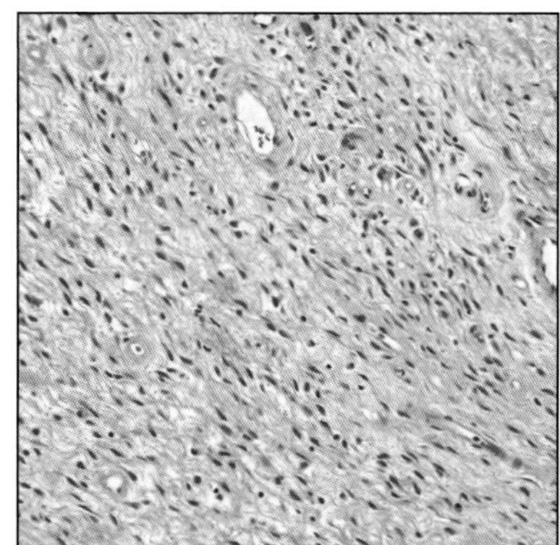
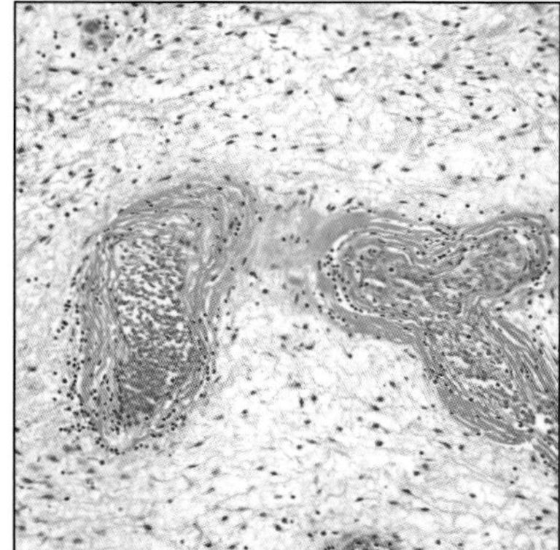
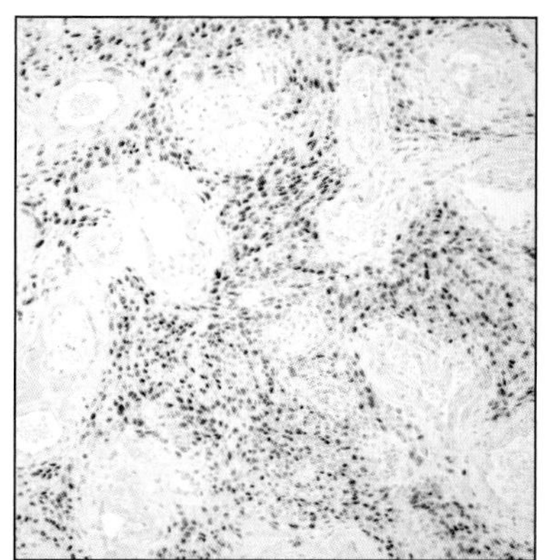

(Left) *This cellular angiofibroma is somewhat myxoid/edematous but composed of uniform spindle cells and wispy collagen.* ***(Center)*** *Prominent thick-walled hyalinized vessels are shown in a hypocellular portion of a cellular angiofibroma.* ***(Right)*** *This cellular angiofibroma shows strong nuclear expression of estrogen receptor (ER). ER expression is common in these lesions, especially in women, but this characteristic does not help distinguish cellular angiofibroma from other tumors of the genital area stroma.*

SUPERFICIAL CERVICOVAGINAL MYOFIBROBLASTOMA

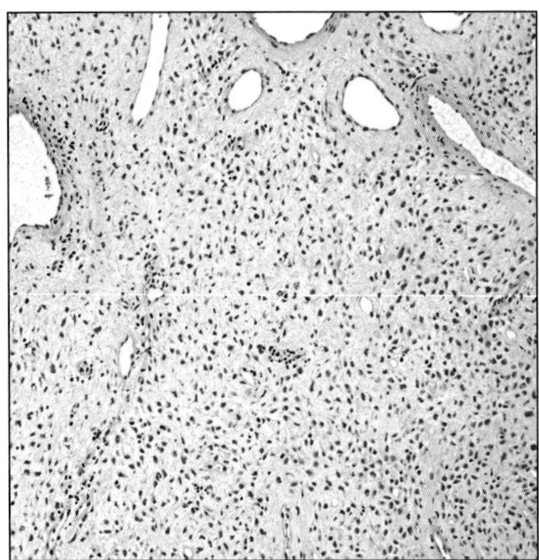

Superficial cervicovaginal myofibroblastoma is characterized by a monotonous proliferation of bland ovoid, spindle, or stellate cells arranged in a monotonous pattern.

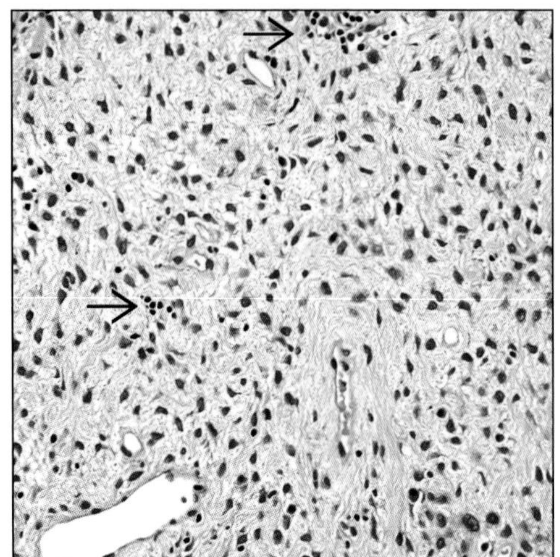

Note the bland appearance of the stellate cells in this image. The lesion is moderately cellular, and there is a background of delicate wavy collagen. Note the scattered background lymphocytes ⇒.

TERMINOLOGY

Synonyms

- Myofibroblastoma of lower female genital tract

Definitions

- Polypoid or nodular benign lesions of vagina, cervix, or vulva, composed of bland mesenchymal cells

CLINICAL ISSUES

Epidemiology

- Age
  - Adults
    - Mean: About 60 years
- Gender
  - Women

Presentation

- Polypoid or nodular mass
  - Vagina, cervix, or vulva

Treatment

- Excision

Prognosis

- Excellent; benign lesions

MACROSCOPIC FEATURES

General Features

- Well marginated
- Unencapsulated
- Covered by overlying mucosa or skin

Size

- Mean: About 3 cm

MICROSCOPIC PATHOLOGY

Histologic Features

- Uninvolved Grenz zone between lesion and overlying mucosa or skin
- Moderately cellular
- Bland ovoid to spindle or stellate cells
- Some cells with wavy nuclear appearance
- Multiple patterns possible
  - Lace-like, sieve-like, fascicular
  - Several patterns can be seen in same lesion
- Finely collagenous stroma
  - Occasional cases with coarser collagen
- Occasional mitotic figures
- Richer vascularity toward center of lesions
- No aggregation of cells around vessels
- Minimal background inflammation

DIFFERENTIAL DIAGNOSIS

Fibroepithelial Stromal Polyp

- Polypoid appearance
- No Grenz zone between lesion and overlying mucosa or skin
- Monomorphic architecture
  - Spindled to stellate cells
  - Multinucleated cells common
    - Some can be atypical
  - Scattered mitoses
- Immunoprofile overlaps with that of superficial cervicovaginal myofibroblastoma

Angiomyofibroblastoma

- Mass rather than polyp
  - Usually deeper than fibroepithelial polyp or superficial cervicovaginal myofibroblastoma
- Aggregation of cells around vessels
- Ovoid to spindle-shaped cells
  - Abundant cytoplasm; plasmacytoid appearance

SUPERFICIAL CERVICOVAGINAL MYOFIBROBLASTOMA

Key Facts

Clinical Issues

- Adults; mean age about 60 years
- Polypoid or nodular mass of vagina, cervix, or vulva
- Treatment: Excision
- Prognosis: Excellent; benign lesions

Microscopic Pathology

- Uninvolved Grenz zone between lesion and overlying mucosa or skin
- Moderately cellular
- Bland ovoid to spindle or stellate cells
- Some cells with wavy appearance
- Multiple patterns possible
  - Lace-like, sieve-like, fascicular
  - Several patterns can be seen in same lesion
- Finely collagenous stroma
- Occasional mitotic figures
- Desmin(+), ER(+), PR(+), CD34(+)

Immunohistochemistry

Antibody	Reactivity	Staining Pattern	Comment
Vimentin	Positive	Cytoplasmic	Virtually all cases reactive
Desmin	Positive	Cytoplasmic	Most cases positive
CD34	Positive	Cytoplasmic	Most cases positive
Actin-sm	Positive	Cytoplasmic	About half of cases
ERP	Positive	Nuclear	Most cases express estrogen receptor
PRP	Positive	Nuclear	Most cases express progesterone receptor
S100	Negative		
CK-PAN	Negative		

- Immunoprofile overlaps with that of superficial cervicovaginal myofibroblastoma

Cellular Angiofibroma

- Well-circumscribed mass lesions
  - Immunoprofile overlaps with that of superficial cervicovaginal myofibroblastoma
- Uniform bland spindle cells in fibrous stroma with wavy collagen
- Prominent vessels with thick and hyalinized walls
- Stromal mast cells and other inflammatory cells
- Immunoprofile overlaps with that of superficial cervicovaginal myofibroblastoma

Neurofibroma

- Spindle cells
- Variably myxoid stroma
- Wavy dense collagen
- Sometimes surrounded by rim of perineurium
- Prominent mast cells
- S100 protein(+)

SELECTED REFERENCES

1. Ganesan R et al: Superficial myofibroblastoma of the lower female genital tract: report of a series including tumours with a vulval location. Histopathology. 46(2):137-43, 2005
2. McCluggage WG: A review and update of morphologically bland vulvovaginal mesenchymal lesions. Int J Gynecol Pathol. 24(1):26-38, 2005
3. Laskin WB et al: Superficial cervicovaginal myofibroblastoma: fourteen cases of a distinctive mesenchymal tumor arising from the specialized subepithelial stroma of the lower female genital tract. Hum Pathol. 32(7):715-25, 2001

IMAGE GALLERY

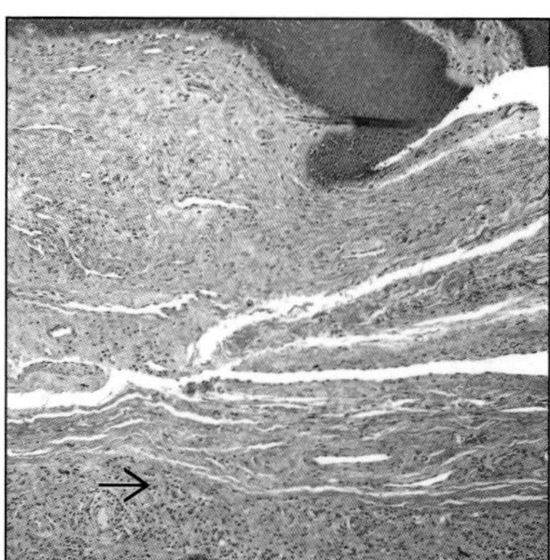

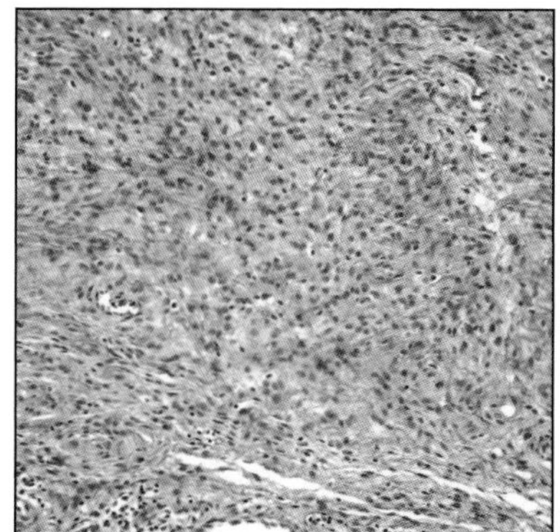

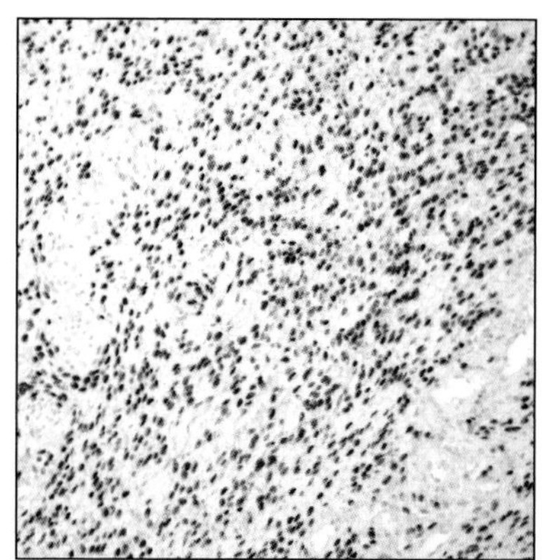

(Left) *Superficial cervicovaginal myofibroblastoma has a Grenz zone between the border of the lesion and the overlying epithelium* ⇒. *This differs from fibroepithelial stromal polyps, which abut the overlying epithelium.* ***(Center)*** *Superficial cervicovaginal myofibroblastoma consists of rounded to wavy nuclei. The lesion lacks the perivascular aggregation of cells seen in angiomyofibroblastoma.* ***(Right)*** *There is ER expression in this superficial cervicovaginal angiomyofibroblastoma.*

Mesothelial Lesions

Benign

Malignant

Examination of Mesothelioma Specimens

ADENOMATOID TUMOR

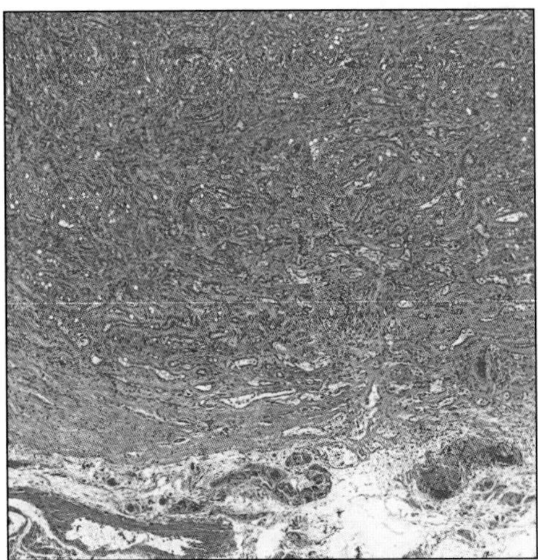

Hematoxylin & eosin shows a well-marginated lesion without a capsule. The cellular component is evenly distributed within a collagenous stroma.

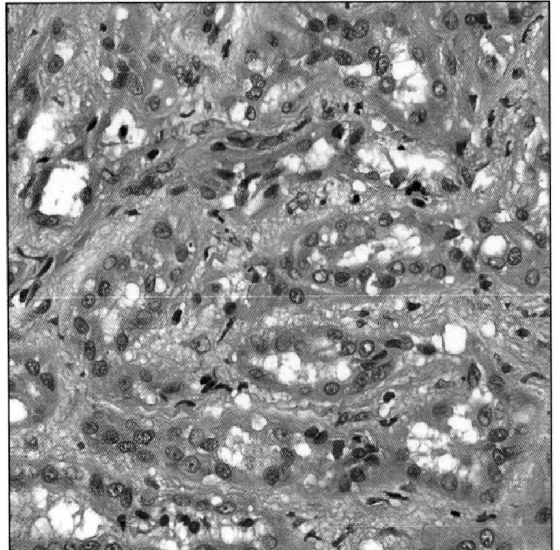

Hematoxylin & eosin shows variably sized tubules randomly orientated in fibrous stroma with a sprinkling of lymphocytes. The tubules are composed of cuboidal mesothelial cells with rounded uniform nuclei.

TERMINOLOGY

Definitions

- Benign mesothelial tumor
- Most common in male and female genital organs

ETIOLOGY/PATHOGENESIS

Benign Neoplasm

- No causal factors known

Antecedent or Associated Conditions

- Can coexist with multicystic peritoneal mesothelioma

CLINICAL ISSUES

Epidemiology

- Incidence
  - Relatively uncommon
    - Usually solitary, rarely multiple
- Age
  - Most common in 4th-7th decades
  - Rare in 1st 2 decades
- Gender
  - Occurs in both males and females

Site

- In males
  - Epididymis, spermatic cord
  - Testis (tunica albuginea, body of testis)
  - Prostate
- In females
  - Uterus
  - Fallopian tube
  - Ovary
- In either sex
  - Adrenal gland
  - Mesentery, pancreas
  - Pleura, mediastinum
  - Lymph node

Presentation

- Painless mass
  - Occasionally causes hydrocele

Treatment

- Surgical approaches
  - Excision is curative

Prognosis

- Malignant change does not occur

MACROSCOPIC FEATURES

General Features

- Circumscribed nodule
- Rarely larger than 2 cm in diameter
- Occasionally cystic

MICROSCOPIC PATHOLOGY

Histologic Features

- Gland-like tubules
- Thin-walled spaces
- Cubical or flattened lining cells
  - Lining cells present within lumen
- Variable fibrous stroma
  - Can have smooth muscle component
- Lymphocytic infiltrate
- Occasional infarction

Predominant Pattern/Injury Type

- Glandular

Predominant Cell/Compartment Type

- Mesothelial

ADENOMATOID TUMOR

Key Facts

Terminology
- Benign mesothelial tumor

Clinical Issues
- Usually solitary, rarely multiple
- Most common in 4th-7th decades
- Most common in male and female genital organs
  - Epididymis, spermatic cord
  - Uterus, fallopian tube
  - Adrenal gland
- Painless mass
- Malignant change does not occur

Macroscopic Features
- Rarely larger than 2 cm in diameter
- Occasionally cystic

Microscopic Pathology
- Gland-like tubules
- Thin-walled spaces

ANCILLARY TESTS

Immunohistochemistry
- Expresses mesothelial markers calretinin, EMA, CK5/6, D2-40, WT1
- Lacks CEA (but some express BER-EP4)

Electron Microscopy
- Transmission
  - Mesothelial features: Long slender microvilli, desmosomes, tonofilaments

DIFFERENTIAL DIAGNOSIS

Well-Differentiated Papillary Mesothelioma
- Different location and clinical picture
- Papillary architecture

Multicystic Peritoneal Mesothelioma
- Usually involves peritoneal surface
- Larger cysts, but features can overlap

Malignant Mesothelioma
- Larger, more diffuse, or multiple lesions
- Infiltrates adjacent tissues
- Nuclear atypia, mitoses, necrosis

Metastatic Adenocarcinoma
- Clinical setting
- Pleomorphism and mitotic activity
- Absence of mesothelial immunohistochemical markers
- Presence of specific antigens, e.g., PSA

DIAGNOSTIC CHECKLIST

Clinically Relevant Pathologic Features
- Gross appearance

Pathologic Interpretation Pearls
- Small circumscribed nodule
- No atypical features
- Mesothelial antigens expressed

SELECTED REFERENCES

1. Timonera ER et al: Composite adenomatoid tumor and myelolipoma of adrenal gland: report of 2 cases. Arch Pathol Lab Med. 132(2):265-7, 2008
2. Skinnider BF et al: Infarcted adenomatoid tumor: a report of five cases of a facet of a benign neoplasm that may cause diagnostic difficulty. Am J Surg Pathol. 28(1):77-83, 2004
3. Isotalo PA et al: Adenomatoid tumor of the adrenal gland: a clinicopathologic study of five cases and review of the literature. Am J Surg Pathol. 27(7):969-77, 2003
4. Nogales FF et al: Adenomatoid tumors of the uterus: an analysis of 60 cases. Int J Gynecol Pathol. 21(1):34-40, 2002
5. Huang CC et al: Adenomatoid tumor of the female genital tract. Int J Gynaecol Obstet. 50(3):275-80, 1995
6. Gaffey MJ et al: Immunoreactivity for BER-EP4 in adenocarcinomas, adenomatoid tumors, and malignant mesotheliomas. Am J Surg Pathol. 16(6):593-9, 1992

IMAGE GALLERY

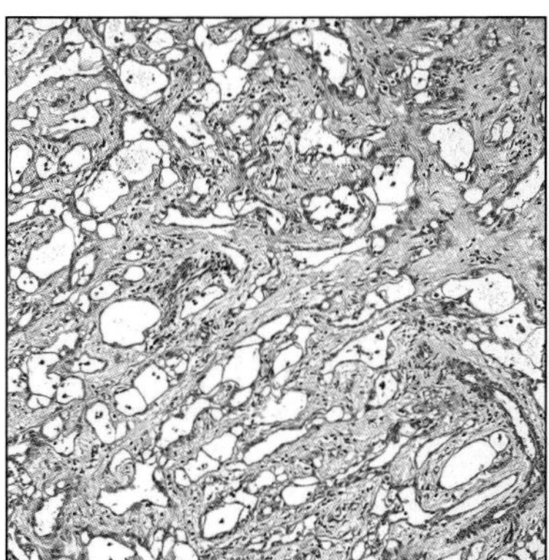
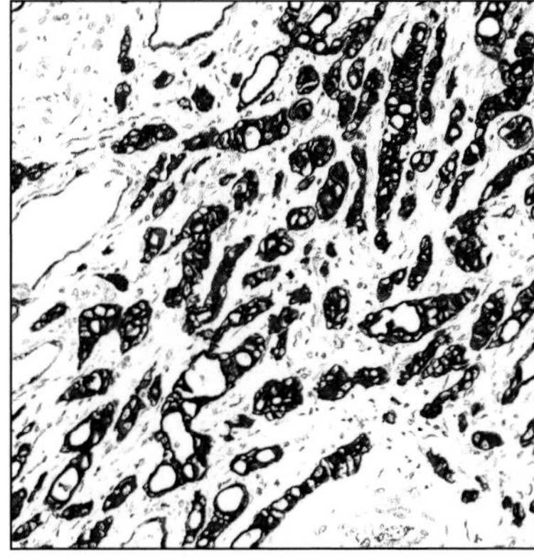
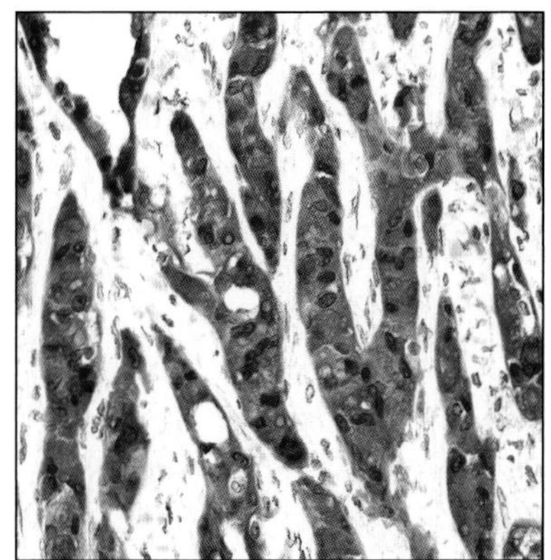

(Left) *Hematoxylin & eosin shows gland-like spaces lined by a flattened layer of mesothelial cells. Note the shedding of the cells into the lumina and focally myxoid inflamed stroma.* ***(Center)*** *Positive CAM5.2 shows diffuse immunoreactivity in lining cells. In some places, these appear multilayered.* ***(Right)*** *Positive Calretinin shows diffuse nuclear and cytoplasmic staining. The lesional mesothelial cells focally form branching solid cords.*

MULTICYSTIC PERITONEAL MESOTHELIOMA

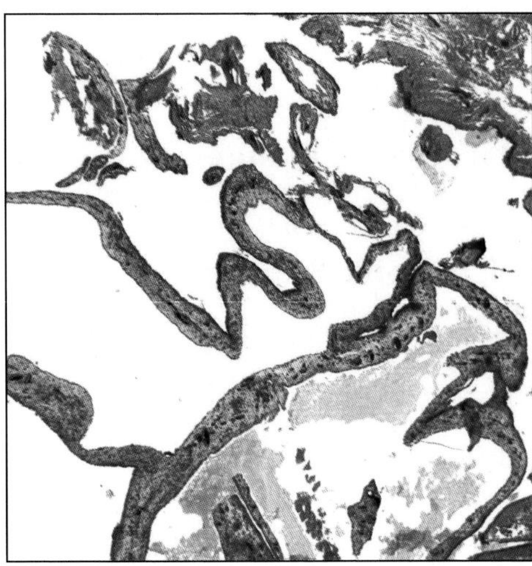

Hematoxylin & eosin shows multiple large cysts separated by connective tissue septa. Cysts vary in size and contain proteinaceous secretion. Note that the cyst lining lacks tufting or papilla formation.

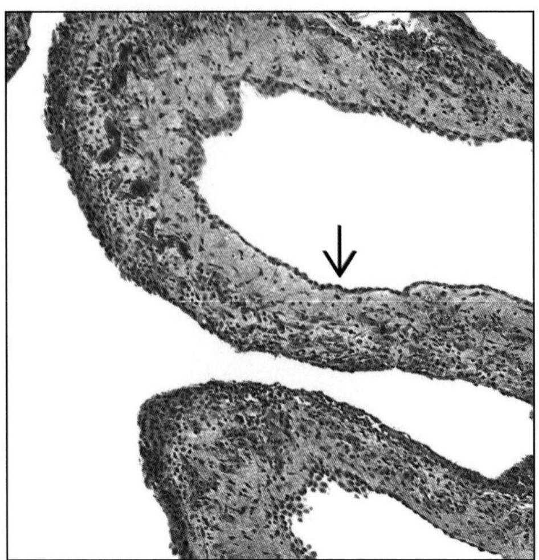

Hematoxylin & eosin shows that the cyst is lined by a single layer of flattened or cuboidal cells ⇒. Hobnail pattern, tufts, or papillae are sometimes seen. The septa are composed of vascular fibrous tissue.

TERMINOLOGY

Abbreviations
- Multicystic peritoneal mesothelioma (MPM)

Synonyms
- Benign cystic mesothelioma
- Peritoneal inclusion cyst

Definitions
- Benign intraabdominal or pelvic lesion of parietal or serosal peritoneal mesothelium
  - Can be multicystic or composed of several separate cystic lesions

ETIOLOGY/PATHOGENESIS

Developmental Anomaly
- Very rare familial cases described

Environmental Exposure
- Rarely associated with previous exposure to asbestos

Antecedent or Associated Conditions
- Previous abdominal or pelvic surgery
- Endometriosis
- Pelvic inflammatory disease
- Adenomatoid tumor in ovary and other sites
  - Some examples have features of both tumors

CLINICAL ISSUES

Epidemiology
- Incidence
  - Rare
- Age
  - Predominantly in 2nd-6th decades
- Gender
  - More common in females

Site
- Mostly on visceral peritoneum including surfaces of pelvic organs
  - Uterus, bladder, rectum
  - Rarely involves other viscera, mesentery, omentum
- Can form detached intraperitoneal mass
- Extraperitoneal sites very rare
  - Pericardium, pleura, cesarean section scar

Presentation
- Incidental finding
- Painful or painless mass

Treatment
- Surgical approaches
  - Complete excision where feasible
  - In situ ablation
    - Sclerosing agents or laser ablation
- Adjuvant therapy
  - Intraperitoneal chemotherapy for intractable cases

Prognosis
- Majority are benign
- Small number recur, or spread, especially if incompletely excised
- Rare single examples have been associated with diffuse epithelioid malignant mesothelioma

IMAGE FINDINGS

CT Findings
- Characteristic pattern of thin-walled cysts

MACROSCOPIC FEATURES

General Features
- Thin-walled cysts in subserosa or as mass
  - Cysts contain clear or hemorrhagic fluid

MULTICYSTIC PERITONEAL MESOTHELIOMA

Key Facts

Terminology
- Benign intraabdominal or pelvic lesion of parietal or serosal peritoneal mesothelium

Etiology/Pathogenesis
- Minimal association with previous exposure to asbestos
- Previous abdominal or pelvic surgery
- Endometriosis
- Adenomatoid tumor in ovary and other sites

Clinical Issues
- More common in females
- Incidental finding
- Small number recur or spread

Microscopic Pathology
- Cysts are lined by cuboidal or flattened epithelium
- No cytological atypia
- Mesothelial cell nests or pseudoglandular spaces in stroma of septa

Size
- Individual lesions vary from 1 mm to > 5 cm

MICROSCOPIC PATHOLOGY

Histologic Features
- Cysts lined by cuboidal or flattened epithelium
- Uniform but variably orientated nuclei
- Scanty, darkly eosinophilic cytoplasm
- Usually single layer of cells with brush border
  - Hobnailing, tufting, or papillation sometimes present
- Stroma between cysts
  - Contains fibroblast, capillaries, collagen, and lymphocytes
  - Occasionally has mesothelial cell clusters that mimic invasive carcinoma
- No cytological atypia
- Rare focal calcifications or hyaline globules

Predominant Pattern/Injury Type
- Cystic, complex

Predominant Cell/Compartment Type
- Mesenchymal

ANCILLARY TESTS

Immunohistochemistry
- Cells express CK, EMA, and calretinin
- CD34 and CD31 are negative

DIFFERENTIAL DIAGNOSIS

Cystic Lymphangioma
- Male predominance, younger age
- Cysts contain milky fluid
- Lining cells express CD34 and CD31, lack CK

Malignant Mesothelioma
- Solid or papillary, rarely cystic
- Cytological atypia, mitotic activity, invasion of stroma

Adenomatoid Tumor
- Circumscribed
- Pattern of tubules within fibrous stroma
- Cuboidal or flattened epithelium
- Features can overlap with those of MPM

SELECTED REFERENCES

1. Muscarella P et al: Retroperitoneal benign cystic peritoneal mesothelioma. Surgery. 135(2):228-31, 2004
2. Sawh RN et al: Benign cystic mesothelioma of the peritoneum: a clinicopathologic study of 17 cases and immunohistochemical analysis of estrogen and progesterone receptor status. Hum Pathol. 34(4):369-74, 2003
3. Weiss SW et al: Multicystic mesothelioma. An analysis of pathologic findings and biologic behavior in 37 cases. Am J Surg Pathol. 12(10):737-46, 1988

IMAGE GALLERY

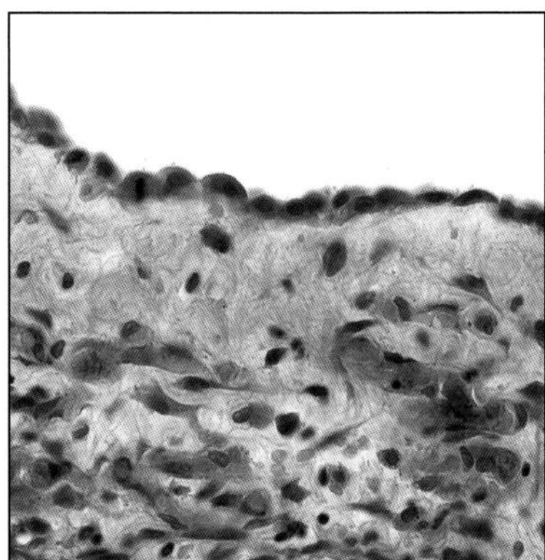
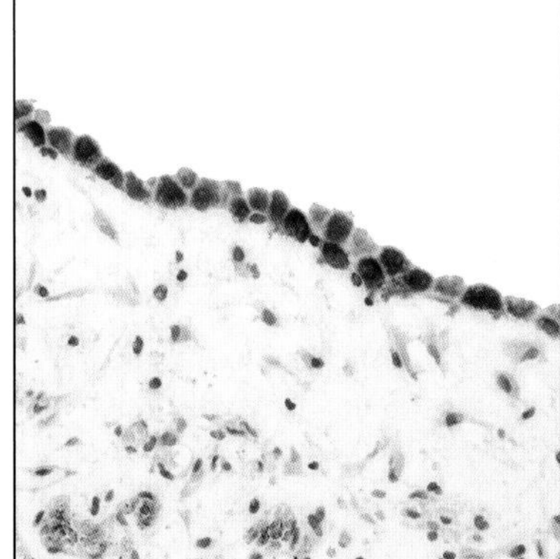
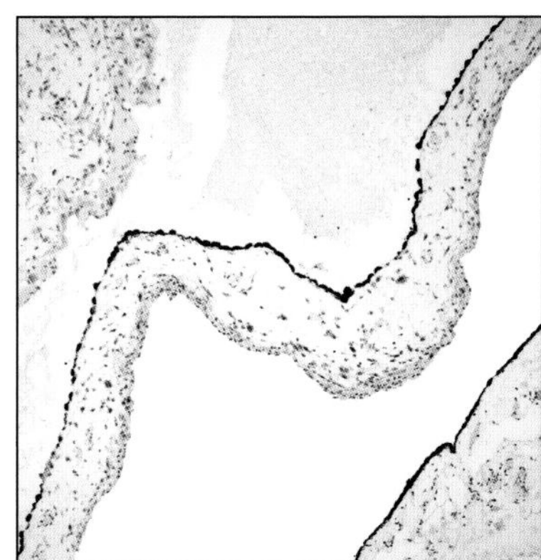

*(**Left**) Hematoxylin & eosin shows a single layer of mesothelial cells with uniform but variably orientated nuclei and scanty cytoplasm. Rarely there is squamous metaplasia. The cyst wall can occasionally contain clusters of mesothelial cells, mimicking carcinoma. (**Center**) Positive CK5/6 shows diffuse distribution in lining cells. Endothelial markers are negative, excluding cystic lymphangioma. (**Right**) Positive calretinin shows a line of highlighted nuclei in the layer of cuboidal cells lining the cyst. This confirms the mesothelial nature of the cells.*

WELL-DIFFERENTIATED PAPILLARY MESOTHELIOMA

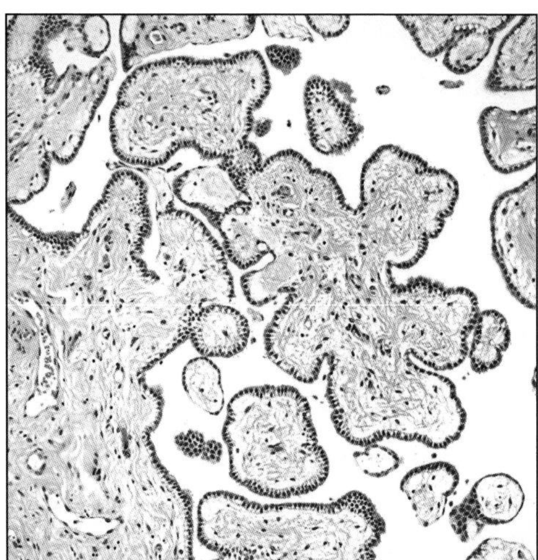

Hematoxylin & eosin shows well-formed branching papillary structures or blunt processes arising from the peritoneal surface.

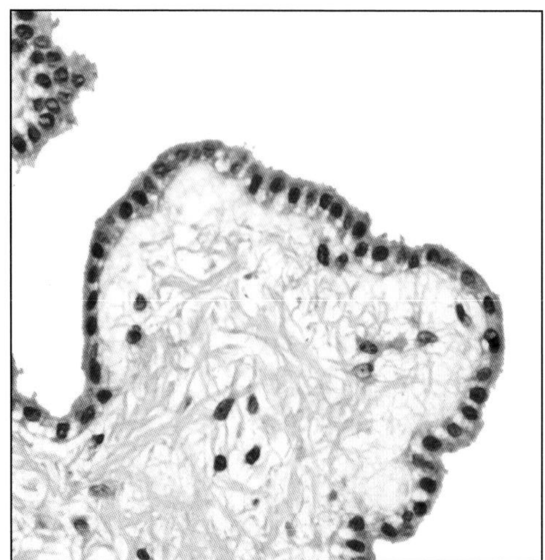

Hematoxylin & eosin shows papillae covered by a single layer of uniform cuboidal mesothelial cells with rounded central nuclei and eosinophilic cytoplasm. Note collagen fibers in the papillary core.

TERMINOLOGY

Synonyms

- Benign mesothelioma
- Mesothelioma of low malignant potential

ETIOLOGY/PATHOGENESIS

Environmental Exposure

- Some patients have history of asbestos exposure

CLINICAL ISSUES

Epidemiology

- Incidence
  - Rare
    - Peritoneum, omentum, pleura, pericardium
    - Paratesticular (tunica vaginalis)
- Age
  - Predominantly 30-50 years
- Gender
  - Peritoneal lesions mostly in females
  - Pleural lesions M = F

Presentation

- Incidental finding

Treatment

- Surgical approaches
  - Excision of localized lesion
- Adjuvant therapy
  - Chemotherapy for multiple or widespread lesions

Prognosis

- Solitary lesions generally benign
  - Some recur after long period as frank malignant mesothelioma with atypia and invasion
- Multiple or widespread lesions can be progressive

MICROSCOPIC PATHOLOGY

Histologic Features

- Well-formed papillary structures
  - Uniform cuboidal cells with central rounded nuclei
  - Single layer of cells on surface
  - Occasionally solid nests, tubules, cords
- Loose fibrous core
  - Occasionally myxoid
  - Multinucleated giant cells

Predominant Pattern/Injury Type

- Papillary

Predominant Cell/Compartment Type

- Mesothelial

DIFFERENTIAL DIAGNOSIS

Malignant Mesothelioma

- Multilayering
- Nuclear atypia, prominent nucleoli, mitoses, necrosis
- Stromal invasion

Primary Peritoneal Serous Carcinoma

- Cytologically malignant
- ER(+)
- BER-EP4(+)
- MOC-31(+)
- Calretinin(-)

Metastatic Ovarian Serous Carcinoma

- Cytologically malignant
- Invades stroma
- ER(+)
- BER-EP4(+)
- MOC-31(+)
- Calretinin usually negative (80%)

WELL-DIFFERENTIATED PAPILLARY MESOTHELIOMA

Key Facts

Clinical Issues

- Rare
- Peritoneal lesions mostly in females
- Occasionally paratesticular in males
- Solitary or multiple
- Rarely recur after long period as malignant mesothelioma with atypia and invasion

Microscopic Pathology

- Well-formed papillary structures
- Uniform cuboidal or epithelioid cells with central rounded nuclei
- Multinucleated cells in stroma

Top Differential Diagnoses

- Malignant mesothelioma
  - Nuclear atypia, nucleoli, mitoses, necrosis
- Metastatic ovarian serous carcinoma
  - Cytological atypia
  - ER, BER-EP4, MOC-31 positive

Immunohistochemistry

Antibody	Reactivity	Staining Pattern	Comment
AE1/AE3	Positive	Cytoplasmic	Diffuse (100%)
Calretinin	Positive	Nuclear	Diffuse (96%)
WT1	Positive	Nuclear	Diffuse (100%)
Podoplanin	Positive	Cell membrane	Diffuse (99%)
EpCAM/BER-EP4/ CD326	Negative		
CEA-M	Negative		
MOC-31	Negative		
ER	Negative		
EMA/MUC1	Equivocal	Cell membrane	Focal (15%)

SELECTED REFERENCES

1. Ikeda K et al: Cytomorphologic features of well-differentiated papillary mesothelioma in peritoneal effusion: a case report. Diagn Cytopathol. 36(7):512-5, 2008
2. Ordonez NG: Value of immunohistochemistry in distinguishing peritoneal mesothelioma from serous carcinoma of the ovary and peritoneum: a review and update. Adv Anat Pathol. 13(1):16-25, 2006
3. Tolhurst SR et al: Well-differentiated papillary mesothelioma occurring in the tunica vaginalis of the testis with contralateral atypical mesothelial hyperplasia. Urol Oncol. 24(1):36-9, 2006
4. Baker PM et al: Malignant peritoneal mesothelioma in women: a study of 75 cases with emphasis on their morphologic spectrum and differential diagnosis. Am J Clin Pathol. 123(5):724-37, 2005
5. Hoekstra AV et al: Well-differentiated papillary mesothelioma of the peritoneum: a pathological analysis and review of the literature. Gynecol Oncol. 98(1):161-7, 2005
6. Churg A: Paratesticular mesothelial proliferations. Semin Diagn Pathol. 20(4):272-8, 2003
7. Butnor KJ et al: Well-differentiated papillary mesothelioma. Am J Surg Pathol. 25(10):1304-9, 2001
8. Perez-Ordonez B et al: Mesothelial lesions of the paratesticular region. Semin Diagn Pathol. 17(4):294-306, 2000
9. Xiao SY et al: Benign papillary mesothelioma of the tunica vaginalis testis. Arch Pathol Lab Med. 124(1):143-7, 2000

IMAGE GALLERY

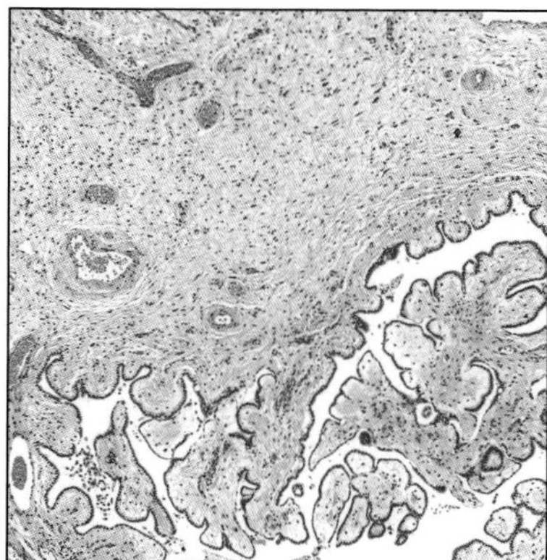

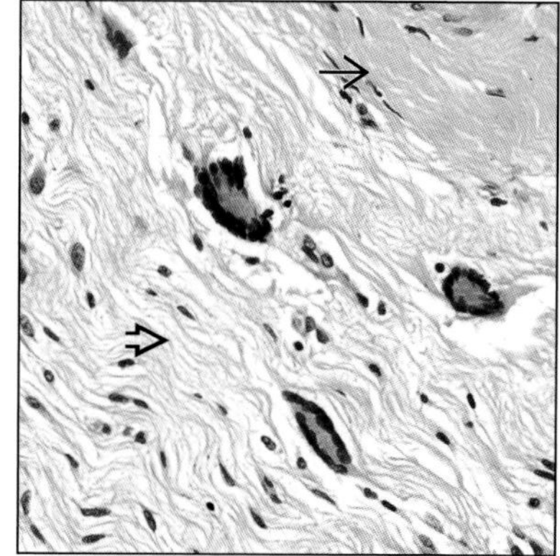

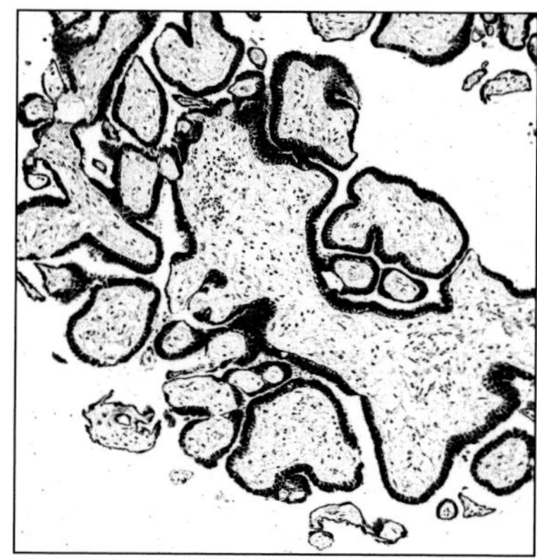

(Left) *Hematoxylin & eosin shows loose fibrous or fibromyxoid stroma with scattered fibroblasts and a few blood vessels.* ***(Center)*** *Hematoxylin & eosin shows multinucleated cells that are a feature of the stroma of papillae and base of lesion. Note both collagenous ⇒ and more myxoid ⇨ areas.* ***(Right)*** *Positive calretinin shows diffuse nuclear positivity in lesional (mesothelial) cells.*

MALIGNANT MESOTHELIOMA

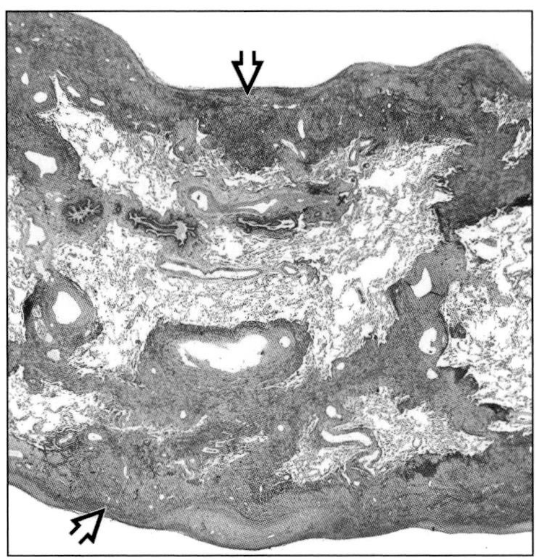

Low magnification of a section of the lung shows pleural thickening ⇒ by malignant mesothelioma. The tumor also extends along fissures and septa.

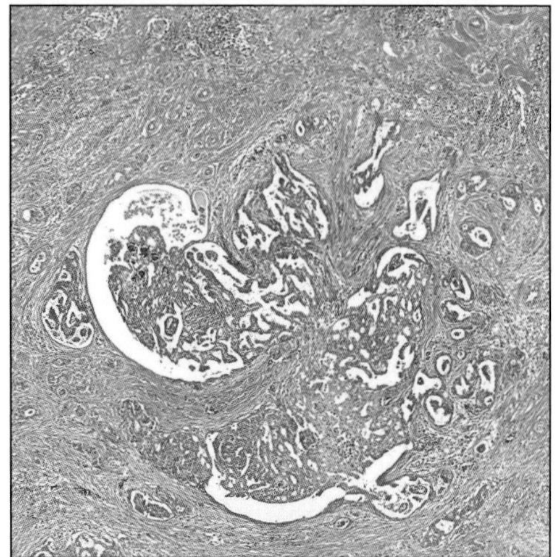

Hematoxylin & eosin shows microglandular, tubular, and papillary patterns of malignant mesothelioma with papillae growing within cystic spaces.

TERMINOLOGY

Abbreviations

- Malignant mesothelioma (MM)

Synonyms

- Diffuse mesothelioma

Definitions

- Malignant tumor of mesothelial cells arising in pleura, peritoneum, or pericardium

ETIOLOGY/PATHOGENESIS

Environmental Exposure

- Asbestos
  - Occupational exposure
    - Mining, construction, vehicle maintenance, shipbuilding
    - Risk relates to intensity and duration of exposure
  - Amphibole fiber types most carcinogenic
    - Persist in lung with or without tissue reaction
    - Crocidolite and amosite have highest risk
    - Longer, thinner fibers more oncogenic
  - Latent period: 15-40 years
- Occasionally other fiber types implicated, e.g., erionite

Infectious Agents

- SV40 DNA oncogenic virus
  - Viral sequences found in some mesotheliomas
  - Contaminated polio vaccine unproven association

Radiation

- Therapeutic
- Contrast media, e.g., thorium dioxide

Chronic Inflammation

- Rarely after prolonged fibrosing inflammation, e.g., empyema

CLINICAL ISSUES

Epidemiology

- Incidence
  - Geographic variation
    - In USA, ~ 20 cases per million of population in males, now peaked and declining
    - In UK, Australia, incidence higher and increasing
    - In Europe, incidence beginning to plateau
- Age
  - Most > 60 years
  - Occasional cases at any age
- Gender
  - 5-10x more common in males
  - Only 20% of cases in females are asbestos-related

Presentation

- Dyspnea, chest pain, cough, weight loss
- Abdominal pain, distension, vague mass

Natural History

- Multiple small lesions fuse to form diffuse sheet
- Invades underlying organs and adjacent structures
  - Lung, mediastinum, through diaphragm, chest wall
  - Viscera, abdominal wall
- Metastasizes
  - To lung, lymph nodes
  - Rarely to liver, bone, brain, kidney, adrenal

Treatment

- Options, risks, complications
  - Multimodal therapy more effective than single
- Surgical approaches
  - Extrapleural pneumonectomy
  - Decortication
- Adjuvant therapy
  - Chemotherapy and radiotherapy can prolong survival
  - More often palliative

MALIGNANT MESOTHELIOMA

Key Facts

Terminology
- Malignant tumor of mesothelial cells arising in pleura, peritoneum, or pericardium

Etiology/Pathogenesis
- Asbestos exposure
  - Amphibole: Crocidolite, amosite
  - Thin long fibers most oncogenic

Clinical Issues
- 5-10x more common in males
- Invades underlying organs and adjacent structures
- Metastasizes

Microscopic Pathology
- Sheet-like, tubular, papillary, microglandular, or mixed patterns
- Fibrosarcoma-like fascicles

Top Differential Diagnoses
- Reactive mesothelial proliferation
  - No atypia, necrosis, invasion
  - Desmin(+), EMA(-)
- Adenocarcinoma of lung
  - BER-EP4, MOC-31, CEA, CD15, TTF-1 (some) typically positive
  - Calretinin, thrombomodulin, CK5/6, WT1 typically negative
- Synovial sarcoma
- Solitary fibrous tumor
  - No pattern
  - CD34(+)
  - Cytokeratin, EMA typically negative
- Angiosarcoma
  - CD34, CD31, FLI-1 positive

Prognosis
- Poor
  - Median survival: 7 months; mortality: 100%
- Desmoplastic sarcomatoid variant is most aggressive

IMAGE FINDINGS

General Features
- Pleural effusion
- Diffuse pleural thickening extending into fissures
- Peritoneal thickening
- Mass

MACROSCOPIC FEATURES

General Features
- Multiple small nodules grow and coalesce
- Firm diffuse white tumor
  - Encases lung
  - Locules contain fluid
  - Invades adjacent structures
    - Lung, mediastinum, diaphragm
    - Chest wall, abdominal wall

MICROSCOPIC PATHOLOGY

Histologic Features
- Epithelioid malignant mesothelioma
  - Polygonal, cuboidal, or flattened discohesive cells
  - Cytoplasm eosinophilic, rarely clear
  - Mild nuclear pleomorphism, variable mitoses
  - Sheet-like, tubular, papillary, microglandular, or mixed patterns
  - Psammoma bodies
  - Variable stromal collagen, inflammation, rare myxoid change
  - Asbestos bodies in adjacent tissues
- Sarcomatoid malignant mesothelioma
  - Fibrosarcoma-like fascicles
  - Variably pleomorphic spindle cells
  - Giant cells
  - Fibrosis, hyalinization (desmoplastic variant)
  - Necrosis
  - Heterologous osteosarcoma, chondrosarcoma, rhabdomyosarcoma
- Biphasic malignant mesothelioma
  - Mixed epithelioid and sarcomatoid morphology
- Other histological variants of malignant mesothelioma
  - Small cell
  - Clear cell
  - Deciduoid
  - Lymphohistiocytoid
  - Pleomorphic

Predominant Pattern/Injury Type
- Diffuse

Predominant Cell/Compartment Type
- Mesothelial

ANCILLARY TESTS

Histochemistry
- PAS-diastase
  - Reactivity: Negative
  - Staining pattern
    - Rare cases mucin(+)

Cytogenetics
- Del 1p21-22, 3p21, 4q, 6q, 9p21, 13q13-14, and 14q
- Allelic loss at 4q33-34, 6q, 14q

PCR
- Inactivation of *CDKN2A/ARF* at 9p21
  - Loss of *p16INK4*, *p14ARF* tumor suppressor genes
- Methylation of *RASSF1A* tumor suppressor gene

Array CGH
- Loss of 4q and proximal 15q

MALIGNANT MESOTHELIOMA

Immunohistochemistry

Antibody	Reactivity	Staining Pattern	Comment
AE1/AE3	Positive	Cytoplasmic	Diffuse (100%)
CK19	Positive	Cytoplasmic	Diffuse (100%)
CK5/6	Positive	Cytoplasmic	Epithelioid MM (92%), sarcomatoid MM (28%)
CK7	Positive	Cytoplasmic	Epithelioid MM (80%), sarcomatoid MM (100%)
EMA/MUC1	Positive	Cell membrane & cytoplasm	Diffuse (78%)
Podoplanin	Positive	Cytoplasmic	Epithelioid MM (88%), sarcomatoid MM (55%)
Calretinin	Positive	Nuclear & cytoplasmic	Epithelioid MM (96%), sarcomatoid MM (55%)
Mesothelin	Positive	Cell membrane	Epithelioid MM (72-100%), sarcomatoid MM (0%)
Thrombomodulin	Positive	Cell membrane	In 66% of cases
WT1	Positive	Nuclear & cytoplasmic	Epithelioid MM (68%), sarcomatoid MM (21%)
HCAD	Positive	Cytoplasmic	Diffuse (98%)
CK20	Positive	Cytoplasmic	Epithelioid and sarcomatoid MM (75-100%)
SNF5	Positive	Nuclear	Epithelioid MM (100%)
CEA-M	Negative		Focal (2%)
TTF-1	Negative		
CD34	Negative		
ER	Negative		
EpCAM/BER-EP4/ CD326	Equivocal	Cell membrane	Focal (11%)
Desmin	Equivocal	Cytoplasmic	Diffuse (9-12%)
MOC-31	Equivocal	Cell membrane	Focal (8-20%)
Actin-sm	Equivocal	Cytoplasmic	Focal (24% of sarcomatoid MM)

DIFFERENTIAL DIAGNOSIS

Reactive Mesothelial Proliferation

- Absence of atypia, necrosis, invasion
- Desmin(+), EMA(-) in most cases

Adenocarcinoma of Lung

- BER-EP4, MOC-31, CEA, CD15, TTF-1 positive
- Calretinin, thrombomodulin, CK5/6, WT1 negative

Peritoneal and Ovarian Serous Carcinoma

- ER, PR, BER-EP4, MOC-31 positive
- Thrombomodulin(-)

Synovial Sarcoma

- Highly cellular in spindle areas, with mast cells
- Absence of pleomorphism
- Mucin in glandular areas
- Specific t(x;18) translocation

Epithelioid Endothelial Tumors

- Hemangioendothelioma
  - Cords or nests of cells in chondromyxoid stroma
  - Intracytoplasmic vacuoles
  - CD34, CD31 positive
- Angiosarcoma
  - Sheets of atypical cells with hemorrhage
  - CD34, CD31, FVIIIRAg, FLI-1 variably positive

Solitary Fibrous Tumor

- Patternless cellular and fibrous areas
- CD34 and Bcl-2 positive
- Cytokeratin, EMA mostly negative

DIAGNOSTIC CHECKLIST

Clinically Relevant Pathologic Features

- Tissue distribution

Pathologic Interpretation Pearls

- Calretinin(+), CEA and BER-EP4(-)

SELECTED REFERENCES

1. Galateau-Sallé F et al: Lymphohistiocytoid variant of malignant mesothelioma of the pleura: a series of 22 cases. Am J Surg Pathol. 31(5):711-6, 2007
2. Weinbreck N et al: SYT-SSX fusion is absent in sarcomatoid mesothelioma allowing its distinction from synovial sarcoma of the pleura. Mod Pathol. 20(6):617-21, 2007
3. Butnor KJ: My approach to the diagnosis of mesothelial lesions. J Clin Pathol. 59(6):564-74, 2006
4. Rdzanek M et al: Spindle cell tumors of the pleura: differential diagnosis. Semin Diagn Pathol. 23(1):44-55, 2006
5. Winstanley AM et al: The immunohistochemical profile of malignant mesotheliomas of the tunica vaginalis: a study of 20 cases. Am J Surg Pathol. 30(1):1-6, 2006
6. Baker PM et al: Malignant peritoneal mesothelioma in women: a study of 75 cases with emphasis on their morphologic spectrum and differential diagnosis. Am J Clin Pathol. 123(5):724-37, 2005
7. Nonaka D et al: Diffuse malignant mesothelioma of the peritoneum: a clinicopathological study of 35 patients treated locoregionally at a single institution. Cancer. 104(10):2181-8, 2005
8. Ordóñez NG: Immunohistochemical diagnosis of epithelioid mesothelioma: an update. Arch Pathol Lab Med. 129(11):1407-14, 2005

Radiographic and Microscopic Features

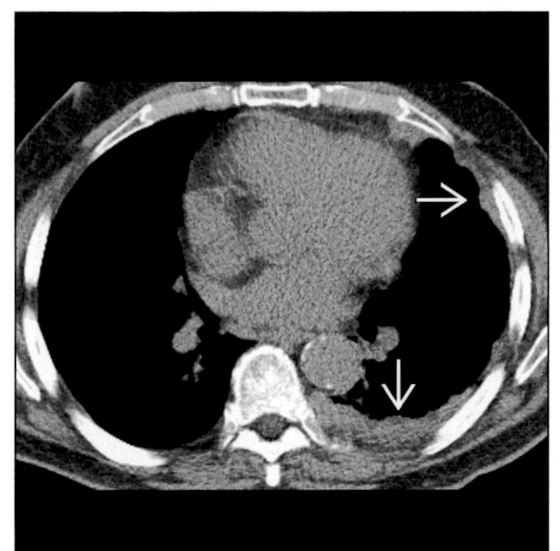

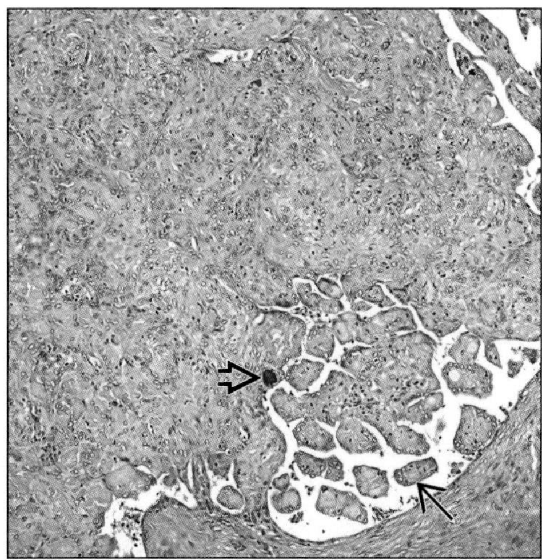

(Left) *Unenhanced CT of the chest shows typical increased thickness of the pleura ➡ from malignant mesothelioma. It will frequently have a multifocal appearance, as in this case.* ***(Right)*** *Hematoxylin & eosin shows solid sheets of cells and papillae with fibrous cores ⇨. Note psammoma body ⇨.*

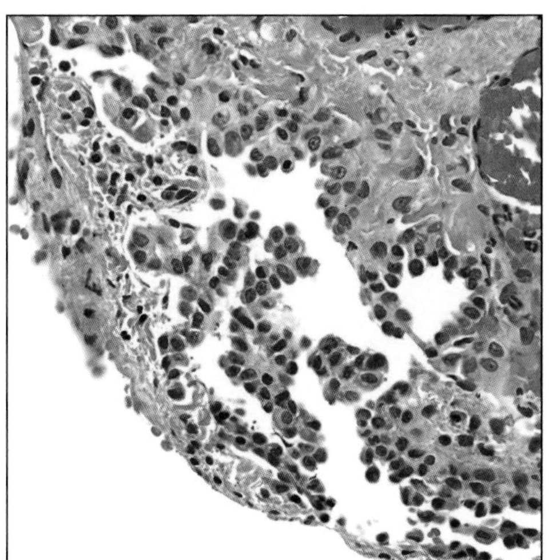

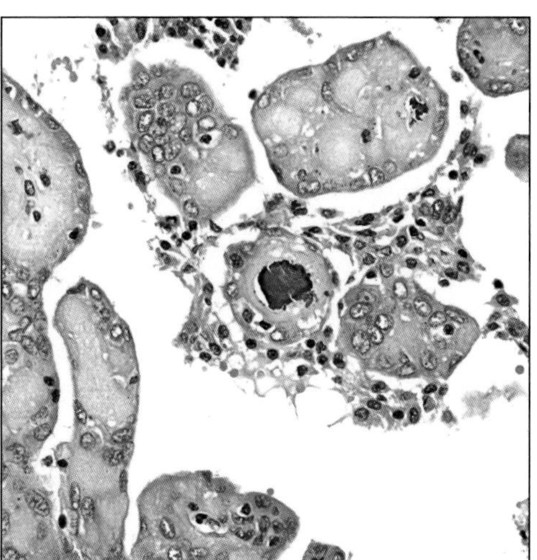

(Left) *Hematoxylin & eosin shows proliferation of mesothelioma cells on the pleural surface.* ***(Right)*** *Hematoxylin & eosin shows psammoma body in the core of the tumor papilla. Psammoma bodies are one of the histiologic features of malignant mesothelioma.*

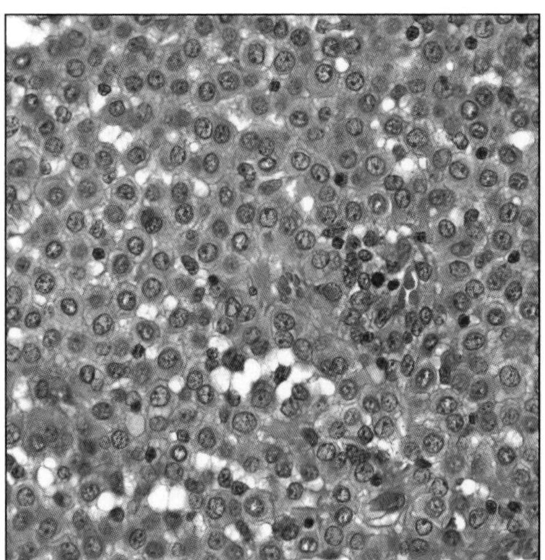

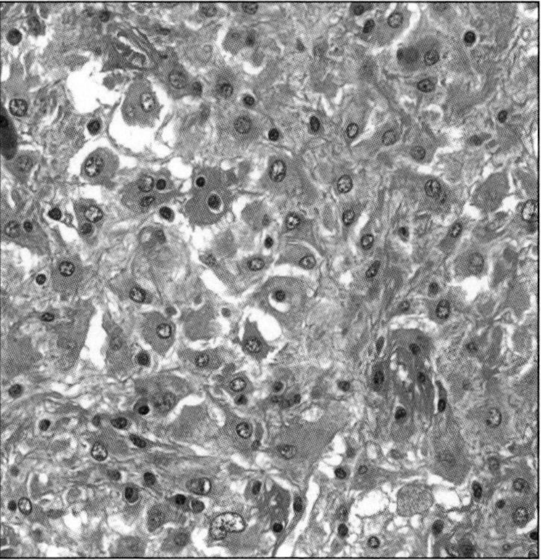

(Left) *Hematoxylin & eosin shows typical epithelioid mesothelioma with sheets of polygonal cells and a sprinkling of lymphocytes.* ***(Right)*** *Hematoxylin & eosin shows epithelioid mesothelioma cells with rounded pale nuclei and relatively abundant eosinophilic cytoplasm.*

MALIGNANT MESOTHELIOMA

Microscopic and Ultrastructural Features

(Left) *Hematoxylin & eosin shows paratesticular mesothelioma in tunica vaginalis with a layer of enlarged atypical mesothelial cells on the surface →. Compare with normal flattened mesothelial layer ⇨. Small foci of superficial invasion are seen ↗.* ***(Right)*** *Hematoxylin & eosin shows ill-defined glandular formations → in the paratesticular mesothelioma.*

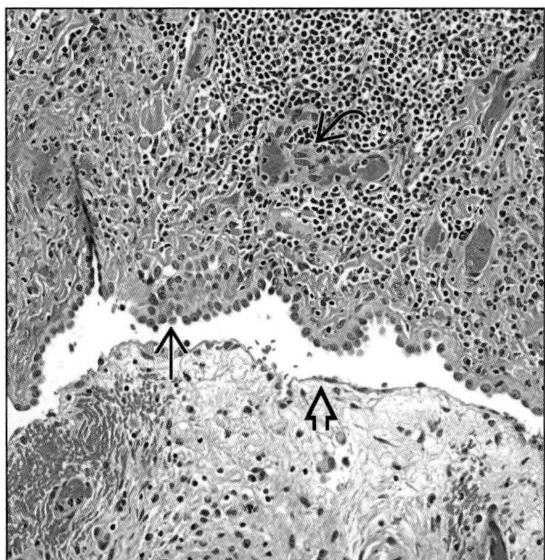

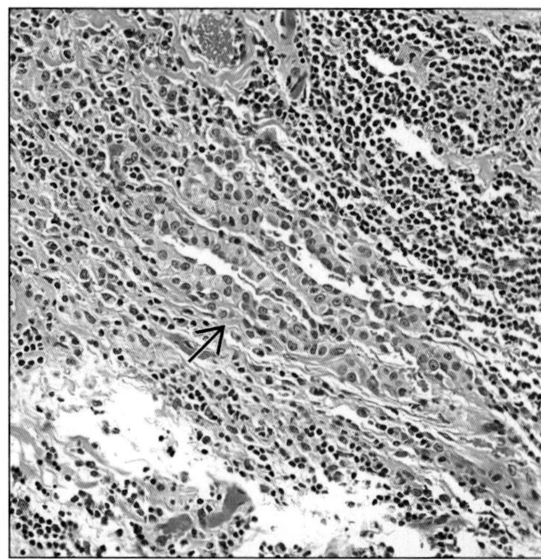

(Left) *Hematoxylin & eosin shows asbestos body → in the interalveolar septum of the lung.* ***(Right)*** *Hematoxylin & eosin at higher magnification shows ferruginous asbestos body. Note the thin straight asbestos fiber → coated with hemosiderin granules of varying size.*

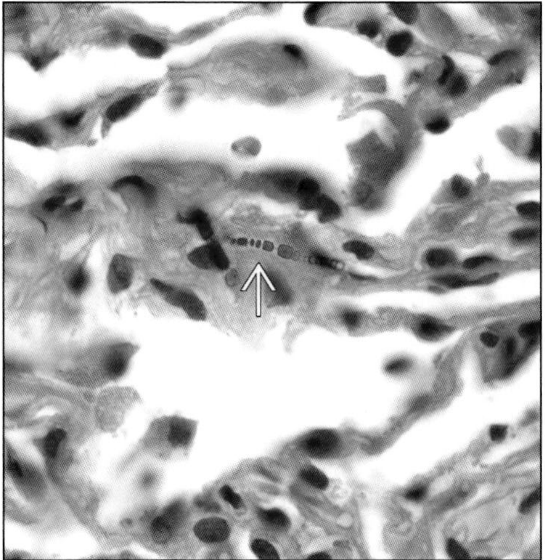

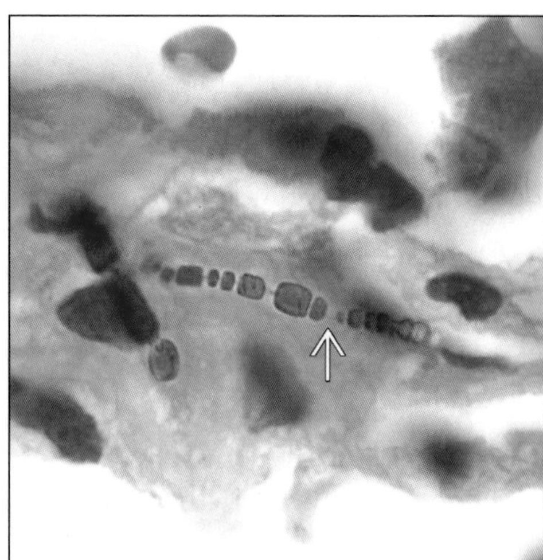

(Left) *Transmission electron microscopy low-power image shows mesothelioma cells with long slender microvilli involving several cell surfaces →.* ***(Right)*** *Transmission electron microscopy high-power image of mesothelioma cells exhibits the classic features of zonula adherens junctions ⇨ joining otherwise separated cells surfaces on which are microvilli of various lengths →. Cells are oriented on basal lamina ↗.*

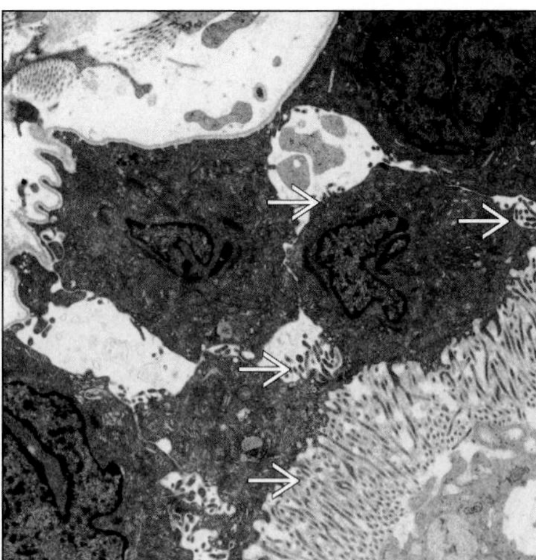

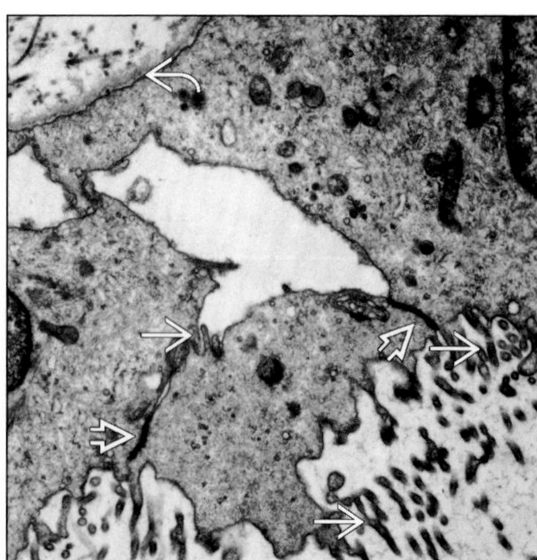

Microscopic and Immunohistochemical Features

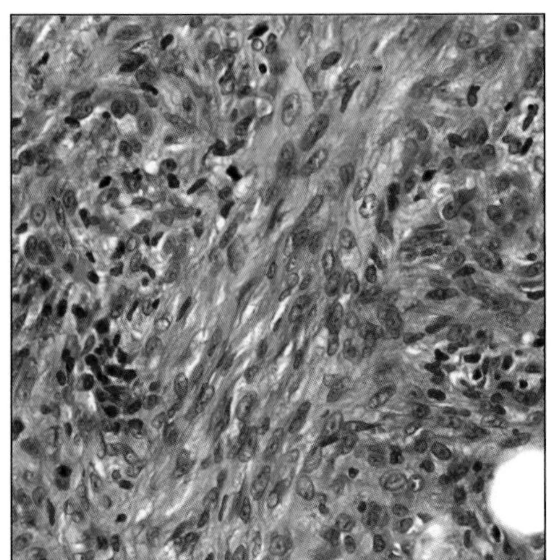

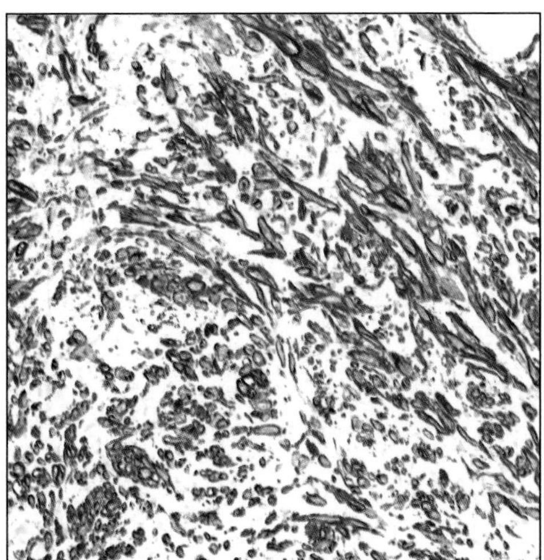

(Left) *Hematoxylin & eosin shows sarcomatoid mesothelioma of pleura with closely packed, elongated, uniform spindle cells and focal chronic inflammatory infiltrate. This can be indistinguishable from other spindle cell sarcomas without use of ancillary techniques.* ***(Right)*** *Positive AE1/AE3 shows diffuse cytokeratin positivity in sarcomatoid mesothelioma.*

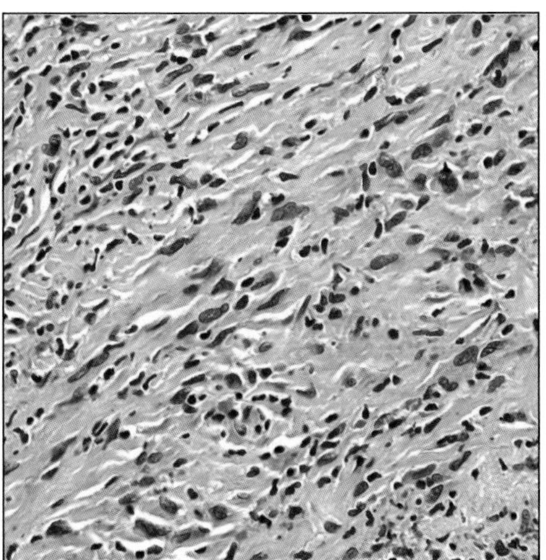

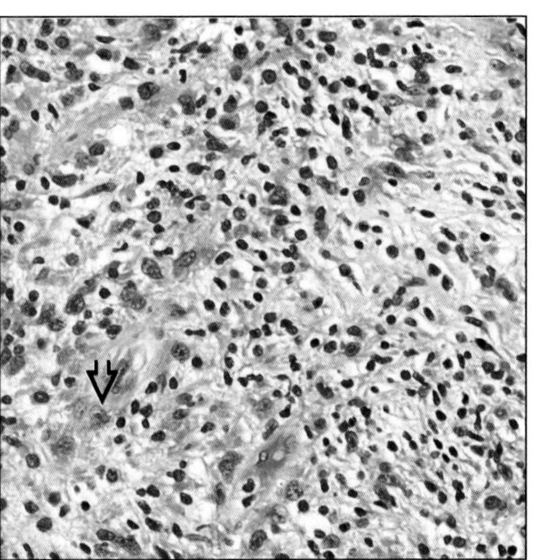

(Left) *Hematoxylin & eosin shows desmoplastic mesothelioma with atypical cells in fibrous stroma. This can be markedly hypocellular.* ***(Right)*** *Hematoxylin & eosin shows lymphohistiocytoid mesothelioma with mixed chronic inflammatory cells obscuring scattered malignant cells ⇨.*

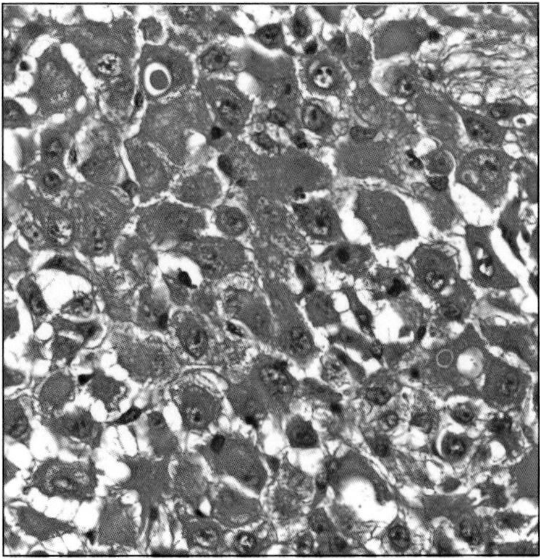

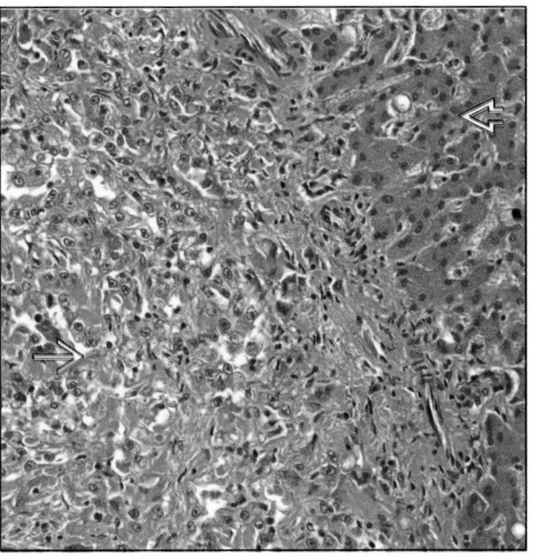

(Left) *Hematoxylin & eosin shows deciduoid variant of mesothelioma characterized by large polygonal cells with abundant glassy eosinophilic cytoplasm.* ***(Right)*** *Hematoxylin & eosin shows a liver ➡ infiltrated by metastatic malignant mesothelioma ➡. This patient had primary peritoneal mesothelioma.*

PROTOCOL FOR THE EXAMINATION OF MESOTHELIOMA SPECIMENS

Pleura: Resection

Surgical Pathology Cancer Case Summary (Checklist)

Specimen

___ Pleura

___ Other (specify): ______________________

___ Not specified

Procedure

___ Pleural decortication

___ Pleurectomy

___ Extrapleural pneumonectomy

___ Other (specify): ______________________

___ Not specified

Specimen Integrity

___ Intact

___ Disrupted

___ Indeterminate

Specimen Laterality

___ Right

___ Left

___ Not specified

Tumor Site (select all that apply)

___ Parietal pleura

___ Visceral pleura

___ Diaphragm

___ Other (specify): ______________________

___ Not specified

****Tumor Size (for localized tumors only)***

*Greatest dimension: ________ cm

*Additional dimensions: ________ x ________ cm

*___ Cannot be determined

Tumor Focality

___ Localized

___ Diffuse

___ Cannot be determined

Histologic Type

___ Epithelioid mesothelioma

___ Sarcomatoid mesothelioma

___ Biphasic mesothelioma

___ Desmoplastic mesothelioma

___ Other (specify): ______________________

Tumor Extension (select all that apply)

___ Parietal pleura without involvement of ipsilateral visceral pleura

___ Parietal pleura with focal involvement of ipsilateral visceral pleura

___ Confluent visceral pleural tumor (including fissure)

___ Into but not through diaphragm

___ Lung parenchyma

___ Endothoracic fascia

___ Into mediastinal fat

___ Solitary focus invading soft tissue of the chest wall

___ Diffuse or multiple foci invading soft tissue of the chest wall

___ Into but not through pericardium

___ Rib(s)

___ Mediastinal organ(s) (specify): ___________________________

___ Other (specify): ___________________________

Margins

___ Not applicable

___ Cannot be assessed

___ Margins negative for mesothelioma

___ Margin(s) involved by mesothelioma

Specify margin(s): ___________________________

Treatment Effect

___ Not applicable

___ Cannot be determined

___ > 50% residual viable tumor

___ < 50% residual viable tumor

Pathologic Staging (pTNM)

TNM descriptors (required only if applicable) (select all that apply)

___ m (multiple primary tumors)

___ r (recurrent)

___ y (post-treatment)

Primary tumor (pT)

___ pTX: Primary tumor cannot be assessed

___ pT0: No evidence of primary tumor

___ pT1a: Tumor limited to ipsilateral parietal pleura ± mediastinal or diaphragmatic pleural involvement; no involvement of visceral pleura

___ pT1b: Tumor involves ipsilateral parietal pleura ± mediastinal or diaphragmatic pleural involvement; tumor also involving visceral pleura

___ pT2: Tumor involves each of the ipsilateral pleural surfaces (parietal, mediastinal, diaphragmatic, and visceral pleura) with at least 1 of the following features

Involvement of diaphragmatic muscle

Extension of tumor from visceral pleura into the underlying pulmonary parenchyma

___ pT3: Locally advanced but potentially resectable tumor that involves all of the ipsilateral pleural surfaces (parietal, mediastinal, diaphragmatic, and visceral pleura), with at least 1 of the following features

Involvement of the endothoracic fascia

Extension into mediastinal fat

Solitary, completely resectable focus of tumor extending into the soft tissues of the chest wall

Nontransmural involvement of the pericardium

___ pT4: Locally advanced, technically unresectable tumor involving all of the ipsilateral pleural surfaces (parietal, mediastinal, diaphragmatic, and visceral pleura), with at least 1 of the following features

Diffuse extension or multifocal masses of tumor in the chest wall ± associated rib destruction

Direct transdiaphragmatic extension to the peritoneum

Direct extension to the contralateral pleura

Direct extension to mediastinal organs

Direct extension into the spine

Extension through the internal surface of the pericardium ± pericardial effusion

Tumor involving the myocardium

Regional lymph nodes (pN)

___ pNX: Regional lymph nodes cannot be assessed

___ pN0: No regional lymph node metastases

___ pN1: Metastases in the ipsilateral bronchopulmonary or hilar lymph nodes

___ pN2: Metastases in the subcarinal or ipsilateral mediastinal lymph nodes including the ipsilateral internal mammary and peridiaphragmatic nodes

___ pN3: Metastases in the contralateral mediastinal, contralateral internal mammary, ipsilateral, or contralateral supraclavicular lymph nodes

Specify: Number examined: _________

Number involved: _________

___ Number cannot be determined

Distant metastasis (pM)

PROTOCOL FOR THE EXAMINATION OF MESOTHELIOMA SPECIMENS

____ Not applicable

____ pM1: Distant metastasis

*Specify site(s), if known: __________________________

*Additional Pathologic Findings (select all that apply)

*____ None identified

*____ Asbestos bodies

*____ Pleural plaque

*____ Pulmonary interstitial fibrosis

*____ Inflammation (type): __________________________

*____ Other (specify): __________________________

*Ancillary Studies (select all that apply)

*____ Immunohistochemical stain(s) result(s) (specify stains): __________________________

*____ Histochemical stain(s) result(s) (specify stains): __________________________

*____ Electron microscopy results: __________________________

*____ Other (specify): __________________________

*Clinical History (select all that apply)

*____ Neoadjuvant therapy

*____ Other (specify): __________________________

*Data elements with asterisks are not required. However, these elements may be clinically important but are not yet validated or regularly used in patient management. Adapted with permission from College of American Pathologists, "Protocol for the Examination of Specimens from Patients with Malignant Pleural Mesothelioma." Web posting date October 2009, www.cap.org.

Myoepithelial Lesions

Intermediate

MYOEPITHELIOMA/MIXED TUMOR/PARACHORDOMA

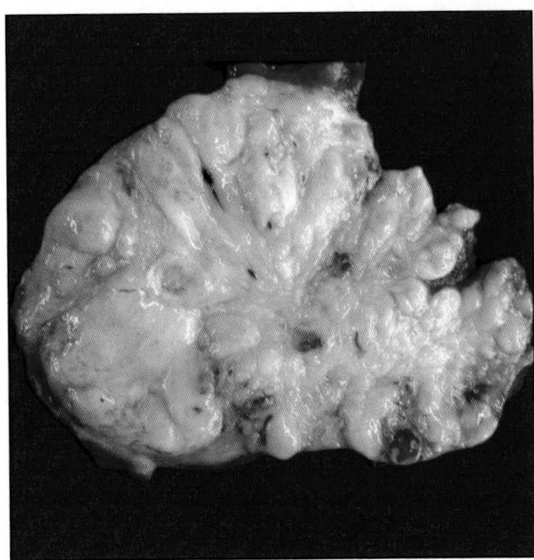

Grossly, this myoepithelioma arising in deep soft tissues represents a rather well-circumscribed, nodular neoplasm with gray-white cut surfaces.

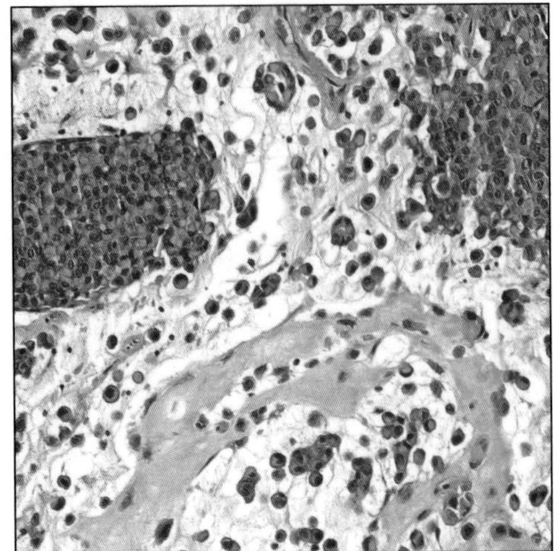

Plasmacytoid myoepithelial tumor cells are arranged in clusters and solid areas and set in a myxohyaline stroma in this example of myoepithelioma of deep soft tissues.

TERMINOLOGY

Synonyms

- Ectomesenchymal chondromyxoid tumor (of tongue)

Definitions

- Neoplasms composed of epithelial &/or myoepithelial cellular elements in varying proportions
  - Tumor cells are set in hyalinized to chondromyxoid stroma and may show foci of ductal differentiation
- Show overlap with mixed tumor of skin and soft tissues
- Show overlap with myoepithelial carcinoma (malignant myoepithelioma) of skin and soft tissues

CLINICAL ISSUES

Epidemiology

- Incidence
  - Rare neoplasms
  - Increasingly reported
- Age
  - Arise usually in adults
  - Significant number of cases arise in children < 10 years old
- Gender
  - Slight male predominance

Site

- Subcutaneous and deep soft tissue
- Rare in skin
- Very rare in bone
- Upper > lower extremities > head/neck region > trunk
- Less commonly on trunk and in head/neck region

Presentation

- Painless mass

Treatment

- Surgical approaches
  - Complete excision

Prognosis

- Most neoplasms behave in benign fashion
- Minority of cases may recur locally and metastasize
  - Benign-appearing neoplasms recur in < 20% of cases and do not metastasize
- At present, no morphologic features reliably predict prognosis
- Cytologic atypia represents most reliable prognostic parameter
- Obvious malignant neoplasms behave aggressively
  - Metastases have been reported in up to 30% of cases

MACROSCOPIC FEATURES

General Features

- Usually well-circumscribed neoplasms

MICROSCOPIC PATHOLOGY

Histologic Features

- Nodular or lobular growth
- Characterized by variable morphology
- Varying proportions of epithelioid cells, spindled cells, plasmacytoid cells, clear cells
- Cytoplasmic vacuolation is prominent in parachordoma-like cases
- Neoplastic cells are arranged in nests, cords, solid formations
- Ductal structures are not or only focally present
- Tumor cells are embedded in hyalinized to chondromyxoid stroma
- Divergent differentiation (squamous, adipocytic, cartilaginous, osseous) may be present
- Nuclear pleomorphism is generally minimal
- Few mitoses are usually present (< 2 mitoses per 10 high-power fields)

Key Facts

Terminology
- Neoplasms that are composed of epithelial &/ or myoepithelial cellular elements in varying proportions
  - Tumor cells are set in hyalinized to chondromyxoid stroma and may show foci of ductal differentiation

Clinical Issues
- Arise usually in adults
- Significant number of cases arise in children < 10 years old
- Subcutaneous and deep soft tissue
- Rare in skin
- Upper > lower extremities
- Most neoplasms behave in benign fashion
- Cytologic atypia represents most reliable prognostic parameter
- Treatment: Complete excision

Microscopic Pathology
- Characterized by variable morphology
- Varying proportions of epithelioid cells, spindled cells, plasmacytoid cells, clear cells
- Neoplastic cells are arranged in nests, cords, ductules
- Tumor cells are embedded in hyalinized to chondromyxoid stroma
- Divergent differentiation (squamous, adipocytic, cartilaginous, osseous) may be present
- Nuclear pleomorphism is generally minimal
- Few mitoses are usually present (< 2 mitoses per 10 high-power fields)
- Dedifferentiation (progression) into frank myoepithelial carcinoma or sarcoma is seen rarely

- Dedifferentiation (progression) into frank myoepithelial carcinoma or sarcoma is seen rarely
- May show loss of INI1 expression in considerable number of cases
- Cutaneous myoepithelioma
  - Rare neoplasms
  - No ductal differentiation (vs. chondroid syringoma)
  - Form spectrum with chondroid syringoma and malignant myoepithelioma of skin
  - No connection with overlying epidermis
  - May infiltrate into subcutis
  - Broad variation in regard to growth patterns and cytomorphology
  - Local recurrences are rare
  - Lymph node metastases are very rare
    - Show increased atypia and proliferative activity
- Malignant myoepithelioma (myoepithelial carcinoma)
  - Very rare neoplasms
  - Tend to be large
  - Severe cytologic atypia
  - Pleomorphic tumor cells
  - Increased proliferative activity
  - Tumor necrosis
  - Metastasize in up to 30% of cases (pulmonary and nodal metastases)

Cytologic Features
- Epithelioid cells
  - Round cells, abundant eosinophilic cytoplasm, round vesicular nuclei
- Spindled cells
  - Spindle-shaped tumor cells with fusiform nuclei
- Plasmacytoid cells
  - Abundant eosinophilic cytoplasm, nuclei are located in periphery of cells
- Clear cells
  - Abundant clear cytoplasm

ANCILLARY TESTS

Molecular Genetics
- Recurrent deletion of *CDKN2A* suggests inactivation of this tumor suppressor gene
- t(1;22)(q23;q12) translocation with *EWSR1-PBX1* fusion has been reported

Electron Microscopy
- Cytoplasmic myofilaments
- Subplasmalemmal attachment plaques
- Desmosomes
- Pinocytic vesicles
- Basal lamina

DIFFERENTIAL DIAGNOSIS

Epithelioid Dermatofibroma
- Polypoid lesions
- No expression of epithelial markers

Spitz Nevi
- Often junctional component
- Nest-like growth
- Prominent nucleoli
- Expression of melanocytic markers (Melan-A, HMB-45)
- No expression of epithelial and myogenic markers

Epithelioid Sarcoma
- Distal extremities
- Diffuse infiltration along fascial and neurovascular structures
- Granulomatous growth pattern
- Rather homogeneous epithelioid cytomorphology
- No ductal structures
- Usually no expression of S100

Cellular Neurothekeoma
- Epithelioid tumor cells are arranged in bands and nests
- Net-like hyalinization of collagen bundles
- Homogeneous expression of NKI/C3
- No expression of epithelial markers

MYOEPITHELIOMA/MIXED TUMOR/PARACHORDOMA

Immunohistochemistry			
Antibody	**Reactivity**	**Staining Pattern**	**Comment**
Vimentin	Positive	Cytoplasmic	
S100	Positive	Cytoplasmic	Positive in most cases (90%)
CK-PAN	Positive	Cytoplasmic	Positive in most cases (90%)
EMA	Positive	Cytoplasmic	Often positive in spindle cells (60%)
Calponin	Positive	Cytoplasmic	Positive in most cases (80%)
GFAP	Positive	Cytoplasmic	Positive in about 1/2 of cases
Actin-sm	Positive	Cytoplasmic	Positive in about 1/2 of cases
p63	Positive	Cytoplasmic	Positive in some cases (30%)
Desmin	Positive	Cytoplasmic	Positive in few cases only (15%)
melan-A103	Negative		

- No expression of S100 protein

Pilar Leiomyoma/Leiomyosarcoma

- Deep eosinophilic cytoplasm
- Coexpression of actin, H-caldesmon, and desmin
- No expression of S100 protein and epithelial markers

Extraskeletal Myxoid Chondrosarcoma

- Multinodular growth
- Uniform tumor cells
- No epithelioid tumor cells
- No expression of epithelial and myogenic markers

Ossifying Fibromyxoid Tumor

- Uniform oval round tumor cells
- Pale eosinophilic cytoplasm
- Incomplete peripheral rim of bone
- No expression of epithelial markers

Epithelioid Myxofibrosarcoma

- Atypical fibroblastic tumor cells
- Enlarged hyperchromatic nuclei
- Often scattered pseudolipoblasts are present
- Abundant myxoid stroma
- Elongated curvilinear blood vessels
- No expression of S100 protein and epithelial markers

Metastatic Malignant Melanoma

- No expression of epithelial immunohistochemical markers
- Expression of further melanocytic markers

Metastatic Carcinoma

- No nodular, lobular growth
- Lack of chondromyxoid stroma

DIAGNOSTIC CHECKLIST

Pathologic Interpretation Pearls

- Variable growth pattern
- Variable cytomorphology
- Variable immunophenotype

SELECTED REFERENCES

1. Balogh Z et al: Malignant myoepithelioma of soft tissue: a case report with cytogenetic findings. Cancer Genet Cytogenet. 183(2):121-4, 2008
2. Brandal P et al: Detection of a t(1;22)(q23;q12) translocation leading to an EWSR1-PBX1 fusion gene in a myoepithelioma. Genes Chromosomes Cancer. 47(7):558-64, 2008
3. Hallor KH et al: Heterogeneous genetic profiles in soft tissue myoepitheliomas. Mod Pathol. 21(11):1311-9, 2008
4. Gleason BC et al: Myoepithelial carcinoma of soft tissue in children: an aggressive neoplasm analyzed in a series of 29 cases. Am J Surg Pathol. 31(12):1813-24, 2007
5. Harada O et al: Malignant myoepithelioma (myoepithelial carcinoma) of soft tissue. Pathol Int. 55(8):510-3, 2005
6. Hornick JL et al: Cutaneous myoepithelioma: a clinicopathologic and immunohistochemical study of 14 cases. Hum Pathol. 35(1):14-24, 2004
7. Neto AG et al: Myoepithelioma of the soft tissue of the head and neck: a case report and review of the literature. Head Neck. 26(5):470-3, 2004
8. van den Berg E et al: Cytogenetics of a soft tissue malignant myoepithelioma. Cancer Genet Cytogenet. 151(1):87-9, 2004
9. Hornick JL et al: Myoepithelial tumors of soft tissue: a clinicopathologic and immunohistochemical study of 101 cases with evaluation of prognostic parameters. Am J Surg Pathol. 27(9):1183-96, 2003
10. Mentzel T et al: Cutaneous myoepithelial neoplasms: clinicopathologic and immunohistochemical study of 20 cases suggesting a continuous spectrum ranging from benign mixed tumor of the skin to cutaneous myoepithelioma and myoepithelial carcinoma. J Cutan Pathol. 30(5):294-302, 2003
11. Kutzner H et al: Cutaneous myoepithelioma: an under-recognized cutaneous neoplasm composed of myoepithelial cells. Am J Surg Pathol. 25(3):348-55, 2001
12. Michal M et al: Myoepitheliomas of the skin and soft tissues. Report of 12 cases. Virchows Arch. 434(5):393-400, 1999
13. Kilpatrick SE et al: Mixed tumors and myoepitheliomas of soft tissue: a clinicopathologic study of 19 cases with a unifying concept. Am J Surg Pathol. 21(1):13-22, 1997
14. Smith BC et al: Ectomesenchymal chondromyxoid tumor of the anterior tongue. Nineteen cases of a new clinicopathologic entity. Am J Surg Pathol. 19(5):519-30, 1995

Microscopic and Immunohistochemical Features

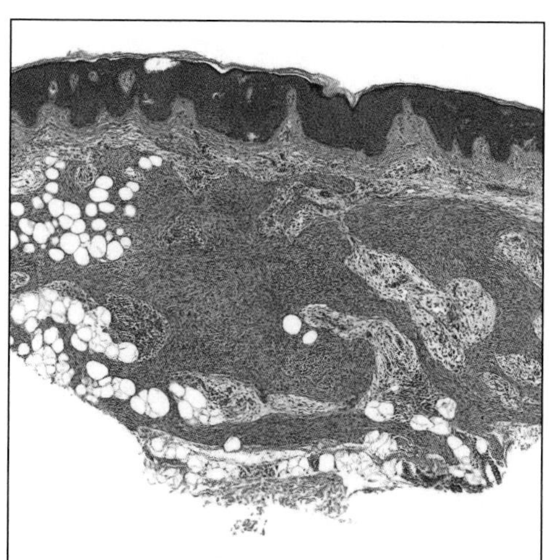
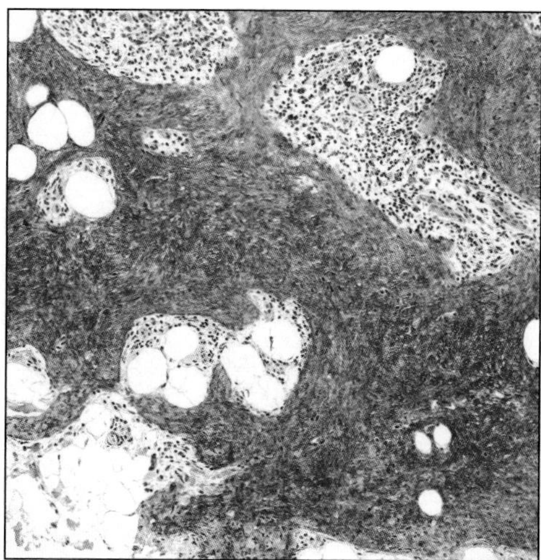

(Left) *This case of cutaneous myoepithelioma is composed predominantly of spindle-shaped tumor cells. Note focal lipomatous stromal changes and scattered inflammatory cells.* ***(Right)*** *Immunohistochemically, an expression of EMA by neoplastic cells was seen, whereas pancytokeratin was negative, a frequent finding in spindle cell myoepithelioma.*

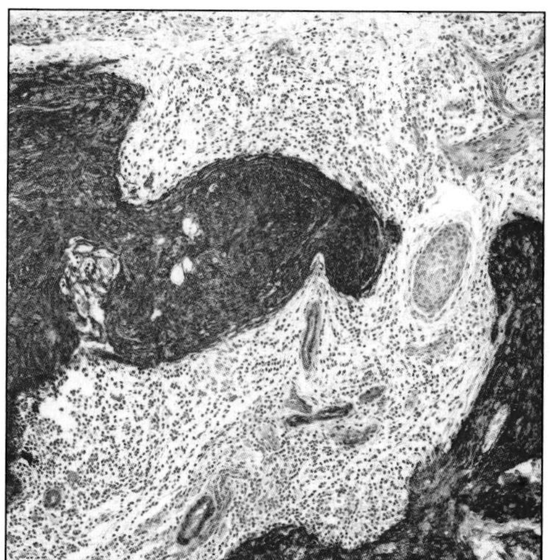
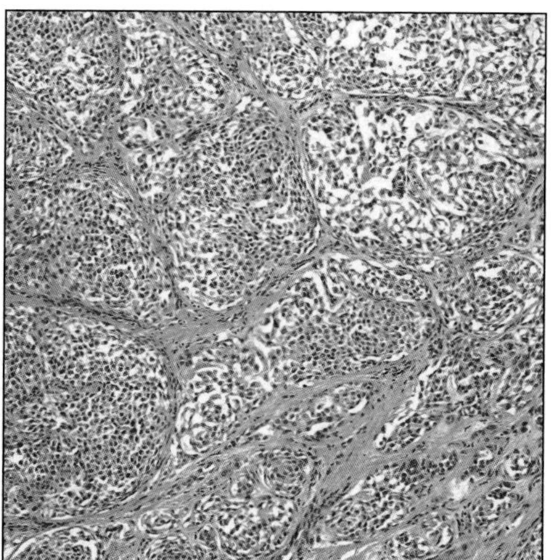

(Left) *In addition, neoplastic cells of this example of cutaneous myoepithelioma stain positively for calponin.* ***(Right)*** *This example of cutaneous myoepithelioma is composed of densely packed epithelioid and plump spindled myoepithelial tumor cells without ductal differentiation.*

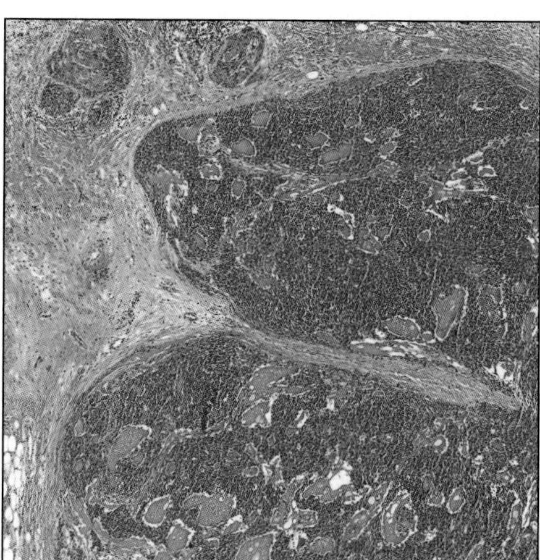
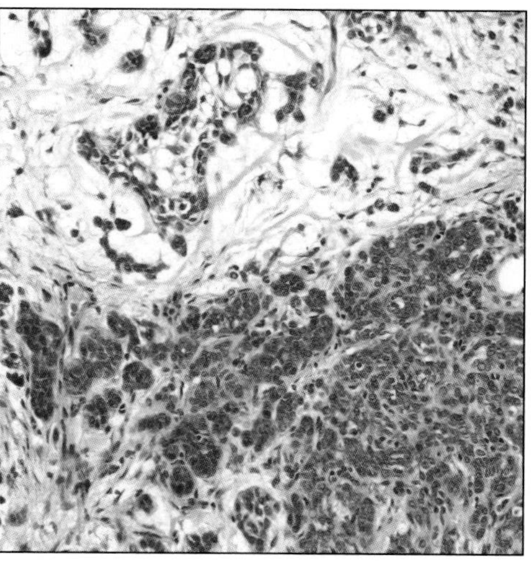

(Left) *A cellular example of a subcutaneously located myoepithelioma is seen. The neoplasm shows a lobular as well as multinodular growth pattern, and neoplastic cells are set in a hyalinized stroma.* ***(Right)*** *Higher power view reveals relatively uniform neoplastic cells and focal myxoid stromal changes. Neoplastic cells contain a pale eosinophilic cytoplasm and mainly round nuclei.*

MYOEPITHELIOMA/MIXED TUMOR/PARACHORDOMA

Microscopic and Immunohistochemical Features

*(**Left**) Neoplastic cells in this example of myoepithelioma of deep soft tissues stain homogeneously positive for pancytokeratin. (**Right**) In addition, a strong expression of S100 protein that represents the most sensitive myoepithelial marker is seen in this case.*

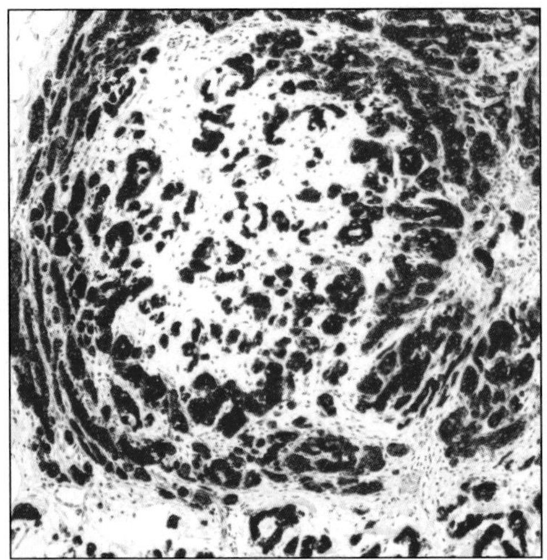

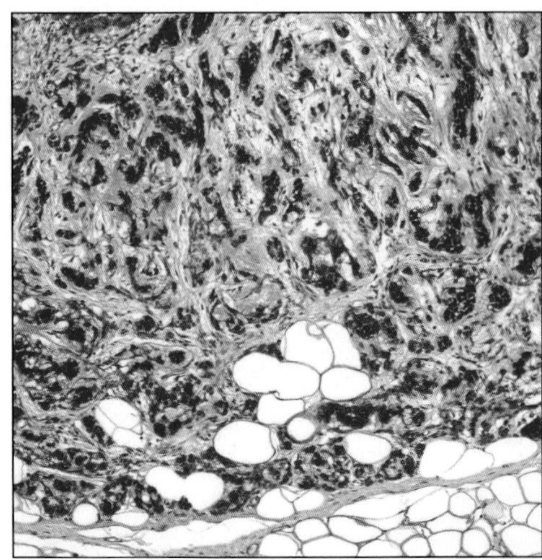

*(**Left**) Neoplastic cells in this example of a myoepithelioma of deep soft tissues show clear cell changes. (**Right**) At least focally, a prominent spindle cell differentiation is noted in this example of myoepithelioma of deep soft tissues. Note prominent myxoid stromal changes ⇨.*

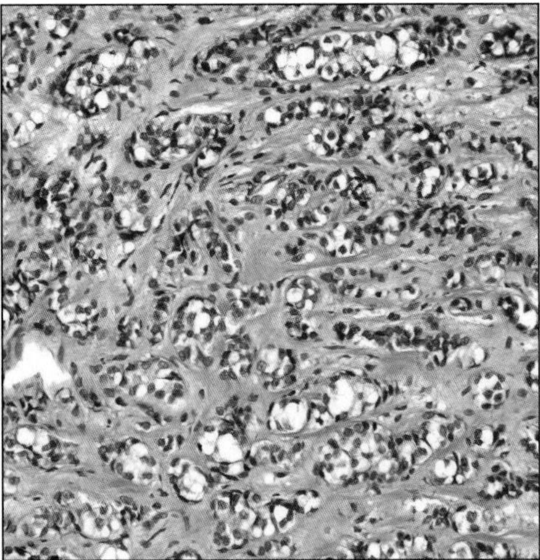

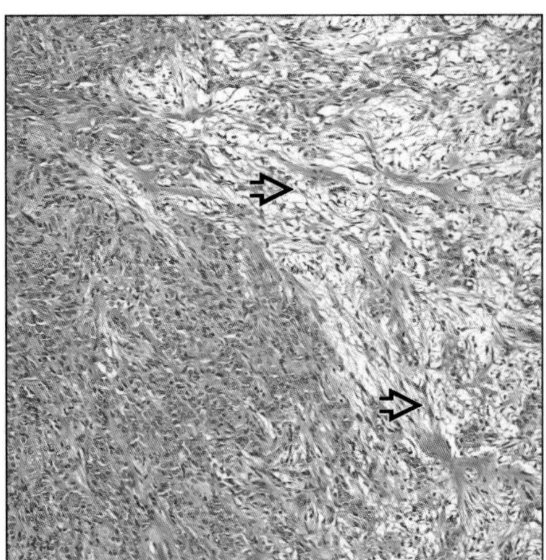

*(**Left**) Spindled tumor cells stain homogeneously positive for pancytokeratin in this example of myoepithelioma. (**Right**) This myoepithelioma of deep soft tissues shows prominent myxoid stromal changes creating a reticular growth pattern of neoplastic cells.*

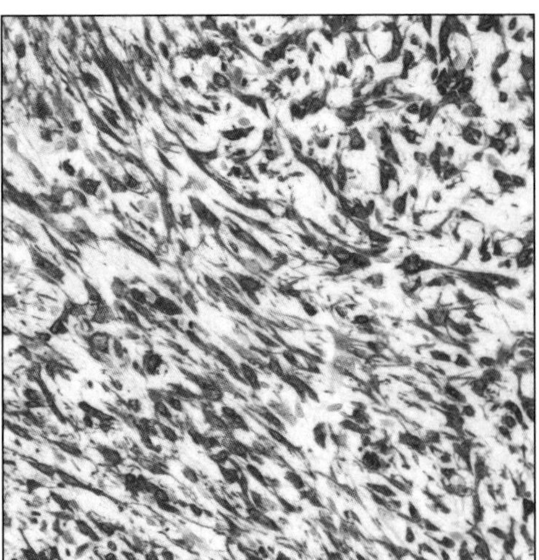

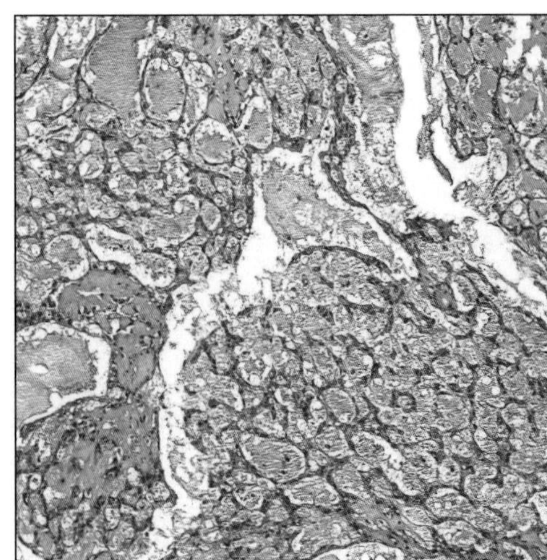

Microscopic, Gross, and Immunohistochemical Features

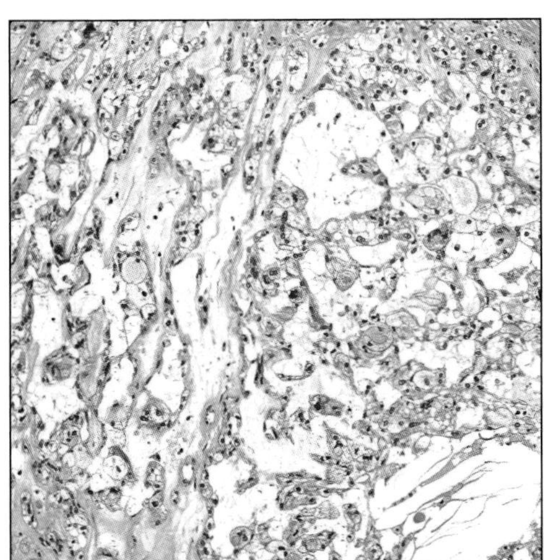

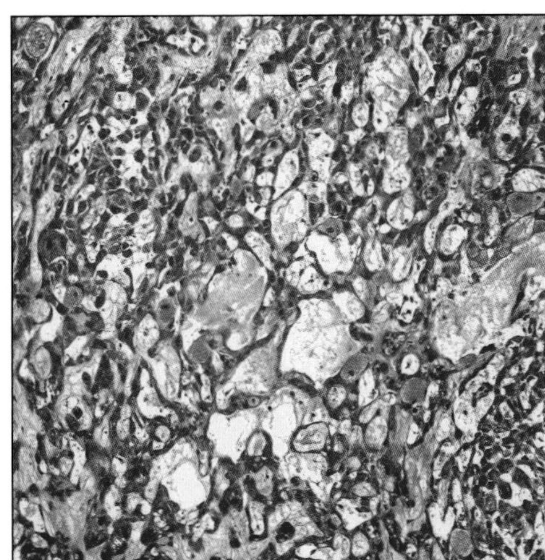

(Left) *This example of myoepithelioma of deep soft tissues is composed of vacuolated tumor cells resembling neoplastic cells in so-called parachordoma. Parachordoma most likely does not represent a distinct entity but rather belongs to the spectrum of myoepithelioma.* ***(Right)*** *Immunohistochemically, neoplastic cells in this parachordoma-like myoepithelioma stain positively for S100 protein.*

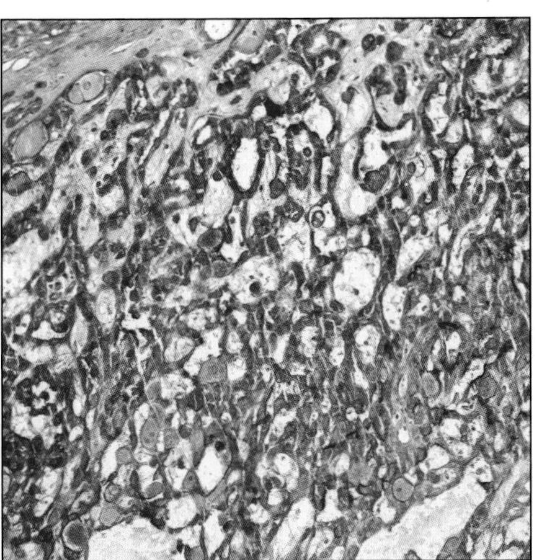

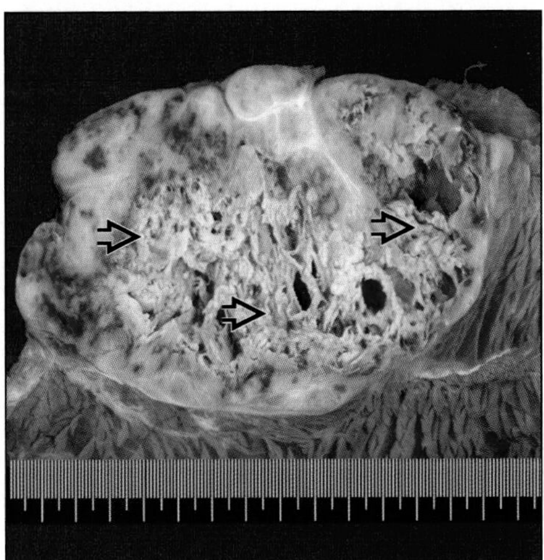

(Left) *In addition, a homogeneous expression of EMA is seen.* ***(Right)*** *A rare case of malignant myoepithelioma of deep soft tissues with gray-white cut surfaces and extensive areas of tumor necrosis ⇨ is shown.*

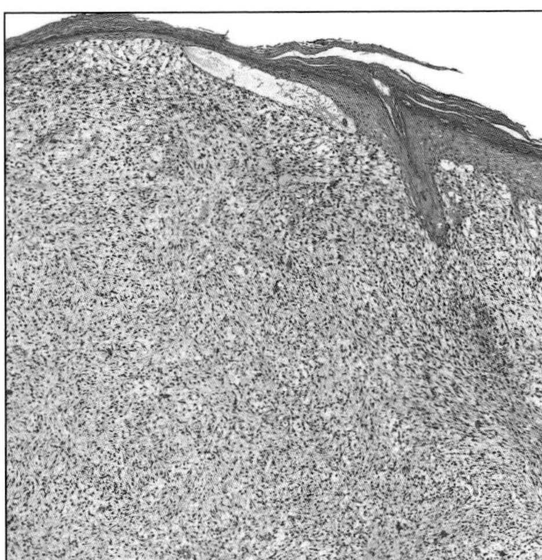

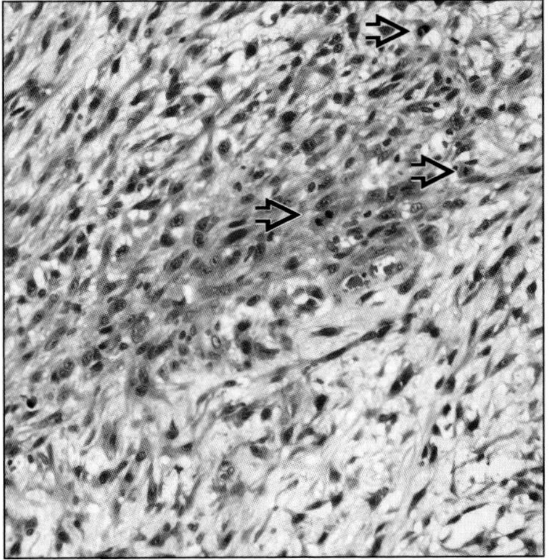

(Left) *This is a rare case of cutaneous malignant myoepithelioma (myoepithelial carcinoma) arising on the face of an elderly male patient.* ***(Right)*** *The neoplasm is composed of atypical spindled tumor cells with enlarged nuclei, and numerous mitoses are seen ⇨. Neoplastic cells are set in a prominent myxoid stroma.*

Nerve Sheath Lesions

Benign

Benign/Malignant

Malignant

FIBROLIPOMATOUS HAMARTOMA

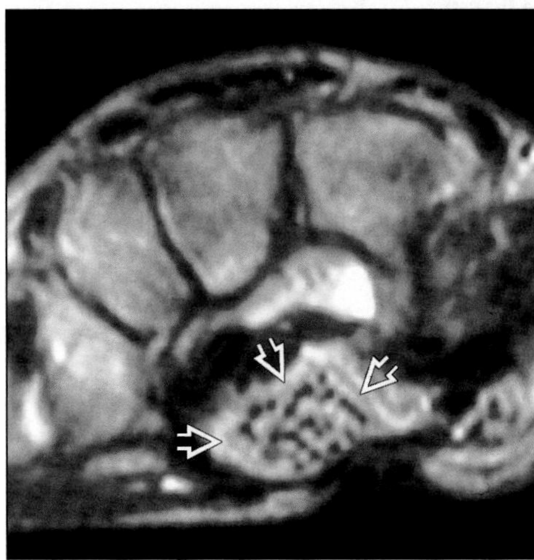

MR of the wrist shows abnormal fat signal ➡ in the stroma between the nerve fascicles (black dots) of an enlarged median nerve.

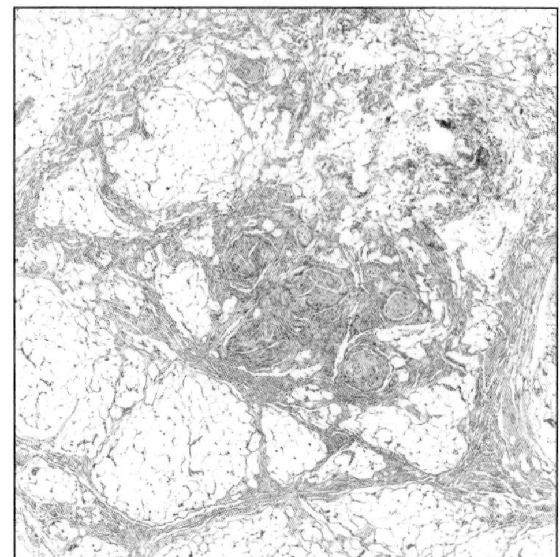

Hematoxylin & eosin shows accumulation of mature adipose tissue with hypocellular fibrous septa around and between nerve bundles.

TERMINOLOGY

Synonyms
- Fibrolipomatous hamartoma of nerve
- Lipofibromatous hamartoma of nerve
- Neural fibrolipoma
- Neurolipomatosis, lipomatosis of nerve

Definitions
- Increased fibrofatty tissue infiltrating and surrounding nerves

CLINICAL ISSUES

Epidemiology
- Age
  - Predominantly in children, including congenital lesions
  - Some cases in young adults up to 30 years of age
  - Rarely in older adults

Site
- Affects palmar surface of hand, wrist, forearm
- Median nerve and branches most commonly affected
- Rarely involves ulnar or radial nerve
- Involves left arm more often than right arm
- Very rarely involves sciatic, peroneal, or cranial nerve

Presentation
- Subcutaneous mass
  - Slow growing
- Paresthesia
- Macrodactyly (digital gigantism, macrodystrophia lipomatosa)
  - In 27% of cases
  - Can be congenital and progressive
  - Increased growth of bone and soft tissue of affected digit

Treatment
- Options, risks, complications
  - Complete excision contraindicated because of nerve damage
- Surgical approaches
  - Biopsy confirms diagnosis
  - Debulking or carpal tunnel release for symptomatic control
  - Removal of deformed digit

Prognosis
- Usually stabilizes if incompletely excised

IMAGE FINDINGS

MR Findings
- Fusiform enlargement of affected nerve segment
- "Telephone cable" sign

MACROSCOPIC FEATURES

General Features
- Sausage-shaped mass
- Yellow-white tissue
- Surrounds and expands nerve
- Can extend into adjacent soft tissue of hand and wrist

Size
- Variable, up to 10 cm length of nerve involved

MICROSCOPIC PATHOLOGY

Histologic Features
- Adipose tissue and fibrous tissue
  - Infiltrate around and between nerve branches and along perineurium
- Epineurial and perineurial fibrous thickening
- Perineurium can become hyperplastic

FIBROLIPOMATOUS HAMARTOMA

Key Facts

Terminology
- Increased fibrofatty tissue infiltrating and surrounding nerves

Clinical Issues
- Median nerve most commonly affected
- Predominantly in children, including congenitally
- Macrodactyly
- Complete excision contraindicated because of nerve damage

Macroscopic Features
- Sausage-shaped mass
- Can extend into adjacent soft tissue of hand and wrist

Microscopic Pathology
- Adipose tissue and fibrous tissue
- Perineurium can become hyperplastic
- Nerve bundles become separated

  - Concentric layers
  - "Onion bulb" intraneural hyperplasia
- Nerve bundles become separated
- Nerves can become atrophic in longstanding cases
- Rare metaplastic bone formation

Predominant Pattern/Injury Type
- Diffuse, interstitial
- Fibrosis

Predominant Cell/Compartment Type
- Adipocyte
- Fibroblast

DIFFERENTIAL DIAGNOSIS

Lipoma of Nerve
- Circumscribed
- Confined within nerve

Neurofibroma
- Proliferation of neural elements
- No fatty component

Neuroma
- Increased number of nerve bundles
- No fatty component

Lipomatosis
- Histologically similar
- Usually affects skin and subcutis
- Spares nerves

Other Causes of Macrodactyly
- Neurofibromatosis type 1
- Ollier disease
- Maffucci syndrome
- Klippel-Trenaunay-Weber syndrome
- Congenital lymphedema
- Proteus syndrome
  - Mutations in *PTEN* tumor suppressor gene
  - Localized gigantism and lipomatous masses

SELECTED REFERENCES

1. Bisceglia M et al: Neural lipofibromatous hamartoma: a report of two cases and review of the literature. Adv Anat Pathol. 14(1):46-52, 2007
2. Razzaghi A et al: Lipofibromatous hamartoma: review of early diagnosis and treatment. Can J Surg. 48(5):394-9, 2005
3. Al-Qattan MM: Lipofibromatous hamartoma of the median nerve and its associated conditions. J Hand Surg [Br]. 26(4):368-72, 2001
4. Marom EM et al: Fibrolipomatous hamartoma: pathognomonic on MR imaging. Skeletal Radiol. 28(5):260-4, 1999
5. Berti E et al: Fibrolipomatous hamartoma of a cranial nerve. Histopathology. 24(4):391-2, 1994
6. Amadio PC et al: Lipofibromatous hamartoma of nerve. J Hand Surg [Am]. 13(1):67-75, 1988
7. Dell PC: Macrodactyly. Hand Clin. 1(3):511-24, 1985
8. Silverman TA et al: Fibrolipomatous hamartoma of nerve. A clinicopathologic analysis of 26 cases. Am J Surg Pathol. 9(1):7-14, 1985

IMAGE GALLERY

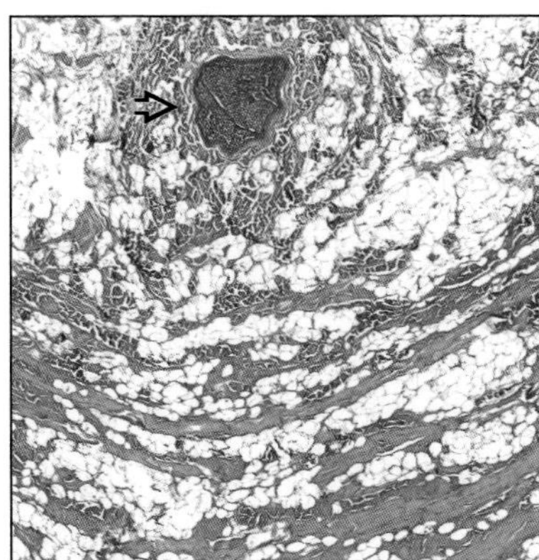
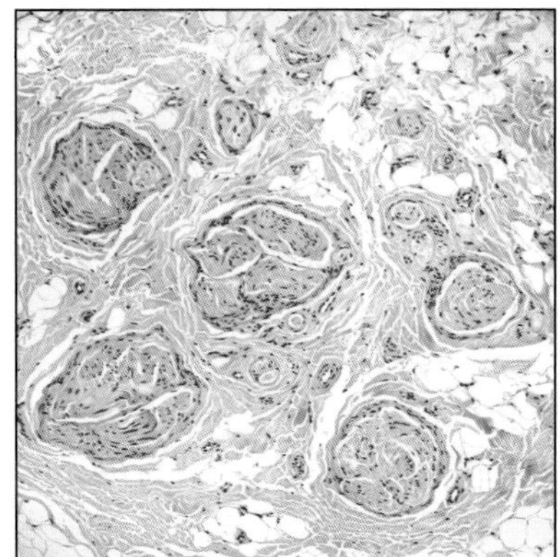
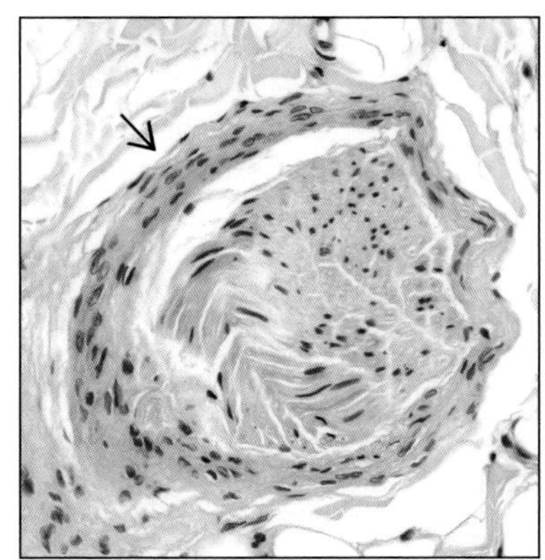

(Left) *Hematoxylin & eosin shows fibrous bands and adipose tissue in subcutis adjacent to nerve ⇨. Note prominent extension of lesional tissue beyond nerve.* ***(Center)*** *Hematoxylin & eosin shows nerve bundles separated by fibrous tissue within fat.* ***(Right)*** *Hematoxylin & eosin shows perineurial cell hyperplasia with several layers of elongated spindle cells ⇨. These demonstrate immunoreactivity for epithelial membrane antigen (EMA).*

NEUROMA

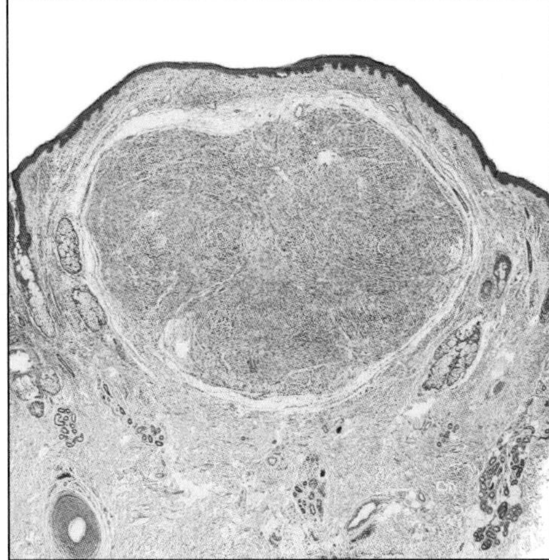

Solitary circumscribed neuroma ("palisaded encapsulated neuroma") represents a well-circumscribed, partly encapsulated, dermal, neural neoplasm.

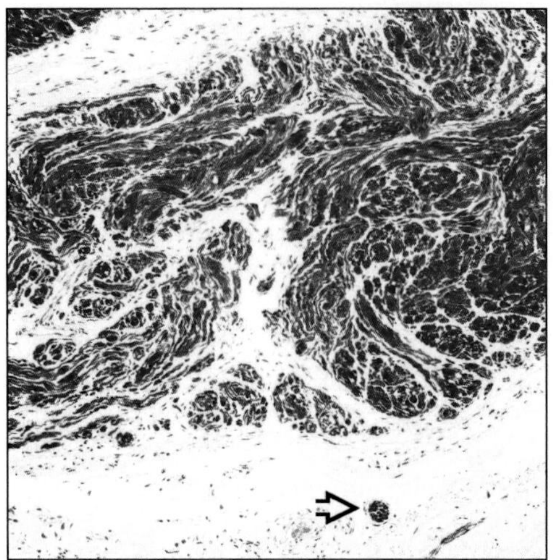

Solitary circumscribed neuroma is composed of S100 positive Schwann cells. Often preexisting peripheral nerves ➪ are seen on the base of these lesions.

TERMINOLOGY

Definitions

- Represents proliferation of peripheral nerve fibers in which ratio of axons to Schwann cell fascicles approaches 1:1
  - Solitary circumscribed neuroma ("palisaded encapsulated neuroma") represents spontaneous proliferation of peripheral nerve fibers
  - Multiple mucosal neuromas associated with multiple endocrine neoplasia syndrome (type 2B) represent rare autosomal dominant condition
  - Traumatic neuroma represents post-traumatic proliferation of peripheral nerve fibers
  - Morton neuroma represents degenerative neural change with reactive fibrosis on the foot
  - Pacinian neuroma represents painful hyperplasia of pacinian bodies on finger
  - Epithelial sheath neuroma represents proliferation of enlarged dermal nerves ensheathed by squamous epithelium

ETIOLOGY/PATHOGENESIS

Developmental Anomaly

- Multiple mucosal neuromas in multiple endocrine neoplasia syndrome
  - Represents rare autosomal dominant condition
  - Also includes medullary carcinoma of thyroid, pheochromocytoma, and somatic abnormalities
  - Mucosal neuromas have been rarely reported without any other systemic features of the syndrome

Environmental Exposure

- Traumatic neuroma
  - Amputation neuroma represents painful, reactive proliferation of nerve fibers after amputation
  - Supernumerary digit represents proliferation of nonencapsulated nerve fibers after intrauterine or perinatal amputation of supernumerary digits
  - Lesion on penis may occur after circumcision
- Morton neuroma
  - Degenerative damage of peripheral nerves

CLINICAL ISSUES

Epidemiology

- Age
  - Solitary circumscribed neuroma is most common in 5th and 7th decades
- Gender
  - Solitary circumscribed neuroma occurs in equal ratio in both genders

Site

- Solitary circumscribed neuroma
  - Majority (90%) located on face
  - Rare in other anatomic locations
  - Mucosal involvement has been reported rarely
- Morton neuroma
  - Usually in distal parts of peripheral nerves of 3rd and 4th os metatarsale
- Pacinian neuroma
  - Usually on fingers

Presentation

- Painful or painless mass
- Slow growing

Treatment

- Surgical approaches
  - Simple excision is curative

Prognosis

- Biologically benign lesions

NEURONA

Key Facts

Terminology

- Neuroma represents proliferation of peripheral nerve fibers in which ratio of axons to Schwann cell fascicles approaches 1:1
- Solitary circumscribed neuroma ("palisaded encapsulated neuroma") represents spontaneous proliferation of peripheral nerve fibers
- Multiple mucosal neuromas associated with multiple endocrine neoplasia syndrome (type 2B) represents rare autosomal dominant condition
- Traumatic neuroma represents post-traumatic proliferation of peripheral nerve fibers
- Morton neuroma represents degenerative neural change with reactive fibrosis on foot
- Pacinian neuroma represents painful hyperplasia of Pacinian bodies on finger
- Epithelial sheath neuroma represents proliferation of enlarged dermal nerves ensheathed by squamous epithelium

Clinical Issues

- Solitary circumscribed neuroma occurs predominantly on face
- Morton neuroma arises usually in distal parts of peripheral nerves of 3rd and 4th os metatarsale

Microscopic Pathology

- Proliferation of peripheral nerve fibers
- Proliferation of S100(+) Schwann cells
- Proliferation of neurofilament(+) axons
- No cytologic atypia
- No increased proliferative activity
- Perineural fibrosis in traumatic neuroma

MACROSCOPIC FEATURES

General Features

- Raised dermal lesions

MICROSCOPIC PATHOLOGY

Histologic Features

- Solitary circumscribed neuroma
  - Single dermal nodule
  - Multinodular &/or plexiform growth are very uncommon
  - Well-developed fascicles of Schwann cells
  - Numerous associated axons
  - Characteristic clefts
  - Superficial part is rather loosely arranged
  - Capsule-like fibroblasts and perineurial cells are seen in deeper parts
  - Small nerve can grow into lesion from below
  - Epithelioid cytomorphology is seen very rarely
  - Vascular variant has been reported rarely
- Multiple mucosal neuromas associated with multiple endocrine neoplasia syndrome
  - Morphology resembles features of solitary circumscribed neuroma
- Traumatic neuroma
  - Irregular arrangement of proliferating nerve fascicles embedded in fibrous scar tissue
  - Perineural fibrosis
  - Perineurial cells surround each small nerve fascicle
- Morton neuroma
  - Enlargement of plantar digital nerves
  - Edema of the nerve
  - Perineural fibrosis
- Pacinian neuroma
  - Hyperplasia of pacinian bodies
- Epithelial sheath neuroma
  - Large hyperplastic peripheral nerves in upper parts of dermis
  - Nerve fibers are surrounded by mature squamous epithelium
  - Associated fibroplasia and scattered inflammatory cells

Cytologic Features

- Elongated spindled cells
- Ill-defined, pale eosinophilic cytoplasm
- Bland, elongated fusiform nuclei
- No cytologic atypia

DIFFERENTIAL DIAGNOSIS

Schwannoma

- Encapsulated neoplasms
- Composed of Schwann cells
- Antoni-A and Antoni-B growth pattern
- Usually no neurofilament(+) axons
- Contains blood vessels

Neurofibroma

- Often poorly circumscribed lesions
- Often myxoid stroma
- No proliferation of peripheral nerve fibers

Perineurioma

- Composed of EMA(+) perineurial cells
- Spindled tumor cells with elongated nuclei and long, thin cytoplasmic processes
- No S100(+) Schwann cells
- No neurofilament(+) axons

Dermal Melanocytic Nevus

- Round nevus cells
- At least focal presence of melanin pigment
- Expression of melanocytic IHC markers

Dermatofibroma

- Rather ill-defined dermal lesions
- Composed of fibrohistiocytic cells
- S100(-)

Dermatomyofibroma

- Plaque-like dermal lesions
- Composed of spindled myofibroblasts

NEUROMA

Immunohistochemistry

Antibody	Reactivity	Staining Pattern	Comment
S100	Positive	Nuclear & cytoplasmic	Schwann cells are positive
NFP	Positive	Cytoplasmic	Axons are positive
EMA	Positive	Cytoplasmic	Perineurial cells are positive
Actin-sm	Negative		
GFAP	Negative		
CK-PAN	Negative		

- S100(-)

Pilar Leiomyoma

- Ill-defined dermal neoplasms
- Composed of spindled eosinophilic tumor cells
- S100(-)
- Expression of muscle markers

Ganglioneuroma

- Very rare neoplasms
- Composed of mature ganglion cells intermixed with fascicles of spindled S100(+) cells

Dermatofibrosarcoma Protuberans

- Diffuse infiltrative growth
- Storiform growth pattern
- CD34(+) spindled cells
- S100(-)

Superficial Acral Fibromyxoma

- Fascicles of spindled tumor cells
- Collagenous and myxoid stroma
- S100 negative
- Often focal expression of EMA &/or CD34

Sclerosing Fibroma (Plywood Fibroma)

- Collagenous stroma with lamellar clefts
- S100(-)
- CD34(+)

DIAGNOSTIC CHECKLIST

Clinically Relevant Pathologic Features

- Organ distribution

Pathologic Interpretation Pearls

- Solitary lesions
- Painful or painless lesions
- Biologically benign lesions
- Proliferation of peripheral nerve fascicles
- Proliferation of axons
- Perineural fibrosis

SELECTED REFERENCES

1. Salcedo E et al: Traumatic neuromas of the penis: a clinical, histopathological and immunohistochemical study of 17 cases. J Cutan Pathol. 36(2):229-33, 2009
2. Misago N et al: Unusual benign myxoid nerve sheath lesion: myxoid palisaded encapsulated neuroma (PEN) or nerve sheath myxoma with PEN/PEN-like features? Am J Dermatopathol. 29(2):160-4, 2007
3. Lombardi T et al: [Solitary circumscribed neuroma (palisaded encapsulated neuroma) of the oral mucosa.] Ann Dermatol Venereol. 129(2):229-32, 2002
4. Dubovy SR et al: Palisaded encapsulated neuroma (solitary circumscribed neuroma of skin) of the eyelid: report of two cases and review of the literature. Br J Ophthalmol. 85(8):949-51, 2001
5. Navarro M et al: Palisaded encapsulated neuroma (solitary circumscribed neuroma) of the glans penis. Br J Dermatol. 142(5):1061-2, 2000
6. Requena L et al: Epithelial sheath neuroma: a new entity. Am J Surg Pathol. 24(2):190-6, 2000
7. Magnusson B: Palisaded encapsulated neuroma (solitary circumscribed neuroma) of the oral mucosa. Oral Surg Oral Med Oral Pathol Oral Radiol Endod. 82(3):302-4, 1996
8. Bennett GL et al: Morton's interdigital neuroma: a comprehensive treatment protocol. Foot Ankle Int. 16(12):760-3, 1995
9. Megahed M: Palisaded encapsulated neuroma (solitary circumscribed neuroma). A clinicopathologic and immunohistochemical study. Am J Dermatopathol. 16(2):120-5, 1994
10. Argenyi ZB et al: Plexiform and other unusual variants of palisaded encapsulated neuroma. J Cutan Pathol. 20(1):34-9, 1993
11. Argenyi ZB et al: Vascular variant of palisaded encapsulated neuroma. J Cutan Pathol. 20(1):92-3, 1993
12. Dakin MC et al: The palisaded, encapsulated neuroma (solitary circumscribed neuroma). Histopathology. 20(5):405-10, 1992
13. Tsang WY et al: Epithelioid variant of solitary circumscribed neuroma of the skin. Histopathology. 20(5):439-41, 1992
14. Alexander J et al: An unusual solitary circumscribed neuroma (palisaded encapsulated neuroma) of the skin--with observations on the nature of pseudo-epitheliomatous hyperplasia. Histopathology. 18(2):175-7, 1991
15. Butterworth DM et al: Solitary circumscribed neuroma of the skin. Histopathology. 19(6):577-9, 1991
16. Eckert F et al: [Encapsulated neuroma of the skin. A clinical, histologic and immunohistologic study.] Hautarzt. 41(7):378-83, 1990
17. Albrecht S et al: Palisaded encapsulated neuroma: an immunohistochemical study. Mod Pathol. 2(4):403-6, 1989
18. Dover JS et al: Palisaded encapsulated neuromas. A clinicopathologic study. Arch Dermatol. 125(3):386-9, 1989
19. Fletcher CD et al: Digital pacinian neuroma: a distinctive hyperplastic lesion. Histopathology. 15(3):249-56, 1989
20. Fletcher CD. Solitary circumscribed neuroma of the skin (so-called palisaded et al: A clinicopathologic and immunohistochemical study. Am J Surg Pathol. 13(7):574-80, 1989
21. Reed RJ et al: Palisaded, encapsulated neuromas of the skin. Arch Dermatol. 106(6):865-70, 1972

Microscopic Features

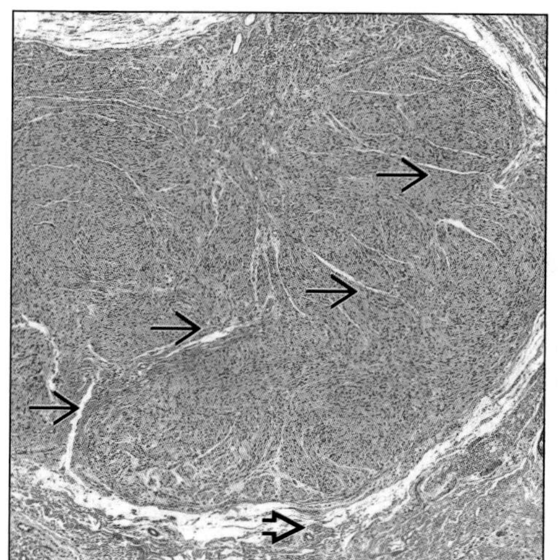

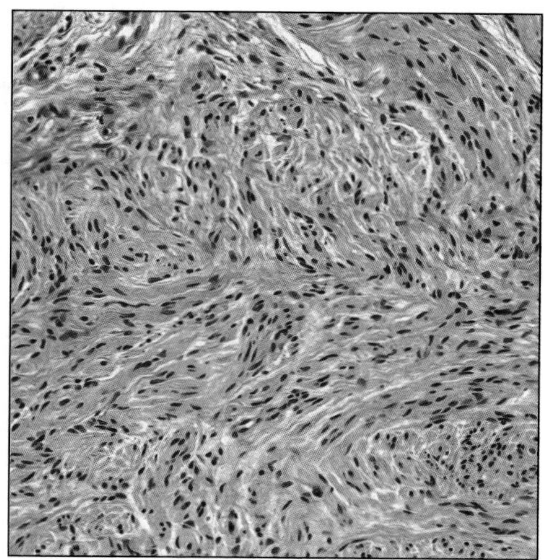

(Left) *Solitary circumscribed neuroma represents a well-circumscribed, partly encapsulated dermal neoplasm that is composed of Schwann cells and associated axons. Note characteristic clefts ➔ and a small preexisting nerve on the base of the lesion ⇨.* **(Right)** *Neoplastic Schwann cells contain an ill-defined, pale eosinophilic cytoplasm and cytologically bland spindled nuclei with evenly distributed chromatin. No prominent cytologic atypia and no increased mitoses are present.*

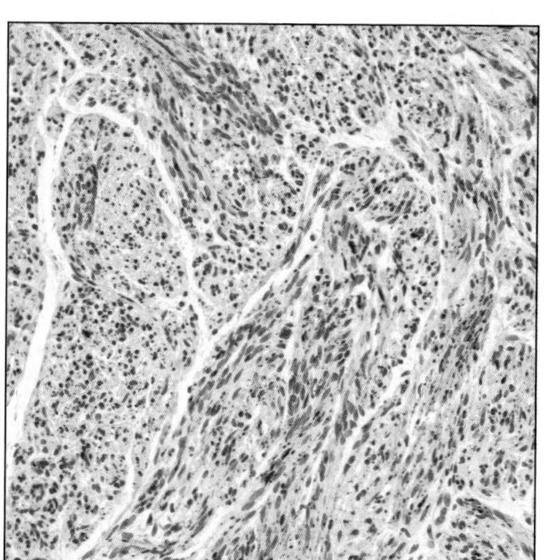

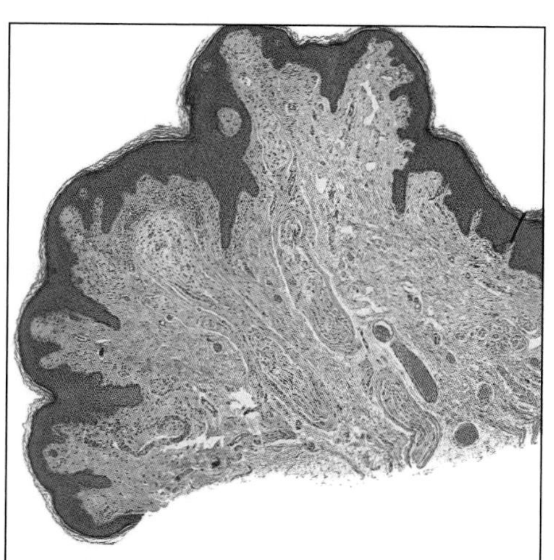

(Left) *In addition to S100(+) Schwann cells, numerous neurofilament(+) axons are seen in solitary circumscribed neuroma.* **(Right)** *Traumatic neuroma after circumcision reveals superficially located hyperplastic nerve fibers with slight perineural fibrosis. These lesions may clinically mimic a condyloma.*

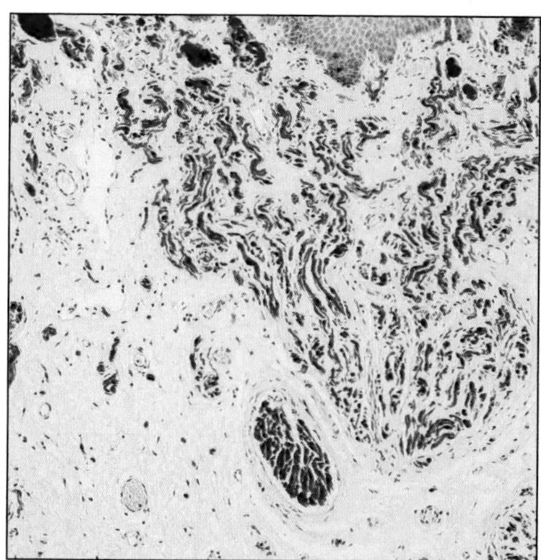

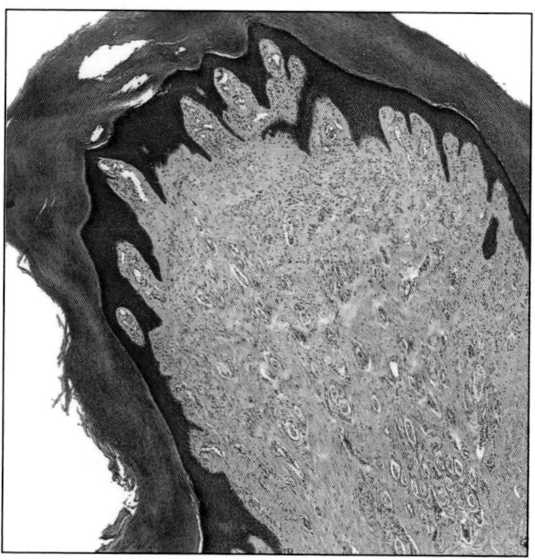

(Left) *S100 immunohistochemical antibodies reveal hyperplastic peripheral nerve fibers in this traumatic neuroma (after circumcision).* **(Right)** *Numerous small, hyperplastic nerve fibers are seen in this raised dermal lesion that represents a supernumerary digit. The fibrosed stroma contains scattered inflammatory cells.*

DERMAL NERVE SHEATH MYXOMA

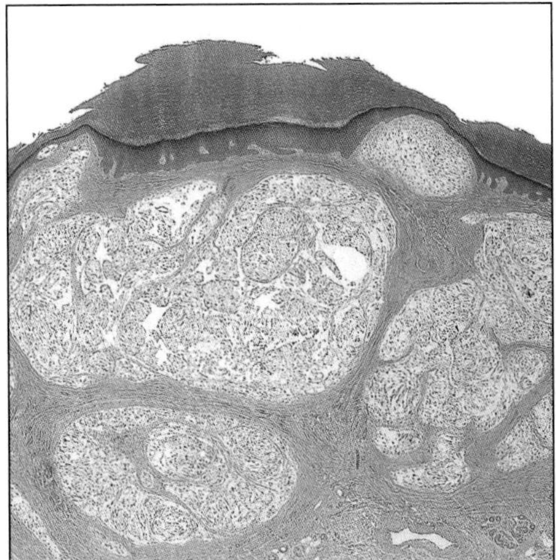

Dermal nerve sheath myxoma is composed of well-defined myxoid lobules. It involves the dermis and often the underlying subcutis. The most common sites are fingers and the hand.

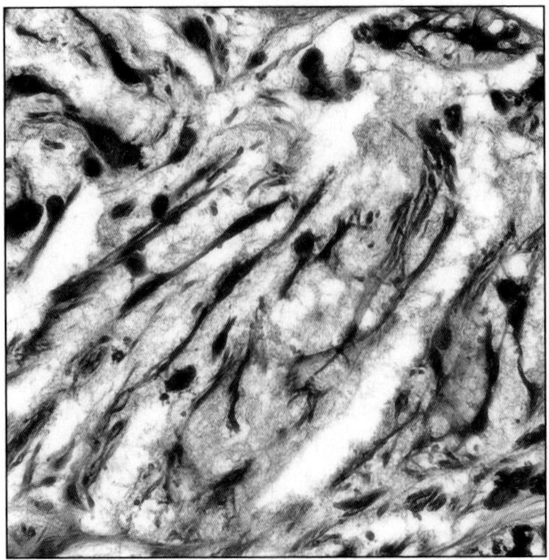

Nerve sheath myxomas are strongly S100(+) consonant with Schwann cell differentiation. This immunohistochemically stained section depicts diffuse but intense nuclear and cytoplasmic reactivity.

TERMINOLOGY

Synonyms

- Cutaneous lobular neuromyxoma, perineurial myxoma, pacinian neurofibroma, myxoid tumor of nerve sheath

Definitions

- Benign cutaneous nerve sheath tumor characterized by Schwann cell differentiation, abundant myxoid matrix, and well-defined lobular architecture

CLINICAL ISSUES

Epidemiology

- Incidence
  - Rare; fewer than 100 reports
- Age
  - Mostly adults; median age: 34 years

Site

- Extremities
  - Fingers and hand most common
  - Pretibial skin common
- Rare intraoral cases
- Uncommon on face

Presentation

- Painless mass
  - Slow growth

Treatment

- Surgical approaches
  - Simple excision

Prognosis

- Benign and nonaggressive but often excised with positive margins
  - Up to 50% recur

MACROSCOPIC FEATURES

Size

- 0.5-4.5 cm

MICROSCOPIC PATHOLOGY

Histologic Features

- Multiple myxoid lobules
  - Well-defined borders separated by dense fibrous septa
- Usually limited to dermis and subcutis
- Paucicellular proliferation of epithelioid and spindle Schwann cells
  - Interconnecting cords/networks, syncytial nests, ring-like structures, Verocay-like structures (rare)
  - Stellate and vacuolated cells common
  - No atypia, very low mitotic rate

Predominant Pattern/Injury Type

- Myxoid

Predominant Cell/Compartment Type

- Spindle and epithelioid

ANCILLARY TESTS

Immunohistochemistry

- S100 diffusely (+) in 100% of cases; GFAP(+) in most
- Negative for SMA, desmin, CD68, HMB-45, synaptophysin, chromogranin-A, CD31

DIFFERENTIAL DIAGNOSIS

Neurothekeoma

- Multinodular, but less myxoid matrix and less defined border
- Whorling pattern common

DERMAL NERVE SHEATH MYXOMA

Key Facts

Terminology
- Benign myxoid nerve sheath tumor with well-defined lobular architecture and Schwann cell differentiation

Clinical Issues
- Fingers and hand most common site
  - Pretibial skin also common
  - Uncommon on face
- Benign, but up to 50% recur

Microscopic Pathology
- Multiple myxoid lobules with well-defined borders
- Epithelioid and spindle Schwann cells
- Interconnecting cords/networks, syncytial nests, ring-like structures
- Stellate and vacuolated cells common
- No atypia, very low mitotic rate

Ancillary Tests
- S100 diffusely positive in 100%, GFAP(+) in most
- Negative for SMA, desmin, CD68, HMB-45, synaptophysin, chromogranin-A, CD31

Top Differential Diagnoses
- Neurothekeoma
- Superficial angiomyxoma
- Digital mucoid cyst
- Myxoid neurofibroma
- Superficial acral fibromyxoma
- Myxoid dermatofibrosarcoma protuberans
- Low-grade myxofibrosarcoma

- Spindle and large plump epithelioid cells, ill-defined cytoplasm
- Greater nuclear variability and mitotic activity
- Lacks cords, syncytial aggregates, and vacuolated cells
- S100(-)
- Predilection for face

Superficial Angiomyxoma
- Poorly circumscribed, extends into adjacent tissue
- Fibroblastic cells, often bi- or multinucleated
- Prominent vascularity; small, thin-walled, curvilinear, congested vessels
- Sparse dispersed inflammation, often neutrophils
- S100(-)
- Predilection for trunk and head and neck

Cutaneous Myxoma in Carney Complex
- Indistinguishable from superficial angiomyxoma
- Wide anatomic distribution; predilection for ear, eyelid, nipple
- Spotty pigmentation, endocrine overactivity, psammomatous melanotic schwannoma

Digital Mucoid Cyst
- Extruded myxoid material, possibly from underlying joint
- Fibroblastic cells can be either spindled or stellate
- Limited to fingers over dorsal aspect of distal interphalangeal joints

Myxoid Neurofibroma
- Small spindle cells with buckled, wavy nuclei and ill-defined cytoplasm
- Lacks lobular architecture, may be plexiform or diffuse
- Collagen bundles within myxoid stroma

Superficial Acral Fibromyxoma
- Variable amount of fibrous and myxoid stroma
- Lacks well-defined lobules
- CD34(+), S100(-)
- Acral extremities, often periungual

Myxoid Dermatofibrosarcoma Protuberans
- Storiform or fascicular, lacks lobular architecture
- Infiltrates subcutis, classic "honeycomb" pattern
- Spindle cells with ill-defined cytoplasm, mitotically active
- CD34(+), S100(-)

Low-Grade Myxofibrosarcoma
- Variable lobular architecture, infiltrative growth into dermis and subcutis
- Pleomorphism and mitotic figures in most cases
- S100(-)

SELECTED REFERENCES

1. Nishioka M et al: Nerve sheath myxoma (neurothekeoma) arising in the oral cavity: histological and immunohistochemical features of 3 cases. Oral Surg Oral Med Oral Pathol Oral Radiol Endod. 107(5):e28-33, 2009
2. Fetsch JF et al: Neurothekeoma: an analysis of 178 tumors with detailed immunohistochemical data and long-term patient follow-up information. Am J Surg Pathol. 31(7):1103-14, 2007
3. Reimann JD et al: Myxoid dermatofibrosarcoma protuberans: a rare variant analyzed in a series of 23 cases. Am J Surg Pathol. 31(9):1371-7, 2007
4. Fetsch JF et al: Nerve sheath myxoma: a clinicopathologic and immunohistochemical analysis of 57 morphologically distinctive, S-100 protein- and GFAP-positive, myxoid peripheral nerve sheath tumors with a predilection for the extremities and a high local recurrence rate. Am J Surg Pathol. 29(12):1615-24, 2005
5. Fetsch JF et al: Superficial acral fibromyxoma: a clinicopathologic and immunohistochemical analysis of 37 cases of a distinctive soft tissue tumor with a predilection for the fingers and toes. Hum Pathol. 32(7):704-14, 2001
6. Calonje E et al: Superficial angiomyxoma: clinicopathologic analysis of a series of distinctive but poorly recognized cutaneous tumors with tendency for recurrence. Am J Surg Pathol. 23(8):910-7, 1999
7. Mentzel T et al: Myxofibrosarcoma. Clinicopathologic analysis of 75 cases with emphasis on the low-grade variant. Am J Surg Pathol. 20(4):391-405, 1996
8. Carney JA et al: Cutaneous myxomas. A major component of the complex of myxomas, spotty pigmentation, and endocrine overactivity. Arch Dermatol. 122(7):790-8, 1986

DERMAL NERVE SHEATH MYXOMA

Microscopic Features

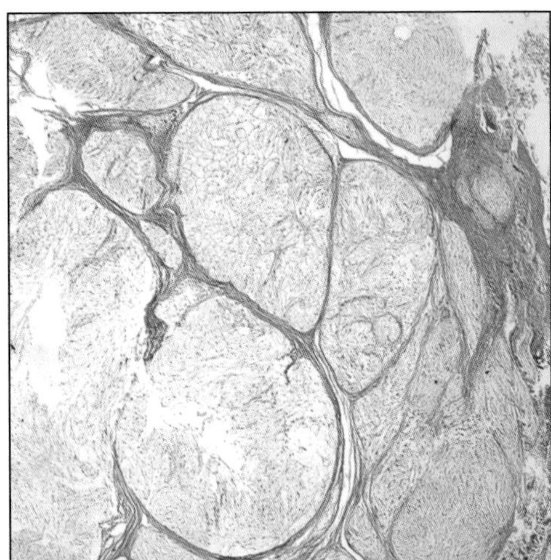
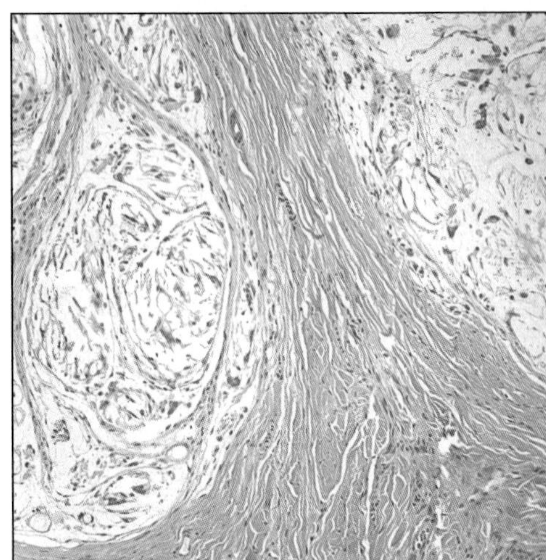

(Left) *On low power, nerve sheath myxoma has a well-defined lobular architecture composed of rounded lobules containing a copious myxoid matrix.* ***(Right)*** *The lobules are typically bordered by thick fibrous septa. Unlike many other cutaneous myxoid lesions, nerve sheath myxomas have a peripheral fibrous border and do not tend to infiltrate adjacent structures or entrap dermal collagen.*

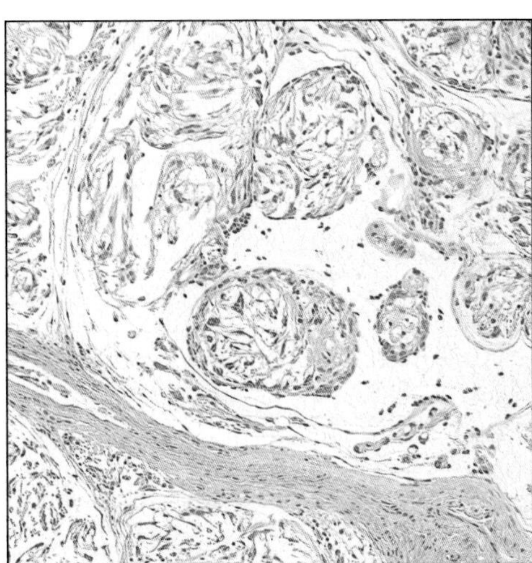
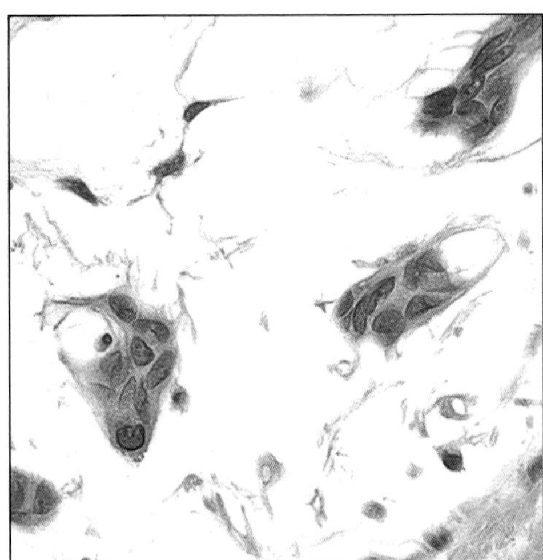

(Left) *Nerve sheath myxomas often form cohesive structures and interconnecting networks of cells. Note the thick fibrous septa at the bottom, which divide adjacent lobules.* ***(Right)*** *The neoplastic cells of nerve sheath myxoma consist of spindle and epithelioid cells with uniform, bland, ovoid nuclei and abundant eosinophilic cytoplasm. They are frequently arranged in syncytial nests and often have intracytoplasmic vacuoles as depicted.*

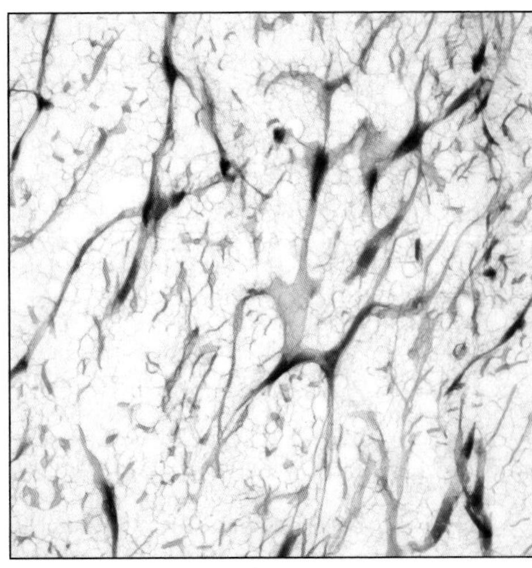
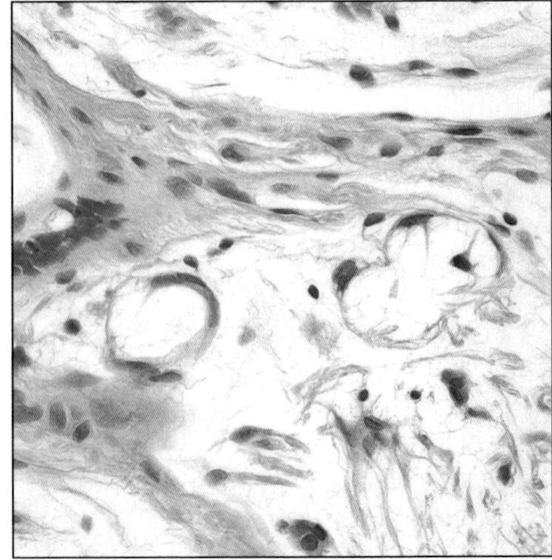

(Left) *This micrograph shows spindle and stellate Schwann cells in a nerve sheath myxoma with abundant eosinophilic cytoplasm and long, interconnecting cell processes, forming a reticulated pattern.* ***(Right)*** *The neoplastic cells often interconnect to form ring-like structures as depicted in this micrograph.*

Microscopic Features and Differential Diagnosis

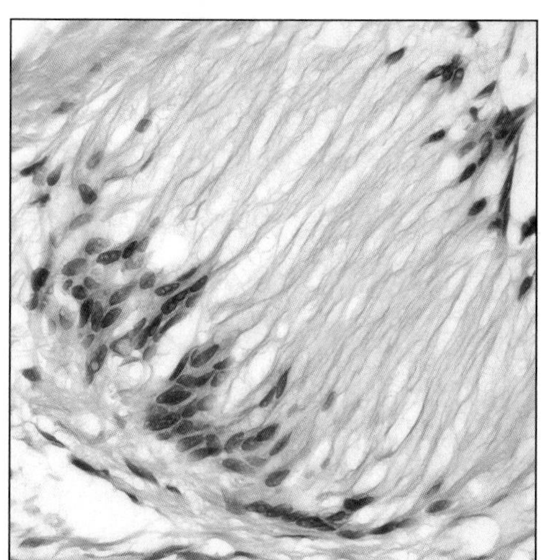

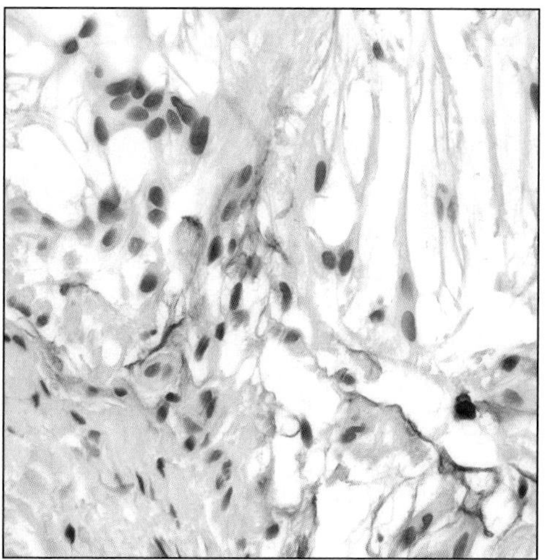

(Left) *Verocay-like bodies are rarely seen in nerve sheath myxomas. These provide additional evidence for Schwann cell differentiation.* ***(Right)*** *This immunohistochemical stain for CD34 highlights long, thin cell processes of intraneural fibroblasts, which are frequently detected in nerve sheath myxoma. In addition, EMA(+) perineurial cells (not depicted) are also detected in most tumors.*

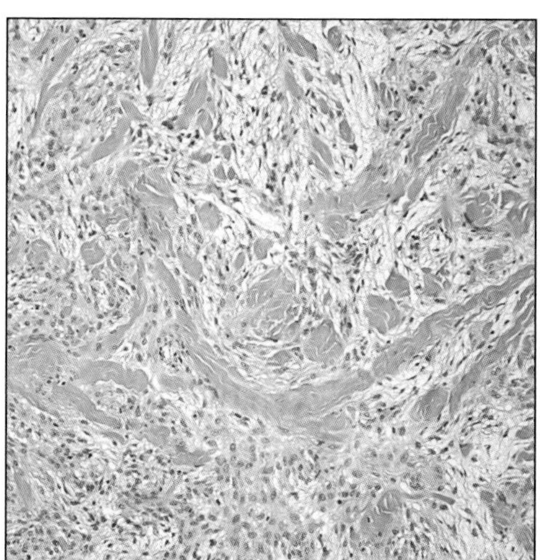

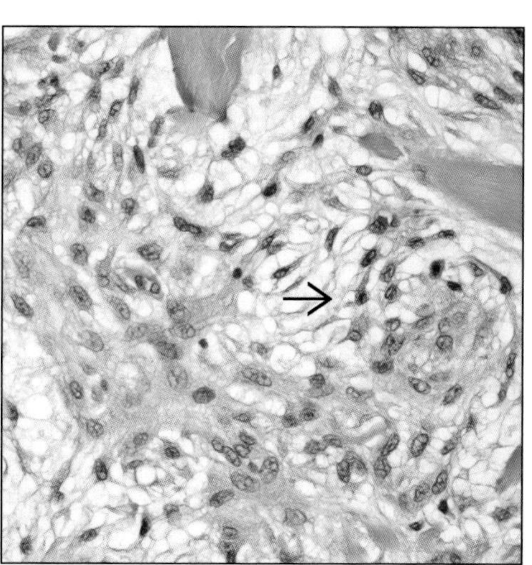

(Left) *Neurothekeoma is an important differential diagnosis. Compared to nerve sheath myxoma, neurothekeoma has a less defined lobular architecture, less myxoid matrix, and a more infiltrative growth pattern as illustrated by entrapment of dermal collagen fibers.* ***(Right)*** *Like nerve sheath myxoma, neurothekeoma has both spindle and epithelioid cells. However, epithelioid cells are larger and plumper, with a tendency to form whorl structures* ➔. *Neurothekeoma is S100(-).*

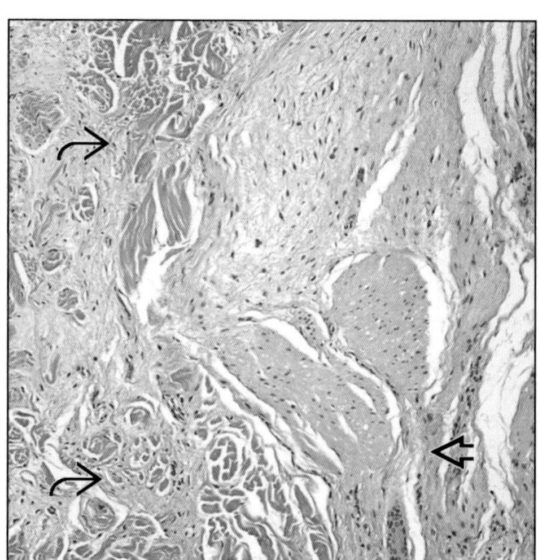

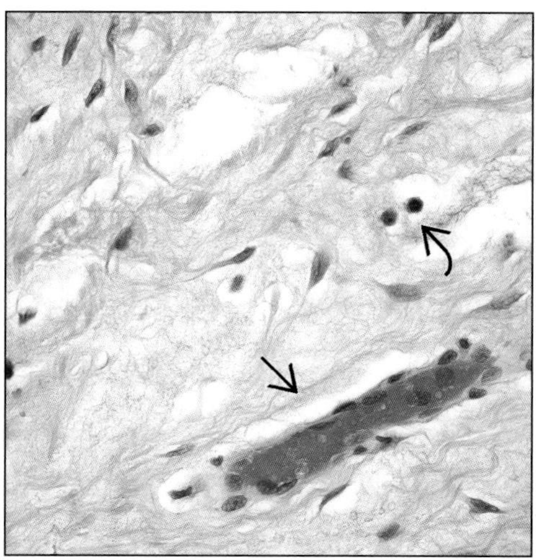

(Left) *Superficial angiomyxoma differs from nerve sheath myxoma by having a less defined lobular architecture and an infiltrative growth pattern, which includes frequent entrapment of adnexal structures* ⇨ *and dermal collagen* ↗. ***(Right)*** *The proliferating cells in superficial angiomyxoma are fibroblastic with spindle-shaped nuclei and are S100(-). Other distinctive features include numerous thin-walled congested vessels* ➔ *and a smattering of inflammatory cells* ↗.

SCHWANNOMA

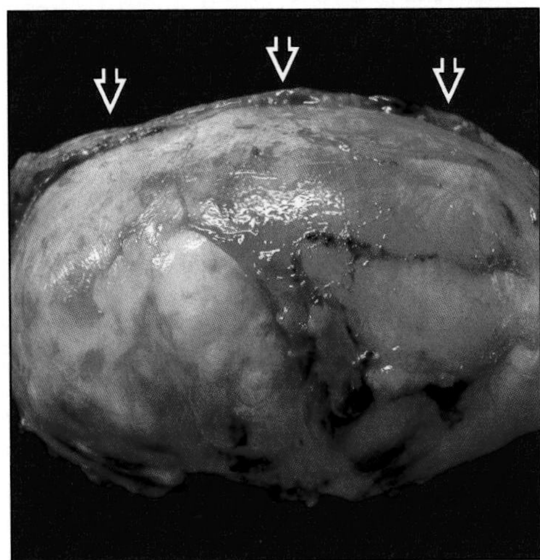

Schwannomas are well-circumscribed, encapsulated tumors and often arise as an eccentric mass loosely attached to an underlying nerve. The underlying nerve ⇨ wraps around the tumor in this example.

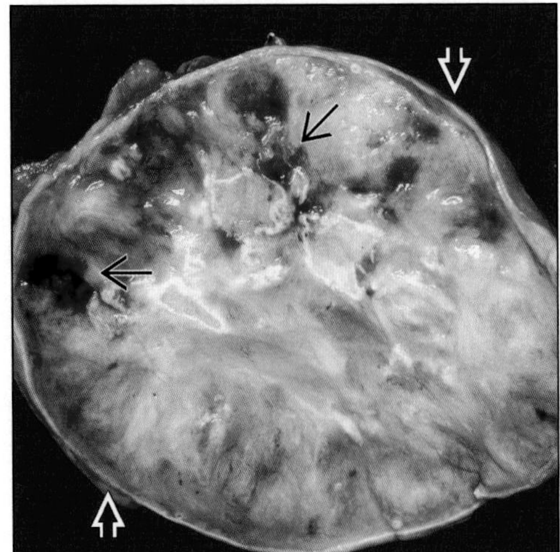

This tumor shows a thick peripheral capsule ⇨ and a yellow-white cut surface with foci of hemorrhage →.

TERMINOLOGY

Definitions

- Encapsulated, benign peripheral nerve sheath tumor composed predominantly of Schwann cells

ETIOLOGY/PATHOGENESIS

Molecular Aberrations

- Somatic *NF2* gene mutations present in most tumors
- Bilateral vestibular schwannomas occur in setting of germline *NF2* gene mutations

CLINICAL ISSUES

Epidemiology

- Incidence
  - 90% are sporadic
  - 10% are syndromic
    - About 3% with neurofibromatosis type 2 (NF2)
    - 2% with schwannomatosis
    - 5% with multiple meningiomas
    - Rarely in association with neurofibromatosis type 1 (NF1)
- Age
  - All ages
  - Common between 20-50 years of age
- Gender
  - Affects males and females equally

Site

- Head & neck
- Upper and lower extremities
- Deep-seated tumors occur in mediastinum and retroperitoneum

Presentation

- Slow growing
- Painless mass
  - Large tumors may be painful
- Cystic tumors may show fluctuation in size

Treatment

- Surgical excision is curative

Prognosis

- Excellent

Multiple Schwannoma Syndromes

- Neurofibromatosis type 2
  - Autosomal dominant condition
  - Incidence around 1:30,000-40,000
  - Inactivating germline mutations of *NF2* gene on chromosome 22
  - Bilateral vestibular schwannomas are characteristic
  - Schwannomas involving other cranial nerves may be present
  - CNS tumors like meningioma, ependymoma, and gliomas are also part of disease spectrum
  - Schwannomas in NF2 resemble their sporadic counterparts
- Schwannomatosis
  - Not associated with germline mutations in *NF1* or *NF2* genes
  - Autosomal dominant inheritance with incomplete penetrance
  - Both sexes affected equally
  - Patients do not develop bilateral vestibular schwannomas or CNS tumors seen in NF2
  - Locus of disease mapped to chromosome 22 proximal to *NF2* gene
  - Morphology similar to sporadic schwannomas

MACROSCOPIC FEATURES

General Features

- Surrounded by true capsule consisting of epineurium
- Eccentric mass loosely attached to underlying nerve

SCHWANNOMA

Key Facts

Terminology

- Encapsulated, benign peripheral nerve sheath tumor composed predominantly of Schwann cells

Clinical Issues

- Common between 20-50 years of age
- Affects males and females equally
- Surgical excision is curative

Macroscopic Features

- Typically presents as eccentric mass loosely attached to underlying nerve

Microscopic Pathology

- Hallmark: Variable amounts of hypercellular Antoni A and hypocellular Antoni B areas
- Spindle cells in short fascicles in Antoni A areas
- Loose matrix with cystic change and inflammatory cells in Antoni B areas
- Bland nuclear features in most instances; degenerative nuclear atypia in "ancient" schwannoma
- Cellular schwannoma may mimic MPNST
- Plexiform schwannoma usually seen in children
- Epithelioid schwannoma may be mistaken for smooth muscle tumor
- Melanotic/psammomatous schwannoma often associated with Carney syndrome
- Schwannomas in NF2 and schwannomatosis similar to sporadic tumors
- Microcystic/reticular schwannoma has predilection for visceral location

Ancillary Tests

- Diffuse, strong S100 positivity is characteristic

- Small tumors may be fusiform in shape and mimic neurofibroma
- Dumbbell-shaped tumors occur in vertebral canal usually in posterior mediastinum
- Cut surface is pink, white-yellow
- Large tumors may show cystic change, hemorrhage, or calcification

Size

- Variable

MICROSCOPIC PATHOLOGY

Histologic Features

- Uninodular mass with fibrous capsule
- Hallmark: Variable amounts of hypercellular Antoni A and hypocellular Antoni B areas
- Antoni A
  - Spindle cells in short fascicles
  - Plump nuclei, indistinct cytoplasmic borders
  - Intranuclear vacuoles in some tumors
  - Nuclear palisading or whorling
  - Verocay bodies
    - Compact rows of palisaded nuclei separated by fibrillary processes
- Antoni B
  - Spindle or oval cells
  - Loose matrix with cystic change and inflammatory cells
  - Large vessels with thick hyalinized walls and luminal thrombi
- Benign epithelial structures and glands may be present in rare instances

Cytologic Features

- Bland nuclear features in most instances

Variants

- **"Ancient" schwannoma**
  - Marked nuclear atypia of degenerative type
  - Usually seen in deep-seated large tumors of long duration
  - Cystic change, hemorrhage, calcification, and hyalinization present
  - Lacks mitotic activity
  - Behavior is similar to ordinary schwannoma
- **Cellular schwannoma**
  - Composed almost exclusively of hypercellular Antoni A areas, which lack Verocay bodies
  - More common in mediastinum and retroperitoneum
  - Encapsulated tumors; some may be multinodular or plexiform in architecture
  - Long sweeping fascicles of spindle-shaped cells
  - Mitotic activity is low (< 4/10 HPF)
  - Small foci of necrosis may be present
  - Diffuse strong S100 positivity distinguishes cellular schwannoma from malignant peripheral nerve sheath tumors (MPNSTs)
- **Plexiform schwannoma**
  - Usually involves skin
  - Infrequent in deeper locations
  - Encapsulated tumors with multinodular or plexiform architecture
  - Often more cellular than ordinary schwannoma
  - Association with neurofibromatosis is weak (unlike plexiform neurofibroma, which is almost pathognomonic of NF1)
- **Epithelioid schwannoma**
  - Small round Schwann cells with eosinophilic cytoplasm and sharp cell borders
  - Arranged in clusters, cords, or as single cells
  - Stroma is collagenous or myxoid
  - Foci of typical schwannoma may be present
  - Degenerative nuclear atypia may be seen
  - Lacks mitotic activity
  - Immunostains for S100 and type IV collagen are positive
- **Melanotic/psammomatous schwannoma**
  - Distinctive tumor of adults (average age around 33 years) that often arises in spinal or autonomic nerves near midline
  - About 50% of patients have evidence of Carney syndrome (cardiac myxoma, spotty pigmentation,

endocrine overactivity, acromegaly, or sexual precocity)
  - Multiple tumors may be present in 20% of patients
  - Pigmentation may be heavy and mask underlying tumor morphology
  - Syncytial arrangement of spindle to ovoid cells with prominent nucleoli and intranuclear inclusions
  - Psammoma bodies are present in most cases
  - Tumors express not only S100 but also HMB-45
  - Difficult to predict behavior since bland-appearing tumors have also been known to metastasize
  - Overall, metastasis occurs in about 26% of cases
- **Neuroblastoma-like schwannoma**
  - Schwann cells are round and small in this variant and cluster around large collagen cores
  - Mimics rosettes seen in neuroblastoma
- **Pseudoglandular schwannoma**
  - Prominent cystic change
  - Cystic spaces are lined by small round tumor cells
  - Mimics epithelial neoplasm
- **Microcystic/reticular schwannoma**
  - Anastomosing strands of spindle cells in myxoid, fibrillary, or collagenous matrix
  - Predilection for visceral location
  - Mimics reticular perineurioma
- **Malignant transformation in schwannomas**
  - Extremely rare
  - Malignant change in schwannomas usually resembles epithelioid MPNST

ANCILLARY TESTS

Immunohistochemistry

- Diffuse, strong S100 positivity is characteristic
- LEU-7 and GFAP may be positive in some tumors

Electron Microscopy

- Transmission
  - Almost exclusively composed of Schwann cells
  - Basal lamina with electron dense material lines surface of Schwann cells
  - Flat invaginated nucleus and attenuated cell processes
  - Increased lysosomes in Schwann cells in Antoni B areas

DIFFERENTIAL DIAGNOSIS

Leiomyoma

- Nuclear palisading is also seen in smooth muscle tumors and may mimic schwannoma
- Leiomyomas lack Antoni A and Antoni B areas
- Leiomyomas are positive for desmin and smooth muscle actin and are negative for S100

Malignant Peripheral Nerve Sheath Tumor (MPNST)

- Cellular schwannomas may be mistaken for MPNST
- Plexiform schwannomas are also cellular and may be mistaken for MPNST arising in plexiform neurofibroma
- MPNSTs show greater nuclear atypia, necrosis, and only focal S100 positivity, unlike benign schwannoma variants, which are diffusely S100 positive

Malignant Melanoma

- Melanotic schwannomas may be mistaken for melanoma due to coexpression of S100 and HMB-45
- Melanotic schwannomas do not have degree of nuclear atypia or mitotic activity seen in malignant melanoma
- Psammoma bodies are present in melanotic schwannoma but not in metastatic melanomas

DIAGNOSTIC CHECKLIST

Pathologic Interpretation Pearls

- Encapsulated tumor with alternating hypercellular and hypocellular areas with diffuse strong S100 positivity

SELECTED REFERENCES

1. Liegl B et al: Microcystic/reticular schwannoma: a distinct variant with predilection for visceral locations. Am J Surg Pathol. 32(7):1080-7, 2008
2. MacCollin M et al: Diagnostic criteria for schwannomatosis. Neurology. 64(11):1838-45, 2005
3. Woodruff JM et al: Congenital and childhood plexiform (multinodular) cellular schwannoma: a troublesome mimic of malignant peripheral nerve sheath tumor. Am J Surg Pathol. 27(10):1321-9, 2003
4. McMenamin ME et al: Expanding the spectrum of malignant change in schwannomas: epithelioid malignant change, epithelioid malignant peripheral nerve sheath tumor, and epithelioid angiosarcoma: a study of 17 cases. Am J Surg Pathol. 25(1):13-25, 2001
5. Antinheimo J et al: Population-based analysis of sporadic and type 2 neurofibromatosis-associated meningiomas and schwannomas. Neurology. 54(1):71-6, 2000
6. Kindblom LG et al: Benign epithelioid schwannoma. Am J Surg Pathol. 22(6):762-70, 1998
7. Chan JK et al: Pseudoglandular schwannoma. Histopathology. 29(5):481-3, 1996
8. Goldblum JR et al: Neuroblastoma-like neurilemoma. Am J Surg Pathol. 18(3):266-73, 1994
9. Brooks JJ et al: Benign glandular schwannoma. Arch Pathol Lab Med. 116(2):192-5, 1992
10. Carney JA: Psammomatous melanotic schwannoma. A distinctive, heritable tumor with special associations, including cardiac myxoma and the Cushing syndrome. Am J Surg Pathol. 14(3):206-22, 1990
11. Fletcher CD et al: Cellular schwannoma: a distinct pseudosarcomatous entity. Histopathology. 11(1):21-35, 1987
12. Fletcher CD et al: Benign plexiform (multinodular) schwannoma: a rare tumour unassociated with neurofibromatosis. Histopathology. 10(9):971-80, 1986

SCHWANNOMA

Gross, Radiographic, and Microscopic Features

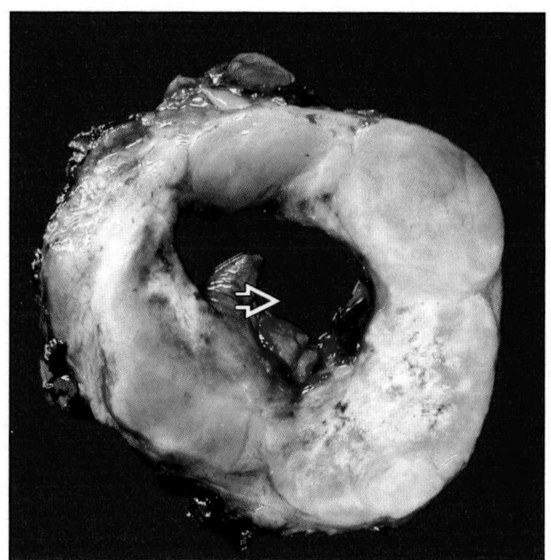

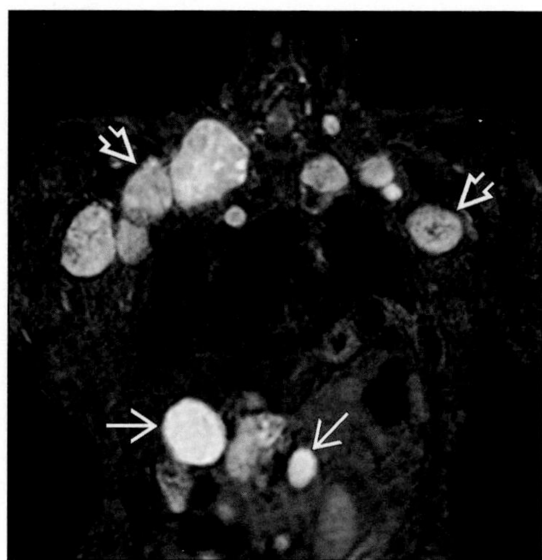

(Left) *Large, deep-seated schwannomas of long duration often undergo degenerative changes. Marked central cystic change is present in this example* ➲. ***(Right)*** *MR in a patient with schwannomatosis shows multiple T2 hyperintense nodular masses involving bilateral branchial plexus* ➲ *and additional intraabdominal lesions* ➔. *No vestibular schwannomas were present in this case.*

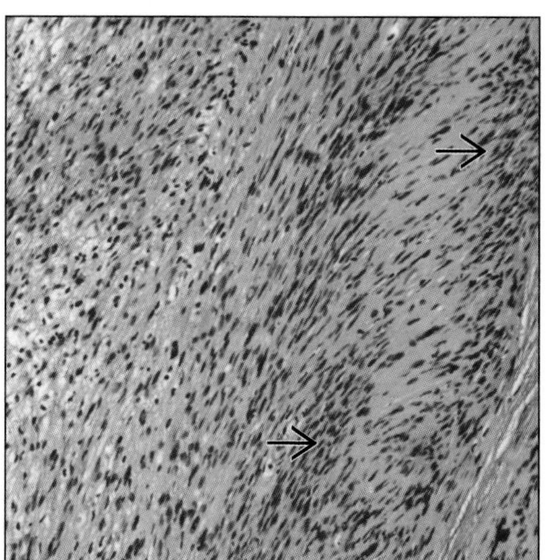

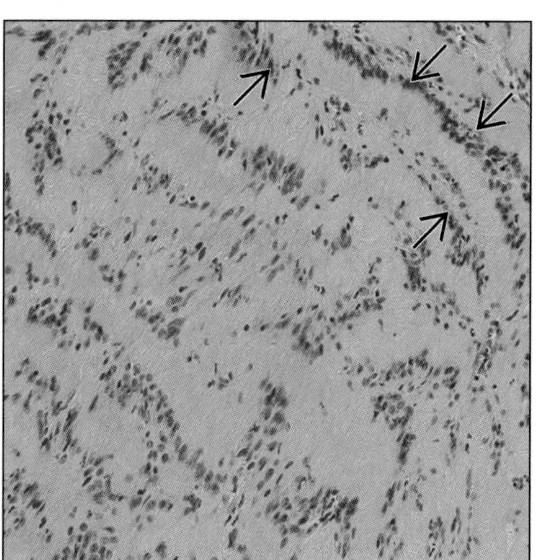

(Left) *Schwannomas are composed of alternating hypercellular spindle cell areas (Antoni A, right) and hypocellular round cell areas (Antoni B, left). Nuclear palisading is often present in Antoni A areas* ➔. ***(Right)*** *Nuclear palisading in Antoni A areas may be prominent and form nuclear palisades around a collagenous hyalinized core (Verocay bodies)* ➔. *Verocay bodies can be quite variable in number from case to case.*

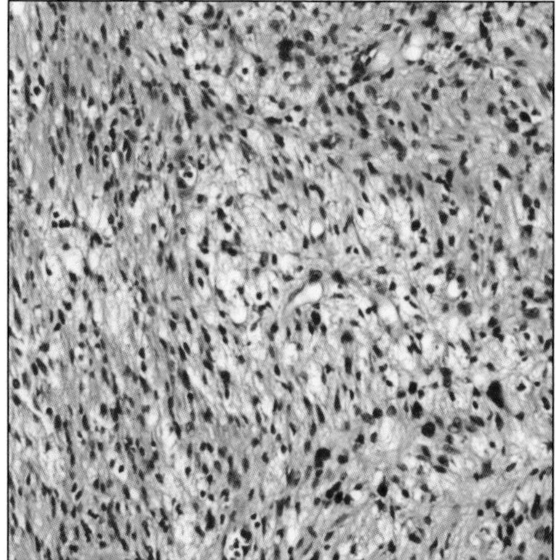

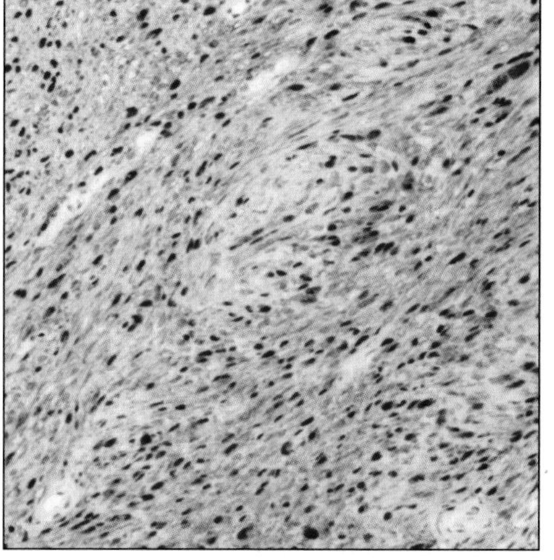

(Left) *Antoni B areas are paucicellular with small, round to ovoid tumor cells and may contain foamy macrophages and inflammatory cells. The background stroma is loose, myxoid in contrast to the more collagenized stroma in Antoni A areas of the tumor.* ***(Right)*** *Schwannomas are characterized by diffuse and strong immunoreactivity for S100 protein. The presence of diffuse positivity is a useful clue to the benign nature of some schwannoma variants that may otherwise be mistaken for a MPNST.*

SCHWANNOMA

Variant Microscopic Features

*(**Left**) "Ancient" schwannomas are longstanding tumors with degenerative nuclear atypia ⇨. The smudgy nuclear chromatin and lack of mitotic activity are useful in excluding the diagnosis of MPNST. (**Right**) Cystic change can be prominent in some cases and mimic an epithelial tumor. Such tumors have been described as "pseudoglandular" schwannomas. This appearance may also overlap with the recently described microcystic/reticular variant of schwannoma.*

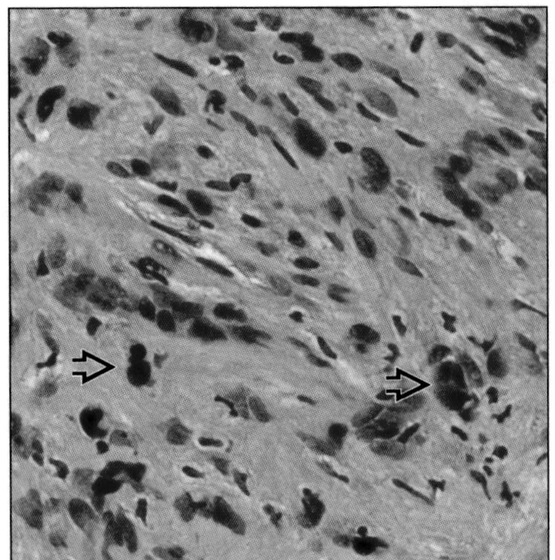

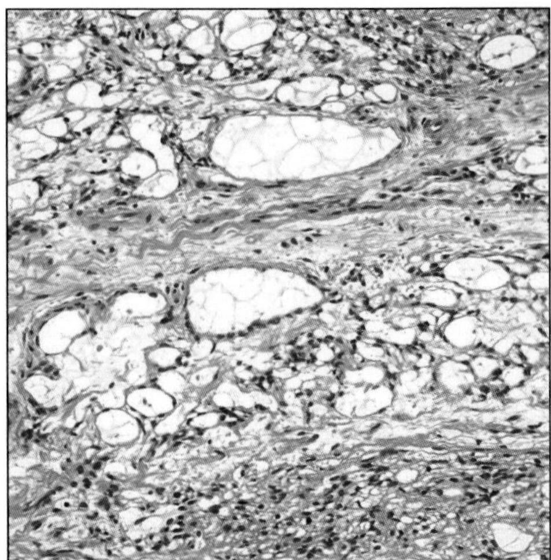

*(**Left**) Cellular schwannomas are encapsulated tumors ⇨ just like typical schwannomas but are composed almost exclusively of Antoni A areas. (**Right**) The hypercellular, fascicular spindle cell proliferation in cellular schwannomas may be mistaken for MPNST. Diffuse S100 positivity is a helpful indicator of the benign nature of this schwannoma variant.*

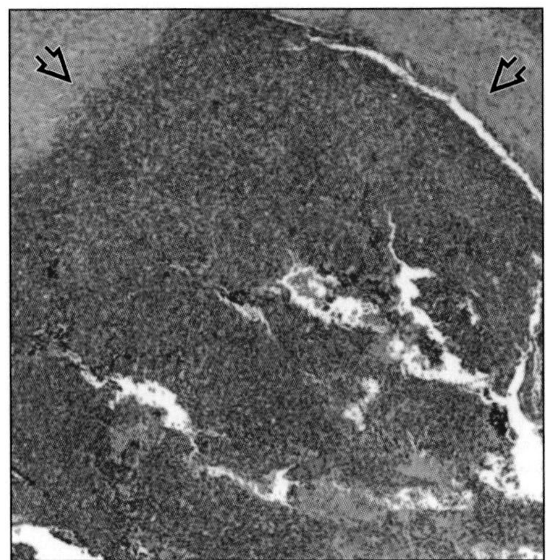

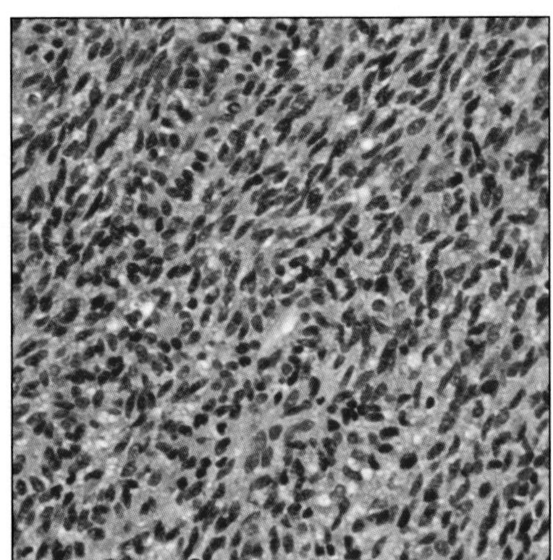

*(**Left**) Plexiform schwannomas are characterized by a multinodular/plexiform architecture. These variants may be quite cellular, as in this example, and can be mistaken for sarcomatous transformation in a plexiform neurofibroma. (**Right**) Neuroblastoma-like schwannoma shows central collagenous cores surrounded by small, round to oval Schwann cells. This appearance mimics the rosettes seen in neuroblastoma.*

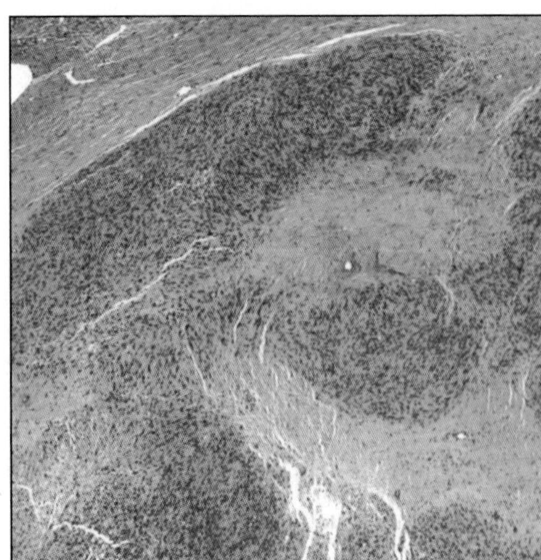

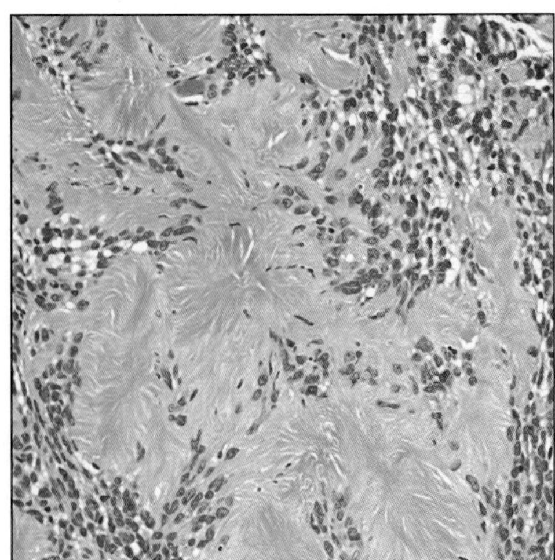

Variant Microscopic Features

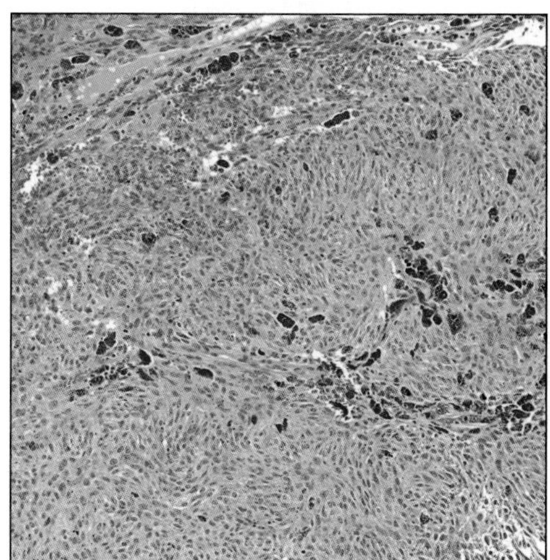

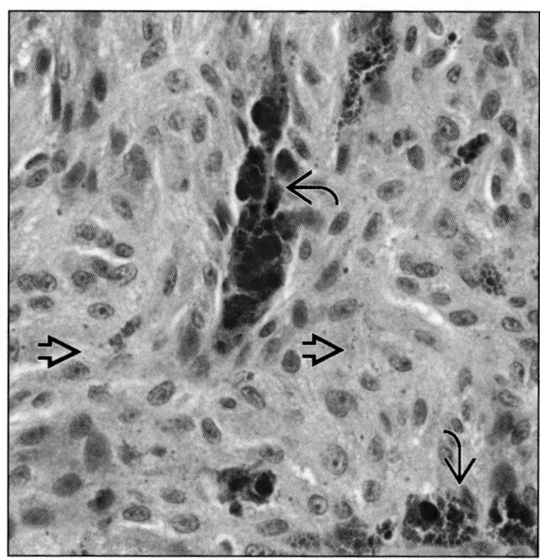

(Left) *Melanotic schwannoma occurs sporadically and in association with Carney syndrome. Syncytial arrangement of spindle cells with prominent melanin pigmentation is characteristic of this variant.* **(Right)** *The tumor cells are spindle-ovoid in shape and show a vesicular nuclear chromatin with prominent nucleoli and finely granular* ⇨ *to coarsely clumped* ↷ *melanin pigmentation.*

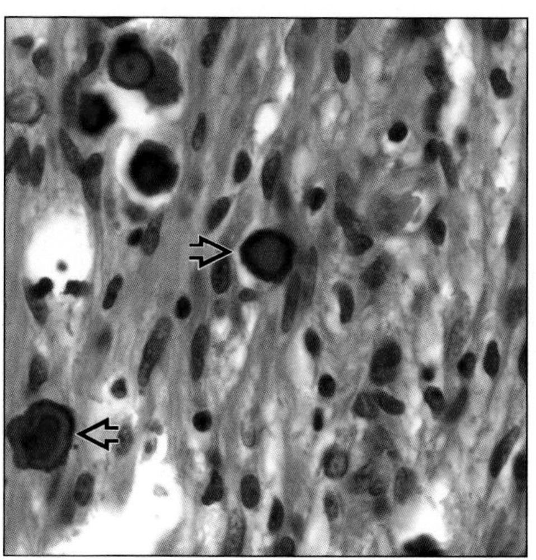

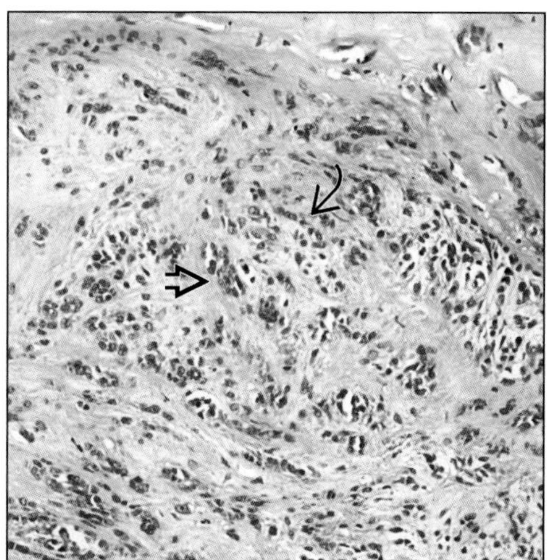

(Left) *Psammomatous calcification* ⇨ *is present in most cases of melanotic schwannoma and is a helpful clue in distinguishing this schwannoma variant from metastatic malignant melanoma.* **(Right)** *Epithelioid schwannomas are characterized by small clusters* ⇨ *and cords* ↷ *of round to oval tumor cells with eosinophilic cytoplasm set in a myxoid or collagenous matrix.*

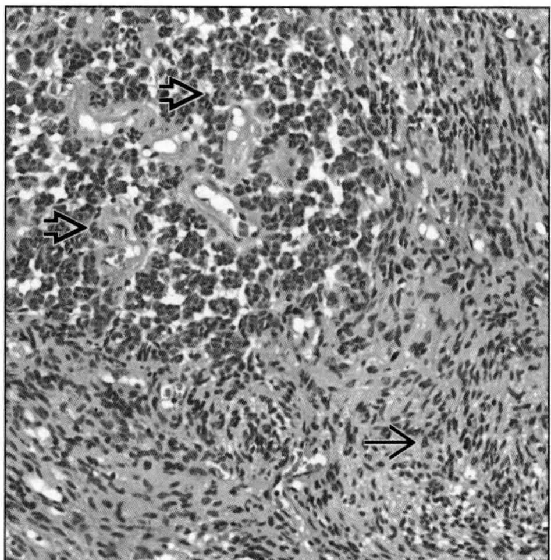

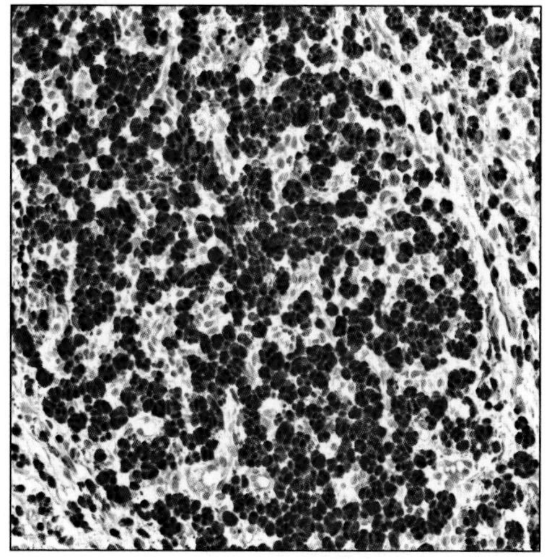

(Left) *Epithelioid schwannomas* ⇨ *may also show spindle cell areas* → *characteristic of a conventional schwannoma in some instances.* **(Right)** *Similar to conventional schwannomas, diffuse, strong S100 positivity is typically seen in the epithelioid variant.*

NEUROFIBROMA

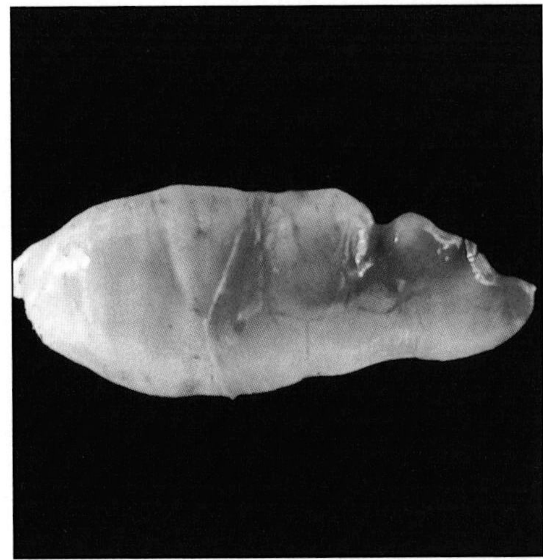

Neurofibromas present as fusiform, uninodular or multinodular, well-circumscribed, but unencapsulated tumors.

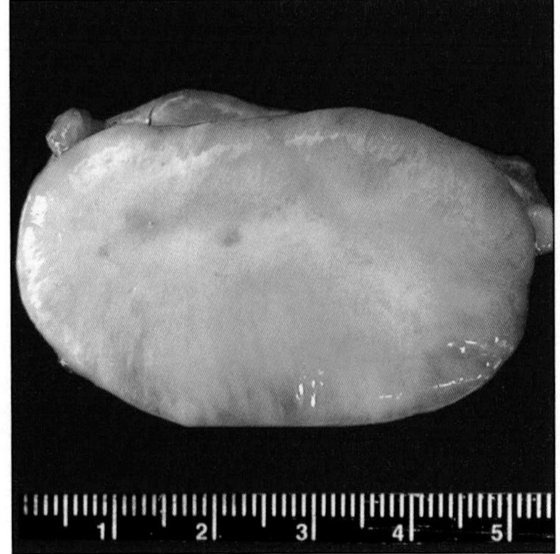

The cut surface of neurofibroma is pale, homogeneous, waxy, and often myxoid in appearance. Degenerative changes typically seen in schwannomas are seldom present in neurofibroma.

TERMINOLOGY

Abbreviations

- Neurofibroma (NF)
- Neurofibromatosis type 1 (NF1)

Synonyms

- Von Recklinghausen disease = neurofibromatosis type 1

Definitions

- Benign peripheral nerve sheath tumor composed of Schwann cells, fibroblasts, perineurial-like cells, and residual nerves in myxoid/collagen matrix

ETIOLOGY/PATHOGENESIS

Histogenesis

- Neurofibromas are sporadic in about 90% of cases; others are syndromic in association with NF1
  - NF1 results from germline mutation in *NF1* gene on chromosome 17q11.2
    - *NF1* gene encodes for neurofibromin protein, which is a GTPase-activating protein
    - Neurofibromin also acts as a tumor suppressor by downregulating *Ras* and *cAMP*
  - Sporadic tumors arise from somatic mutations in *NF1*
- Evidence supporting neoplastic nature of NF
  - Sporadic tumors are histologically similar to NF1-associated neurofibromas
  - Tumors are monoclonal on X chromosome inactivation studies
  - Lesional cells carry *NF1* gene deletion

CLINICAL ISSUES

Epidemiology

- Incidence
  - Most common tumor of peripheral nerve
  - NF1 incidence: 1 in 2,500-4,000 births
- Age
  - Solitary, sporadic lesions: In patients 20-30 years old
  - Tumors in setting of NF1 present during puberty
  - Plexiform NF may be congenital
- Gender
  - Affects both sexes equally

Presentation

- Most tumors are solitary and sporadic
- Superficial cutaneous or localized intraneural NF present as painless, palpable mass
- Deep intraneural tumors may present with pain or dysesthesia
- Intraspinal (nerve root) NF may show signs of spinal cord compression

Natural History

- Slow-growing tumors in most instances
  - Increased rates of growth may be seen in puberty and pregnancy
- Malignant transformation in NF
  - Rare in sporadic tumors; usually occurs in setting of NF1
  - Rare in cutaneous NF (0.001%)
  - More common in plexiform NF (2-10%)
  - Clinical suspicion for malignant transformation
    - Rapid enlargement of preexisting NF
    - Pain or change in neurological symptoms

Treatment

- Surgical approaches
  - Complete resection is curative
  - Decompression of spinal cord in symptomatic tumors

Prognosis

- Recurrence rare, even after partial removal

NEUROFIBROMA

Key Facts

Terminology
- Benign peripheral nerve sheath tumor with heterogeneous admixture of axons, Schwann cells, perineurial cells, and fibroblasts
- Most are sporadic; NF1 associated with multiple, large, or plexiform tumors

Clinical Issues
- Localized cutaneous NF most common subtype
- Diffuse cutaneous NF infiltrate dermis and subcutis
- Localized intraneural NF are deep seated and involve larger nerves
- Plexiform NF involves multiple nerve fascicles or branches ("bag of worms")
- Massive soft tissue NF involves pelvis, shoulder, or extremities ("localized gigantism")

Macroscopic Features
- Variable size and consistency
- Lack degenerative changes seen in schwannomas

Microscopic Pathology
- Bundles of spindle cells with angulated or wavy nuclei
- Loose, myxoid or thick collagenous matrix
- Coarse collagen bundles resemble "shredded carrots"
- Residual, central, neurofilament-positive axon fibers present
- Atypical NF behave in benign manner

Diagnostic Checklist
- Malignant transformation occurs in about 2-10% of plexiform NF
  - ↑ cellularity, atypia, hyperchromasia, mitoses

Subtypes
- **Localized cutaneous NF**
  - Most common type
  - Nodular or polypoid, usually well circumscribed
  - Freely movable, soft, round lesions that elevate skin
  - Generally not associated with peripheral nerve
- **Diffuse cutaneous NF**
  - Typically affects children and young adults
  - Large plaque-like tumors that often affect head and neck region
  - 10% associated with NF1
  - Diffuse infiltration of dermis and subcutaneous adipose tissue
  - Entraps dermal vessels, nerves, and adnexa
  - Spreads along subcutaneous connective tissue septa
- **Plexiform NF**
  - Usually presents in early childhood
  - Pathognomonic of NF1 if plexiform architecture is strictly defined
  - Multinodular lesions involving multiple nerves or nerve branches
  - "Bag of worms" appearance is characteristic
  - Generally affects small nerves
  - Entire extremity may be involved ("elephantiasis neuromatosa")
- **Massive soft tissue NF**
  - Tend to be very large, diffuse, or plexiform
  - Widespread infiltration of adipose tissue and muscle
  - Result in large pendulous folds of neurofibromatous tissue ("localized gigantism")

IMAGE FINDINGS

MR Findings
- Irregular or bright on T2WI MR
- Gadolinium enhancing on T1WI
- "Target" sign due to reduced signal in intraneural NF
- "Dumbbell" tumors: Intradural and extradural portions of paraspinal tumor acquire shape of dumbbell

MACROSCOPIC FEATURES

General Features
- Gray to tan cut surface
- Glistening, gelatinous to firm/fibrous consistency
- Relatively well circumscribed but not encapsulated
  - Intraneural NF may be covered by epineurium
- Lack degeneration (hemorrhage, cystic change) commonly seen in schwannomas

Size
- Localized cutaneous lesions: Up to 2 cm
- May reach much larger size (e.g., massive soft tissue NF)

MICROSCOPIC PATHOLOGY

Histologic Features
- Irregular interlacing bundles or fascicles of spindle cells
- Ovoid to spindled, wavy, dark nuclei with thin cell processes
- Variable proportions of loose myxoid matrix and coarse collagen bundles
- Collagen bundles impart "shredded carrot" appearance
- Residual axons usually present within tumor
- Mast cells, lymphocytes, and even xanthoma cells may be present
- Some tumors may be more cellular with uniform collagenous matrix ("cellular neurofibroma")
- Nuclear atypia may be present in some cases
  - Atypia in absence of increased cellularity, mitotic activity, and necrosis is not feature of malignancy in NF
- Rare morphological findings
  - Epithelioid Schwann cells
  - Skeletal muscle
  - Glandular epithelium or rosettes
- NF subtypes
  - **Localized NF**

- Dense collagenized stroma is typical; cutaneous NF separated from epidermis by Grenz zone
  - **Diffuse NF**
    - Uniformly fine fibrillary collagenous matrix
    - Clusters of Meissner body-like structures are often present
  - **Plexiform NF**
    - Tortuous mass of multinodular tumor tissue
    - Early stages of tumor may show only increased endoneurial matrix
    - Large tumors may also have intermixed areas of diffuse NF
    - Nuclear atypia may be present

Cytologic Features

- Bland nuclear features in most cases

Histologic Variants

- Pigmented NF
  - Rare (< 1% of all NF)
  - Melanin pigment present in dendritic or epithelioid tumor cells
  - Pigmented cells cluster in superficial parts of tumor
  - Stain positively with S100 and melanocytic markers, such as HMB-45
  - May recur but do not metastasize
- Atypical NF
  - Tumors in which features fall short of diagnosis of low-grade malignant peripheral nerve sheath tumor (MPNST)
  - Nuclear atypia or rare mitotic figures in isolation should not be construed as signs of malignancy
  - Atypical NF shows variable number of large hyperchromatic nuclei
  - Mitotic activity is low or absent

ANCILLARY TESTS

Immunohistochemistry

- S100 stains subset of tumor cells; may also be positive for GFAP
- Perineurial cells positive for EMA and axons in tumor for neurofilament protein

Electron Microscopy

- Heterogeneous mixture of cell types, including Schwann cells, small neurites, perineurial cells, and fibroblasts

DIFFERENTIAL DIAGNOSIS

Plexiform Schwannoma

- Biphasic tumor with Antoni A and Antoni B areas
- Verocay bodies, perivascular hyalinization, and hemosiderin deposits present in schwannoma
- S100 positivity is more diffuse and uniform
- Cellular plexiform schwannoma may be mistaken for MPNST arising in plexiform neurofibroma

Perineurioma

- Concentric "onion bulb" or whorled proliferations around nerve fibers
- Diffuse and strongly positive for EMA

Ganglioneuroma (GN)

- Large neoplastic ganglion cells interspersed with neurofibroma-like areas
- GN shows abundant unmyelinated axons

Malignant Peripheral Nerve Sheath Tumor

- Cellular NF may be mistaken for MPNST
- Pleomorphism, nuclear enlargement, necrosis, and high mitotic activity (> 4/10 HPF) favors MPNST

Plexiform Fibrohistiocytic Tumors (PFHT)

- PFHT may be mistaken for plexiform NF
- Female predilection; myofibroblastic proliferation with multinucleated histiocytic giant cells in PFHT
- PFHT is actin-HHF-35(+), CD68(+), S100(-)

Dermatofibrosarcoma Protuberans (DFSP)

- Infiltration into subcutaneous adipose tissue in diffuse NF may be mistaken for DFSP
- DFSP is more cellular with uniformly storiform architecture and CD34 positivity

DIAGNOSTIC CHECKLIST

Clinically Relevant Pathologic Features

- Features pathognomonic for NF1
  - Multiple intraneural or cutaneous involvement
  - Plexiform architecture
  - Large (massive) soft tissue lesions
- Cutaneous NF associated with NF1
  - Overlying café au lait spots (pigmented macules)

Pathologic Interpretation Pearls

- Transformation to MPNST evident by increased cellularity, atypia, necrosis, and high mitotic activity

SELECTED REFERENCES

1. Skovronsky DM et al: Pathologic classification of peripheral nerve tumors. Neurosurg Clin N Am. 15(2):157-66, 2004
2. Evans DG et al: Malignant peripheral nerve sheath tumours in neurofibromatosis 1. J Med Genet. 39(5):311-4, 2002
3. Ferner RE et al: Neurofibroma and schwannoma. Curr Opin Neurol. 15(6):679-84, 2002
4. Fetsch JF et al: Pigmented (melanotic) neurofibroma: a clinicopathologic and immunohistochemical analysis of 19 lesions from 17 patients. Am J Surg Pathol. 24(3):331-43, 2000
5. Rasmussen SA et al: NF1 gene and neurofibromatosis 1. Am J Epidemiol. 151(1):33-40, 2000
6. Woodruff JM: Pathology of tumors of the peripheral nerve sheath in type 1 neurofibromatosis. Am J Med Genet. 89(1):23-30, 1999
7. Lin BT et al: Neurofibroma and cellular neurofibroma with atypia: a report of 14 tumors. Am J Surg Pathol. 21(12):1443-9, 1997
8. Lassmann H et al: Different types of benign nerve sheath tumors. Light microscopy, electron microscopy and autoradiography. Virchows Arch A Pathol Anat Histol. 375(3):197-210, 1977

Radiographic, Gross, and Microscopic Features

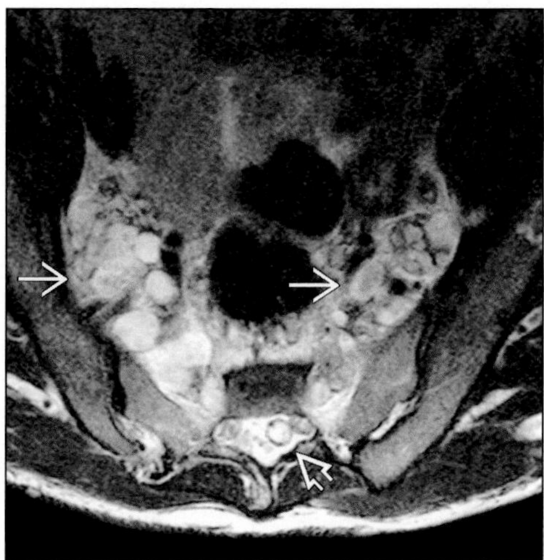

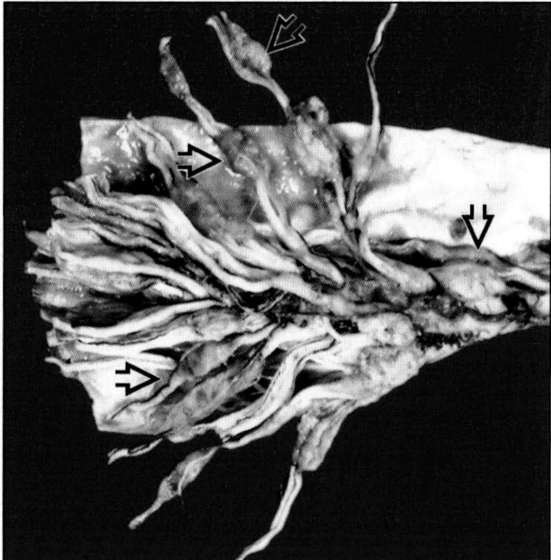

(Left) *Axial T2WI MR shows bilateral plexiform neurofibromas ➔ involving the sacral plexus with a characteristic "bag of worms" appearance. There is intraspinal extension ➔.* ***(Right)*** *Gross photograph shows multiple small fusiform tumors ➔ involving spinal nerve roots around the sacral plexus in a patient with neurofibromatosis type 1.*

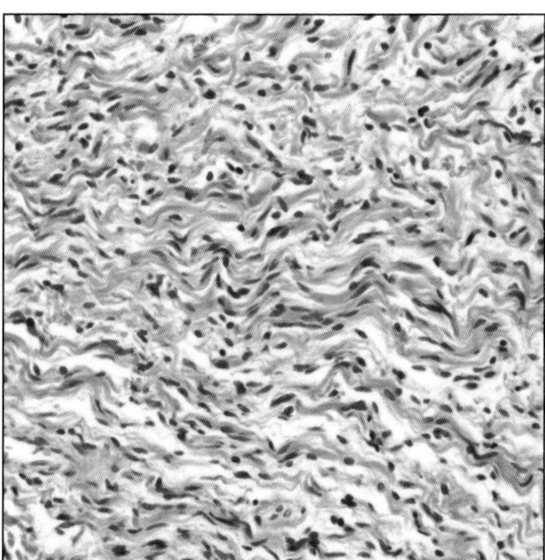

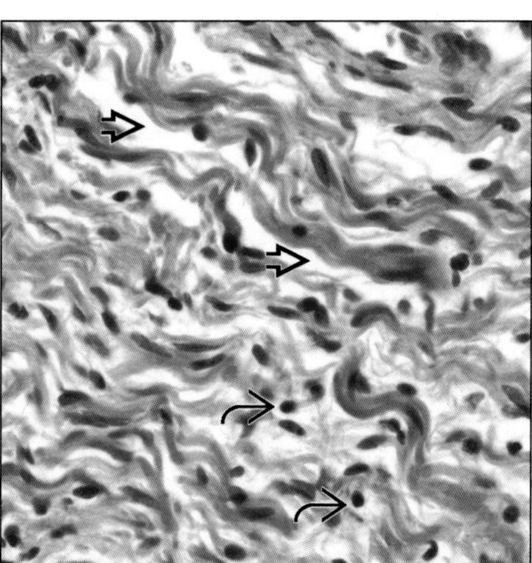

(Left) *Neurofibromas are composed of small ovoid to spindled cells with dark wavy nuclei in a variably myxoid or collagenous background.* ***(Right)*** *They also show thick coarse collagen bundles ➔ and an inflammatory component consisting of lymphocytes ➔ or mast cells.*

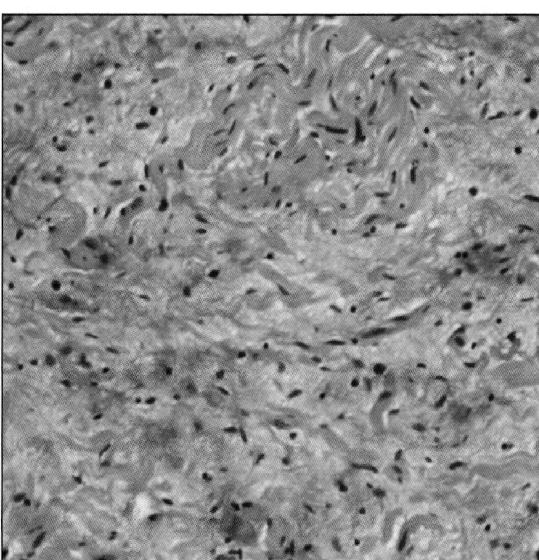

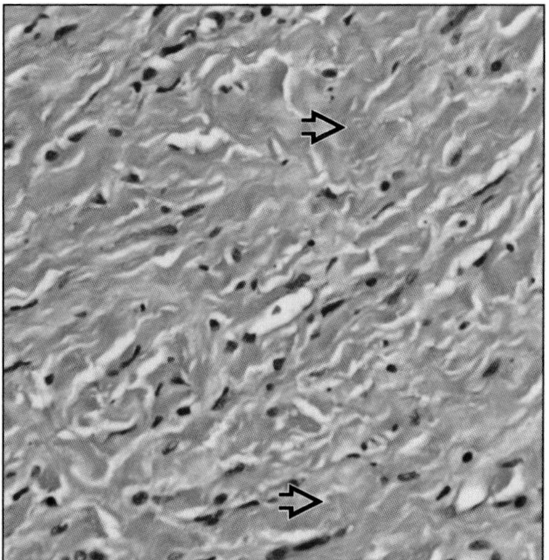

(Left) *Some neurofibromas may show prominent myxoid stromal change. When this change is prominent, these tumors may be mistaken for a myxoma.* ***(Right)*** *Other tumors may be extremely hypocellular and show a densely collagenized stroma ➔.*

NEUROFIBROMA

Microscopic Features

(Left) Coarse stromal collagen bundles ⇒, which usually occur in localized NF, have been likened to a "shredded carrot" appearance. *(Right)* Whorled structures ⇒ resembling Meissner or pacinian corpuscles are commonly present in diffuse neurofibromas.

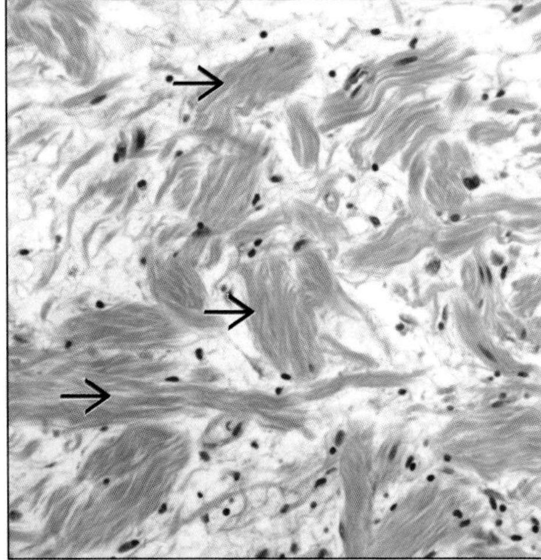

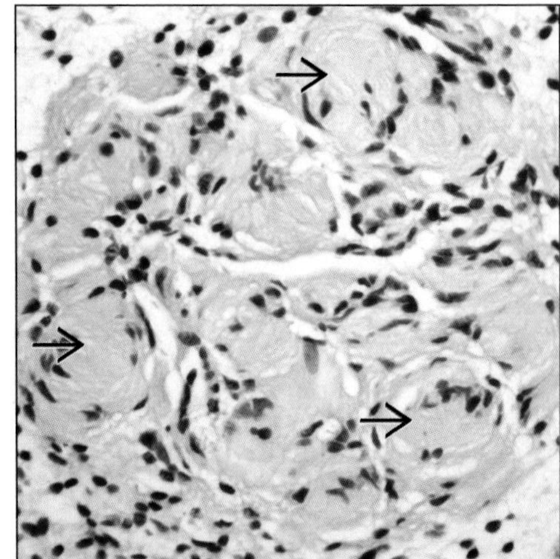

(Left) Neurofibromas consist of a heterogeneous population of tumor cells. Therefore, in contrast to schwannomas, S100 protein stains only a subset of tumor cells in neurofibroma. *(Right)* Scattered EMA(+) cells may also be present in a neurofibroma, usually at the periphery of the tumor mass. This corresponds to perineurial cells within the tumor seen on ultrastructural examination.

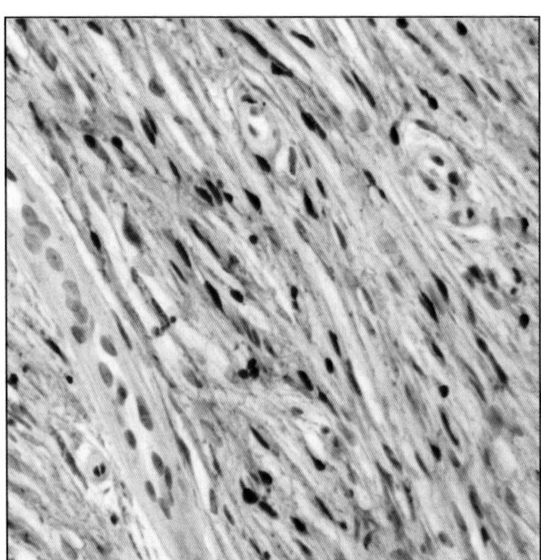

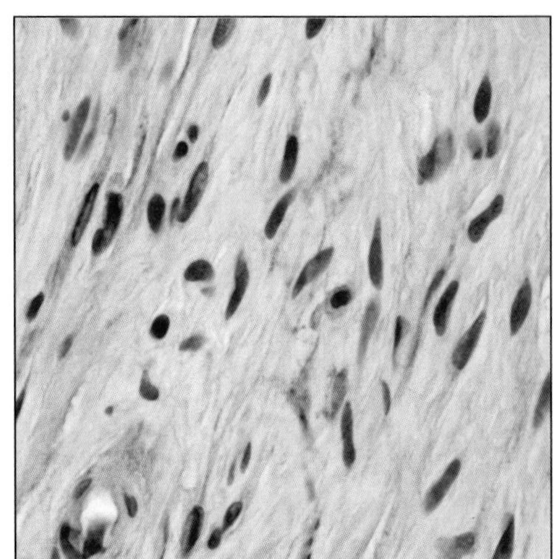

(Left) Localized cutaneous neurofibromas are fairly well circumscribed ⇒ but unencapsulated tumors. Although they may occur in NF1, the majority of localized cutaneous tumors are sporadic in nature. *(Right)* Localized cutaneous neurofibromas typically show a uniformly collagenous stroma and are separated from the overlying dermis by a Grenz zone ⇒.

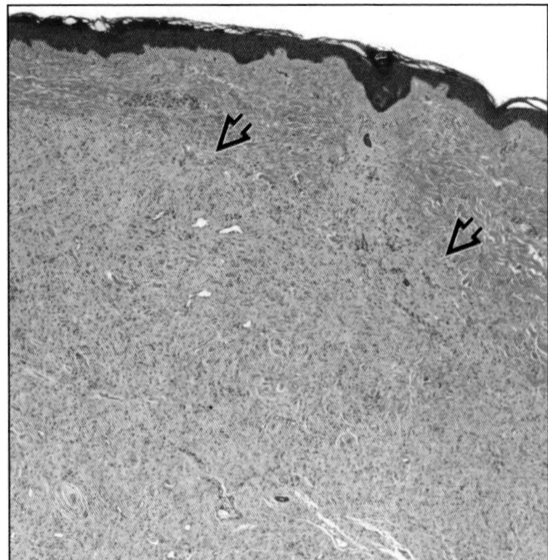

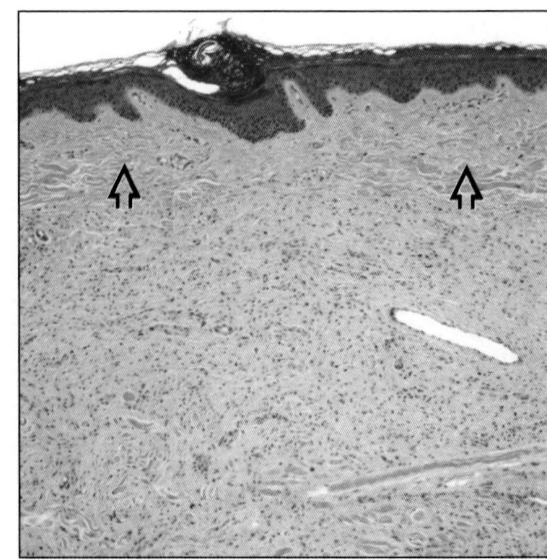

Variant Microscopic Features

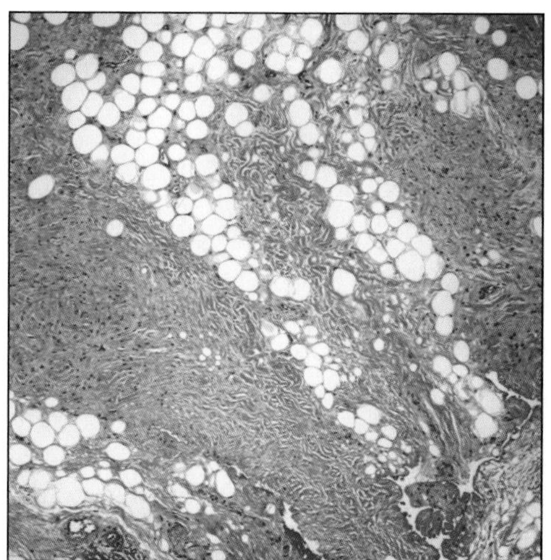

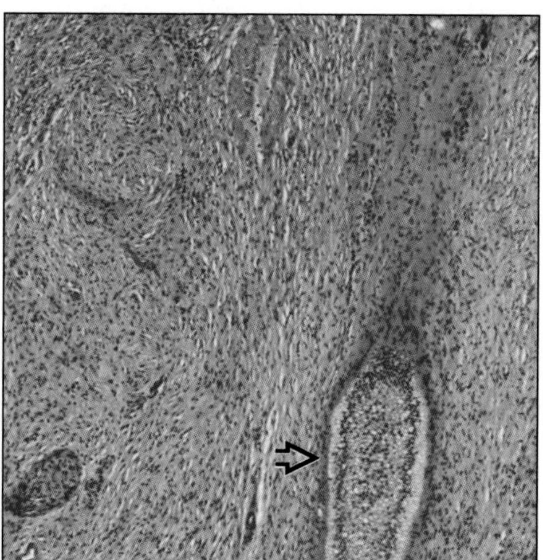

(Left) *Diffuse neurofibromas infiltrate deep into subcutaneous adipose tissue and may occur sporadically or in association with NF1. The collagenous matrix is usually fine and fibrillary in diffuse neurofibroma.* ***(Right)*** *Dermal appendages ➩ are often entrapped within a diffuse neurofibroma. The tumor cells typically wrap around these preexisting structures but do not replace them.*

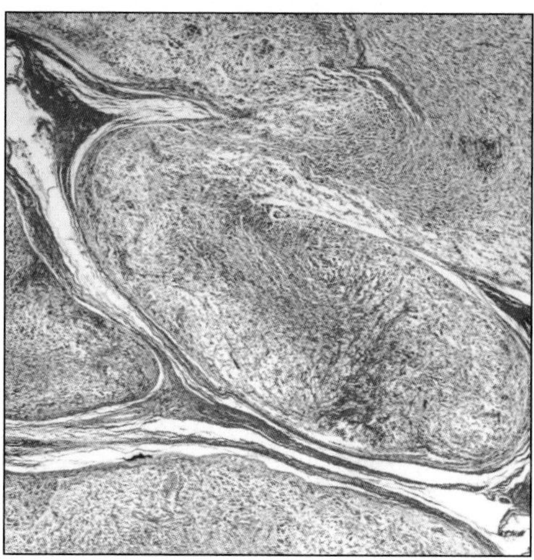

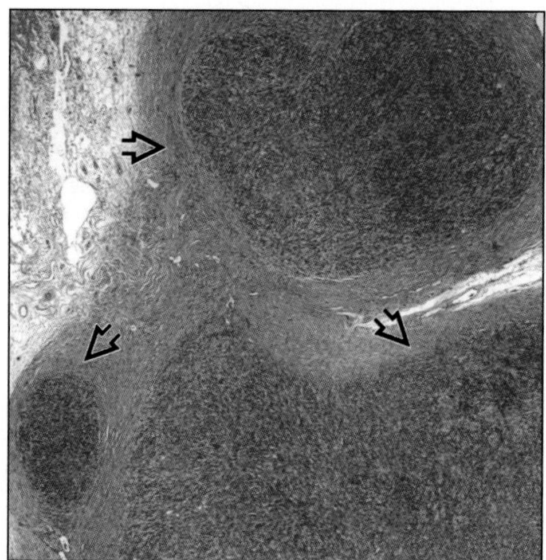

(Left) *Plexiform neurofibromas are cytologically similar to their localized and diffuse counterparts but differ in their multinodular and plexiform architecture, which imparts a "bag of worms" appearance.* ***(Right)*** *Plexiform neurofibromas in NF1 may undergo malignant transformation, as in this example. The multinodular architecture is still apparent ➩, but there is marked increase in cellularity and nuclear hyperchromasia. Increased mitotic activity was also present.*

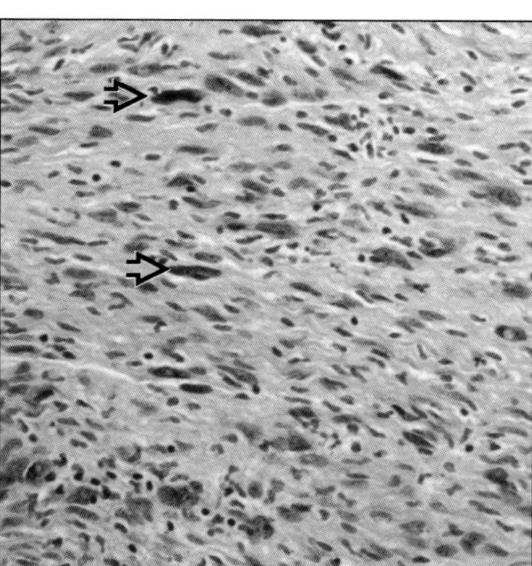

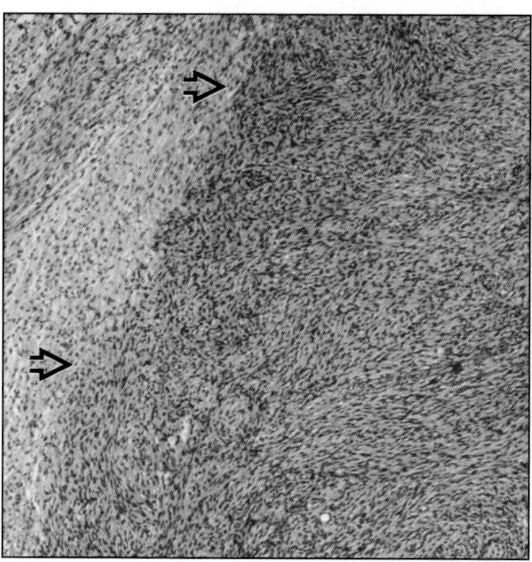

(Left) *Atypical neurofibromas show increased foci of cellularity with scattered large hyperchromatic nuclei ➩. Mitotic activity is low. Usually seen in NF1 patients, these tumors may be precursors of MPNST.* ***(Right)*** *Abrupt change in cellularity ➩ heralds the onset of malignant transformation in neurofibromas. The precursor hypocellular lesion is apparent on the left.*

PERINEURIOMA

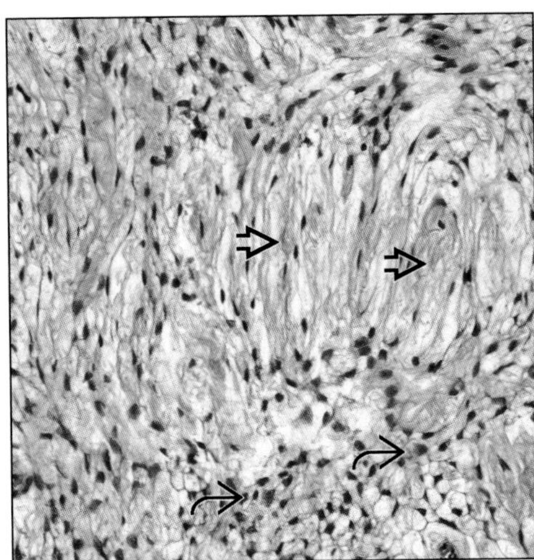

Perineurioma is composed of spindled tumor cells containing uniform fusiform nuclei and thin, elongated cell processes ⇒. In addition, plump tumor cells with round nuclei are seen ↗.

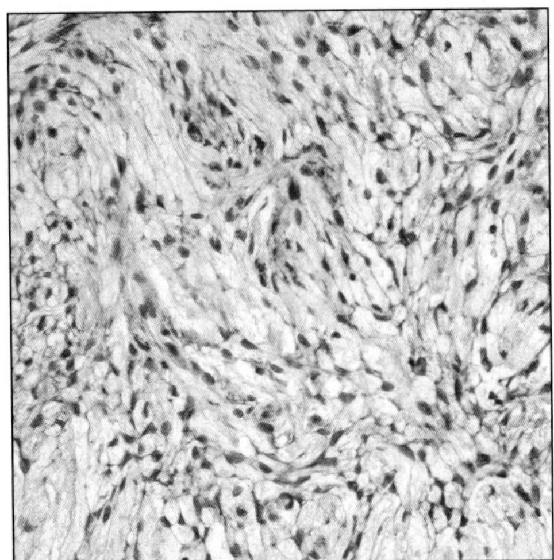

Immunohistochemical staining for perineural markers (e.g., claudin-1) highlights the presence of thin and elongated cell processes in neoplastic perineural cells.

TERMINOLOGY

Synonyms

- Intraneural perineurioma (localized hypertrophic neuropathy of the limbs)
- Extraneural perineurioma (storiform perineural fibroma)
- Sclerosing perineurioma

Definitions

- Benign mesenchymal neoplasm composed of neoplastic perineural cells

CLINICAL ISSUES

Epidemiology

- Incidence
  - Very rare neoplasms
- Age
  - Intraneural perineuriomas occur in adolescents and in early adulthood
  - Extraneural perineuriomas occur in adults of all ages
  - Children are only rarely affected
- Gender
  - Intraneural perineurioma shows no sex predilection
  - Extraneural perineurioma shows slight female predominance

Site

- Intraneural perineurioma is seen in peripheral nerves of limbs
- Extraneural perineurioma arises most frequently on trunk and extremities
- Sclerosing perineurioma tends to occur in superficial tissue of hands

Natural History

- Progressive muscle weakness &/or sensory disturbances are seen in intraneural perineurioma
- Extraneural perineurioma is not associated with neurofibromatosis

Treatment

- Surgical approaches
  - Resection of affected nerves should be avoided as long as possible in intraneural perineurioma
  - Complete excision is advised in extraneural perineurioma

Prognosis

- Intraneural perineuriomas are benign mesenchymal neoplasms
- Malignant peripheral nerve sheath tumors with perineural differentiation (malignant perineuriomas) are extremely rare

MACROSCOPIC FEATURES

General Features

- Intraneural perineurioma
  - Characterized by fusiform swelling of affected nerves
  - Segmental enlargement of affected nerve
- Extraneural perineurioma
  - Solitary, well-circumscribed, unencapsulated, nodular neoplasms
  - Frequently in subcutaneous tissue, whereas deep soft tissue and dermis are more rarely affected
- Sclerosing perineurioma
  - Arises more frequently in superficial dermal location

MICROSCOPIC PATHOLOGY

Histologic Features

- Intraneural perineurioma
  - Residual S100 protein(+) nerve fibers are surrounded by EMA(+) perineural tumor cells

PERINEURIOMA

Key Facts

Terminology

- Benign mesenchymal neoplasm composed of neoplastic perineural cells

Clinical Issues

- Progressive muscle weakness &/or sensory disturbances are seen in intraneural perineurioma
- Extraneural perineurioma is not associated with neurofibromatosis

Macroscopic Features

- Intraneural perineurioma is characterized by fusiform swelling of affected nerves
- Extraneural perineuriomas are solitary, well-circumscribed, unencapsulated, nodular neoplasms

Microscopic Pathology

- Residual S100 protein(+) nerve fibers are surrounded by EMA(+) perineural tumor cells in intraneural perineurioma
- Different growth patterns (storiform, lamellar, fascicular) are present in extraneural perineurioma
- Spindled tumor cells with elongated spindled nuclei and long and very thin cell processes
- In addition, round, slightly enlarged tumor cells are seen
- Sclerosing perineurioma is composed of plump spindled and epithelioid tumor cells
- Prominent degenerative myxoid &/or edematous stromal changes are present in reticular perineurioma

---

 - EMA(+) perineural cells form concentric layers around nerve fibers with characteristic pseudo-onion bulbs
- Extraneural spindle cell perineurioma
  - Variable cellularity
  - Different growth patterns (storiform, lamellar, fascicular)
  - Spindled tumor cells with elongated spindled nuclei
  - Round, slightly enlarged tumor cells
  - Collagenous stroma may show focal hyalinization
  - Presence of focal infiltration and cytologic atypia does not affect benign biologic behavior
  - Rare hybrid forms of perineurioma/schwannoma and perineurioma/neurofibroma have been reported
- Sclerosing perineurioma
  - Composed of plump spindled and epithelioid tumor cells
  - Hyalinized stroma containing numerous thin-walled blood vessels
  - Perivascular and lace-like arrangement of neoplastic cells often seen
  - Neoplasms showing combination of extraneural spindle cell and sclerosing perineurioma have been reported
- Reticular perineurioma
  - Prominent degenerative myxoid &/or edematous stromal changes
  - Pseudocystic spaces may be present
  - Tumor cells with thin and elongated cell processes anastomose in lace-like, reticular pattern
  - Occasionally degenerative cytologic atypia is noted
- Plexiform perineurioma
  - Extremely rare morphologic variant
  - Plexiform architecture of neoplastic perineural cells
- Sclerosing pacinian-like perineurioma, lipomatous perineurioma, ossifying perineurioma, and perineurioma with granular cells represent very rare morphologic variants
- Malignant perineurioma
  - Exceedingly rare sarcomas
  - Infiltrative growth
  - Prominent cytologic atypia
  - Increased number of mitoses
  - Presence of tumor necrosis

Cytologic Features

- Spindle-shaped tumor cells
- Bipolar, pale eosinophilic cytoplasm
- Fusiform nuclei with finely distributed chromatin
- Long and very thin cell processes

ANCILLARY TESTS

Molecular Genetics

- Monosomy of chromosome 22

Electron Microscopy

- Elongated bipolar cell processes
- Cells processes are surrounded incompletely by external lamina
- Numerous pinocytic vesicles
- Well-formed tight junctions

DIFFERENTIAL DIAGNOSIS

Dermatofibroma

- Hyperplastic epidermis
- Stellate growth
- Proliferation of plump spindled and histiocytoid cells
- EMA may be focal and weakly positive

Superficial Acral Fibromyxoma

- Arises usually on hands and feet and often in periungual location
- Bundles of spindled cells set in variable myxoid and collagenous stroma
- Claudin-1(-)

Neurofibroma

- Rather ill-defined neoplasms
- Expression of S100 protein

Schwannoma

- Usually encapsulated neoplasms

PERINEURIOMA

Immunohistochemistry

Antibody	Reactivity	Staining Pattern	Comment
EMA	Positive	Cell membrane & cytoplasm	Can be very weak
Claudin-1	Positive	Cell membrane & cytoplasm	
GLUT1	Positive	Cell membrane & cytoplasm	
CD34	Positive	Cell membrane & cytoplasm	Variable positivity
S100	Negative		
AE1/AE3	Negative		
Desmin	Negative		
Actin-sm	Equivocal	Cytoplasmic	May be positive in sclerosing perineurioma

- Expression of S100 protein

Solitary Fibrous Tumor
- Characteristic hemangiopericytoma-like vascular pattern
- EMA may be focal and weakly positive

Desmoid Fibromatosis
- Ill-defined, infiltrative neoplasms
- Bundles of bland spindled tumor cells
- Perivascular edema
- Nuclear expression of β-catenin in majority of cases

Dermatofibrosarcoma Protuberans
- Diffuse infiltration of dermis and subcutis
- Storiform growth pattern
- Homogeneous expression of CD34
- EMA may be focal and weakly positive
- Characteristic *COL1A1-PDGFB* gene fusion

Low-Grade Fibromyxoid Sarcoma
- Deep-seated, infiltrative neoplasms
- Variable myxoid and collagenous stroma
- Whorling and swirling of spindled tumor cells
- Arcades of blood vessels
- EMA may be focal and weakly positive
- Characteristic translocation (7;16)(q34;p11)

Epithelioid Dermatofibroma
- Polypoid growth
- Hyperplastic epidermis
- EMA may be focal and weakly positive

Sclerosing Melanocytic Neoplasms
- Expression of melanocytic immunohistochemical markers
- No expression of perineural immunohistochemical markers

Intramuscular Myxoma
- Fibroblastic tumor cell
- Tumor cells do not contain very thin and elongated cell processes
- EMA(-) or only focal positive

Myoepithelioma
- Tumor cells are arranged in nests and clusters
- Ductal differentiation is often present
- Expression of S100 protein in majority of cases
- EMA(-)

Extraskeletal Myxoid Chondrosarcoma
- Rather round tumor cells
- EMA is usually negative

SELECTED REFERENCES

1. Hornick JL et al: Hybrid schwannoma/perineurioma: clinicopathologic analysis of 42 distinctive benign nerve sheath tumors. Am J Surg Pathol. 33(10):1554-61, 2009
2. Brock JE et al: Cytogenetic aberrations in perineurioma: variation with subtype. Am J Surg Pathol. 29(9):1164-9, 2005
3. Hornick JL et al: Soft tissue perineurioma: clinicopathologic analysis of 81 cases including those with atypical histologic features. Am J Surg Pathol. 29(7):845-58, 2005
4. Mentzel T et al: Reticular and plexiform perineurioma: clinicopathological and immunohistochemical analysis of two cases and review of perineurial neoplasms of skin and soft tissues. Virchows Arch. 447(4):677-82, 2005
5. Michal M et al: A benign neoplasm with histopathological features of both schwannoma and retiform perineurioma (benign schwannoma-perineurioma): a report of six cases of a distinctive soft tissue tumor with a predilection for the fingers. Virchows Arch. 445(4):347-53, 2004
6. Rankine AJ et al: Perineurioma: a clinicopathological study of eight cases. Pathology. 36(4):309-15, 2004
7. Yamaguchi U et al: Sclerosing perineurioma: a clinicopathological study of five cases and diagnostic utility of immunohistochemical staining for GLUT1. Virchows Arch. 443(2):159-63, 2003
8. Folpe AL et al: Expression of claudin-1, a recently described tight junction-associated protein, distinguishes soft tissue perineurioma from potential mimics. Am J Surg Pathol. 26(12):1620-6, 2002
9. Graadt van Roggen JF et al: Reticular perineurioma: a distinctive variant of soft tissue perineurioma. Am J Surg Pathol. 25(4):485-93, 2001
10. Fetsch JF et al: Sclerosing perineurioma: a clinicopathologic study of 19 cases of a distinctive soft tissue lesion with a predilection for the fingers and palms of young adults. Am J Surg Pathol. 21(12):1433-42, 1997
11. Giannini C et al: Soft-tissue perineurioma. Evidence for an abnormality of chromosome 22, criteria for diagnosis, and review of the literature. Am J Surg Pathol. 21(2):164-73, 1997
12. Mentzel T et al: Perineurioma (storiform perineurial fibroma): clinico-pathological analysis of four cases. Histopathology. 25(3):261-7, 1994
13. Tsang WY et al: Perineurioma: an uncommon soft tissue neoplasm distinct from localized hypertrophic neuropathy and neurofibroma. Am J Surg Pathol. 16(8):756-63, 1992

Gross, Microscopic, and Immunohistochemical Features

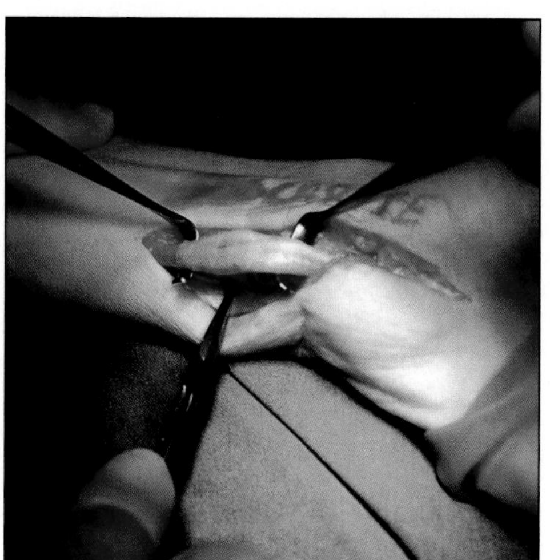

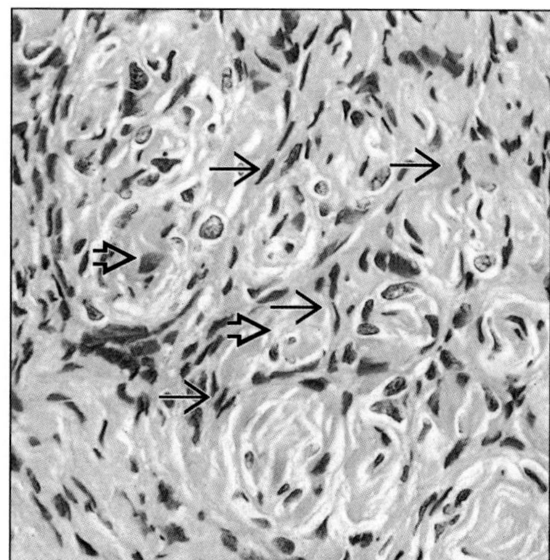

(Left) *A fusiform swelling of the affected peripheral nerve is seen in this case of an intraneural spindle cell perineurioma.* ***(Right)*** *Preexisting axons of the affected peripheral nerve ⇨ are surrounded by uniform spindled perineural tumor cells containing fusiform nuclei →.*

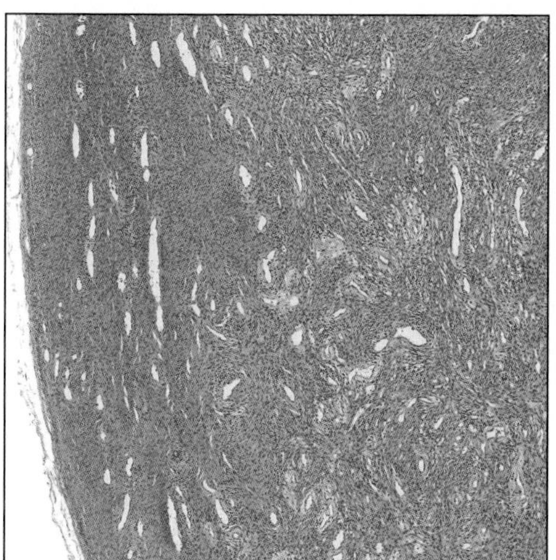

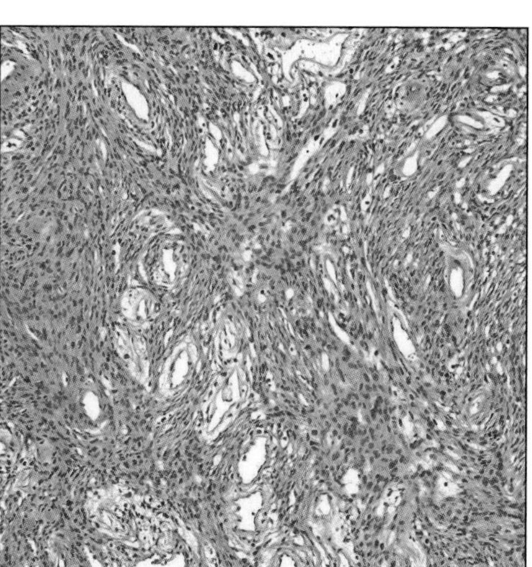

(Left) *A cellular example of extraneural spindle cell perineurioma is shown. The well-circumscribed nodular neoplasm is composed of spindled tumor cells and contains numerous thin-walled blood vessels.* ***(Right)*** *Spindled tumor cells contain an ill-defined, pale eosinophilic cytoplasm and uniform spindle-shaped nuclei.*

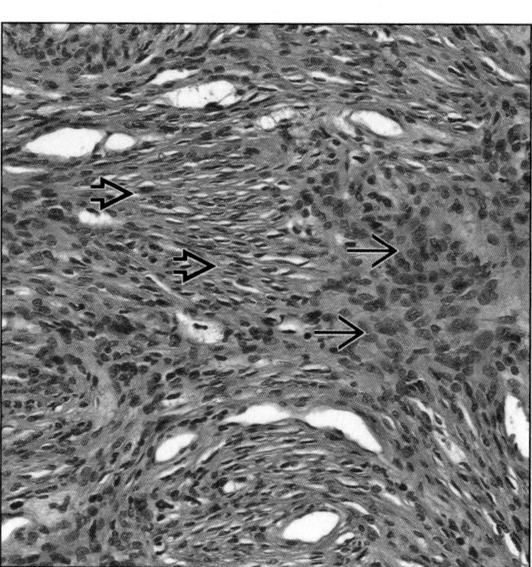

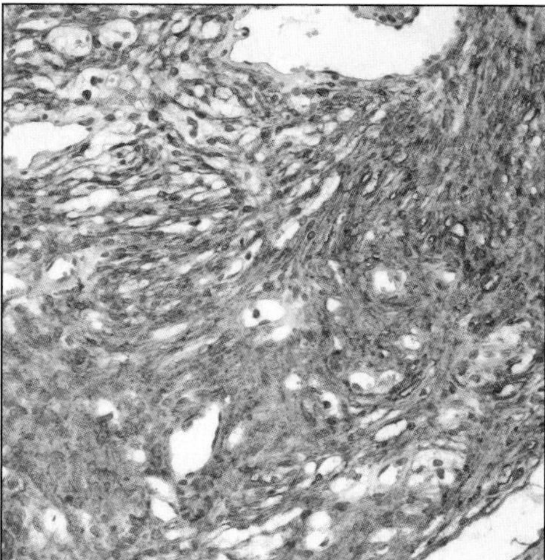

(Left) *Neoplastic spindled cells in perineurioma contain thin and elongated cell processes ⇨ and are admixed with plumper tumor cells with rather round nuclei →.* ***(Right)*** *Tumor cells in perineurioma stain positively for EMA. Given the presence of very thin and elongated cell processes, this staining can be very weak.*

Microscopic, IHC, and Ultrastructural Features

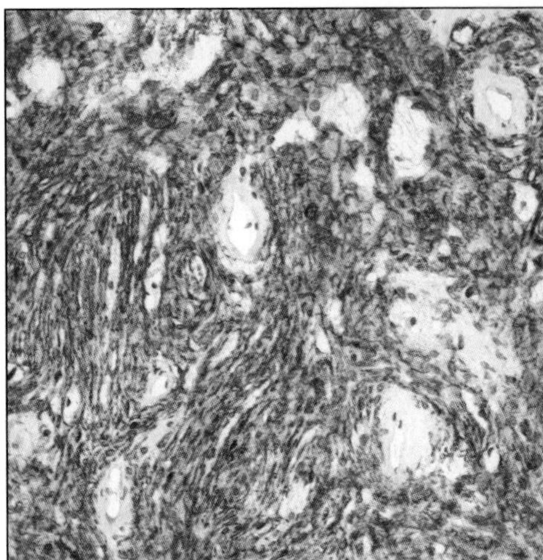

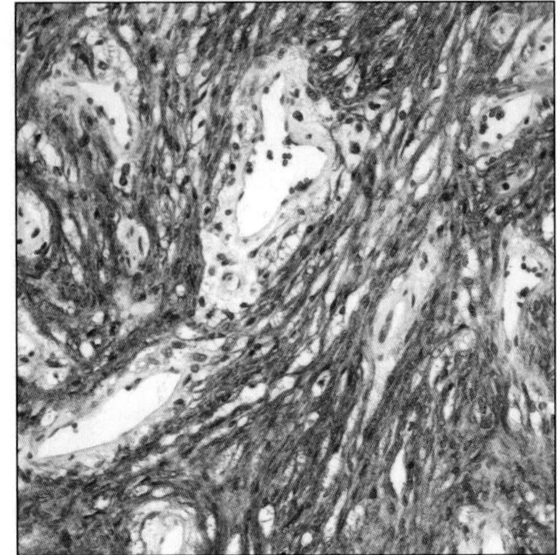

(Left) *Tumor cells in this case of an extraneural spindle cell perineurioma stain positively for claudin-1, which represents another sensitive perineural immunohistochemical marker.* ***(Right)*** *Although not specific, GLUT1 represents a further sensitive perineural immunohistochemical marker. Note the positive erythrocytes as a positive internal control.*

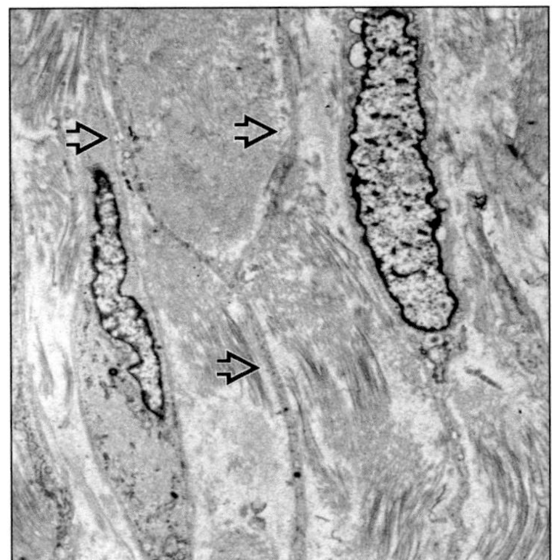

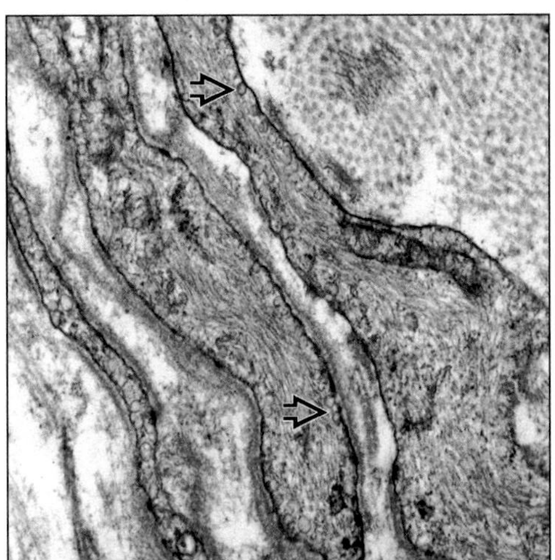

(Left) *Spindle-shaped perineural tumor cells contain spindled nuclei and very thin and elongated cell processes* ➩. ***(Right)*** *Thin and elongated cell processes in neoplastic perineural cells are surrounded by a basal lamina. Usually, numerous micropinocytotic vesicles are seen* ➩.

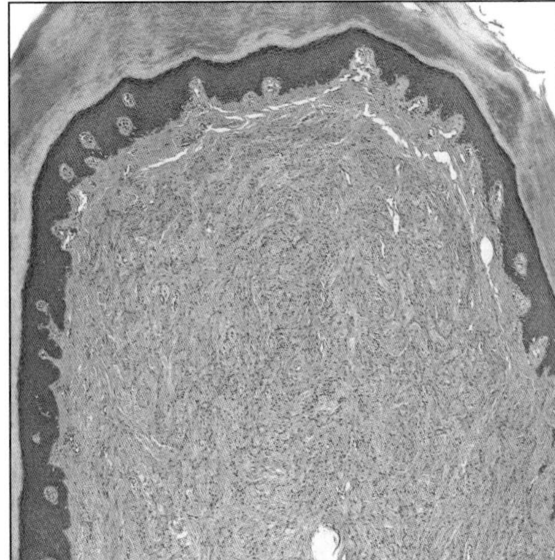

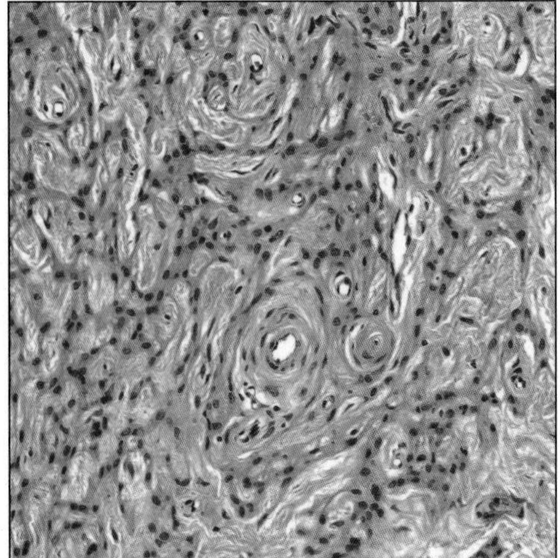

(Left) *Cases of sclerosing perineurioma arise frequently in acral skin, as in this male patient who presented with a raised, firm, dermal nodule.* ***(Right)*** *Sclerosing perineurioma is composed of rather plump, epithelioid tumor cells set in collagenous sclerosing stroma. Note the net-like and perivascular arrangement of neoplastic cells.*

Variant Microscopic and Immunohistochemical Features

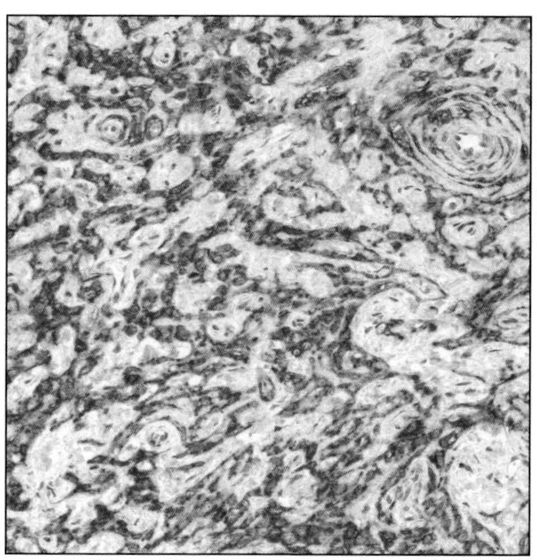

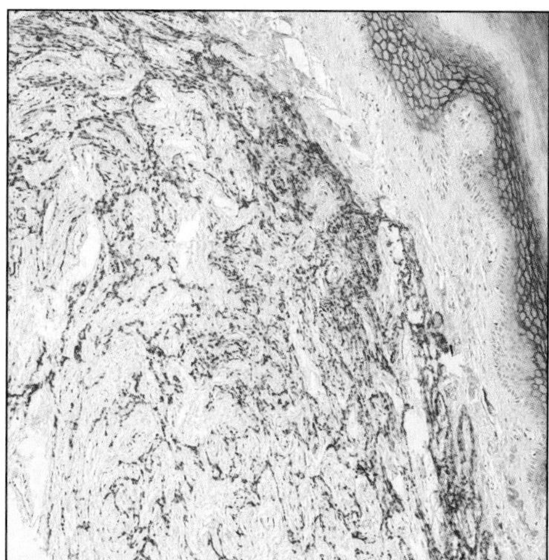

(Left) *Note the net-like arrangement of EMA(+) neoplastic cells in this example of a sclerosing perineurioma.* ***(Right)*** *A homogeneous expression of claudin-1 is seen in this example of sclerosing perineurioma. Note the positive internal control in the overlying epidermis.*

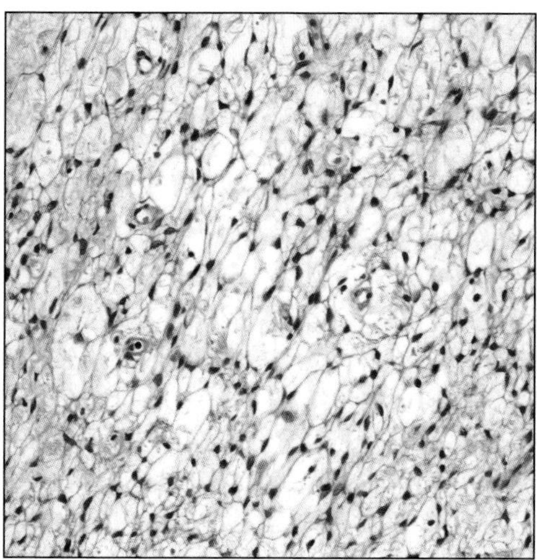

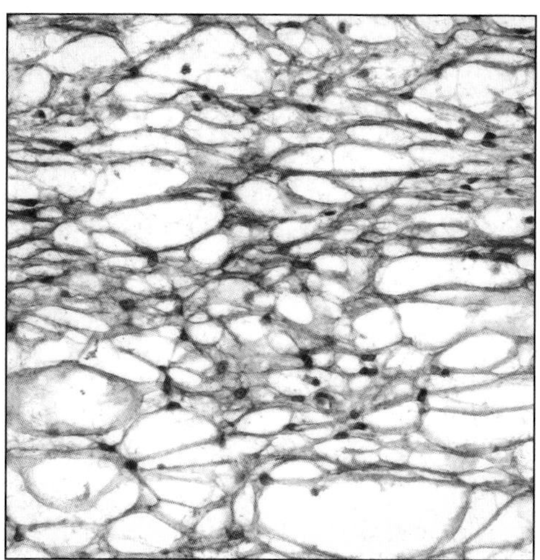

(Left) *Rare cases of reticular perineurioma are characterized by prominent myxoid stromal changes. The neoplastic cells contain very thin and elongated cell processes and are arranged in a net-like, reticular fashion.* ***(Right)*** *Immunohistochemical staining for EMA highlights the presence of elongated and very thin cell processes in this example of a reticular perineurioma, which arose in the deep soft tissues of the right upper arm of a female patient.*

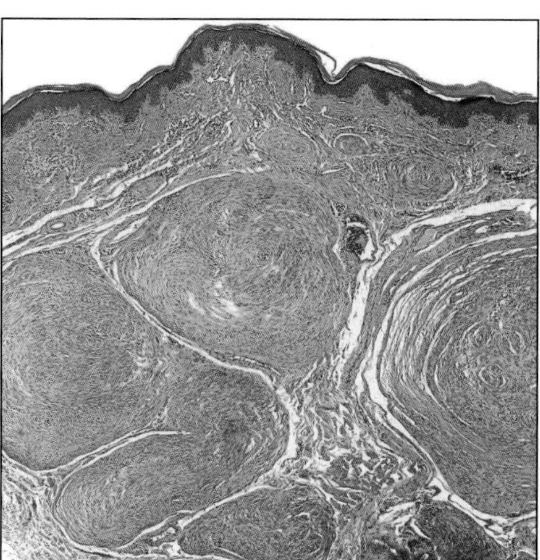

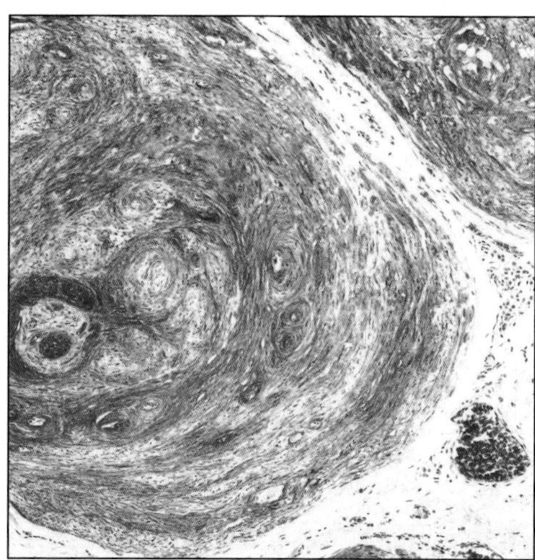

(Left) *A rare case of a plexiform perineurioma, arising on the lower lip of a 60-year-old woman, shows a dermal neoplasm with a plexiform growth of spindled tumor cells.* ***(Right)*** *Neoplastic cells in this plexiform perineurioma stain homogeneously positive for GLUT1.*

GRANULAR CELL TUMOR

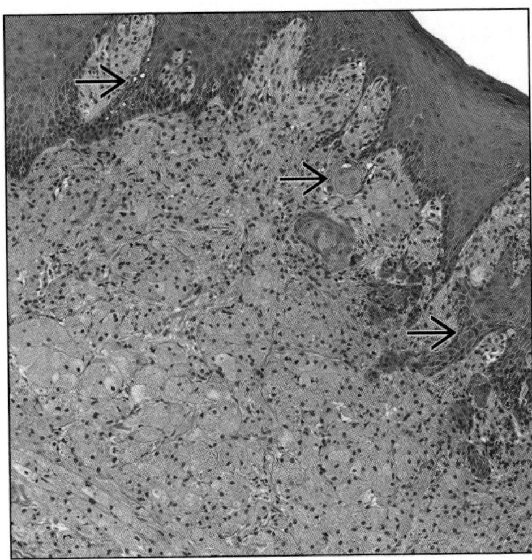

Prominent pseudoepitheliomatous hyperplasia ➔ is noted overlying the granular cell tumor. The tumor is unencapsulated, creating a sheet-like distribution of neoplastic granular cells.

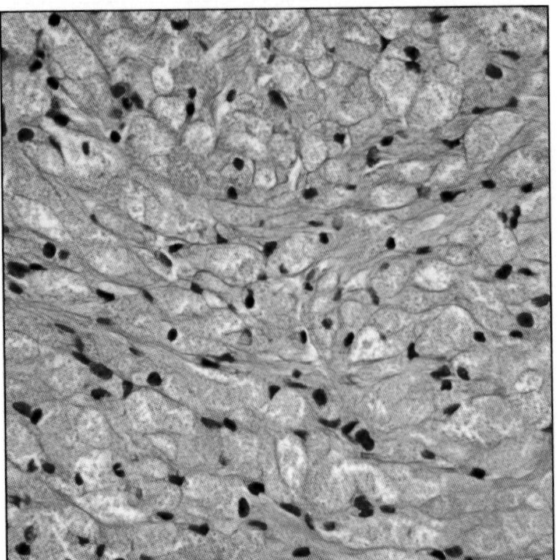

The granular cells are polygonal, showing a slightly spindled appearance. The cytoplasm contains numerous eosinophilic granules. The nuclei are small, round to oval, and hyperchromatic.

TERMINOLOGY

Abbreviations

- Granular cell tumor (GCT)

Synonyms

- Granular cell myoblastoma
- Abrikossoff tumor

Definitions

- Benign tumor composed of poorly demarcated accumulation of plump granular cells
  - Distinct from congenital epulis of newborn (gingival granular cell tumor of infancy)

ETIOLOGY/PATHOGENESIS

Schwann Cell Derivation

- Thought to arise from Schwann cells
  - Positive with neural-associated antibodies
  - Granules represent senescent change with accumulation of autophagocytic lysosomes

CLINICAL ISSUES

Epidemiology

- Incidence
  - Rare
    - About 50% of GCTs develop in head and neck
- Age
  - All ages
    - Peak between 40-60 years
- Gender
  - Female > male (2:1)
- Ethnicity
  - Blacks affected more often than whites

Site

- Over 50% involve head and neck
  - Up to 70% of these develop in oral cavity (tongue, oral mucosa, hard palate)
  - Tongue is most common single site (> 50% of head and neck GCTs)
    - Dorsum > > lateral margin
- Skin
- Nerve
- Esophagus
- Biliary tract
- Neurohypophysis
- Up to 20% of patients have multiple lesions

Presentation

- Most present as painless mass
  - Usually have symptoms for < 12 months
- Rarely, may present with Eagle syndrome
  - Elicitation of pain on swallowing, turning head, or extending tongue
    - Syndrome is thought to be caused by irritation of glossopharyngeal nerve

Endoscopic Findings

- Overlying epithelium may be slightly pale
- Concurrent *Candida* infections in some

Treatment

- Surgical approaches
  - Complete excision with narrow margins yields best outcome
  - Laser excision can be performed

Prognosis

- Excellent long-term prognosis
- Recurrence/relapse/persistence is uncommon (~ 10%)
- Malignant GCTs very rare

MACROSCOPIC FEATURES

General Features

- Smooth surfaced submucosal or subcutaneous nodule

GRANULAR CELL TUMOR

Key Facts

Terminology
- Benign tumor composed of poorly demarcated accumulation of plump granular cells
- Thought to arise from Schwann cells

Clinical Issues
- Female > male (2:1)
- Blacks affected more often than whites
- Up to 70% of head and neck lesions develop in oral cavity (tongue most common)
- Up to 20% of patients will have multifocal disease
- Recurrence/relapse/persistence is uncommon (~ 10%)

Macroscopic Features
- Cut surface is firm, pale-cream

Microscopic Pathology
- Unencapsulated plump, polygonal to elongated granular cells blending with adjacent soft tissues, especially skeletal muscle
- Indistinct cell membranes surround abundant granular, eosinophilic cytoplasm
- Overlying pseudoepitheliomatous hyperplasia is common

Ancillary Tests
- Granules are PAS(+), diastase-resistant
- Strongly and uniformly positive for S100 protein

Top Differential Diagnoses
- Squamous cell carcinoma, rhabdomyoma, schwannoma, congenital epulis of newborn

  - Poorly demarcated
- Cut surface firm, pale yellow or cream
- In mouth, concurrent *Candida* infection can form a discrete, white plaque

Size
- Mean: 1-2 cm

MICROSCOPIC PATHOLOGY

Histologic Features
- Nonencapsulated
  - Blending with adjacent soft tissues, especially skeletal muscle, is common
  - May extend up to epithelium
  - Satellite nodules can develop
    - Rarely plexiform pattern
- Plump, polygonal to elongated eosinophilic cells
- Indistinct cell membranes, creating a syncytium
- Abundant granular eosinophilic cytoplasm
  - Represents lysosomes
- Contains central small, dark to vesicular nuclei
- Overlying pseudoepitheliomatous hyperplasia
  - Usually limited to epithelium immediately overlying tumor
  - Seen in ~ 30% of cases
- Rarely, marked stroma desmoplasia may be seen
- Malignant GCT has 3 or more atypical features
  - Mitoses > 2 per 10 high-power fields
  - Prominent nucleoli
  - High nuclear/cytoplasmic ratio
  - Pleomorphism
  - Necrosis
  - Spindling of cells

ANCILLARY TESTS

Frozen Sections
- Pseudoepitheliomatous hyperplasia can mask tumor
- Granular eosinophilic cytoplasm usually easy to detect

Histochemistry
- PAS-diastase
  - Staining pattern
    - Granules are periodic acid-Schiff (PAS) positive, diastase-resistant

Immunohistochemistry
- Strongly and uniformly positive for S100 protein (nuclear and cytoplasmic) and CD68

Electron Microscopy
- Continuous external lamina around cell nests
- Rare rudimentary intercellular junctions
- Pleomorphic secondary lysosomes
    - Autophagosomes
    - Residual bodies
    - Myelin-like figures
    - Angulate lysosomes

DIFFERENTIAL DIAGNOSIS

Squamous Cell Carcinoma
- Pseudoepitheliomatous hyperplasia (PEH) can mimic squamous cell carcinoma (SCC)
  - Especially in oral cavity, tongue
  - Small, superficial surface biopsy specimens can be difficult
  - Must be properly oriented
- SCC usually shows p53 and E-cadherin immunoreactivity, a finding not seen in PEH
- Immunohistochemistry does not replace properly oriented H&E section

Rhabdomyoma
- Sheet-like distribution of polygonal cells with homogeneous, eosinophilic cytoplasm
- Cytoplasmic clearing with "spider web" cells is characteristic
- PTAH highlights cross striations in cytoplasm
- Expresses desmin and myogenin (in nuclei)

GRANULAR CELL TUMOR

Immunohistochemistry

Antibody	Reactivity	Staining Pattern	Comment
S100	Positive	Nuclear & cytoplasmic	Nearly all tumor cells
CD68	Positive	Cytoplasmic	Schwann cells and histiocytes
Vimentin	Positive	Cytoplasmic	Strong and diffuse in all tumor cells
NSE	Positive	Cytoplasmic	Weak to strong in most tumor cells
CD57	Positive	Cytoplasmic	Weak reaction but in nearly all tumor cells
PGP9.5	Positive	Cytoplasmic	Most tumor cells
Inhibin-α	Positive	Cytoplasmic	Variably positive in most tumor cells
Calretinin	Positive	Nuclear & cytoplasmic	Variable in most tumor cells
NGFR	Positive	Cell membrane	Same as p75/NGFR
Collagen IV	Positive	Stromal matrix	Basement membrane around tumor cells is positive
Ki-67	Positive	Nuclear	< 2% of nuclei in general
GFAP	Negative		
CK-PAN	Negative		
α1-antitrypsin	Negative		
Desmin	Negative		

Schwannoma
- Often encapsulated, with well-defined border
- Has Antoni A and Antoni B areas, with Verocay bodies
- More spindled cellular arrangement
- Not associated with PEH
- Shows strong S100 protein staining, capsular EMA staining while lacking CD68

Congenital Epulis of Newborn
- Can be histologically indistinguishable from GCT
- Develops in newborns or infants only
- Lacks S100 protein
- Positive for NSE

Leiomyoma
- Short to long, sweeping, and interlacing fascicles
- Granular cells rarely seen
- SMA(+) and desmin(+)
- S100 protein(-)

Nonneural Granular Cell Tumor
- Cutaneous lesion, often polypoid
- Histologically similar but lacks S100 protein
- Mild focal to rare moderate nuclear atypia
- Benign

Lichen Planus Reaction
- Significant granular cells can be seen in association with oral lichen planus
  - Also called oral ceroid granuloma
- Characteristic inflammatory infiltrate with Civatte bodies at interface
- Direct immunofluorescence characteristic for lichen planus
- Cells are positive with S100 protein
- Can coexist with granular cell tumor

Granular Cell Change in Other Tumors
- Cutaneous fibrous histiocytoma
  - Typical features present elsewhere in lesion
  - S100 protein(-)
- Dermatofibrosarcoma
  - CD34(+), S100(-)
- Leiomyoma and leiomyosarcoma
  - Smooth muscle markers(+), S100 protein(-)

DIAGNOSTIC CHECKLIST

Pathologic Interpretation Pearls
- Large granular cells
- Diffuse S100 protein positivity

SELECTED REFERENCES

1. Papalas JA et al: Isolated and synchronous vulvar granular cell tumors: a clinicopathologic study of 17 cases in 13 patients. Int J Gynecol Pathol. 29(2):173-80, 2010
2. Aldabagh B et al: Plexiform pattern in cutaneous granular cell tumors. J Cutan Pathol. 36(11):1174-6, 2009
3. Rose B et al: Granular cell tumours: a rare entity in the musculoskeletal system. Sarcoma. 2009:765927, 2009
4. Vered M et al: Granular cell tumor of the oral cavity: updated immunohistochemical profile. J Oral Pathol Med. 38(1):150-9, 2009
5. Zarovnaya E et al: Distinguishing pseudoepitheliomatous hyperplasia from squamous cell carcinoma in mucosal biopsy specimens from the head and neck. Arch Pathol Lab Med. 129(8):1032-6, 2005
6. van der Meij EH et al: Granular cells in oral lichen planus. Oral Dis. 7(2):116-8, 2001
7. Fanburg-Smith JC et al: Malignant granular cell tumor of soft tissue: diagnostic criteria and clinicopathologic correlation. Am J Surg Pathol. 22(7):779-94, 1998
8. Junquera LM et al: Granular-cell tumours: an immunohistochemical study. Br J Oral Maxillofac Surg. 35(3):180-4, 1997
9. Collins BM et al: Multiple granular cell tumors of the oral cavity: report of a case and review of the literature. J Oral Maxillofac Surg. 53(6):707-11, 1995
10. Gordon AB et al: Granular cell tumour of the breast. Eur J Surg Oncol. 11(3):269-73, 1985

Clinical, Microscopic, and Ancillary Features

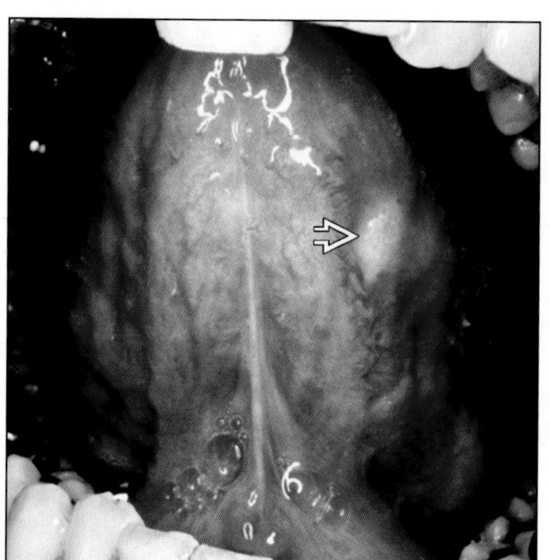
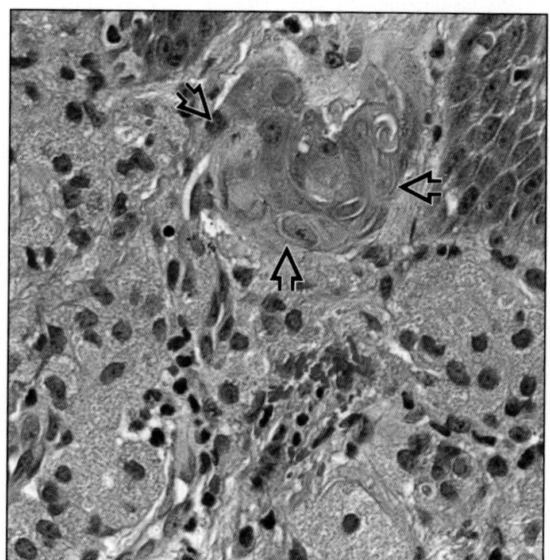

(Left) *Granular cell tumors present clinically as either a smooth-surfaced, submucosal swelling or nodule or as a pale to white, discrete, plaque-like lesion ➡. The overlying epithelium may be pale. Secondary candidiasis may be present* ***(Right)*** *Pseudoepitheliomatous hyperplasia can mimic squamous cell carcinoma ⇨, as seen here. Note the dyskeratosis and paradoxical maturation. The cells of granular cell tumor have granular cytoplasm with central round nuclei.*

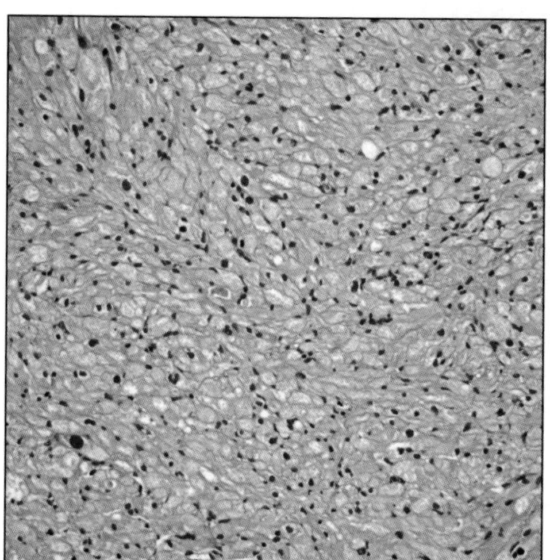
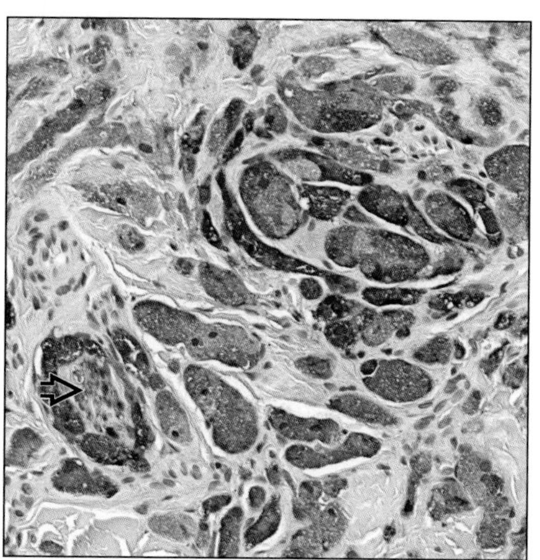

(Left) *There is a vaguely fascicular arrangement to these polygonal granular cells. Note abundant granular cytoplasm. The nuclei are small with hyperchromatic appearance on this intermediate-power view.* ***(Right)*** *S100 protein strongly stains the cytoplasm and the nuclei of the granular cells. Note the entrapped peripheral nerve ⇨. The tumor is derived from Schwann cells, so nerve association is common.*

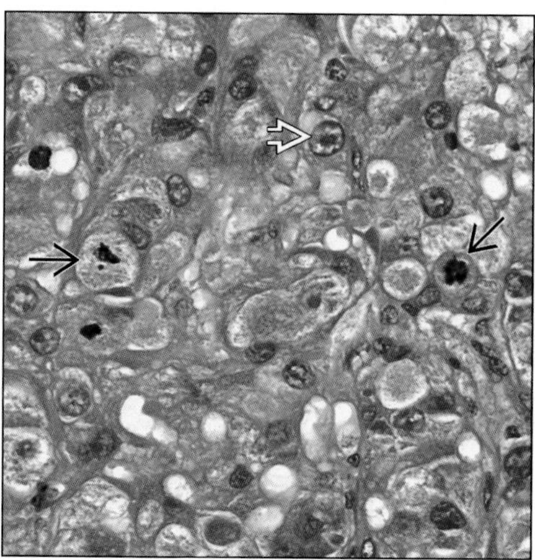
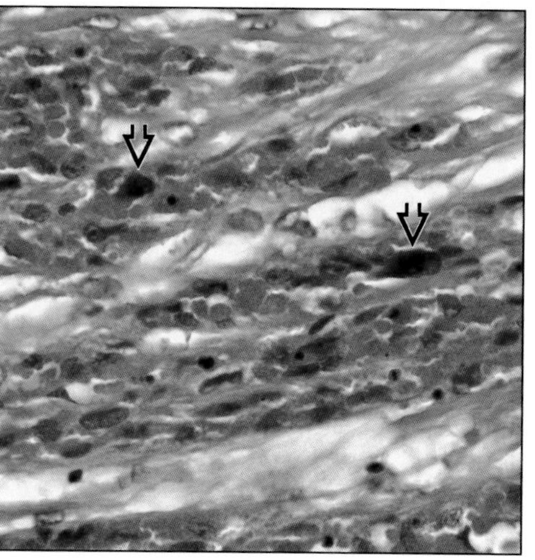

(Left) *Malignant granular cell tumor shows enlarged nuclei, prominent nucleoli ➡, and mitotic activity →. Cases can be regarded as malignant if 3 or more of the following factors are present: Pleomorphism, high nuclear/ cytoplasmic ratio, prominent nucleoli, mitoses > 2 per 10 high-power fields, spindling, and necrosis. Atypical GCTs have 1 or 2 of these features.* ***(Right)*** *Atypical granular cell tumor shows focal spindling of cells and enlarged hyperchromatic nuclei ⇨.*

MALIGNANT PERIPHERAL NERVE SHEATH TUMOR

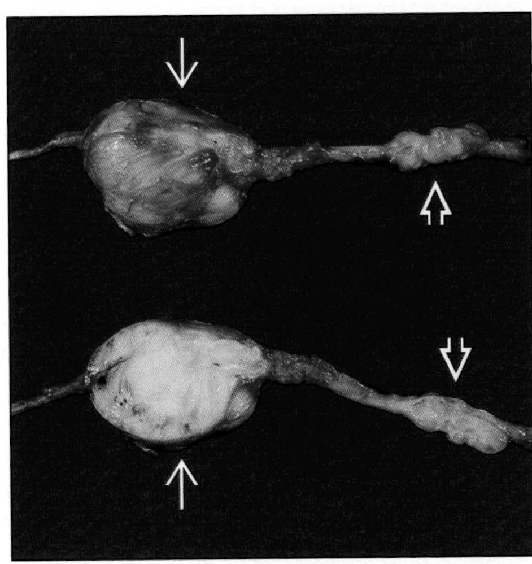

MPNSTs often arise from a major nerve trunk, such as this sciatic nerve tumor forming a fusiform, lobulated, intraneural mass ➡. MPNSTs can extend along the nerve to form satellite nodules ➡.

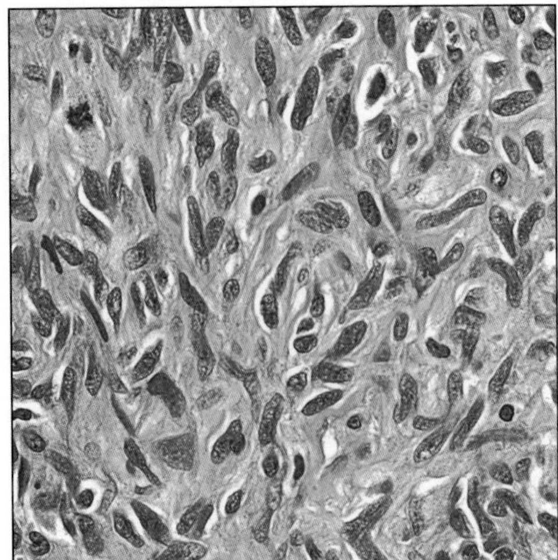

Microscopically, MPNSTs are highly variable in appearance and degree of differentiation. Well-differentiated tumors have spindle cells with tapered and wavy nuclei and indistinct cytoplasm, as shown.

TERMINOLOGY

Abbreviations

- Malignant peripheral nerve sheath tumor (MPNST)

Synonyms

- Neurofibrosarcoma, malignant schwannoma, neurogenic sarcoma

Definitions

- Sarcoma arising from a nerve or benign nerve sheath tumor or showing nerve sheath cellular differentiation
  - Diagnostic criteria
    - Arises from a nerve or benign nerve sheath tumor
    - Or shows histological evidence of nerve sheath differentiation in a NF1 patient
    - Or shows histological plus immunohistochemical or ultrastructural evidence of nerve sheath differentiation in non-NF1 patient

ETIOLOGY/PATHOGENESIS

Genetic Predisposition

- 50% associated with neurofibromatosis type 1 (NF1)
  - Lifetime incidence: 2-16%
- 40% sporadic

Environmental Exposure

- 10% associated with radiation

Molecular Pathogenesis

- NF1 caused by germline mutation of *NF1* tumor suppressor gene
  - Somatic loss of 2nd *NF1* allele required for tumorigenesis
- Malignant transformation in both NF1-associated and sporadic MPNST often involves *INK4A* and *P53* and their downstream pathways

CLINICAL ISSUES

Epidemiology

- Incidence
  - Rare: 5-10% of soft tissue sarcomas
- Age
  - Mostly adults (20-50 years)
    - Wide age range: 10-70 years
    - Average age in NF1: 30 years
    - Average age in sporadic MPNST: 40 years
- Gender
  - Women and men roughly equal

Site

- Common sites: Thigh, buttock, trunk, upper arm, retroperitoneum, head and neck
  - Mostly deep-seated
  - Central body axis more common in NF1
- Most (70%) arise in major nerve trunks
  - Sciatic nerve most common
  - Brachial plexus, sacral plexus, paraspinal nerves

Presentation

- Painful mass
- Neurological deficit in some

Treatment

- Surgical approaches
  - Wide excision/resection
  - Amputation
- Adjuvant therapy
  - Radiation
- Drugs
  - Generally poor response to chemotherapy

Prognosis

- Poor
  - Local recurrence: > 40%
  - Metastasis: 30-60%
    - Lungs, bone, pleura most common

MALIGNANT PERIPHERAL NERVE SHEATH TUMOR

Key Facts

Terminology
- Sarcoma arising from a nerve or benign nerve sheath tumor or showing nerve sheath cellular differentiation

Etiology/Pathogenesis
- 50% associated with NF1
- 10% associated with radiation

Clinical Issues
- Mostly adults (20-50 years)
- Most (70%) arise in major nerve trunks
- Local recurrence: > 40%
- Metastasis: 30-60%
- 5-year survival: 15-34%

Microscopic Pathology
- Mostly high-grade sarcomas
- Spindle cell MPNST (80%)
  - Long fascicles of closely spaced hyperchromatic spindle cells
  - Small round blue cells
  - Pleomorphic cells
  - Extensive necrosis with perivascular preservation
- Epithelioid MPNST (5%)
- Heterologous differentiation (15%)

Ancillary Tests
- S100: 50-60%

Top Differential Diagnoses
- Synovial sarcoma
- Cellular schwannoma
- Atypical neurofibroma
- Malignant melanoma

- > 60% die of disease
- 5-year survival: 15-34%
- NF1 patients have worse overall prognosis
  - Probably due to higher incidence of large, central axis tumors

IMAGE FINDINGS

General Features
- Morphology
  - Large heterogeneous mass
  - Fusiform mass within major nerve trunk

MACROSCOPIC FEATURES

General Features
- Similar to other soft tissue sarcomas
  - Pseudoencapsulated
  - Gray-tan
  - Firm to fleshy
  - Necrosis and hemorrhage common
- Fusiform or eccentric mass when arising in major nerve trunk
- Coexisting neurofibroma in some
  - Solitary or plexiform

Size
- Most > 5 cm
- Sometimes very massive

MICROSCOPIC PATHOLOGY

Histologic Features
- Wide spectrum of cytoarchitectural patterns
  - Mostly high-grade sarcomas
    - High mitotic rate and necrosis
    - Only around 15% are low grade
  - Nerve sheath differentiation
    - Nuclear palisading uncommon (15%), usually focal
    - Tactoid differentiation with whorling or Wagner-Meissner-like features
  - Intraneural tumors
    - Plexiform architecture
    - Microscopic extension within nerve fascicle
  - Tumors arising from preexisting benign nerve sheath tumor
    - Neurofibroma most common, transitional areas, usually in NF1 patients
    - Schwannoma, ganglioneuroma, ganglioneuroblastoma, or pheochromocytoma; very rare
  - Diffuse sarcomatous proliferation with no evidence of nerve or nerve sheath origin
- Spindle cell MPNST (80%)
  - Long fascicles of uniform, closely spaced, hyperchromatic spindle cells
  - Alternating cellular fascicles and hypocellular areas ("tapestry" or "marbled" pattern)
  - Storiform arrays
  - Small round blue cells
  - Pleomorphic cells
    - Multinucleated giant cells
  - Extensive necrosis with perivascular preservation
  - Hemangiopericytoma-like vascular pattern in some
- Epithelioid MPNST (5%)
  - Multinodular architecture
  - Cords and clusters in some
  - Large epithelioid cells
    - Abundant eosinophilic cytoplasm
    - Large vesicular nuclei with macronucleoli
    - Clear cytoplasm in some
  - Often mixed with spindle cells
- Heterologous differentiation (15%)
  - Osseous and osteosarcomatous
  - Chondroid and chondrosarcomatous
  - Rhabdomyosarcomatous (Triton tumor)
  - Angiosarcomatous
  - Glandular
  - Neuroepithelial (rosettes)

MALIGNANT PERIPHERAL NERVE SHEATH TUMOR

Cytologic Features

- Spindle cells
  - Ill-defined cytoplasm
  - Hyperchromatic nucleus with dispersed coarse chromatin
  - Tapered and wavy nuclei in well-differentiated tumors
  - Very brisk mitotic activity in high-grade tumors
- Epithelioid cells
  - Abundant eosinophilic or clear cytoplasm
  - Vesicular nucleus with prominent inclusion-like nucleolus

ANCILLARY TESTS

Immunohistochemistry

- S100 protein(+) in about 60%, usually focal
- Nestin(+) in 50-80%

Cytogenetics

- Complex structural and numeric chromosomal abnormalities
  - Frequent loss of *NF1* at 17q11
  - Frequent loss of *P53* at 17q13

DIFFERENTIAL DIAGNOSIS

Monophasic or Poorly Differentiated Synovial Sarcoma

- Nuclei have softer, less coarse chromatin
- Usually has lower mitotic rate
- TLE1(+)
  - MPNST rarely (2%) positive
- Usually cytokeratin(+) and EMA(+)
  - MPNST usually negative
- Usually S100(-)
- t(X:18) by cytogenetics
- *SYT* break apart by FISH
- *SSX-SYT* fusion by RT-PCR

Cellular Schwannoma

- Usually located in retroperitoneum, pelvis, posterior mediastinum
- Exclusively Antoni A areas; often lacks Verocay bodies
- Necrosis and mitotic figures present
- Can erode/destroy bone
- Lacks malignant cytological atypia
- Strong, diffuse S100 staining
  - MPNST usually has only focal staining

Atypical Neurofibroma

- Large, hyperchromatic spindle cells
- Degenerated (smudged) chromatin
- Low miotic rate
- Usually retains cytoarchitectural features of neurofibroma
  - Edematous fibrillary or myxoid matrix with collagen bundles ("shredded carrots" pattern)

Malignant Melanoma

- Spindle cell/sarcomatoid melanoma
  - May have clustered or thèque-like areas
  - Diffusely S100(+)
    - MPNST often S100(-) (50%) or with only focal staining
  - Usually HMB-45(-) and Melan-A(-)
- Epithelioid melanoma
  - Amelanotic melanoma may be indistinguishable from epithelioid MPNST
  - Usually HMB-45(+) and Melan-A(+)
    - MPNST negative for these markers

Clear Cell Sarcoma

- Predilection for acral extremities
- Multinodular, vague nested architecture
- Uniform epithelioid and spindle cells
- Prominent nucleoli
- Diffuse S100, HMB-45 and Melan-A staining in most
- t(12:22) by cytogenetics
- *EWSR1* break apart by FISH
- *EWS-ATF1* or *EWS-CREB1* by RT-PCR

Ewing Sarcoma

- Usually a primary bone tumor but may present as soft tissue primary
  - MPNST exceedingly rare as primary bone tumor
- Small round blue cell tumor
  - Often with glycogenated (clear) cytoplasm
  - Diffusely CD99(+), usually S100(-)
    - MPNST sometimes CD99(+) but usually weak/focal and nonmembranous
  - t(11:22), t(7:22), t(21:22), or t(2:22) by cytogenetics
  - *EWSR1* break apart by FISH
  - *EWS-FLI1* or *EWS-ERG* fusion by RT-PCR

Embryonal Rhabdomyosarcoma

- Small round blue cells and spindle cells
- Scattered rhabdomyoblasts
- S100(-), Desmin(+) and myogenin(+)

SELECTED REFERENCES

1. Gottfried ON et al: Neurofibromatosis Type 1 and tumorigenesis: molecular mechanisms and therapeutic implications. Neurosurg Focus. 28(1):E8, 2010
2. Jagdis A et al: Prospective evaluation of TLE1 as a diagnostic immunohistochemical marker in synovial sarcoma. Am J Surg Pathol. 33(12):1743-51, 2009
3. Olsen SH et al: Cluster analysis of immunohistochemical profiles in synovial sarcoma, malignant peripheral nerve sheath tumor, and Ewing sarcoma. Mod Pathol. 19(5):659-68, 2006
4. Birindelli S et al: Rb and TP53 pathway alterations in sporadic and NF1-related malignant peripheral nerve sheath tumors. Lab Invest. 81(6):833-44, 2001
5. Hruban RH et al: Malignant peripheral nerve sheath tumors of the buttock and lower extremity. A study of 43 cases. Cancer. 66(6):1253-65, 1990
6. Ducatman BS et al: Malignant peripheral nerve sheath tumors. A clinicopathologic study of 120 cases. Cancer. 57(10):2006-21, 1986
7. Guccion JG et al: Malignant Schwannoma associated with von Recklinghausen's neurofibromatosis. Virchows Arch A Pathol Anat Histol. 383(1):43-57, 1979

Radiographic and Gross Features

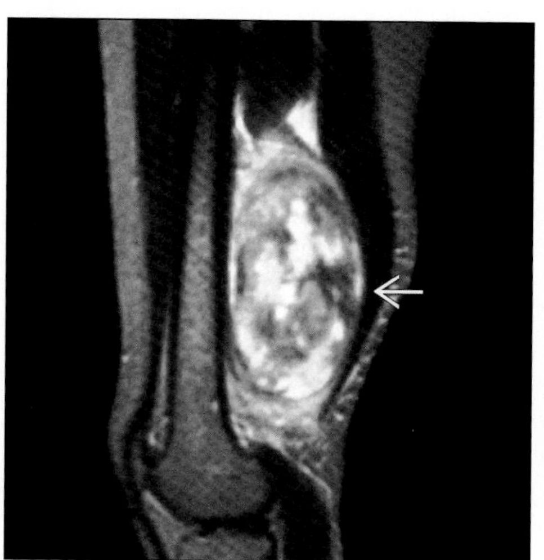

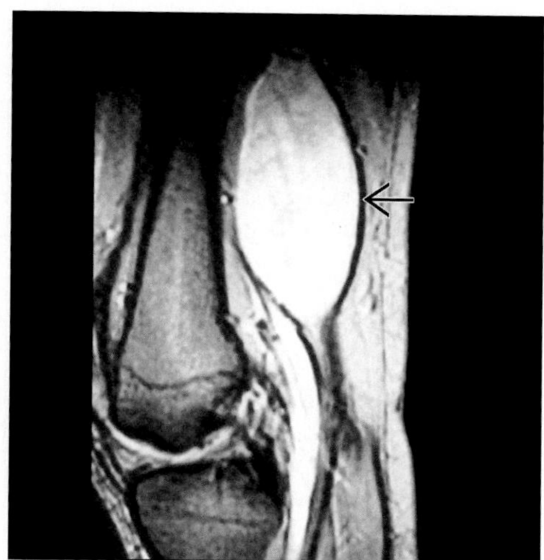

*(**Left**) The sciatic nerve is the nerve most affected by MPNST, followed by the brachial or sacral plexus. In this case the femoral nerve was involved. In many cases, however, nerve origin cannot be demonstrated. MPNSTs are often necrotizing sarcomas that show heterogeneous signal ➔ on MR. (**Right**) Sagittal T2 FSE MR show fusiform hyperintense tumor ➔ arising from the femoral nerve. This was found to represent a malignant schwannoma at surgery.*

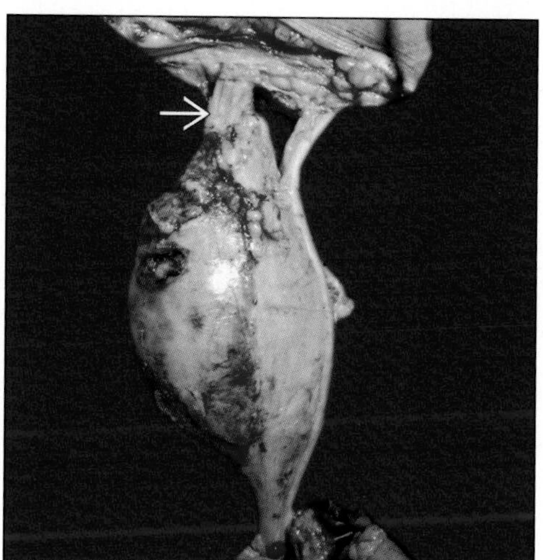

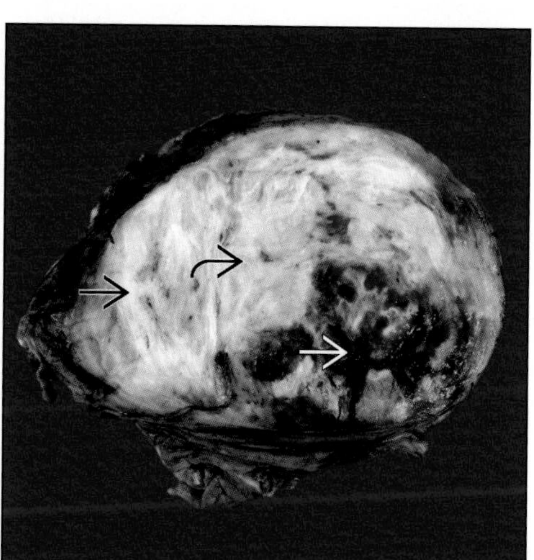

*(**Left**) This intraoperative photograph of MPNST shows a large fusiform tumor mass arising from and incorporating the femoral nerve. Note the enlarged nerve ➔ entering and exiting the tumor. (**Right**) MPNSTs tend to form bulky, circumscribed, and pseudoencapsulated masses often with a variegated cut surface, including firm white-tan fascicular areas of viable tumor ➔, yellow necrotic areas ➔, and cystic hemorrhagic foci ➔.*

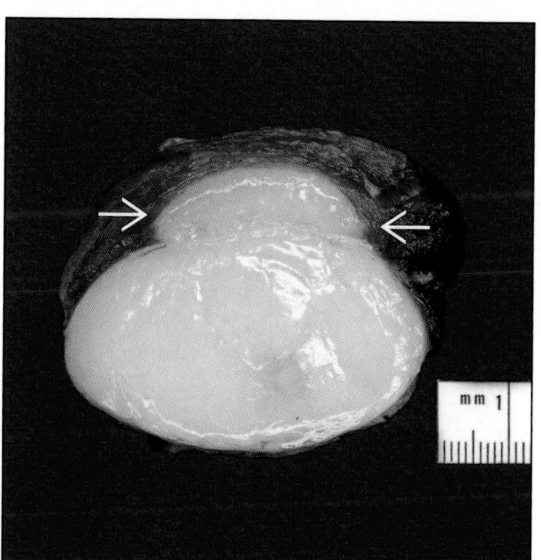

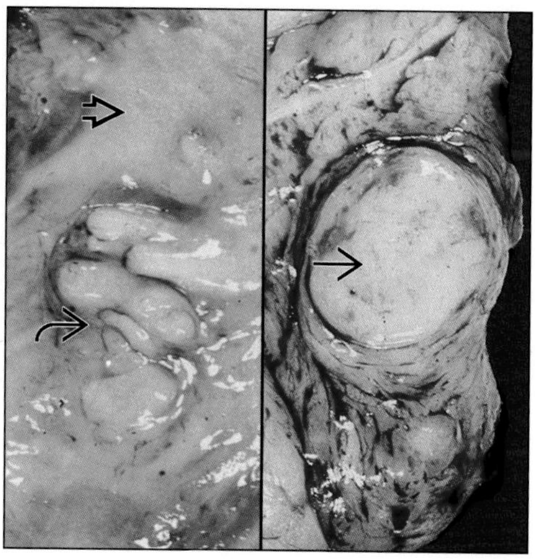

*(**Left**) This well-differentiated MPNST excised from the calf of a 17-year-old girl has a uniform gray-tan, fleshy cut surface. A definite nerve origin was not appreciated grossly. Note invasion beyond its pseudocapsule into adjacent skeletal muscle ➔. (**Right**) Approximately half of MPNSTs are associated with NF1. This composite gross photograph depicts a discrete fleshy mass of MPNST ➔ arising within a background of diffuse ➔ and plexiform ➔ neurofibromatosis.*

MALIGNANT PERIPHERAL NERVE SHEATH TUMOR

Microscopic Features

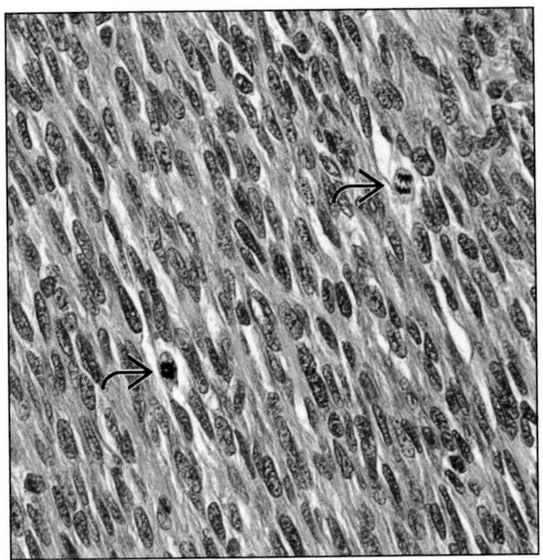

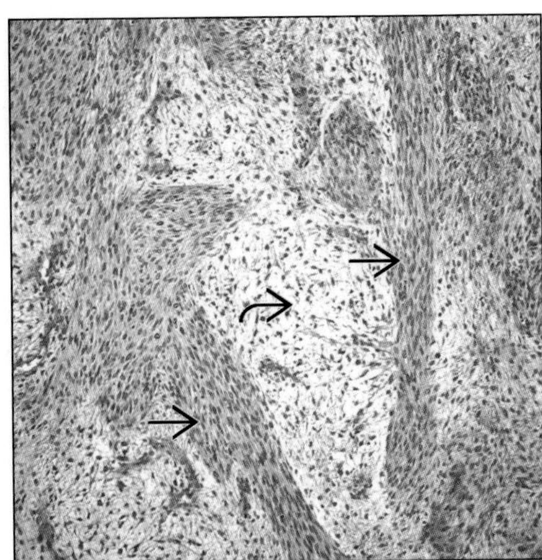

(Left) *The most common pattern of MPNST is a high-grade spindle cell sarcoma composed of long fascicles of closely spaced, uniform spindle cells with ill-defined cytoplasmic borders, coarse nuclear hyperchromasia, and very brisk mitotic activity ⮫.* ***(Right)*** *A distinctive pattern seen in spindle cell MPNST consists of alternating hypercellular fascicles → and less cellular edematous regions ⮫, sometimes referred to as a "tapestry" or "marbled" pattern.*

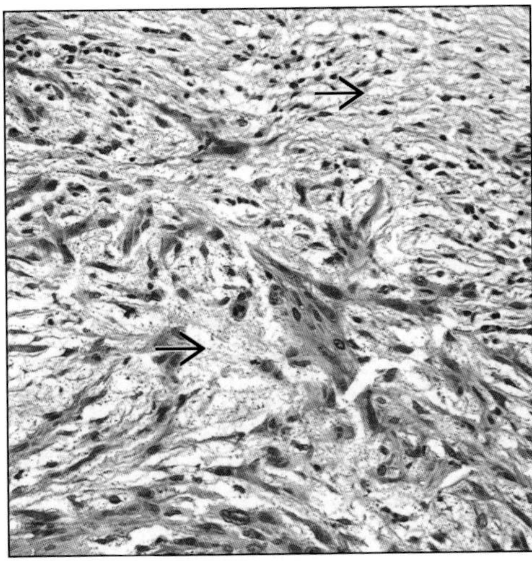

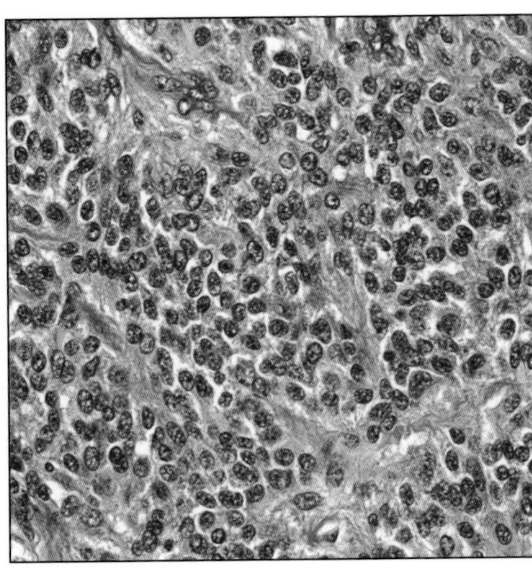

(Left) *Myxoid stroma → is common in MPNST. It usually accounts for only a portion of a given tumor with solid areas predominating, but this can occasionally lead to diagnostic difficulty in a core biopsy.* ***(Right)*** *MPNST can have prominent small round blue cell areas mimicking Ewing sarcoma or poorly differentiated synovial sarcoma. Appropriate immunohistochemistry and molecular genetic investigation can resolve these differential diagnoses in most instances.*

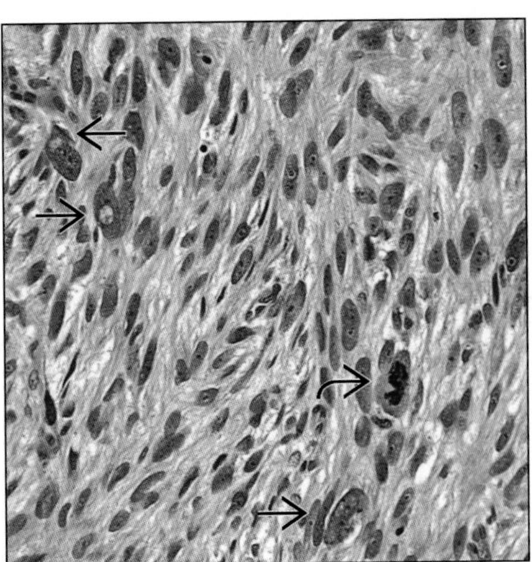

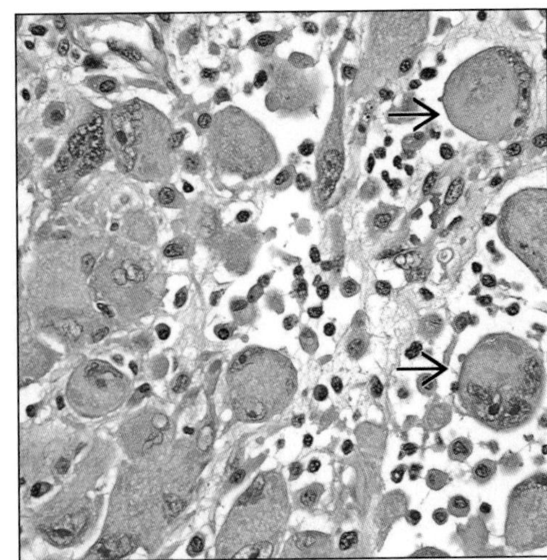

(Left) *MPNST can sometimes have a pleomorphic spindle cell pattern with marked nuclear enlargement → and atypical mitotic figures ⮫, mimicking pleomorphic undifferentiated sarcoma. More typical areas or neural connection are helpful for diagnosis.* ***(Right)*** *Markedly enlarged pleomorphic cells, including multinucleated giant cells →, are occasionally seen in MPNST, exemplified in this thigh tumor resected from a neurofibromatosis patient.*

Microscopic Features

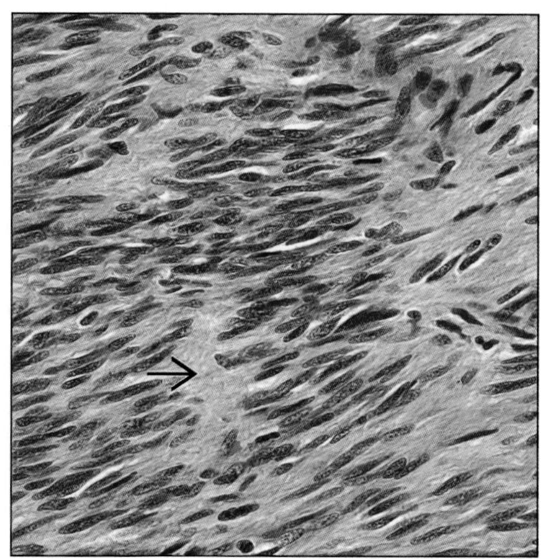

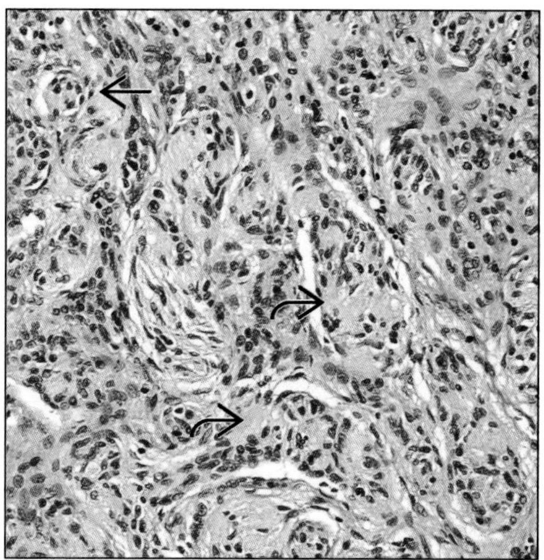

(Left) *Microscopic evidence of nerve sheath differentiation is uncommon in MPNST. For example, nuclear palisading with Verocay body formation ➔ is seen in only 15% of MPNSTs, and it is usually a focal finding.* ***(Right)*** *Tactoid differentiation is also uncommon in MPNST. This micrograph depicts cell clusters with a vague whorling growth pattern ➔ and hyaline matrix ➚ mimicking tactoid or Wagner-Meissner-like bodies.*

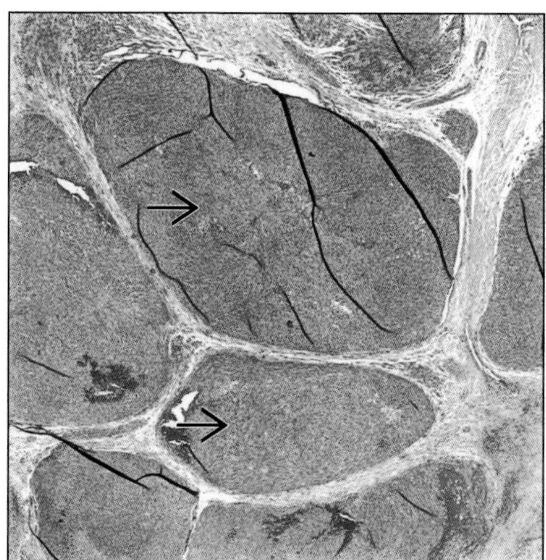

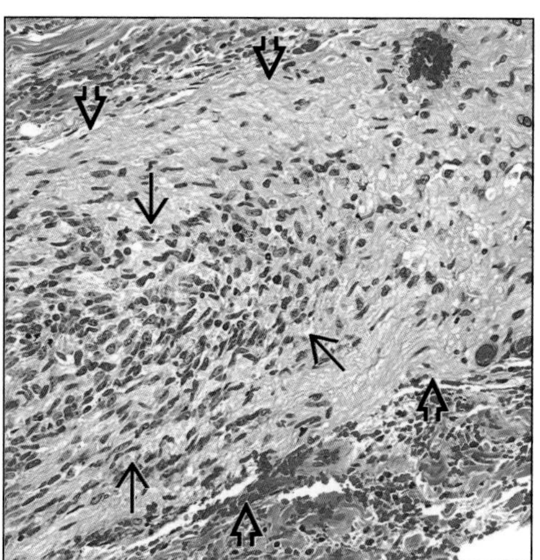

(Left) *MPNSTs that arise within large nerve trunks frequently have a plexiform architecture, which is formed by enlarged nerve fascicles ➔ expanded by malignant cells. Rarely, wide intraneural extension can result in spinal cord involvement.* ***(Right)*** *Microscopic intraneural extension beyond the grossly visible mass is depicted here by hyperchromatic spindle cells ➔ infiltrating within a peripheral nerve ➲. This can result in a positive surgical margin and local recurrence.*

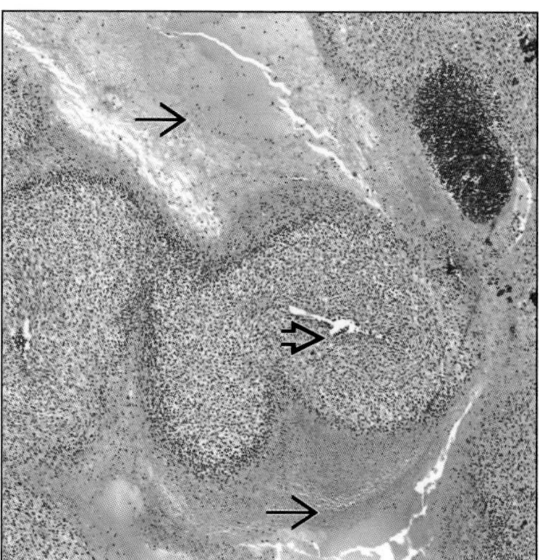

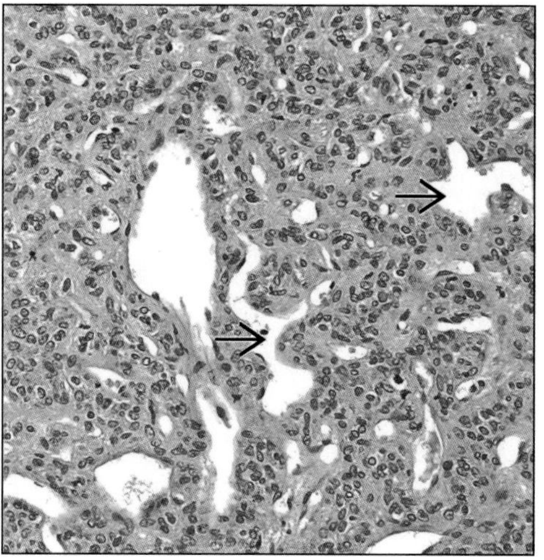

(Left) *Large geographic zones of necrosis ➔ are a common and characteristic feature of high-grade MPNSTs. In this example, a cuff of viable malignant cells surrounds a blood vessel ➲ ("perivascular preservation").* ***(Right)*** *Although a thin-walled branching or pericytic vascular pattern ➔ is more characteristic of other tumors, such as synovial sarcoma and solitary fibrous tumor, it can occasionally be a prominent focal feature in MPNST as shown here.*

MALIGNANT PERIPHERAL NERVE SHEATH TUMOR

Microscopic and Immunohistochemical Features

(Left) Only around 50-60% of MPNSTs are positive for S100 immunohistochemically, and in most cases the staining reaction is focal as shown. Well-differentiated tumors can show more diffuse staining. (Right) Epithelioid MPNST accounts for ~ 5% of tumors. It is characterized by sheets of epithelioid cells with abundant eosinophilic cytoplasm arranged in a vaguely nodular pattern. It usually arises from a major nerve trunk in an extremity and is not associated with NF1.

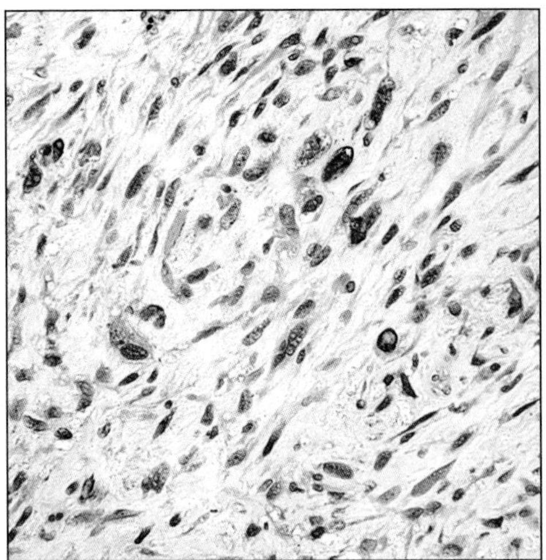

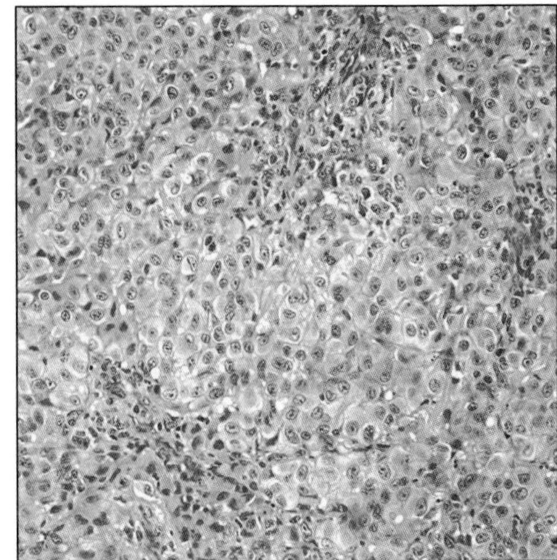

(Left) Cytologically, epithelioid MPNST is characterized by large polygonal cells with abundant eosinophilic cytoplasm and vesicular nuclei with prominent, inclusion-like nucleoli. Although most are S100(+), it is negative for HMB-45 and Melan-A, which distinguishes it from malignant melanoma. (Right) In some epithelioid MPNSTs, the cells are arranged in single file cords ⇒ and small clusters ⇒, mimicking carcinoma. However, immunostaining for cytokeratins is negative.

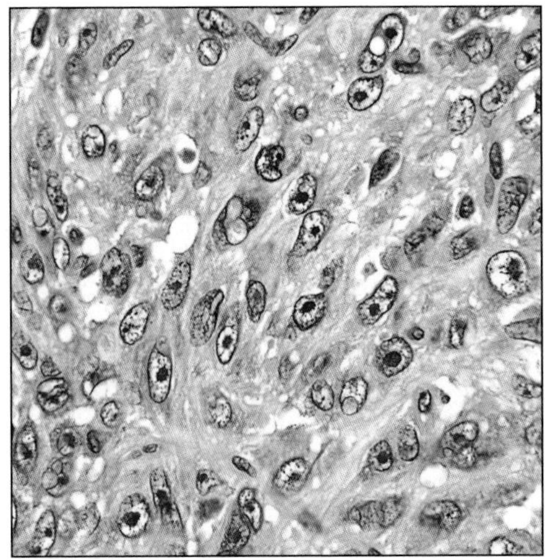

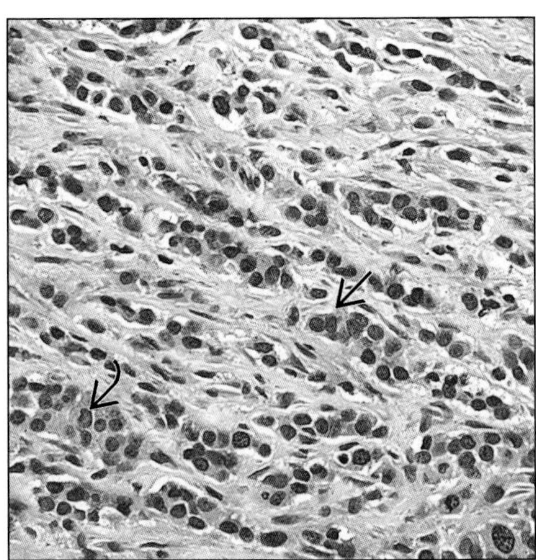

(Left) Occasionally, epithelioid MPNST shows prominent clear cell features ⇒ as in this image. (Right) Heterologous differentiation is present in 15% of MPNSTs, usually composed of histologically malignant elements. Rhabdomyosarcomatous differentiation consists of malignant rhabdomyoblasts with deeply eosinophilic cytoplasm ⇒ in a spindle cell MPNST. Such tumors are sometimes called "Triton tumors" and should be distinguished from embryonal rhabdomyosarcoma.

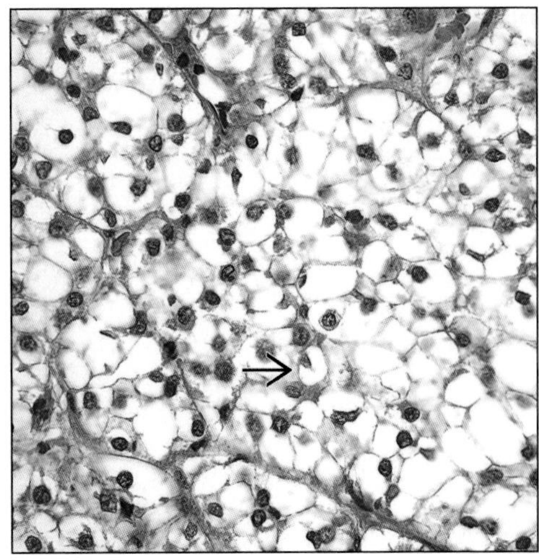

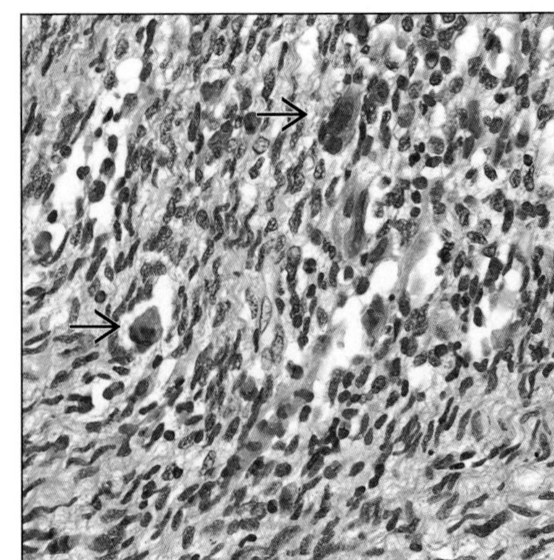

Microscopic and Immunohistochemical Features

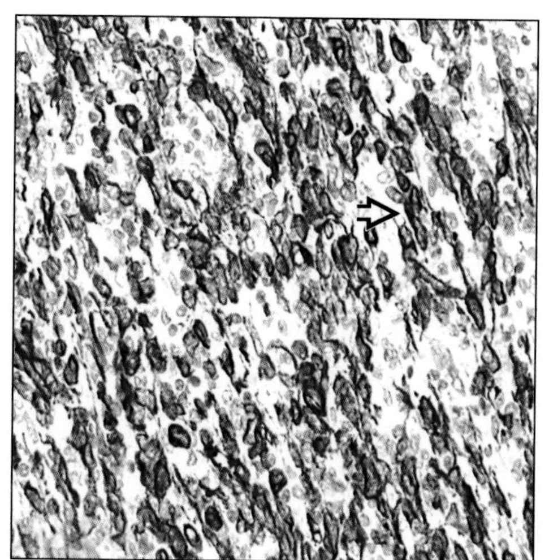
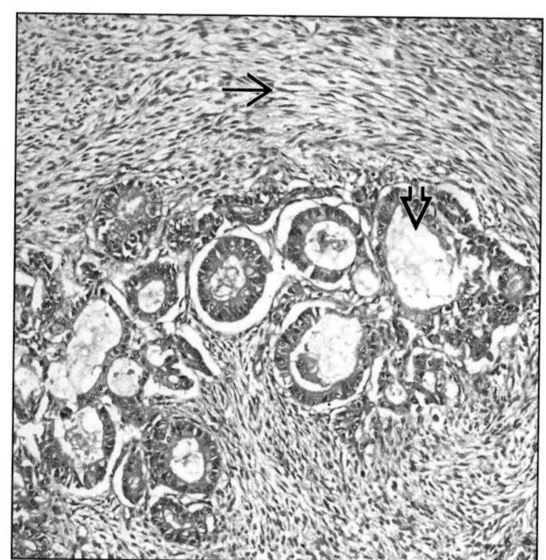

*(**Left**) In malignant Triton tumor, rounded rhabdomyoblasts are easily seen, but areas with spindled rhabdomyoblasts can be overlooked. However, they can be distinguished from background MPNST by immunoreactivity for desmin ➯ and by showing myogenin positivity in nuclei. (**Right**) MPNST ➔ rarely can have heterologous glandular elements. The glands secrete mucin ➯ and can have focal neuroendocrine differentiation. This tumor must not be mistaken for biphasic synovial sarcoma.*

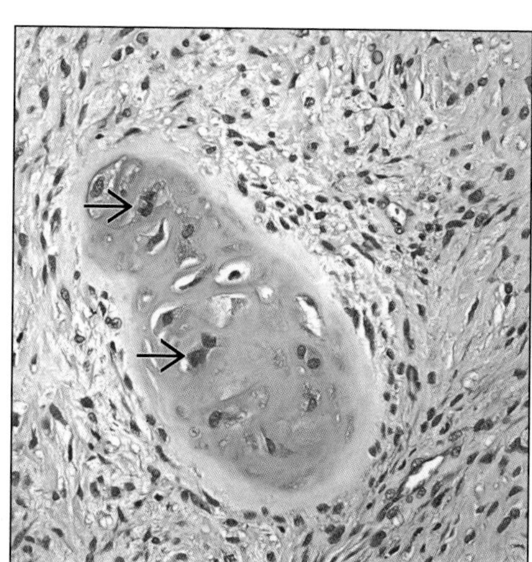
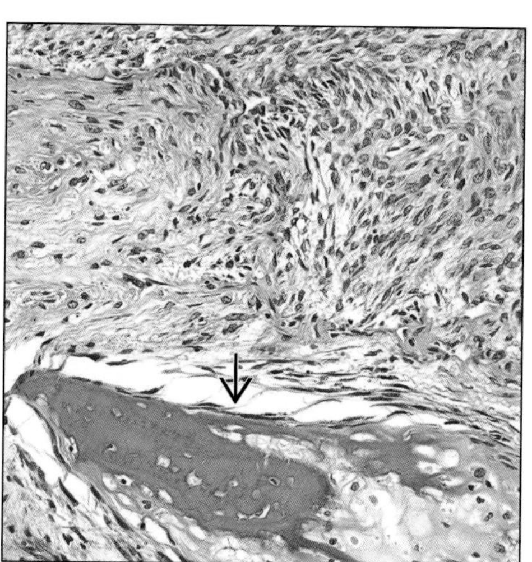

*(**Left**) Cartilaginous differentiation in MPNST can be benign or malignant (chondrosarcomatous) as indicated in this case by cytological atypia ➔. (**Right**) Heterologous osseous differentiation also occurs in MPNST, represented in this example by benign-appearing woven bone ➔. However, osteosarcomatous differentiation as well as other rare forms of heterologous differentiation, such as angiosarcomatous, glandular, and neuroepithelial, also occur.*

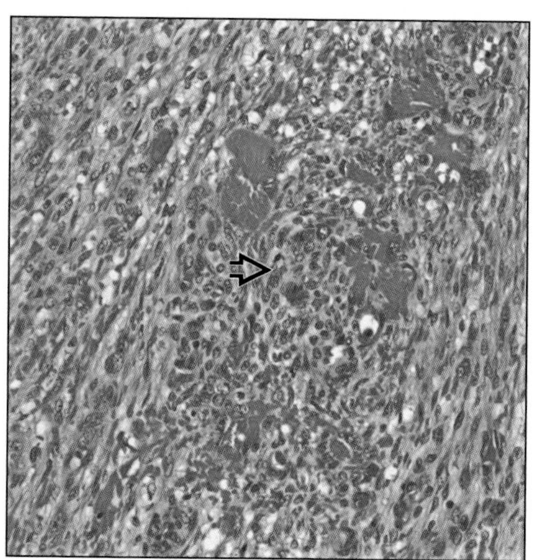
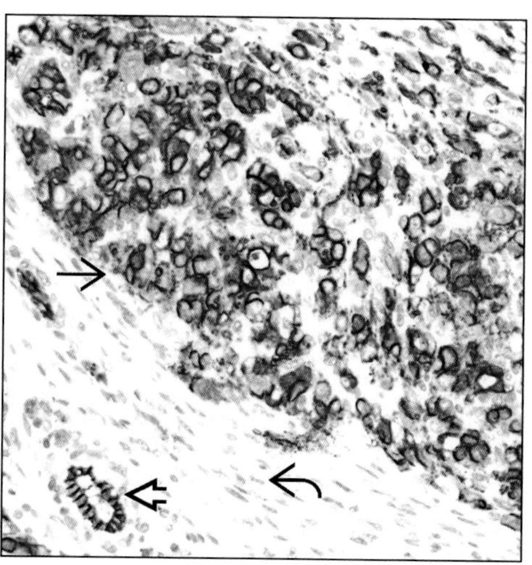

*(**Left**) Angiosarcoma can rarely arise in MPNST in patients with neurofibromatosis type 1. Here it forms a cellular area ➯ with atypical polygonal or spindle cells and hemorrhage, with or without vasoformation. (**Right**) Immunostaining for CD31 highlights angiosarcoma ➔ arising in MPNST. CD31 is more specific than CD34, which can also be expressed in nerve sheath tumors. Normal endothelium ➯ is also positive for CD31, but spindle cells of the adjacent MPNST ➦ are negative.*

Neural and Neuroectodermal Lesions

Benign

Benign/Malignant

Malignant

Examination of PNET/Ewing Sarcoma Specimens

NASAL GLIOMA

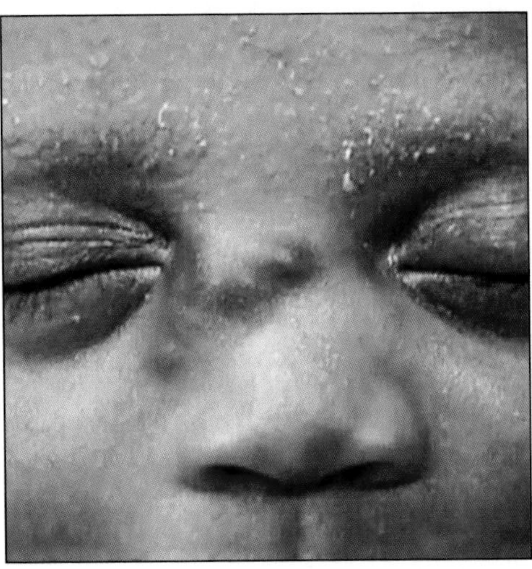

Clinical photograph shows a nodular lesion on the bridge of the nose in this infant. This is a common site, but a nasal glioma can also form a polypoid intranasal mass.

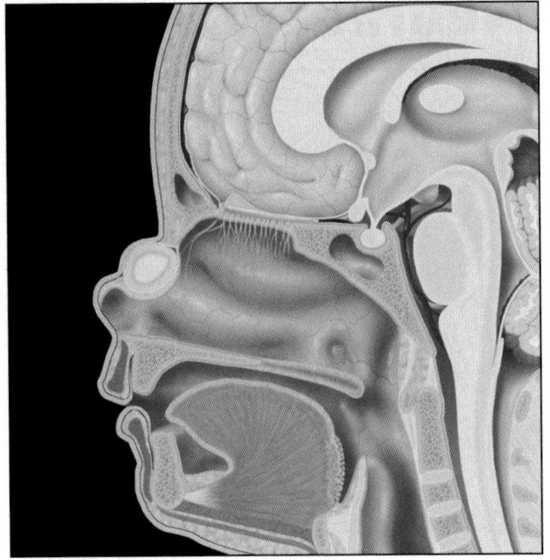

Graphic of a nasal glioma shows a mass of dysplastic glial tissue at the nasal dorsum. Note the absence of a connection to the intracranial contents.

TERMINOLOGY

Abbreviations

- Nasal glioma (NG)

Synonyms

- Heterotopic glial tissue
- Glial heterotopia

Definitions

- Rare congenital anomaly
  - Heterotopic glial tissue
    - "Glioma" is misnomer as nasal glioma is nonneoplastic tissue
  - Well-circumscribed round, ovoid, or polypoid mass
  - Not locally invasive

CLINICAL ISSUES

Epidemiology

- Incidence
  - Very rare
    - Rarely associated with other brain or systemic anomalies
- Age
  - Newborns
    - Identified at birth or within 1st few years of life

Site

- In and around nasal cavity
  - Bridge of nose is most common site
  - 1/3 are intranasal
    - Can be attached to septum

Presentation

- Subcutaneous mass
  - 20% associated with communication to frontal lobes
    - Usually communication is fibrous cord
    - Occasionally represents true encephalocele

Treatment

- Options, risks, complications
  - Mandatory to exclude communication with brain prior to excision
    - MR usually preferred over CT scan
- Surgical approaches
  - Simple excision is curative
    - 10% recurrence rate with incomplete resection

MACROSCOPIC FEATURES

General Features

- Firm, smooth mass

Size

- 1-3 cm in diameter (can reach 7 cm)
  - Grows slowly in proportion to adjacent tissue

MICROSCOPIC PATHOLOGY

Histologic Features

- Astrocytes and oligodendrocytes
- Loose fibrillary stroma
- Rarely may be associated with proliferation of eccrine ducts
- In older patients, lesions may be more fibrotic
  - Immunohistochemistry for GFAP crucial for diagnosis in this histologic setting

Predominant Pattern/Injury Type

- Nonencapsulated

Predominant Cell/Compartment Type

- Nervous, glial

ANCILLARY TESTS

Immunohistochemistry

- Positive for GFAP, S100 protein

NASAL GLIOMA

Key Facts

Terminology
- Rare congenital anomaly

Clinical Issues
- Subcutaneous mass
- Bridge of nose most common site
- 1/3 are intranasal
- 20% associated with communication to frontal lobes
- Mandatory to exclude communication with brain prior to excision
- Nodule or polyp

Microscopic Pathology
- Astrocytes and oligodendrocytes
- Loose fibrillary stroma
- Immunoreactive for GFAP

Ancillary Tests
- Positive for GFAP, S100 protein
- Negative for EMA, CD34, SMA, desmin

DIFFERENTIAL DIAGNOSIS

Neurofibroma
- Spindled cells with comma-shaped nuclei
- Collagenous rather than fibrillary stroma
- Negative for GFAP

True Encephalocele
- Histologically indistinguishable
- Differential diagnosis requires imaging studies

Cutaneous Meningioma
- Type 1
  - Congenital lesion
  - Scalp most common location
  - Dilated spaces lined by meningothelial cells
  - Thickened collagen bundles rather than delicate fibrillary glial tissue
- Type 2
  - Presents in adults
  - Head and neck
  - Nests of meningothelial cells
- Type 3
  - Extension from intracranial meningioma
  - Spindled and oval meningothelial cells
  - Collagenous stroma
- All types
  - Positive for EMA

DIAGNOSTIC CHECKLIST

Clinically Relevant Pathologic Features
- Age distribution
  - Almost always present in newborn infants
- Nasal bridge most common site
- Can also be intranasal
  - Polypoid
- May present along other cranial closure lines

Pathologic Interpretation Pearls
- Delicate fibrillary matrix important clue to diagnosis
- Presence of glial elements key to diagnosis
- Immunoreactive for GFAP

SELECTED REFERENCES

1. Penner CR et al: Nasal glial heterotopia: a clinicopathologic and immunophenotypic analysis of 10 cases with a review of the literature. Ann Diagn Pathol. 7(6):354-9, 2003
2. Cerdá-Nicolás M et al: Nasal glioma or nasal glial heterotopia? Morphological, immunohistochemical and ultrastructural study of two cases. Clin Neuropathol. 21(2):66-71, 2002
3. Jartti PH et al: MR of a nasal glioma in a young infant. Acta Radiol. 43(2):141-3, 2002

IMAGE GALLERY

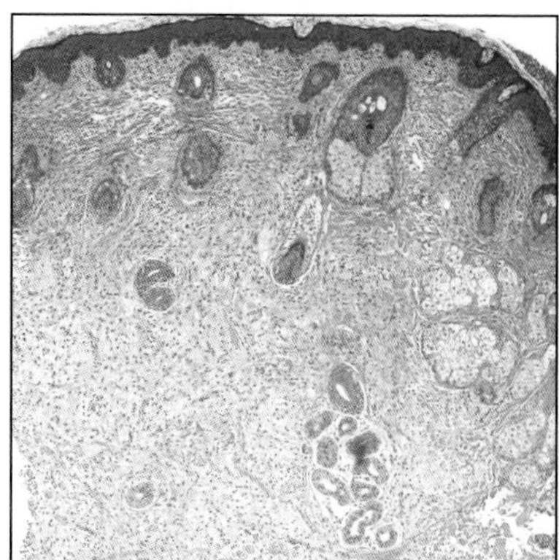
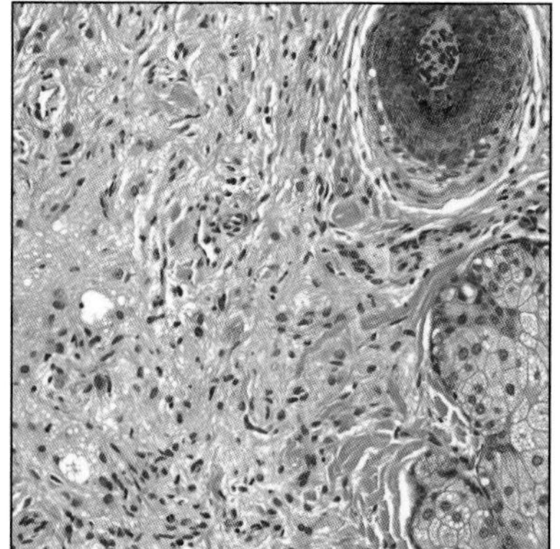
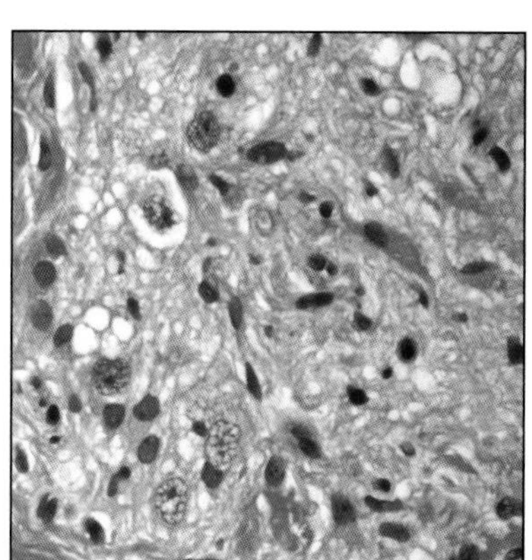

(Left) *Hematoxylin & eosin at low power demonstrates diffuse proliferation of glial tissue in the dermis. The lesion is poorly defined.* ***(Center)*** *Medium-power view shows a nasal glioma with characteristic fibrillary glial stroma. This is unencapsulated but can sometimes have a fibrous pseudocapsule or fibrous septa subdividing the lesion.* ***(Right)*** *Hematoxylin & eosin shows astrocytes and oligodendrocytes within loose fibrillary stroma.*

ECTOPIC MENINGIOMA

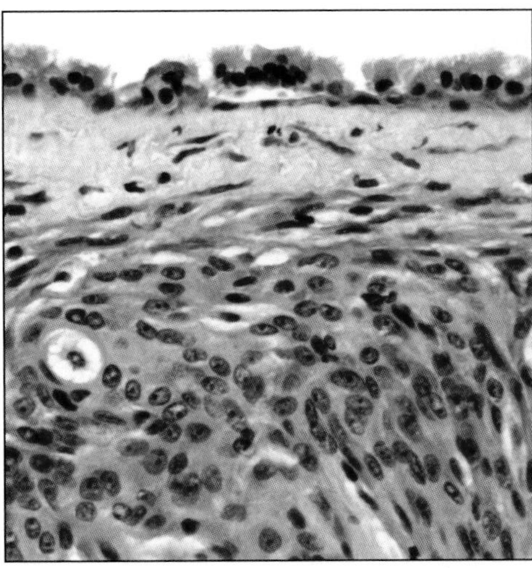

Hematoxylin & eosin shows intact respiratory mucosa overlying a syncytial-like neoplastic proliferation of meningothelial cells. The nuclei are uniform, and there are moderate amounts of cytoplasm.

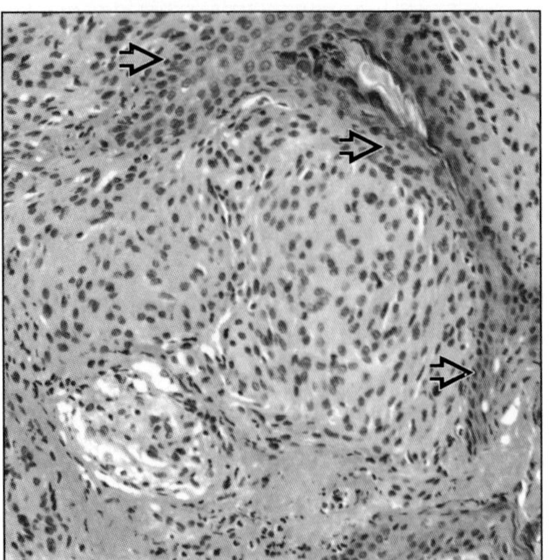

The meningothelial cells are arranged in a distinctive whorled pattern, with uninvolved surface squamous epithelium ➲. Cell boundaries are indistinct.

TERMINOLOGY

Definitions

- Benign neoplasm of meningothelial cells within nasal cavity, sinonasal tract, nasopharynx, or lung

ETIOLOGY/PATHOGENESIS

Pathogenesis

- Arachnoid cells from arachnoid granulations or pacchionian bodies lining sheaths of nerves and vessels through skull foramina

CLINICAL ISSUES

Epidemiology

- Incidence
  - Approximately 0.2% of sinonasal tract and nasopharynx tumors
    - 20% of meningiomas have extracranial extension
  - Very rare examples occur outside head and neck
- Age
  - Mean: 40-48 years old
  - Women older than men by over a decade
- Gender
  - M:F = 1:1.2

Site

- Mixed nasal cavity and paranasal sinuses (majority)
  - Nasal cavity alone (~ 25%)
  - Frontal sinus most commonly affected in isolation
  - Majority are left-sided
- Rare examples in lung, brachial plexus, soft tissue, skin

Presentation

- Mass, obstruction, discharge, and epistaxis
- Sinusitis, pain, headache, seizure activity
- Exophthalmos, periorbital edema, visual changes, ptosis

Treatment

- Surgical approaches
  - Excision (although difficult at times)

Prognosis

- Good outcome: 10-year survival (80%)
- Recurrences develop (usually < 5 years after primary)

IMAGE FINDINGS

Radiographic Findings

- Must exclude direct CNS extension from en plaque tumor
- Bony sclerosis with focal destruction of bony tissues
- Widening of suture lines and foramina at base of skull

MACROSCOPIC FEATURES

General Features

- Intact surface mucosa but infiltrative into bone
- Multiple fragments of grayish, white-tan, gritty, firm to rubbery masses
- Many in head and neck sites are polypoid

Size

- Range: 1-8 cm, mean: 3.5 cm

MICROSCOPIC PATHOLOGY

Histologic Features

- Infiltrative growth of neoplastic cells, including soft tissue and bone
- Meningothelial (syncytial) lobules of neoplastic cells without distinct borders
- Whorled architecture
- Psammoma bodies or "pre-psammoma" bodies
- Epithelioid cells with round to regular nuclei and even nuclear chromatin

ECTOPIC MENINGIOMA

Key Facts

Terminology
- Benign neoplasm of meningothelial cells

Clinical Issues
- Approximately 0.2% of sinonasal tract and nasopharynx tumors
- M:F = 1:1.2
  - Women older by over a decade
- Good outcome: 10-year survival (80%)

Image Findings
- Must exclude direct CNS extension

Microscopic Pathology
- Infiltrative growth of neoplastic cells, including soft tissue and bone
- Meningothelial (syncytial) lobules of neoplastic cells without distinct borders
- Whorled architecture, psammoma bodies
- Intranuclear cytoplasmic inclusions
- Histologic subtypes of meningioma can be seen
  - Transitional, metaplastic, atypical

ANCILLARY TESTS

Immunohistochemistry
- Positive: EMA, keratin ("pre-psammoma" body pattern), CAM5.2, claudin-1
- Weak positive: S100 protein
- Negative: Chromogranin, synaptophysin

DIFFERENTIAL DIAGNOSIS

Angiofibroma
- Males, in nasopharynx
- Stellate cells in fibrous stroma
  - Nuclei positive for β-catenin
- "Staghorn" vessels

Aggressive Psammomatoid Ossifying Fibroma
- Young age
- Abundant psammoma bodies
- Osteoclasts and osteoblasts

Olfactory Neuroblastoma
- Cribriform plate
- Lobules of small cells with scanty cytoplasm in fibrillary background
- Rosette/pseudorosette formation

Paraganglioma
- Nested architecture
- Chromogranin(+)
- Sustentacular cells S100 protein(+)

Perineurioma
- Long thin cells
- Perivascular whorls

SELECTED REFERENCES

1. Dekker G et al: Meningioma presenting as an oropharyngeal mass--an unusual presentation. S Afr Med J. 97(5):342, 2007
2. Petrulionis M et al: Primary extracranial meningioma of the sinonasal tract. Acta Radiol. 46(4):415-8, 2005
3. Thompson LD et al: Extracranial sinonasal tract meningiomas: a clinicopathologic study of 30 cases with a review of the literature. Am J Surg Pathol. 24(5):640-50, 2000
4. Moulin G et al: Plaque-like meningioma involving the temporal bone, sinonasal cavities and both parapharyngeal spaces: CT and MRI. Neuroradiology. 36(8):629-31, 1994
5. Gabibov GA et al: Meningiomas of the anterior skull base expanding into the orbit, paranasal sinuses, nasopharynx, and oropharynx. J Craniofac Surg. 4(3):124-7; discussion 134, 1993
6. Perzin KH et al: Nonepithelial tumors of the nasal cavity, paranasal sinuses, and nasopharynx. A clinicopathologic study. XIII: Meningiomas. Cancer. 54(9):1860-9, 1984

IMAGE GALLERY

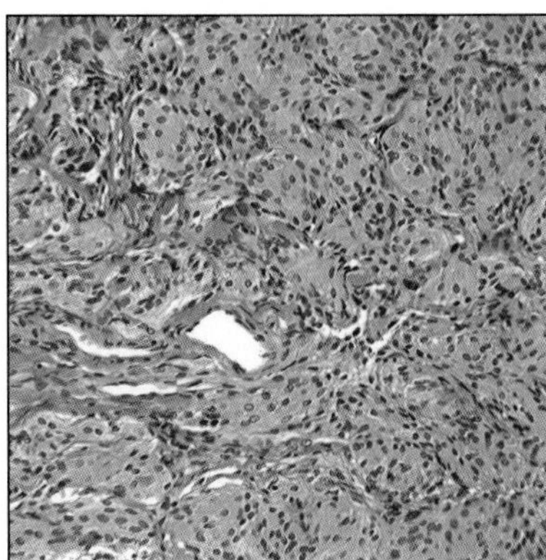
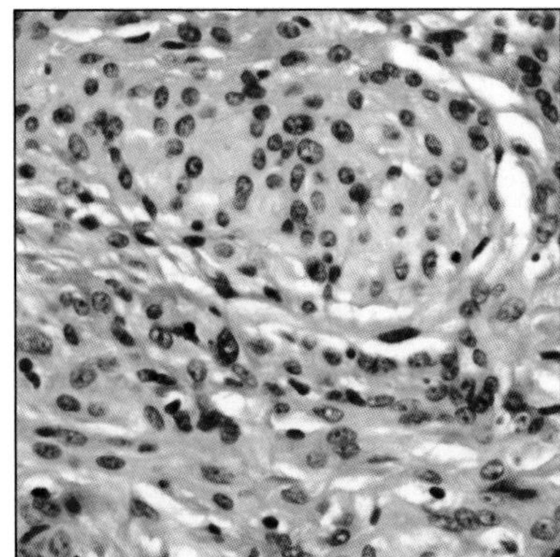
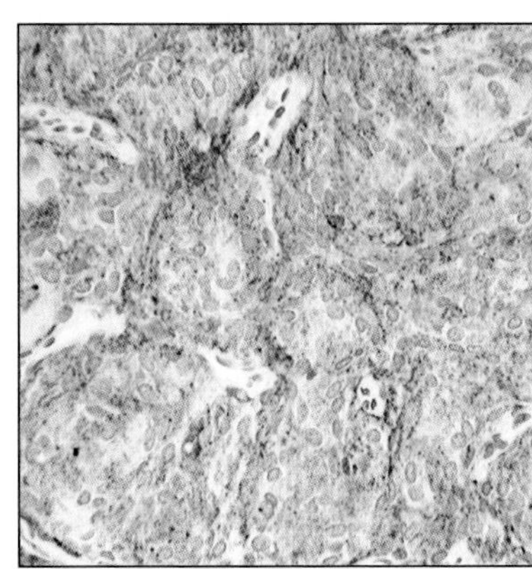

(Left) *This example shows multiple small nests of meningothelial cells with a slightly whorled appearance. This appearance resembles paraganglioma, but the latter has sustentacular cells (which can be demonstrated by immunoreactivity for S100 protein).* ***(Center)*** *Hematoxylin & eosin demonstrates a nest of cells without cell borders, showing focal nuclear hyperchromasia.* ***(Right)*** *Immunostaining for epithelial membrane antigen is positive on cell membranes or in cytoplasm.*

EPENDYMOMA

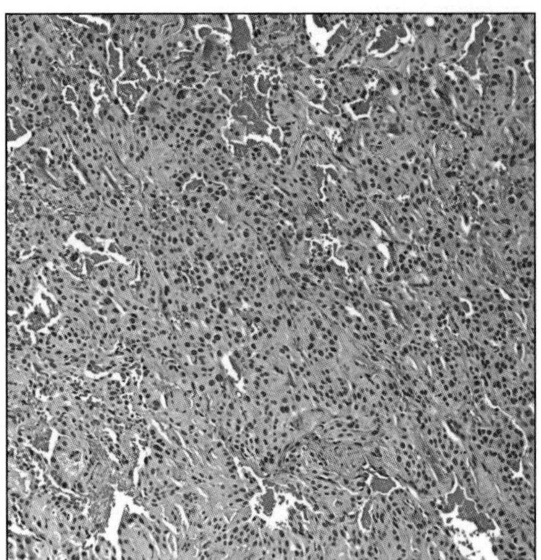

Extraspinal ependymoma appears identical to those lesions arising in the neuraxis (4th ventricle, spinal cord central canal). Note the prominent vascularity at low magnification.

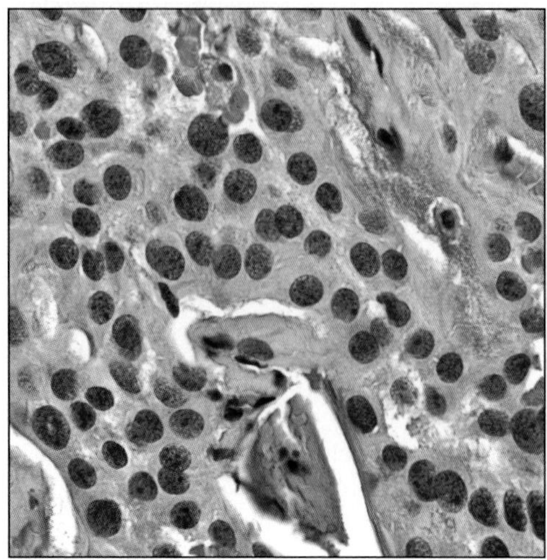

At high magnification, ependymomas are composed of cells with round nuclei and indistinct but fibrillary cytoplasm. Nucleoli are inconspicuous.

TERMINOLOGY

Synonyms

- Extraspinal ependymoma, sacrococcygeal ependymoma

Definitions

- Cellular glial or epithelial-appearing neoplasm manifesting ependymal differentiation as either perivascular rosettes or true rosettes
  - Myxopapillary variant has pseudopapillary architecture and intercellular myxoid matrix

ETIOLOGY/PATHOGENESIS

Subcutaneous Sacrococcygeal Ependymomas

- Believed to arise from coccygeal medullary vestige
  - Ependymal-lined cavity composed of remnant of caudal portion of neural tube

Presacral Ependymomas

- Believed to arise from extradural remnants of filum terminale

Ependymomas of Ovary and Mediastinum

- Germ cell origin postulated

CLINICAL ISSUES

Epidemiology

- Incidence
  - Rare
- Age
  - Usually children and young adults
    - Wide range: Months to > 65 years
- Gender
  - No preference

Presentation

- Subcutaneous, usually in coccygeal area
  - Can be mistaken for pilonidal cyst
- Presacral area

Treatment

- Surgical excision

Prognosis

- Generally favorable
  - Recurrences common; occasional local and distant metastases (lungs)

MICROSCOPIC PATHOLOGY

Histologic Features

- Well-marginated lesions
  - Less circumscribed than central nervous system examples
- Range of cellularity
  - Depends on ratio of fibrillary stroma to nuclei
    - Hypocellular to "blue"
- Nuclei round
  - Respect blood vessels
  - Anuclear zone around vessels composed of cell processes (pseudorosettes)
- Perivascular rosettes often inconspicuous in extraspinal lesions
- Myxopapillary ependymoma
  - Pseudopapillary architecture
  - Perivascular and intercellular myxoid matrix
    - Microcystic change
  - Nuclei more elongated than round

DIFFERENTIAL DIAGNOSIS

Chordoma

- Sacrococcygeal
- Usually involves bone

Key Facts

Terminology

- Cellular glial or epithelial-appearing neoplasm manifesting ependymal differentiation as either perivascular rosettes or true rosettes
  - Myxopapillary variant has pseudopapillary architecture and intercellular myxoid matrix
- Synonyms: Extraspinal ependymoma, sacrococcygeal ependymoma

Microscopic Pathology

- Range of cellularity
  - Hypocellular to "blue"
- Nuclei round
  - Respect blood vessels
  - Anuclear zone around vessels composed of cell processes (pseudorosettes)
- Perivascular rosettes often inconspicuous in extraspinal lesions

Immunohistochemistry

Antibody	Reactivity	Staining Pattern	Comment
GFAP	Positive	Cytoplasmic	Essentially all cases positive
S100	Positive	Nuclear & cytoplasmic	Most cases positive; not as intense as schwannomas
EMA	Positive	Cell membrane	Variable; highlights intracytoplasmic microlumina in some cases
CD99	Positive	Cell membrane	Variable; highlights intracytoplasmic microlumina in some cases
AE1/AE3	Positive	Cytoplasmic	Variable
CK20	Equivocal		Usually negative; focal if positive
CK7	Equivocal		Usually negative; focal if positive
34bE12	Equivocal		Usually negative; focal if positive

- Large "bubbly" cells (physaliferous cells)
  - Abundant mucopolysaccharide matrix in cytoplasm and between cells
- Inconspicuous vascularity
- CK(+), S100 protein(+), brachyury(+), GFAP(-), D2-40(-)

Schwannoma

- Anywhere in body
  - Head and neck favored
- Spindle cell lesions with hypercellular (Antoni A) and hypocellular myxoid (Antoni B) zones
- No vascular pseudorosettes
  - Thick-walled vessels, hemosiderin deposition, foam cells, and lymphocytes
- Strong S100 protein labeling, negative keratin
  - Exception: Retroperitoneal schwannomas sometimes have strong keratin expression

SELECTED REFERENCES

1. Ma YT et al: Case report: primary subcutaneous sacrococcygeal ependymoma: a case report and review of the literature. Br J Radiol. 79(941):445-7, 2006
2. Takano T et al: Primary ependymoma of the ovary: a case report and literature review. Int J Gynecol Cancer. 15(6):1138-41, 2005
3. Chou S et al: Extraspinal ependymoma. J Pediatr Surg. 22(9):802-3, 1987
4. Helwig EB et al: Subcutaneous sacrococcygeal myxopapillary ependymoma. A clinicopathologic study of 32 cases. Am J Clin Pathol. 81(2):156-61, 1984
5. Morantz RA et al: Extraspinal ependymomas. Report of three cases. J Neurosurg. 51(3):383-91, 1979

IMAGE GALLERY

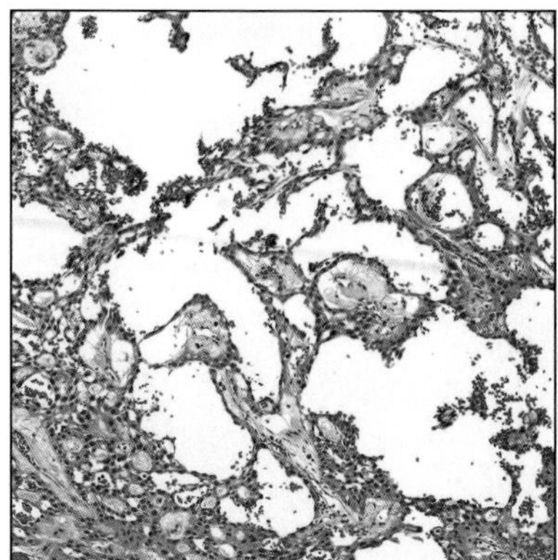

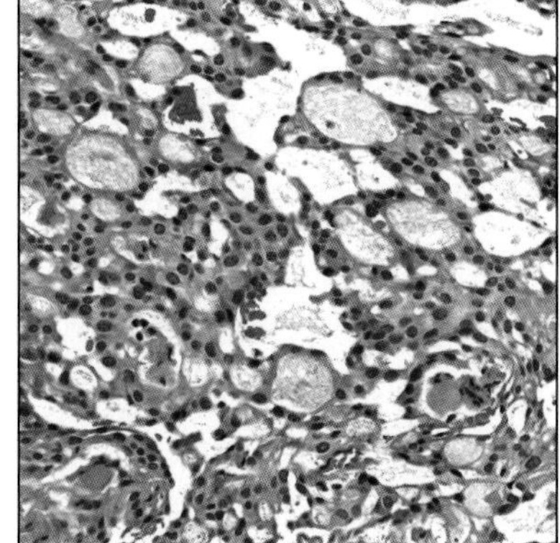

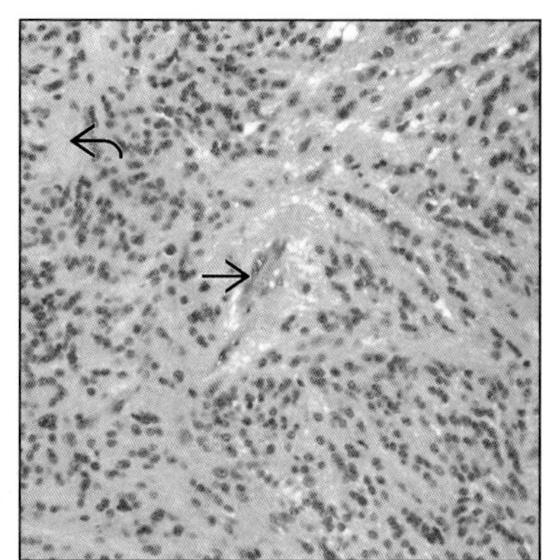

(Left) *This sacrococcygeal ependymoma has myxopapillary features; indeed, myxopapillary ependymoma is more common in the sacrococcygeal area than classic cellular ependymoma.* ***(Center)*** *Sacrococcygeal ependymoma shows uniform rounded cells and myxoid stroma.* ***(Right)*** *This sacrococcygeal ependymoma has fibrillary stroma ⇗. A vascular pseudorosette is present in the center of the field. The vessel → is surrounded by a fibrillary zone that lacks nuclei.*

GANGLIONEUROMA

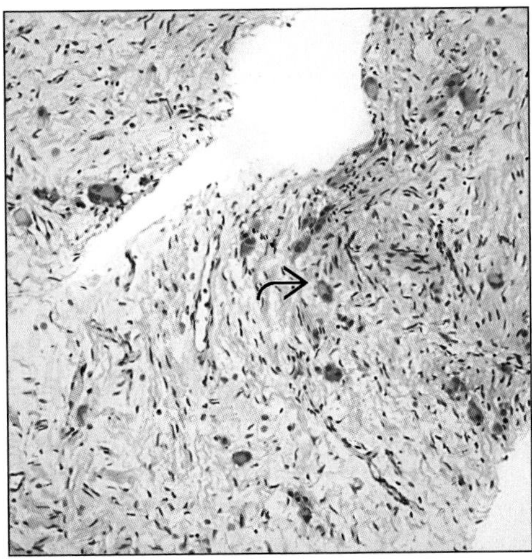

Needle core biopsy specimen of ganglioneuroma shows small numbers of mature ganglion cells singly ➔ and in clusters, within a moderately cellular schwannian stroma-rich background.

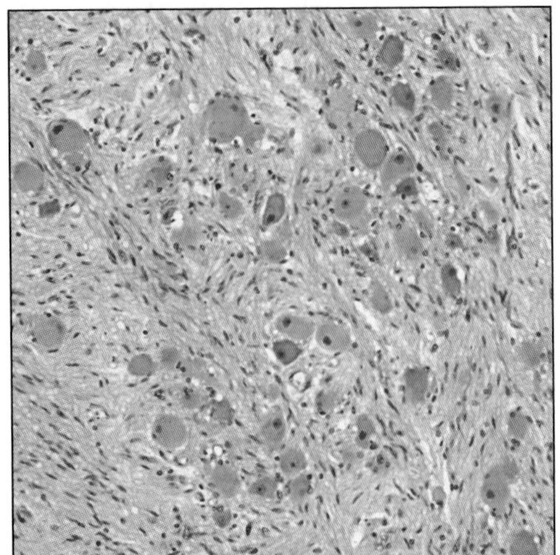

The number of ganglion cells varies in this case of ganglioneuroma. They are numerous and mature with abundant cytoplasm. The stroma is composed of bland, Schwann cell-like spindle cells.

TERMINOLOGY

Abbreviations

- Ganglioneuroma (GN)

Definitions

- Benign, well-differentiated tumor of neural crest origin
- Arises from sympathetic or peripheral nerves

ETIOLOGY/PATHOGENESIS

Associated Conditions

- Within intestinal tract, lesions often associated with tumor syndromes
  - Polypoid GN in GI tract has associations with Cowden syndrome, juvenile polyposis, and tuberous sclerosis
  - Ganglioneuromatous polyposis reported in patients with neurofibromatosis type 1 and MEN2B
- Most develop de novo
  - Some develop from maturation of neuroblastoma

CLINICAL ISSUES

Epidemiology

- Incidence
  - Rare compared to other benign nerve sheath tumors
- Age
  - Significantly older population than in neuroblastoma
    - Usually patients < 30 years
    - Mostly children > 10 years
- Gender
  - M = F

Site

- Posterior mediastinum (most common site)
- Retroperitoneum (extraadrenal)
- Rarer in adrenal gland
- Rarely in skin, parapharynx, GI tract, and paratestis
- Usually solitary

Presentation

- Painless mass
- Large tumors can rarely present with urinary catecholamine secretion

Treatment

- Surgical approaches
  - Conservative treatment
  - Follow-up indicated for recurrence

Prognosis

- Vast majority behave in benign fashion
- Rare "metastatic" GN foci described in lymph nodes
  - Presumably represent metastatic neuroblastoma in which metastatic primary tumor matured
- Malignant transformation described in rare cases
  - In both de novo GN and those developing from maturation in neuroblastoma
  - Some in previously irradiated sites of neuroblastoma

IMAGE FINDINGS

General Features

- Radiologic calcification in 1/3 of cases

MACROSCOPIC FEATURES

General Features

- Well-defined, smooth, encapsulated mass
- Gray-white or yellow cut surface
- May have calcification
- Hemorrhage and necrosis absent

GANGLIONEUROMA

Key Facts

Terminology
- Benign, well-differentiated tumor of neurogenic origin

Etiology/Pathogenesis
- Usually develop de novo

Clinical Issues
- Most commonly located in posterior mediastinum
- Also in retroperitoneum (extraadrenal)
- Affects older population than in neuroblastoma
- Mostly children > 10 years

Microscopic Pathology
- Abundant moderately cellular, uniform spindle cell matrix
- Intermixed ganglion cells of variable number and maturation
- Primitive neuroblasts absent

MICROSCOPIC PATHOLOGY

Histologic Features
- Abundant uniform spindle cell matrix
- Schwann cell-like spindle cells
  - Fascicles or patternless arrays
  - Elongated or wavy nuclei
  - Matrix resembles neurofibroma or schwannoma
- Intermixed ganglion cells
  - Variable size and number
  - Clusters, nests, and singly
    - Round vesicular, sometimes multiple nuclei
    - May show mild to moderate atypia
    - Abundant eosinophilic or amphophilic cytoplasm
    - May contain fine granular cytoplasmic pigment, thought to represent catecholamine products
  - Maturation varies
  - Primitive neuroblasts absent
- May show calcification or cystic change
- Rarely fat can be present
- Rare mixed ganglioneuroma and pheochromocytoma

ANCILLARY TESTS

Immunohistochemistry
- S100 protein in neuromatous matrix
- Neurofilament protein and NSE in ganglion cells and nerve fascicles

DIFFERENTIAL DIAGNOSIS

Neurofibroma
- Ganglion cells absent

Schwannoma
- Diffuse and strong S100 protein positivity
- Antoni A and B areas
- Ganglion cells absent

Ganglioneuroblastoma
- Islands of immature neuroblasts

SELECTED REFERENCES

1. Thway K et al: Diffuse ganglioneuromatosis in small intestine associated with neurofibromatosis type 1. Ann Diagn Pathol. 13(1):50-4, 2009
2. Geoerger B et al: Metabolic activity and clinical features of primary ganglioneuromas. Cancer. 91(10):1905-13, 2001
3. Shekitka KM et al: Ganglioneuromas of the gastrointestinal tract. Relation to Von Recklinghausen disease and other multiple tumor syndromes. Am J Surg Pathol. 18(3):250-7, 1994
4. Ghali VS et al: Malignant peripheral nerve sheath tumor arising spontaneously from retroperitoneal ganglioneuroma: a case report, review of the literature, and immunohistochemical study. Hum Pathol. 23(1):72-5, 1992
5. Ricci A Jr et al: Malignant peripheral nerve sheath tumors arising from ganglioneuromas. Am J Surg Pathol. 8(1):19-29, 1984

IMAGE GALLERY

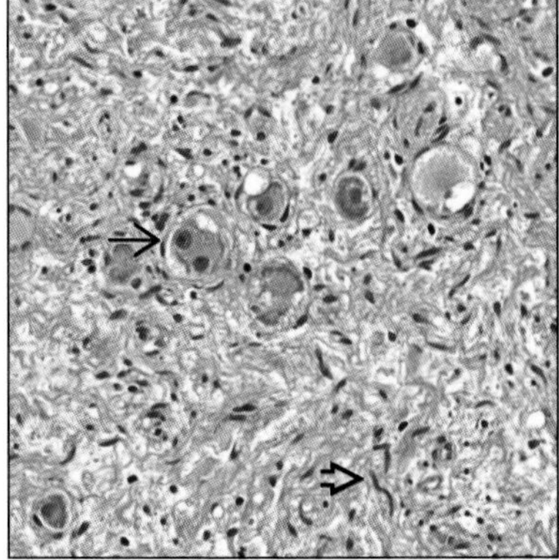

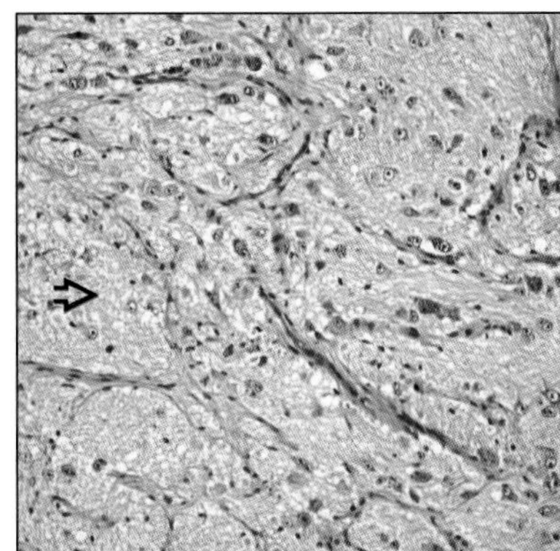

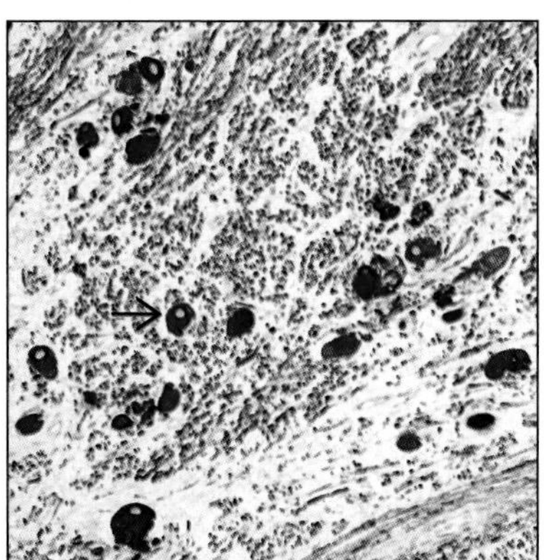

(Left) *The ganglion cells are often binucleate ➡. Note the typical "neurofibromatous" background, with tapered, wavy, nerve sheath-type spindle nuclei ➡.* ***(Center)*** *Here the ganglion cells display a slightly more immature phenotype, with less cytoplasm. Note the abundant neurofibrillary matrix ➡.* ***(Right)*** *Ganglion cells strongly express neurofilament protein ➡, as do the small nerve trunks within the background stroma.*

PARAGANGLIOMA

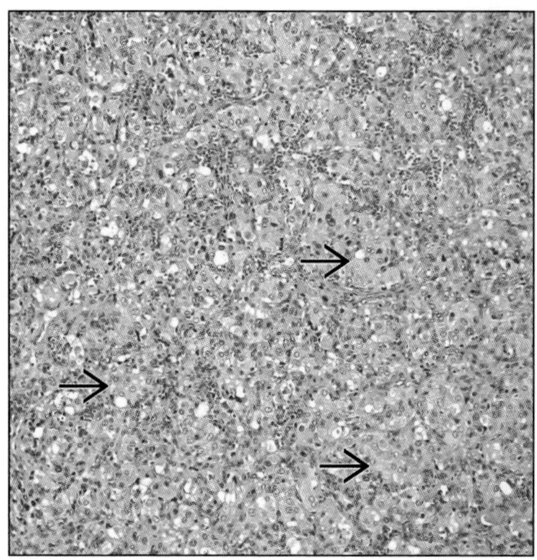

Hematoxylin & eosin shows the characteristic alveolar pattern (zellballen) of paraganglioma. Small nests of cells ⇒ are surrounded by a fibrovascular, richly vascularized stroma.

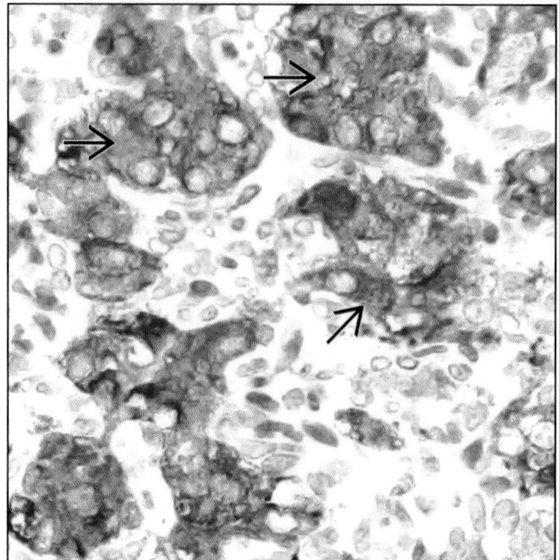

Synaptophysin shows strong and diffuse immunoreactivity of the chief cells ⇒. There is no reactivity of the supporting sustentacular cells (which would stain with S100 protein).

TERMINOLOGY

Synonyms

- Chemodectoma
- Glomus (do not confuse with soft tissue glomus)

Definitions

- Neuroendocrine tumor arising from paraganglia at specified locations
- Chromaffin(+) tumors resemble pheochromocytoma
  - Aorticosympathetic, can be functional
- Chemoreceptor (branchiomeric) type are nonchromaffin
  - Usually nonfunctional
- Chief and sustentacular cells arranged in organoid pattern

CLINICAL ISSUES

Epidemiology

- Incidence
  - Sporadic or familial
    - Germline mutations include succinate dehydrogenase gene *SDH*
    - Can be part of MEN2, Carney triad, or NF1
    - Many familial lesions are multifocal
- Age
  - Any age but mostly adults
- Gender
  - M > F for carotid body tumors
  - Slight female predominance in other sites

Site

- Head and neck
  - Carotid body is most common site
    - > 1/2 of head and neck paragangliomas
    - More common in high-altitude habitat
  - Jugular bulb, middle ear
  - Vagus nerve
- Mediastinum (aorticopulmonary)
- Retroperitoneum (from aorticosympathetic paraganglia or organ of Zuckerkandl)
- Organ-based
  - Duodenum (gangliocytic paraganglioma)
  - Bladder, heart, larynx

Presentation

- Painless mass
  - Pressure effect
- Vagal symptoms

Treatment

- Surgical approaches
  - Surgical excision with external approach
    - Intraoperative bleeding may be significant

Prognosis

- Most benign but can recur
- Rare malignant examples
  - Metastasize to lymph nodes, lung, bone

MACROSCOPIC FEATURES

General Features

- Circumscribed mass
- Cut surface is pink to tan and dark red

Size

- Range: 0.5-6 cm

MICROSCOPIC PATHOLOGY

Histologic Features

- Nests of tumor cells in highly vascular fibrous tissue
- Chief cells have eosinophilic, finely granular cytoplasm and central nuclei
  - Nuclear pleomorphism may be present but is prognostically unimportant
- Clear cells change focally or diffusely

PARAGANGLIOMA

Key Facts

Terminology
- Tumor arising from paraganglia

Clinical Issues
- Variety of sites
  - More frequent in head and neck
  - Thorax, abdomen, larynx, bladder
- Functional or nonfunctional
- Mostly benign

Microscopic Pathology
- Circumscribed tumor
- Nested alveolar (zellballen) pattern
- Chief cells with granular cytoplasm
- Clear cells in some
- Nuclear pleomorphism not uncommon
- Sustentacular cell processes around nests
- Highly vascular stroma
- Focal fibrosis
- Malignant variants have mitoses, necrosis, vascular invasion, fewer sustentacular cells
  - Histology does not predict behavior

Ancillary Tests
- CD56(+), chromogranin(+), neurofilament(+)
- S100 protein(+) in sustentacular cells
- Cytokeratin(-) and EMA(-)
- Electron microscopy shows dense-core granules

Top Differential Diagnoses
- Neuroendocrine carcinoma
- Alveolar soft part sarcoma
- Metastatic renal cell carcinoma
- Adrenal cortical carcinoma

Immunohistochemistry

Antibody	Reactivity	Staining Pattern	Comment
Chromogranin-A	Positive	Cytoplasmic	Chief, paraganglia cells
Synaptophysin	Positive	Cytoplasmic	Chief, paraganglia cells
CD56	Positive	Cell membrane	Chief, paraganglia cells
NSE	Positive	Cytoplasmic	Chief, paraganglia cells
S100	Positive	Nuclear & cytoplasmic	Sustentacular cells
GFAP	Positive	Cytoplasmic	Sustentacular cells
CK-PAN	Negative		

- Sustentacular cells at periphery of nests
  - Modified Schwann cells
- Rare mitoses
- Sinusoidal vascular pattern
- Malignant features include
  - Marked nuclear pleomorphism, mitotic activity
  - Necrosis, vascular invasion
  - Paucity of sustentacular cells
  - Occurrence of metastasis
- Hyalinizing variant

ANCILLARY TESTS

Electron Microscopy
- Chief cells have dense core granules 100-400 nm
- Sustentacular cells have continuous external lamina

DIFFERENTIAL DIAGNOSIS

Neuroendocrine Tumors
- Both typical and atypical carcinoid
- Organoid, trabecular, or glandular patterns
- Express cytokeratin and neuroendocrine markers
- Absence of sustentacular cells

Alveolar Soft Part Sarcoma
- Deep soft tissue of extremities
- Large polygonal cells with abundant cytoplasm
- Lacks neural markers; some are desmin(+)
- Nuclear TFE3 positivity
- t(X;17)(p11.q25), with *ASPL-TFE3* fusion

Metastatic Renal Cell Carcinoma
- Organoid pattern
- Cytokeratin(+)

Adrenal Cortical Carcinoma
- Sheets of clear cells
- Absence of sustentacular cells
- Cytokeratin(+)

Melanoma
- S100 protein(+), HMB-45 and Melan-A variable

SELECTED REFERENCES

1. Sangoi AR et al: A tissue microarray-based comparative analysis of novel and traditional immunohistochemical markers in the distinction between adrenal cortical lesions and pheochromocytoma. Am J Surg Pathol. 34(3):423-32, 2010
2. Petri BJ et al: Phaeochromocytomas and sympathetic paragangliomas. Br J Surg. 96(12):1381-92, 2009
3. Plaza JA et al: Sclerosing paraganglioma: report of 19 cases of an unusual variant of neuroendocrine tumor that may be mistaken for an aggressive malignant neoplasm. Am J Surg Pathol. 30(1):7-12, 2006
4. Wasserman PG et al: Paragangliomas: classification, pathology, and differential diagnosis. Otolaryngol Clin North Am. 34(5):845-62, v-vi, 2001

PARAGANGLIOMA

Diagrammatic and Microscopic Features

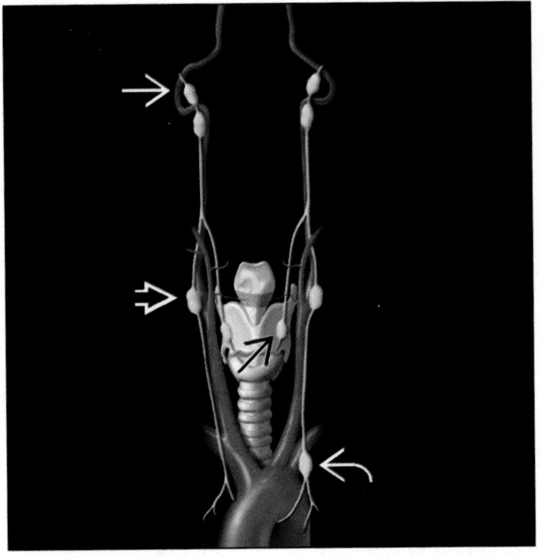

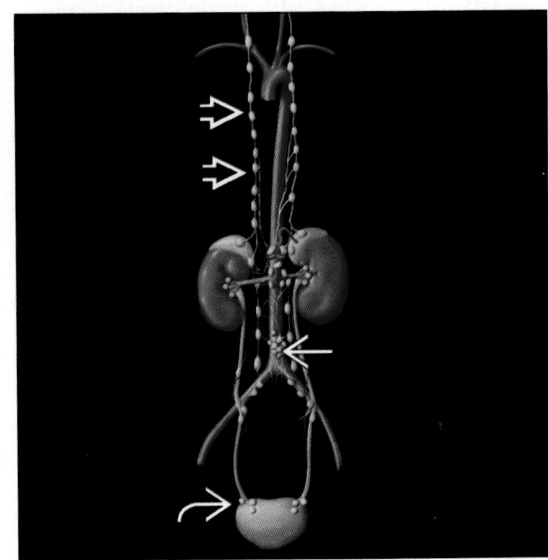

(Left) *Graphic shows paraganglia in head, neck, & upper thorax associated with arteries or cranial nerves. They include aortic & carotid bodies, & jugulotympanic, vagal, & laryngeal paraganglia.* ***(Right)*** *Graphic shows aorticosympathetic paraganglia in thorax and abdomen. These are associated with sympathetic chain and arterial plexuses and include adrenal medulla and organ of Zuckerkandl near aortic bifurcation. Paraganglia in bladder can be the site of paraganglioma.*

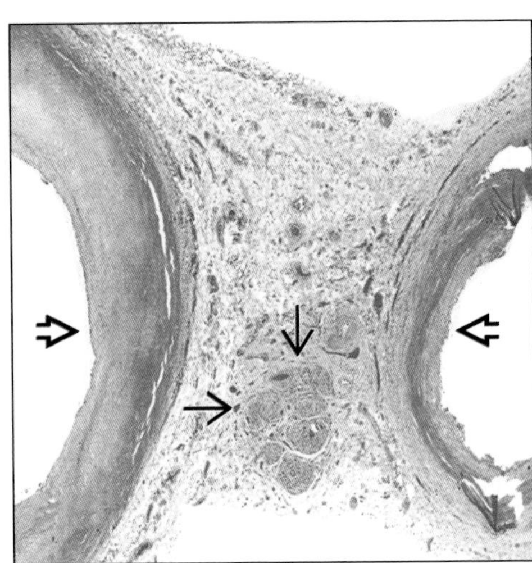

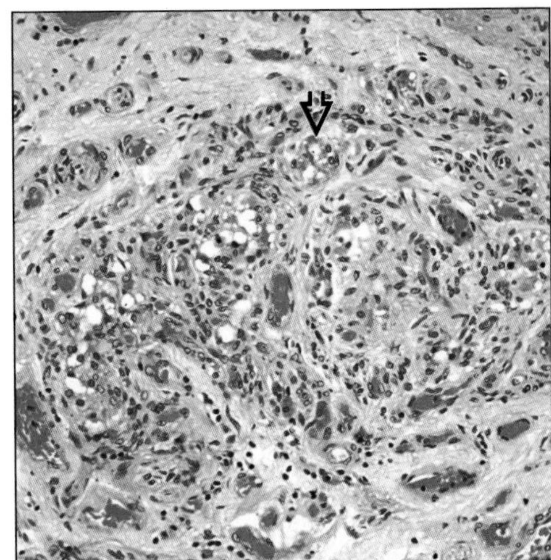

(Left) *This low-power image shows a normal carotid body in connective tissue at the bifurcation of the carotid artery in the neck. The organ represents an aggregate of chemoreceptor tissue that is not encapsulated.* ***(Right)*** *Higher magnification of carotid body shows "organoid" appearance with small nests of chief cells intimately admixed with thin-walled blood vessels. Note the absence of nuclear pleomorphism.*

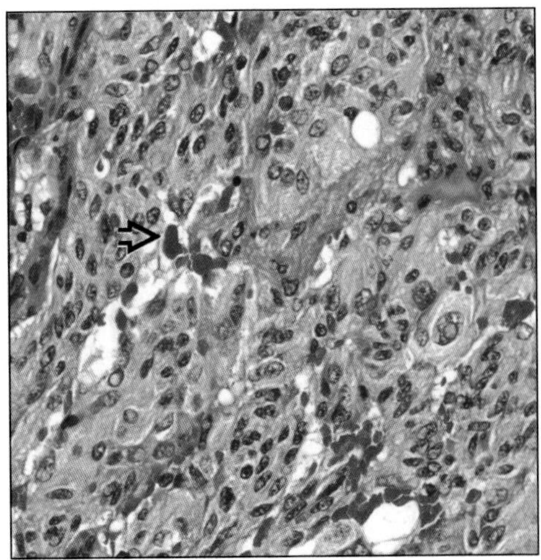

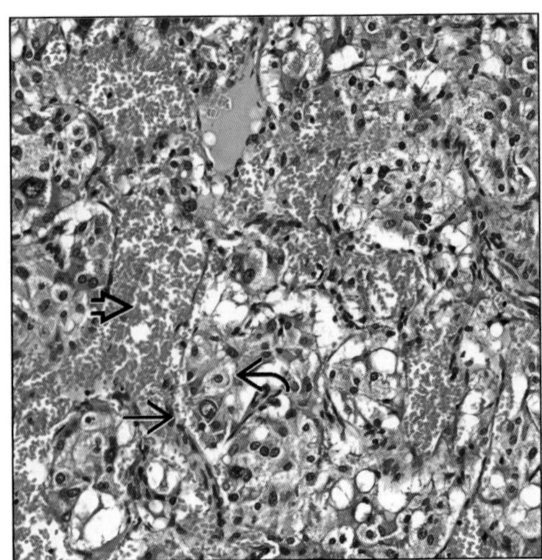

(Left) *Typical architecture of paraganglioma is seen with variably sized nests of rounded chief cells with moderate amounts of amphophilic cytoplasm and distinct cell membranes. Note thin-walled vessels containing red blood cells.* ***(Right)*** *This paraganglioma is dissected by dilated or congested sinusoidal blood spaces lined by a single layer of endothelium. Some of the chief cells demonstrate cytoplasmic clear cell change, while most have slightly granular cytoplasm.*

Microscopic Features, Variants, and Ancillary Techniques

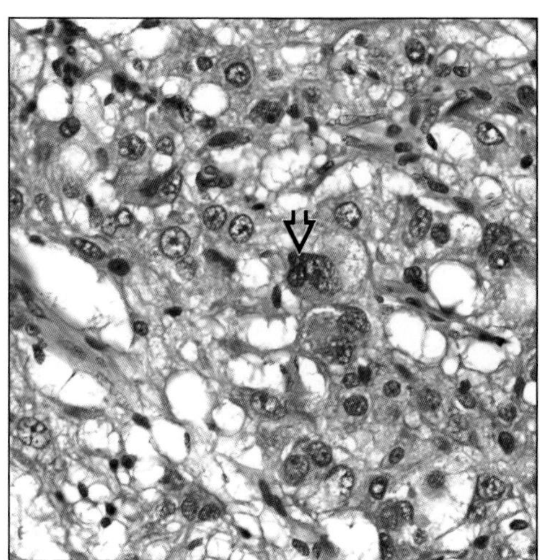

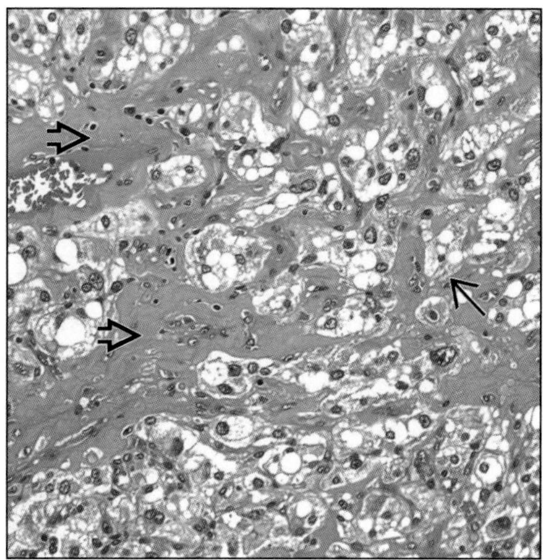

*(**Left**) Variation in nuclear size, prominent nucleoli, and nuclear pleomorphism ⊳ are common features in paragangliomas and do not indicate malignant potential. Malignant paragangliomas can have mitoses, necrosis, vascular invasion, and loss of sustentacular cells. (**Right**) This paraganglioma is traversed by bands of collagen ⊳ of variable width. Sclerosis can be marked with only a few scattered nests of lesional cells, some of which show clear cytoplasm → in this case.*

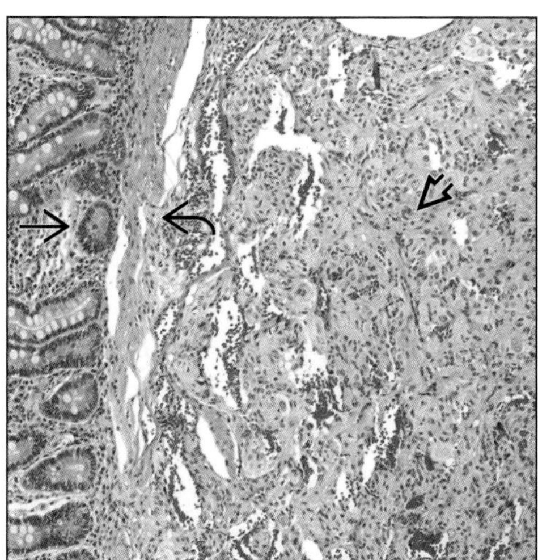

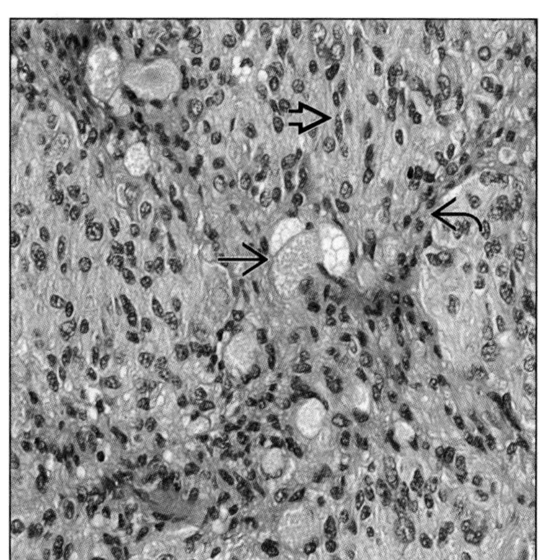

*(**Left**) This is an example of gangliocytic paraganglioma arising in 2nd part of duodenum. The intact intestinal mucosa → overlies the tumor ⊳, which is located in the submucosa and infiltrates between fibers of muscularis mucosae ⇗. (**Right**) Gangliocytic paraganglioma is composed of a mixture of ganglion cells →, carcinoid-like cells ⊳, and spindly Schwann cells ⇗, each of which can be demonstrated by NSE, CD56, or S100 protein immunostain.*

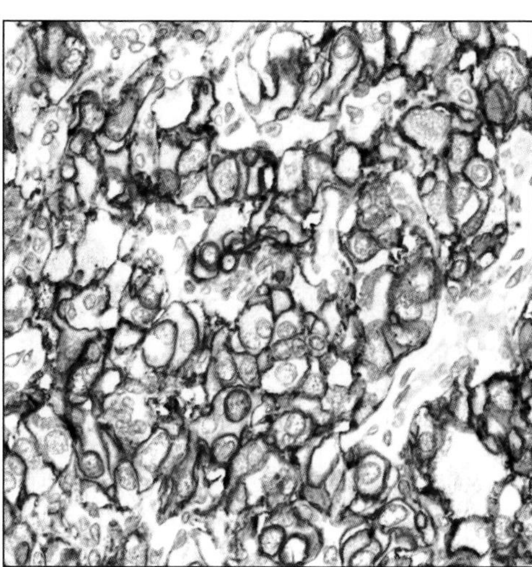

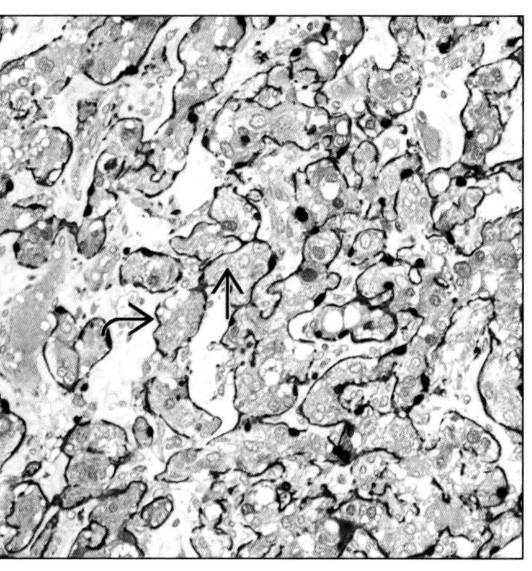

*(**Left**) Immunostaining for CD56 (N-CAM) shows diffuse membranous staining on chief cells. Although a nonspecific neural or neuroendocrine marker, CD56 is useful in this context for supporting the diagnosis of paraganglioma. (**Right**) Immunostain for S100 protein shows sustentacular cell nuclei and processes ⇗. The long cytoplasmic processes of these modified Schwann cells embrace and delineate the nest of chief cells →, which are negative.*

MELANOTIC NEUROECTODERMAL TUMOR OF INFANCY

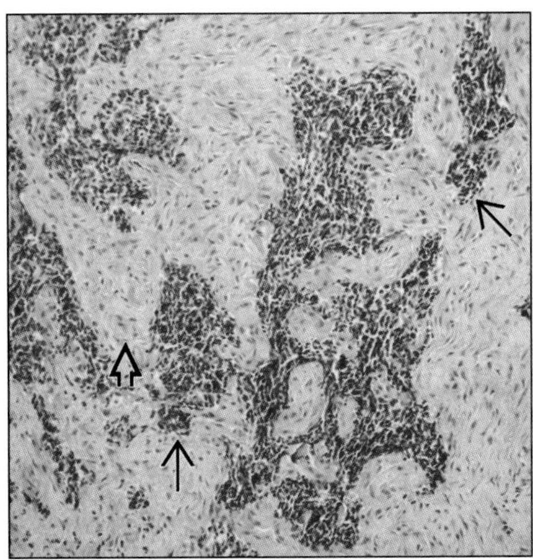

The neuroblastic small cells ⇨ separated by a fibrocollagenous stroma ⇨ demonstrate an alveolar pattern of growth in this melanotic neuroectodermal tumor of infancy (MNTI).

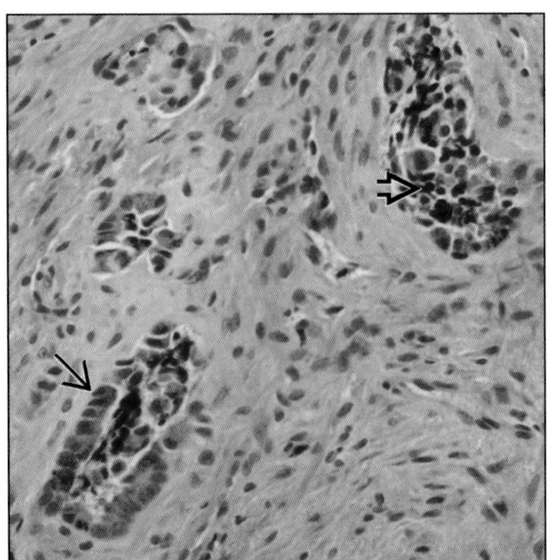

Epithelial cells with abundant eosinophilic cytoplasm and melanin pigment ⇨ form glandular structures with scattered small neuroblastic cells ⇨ in this MNTI.

TERMINOLOGY

Abbreviations

- Melanotic neuroectodermal tumor of infancy (MNTI)

Synonyms

- Retinal anlage tumor
- Melanotic progonoma
- Melanotic ameloblastoma

Definitions

- Rare, fast-growing, pigmented neoplasm, likely of neural crest origin

ETIOLOGY/PATHOGENESIS

Disputed Histogenesis

- Current studies support neural crest (neuroectodermal) origin

CLINICAL ISSUES

Epidemiology

- Age
  - Most present in 1st year of life (> 90%)

Site

- Most involve craniofacial sites
  - Upper and lower jaw
    - Maxilla (69%)
    - Mandible (6%)
  - Skull (11%)
- Unusual sites
  - Epididymis, mediastinum, brain, shoulder, and skin

Presentation

- Rapidly enlarging, firm, expansile mass
- Erosion into adjacent bone
- Nontender
- Intact overlying mucosa
- Bluish discoloration

Laboratory Tests

- Elevated urinary vanillylmandelic acid may be present

Treatment

- Complete local excision
  - Local recurrence rate: 10-15%
  - Usually recurs in 1st postoperative year

Prognosis

- Benign to intermediate clinical course
  - Recurrence rate: 10-15%
  - Metastatic spread in < 5%

IMAGE FINDINGS

General Features

- Well-demarcated radiolucent lesion
- Capacity for local destruction

MACROSCOPIC FEATURES

Gross Features

- Firm
- Well circumscribed
- Gray to blue-black cut surface

MICROSCOPIC PATHOLOGY

Predominant Pattern/Injury Type

- Glandular/alveolar
  - Spaces lined by cuboidal pigmented epithelial cells
  - Small neuroblastic cells found within spaces
- Solid
  - Background of fibrocollagenous stroma

MELANOTIC NEUROECTODERMAL TUMOR OF INFANCY

Key Facts

Terminology
- Rare, fast-growing, pigmented neoplasm, likely of neural crest origin

Clinical Issues
- Most present in 1st year of life
- Commonly involve craniofacial sites
  - Maxilla (69%)
- Rapidly enlarging expansile mass
- Elevated urinary vanillylmandelic acid may be present

Microscopic Pathology
- 3 distinct components
  - Clusters of small round neuroblastic cells
  - Primitive gland-like structures
  - Fibrocollagenous stroma

Top Differential Diagnoses
- Neuroblastoma
  - Sheets and lobules of small round hyperchromatic cells
- Alveolar rhabdomyosarcoma
  - Aggregates and nests of poorly differentiated small hyperchromatic cells
  - Characteristic immunohistochemical and cytogenetic findings
- Primitive neuroectodermal tumor
  - Sheets of small-medium round blue cells
  - Characteristic t(11;22)
- Congenital epulis
  - Characteristic location in labial aspect of dental ridge
  - Protruding round or ovoid nodule

Immunohistochemistry

Antibody	Reactivity	Staining Pattern	Comment
AE1/AE3	Positive	Cell membrane & cytoplasm	Epithelial cells
HMB-45	Positive	Cytoplasmic	Epithelial cells
NSE	Positive	Cytoplasmic	Frequently expressed by neuroblastic cells and epithelial cells
Synaptophysin	Positive	Cytoplasmic	Neuroblastic cells and variably expressed in epithelial cells
CD57	Positive	Cell membrane & cytoplasm	Neuroblastic cells and epithelial cells

Predominant Cell/Compartment Type
- Dual population of cells
  - Flat to cuboidal pigmented epithelial cells
  - Small neuroblastic cells
  - Fibrocollagenous stroma

Microscopic Features
- 3 distinct components
  - Primitive gland-like structures
    - Larger cells with round vesicular nuclei
    - Abundant cytoplasm with melanin granules
    - Alveolar or glandular arrangements
    - May contain neuroblastic cells within gland space
  - Clusters of small round neuroblastic cells
    - Small round hyperchromatic nuclei
    - Scant cytoplasm
    - Arranged in small islands and cords
    - Crush artifact frequently encountered
    - May be found independent from gland-like structures
  - Fibrocollagenous stroma

DIFFERENTIAL DIAGNOSIS

Neuroblastoma
- Predominantly located in retroperitoneum
- Sheets and lobules of small round hyperchromatic cells
- Homer-Wright rosettes

Alveolar Rhabdomyosarcoma
- More commonly located in extremities
- Aggregates and nests of poorly differentiated small hyperchromatic cells
- Separated by fibrous septae
- Characteristic immunohistochemical and cytogenetic findings

Primitive Neuroectodermal Tumor
- Sheets of small-medium round blue cells
- Frequent mitoses and foci of necrosis
- Characteristic t(11;22)

Congenital Epulis
- Characteristic location in labial aspect of dental ridge
- Protruding round or ovoid nodule
- Microscopically resembles adult granular cell tumor
  - Polygonal cells with abundant eosinophilic cytoplasm
  - Lacks pseudoepitheliomatous hyperplasia

SELECTED REFERENCES

1. Chaudhary A et al: Melanotic neuroectodermal tumor of infancy: 2 decades of clinical experience with 18 patients. J Oral Maxillofac Surg. 67(1):47-51, 2009
2. Selim H et al: Melanotic neuroectodermal tumor of infancy: review of literature and case report. J Pediatr Surg. 43(6):E25-9, 2008
3. George JC et al: Melanotic neuroectodermal tumor of infancy. AJNR Am J Neuroradiol. 16(6):1273-5, 1995
4. Borello ED et al: Melanotic neuroectodermal tumor of infancy--a neoplasm of neural crese origin. Report of a case associated with high urinary excretion of vanilmandelic acid. Cancer. 19(2):196-206, 1966

MELANOTIC NEUROECTODERMAL TUMOR OF INFANCY

Clinical, Radiographic, and Microscopic Features

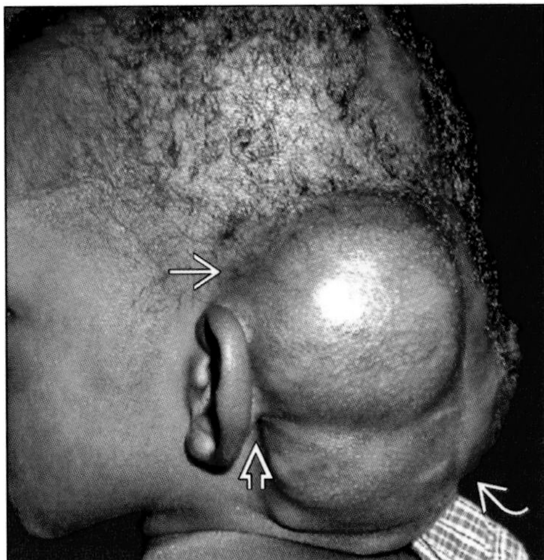

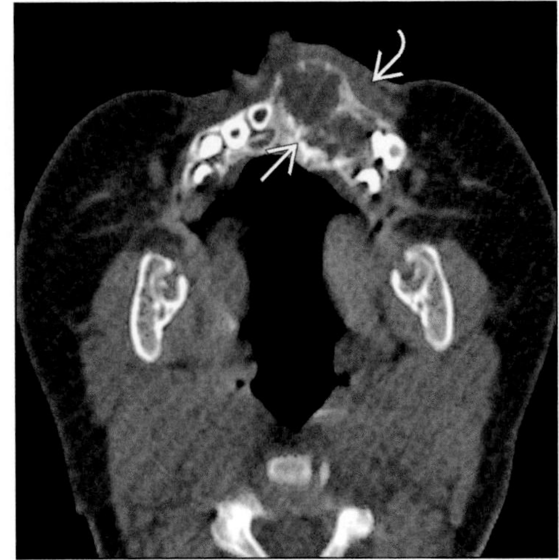

(Left) Clinical photograph shows a huge mass extending toward parietal squama superiorly ➡ and in upper neck inferiorly ➡ behind displaced left ear ➡. The overlying skin looks normal. (Right) Axial bone CT shows most common appearance, location, and patient age for a melanotic neuroectodermal tumor: Maxillary expansion with osteolysis ➡ and adjacent soft tissue changes ➡ in an infant.

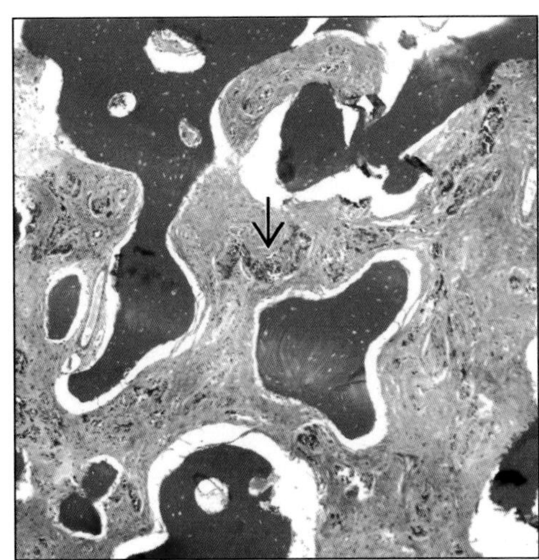

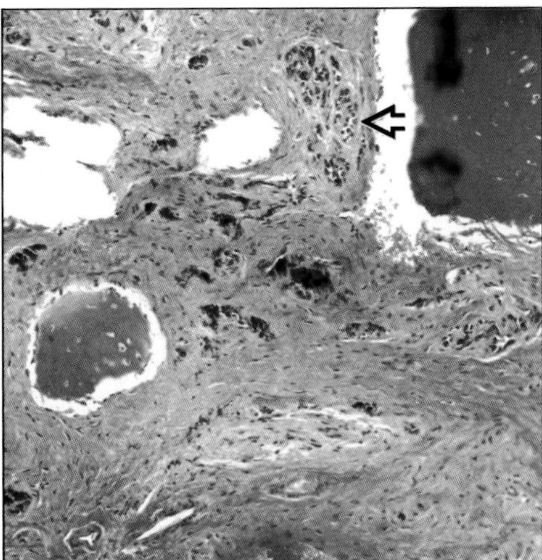

(Left) Pigmented epithelial cells ➡ with focal small neuroblastic cells in a dense fibrous stroma are shown infiltrating the bony trabeculae. (Right) Higher power view shows infiltration of a MNTI infiltrating bone. Note the small scattered pigmented epithelial cells, some of which show glandular formations ➡.

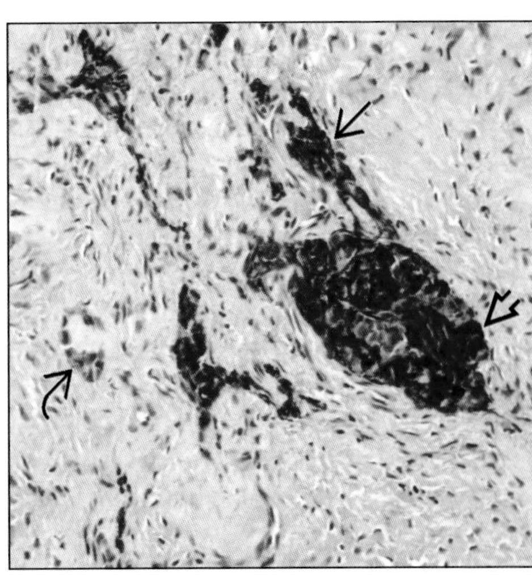

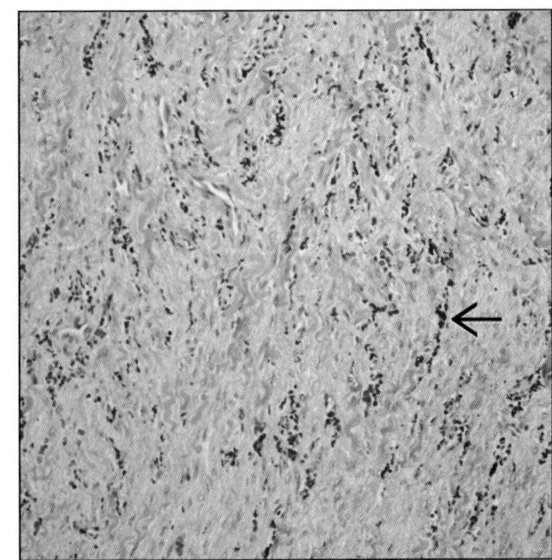

(Left) A mixture of pigmented epithelial cells ➡ and small neuroblastic cells ➡ separated by dense fibrocollagenous stroma show an alveolar pattern of growth in this MNTI. Note the crush artifact in the small hyperchromatic small cells ➡. (Right) H&E shows dense fibrous stroma with scattered small neuroblastic cells arranged individually and in cords ➡ in this MNTI. Note the lack of a prominent epithelial component in this field.

Microscopic Features

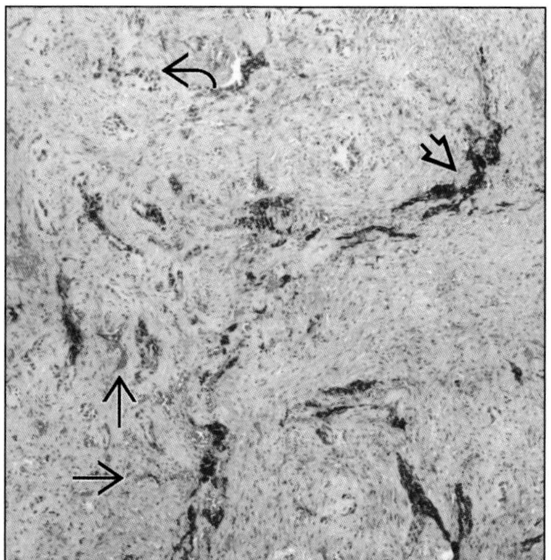

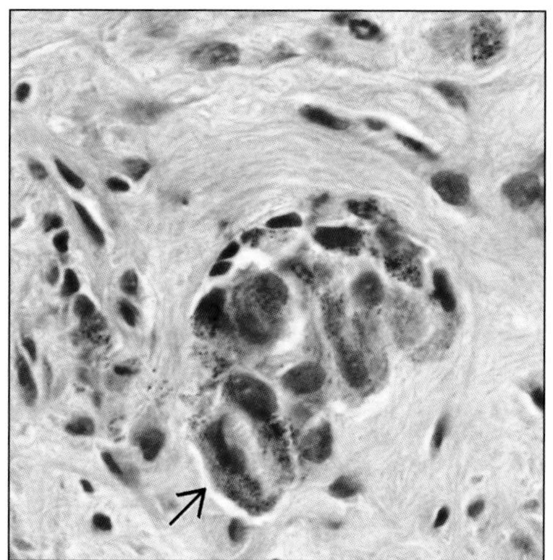

(Left) *Scattered nests of small neuroblastic cells ⇨ show crush artifact and pigmented epithelial cells ⇗. Note the numerous vessels → in the well-vascularized fibrocollagenous stroma that is a frequent feature of MNTI.* ***(Right)*** *High-power view of this MNTI highlights the prominent melanin granules in the abundant eosinophilic cytoplasm of these epithelial cells →. The small neuroblastic cells may or may not be associated with the epithelial cells.*

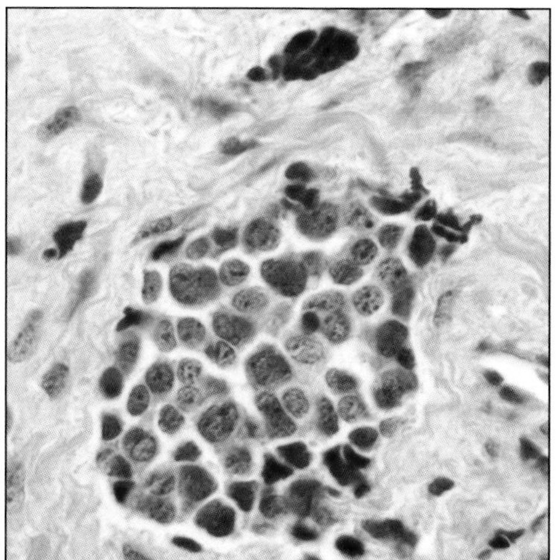

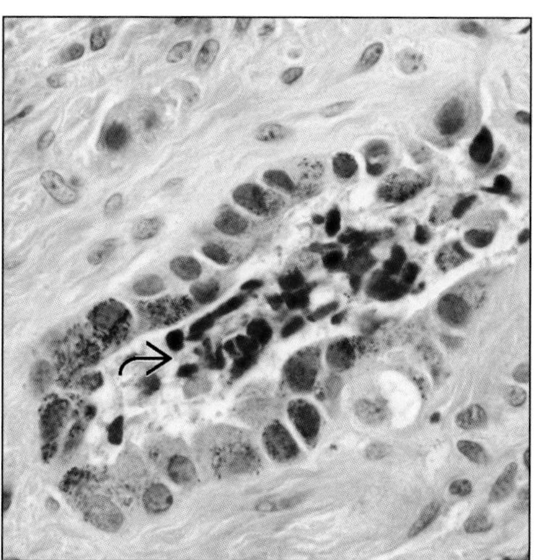

(Left) *High-power view of this nest of small neuroblastic round cells highlights the scant amount of cytoplasm and the small nucleoli with dispersed "salt and pepper" chromatin. Mitotic figures are rarely observed.* ***(Right)*** *High-power view highlights the presence of small neuroblastic cells ⇗ within the lumen of this glandular structure.*

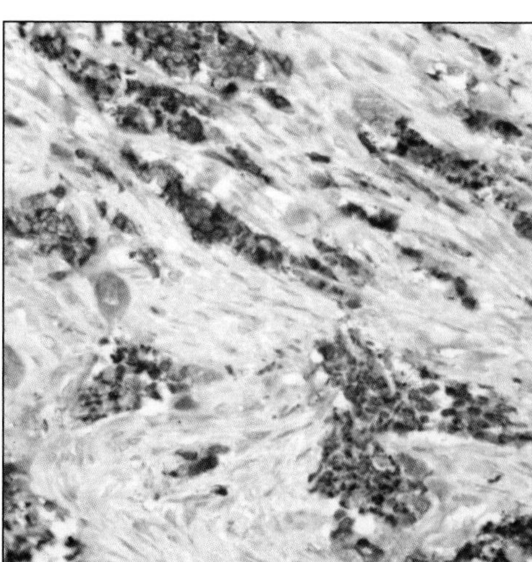

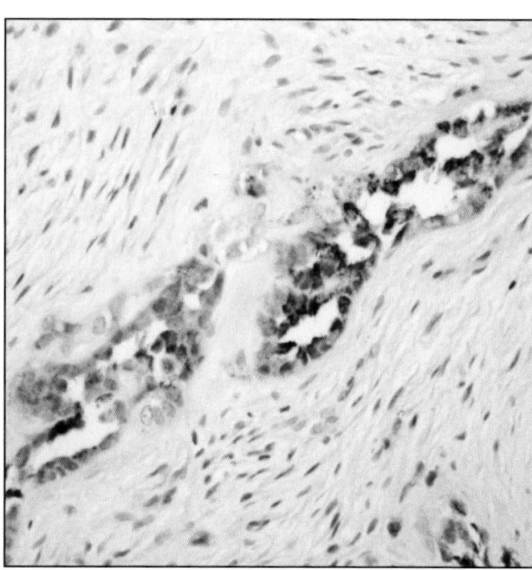

(Left) *Immunohistochemical staining for synaptophysin shows strong cytoplasmic reactivity in both the epithelial and small neuroblastic cellular components.* ***(Right)*** *Immunohistochemical reactivity for HMB-45 is observed in the cytoplasm of the epithelial cells.*

EWING SARCOMA/PNET OF SOFT TISSUE

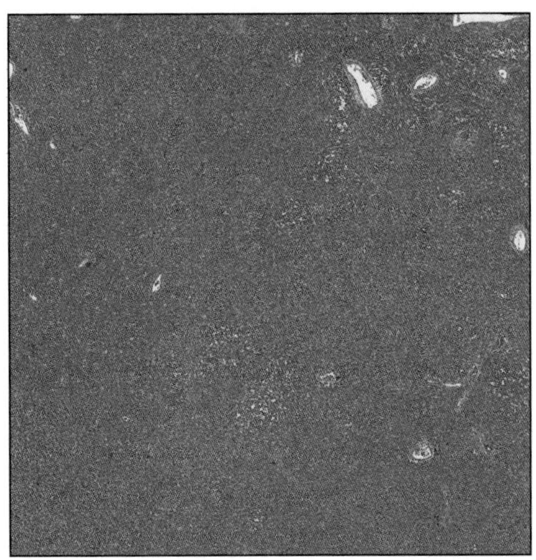

Ewing sarcoma and PNET are usually extremely cellular, with a dense, solid to sheet-like distribution of cells. A delicate vascularity is noted, but overall this is a solid population of cells.

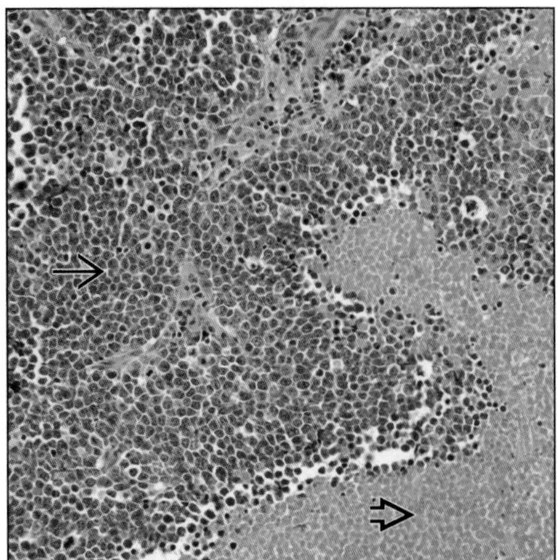

This is a very cellular tumor arranged in a diffuse sheet-like pattern →. Geographic areas of coagulative necrosis are easily identified ⇨. There is often perivascular viable tumor.

TERMINOLOGY

Abbreviations

- Ewing sarcoma (ES)
- Primitive neuroectodermal tumor (PNET)

Definitions

- Family of small round cell translocation-associated sarcomas occurring in bone or soft tissue
  - Extraskeletal ES
  - Small cell tumor of thoracopulmonary region (Askin tumor)
  - PNET of soft tissue
    - Same morphologic spectrum as ES
    - Additionally shows neural differentiation
- Several translocations known
  - Similar changes in all types and sites

CLINICAL ISSUES

Epidemiology

- Incidence
  - Rare
- Age
  - Mostly children and young adults
  - Sporadic cases at any age
- Gender
  - Slight male predominance
- Ethnicity
  - More common in Caucasians
  - Very rare in Africans and African-Americans

Site

- Lung, mediastinum, paravertebral region
- Retroperitoneum, abdominal cavity
- Limbs (deep soft tissue), skin (rare)
  - Primary bone tumor can extend and present in soft tissue
- Rarely in viscera (kidney, uterus, pancreas, larynx)

Presentation

- Painful or painless mass
- Systemic symptoms
  - Fever, anemia, leukocytosis

Treatment

- Options, risks, complications
  - Chemotherapy is treatment of choice
  - Surgical excision of residual masses
  - Irradiation in selected cases
- Drugs
  - Multiagent
    - At least 3 of vincristine, doxorubicin, cyclophosphamide, ifosfamide, etoposide
  - Potential biologic therapies
    - Anti-CD99 antibodies
    - Small interfering RNA against *EWSR1-FLI1* gene product
    - Trastuzumab (against *EGFR2*), figitumumab (against *IGF-1R*)

Prognosis

- 5-year survival: 65-90%
  - 25% in those presenting with metastatic disease
- Locally infiltrative
- Metastasizes to bone, lungs
- Presence of *EWSR1-FLI1* rearrangement is prognostically favorable
- Cutaneous and subcutaneous tumors have improved prognosis

MACROSCOPIC FEATURES

General Features

- Pale friable tumor
- Hemorrhage and necrosis
- Can be cystic

Size

- Variable, up to 20 cm

Key Facts

Terminology
- Family of small round cell translocation-associated sarcomas occurring in bone, soft tissue, or skin
- Additionally, PNET shows neural differentiation

Clinical Issues
- Mostly children and young adults
- Painful or painless mass
- 5-year survival: 65-90%
  - 25% in those presenting with metastatic disease

Microscopic Pathology
- Sheets of closely packed uniform cells
- Round uniform nuclei
  - Scanty cytoplasm, sometimes clear
- Homer-Wright rosette formation in PNET
- Atypical (large cell) variant
  - Conspicuous nucleoli

Ancillary Tests
- PAS stains glycogen in cytoplasm
- Several translocations involving *EWSR1* and *ETS* family genes
  - Most common are *EWSR1-FLI1* (90%) and *EWSR1-ERG* (8-10%)

Top Differential Diagnoses
- Alveolar rhabdomyosarcoma
- Poorly differentiated synovial sarcoma
- Desmoplastic small round cell tumor
- Neuroblastoma
- Small cell carcinoma
- Extraskeletal mesenchymal chondrosarcoma
- Lymphoma

MICROSCOPIC PATHOLOGY

Histologic Features
- Sheets of closely packed uniform cells
- Sometimes divided into lobules
  - Pseudoalveolar pattern
- Round uniform nuclei
- Dispersed fine chromatin, inconspicuous nucleoli
- Scanty cytoplasm
  - Can be clear due to glycogen
- Cells rarely spindled focally
- Homer-Wright rosette formation in PNET
  - Central fibrillary core without lumen
- Minimal intercellular collagen or reticulin
- Rare myxoid change
  - Stromal microcysts sometimes present
- Necrosis frequent
  - Perivascular preservation
- Rare morphologic variants
  - Atypical (large cell) variant
    - Larger, vesicular nuclei
    - Irregular nuclear outline
    - Conspicuous nucleoli
    - Pleomorphism, spindling
  - Adamantinoma-like variant occurs mostly in bone
  - Sclerosing and clear cell variants described

ANCILLARY TESTS

Histochemistry
- PAS
  - Reactivity: Positive for glycogen
  - Staining pattern
    - Cytoplasmic
    - Staining is abolished by pretreatment with diastase
- Reticulin
  - Reactivity: Negative
  - Staining pattern
    - Minimal or no intercellular reticulin except around blood vessels

In Situ Hybridization
- FISH with break-apart probe for *EWSR1* gene (at 22q12) shows rearrangement

Molecular Genetics
- Several balanced translocations and fusions involving *EWSR1* and *ETS* family genes
  - t(11;22)(q24;q12), *EWSR1-FLI* fusion (90% of cases)
  - t(21;22)(q12;q12), *EWSR1-ERG* fusion (5-10% of cases)
  - t(2;22)(q33;q12), *EWSR1-FEV* fusion (< 1% of cases)
  - t(7;22)(p22;q12), *EWSR1-ETV1* (< 1% of cases)
  - t(17;22)(q12;q12), *EWSR1-E1AF* (< 1% of cases)
- Rarely others in occasional cases
- Genetic changes do not correlate with site or morphology

DIFFERENTIAL DIAGNOSIS

Alveolar Rhabdomyosarcoma
- Solid nests
  - Cells with eosinophilic cytoplasm
  - Multinucleated "wreath" cells
- Desmin diffusely positive
- Myogenin positive in nuclei
- *PAX-FOXO1* gene fusions

Poorly Differentiated Synovial Sarcoma
- Nuclei less regular, appear to overlap
- More often a spindle cell component
  - Can be biphasic
- Immunoreactive for TLE1 in nuclei
- t(X;18) with *SS18-SSX* gene fusions

Desmoplastic Small Round Cell Tumor
- Usually intraabdominal, rarely other sites
- Nests of cells in cellular fibrous stroma
- Polyphenotypic
  - Expresses CK, desmin, and neural markers
- CD99(-) in most cases
- WT1(+) (nuclear)
- *EWSR1-WT1* gene fusion

EWING SARCOMA/PNET OF SOFT TISSUE

Immunohistochemistry

Antibody	Reactivity	Staining Pattern	Comment
CD99	Positive	Cell membrane	Positive in almost all cases
Caveolin-1	Positive	Cell membrane & cytoplasm	Positive in 95% of cases, including CD99(-) ones
Bcl-2	Positive	Cytoplasmic	Positive in up to 50% of cases
NSE	Positive	Cytoplasmic	Positive in up to 50% (PNET)
CD57	Positive	Cytoplasmic	Positive (focal dot) in about 55% of cases
Chromogranin-A	Negative	Cytoplasmic	Occasional case shows positivity (PNET)
CD56	Negative	Cytoplasmic	
WT1	Negative	Nuclear & cytoplasmic	
CD45	Negative	Cell membrane	
Myogenin	Negative	Nuclear	
CD34	Negative	Cell membrane	
TLE1	Negative	Nuclear	
CK-PAN	Equivocal	Dot positivity	Occasional dot positivity in up to 20% of cases
Desmin	Equivocal	Cytoplasmic	Positive in about 1% of cases
S100	Equivocal	Nuclear & cytoplasmic	Positive in up to 30% of cases
CD117	Equivocal	Cell membrane	Positive in about 1/3 of cases
Neuroblastoma	Equivocal	Cytoplasmic	Positive in about 25% of cases
NFP	Equivocal	Cytoplasmic	Positive in about 20% (PNET)

Neuroblastoma

- Usually younger than 4 years of age
- Associated with sympathetic ganglia
- Sheets of neuroblasts, variable ganglionic differentiation
- CD99(-)
- Lacks specific translocations of ES

Extraskeletal Mesenchymal Chondrosarcoma

- Marked hemangiopericytomatous pattern
- Focal chondroid formation (can be sparse)
- Lacks specific translocation

Small Cell Carcinoma

- Usually in viscera but can present as metastasis
- Nuclear molding, scanty cytoplasm
- Diffuse (often dot) positivity for CK
- CD56(+)
- TTF1(+) (nuclear)
- CD99(-) in majority of cases
- Lacks specific fusion genes

Lymphoma

- Involvement of lymphoid tissue
  - Lymph node, spleen
- Presence of lymphoid immunohistochemical markers

DIAGNOSTIC CHECKLIST

Clinically Relevant Pathologic Features

- Age distribution
- Symptom complex

Pathologic Interpretation Pearls

- Sheets of uniform rounded cells
- Diffuse membranous positivity for CD99
- Minimal or no intercellular reticulin
- Specific genetic abnormalities

SELECTED REFERENCES

1. Mackintosh C et al: The molecular pathogenesis of Ewing's sarcoma. Cancer Biol Ther. 9(9), 2010
2. Llombart-Bosch A et al: Histological heterogeneity of Ewing's sarcoma/PNET: an immunohistochemical analysis of 415 genetically confirmed cases with clinical support. Virchows Arch. 455(5):397-411, 2009
3. Machado I et al: Molecular diagnosis of Ewing sarcoma family of tumors: a comparative analysis of 560 cases with FISH and RT-PCR. Diagn Mol Pathol. 18(4):189-99, 2009
4. Ordóñez JL et al: Advances in Ewing's sarcoma research: where are we now and what lies ahead? Cancer Res. 69(18):7140-50, 2009
5. Ludwig JA: Ewing sarcoma: historical perspectives, current state-of-the-art, and opportunities for targeted therapy in the future. Curr Opin Oncol. 20(4):412-8, 2008
6. Jambhekar NA et al: Comparative analysis of routine histology, immunohistochemistry, reverse transcriptase polymerase chain reaction, and fluorescence in situ hybridization in diagnosis of Ewing family of tumors. Arch Pathol Lab Med. 130(12):1813-8, 2006
7. Folpe AL et al: Morphologic and immunophenotypic diversity in Ewing family tumors: a study of 66 genetically confirmed cases. Am J Surg Pathol. 29(8):1025-33, 2005
8. Navarro S et al: Atypical pleomorphic extraosseous ewing tumor/peripheral primitive neuroectodermal tumor with unusual phenotypic/genotypic profile. Diagn Mol Pathol. 11(1):9-15, 2002
9. Llombart-Bosch A et al: Immunohistochemical detection of EWS and FLI-1 proteins in Ewing sarcoma and primitive neuroectodermal tumors: comparative analysis with CD99 (MIC-2) expression. Appl Immunohistochem Mol Morphol. 9(3):255-60, 2001
10. Folpe AL et al: Immunohistochemical detection of FLI-1 protein expression: a study of 132 round cell tumors with emphasis on CD99-positive mimics of Ewing's sarcoma/ primitive neuroectodermal tumor. Am J Surg Pathol. 24(12):1657-62, 2000

Microscopic Features

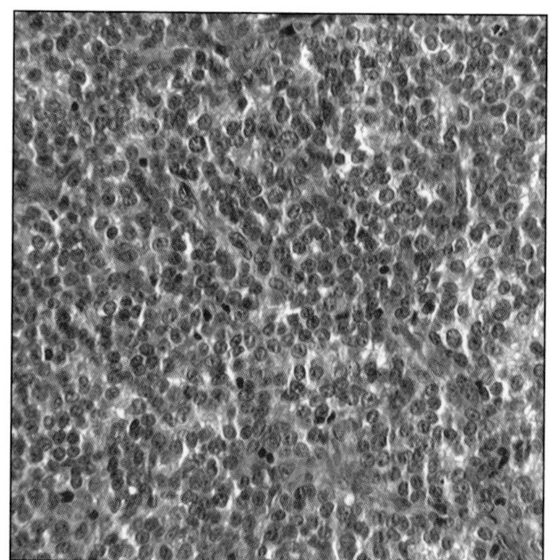

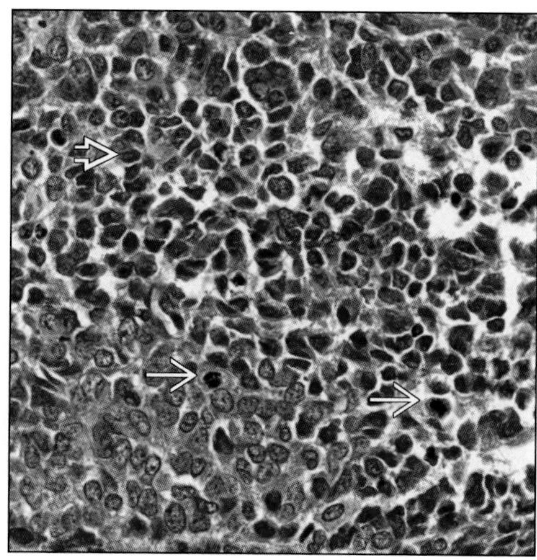

(Left) *There is a vaguely lobular appearance to this monotonous tumor cell population. The cells have round nuclei with small and inconspicuous nucleoli. There are occasional small blood vessels but no prominent pattern.* ***(Right)*** *This tumor is beginning to undergo degeneration with a number of apoptotic bodies ➡. Mitoses ➡ are also easily identified throughout the tumor, which can aid in the diagnostic separation from other tumor types.*

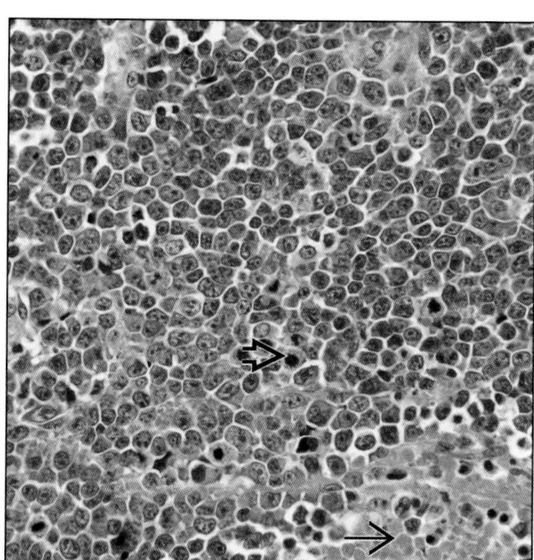

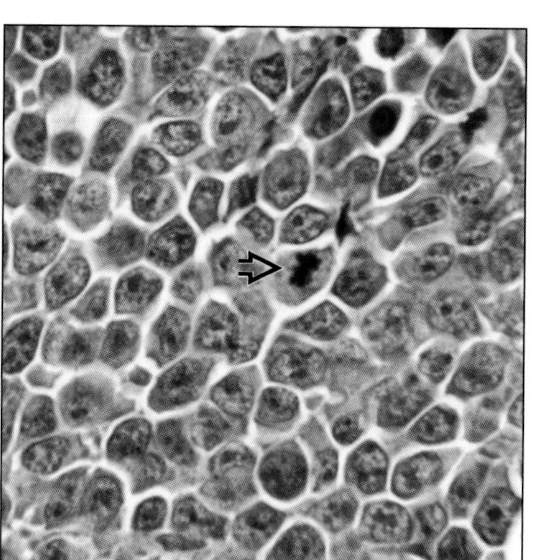

(Left) *The cells do not really show distinct cell borders but are apparently arranged in a syncytium. There are areas of coagulative necrosis ➡ and a number of apoptotic bodies ➡ and mitotic figures.* ***(Right)*** *Higher magnification shows a relatively uniform population of medium cells with high nuclear to cytoplasmic ratio. The nuclei are round to slightly irregular with dispersed, fine chromatin distribution and small nucleoli. Mitotic figures are present ➡.*

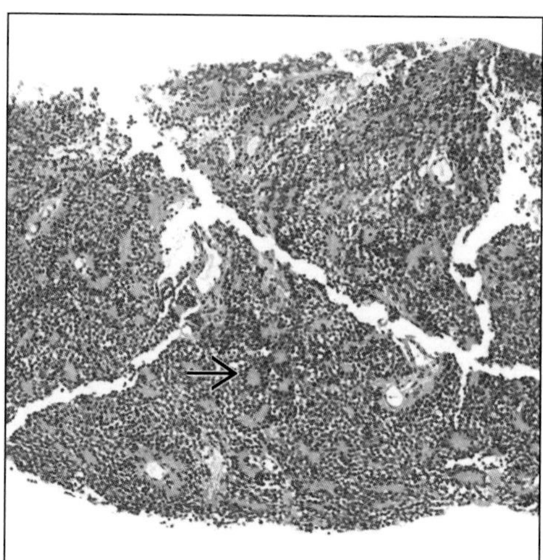

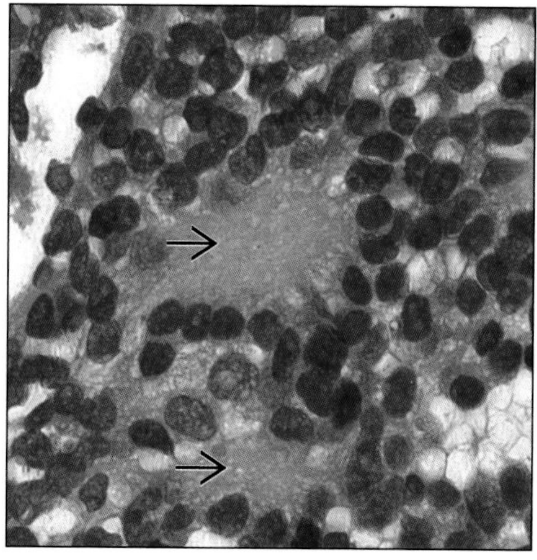

(Left) *Core biopsy specimen of primitive neuroectodermal tumor shows sheets of small round cells with formation of scattered rosettes ➡, a feature of some PNETs. Ewing sarcoma is undifferentiated and lacks neural features.* ***(Right)*** *Higher magnification shows Homer-Wright rosettes, in which the cells are arranged around a core of fibrillary material ➡ without formation of a central lumen. Cell boundaries are indistinct.*

EWING SARCOMA/PNET OF SOFT TISSUE

Variant Microscopic Features

*(**Left**) H&E shows Ewing sarcoma displaying a sheet of neoplastic cells with no particular pattern. The cells are medium-sized and have a high nuclear to cytoplasmic ratio. The nuclear chromatin is evenly distributed, and there are numerous mitotic figures. (**Right**) This is an example of large cell (atypical) Ewing sarcoma, arising at the ankle in a 12-year-old girl. The cells are larger than usual, with some variation in size, and many have prominent nucleoli ⇒.*

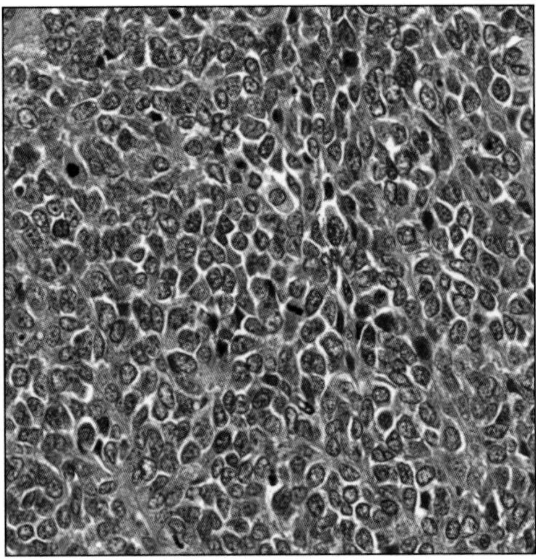

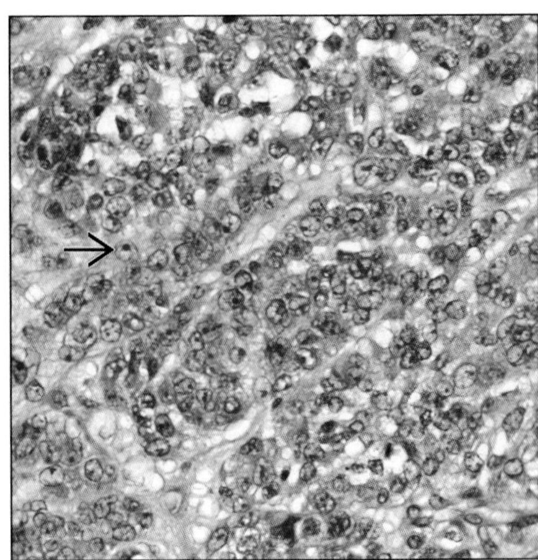

*(**Left**) This section shows an unusual variant of Ewing sarcoma with myxoid change resulting in separation of tumor cells into irregular cords or small nests. (**Right**) A rare feature of Ewing sarcoma is the presence of focal spindle cell morphology ⇒, seen here merging with more typical round cells ⇨ in an area of myxoid stromal change with hemorrhage. Spindling is more frequently seen in the large cell atypical variant.*

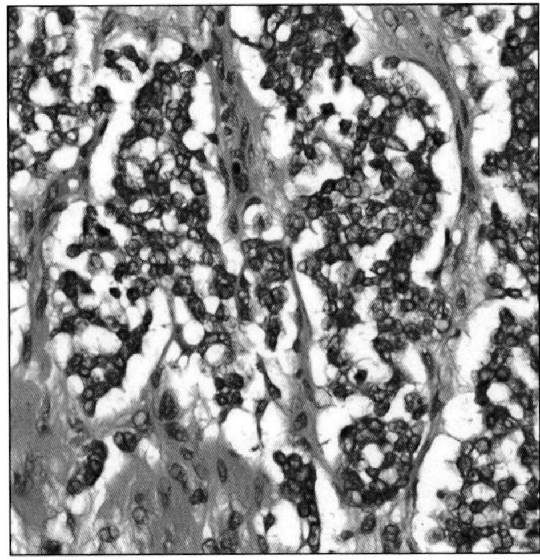

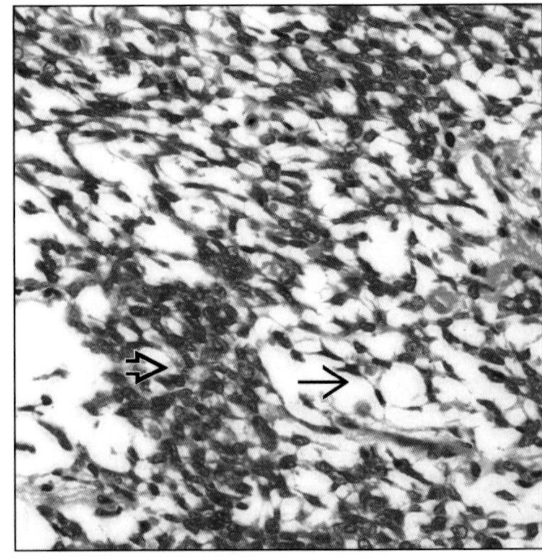

*(**Left**) Clearing of the cytoplasm of tumor cells can be a focal or diffuse feature in some examples of Ewing sarcoma. It reflects the presence of abundant glycogen. (**Right**) After chemotherapy there is shrinkage ⇨ and loss of tumor cells, with edema ⇒ and later fibrosis of the stroma. Large areas of necrosis can also result.*

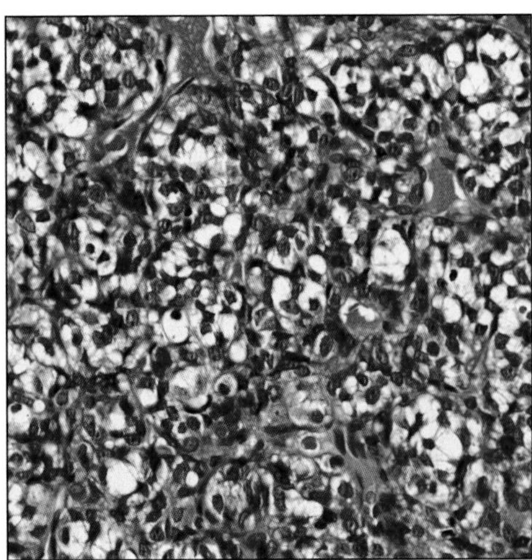

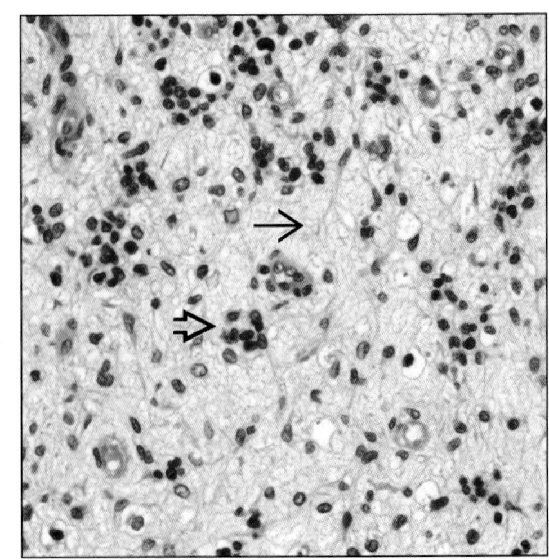

Ancillary Techniques

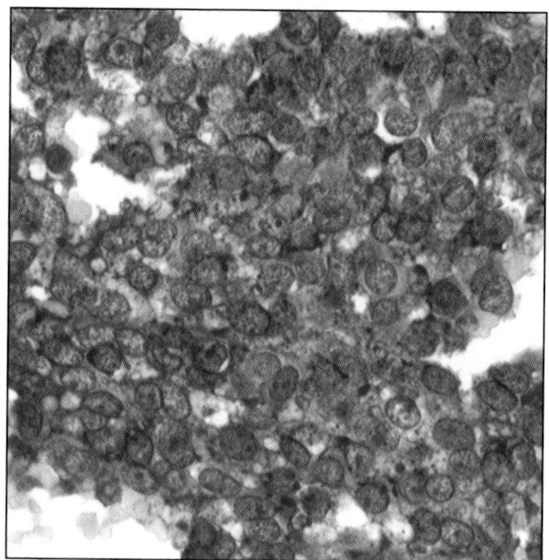

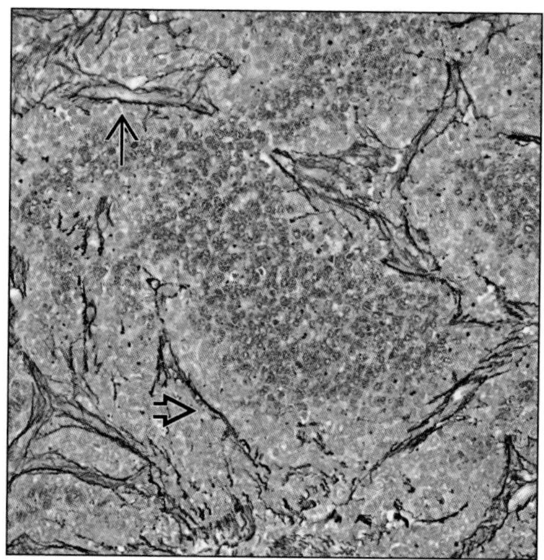

(Left) *The cytoplasm can contain abundant glycogen, demonstrable as magenta staining by PAS and removed by pretreatment with diastase. This is not specific as glycogen occurs in other tumors, notably rhabdomyosarcoma.* ***(Right)*** *This image demonstrates no reticulin deposition between neoplastic cells. Reticulin fibers are seen around blood vessels → or delineating tumor lobules ⇨. In poorly differentiated synovial sarcoma, reticulin often surrounds small groups of cells.*

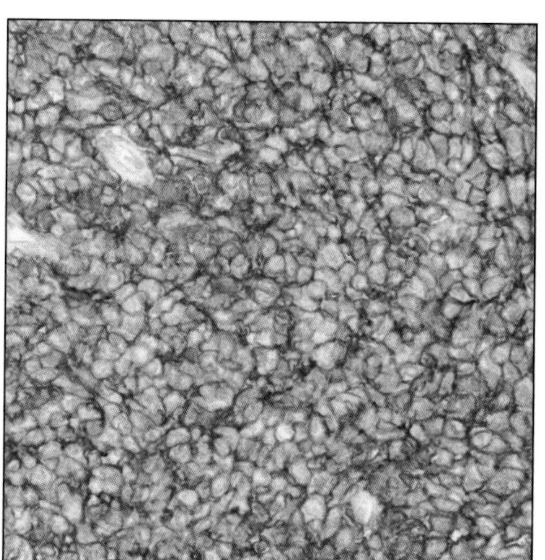

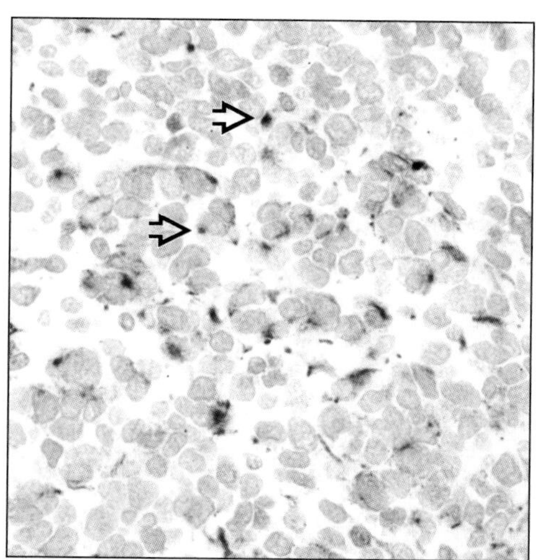

(Left) *There is a strong, diffuse membranous staining for CD99 (MIC2). Although several other small round cell tumors can display focal positivity, this diffuse pattern is typical of Ewing sarcoma.* ***(Right)*** *This PNET has rare focal dot positivity for cytokeratin ⇨. This can also be seen in desmoplastic small round cell tumor, small cell carcinoma, and synovial sarcoma. A panel of immunohistochemical markers should always be used, with molecular analysis where appropriate.*

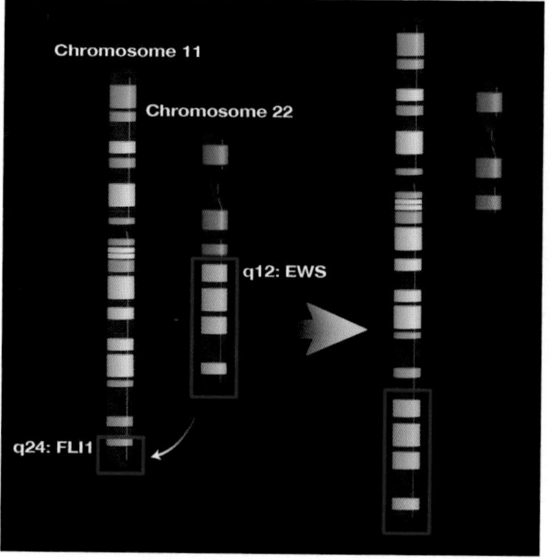

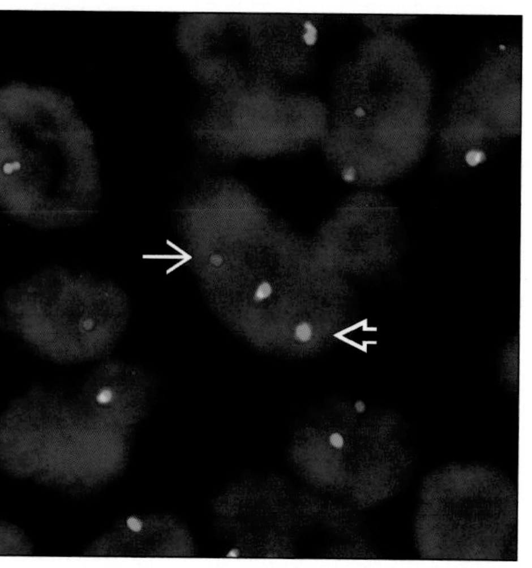

(Left) *Graphic depicts the t(11;22)(q24;q12) translocation between the carboxy-terminal domain of FLI1 (11q24) and the EWS gene amino-terminal domain (22q12), resulting in EWS-FLI1 fusion gene.* ***(Right)*** *In this fluorescence in situ hybridization (FISH) preparation, dual color break-apart probes are used for the EWSR1 gene on chromosome 22. In the nucleus of a tumor cell, split red → & green ⇨ signals, instead of a fused yellow one, indicate a translocation involving EWSR1.*

NEUROBLASTOMA AND GANGLIONEUROBLASTOMA

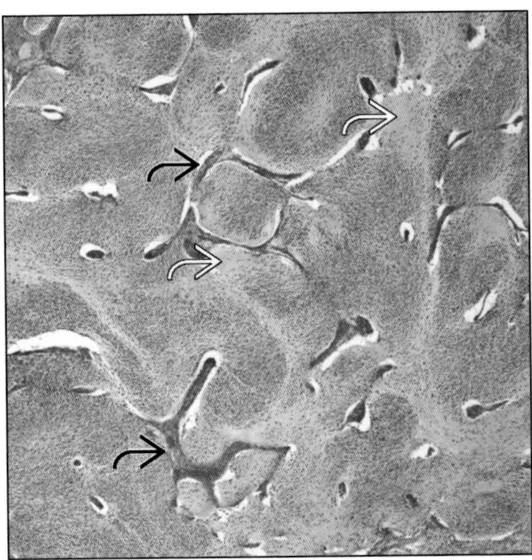

This low-power view of a poorly differentiated neuroblastoma shows thin septa of schwannian stroma ➔. Pale, eosinophilic neuropil ➔ is seen in places between the nodules or nests of neuroblastoma cells.

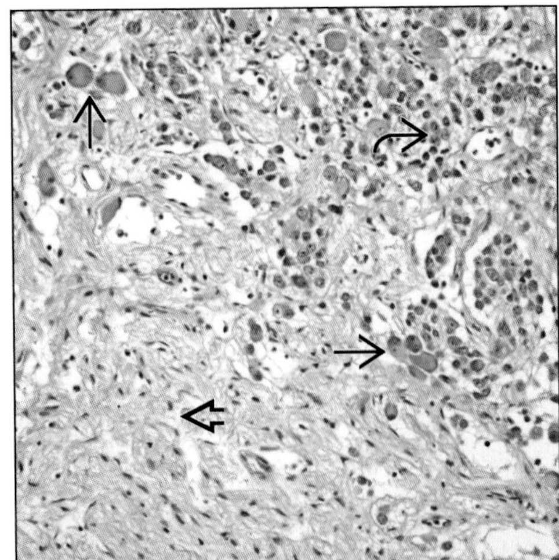

A typical intermixed ganglioneuroblastoma is seen in this image. The tumor is composed of a mixture of maturing ganglion cells ➔, neuroblasts ➔, and abundant schwannian stroma ➔.

TERMINOLOGY

Abbreviations

- Neuroblastoma (NB)
- Ganglioneuroblastoma (GNB)

Synonyms

- Schwannian stroma-poor neuroblastic tumor (neuroblastoma)
- Schwannian stroma-rich neuroblastic tumor (ganglioneuroblastoma)

Definitions

- Malignant tumor derived from primordial neural crest cells
- On maturational spectrum of neuroblastic tumors
  - NB is least differentiated
  - GNB is moderately differentiated
  - Ganglioneuroma (GN) is well-differentiated, benign

ETIOLOGY/PATHOGENESIS

Developmental Anomaly

- Derived from primordial neural crest cells
  - These cells migrate from spinal cord to adrenal medulla and sympathetic ganglia

CLINICAL ISSUES

Epidemiology

- Incidence
  - About 1 in 10,000 children
  - 3rd most common malignant tumor in children
    - Most common extracranial solid tumor in children
  - Usually sporadic
    - Some autosomal dominant familial cases have been seen
  - Screening not recommended
- Age
  - Half of patients diagnosed by age 2 years
  - 90% diagnosed by age 5 years
  - About 1/4 are congenital, with some detected prenatally on ultrasound
- Gender
  - Slight male predominance
- Ethnicity
  - Less common in African-Americans

Site

- Follows distribution of sympathetic ganglia
  - Paramidline from base of skull to pelvis
  - Most common in abdomen and retroperitoneum
- Adrenal medulla
- Dorsal root ganglia
- Metastases
  - Bone
  - Lymph nodes
  - Liver
  - Skin

Presentation

- Depends on age of patient, location of tumor, and associated clinical syndromes
- Most have nonspecific symptoms
  - Fever, weight loss, diarrhea, anemia, hypertension
- Fetuses may have hydrops
- Palpable mass in about half
- About 2/3 have metastases on presentation
- "Blueberry muffin" baby
  - Blue-red cutaneous masses in infants
- Myoclonus-opsoclonus syndrome
  - Associated with good prognosis
  - Rapid, alternating eye movements and myoclonic movements of extremities
  - Resolves with tumor eradication
- Other associated syndromes include
  - Myasthenia gravis
  - Beckwith-Wiedemann syndrome

NEUROBLASTOMA AND GANGLIONEUROBLASTOMA

Key Facts

Terminology

- Malignant tumor derived from primordial neural crest cells

Clinical Issues

- 3rd most common malignant tumor in children
- 90% diagnosed by age 5 years
- Follows distribution of sympathetic ganglia, also adrenal medulla
- Presentation depends on age of patient, location of tumor, and associated clinical syndromes
- Urine catecholamines elevated in 95% of patients with neuroblastoma (NB)

Microscopic Pathology

- International Neuroblastoma Pathology Committee Classification
  - Undifferentiated NB
  - Poorly differentiated NB
  - Differentiating NB
  - Nodular GNB
  - Intermixed GNB
- Mitotic-karyorrhectic index (MKI)

Ancillary Tests

- N-myc amplification is associated with worse prognosis

Top Differential Diagnoses

- Alveolar rhabdomyosarcoma (ARMS)
- Ewing sarcoma/primitive neuroectodermal tumor (PNET)
- Ganglioneuroma
- Lymphoma

  - Cushing syndrome
  - Neurofibromatosis
  - Fetal hydantoin syndrome
  - Hirschsprung disease

Laboratory Tests

- Urine catecholamines (elevated in 95% of patients with NB)
  - Epinephrine
  - Norepinephrine
  - Homovanillic acid (HVA)
  - Vanillylmandelic acid (VMA)
    - VMA/HVA ratio > 1.5 is associated with better prognosis
- Lactate dehydrogenase
  - > 1500 IU/L associated with worse clinical outcome
- Ferritin
  - > 142 ng/mL associated with worse clinical outcome
- Neuron-specific enolase (NSE)
  - > 100 ng/mL associated with worse clinical outcome

Natural History

- 1-2% will spontaneously regress
  - Most in children under age 1 year
- NB can metastasize widely via lymphatics and vessels

Treatment

- Low risk
  - Surgery or observation alone
- Intermediate risk
  - Surgery and adjuvant chemotherapy
- High risk
  - Induction chemotherapy
  - Delayed tumor resection
  - Radiation of primary site
  - Myeloablative chemotherapy with stem cell recovery

Prognosis

- Favorable prognostic factors
  - Age < 1.5 years at diagnosis
  - Favorable histology
  - Stage 1, 2, or 4S
    - Related to location of tumor
  - No N-myc amplification
  - Hyperdiploidy
  - No loss of 1p
  - High expression of TrKA
  - Normal serum ferritin, NSE, and LDH
  - Urinary VMA/HVA ratio > 1.5

IMAGE FINDINGS

General Features

- Extensive radiographic evaluation is required to determine extent of disease and identify metastatic foci
- Calcifications often seen in central portion of tumor

Bone Scan

- Radiolabeled metaiodobenzylguanidine (MIBG) incorporates into catecholamine-secreting cells and can detect neuroblastoma

MACROSCOPIC FEATURES

General Features

- **Neuroblastoma**
  - Fine membranous capsules
  - Cut surface is soft, fleshy, often with hemorrhage and necrosis
- **Ganglioneuroblastoma**
  - Cut surface is firm, gray-white
  - Nodular GNB must have grossly visible, usually hemorrhagic nodules
  - Intermixed GNB can look like NB or GN depending on extent of differentiation

Size

- Average: 6-8 cm diameter

MICROSCOPIC PATHOLOGY

Histologic Features

- Neuroblasts

- Small round blue cells
- Very little cytoplasm
- Homer-Wright pseudorosette
  - Neuroblasts forming a ring around central core of cytoplasmic processes
- Ganglionic differentiation
  - Cells enlarge
  - Increased eosinophilic or amphophilic cytoplasm
  - Nuclear chromatin pattern becomes vesicular
  - Must have synchronous differentiation of cytoplasm and nucleus
- Neuropil
  - Fibrillar eosinophilic matrix
- Mitotic-karyorrhectic index (MKI)
  - Count of cells undergoing mitosis or karyorrhexis, per 5,000 cells
    - Can be estimated
  - Low: < 100 cells per 5,000
  - Intermediate: 100-200 cells per 5,000
  - High: > 200 cells per 5,000

International Neuroblastoma Pathology Committee (INPC) Classification

- a.k.a. Shimada classification
- **Undifferentiated NB**
  - No ganglionic differentiation
  - No neuropil
  - No or minimal schwannian stroma
  - Often requires immunohistochemistry for accurate diagnosis
- **Poorly differentiated NB**
  - < 5% of tumor cells showing ganglionic differentiation
  - Neuropil background
  - No or minimal schwannian stroma
- **Differentiating NB**
  - > 5% of tumor cells showing ganglionic differentiation
  - Usually more abundant neuropil
  - Usually more prominent schwannian stroma
    - Must be < 50%
- **Nodular GNB**
  - Grossly identifiable nodules will be neuroblastoma
  - Abrupt demarcation between stroma-poor neuroblastoma and stroma-rich component
  - Fibrous pseudocapsule often seen surrounding NB component
  - > 50% schwannian stroma
- **Intermixed GNB**
  - Microscopic nests of neuroblastoma within schwannian stroma
  - > 50% schwannian stroma
- Do not classify post-treatment resections
  - "Neuroblastoma with treatment effect" is sufficient
- May classify metastatic disease if resection/biopsy is pre-treatment

ANCILLARY TESTS

Immunohistochemistry

- Neuron-specific enolase (NSE)
  - Most sensitive but least specific
  - Is found at least focally even in very undifferentiated NBs
- NB84(+) in almost all NBs
  - Not specific; occasionally positive in other small round cell tumors
- S100 protein
  - Positive in schwannian stroma
- Other useful positive immunostains include
  - Chromogranin
  - Synaptophysin
  - Protein gene product 9.5 (PGP9.5)
  - CD56

Cytogenetics

- *MYCN*
  - Amplification is associated with worse prognosis
  - Usually seen in advanced disease
- DNA ploidy
  - Near-diploidy or tetraploidy is associated with worse prognosis
  - Hyperdiploidy is associated with better prognosis
- Loss of heterozygosity of 1p and 11q
  - Both associated with worse prognosis
- TrkA (high-affinity nerve growth factor receptor)
  - Increased expression associates with better prognosis

Electron Microscopy

- Wide range of cytologic differentiation
- Dense core of neurosecretory granules
    - Found in elongated cell processes
    - 100 nm in diameter
    - Dense core surrounded by clear halos and delicate outer membranes

DIFFERENTIAL DIAGNOSIS

Alveolar Rhabdomyosarcoma (ARMS)

- Clinical presentations may be similar
- More marked alveolar pattern except in solid variant
- More pleomorphism
- Cells have more abundant cytoplasm than NB
- Diffuse immunoreactivity for desmin in cytoplasm
- Myogenin(+) in nuclei
- Characteristic t(1;13) or t(2;13) with *PAX-FOXO1* fusions

Ewing Sarcoma/Primitive Neuroectodermal Tumor (PNET)

- Usually in older patients
- Cells have finely stippled chromatin and glycogen-filled cytoplasm
- CD99 usually shows diffuse membranous immunoreactivity
- Specific gene fusions, most commonly *EWSR1-FLI1*

Lymphoma

- Lacks NSE, synaptophysin, and chromogranin
- Has confirmatory lymphoid markers
  - CD45, CD3, CD20
  - TdT in lymphoblastic lymphoma

Favorable vs. Unfavorable Histology in Neuroblastic Tumors

Classification	Subclass	MKI	Age at Diagnosis	Histologic Category
Neuroblastoma (NB)	Undifferentiated	Any MKI	Any age	Unfavorable histology
	Poorly differentiated	High MKI	Any age	Unfavorable histology
		Low or intermediate MKI	> 1.5 years	Unfavorable histology
			< 1.5 years	Favorable histology
	Differentiating	High MKI	Any age	Unfavorable histology
		Intermediate MKI	> 1.5 years	Unfavorable histology
			< 1.5 years	Favorable histology
		Low MKI	> 5 years	Unfavorable histology
			< 5 years	Favorable histology
Ganglioneuroblastoma (GNB)	Nodular	**	**	Unfavorable or favorable
	Intermixed	N/A	Any age	Favorable histology
Ganglioneuroma (GN)	Mature or maturing	N/A	Any age	Favorable histology

***The determination of favorable vs. unfavorable histology in nodular GNB is based on the NB component. MKI = mitosis-karyorrhexis index; N/A = not applicable.*

Prognosis Based on N-myc Amplification and Histology

N-myc Amplification	Favorable Histology	Unfavorable Histology
N-myc nonamplified	Excellent prognosis	Poor prognosis
N-myc amplified	Rare	Extremely poor prognosis

Neuroblastoma Staging System

Stage	Definition
1	Localized tumor; complete gross resection; ipsilateral nodes negative
2A	Localized tumor; incomplete gross resection; nonadherent ipsilateral nodes negative
2B	Localized tumor with or without complete gross resection; nonadherent ipsilateral nodes positive
3	Unresectable tumor that crosses midline with or without positive nodes; or localized tumor with positive contralateral nodes
4	Distant metastases to nodes, bone, bone marrow, liver, skin, &/or other organs not stage 4S
4S	Localized primary tumor (stage 1 or 2) with metastases limited to skin, liver, &/or bone marrow

Maturing Ganglioneuroma

- Differs from intermixed GNB in having single cells instead of nests of cells within schwannian stroma

SELECTED REFERENCES

1. Maris JM: Recent advances in neuroblastoma. N Engl J Med. 362(23):2202-11, 2010
2. Ambros PF et al: International consensus for neuroblastoma molecular diagnostics: report from the International Neuroblastoma Risk Group (INRG) Biology Committee. Br J Cancer. 100(9):1471-82, 2009
3. Cohn SL et al: The International Neuroblastoma Risk Group (INRG) classification system: an INRG Task Force report. J Clin Oncol. 27(2):289-97, 2009
4. Chan EL et al: Favorable histology, MYCN-amplified 4S neonatal neuroblastoma. Pediatr Blood Cancer. 48(4):479-82, 2007
5. Tornóczky T et al: Pathology of peripheral neuroblastic tumors: significance of prominent nucleoli in undifferentiated/poorly differentiated neuroblastoma. Pathol Oncol Res. 13(4):269-75, 2007
6. Sano H et al: International neuroblastoma pathology classification adds independent prognostic information beyond the prognostic contribution of age. Eur J Cancer. 42(8):1113-9, 2006
7. Shimada H et al: TrkA expression in peripheral neuroblastic tumors: prognostic significance and biological relevance. Cancer. 101(8):1873-81, 2004
8. Tornóczky T et al: Large cell neuroblastoma: a distinct phenotype of neuroblastoma with aggressive clinical behavior. Cancer. 100(2):390-7, 2004
9. Peuchmaur M et al: Revision of the International Neuroblastoma Pathology Classification: confirmation of favorable and unfavorable prognostic subsets in ganglioneuroblastoma, nodular. Cancer. 98(10):2274-81, 2003
10. Shimada H: The International Neuroblastoma Pathology Classification. Pathologica. 95(5):240-1, 2003
11. Goto S et al: Histopathology (International Neuroblastoma Pathology Classification) and MYCN status in patients with peripheral neuroblastic tumors: a report from the Children's Cancer Group. Cancer. 92(10):2699-708, 2001
12. Shimada H et al: International neuroblastoma pathology classification for prognostic evaluation of patients with peripheral neuroblastic tumors: a report from the Children's Cancer Group. Cancer. 92(9):2451-61, 2001

NEUROBLASTOMA AND GANGLIONEUROBLASTOMA

Diagrammatic, Radiographic, and Gross Features

*(**Left**) This graphic shows the anatomic extent of the sympathetic chain ➡ (including adrenal gland) from cervical region through mediastinum and abdomen to the inferior pelvis. Neuroblastoma can arise anywhere along the sympathetic chain. (**Right**) Coronal T2-weighted MR in a patient with ganglioneuroblastoma shows a mildly hyperintense posterior mediastinal mass ➡ with no abnormality in the adjacent osseous marrow signal.*

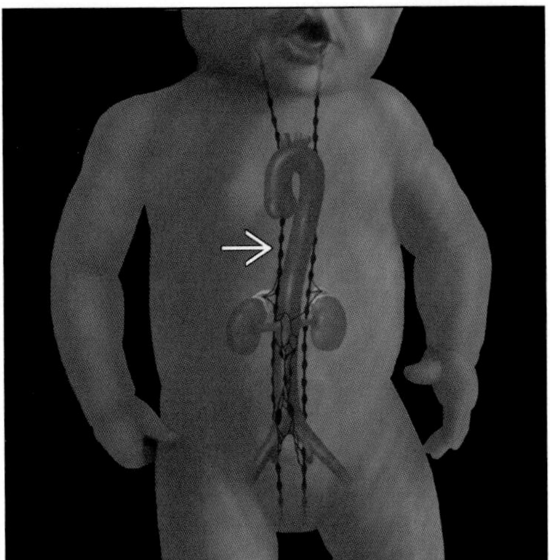

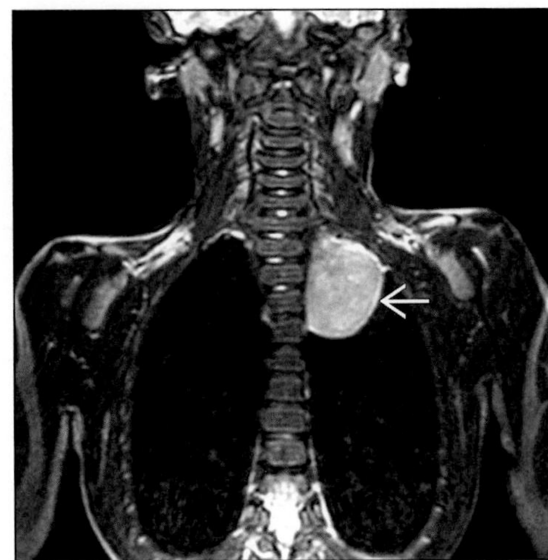

*(**Left**) Gross pathology shows a large circumscribed mass ➡ arising from the adrenal gland and compressing the upper pole of the subjacent kidney ➡. Neuroblastoma is often grossly hemorrhagic with areas of necrosis and calcification seen on sectioning the specimen. (**Right**) This coronal T2-weighted MR shows a neuroblastoma ➡ of the left adrenal gland with an area of central necrosis ➡.*

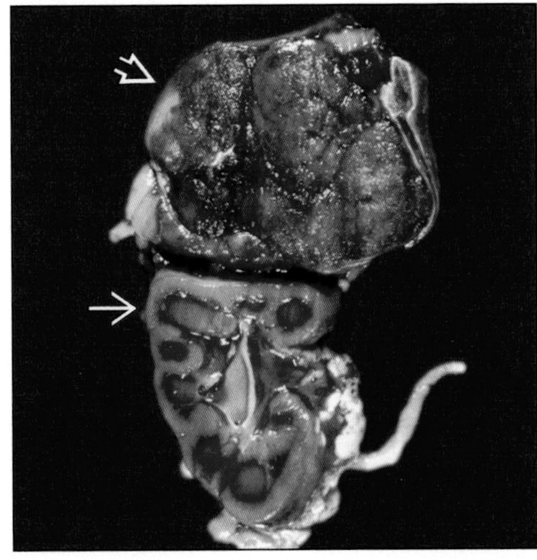

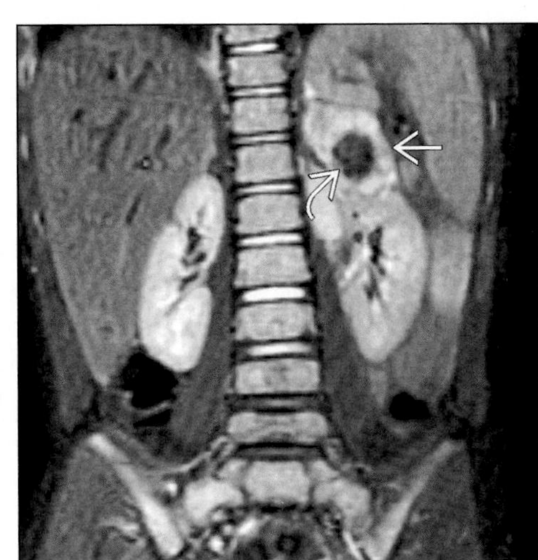

*(**Left**) This specimen of liver shows diffuse involvement and extensive replacement by multiple deposits of metastatic neuroblastoma. There are several foci of hemorrhage. (**Right**) This axial T2-weighted MR shows a left adrenal mass ➡, which proved to be a neuroblastoma. It was widely metastatic; the liver was filled with multiple high signal nodular lesions ➡, with little normal remaining hepatic parenchyma.*

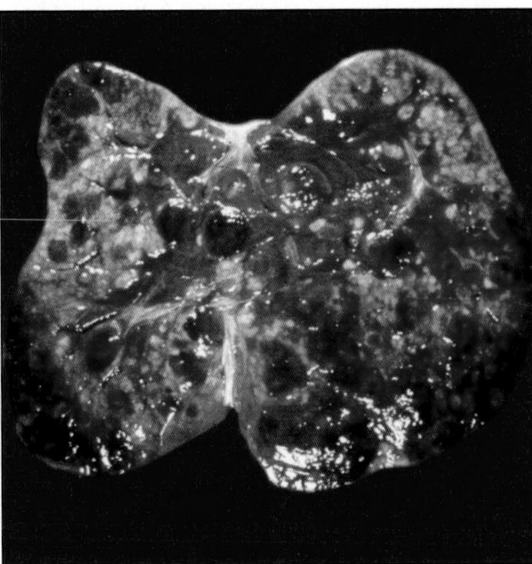

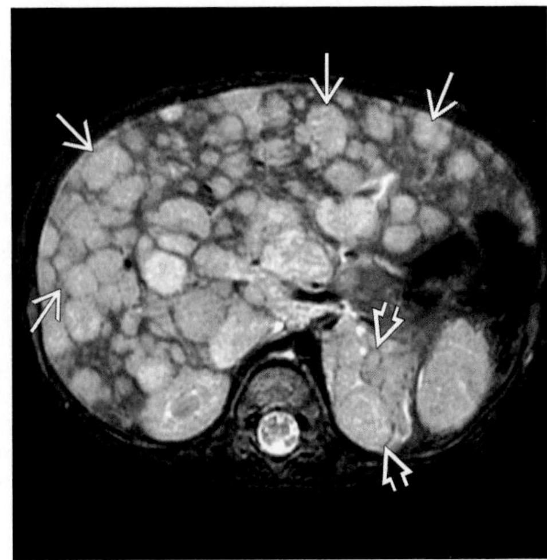

Microscopic Features

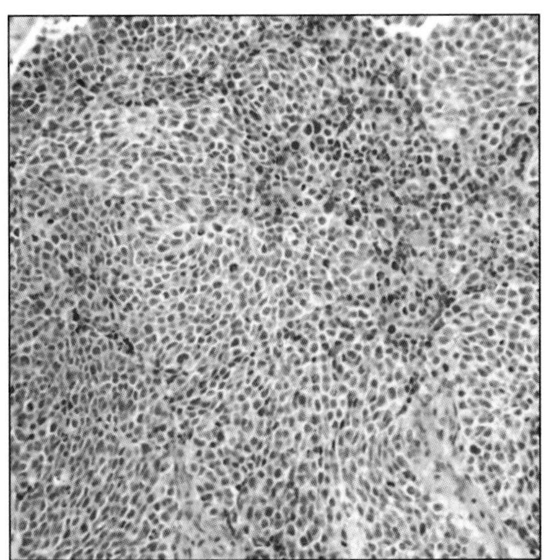

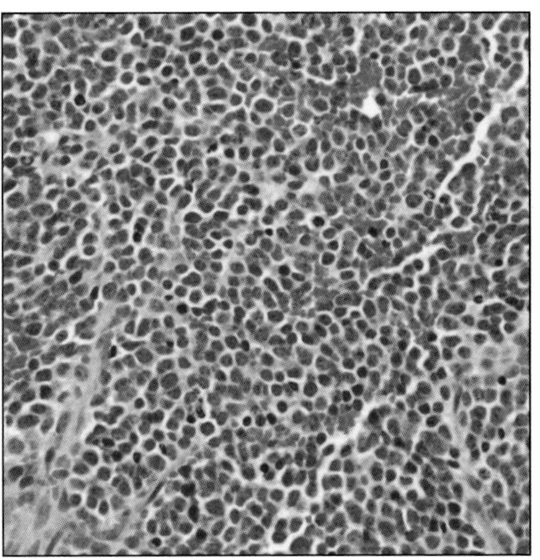

(Left) *The typical appearance of an undifferentiated neuroblastoma is a small round cell tumor without histologic differentiation. Immunohistochemistry is required to make the diagnosis and to exclude other neoplasms.* ***(Right)*** *In undifferentiated neuroblastoma, the cells have scant cytoplasm and rounded, deeply staining nuclei. On H&E, this could be mistaken for Ewing sarcoma, alveolar rhabdomyosarcoma, or lymphoma.*

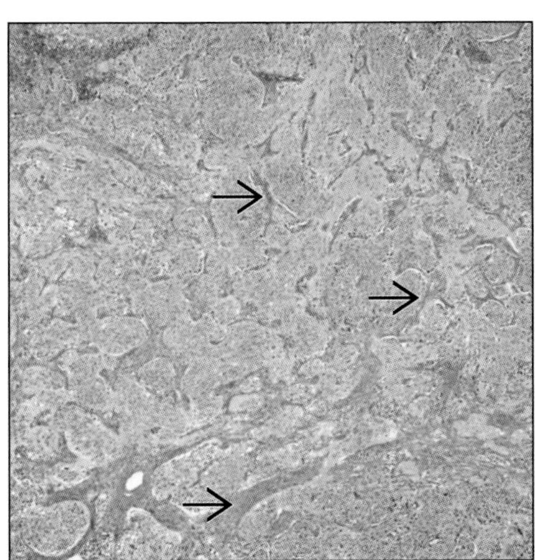

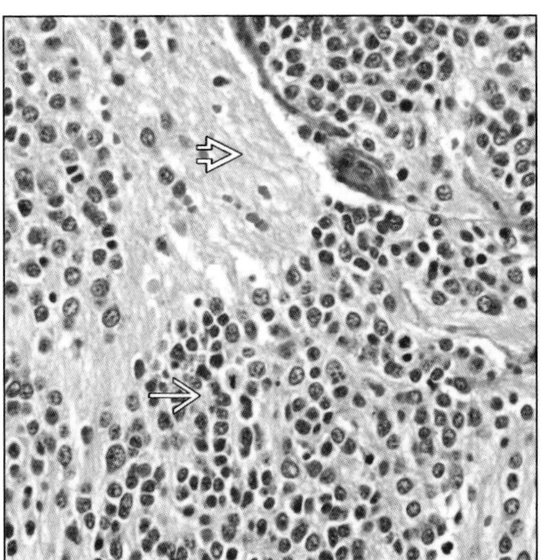

(Left) *This image shows the typical low-power appearance of a poorly differentiated neuroblastoma. Small strips of schwannian stroma* → *separate the neuroblasts and neuropil, imparting a nested or multinodular appearance.* ***(Right)*** *This poorly differentiated neuroblastoma shows sheets of small round cells* → *in aggregates within a background of neuropil* ⇨. *The neuropil is composed of a dense tangle of fibrillary, eosinophilic cytoplasmic processes.*

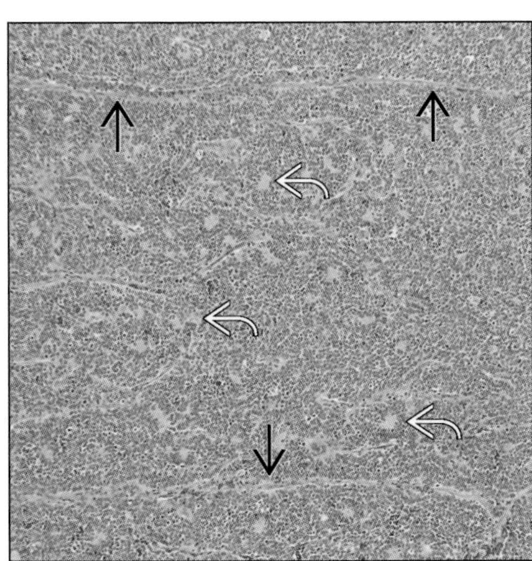

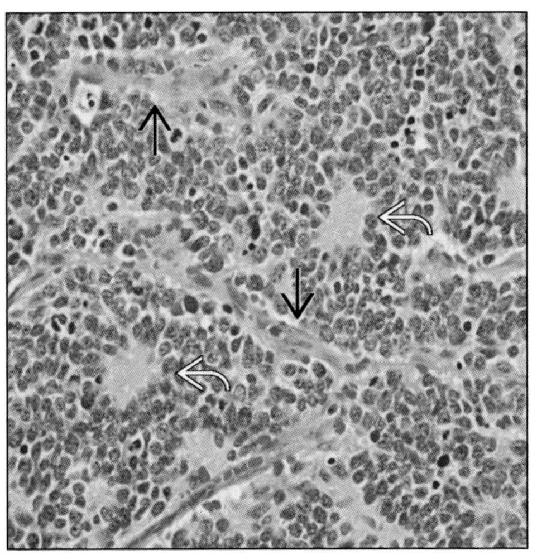

(Left) *This poorly differentiated neuroblastoma shows scattered rosettes* ↪*, an early sign of differentiation. Also seen are thin bands of schwannian stroma* →*.* ***(Right)*** *Homer-Wright rosettes* ↪ *are composed of neuroblasts surrounding a central core of neurites (cytoplasmic processes), without a central lumen. These can be found in varying numbers in poorly differentiated NBs but are not wholly specific. Small foci of schwannian stroma* → *are also seen.*

NEUROBLASTOMA AND GANGLIONEUROBLASTOMA

Microscopic Features

*(**Left**) Schwannian stroma in a NB is often present as thin septa composed of spindled cells, sometimes with wavy nuclei ➔. The Schwann cell component can be demonstrated by immunohistochemistry for S100 protein. (**Right**) Neuroblastomas are commonly hemorrhagic with areas of necrosis ➔. These changes can also be seen after treatment. Neuroblastomas that have undergone treatment should not be classified in the INPC system.*

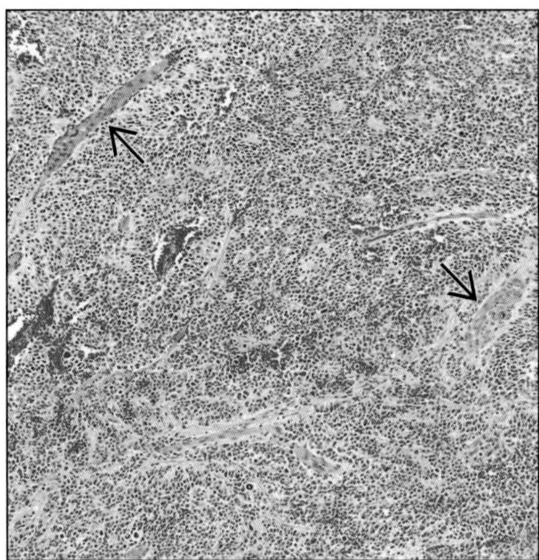

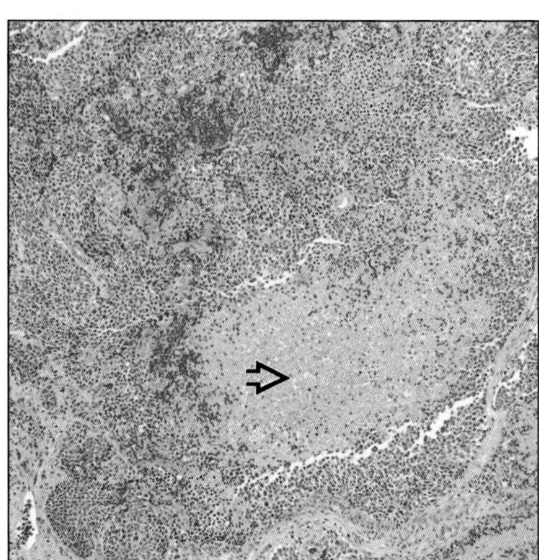

*(**Left**) This is an example of differentiating neuroblastoma, in which more than 5% of the neuroblasts show differentiation with increased cytoplasm and vesicular nuclei ➔. (**Right**) Differentiating neuroblasts ➔ are characterized by an increased amount of eosinophilic cytoplasm, an eccentrically placed nucleus, and vesicular chromatin. These can resemble the cells of alveolar rhabdomyosarcoma but express neural antigens and lack desmin and myogenin.*

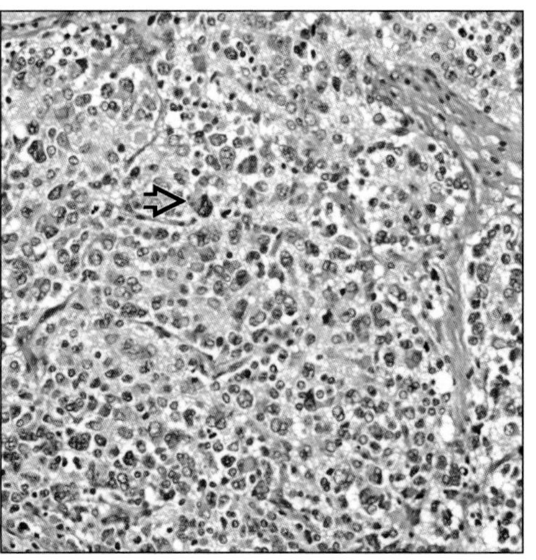

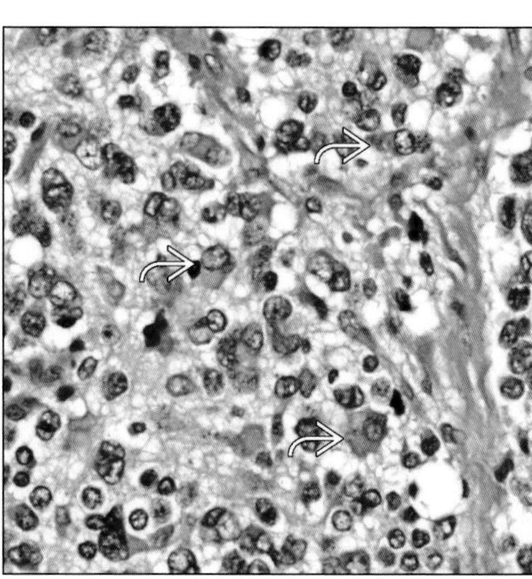

*(**Left**) The mitotic-karyhorrectic index (MKI) is determined by counting the number of mitoses ➔ and karyhorrectic cells ➔ per 5,000 tumor cells. An estimated result is usually considered acceptable, since counting 5,000 cells is tedious. MKI counts should be averaged over the entire tumor and not assessed in only the worst-looking areas. (**Right**) This is an example of a poorly differentiated neuroblastoma, which has an intermediate mitotic-karyhorrectic index.*

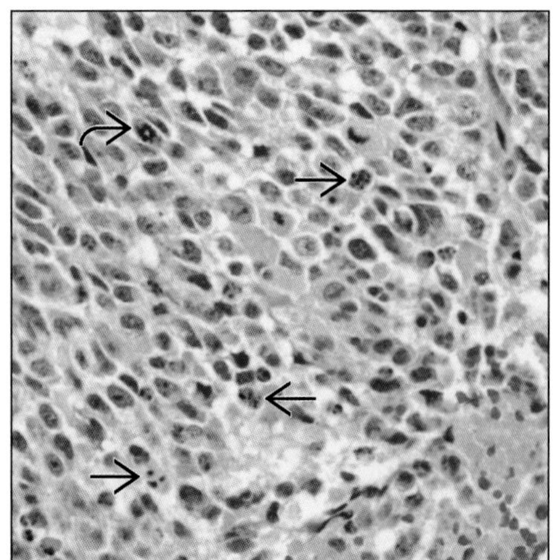

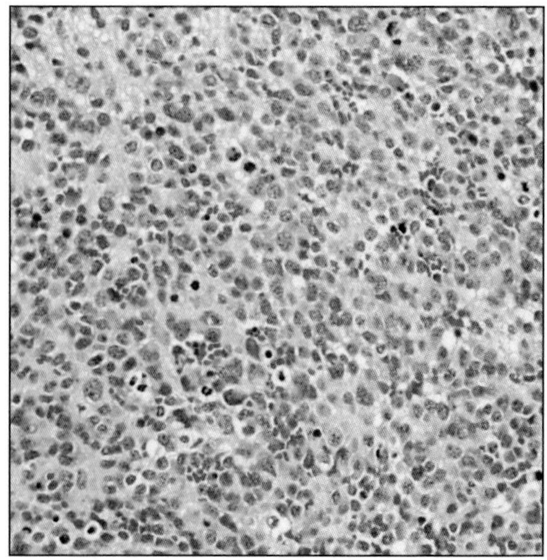

Microscopic Features and Ancillary Techniques

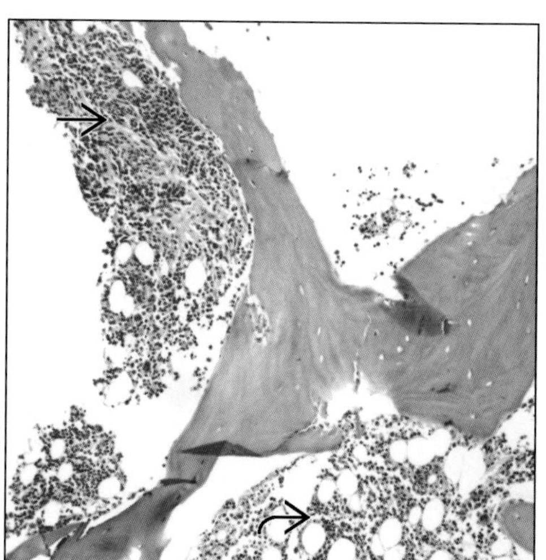
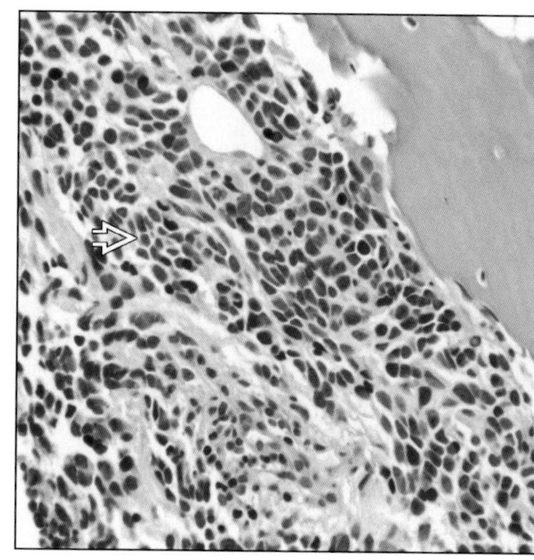

(Left) *This core biopsy specimen of bone marrow shows normal marrow in the lower part of the field ➢ and a focus of metastatic neuroblastoma in the upper part ➔. Notice how the architecture changes in the focus of metastatic tumor* ***(Right)*** *This is a focus of metastatic neuroblastoma in a core biopsy specimen of bone. The marrow has been extensively replaced by sheets of metastatic small round cell tumor ➔ and shows no areas with normal trilineage hematopoiesis.*

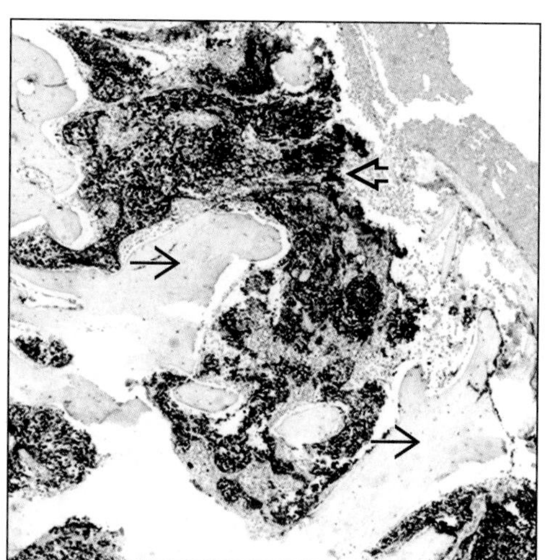
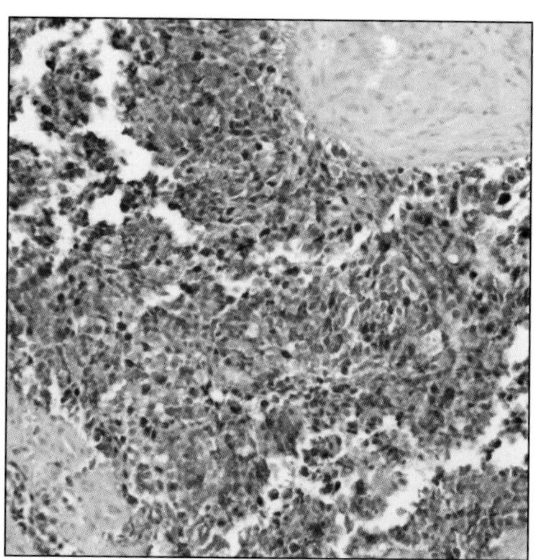

(Left) *In this bone marrow trephine specimen, there is diffuse immunoreactivity for neuroblastoma antigen (NB84) in metastatic deposits of neuroblastoma ➔ that extend between bony trabeculae ➔.* ***(Right)*** *Immunohistochemical staining for NSE shows strong diffuse cytoplasmic staining in neuroblastoma. NSE is a sensitive marker for NB, and although nonspecific, it can usefully be included in a panel of antibodies in the differential diagnosis with other small round cell tumors.*

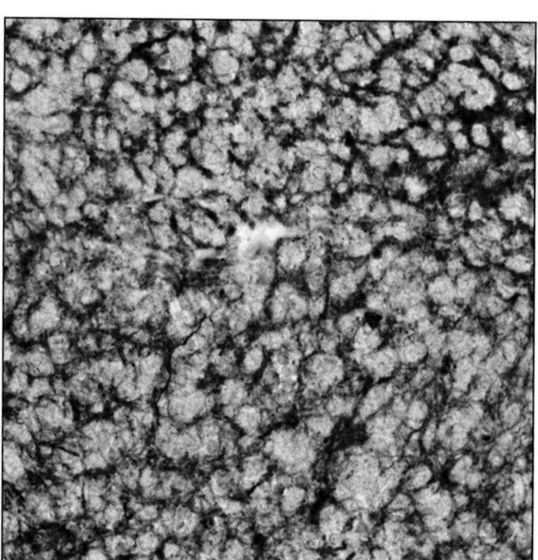
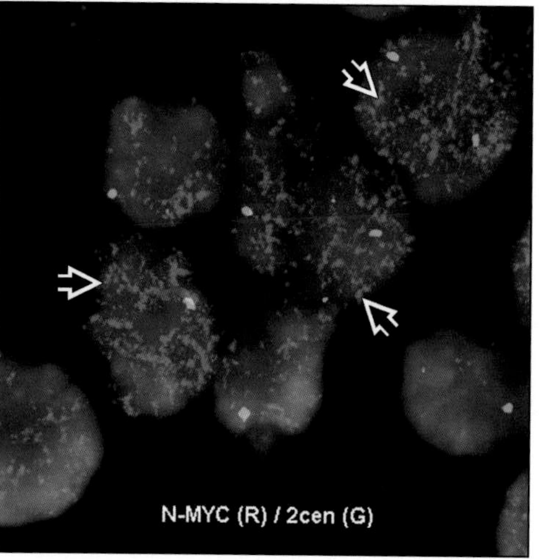

(Left) *Neurofilament protein is demonstrable, diffusely or focally, in cytoplasm of 70% of neuroblastomas. It is negative in most Ewing sarcomas.* ***(Right)*** *Fluorescence in situ hybridization (FISH) of this neuroblastoma shows marked amplification of MYCN demonstrated by numerous red dots ➔. This finding predicts poor prognosis, although the amount of amplification does not relate to outcome. (Courtesy L. McGavran, PhD, and K. Swisshelm, PhD.)*

NEUROBLASTOMA AND GANGLIONEUROBLASTOMA

Gross and Microscopic Features of Ganglioneuroblastoma

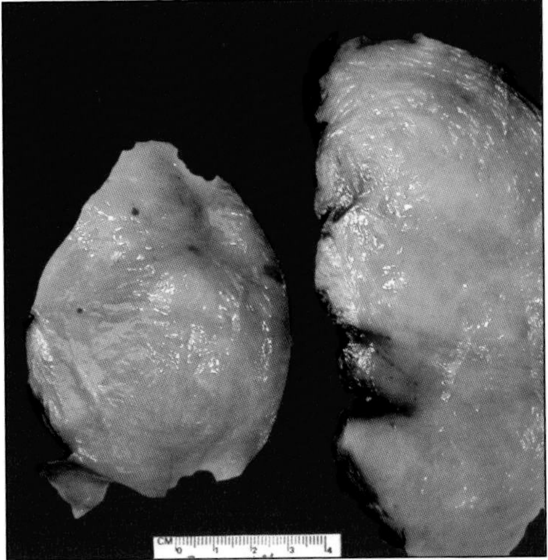
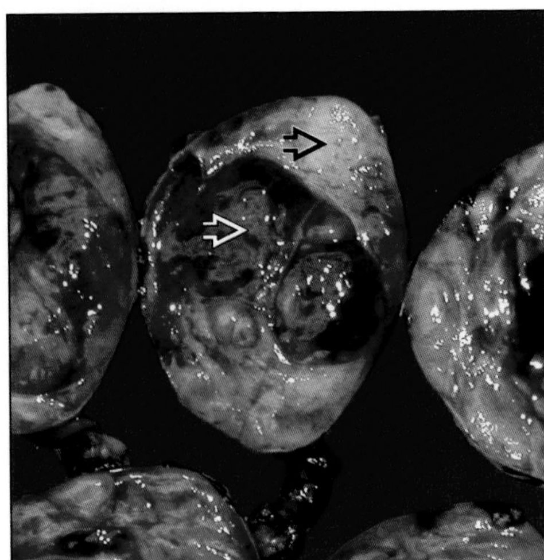

(Left) *This is a ganglioneuroblastoma (GNB) from the mediastinum. This image depicts a tumor with a tan firm cut surface, but the gross appearance of GNB depends on how much of the tumor is neuroblastic.* ***(Right)*** *This is the typical look of a nodular GNB on cut surface. The hemorrhagic nodule in the center ➡ is stroma-poor neuroblastoma, whereas the tan, fleshy rim ➡ is either ganglioneuroma or intermixed GNB. The diagnosis of nodular GNB requires grossly visible nodules.*

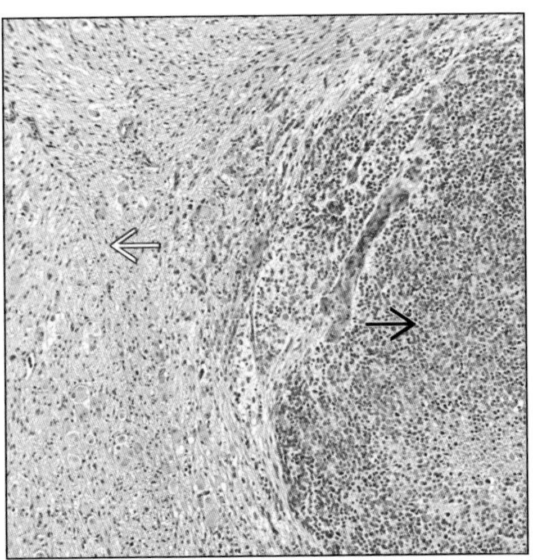
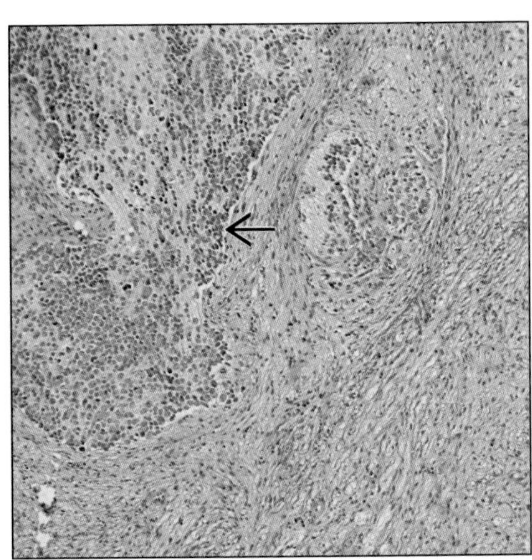

(Left) *This nodular GNB shows the pushing border between the stroma-poor neuroblastoma component → and the ganglioneuroma component ➡. There is often a fibrous pseudocapsule between the 2 components. Even with this histologic picture, a grossly visible nodule is required to diagnose nodular GNB.* ***(Right)*** *In intermixed ganglioneuroblastoma, the nests of neuroblastoma can vary in size and maturation of neuroblasts. Here, a larger nest of immature neuroblasts is seen →.*

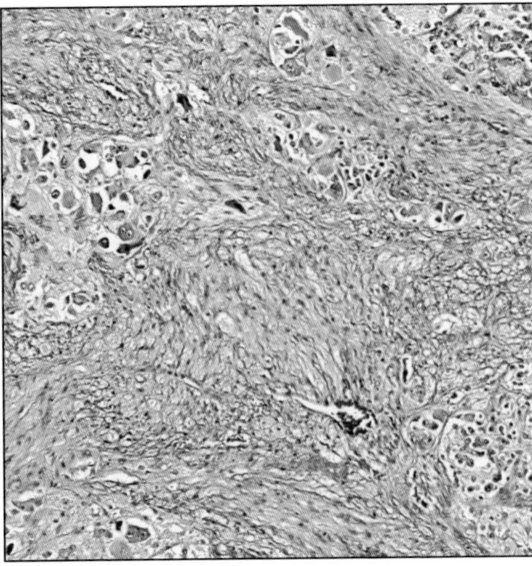
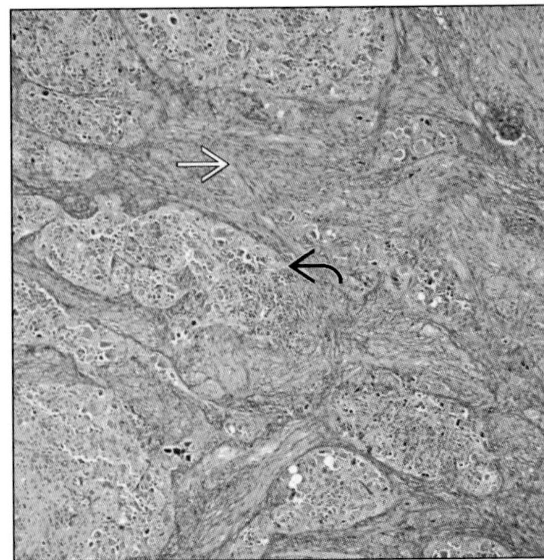

(Left) *To diagnose intermixed ganglioneuroblastoma, at least 50% of the tumor must be composed of schwannian stroma. This is characterized by spindled, wavy cells in bundles of varying cellularity. The Schwann cells lack nuclear atypia and demonstrate nuclear immunoreactivity for S100 protein.* ***(Right)*** *This intermixed ganglioneuroblastoma shows well-defined nests → of maturing neuroblasts, ganglion cells, and neuropil within a schwannian stroma ➡.*

Microscopic Features of Ganglioneuroblastoma

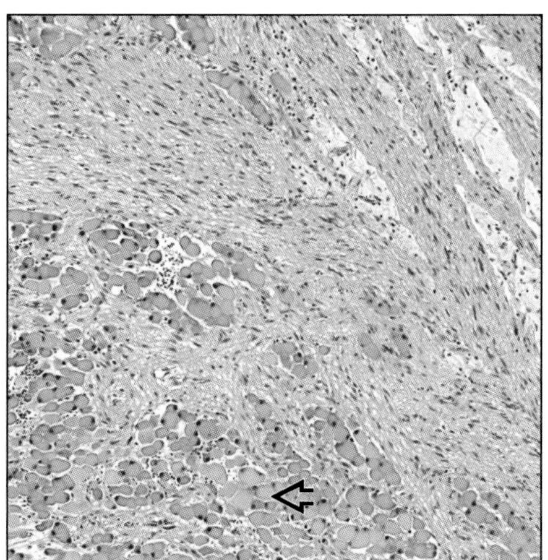

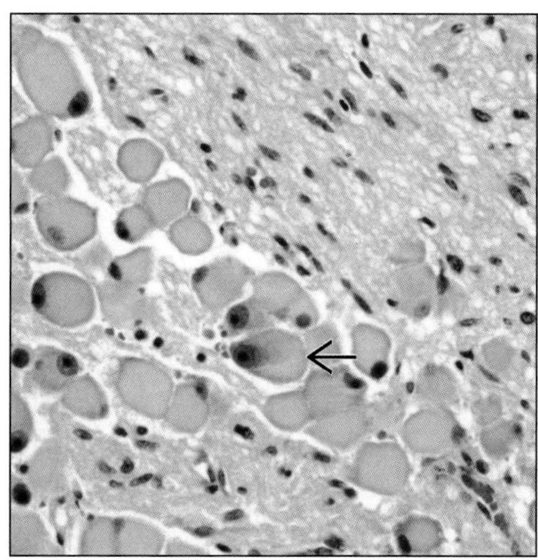

(Left) *The neuroblastomatous component of this intermixed GNB is predominantly mature (or nearly mature) ganglion cells ⇨. The ganglion cells are present in clusters in this tumor, differing from the pattern in maturing ganglioneuroma in which they are present as single cells.* ***(Right)*** *Mature ganglion cells → are characterized by abundant eosinophilic to amphophilic cytoplasm, eccentric nuclei, and prominent nucleoli. Nissl substance may or may not be present.*

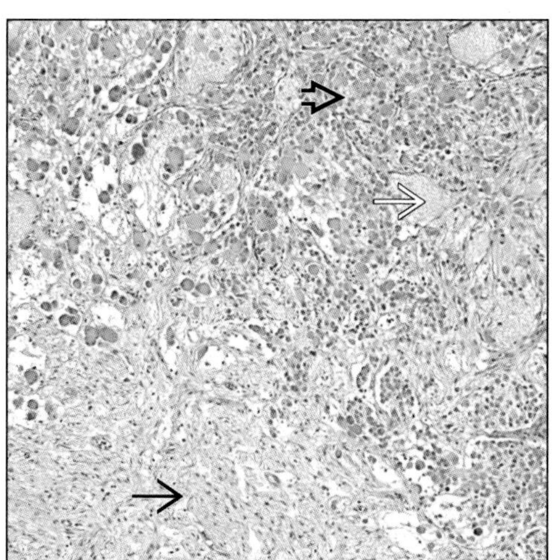

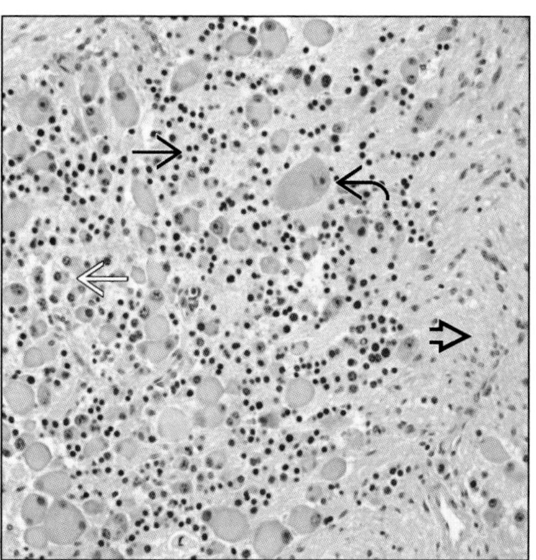

(Left) *This low-magnification field of intermixed ganglioneuroblastoma shows clusters of maturing neuroblasts and ganglion cells ⇨, foci of neuropil ➡, and areas of schwannian stroma →.* ***(Right)*** *Higher magnification of intermixed ganglioneuroblastoma shows details of neuroblasts →, maturing neuroblasts ➡, and ganglion cells ↪ blending into the schwannian stroma ⇨.*

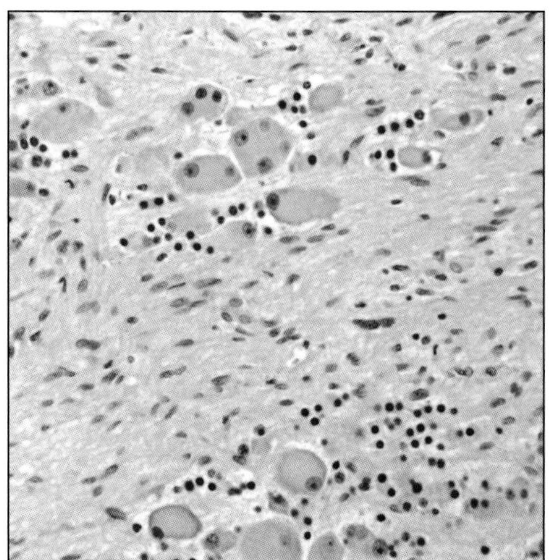

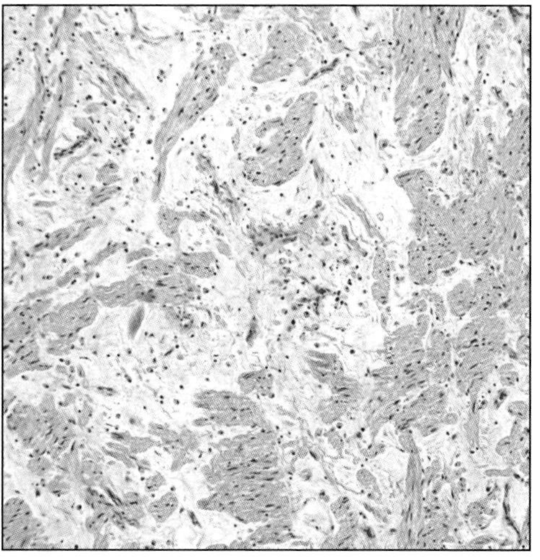

(Left) *This section from an intermixed GNB could be mistaken for a maturing GN. In maturing GN, the tumor is predominantly composed of schwannian stroma, and individual neuroblastic cells merge into the schwannian stroma instead of forming distinct nests.* ***(Right)*** *This field of an intermixed GNB could be mistaken for neurofibroma (spindled wavy cells in a myxoid background). Adequate sampling, generally 1 section per centimeter of tumor, is required to make an accurate diagnosis.*

ECTOMESENCHYMOMA

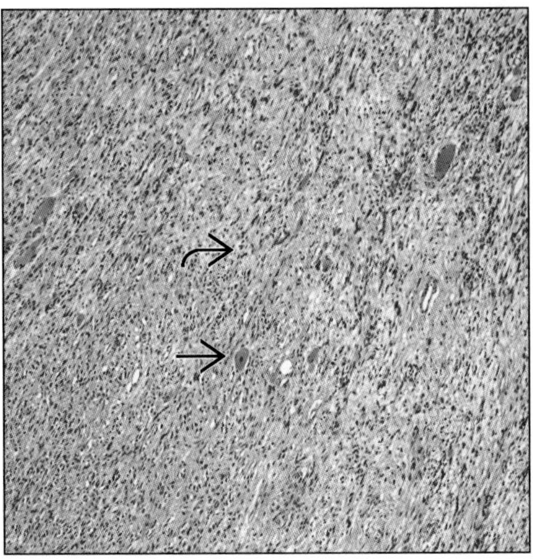

This slide shows ectomesenchymoma with admixed spindle cells, ganglion cells ➙, and small round cells ➙, which can require immunohistochemistry to distinguish neuroblasts from rhabdomyoblasts.

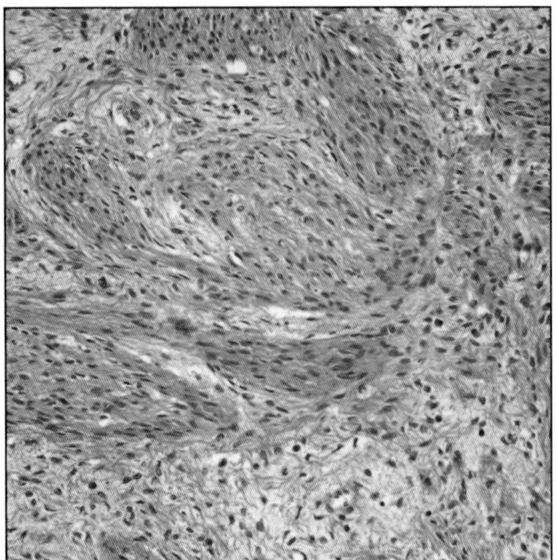

This different area of ectomesenchymoma from the same case is composed of fascicles of differentiated Schwann cells. In a biopsy specimen, this might be indistinguishable from cellular schwannoma.

TERMINOLOGY

Synonyms

- Malignant ectomesenchymoma

Definitions

- Tumor composed of neuroectodermal and mesenchymal elements
  - Usually ganglioneuroma and embryonal rhabdomyosarcoma

ETIOLOGY/PATHOGENESIS

Developmental Anomaly

- No specific molecular genetic abnormality
- Postulated to recapitulate neural crest-derived ectomesenchyme
- Rhabdomyosarcoma can metastasize as ectomesenchymoma

CLINICAL ISSUES

Epidemiology

- Incidence
  - Very rare
- Age
  - Usually childhood
    - Under age of 4 years
  - Exceptionally in adults

Site

- Head and neck
  - Nasal cavity
  - Orbit
  - Central nervous system
- Abdomen
- Genitourinary tract
- Paratesticular region
- Extremities

Presentation

- Rapidly growing mass

Prognosis

- Aggressive neoplasm
- Poor outcome

MACROSCOPIC FEATURES

General Features

- Variably sized
- Infiltrative
- Hemorrhage and necrosis

MICROSCOPIC PATHOLOGY

Histologic Features

- Variable neural component
  - Ganglioneuroma
    - Ganglion cells in variable numbers
    - Differentiated Schwann cells in fascicles or whorls
    - Rarely malignant peripheral nerve sheath cells
  - Rarely neuroblastic element
    - Nodules of small darkly staining cells
- Mesenchymal component
  - Rhabdomyosarcoma
    - Sheets, nests, or cords of small round cells
    - Spindled or rounded rhabdomyoblasts with eosinophilic cytoplasm
  - Rarely other elements, e.g., chondrosarcoma
- Components are typically intermingled, not discrete
- Lacks pleomorphism

ANCILLARY TESTS

Gene Expression Profiling

- Some CNS cases show overlap with malignant peripheral nerve sheath tumor

ECTOMESENCHYMOMA

Key Facts

Terminology
- Tumor composed of neuroectodermal and mesenchymal elements
- Usually variably differentiated neuroblastoma plus rhabdomyosarcoma

Etiology/Pathogenesis
- Postulated to recapitulate neural crest-derived ectomesenchyme

Clinical Issues
- Usually childhood
- Aggressive neoplasm

Microscopic Pathology
- Variable neural element
  - Neuroblasts, ganglion cells, Schwann cells
- Rhabdomyosarcoma
  - Spindled or rounded rhabdomyoblasts

Immunohistochemistry

Antibody	Reactivity	Staining Pattern	Comment
Desmin	Positive	Cytoplasmic	In rhabdomyosarcomatous element
Myogenin	Positive	Nuclear	In rhabdomyosarcomatous element
Neuroblastoma	Positive	Nuclear & cytoplasmic	In neuroblastic element
Chromogranin-A	Positive	Cytoplasmic	In neuroblasts and ganglion cells
NFP	Positive	Cytoplasmic	In neuroblasts and ganglion cells
S100	Positive	Nuclear & cytoplasmic	In Schwann cells
CD56	Positive	Cytoplasmic	Can be positive in both components
CK-PAN	Negative	Not applicable	
CD34	Negative	Not applicable	

DIFFERENTIAL DIAGNOSIS

Rhabdomyosarcoma
- Typical patterns of embryonal or alveolar subtype
- Absence of neural component
- Characteristic genetic findings in alveolar rhabdomyosarcoma

Malignant Triton Tumor
- Malignant nerve sheath cells predominate
- Lacks neuroblastomatous component
- Lacks ganglion cells

Neuroblastoma
- Lacks rhabdomyosarcomatous component

Ganglioneuroma
- Mixture of Schwann cells and mature ganglion cells
- Lacks rhabdomyoblastic component
- Lacks neuroblastomatous component

SELECTED REFERENCES

1. Kleinschmidt-DeMasters BK et al: Molecular array analyses of 51 pediatric tumors shows overlap between malignant intracranial ectomesenchymoma and MPNST but not medulloblastoma or atypical teratoid rhabdoid tumor. Acta Neuropathol. 113(6):695-703, 2007
2. Edwards V et al: Rhabdomyosarcoma metastasizing as a malignant ectomesenchymoma. Ultrastruct Pathol. 23(4):267-73, 1999
3. Mouton SC et al: Malignant ectomesenchymoma in childhood. Pediatr Pathol Lab Med. 16(4):607-24, 1996

IMAGE GALLERY

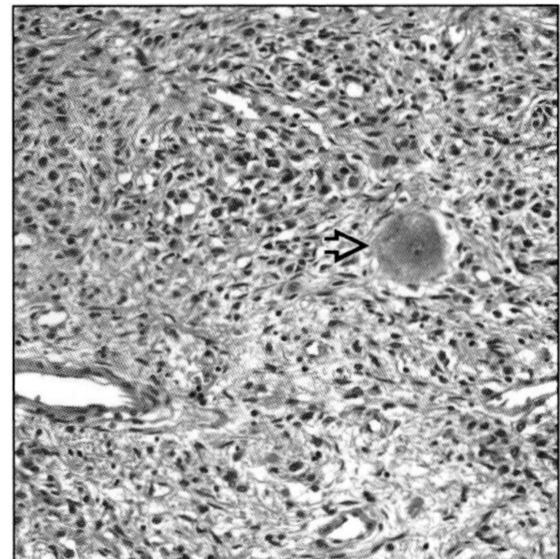

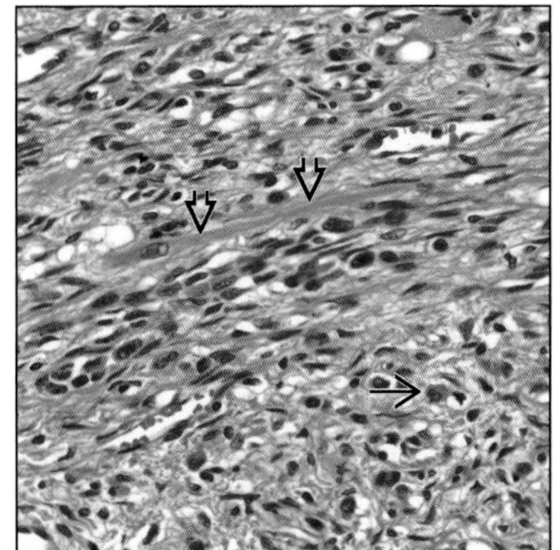

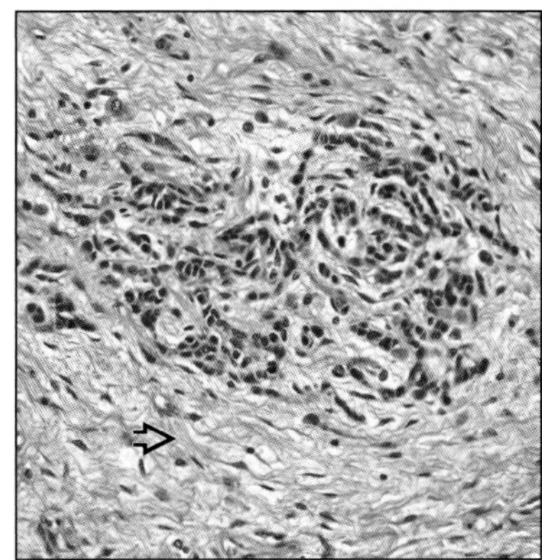

*(**Left**) Higher magnification shows a ganglion cell ⇨ and round cells with small hyperchromatic nuclei dispersed in a fibrillary background. Typically the elements of ectomesenchymoma are randomly intermingled. (**Center**) This image shows ectomesenchymoma with a cellular focus of spindled ⇨ and rounded → rhabdomyoblasts. (**Right**) A focus of small round cells of rhabdomyosarcoma forms nests and cords in a bland spindle cell stroma ⇨.*

PROTOCOL FOR THE EXAMINATION OF PNET/EWING SARCOMA SPECIMENS

Ewing Sarcoma/Primitive Neuroectodermal Tumor: Biopsy

Surgical Pathology Cancer Case Summary (Checklist)

Procedure

___ Core needle biopsy
___ Incisional biopsy
___ Excisional biopsy
___ Other (specify): ______________________
___ Not specified

Tumor Site

Greatest dimension: ________ cm
*Additional dimensions: ________ x ________ cm
___ Cannot be determined

****Extent of Osseous Tumors (select all that apply)***

*___ Diaphysis
*___ Metaphysis
*___ Medullary cavity
*___ Tumor extension into soft tissue
*___ Other (specify): ______________________
*___ Not specified
*___ Cannot be determined

****Extent of Primary Extraosseous Tumors (select all that apply)***

*___ Dermal
*___ Subcutaneous/suprafascial
*___ Subfascial
*___ Intramuscular
*___ Intraabdominal/pelvic
*___ Retroperitoneal
*___ Other (specify): ______________________
*___ Not specified
*___ Cannot be determined

Margins (for excisional biopsy only)

___ Cannot be assessed
___ Margins negative for tumor
Distance of tumor from closest bone margin: ________ cm
Distance of tumor from closest soft tissue margin: ________ cm
___ Margin(s) positive for sarcoma
Specify margin(s) ______________________

****Lymph-Vascular Invasion***

*___ Not identified
*___ Present
*___ Indeterminate

Pre-biopsy Treatment (select all that apply)

___ No therapy
___ Chemotherapy performed
___ Radiation therapy performed
___ Therapy performed, type not specified
___ Unknown

Necrosis Post Chemotherapy

___ Necrosis not identified
___ Necrosis present
*Specify extent of total specimen: ________ %

____ Cannot be determined

____ Not applicable

*Additional Pathologic Findings

*Specify: ______________________

*Ancillary Studies

***Cytogenetics**

*Specify: ______________________

*____ Not performed

***Molecular pathology**

*Specify: ______________________

*____ Not performed

**Data elements with asterisks are not required. However, these elements may be clinically important but are not yet validated or regularly used in patient management. Adapted with permission from College of American Pathologists, "Protocol for the Examination of Specimens from Patients with Primitive Neuroectodermal Tumor (PNET)/Ewing Sarcoma (ES)." Web posting date October 2009, www.cap.org.*

Ewing Sarcoma/Primitive Neuroectodermal Tumor: Resection

Surgical Pathology Cancer Case Summary (Checklist)

Procedure

____ Resection

____ Amputation (specify type): ______________________

____ Other (specify): ______________________

____ Not specified

Tumor Site

Specify site(s): ______________________

____ Not specified

Tumor Size

Greatest dimension: ________ cm

*Additional dimensions: ________ x ________ cm

____ Cannot be determined

*Extent of Primary Osseous Tumors (select all that apply)

*____ Diaphysis

*____ Metaphysis

*____ Medullary cavity

*____ Tumor extension into soft tissue

*____ Other (specify): ______________________

*____ Not specified

*____ Cannot be determined

*Extent of Primary Extraosseous Tumors (select all that apply)

*____ Dermal

*____ Subcutaneous

*____ Subfascial

*____ Intramuscular

*____ Intraabdominal/pelvic

*____ Retroperitoneal

*____ Other (specify): ______________________

*____ Not specified

*____ Cannot be determined

Margins

____ Cannot be assessed

____ Margins negative for tumor

Distance of tumor from closest bone margin: ________ cm

Distance of tumor from closest soft tissue margin: ________ cm

____ Margin(s) positive for sarcoma

PROTOCOL FOR THE EXAMINATION OF PNET/EWING SARCOMA SPECIMENS

Specify margin(s): ______________________

*Lymph-Vascular Invasion

*___ Not identified
*___ Present
*___ Indeterminate

Pre-resection Treatment (select all that apply)

___ No therapy
___ Chemotherapy performed
___ Radiation therapy performed
___ Therapy performed, type not specified
___ Unknown

Necrosis Post Chemotherapy

___ Necrosis not identified
___ Necrosis present
*Specify extent of total mass: ________ %
___ Cannot be determined
___ Not applicable

*Ancillary Studies

***Cytogenetics**
*Specify: ______________________
*___ Not performed

***Molecular pathology**
*Specify: ______________________
*___ Not performed

Pathologic Staging (pTNM)

TNM descriptors (required only if applicable) (select all that apply)
___ m (multiple primary tumors)
___ r (recurrent)
___ y (post-treatment)

Primary tumor (pT)

For primary osseous tumors
___ pTX: Primary tumor cannot be assessed
___ pT0: No evidence of primary tumor
___ pT1: Tumor ≤ 8 cm in greatest dimension
___ pT2: Tumor > 8 cm in greatest dimension
___ pT3: Discontinuous tumors in the primary bone site (not including skip metastases)

For primary extraosseous tumors
___ pTX: Primary tumor cannot be assessed
___ pT0: No evidence of primary tumor
___ pT1a: Tumor ≤ 5 cm in greatest dimension, superficial tumor
___ pT1b: Tumor ≤ 5 cm in greatest dimension, deep tumor
___ pT2a: Tumor > 5 cm in greatest dimension, superficial tumor
___ pT2b: Tumor > 5 cm in greatest dimension, deep tumor

Lymph nodes

Regional lymph nodes (pN)
___ pNX: Cannot be assessed
___ pN0: No regional lymph node metastasis
___ pN1: Regional lymph node metastasis
Specify: Number of lymph nodes examined: ________
Number of lymph nodes involved: ________

Nonregional lymph nodes
___ Cannot be assessed
___ No nonregional lymph node metastasis

___ Nonregional lymph node metastasis

Specify: Number of lymph nodes examined: ________

Number of lymph nodes involved: ________

Distant metastasis

For primary osseous tumors

___ Not applicable

___ pM1a: Lung

___ pM1b: Metastasis involving distant sites other than lung (including skip metastases)

*Specify site(s), if known: ________________________

For primary extraosseous tumors

___ Not applicable

___ pM1: Distant metastasis

*Specify site(s), if known: ________________________

**Data elements with asterisks are not required. However, these elements may be clinically important but are not yet validated or regularly used in patient management. Adapted with permission from College of American Pathologists, "Protocol for the Examination of Specimens from Patients with Primitive Neuroectodermal Tumor (PNET)/Ewing Sarcoma (ES)." Web posting date October 2009, www.cap.org.*

Osseous and Chondroid Lesions

Benign

Malignant

FIBRODYSPLASIA OSSIFICANS PROGRESSIVA

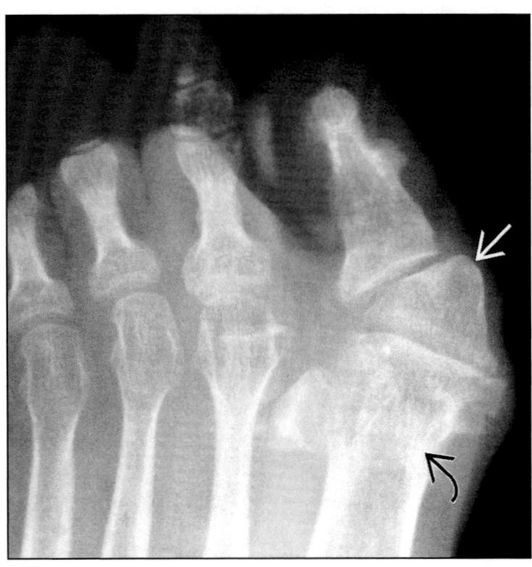

Plain radiograph of the left foot demonstrates a shortened 1st metatarsal ⇗ as well as a large free osseous body ➡ that have resulted in marked hallux valgus.

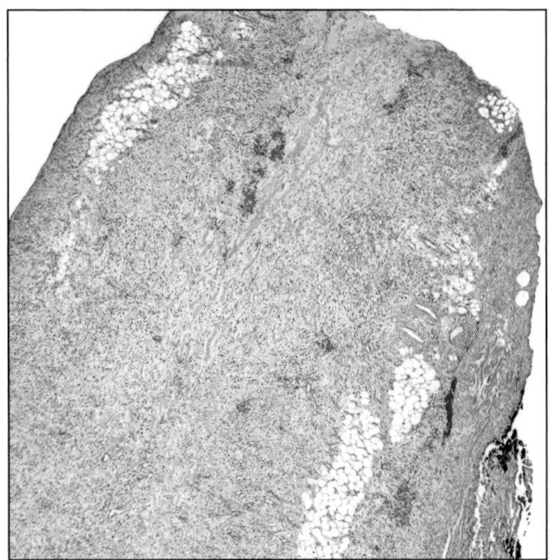

The appearance of the lesions in fibrodysplasia ossificans progressiva is related to the duration of the lesions. This lesion was early, and it appears similar to nodular fasciitis.

TERMINOLOGY

Abbreviations

- Fibrodysplasia ossificans progressiva (FOP, FDOP)

Synonyms

- Myositis ossificans progressiva, stone man disease

Definitions

- Rare disabling genetic disorder of progressive heterotopic ossification

ETIOLOGY/PATHOGENESIS

Genetics

- Heterozygous activating mutation of gene encoding activin receptor A type 1/activin-like kinase 2 (*ACVR1/ALK2*)
  - Bone morphogenic protein (BMP) type 1 receptor

CLINICAL ISSUES

Epidemiology

- Incidence
  - Approximately 1 in 2 million persons
- Age
  - Childhood onset
- Gender
  - No predilection
- Ethnicity
  - No predilection

Presentation

- Hallux valgus
- Short 1st metatarsals
- Rapidly changing swellings in neck or back
- Minor trauma results in progressive heterotopic ossification
  - Ideally diagnosis should be made by clinical presentation and imaging study findings
    - Metatarsal changes occur early
  - Biopsy contraindicated since it will exacerbate lesions, cause new lesions

Treatment

- None exists
  - Supportive care

Prognosis

- Progressive from childhood
- Most patients wheelchair-bound by 3rd decade
- Median lifespan: 56 years
  - Most common cause of death: Cardiorespiratory failure from thoracic insufficiency syndrome
    - Costovertebral malformations
    - Orthotopic ankylosis of costovertebral joints
    - Fusion of ribs
    - Ossification of intercostal muscles, paravertebral muscles, and aponeuroses
    - Progressive spinal deformity (kyphoscoliosis or thoracic lordosis): Surgical correction contraindicated

IMAGE FINDINGS

General Features

- Characteristic appearance of 1st metatarsals on plain radiographs
- MR highlights lesions in muscles of back and neck

MICROSCOPIC PATHOLOGY

Histologic Features

- Early lesions are nodular fasciitis-like
  - Disorganized collagen
  - Large myofibroblastic cells
  - Extravasated erythrocytes

FIBRODYSPLASIA OSSIFICANS PROGRESSIVA

Key Facts

Terminology

- Rare disabling genetic disorder of progressive heterotopic ossification

Etiology/Pathogenesis

- Heterozygous activating mutation of gene encoding activin receptor A type 1/activin-like kinase 2 (*ACVR1/ALK2*)

Clinical Issues

- Approximately 1 in 2 million persons
- Childhood onset
- No treatment exists

Microscopic Pathology

- Early lesions are nodular fasciitis-like
- Progressive ossification similar to that of myositis ossificans

---

  - Mitotic activity
- Progressive ossification similar to that of myositis ossificans
  - Less prominent zonation than in myositis
- Histologic material should not be generally available since biopsy is deleterious for patient

DIFFERENTIAL DIAGNOSIS

Myositis Ossificans

- Presents in individuals in their 30s
- Arises in extremities
  - Elbow, thigh, buttock, shoulder
  - 2-5 cm, well marginated
- No associated skeletal anomalies
- Zonated lesions with cellular central portion and peripheral ossification
  - Central portion consisting of short fascicles of myofibroblastic cells
  - Numerous mitoses
  - Vascular stroma, numerous mitoses
  - Peripheral portion with trabeculae of woven bone rimmed by osteoblasts
    - Older lesions show mature bone
- Benign and nonprogressive

Extraskeletal Osteosarcoma

- Large lesions of deep soft tissue
  - Common in deep soft tissues of thigh
- Older adults
- Marked cytologic atypia
- Irregularly distributed zones of osteoid rimmed by cytologically malignant cells
- Dismal outcome: Death due to widely metastatic disease

Nodular Fasciitis

- Lesions of young adults
- Classically involves forearm
  - Head and neck also common site
- 2-3 cm
- Loose storiform pattern
- Myofibroblasts, myxoid matrix
- Keloid-like collagen, extravasated erythrocytes, lymphocytes
- Benign and nonprogressive

SELECTED REFERENCES

1. Kaplan FS et al: Early mortality and cardiorespiratory failure in patients with fibrodysplasia ossificans progressiva. J Bone Joint Surg Am. 92(3):686-91, 2010
2. Shore EM et al: A recurrent mutation in the BMP type I receptor ACVR1 causes inherited and sporadic fibrodysplasia ossificans progressiva. Nat Genet. 2006 May;38(5):525-7. Epub 2006 Apr 23. Erratum in: Nat Genet. 39(2):276, 2007
3. Maxwell WA et al: Histochemical and ultrastructural studies in fibrodysplasia ossificans progressiva (myositis ossificans progressiva). Am J Pathol. 87(3):483-98, 1977

IMAGE GALLERY

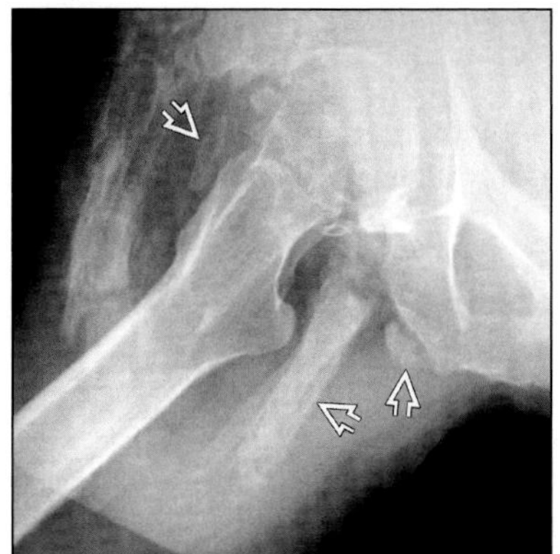

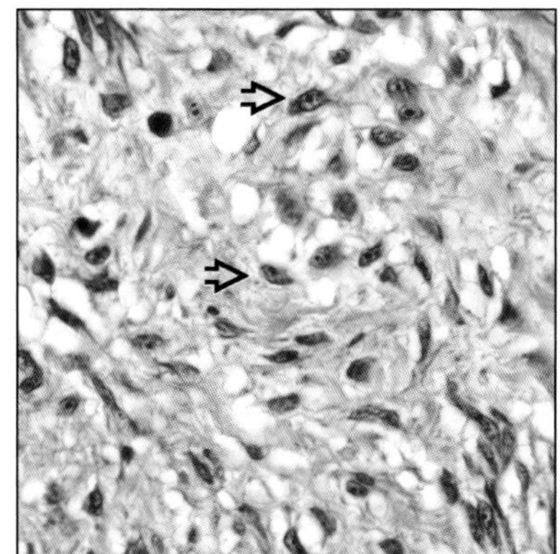

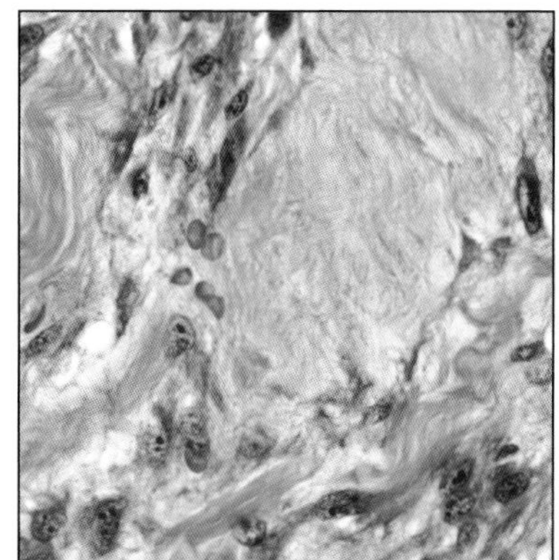

*(**Left**) Radiograph of the right hip demonstrates severe destructive skeletal changes as well as prominent soft tissue ossification ➡. Generally biopsy is not recommended of these lesions since surgical manipulation results in additional lesions. (**Center**) This fibrodysplasia ossificans progressiva lesion is composed of reactive-appearing myofibroblasts ⇨. (**Right**) H&E shows a collagenized area in fibrodysplasia ossificans progressiva.*

MYOSITIS OSSIFICANS

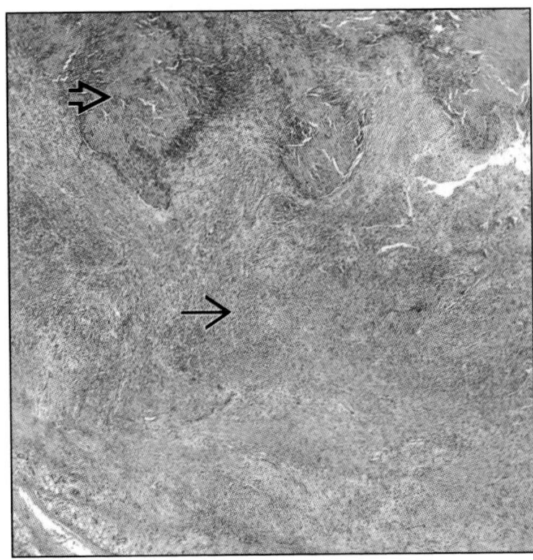

Myositis ossificans is characterized by a zoned proliferation of myofibroblasts with a peripheral rim of woven bone ⇨. This example has a highly cellular central portion →.

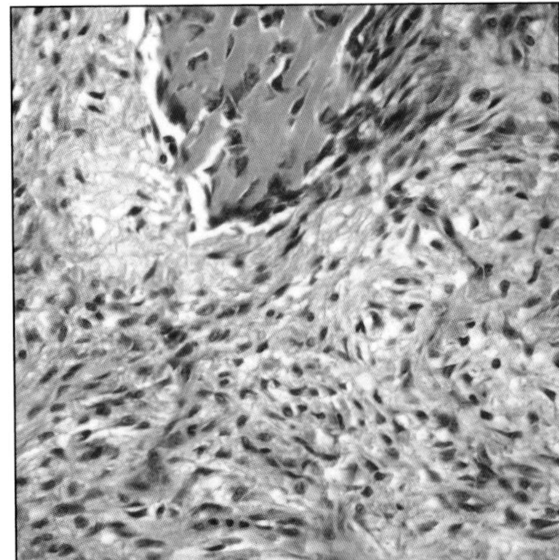

The cytologic features of myositis ossificans are similar to those of nodular fasciitis. The lesional cells are uniform and have bland nuclear features. Mitoses can be present but are not atypical.

TERMINOLOGY

Synonyms

- Fibroosseous pseudotumor of digits (for finger lesions)
- Pseudomalignant osseous tumor of soft tissue

Definitions

- Localized self-limited benign lesions composed of cellular myofibroblastic proliferation with ossification

CLINICAL ISSUES

Epidemiology

- Incidence
  - Rare
- Age
  - Mean age: ~ 30 years
    - Range: 1-95 years
- Gender
  - M > F (~ 3:2) for classic lesions
  - F > M for digital lesions

Presentation

- Arise in areas prone to local trauma
  - Elbow, thigh, buttock, shoulder
- Rapidly growing, variably tender mass

Treatment

- Simple excision

Prognosis

- Benign lesions
  - Occasionally recurrent after incomplete excision

IMAGE FINDINGS

CT Findings

- Early lesions: Soft tissue fullness
- 6 weeks later: Development of bony shell (eggshell-like)
  - More random calcification in digital examples

MACROSCOPIC FEATURES

Size

- Most examples ~ 5 cm (range: 2-12 cm)

MICROSCOPIC PATHOLOGY

Histologic Features

- Zonated appearance with cellular central area with peripheral ossification
  - Digital lesions lack zonation
- Cellular central portion composed of short fascicles of myofibroblasts
  - Faintly eosinophilic cytoplasm
  - Finely granular nuclei with smooth nuclear membranes
  - Numerous mitoses (not atypical)
  - Vascular stroma
    - Myxoid areas, fibrin, extravasated erythrocytes
  - Older lesions are less cellular
- Peripheral portion with bone formation
  - Merges with cellular myofibroblastic portion
  - Trabeculae of woven bone rimmed by osteoblasts
  - Older lesions show mature-appearing bone
  - Cartilage uncommon but occasionally encountered

DIFFERENTIAL DIAGNOSIS

Extraskeletal Osteosarcoma

- Large lesions involving deep soft tissues
  - Older adults
  - Essentially never arises in digits
- Marked cytologic atypia
- No zonation

MYOSITIS OSSIFICANS

Key Facts

Clinical Issues

- Mean age: ~ 30 years (range: 1-95 years)
- M > F (~ 3:2) for classic lesions
- F > M for digital lesions

Microscopic Pathology

- Zonated appearance with cellular central area with peripheral ossification
- Cellular central portion composed of short fascicles of myofibroblasts
- Numerous mitoses (not atypical)
- Vascular stroma with myxoid areas, fibrin, extravasated erythrocytes
- Peripheral portion with bone formation
- Trabeculae of woven bone rimmed by osteoblasts
- Older lesions show mature-appearing bone
- Digital lesions lack zonation
- Cartilage uncommon but occasionally encountered

  - Random collections of osteoid elaborated by cytologically malignant cells
  - Markedly atypical cells embedded within osteoid

Nodular Fasciitis

- Young adults
- Classically arises in forearm
  - Also head and neck, trunk
- 2-3 cm diameter
- Loose storiform pattern of myofibroblasts
- Myxoid stroma
- Small osteoclast-like giant cells
- Keloid-like collagen in older lesions

Calcifying Aponeurotic Fibroma

- Hands of infants and children
- Infiltrative
- Spindle cell fibromatosis-like proliferation
- Chondroid material
- Stippled islands of calcification
- Benign but prone to local recurrences

Proliferative Fasciitis/Myositis

- Older adults
  - Rare pediatric cases
- Distal (usually upper) extremity
- Proliferates along fascia
  - Within muscle (proliferative myositis)
- Large reactive fibroblastic cells with macronucleoli
  - Ganglion-like fibroblasts
- Background appears similar to nodular fasciitis
  - Bland nuclei
  - Myxoid stroma
  - Extravasated erythrocytes
- Pediatric lesions extremely cellular and mistaken for rhabdomyosarcomas in the past
  - Brisk mitotic activity
  - Lack MYOD1, myogenin, desmin

Ossifying Fibromyxoid Tumor

- Adults, extremities, usually 3-5 cm
- Most behave indolently
  - ~ 10% recur, rare metastases
- Uniform rounded cells
- Lace-like patterns
- Fibromyxoid stroma
- Variable shell of bone surrounds lesions
- Most express S100 protein
  - Variable GFAP, desmin, SMA, CK

SELECTED REFERENCES

1. Nuovo MA et al: Myositis ossificans with atypical clinical, radiographic, or pathologic findings: a review of 23 cases. Skeletal Radiol. 21(2):87-101, 1992
2. Dupree WB et al: Fibro-osseous pseudotumor of the digits. Cancer. 58(9):2103-9, 1986
3. Angervall L et al: Pseudomalignant osseous tumour of soft tissue. A clinical, radiological and pathological study of five cases. J Bone Joint Surg Br. 51(4):654-63, 1969
4. Ackerman LV: Extra-osseous localized non-neoplastic bone and cartilage formation (so-called myositis ossificans): clinical and pathological confusion with malignant neoplasms. J Bone Joint Surg Am. 40-A(2):279-98, 1958

IMAGE GALLERY

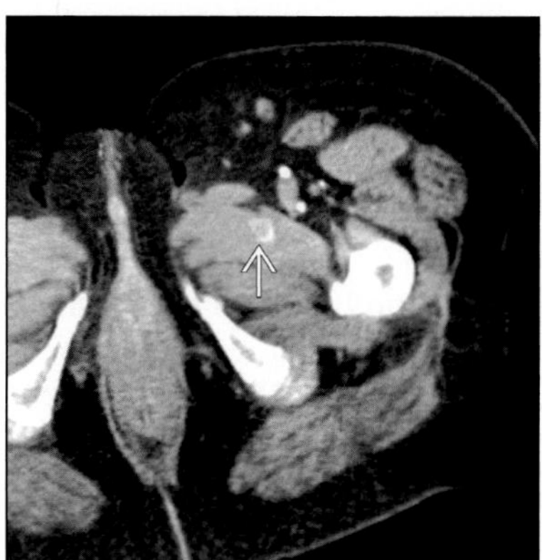

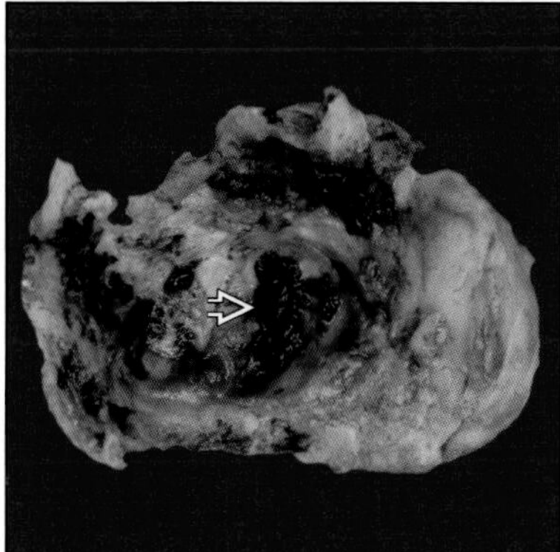

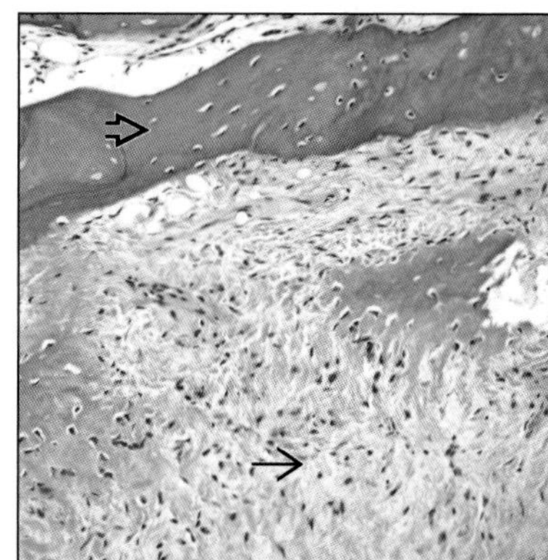

*(**Left**) CT through the left leg shows a partial rim of bone ➡ in this example of well-developed myositis ossificans. (**Center**) Excision specimen is shown with a circumscribed but not encapsulated early lesion. There are foci of hemorrhage ➡, mainly in the center of the lesion, with adjacent firm white-yellow tissue. (**Right**) In later stages, there is reduced cellularity in the central portions of the lesion → compared with earlier stages and more mature bone at the periphery ➡.*

FIBROOSSEOUS PSEUDOTUMOR

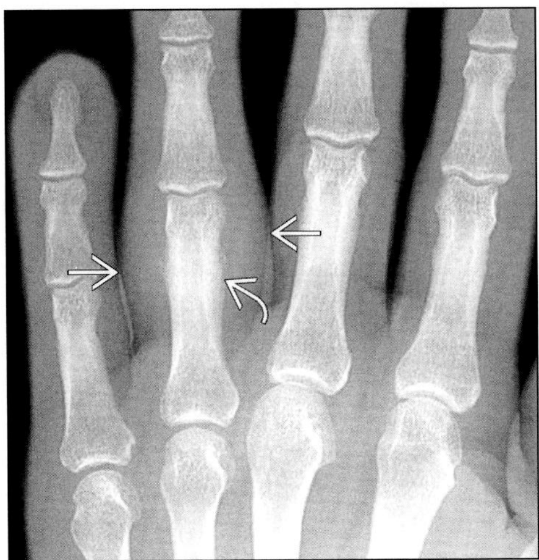

Fibroosseous pseudotumor (FP) typically presents as fusiform swelling in a proximal phalanx of the hand. This radiograph depicts ill-defined soft tissue density ➡ and periosteal reaction ↪.

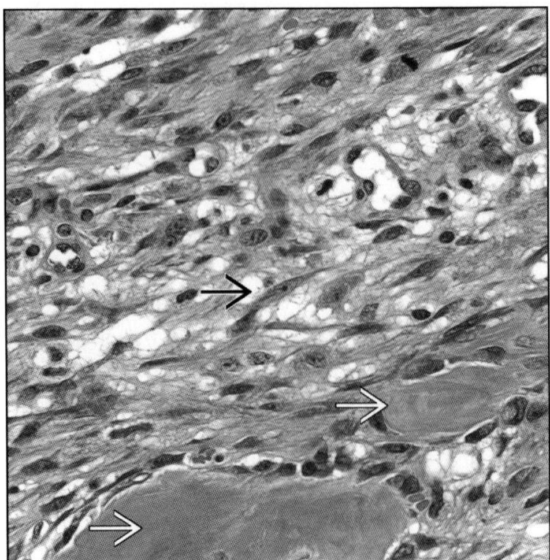

Microscopically, FP consists of a fasciitis-like proliferation of myofibroblasts ➡ admixed with osteoid and reactive bone ➡. FP is regarded as a reactive nonneoplastic process.

TERMINOLOGY

Abbreviations

- Fibroosseous pseudotumor (FP)

Synonyms

- Florid reactive periostitis of tubular bones of hands and feet
- Fasciitis ossificans
- Panniculitis ossificans
- Parosteal fasciitis
- Pseudomalignant osseous tumor of soft tissues

Definitions

- Benign reactive ossifying fibroblastic proliferation most often affecting skin and soft tissue in digits of hands and feet

ETIOLOGY/PATHOGENESIS

Reparative Reaction

- Trauma
- Repetitive injury

CLINICAL ISSUES

Epidemiology

- Incidence
  - Rare, exact incidence unknown
- Age
  - 5-75 years; median: ≈ 35 years
- Gender
  - Slight female predominance

Site

- Hands and feet
  - Proximal phalanx of hand most common site
  - Rarely occurs beyond acral extremities

Presentation

- Fusiform swelling, often with erythema, pain, or ulceration
- Rapid onset, weeks to months

Natural History

- Benign, may be self-limited

Treatment

- Surgical approaches
  - Simple excision usually curative

Prognosis

- Excellent, rarely recurs

IMAGE FINDINGS

General Features

- Early lesions characterized by ill-defined soft tissue density
- Older lesions with intralesional calcification
- Periosteal reaction common

MACROSCOPIC FEATURES

Size

- 0.5-5.6 cm; median: ≈ 2 cm

MICROSCOPIC PATHOLOGY

Histologic Features

- Fasciitis-like spindle cell proliferation with active ossification
- Cellular areas alternate with less cellular fibromyxoid areas in lobular pattern
- Myofibroblastic spindle and stellate cells with vesicular nuclei and amphophilic cytoplasm
- Ossification at various stages of maturation

FIBROOSSEOUS PSEUDOTUMOR

Key Facts

Terminology

- Benign reactive ossifying fibroblastic proliferation most often affecting skin and soft tissue in digits of hands and feet

Clinical Issues

- Proximal phalanx of hand most common site
- Fusiform swelling, often with erythema, pain, or ulceration
- Rapid onset, weeks to months
- Simple excision usually curative

Image Findings

- Early lesions characterized by ill-defined soft tissue density
- Older lesions with intralesional calcification
- Periosteal reaction common

Microscopic Pathology

- Fasciitis-like spindle cell proliferation with active ossification
- Myofibroblastic spindle and stellate cells with vesicular nuclei and granular amphophilic cytoplasm
- Ossification in various stages of maturation
- Peripheral zonal osseous maturation present in 50%

Top Differential Diagnoses

- Extraskeletal osteosarcoma
- Myositis ossificans
- Fracture callus
- Bizarre parosteal osteochondromatous proliferation of hands and feet (Nora lesion)

  - Osteoid and wispy immature woven bone
  - Anastomosing trabeculae of woven bone rimmed by single layer of plump activated osteoblasts
  - Mature lamellar bone
  - Peripheral zonal osseous maturation as in myositis ossificans present in 50%
- Geographic areas of collagenous/osseous stroma in some
- Hyaline cartilage with endochondral ossification in some

DIFFERENTIAL DIAGNOSIS

Extraskeletal Osteosarcoma

- Much larger tumor
- Very rare in digits
- High-grade histology with overtly malignant cytoarchitectural features

Myositis Ossificans

- Reactive fibroosseous tumor similar to FP
- Occurs in skeletal muscle, most often in proximal extremities and trunk
- Larger tumor
- Well-defined peripheral zonal ossification
  - Radiographs disclose peripheral ring of calcification in mature lesions

Fracture Callus

- Reactive proliferation of woven bone, granulation tissue, scar tissue, and reactive cartilage with endochondral ossification
- Clinical or radiographic evidence of fracture in most cases

Bizarre Parosteal Osteochondromatous Proliferation of Hands and Feet (Nora Lesion)

- Ossifying tumor with cartilage cap
  - Large reactive chondrocytes in cartilage cap
  - Fibroosseous lesion with spindle cell stroma, woven bone, and immature basophilic "blue" bone
- Adherent to periosteum/bone surface
- Most common in tubular bones of hands and feet

Giant Cell Tumor of Tendon Sheath

- Soft tissue tumor associated with tendon sheath
- Most common in fingers
- Lobular architecture
- Polymorphous population of ovoid stromal cells, macrophages, xanthoma cells, and osteoclastic giant cells
- May have abundant hyalinized collagenous matrix that mimics osteoid

Giant Cell Tumor of Soft Tissue

- Identical histology to giant cell tumor of bone
- Ovoid or spindled stromal cells and numerous osteoclastic giant cells
- Often with peripheral rim of bone

Ossifying Fibromyxoid Tumor

- Soft tissue tumor often with peripheral rim of bone
- Fibrous capsule
- Ovoid mesenchymal cells arranged in cords and clusters
- Lobular architecture
- Myxohyaline matrix

SELECTED REFERENCES

1. Chaudhry IH et al: Fibro-osseous pseudotumor of the digit: a clinicopathological study of 17 cases. J Cutan Pathol. 37(3):323-9, 2010
2. Moosavi CA et al: Fibroosseous [corrected] pseudotumor of the digit: a clinicopathologic study of 43 new cases. Ann Diagn Pathol. 12(1):21-8, 2008
3. Dupree WB et al: Fibro-osseous pseudotumor of the digits. Cancer. 58(9):2103-9, 1986
4. Spjut HJ et al: Florid reactive periostitis of the tubular bones of the hands and feet. A benign lesion which may simulate osteosarcoma. Am J Surg Pathol. 5(5):423-33, 1981

FIBROOSSEOUS PSEUDOTUMOR

Radiographic and Microscopic Features

(Left) Although the most common site is a proximal phalanx of the hand, FP affects other sites such as the thenar compartment, depicted as ill-defined soft tissue density ➔ on this radiograph. Only rare examples have been reported outside the hands and feet. ***(Right)*** *On low power, FP has a lobular architecture composed of anastomosing cellular trabeculae containing osteoid and immature bone ➔ within a loosely textured, less cellular fibromyxoid background ➔.*

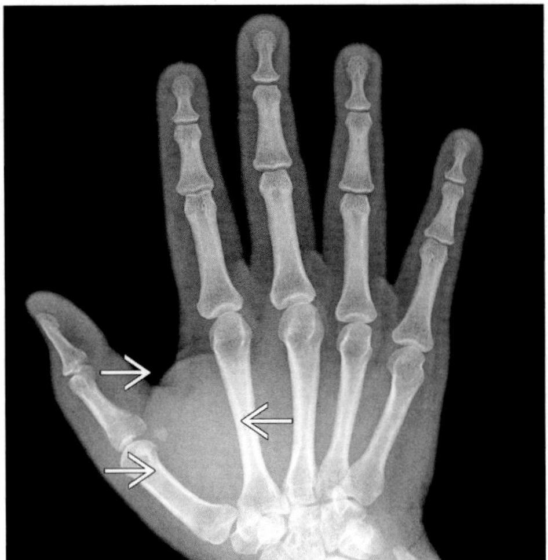

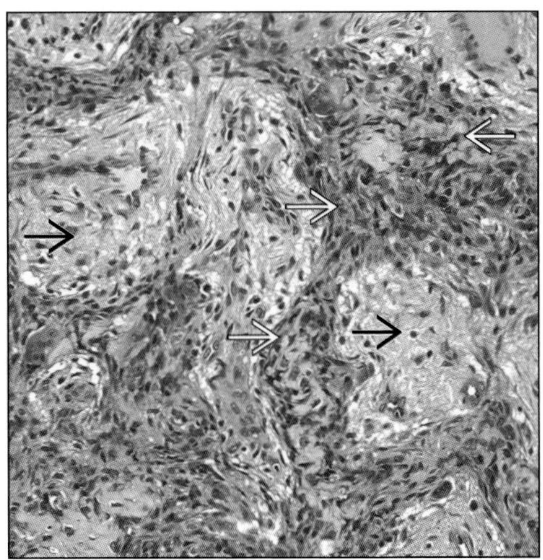

(Left) High-power micrograph depicts very immature ossification, consisting of irregular deposits of osteoid matrix ➔, admixed and numerous plump osteoblastic stromal cells, and scattered osteoclastic giant cells ➔. Note the loosely textured, less cellular areas above and below ➔. ***(Right)*** *Interconnecting trabeculae of hyalinized osteoid matrix ➔ alternate with hypocellular myxoid areas ➔ in this example.*

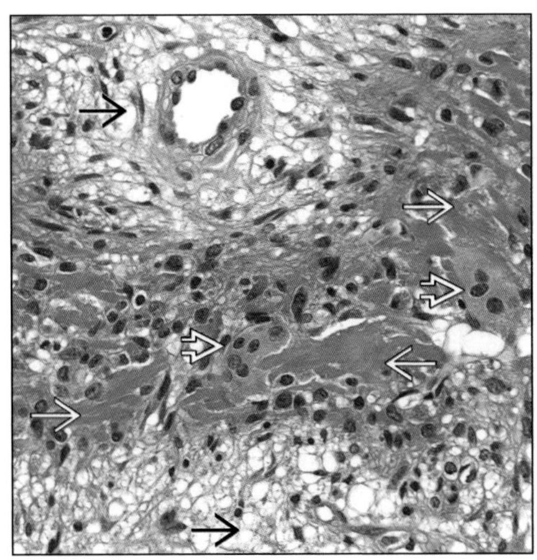

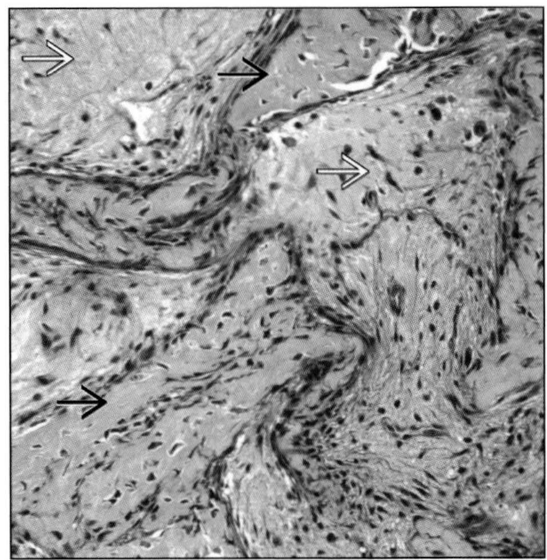

(Left) Low-power micrograph depicts osseous maturation in FP, characterized by osteoid ➔ merging with woven bone ➔. As in myositis ossificans, FP often shows zonal maturation, in which mature bone forms at the periphery of the tumor. In many cases, however, it has a more random, haphazard distribution. ***(Right)*** *FP typically has a large amount of reactive-appearing bone exemplified by a trabecula of immature woven bone, rimmed by a single layer of plump activated osteoblasts.*

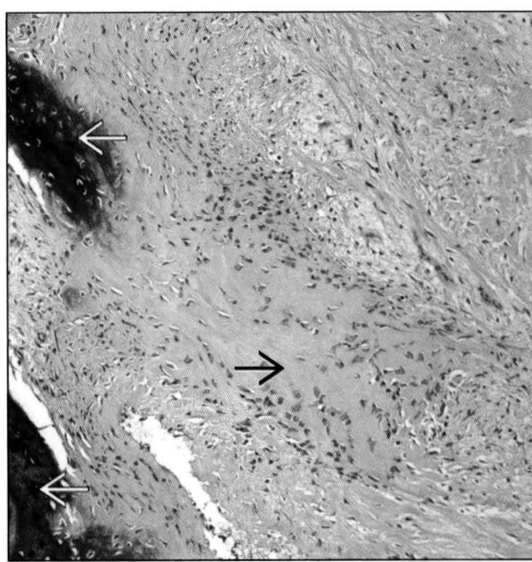

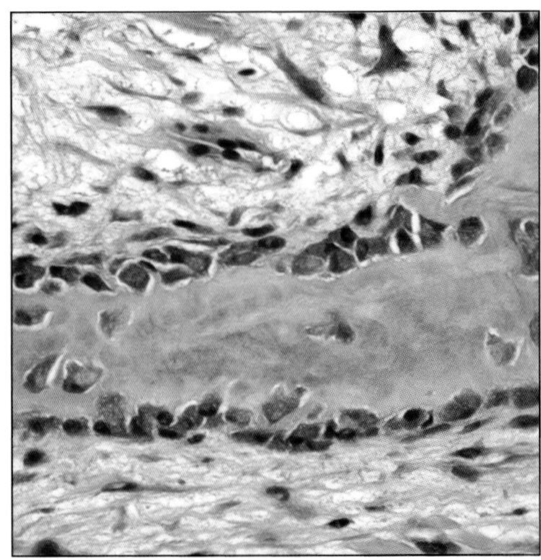

Microscopic Features

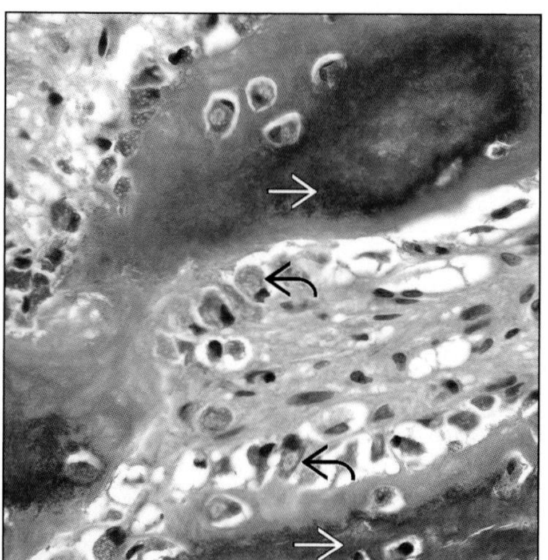

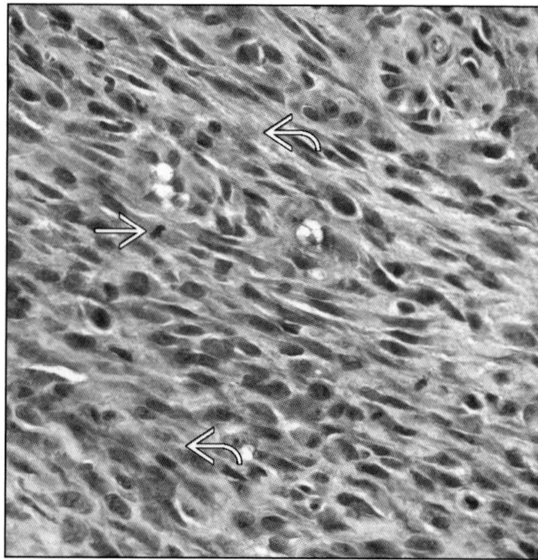

(Left) *This micrograph illustrates woven bone with matrix calcification ➡. The bony trabeculae are lined by single layers of osteoblasts with eccentric nuclei and abundant cytoplasm with perinuclear hofs ⇨ corresponding to the Golgi apparatus.* ***(Right)*** *The spindle cell component of FP resembles nodular fasciitis, consisting of fascicles of myofibroblasts with mitotic activity ➡ and extravasated red blood cells ➡.*

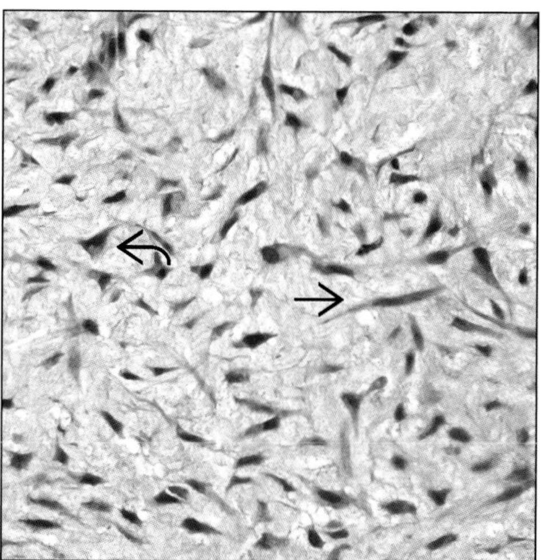

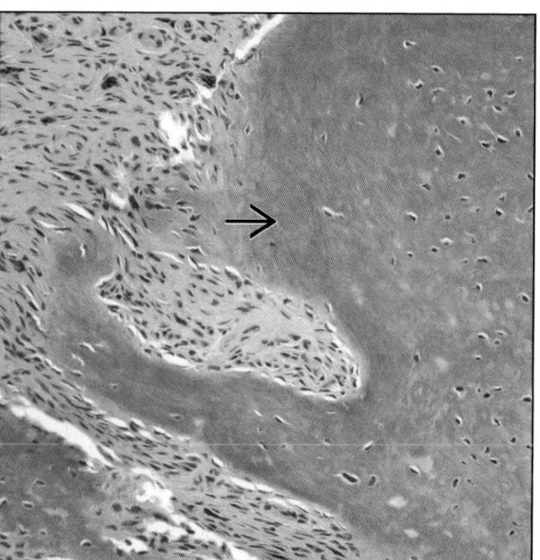

(Left) *The spindle cell areas may be highly myxoid. In this example, myofibroblastic cells with bipolar ⇨ and stellate ⇨ configurations are separated by abundant pale blue myxoid matrix.* ***(Right)*** *Large geographic sheets of collagenous/osseous matrix ⇨ may be seen in FP, as depicted in this low-power micrograph.*

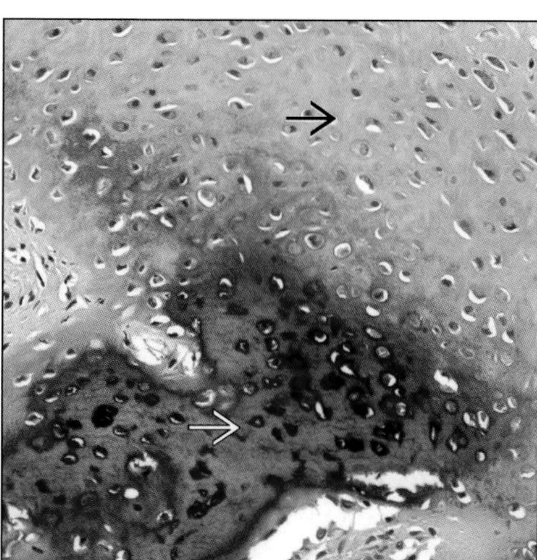

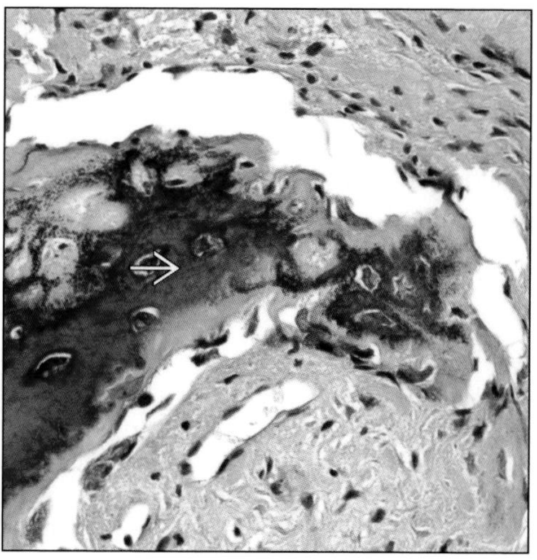

(Left) *Hyaline cartilage is occasionally present in FP. In this example, hyaline cartilage with large reactive chondrocytes ⇨ merges with and becomes transformed into bone ➡ via endochondral ossification.* ***(Right)*** *Immature woven bone with deep basophilic granular calcification ➡ is often present. This irregular pattern of calcification is sometimes referred to as "spiculated blue bone."*

HETEROTOPIC MESENTERIC OSSIFICATION

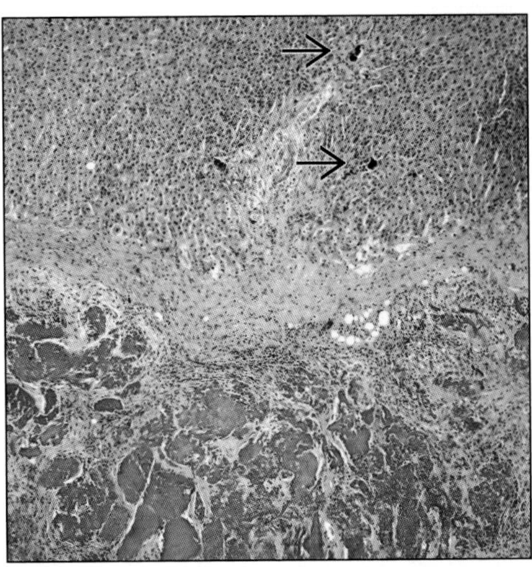

This example of heterotopic mesenteric ossification arose in a patient who had a prior operation. The lesion was adherent to the liver, which shows bile plugs ⇒ from local obstruction.

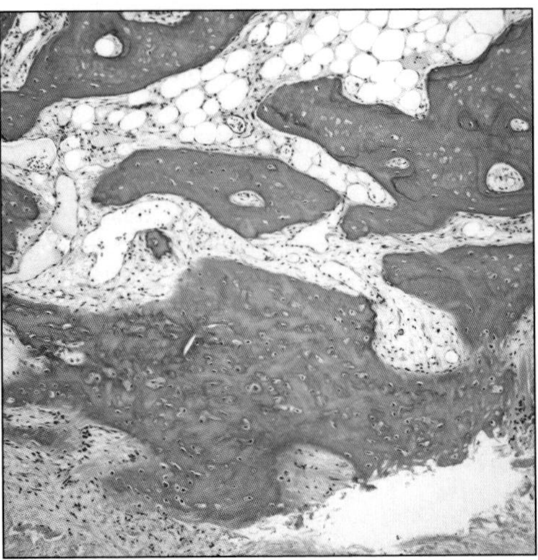

Focus from the same lesion shows mature ossification in this area. The majority of patients with heterotopic mesenteric ossification have had prior surgery.

TERMINOLOGY

Synonyms

- Intraabdominal myositis ossificans

Definitions

- Metaplastic, probably reactive process variably associated with trauma
  - Classically termed "myositis ossificans" when arising in soft tissues

CLINICAL ISSUES

Epidemiology

- Incidence
  - Rare
- Age
  - Adults; mean: 50-60 years

Site

- Small bowel mesentery and omentum most common sites

Presentation

- Bowel obstruction
- Most patients have had prior abdominal surgery

Treatment

- Surgical excision

Prognosis

- Excellent; does not recur after excision

MACROSCOPIC FEATURES

General Features

- Resembles fat necrosis
- Grittiness on cutting

Size

- 3-20 cm; median: 10-15 cm

MICROSCOPIC PATHOLOGY

Predominant Pattern/Injury Type

- Ossification

Predominant Cell/Compartment Type

- Myofibroblast

Key Microscopic Features

- Exuberant myofibroblastic proliferation similar to nodular fasciitis
  - Hemorrhage
  - Collagen deposition
  - Mixed inflammatory infiltrate
  - Proliferating cells all have fine delicate chromatin, smooth nuclear membranes, small nucleoli
  - Loose storiform arrangement of cells
  - Zonation with ossification at margins of lobules
- Fat necrosis
- Abundant lace-like osteoid
  - Matrix-forming cells all have fine delicate chromatin, smooth nuclear membranes, small nucleoli
- Abundant bone
- Plentiful mitotic activity
  - No abnormal mitoses
- Molecular pathogenesis (unstudied)

DIFFERENTIAL DIAGNOSIS

Extraskeletal Osteosarcoma

- No zonation of bone at periphery of nodules
- Cytologic atypia
  - Overtly malignant atypical hyperchromatic cells
- Atypical mitoses
- Necrosis

Key Facts

Terminology
- Intraabdominal myositis ossificans
- Metaplastic, probably reactive process variably associated with trauma

Clinical Issues
- Adults; mean age: 50-60 years
- Small bowel mesentery, omentum most common sites
- Bowel obstruction

Microscopic Pathology
- Exuberant myofibroblastic proliferation similar to nodular fasciitis
- Fat necrosis
- Abundant lace-like osteoid
- Abundant bone
- Plentiful mitotic activity
  - No abnormal mitoses

- Malignant

Mesenteric Fibromatosis
- Long fascicles of myofibroblasts
- Prominent vascular pattern
- Ossification unusual and focal
- β-catenin and *APC* gene mutations
- Recurrences common
- No metastases

Sclerosing Mesenteritis
- Infiltrative sclerosis with fat necrosis
- Lymphoplasmacytic inflammation
- Some cases have venulitis
- Occasional calcification, ossification unusual and focal
- Some cases have increased immunolabeling for IgG4
- Seldom recur following excision

Reactive Nodular Fibrous Pseudotumor of Mesentery
- Predominantly hypocellular fibroblastic proliferation reminiscent of collagenous fibroma
  - Some areas with similar cellularity to fibromatosis
- Frequent hyalinization
- Lymphoid aggregates concentrated toward periphery of lesions
- Not ossified
- Benign

Inflammatory Myofibroblastic Tumor
- Proliferation of myofibroblastic cells
  - Calcification and ossification uncommon and focal
- Lymphoplasmacytic background
  - Scattered eosinophils and macrophages
- Some with *ALK* gene rearrangements and immunolabeling
- Recurrences in subset
- Rare metastases

Calcifying Fibrous Pseudotumor
- Hypocellular lesions composed of fibroblasts
- Plasma cells and lymphocytes
- Dystrophic and psammomatous calcifications
- Ossification unusual and focal
- Benign, does not recur

Gastrointestinal Stromal Tumor
- Cellular spindle and epithelioid cell lesions
- Minimal inflammation
- Seldom calcified or ossified
- *CD117* gene mutations and immunolabeling
- Variable biologic potential
  - Subset is clinically malignant

SELECTED REFERENCES

1. Patel RM et al: Heterotopic mesenteric ossification: a distinctive pseudosarcoma commonly associated with intestinal obstruction. Am J Surg Pathol. 30(1):119-22, 2006
2. Zamolyi RQ et al: Intraabdominal myositis ossificans: a report of 9 new cases. Int J Surg Pathol. 14(1):37-41, 2006

IMAGE GALLERY

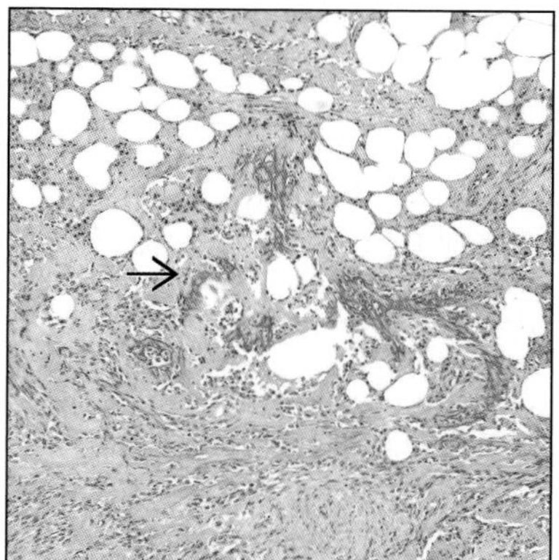

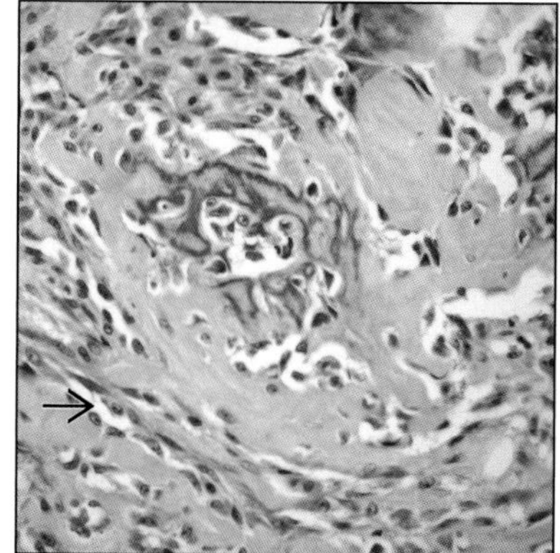

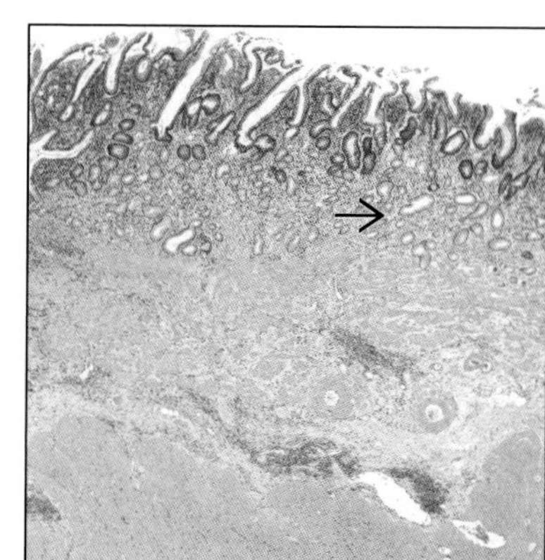

(Left) *This example of heterotopic mesenteric ossification resembles classic myositis ossificans, with maturation toward the periphery of the lesion* ⇒. ***(Center)*** *High magnification of the same lesion shows background myofibroblasts resembling those seen in nodular fasciitis* ⇒. ***(Right)*** *This example of heterotopic mesenteric ossification arose in the ileal mesentery of a Crohn disease patient with fistulizing disease. The small intestinal mucosa from the resection shows active chronic enteritis. There is pyloric gland metaplasia* ⇒, *a feature of chronicity.*

OSTEOMA CUTIS

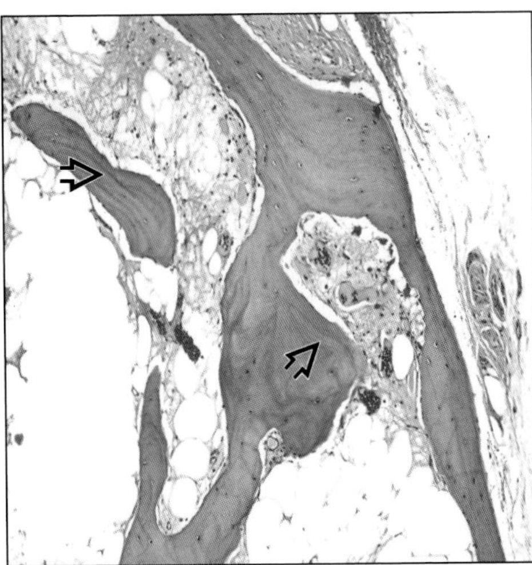

Low-magnification image of an osteoma cutis shows mature bone-forming trabeculae, with cement lines ⇨ surrounding adipocytes and small blood vessels.

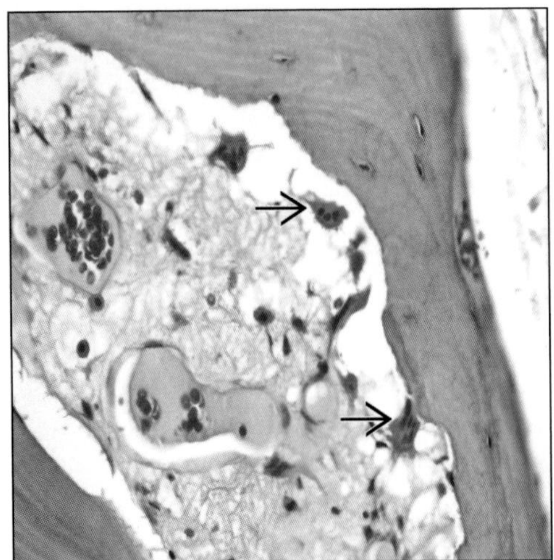

Higher power view shows mature trabeculae composed of lamellar-type bone lined by scattered osteoclasts →.

TERMINOLOGY

Synonyms

- Primary cutaneous osteoma cutis
- Metaplastic (secondary) ossification
- Cutaneous ossification

Definitions

- Primary or secondary cutaneous bone formation

ETIOLOGY/PATHOGENESIS

Primary

- Often genetic or developmental in origin, presents at early age
- May be part of Albright hereditary osteodystrophy or other genetic syndromes
  - Albright: X-linked dominant condition associated with characteristic facies, mental retardation, basal ganglia calcification, and cataracts
  - Other rare syndromes include congenital plaque-like osteomatosis, multiple miliary osteomas of face, progressive osseous heteroplasia, and fibrodysplasia ossificans progressiva

Secondary

- Associated with preexisting lesions, such as nevi, tumors (including adnexal tumors and basal cell carcinoma), scars, acne, and ruptured cysts

CLINICAL ISSUES

Epidemiology

- Age
  - Primary cases often present at birth or in early childhood
  - Secondary cases typically present in adulthood

Site

- Variable, but often involves extremities or face

Presentation

- Dermal papule, plaque, or nodule
  - Multiple lesions more common in primary types

Treatment

- Surgical approaches
  - Complete conservative excision is curative

Prognosis

- Excellent in vast majority of cases; no malignant potential
- Genetic cases may develop numerous debilitating lesions

MACROSCOPIC FEATURES

General Features

- Nodular, dermal-based, solid bony lesion

MICROSCOPIC PATHOLOGY

Histologic Features

- Appearance varies from small spicules to large masses of bone
  - Typically located in deep dermis &/or subcutaneous tissue
  - Mature-appearing bone, often with Haversian systems and cement lines
  - Cartilaginous precursor material usually absent
  - Osteoblastic activity may be present (especially in Albright syndrome), osteoclasts are less common
  - Stromal fat may be present
  - Hematopoietic cells occasionally present
- Bone may extend around adnexal structures
- Transepidermal elimination may be seen, particularly in plaque-like osteomas

OSTEOMA CUTIS

Key Facts

Etiology/Pathogenesis

- Primary: May be part of Albright hereditary osteodystrophy or other genetic syndromes
- Secondary: Associated with preexisting lesions, such as nevi, tumors, scars, and ruptured cysts

Clinical Issues

- Primary cases often present at birth or in early childhood; secondary cases in adults

Microscopic Pathology

- Appearance varies from small spicules to large masses of bone
- Mature-appearing bone, often with Haversian systems and cement lines
- Osteoblastic activity may be present (especially in Albright syndrome), osteoclasts are less common
- Typically located in deep dermis &/or subcutaneous tissue

- Associated/precursor lesions often present in secondary ossification, including
  - Nevi (especially on face)
  - Pilomatrixomas (often ruptured lesions)
  - Basal cell carcinomas
  - Other tumors, including trichoepitheliomas, hemangiomas, schwannomas, lipomas, and dermatofibromas
  - Cysts, including epidermoid and pilar (trichilemmal) cysts, especially ruptured
  - Sites of trauma, scars, injections, and previous infection
- Pigmentation has been reported in patients treated with minocycline or tetracycline

Cytologic Features

- Osteocytes, osteoblasts, and osteoclasts show bland cytologic features without atypia

DIFFERENTIAL DIAGNOSIS

Calcinosis Cutis

- Nodules of dense basophilic material typically lacking well-formed bone
- Peripheral rim of secondary ossification may form

Chondroma

- Very rare dermal or subcutaneous tumor
- Cartilaginous tumor that lacks mature bone formation

Myositis Ossificans

- Subcutaneous tumor showing shell of reactive bone
- Central proliferation of fibroblastic cells with "tissue-culture" appearance (similar to nodular fasciitis)

SELECTED REFERENCES

1. Haro R et al: Plaque-like osteoma cutis with transepidermal elimination. J Cutan Pathol. 36(5):591-3, 2009
2. Kacerovska D et al: Cutaneous and superficial soft tissue lesions associated with Albright hereditary osteodystrophy: clinicopathological and molecular genetic study of 4 cases, including a novel mutation of the GNAS gene. Am J Dermatopathol. 30(5):417-24, 2008
3. Burford C: Pigmented osteoma cutis secondary to long-term tetracyclines. Australas J Dermatol. 48(2):134-6, 2007
4. Thielen AM et al: Multiple cutaneous osteomas of the face associated with chronic inflammatory acne. J Eur Acad Dermatol Venereol. 20(3):321-6, 2006
5. Bergonse FN et al: Miliary osteoma of the face: a report of 4 cases and review of the literature. Cutis. 69(5):383-6, 2002
6. Shoji T et al: Basal cell carcinoma with massive ossification. Am J Dermatopathol. 21(1):34-6, 1999
7. Cottoni F et al: Primary osteoma cutis. Clinical, morphological, and ultrastructural study. Am J Dermatopathol. 15(1):77-81, 1993
8. Prendiville JS et al: Osteoma cutis as a presenting sign of pseudohypoparathyroidism. Pediatr Dermatol. 9(1):11-8, 1992

IMAGE GALLERY

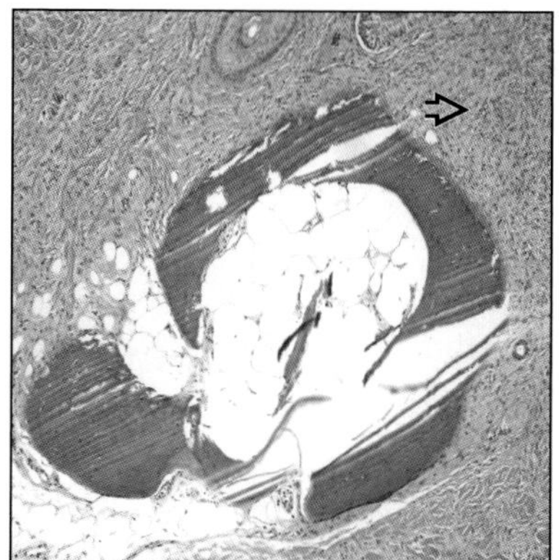

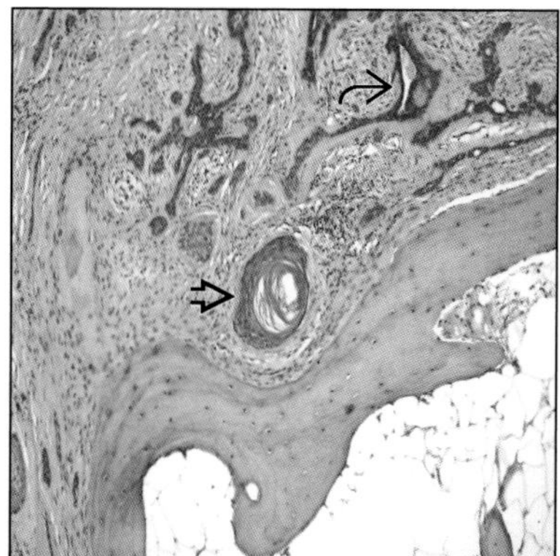

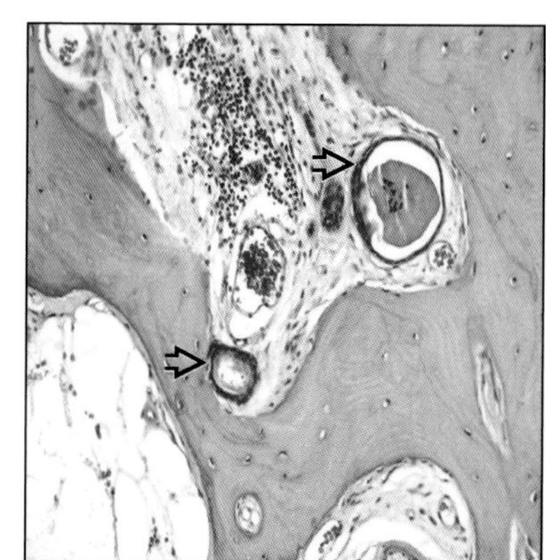

(Left) *Low-power view of an osteoma cutis arising in association with a dermatofibroma ➭ shows a proliferation of mature osteoid surrounding large, bland fat cells.* ***(Center)*** *Hematoxylin & eosin of an osteoma cutis associated with a chondroid syringoma (cutaneous mixed tumor) shows a proliferation of bland ductal ➚ and folliculocystic structures ➭ surrounding the bone.* ***(Right)*** *Higher power examination of the same osteoma cutis shows a few bland adnexal ducts ➭ trapped between the mature bony trabeculae.*

SOFT TISSUE CHONDROMA

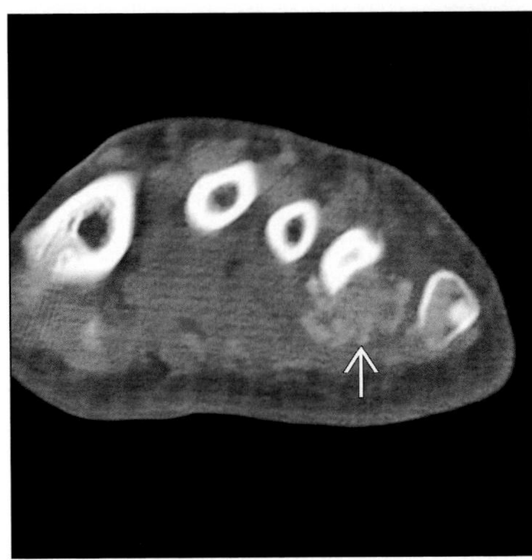

CT depicts a mineralized soft tissue chondroma ➡ adjacent to the 4th metatarsal. Soft tissue chondroma has a predilection for the hands and feet, often near a joint or tendon.

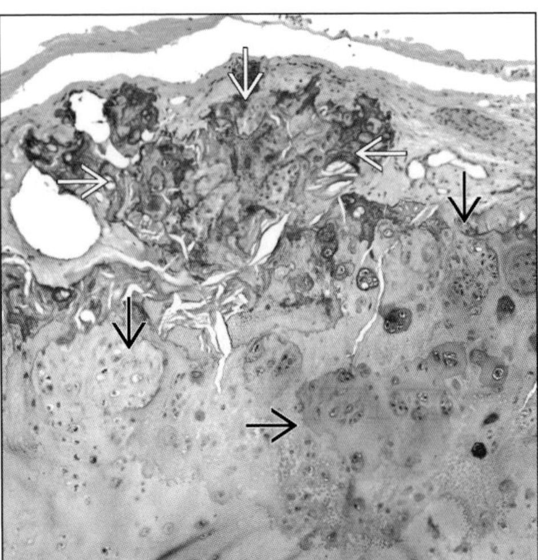

Soft tissue chondroma typically appears as a well-circumscribed tumor composed of hyaline cartilage lobules ⇨ with extensive calcification ➡ and sharp demarcation from adjacent soft tissue (top).

TERMINOLOGY

Synonyms

- Extraskeletal chondroma, chondroma of soft parts, fibrochondroma, osteochondroma, myxochondroma, chondroblastoma-like chondroma of soft tissue

Definitions

- Benign hyaline cartilage neoplasm of soft tissue with predilection for hands and feet

CLINICAL ISSUES

Epidemiology

- Incidence
  - Uncommon; exact incidence unknown
- Age
  - Median: 4th decade; range: Infancy to 9th decade
- Gender
  - Women and men equally affected

Presentation

- Painless mass
- Most common in hands and feet (60-95%), especially fingers (40-50%)
  - Rare reports in proximal extremities, trunk, head and neck, upper aerodigestive tract, dura, skin, fallopian tube

Treatment

- Surgical approaches
  - Simple excision

Prognosis

- Low recurrence rate (15-20%)
  - Recurrences controlled by reexcision
- No reports of malignant degeneration

IMAGE FINDINGS

General Features

- Best diagnostic clue
  - Small, well-demarcated, mineralized soft tissue mass in acral extremity
- Location
  - Hands and feet
  - Often in vicinity of joint or tendon
  - No intraarticular or subperiosteal localization by definition
- Morphology
  - Most are calcified or ossified
  - Sometimes erode and deform underlying bone

MACROSCOPIC FEATURES

General Features

- Well demarcated, spherical or ovoid
- Rubbery or hard
- Sometimes soft, friable, gelatinous, or cystic

Size

- Median: 1.6 cm; range: 0.3-6.5 cm

MICROSCOPIC PATHOLOGY

Histologic Features

- Well circumscribed and lobulated
- Mostly composed of mature hyaline cartilage
- Chondrocytes located in lacunae
  - Arranged diffusely or in small clusters
  - Some have enlarged nuclei and moderate pleomorphism
  - Very low mitotic rate
- Variable amounts of calcification
  - Granular stippled calcification that surrounds chondrocytes in lace-like pattern

Key Facts

Terminology
- Benign hyaline cartilage neoplasm of soft tissue with predilection for hands and feet

Clinical Issues
- Low recurrence rate (15-20%)
- Recurrences controlled by reexcision

Image Findings
- Small, well-demarcated, mineralized soft tissue mass in acral extremity

Macroscopic Features
- Median size: 1.6 cm; range: 0.3-6.5 cm

Microscopic Pathology
- Well circumscribed and lobulated
- Mostly composed of mature hyaline cartilage
- Variable amounts of calcification
- Ossification common
- Granulomatous inflammation in 15% of cases
- Rare tumors with extensive xanthogranulomatous inflammation
- Rare tumors with extensive stromal fibrosis (fibrochondroma)
- Chondroblastoma-like chondroma

Top Differential Diagnoses
- Synovial chondromatosis
- Tophaceous pseudogout
- Tumoral calcinosis
- Extraskeletal myxoid chondrosarcoma
- Calcifying aponeurotic fibroma

- Some have extensive calcification with deep basophilia of matrix
- Ossification common
- Granulomatous inflammation in 15% of cases
  - Epithelioid macrophages and osteoclastic giant cells
  - Most pronounced in heavily calcified tumors
- Rare tumors with extensive xanthogranulomatous inflammation mimicking fibrous histiocytoma or giant cell tumor of tendon sheath
- Rare tumors with extensive stromal fibrosis (fibrochondroma)
- Chondroblastoma-like chondroma
  - Abundant myxoid matrix
  - Immature chondrocytes
    - Polygonal or elongated cells
    - Abundant eosinophilic or vacuolated cytoplasm
    - Eccentrically located nuclei, often grooved or reniform, resembling cells of chondroblastoma

DIFFERENTIAL DIAGNOSIS

Synovial Chondromatosis
- Larger tumors
- Most often in synovium of large joints, especially knee, but also tenosynovium of acral extremities
- More discrete lobular architecture and chondrocyte clusters

Tophaceous Pseudogout
- Wide distribution, including acral extremities, but predilection for temporomandibular joint
- Heavily calcified lesions with metaplastic cartilage formation
- Rhomboid-shaped CPPD crystals with positive birefringence under polarized light

Tumoral Calcinosis
- Predilection for large joints
- Calcium hydroxyapatite crystals (psammomatous)
- Histiocytic giant cells with intracytoplasmic calcifications

Extraskeletal Myxoid Chondrosarcoma
- Large, lobulated soft tissue mass
- Myxoid matrix, thick fibrous septa, and cords of neoplastic cells

Calcifying Aponeurotic Fibroma
- Hands and feet, especially palm of children
- Geographic areas of calcification surrounded by chondrocytic cells
- Extensive fibromatous areas

DIAGNOSTIC CHECKLIST

Clinically Relevant Pathologic Features
- Tissue distribution

Pathologic Interpretation Pearls
- Features that can lead to misdiagnosis
  - Chondrocyte atypia
  - Increased cellularity
  - Extensive calcification and ossification
  - Granulomatous or xanthogranulomatous reaction
  - Fibrous, myxoid, and chondroblastoma-like features

SELECTED REFERENCES

1. Fetsch JF et al: Tenosynovial (extraarticular) chondromatosis: an analysis of 37 cases of an underrecognized clinicopathologic entity with a strong predilection for the hands and feet and a high local recurrence rate. Am J Surg Pathol. 27(9):1260-8, 2003
2. Cates JM et al: Chondroblastoma-like chondroma of soft tissue: an underrecognized variant and its differential diagnosis. Am J Surg Pathol. 25(5):661-6, 2001
3. Ishida T et al: Tophaceous pseudogout (tumoral calcium pyrophosphate dihydrate crystal deposition disease). Hum Pathol. 26(6):587-93, 1995
4. Chung EB et al: Chondroma of soft parts. Cancer. 41(4):1414-24, 1978
5. Dahlin DC et al: Cartilaginous tumors of the soft tissues of the hands and feet. Mayo Clin Proc. 49(10):721-6, 1974

SOFT TISSUE CHONDROMA

Microscopic Features

(Left) Soft tissue chondroma typically has a lobular architecture with islands of hyaline cartilage ➙ separated by fibrous bands ➙. Ossification ➙ is common. *(Right)* High-power micrograph illustrates typical cytological features. The chondrocytes are often arranged in clusters, situated in lacunar spaces within pale blue hyaline matrix, and have uniform round nuclei and abundant eosinophilic cytoplasm. Rare binucleated cells can be seen ➙. Mitoses are rare.

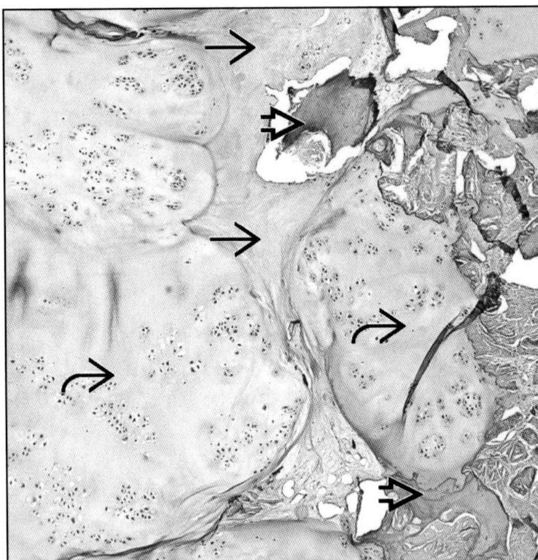

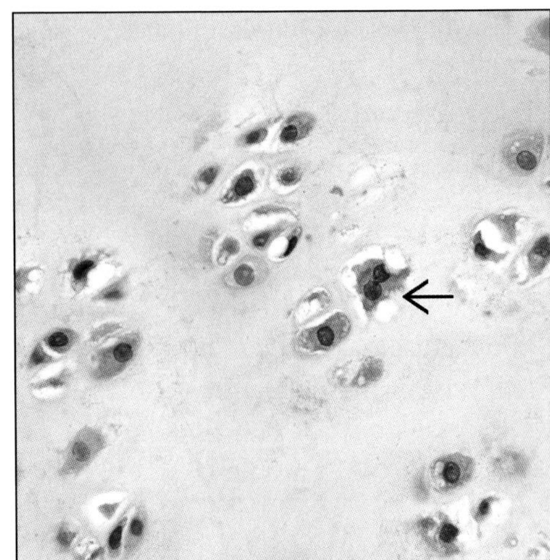

(Left) Calcification is very common in soft tissue chondroma. It appears as granular basophilic stippling of the matrix, which often surrounds individual chondrocytes to form a lace-like pattern ➙. *(Right)* Areas of very dense calcification are also common, illustrated by heavy basophilic staining of the cartilage matrix.

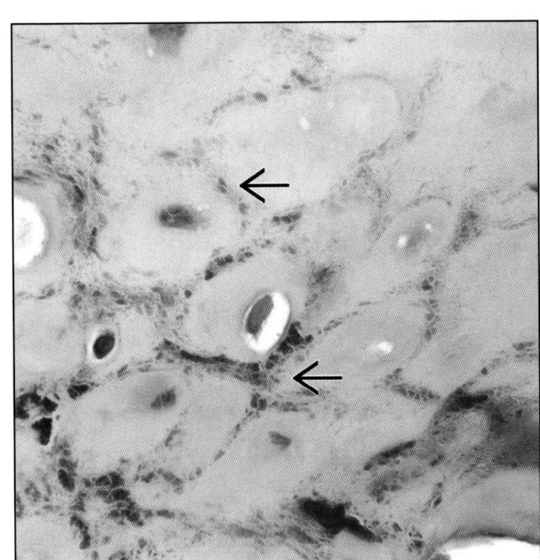

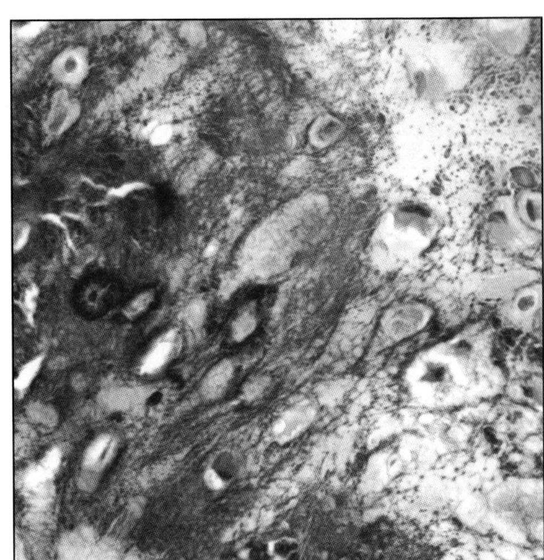

(Left) Ossification ➙ is also common and can sometimes be extensive, as illustrated here. It can be located either at the center or periphery of the tumor and is formed via endochondral ossification of calcified cartilage matrix ➙. *(Right)* Granulomatous inflammation is common, especially in calcified tumors. This micrograph illustrates epithelioid macrophages ➙ and osteoclastic giant cells ➙ in a calcified tumor. When extensive, this mimics giant cell tumor of tendon sheath.

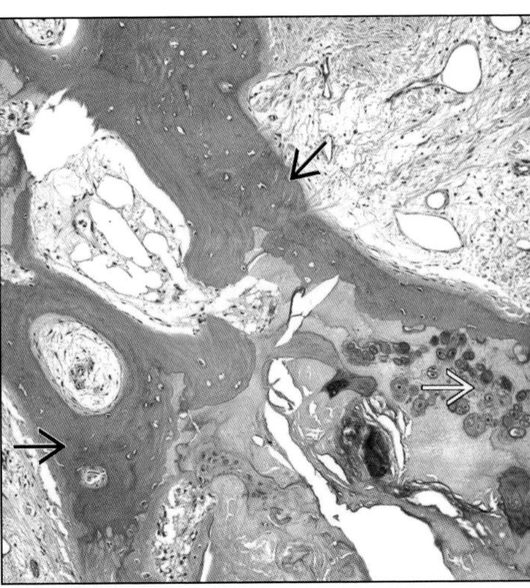

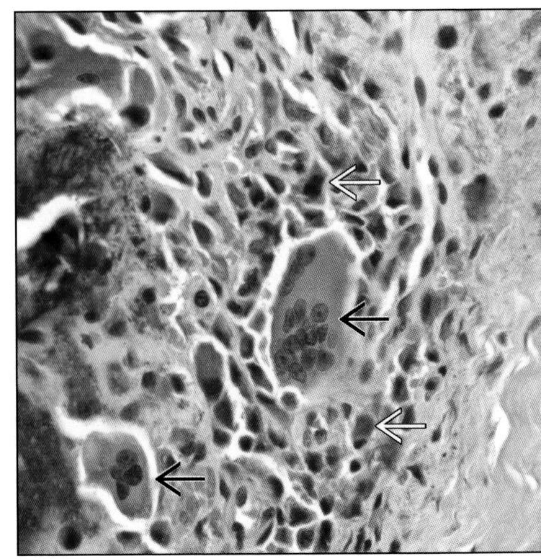

Microscopic Features

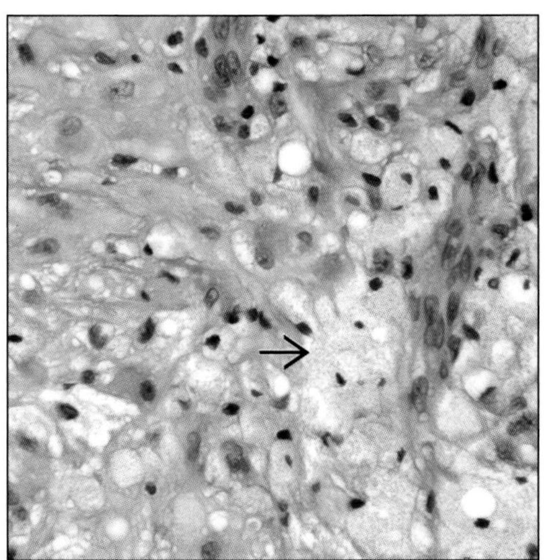

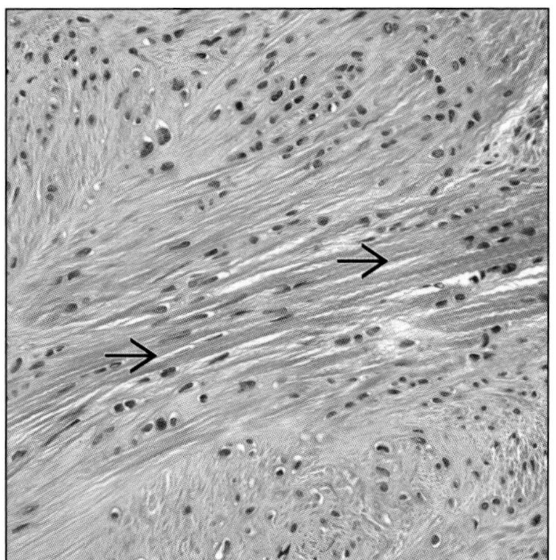

(Left) *Xanthogranulomatous inflammation can be present in soft tissue chondroma, consisting of sheets or clusters of foamy histiocytes* ⇒*. When extensive, such a tumor can be mistaken for fibrous histiocytoma or giant cell tumor of tendon sheath.* **(Right)** *Soft tissue chondroma can have extensive fibrosis exemplified by numerous collagen bundles transversing this tumor* ⇒*. Tumors with extensive fibrosis are sometimes referred to as fibrochondromas.*

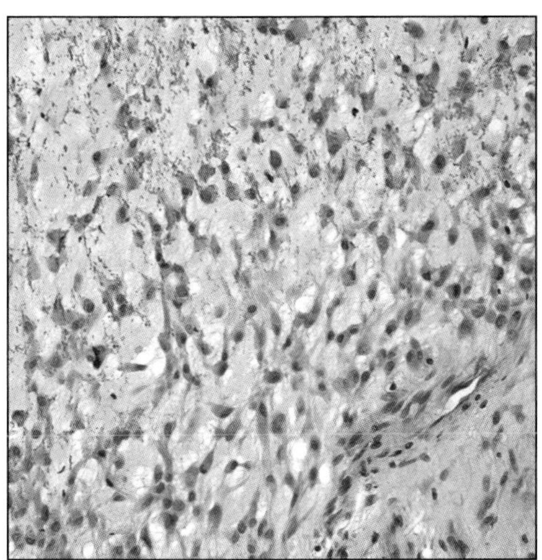

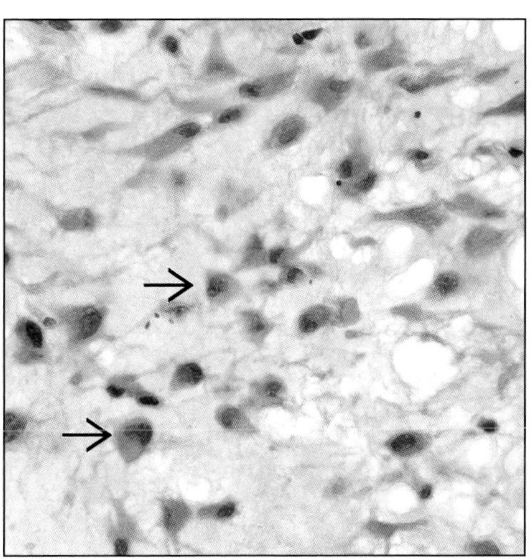

(Left) *Soft tissue chondroma can have extensive myxoid matrix where chondrocytes assume elongated & stellate configurations, sometimes interconnecting with each other to form a fine network, mimicking extraskeletal myxoid chondrosarcoma. Tumors with extensive myxoid matrix are sometimes called myxochondromas.* **(Right)** *Chondrocytes can resemble chondroblasts consisting of rounded cells with abundant eosinophilic cytoplasm & eccentric grooved or reniform nuclei* ⇒*.*

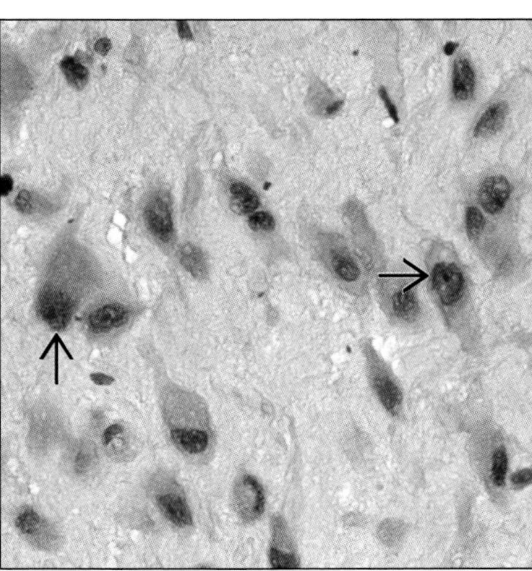

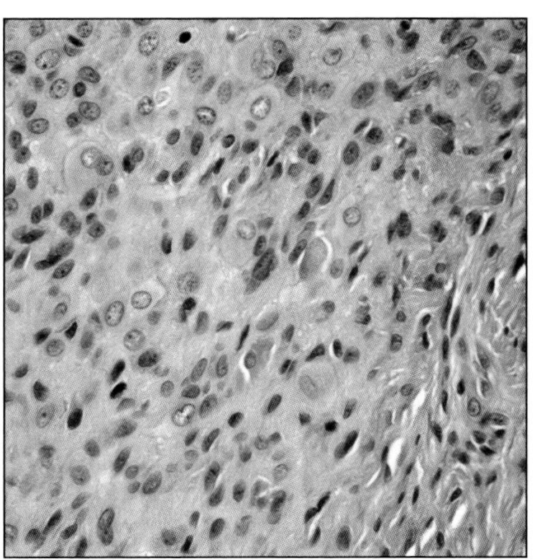

(Left) *Degenerative cytologic atypica is not uncommon in soft tissue chondroma. This high-power micrograph illustrates chondrocytes with nuclear enlargement* ⇒ *and pleomorphism, which out of context would be suspicious for chondrosarcoma.* **(Right)** *Focal areas of increased cellularity can also be present in soft tissue chondroma, as exemplified by this tumor, and should not be regarded as worrisome for malignancy.*

SYNOVIAL CHONDROMATOSIS

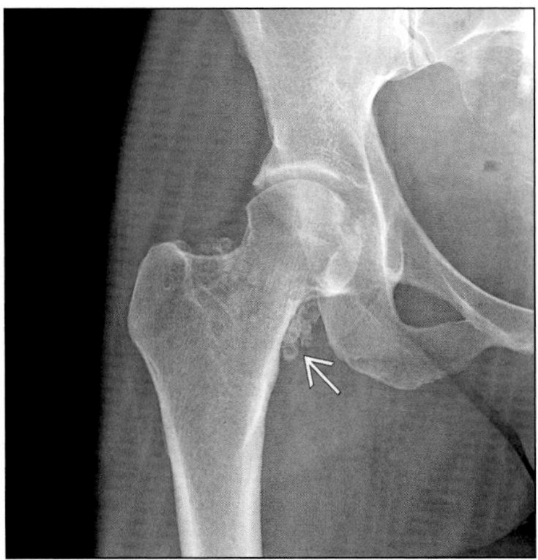

Synovial chondromatosis typically presents as a calcified mass in a large weight-bearing joint, such as the hip. It usually presents as multiple diffuse punctate or ring-like calcifications ➡.

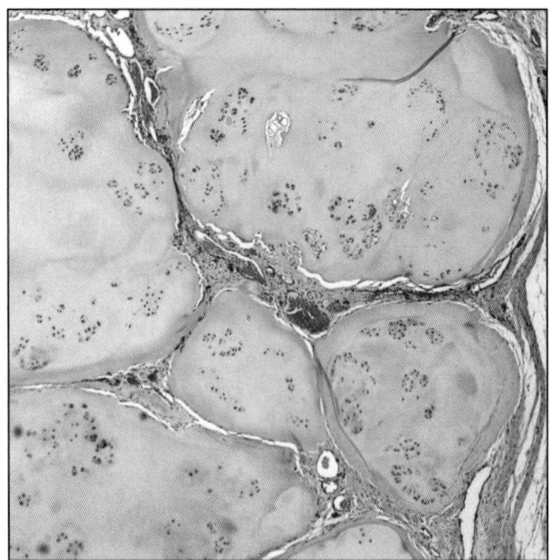

Synovial chondromatosis has a well-defined lobular architecture, characterized by discrete nodules of hyaline cartilage within the subsynovial tissue. The chondrocytes are arranged in small clusters.

TERMINOLOGY

Synonyms

- Primary synovial chondromatosis, synovial osteochondromatosis, synovial chondroma, synovial chondrometaplasia

Definitions

- Benign multinodular proliferation of hyaline cartilage within articular synovium, tendon sheath, or bursa
  - Usually diffuse and associated with loose bodies, with propensity for local recurrence

CLINICAL ISSUES

Epidemiology

- Incidence
  - Rare, but exact incidence unknown
- Age
  - Peak age 5th decade but wide variation (1st-7th decades)
- Gender
  - M:F = 2:1

Site

- Virtually any joint may be involved
  - Knee is most common site
  - Hip, elbow, and shoulder common
  - Temporomandibular joint
- Soft tissue around joints
  - Tenosynovium of acral extremities most common
  - Bursa

Presentation

- Painful or painless mass
- Impaired range of motion

Treatment

- Surgical approaches
  - Synovectomy and removal of loose bodies

Prognosis

- Benign but high local recurrence rate

IMAGE FINDINGS

Radiographic Findings

- Multifocal punctate and ring-like calcifications involving joint, tendon sheath, or bursa
  - Early lesions lack calcification
  - Older lesions may become heavily mineralized with ossified bodies

MR Findings

- Lobulated mass
- Intense T2 signal

MACROSCOPIC FEATURES

General Features

- Multiple small cartilaginous nodules (0.1-1 cm) that coalesce into larger conglomerates
  - Diffuse lesions stud synovial membrane
  - Detached loose bodies
  - Ossified nodules in older lesions
  - May erode adjacent bone

MICROSCOPIC PATHOLOGY

Histologic Features

- Multiple nodules of hyaline cartilage
- Nodules underlie flattened synovium
- Chondrocytes arranged in small clusters
  - Binucleation common
  - Cytological atypia and increased cellularity in some lesions
- Hyaline cartilage matrix
  - Can be focally myxoid
  - Calcification common

SYNOVIAL CHONDROMATOSIS

Key Facts

Terminology

- Benign multinodular proliferation of hyaline cartilage within articular synovium, tendon sheath, or bursa
  - Usually diffuse and associated with loose bodies, with propensity for local recurrence

Clinical Issues

- Site
  - Knee, hip, and elbow most common
  - Temporomandibular joint
  - Tenosynovium of acral extremities
  - Benign but high local recurrence rate

Image Findings

- Diffuse punctate and ring-like calcifications
- Intense T2 signal on MR

Macroscopic Features

- Multiple small cartilaginous nodules (0.1-1 cm) that coalesce into larger conglomerates
- Diffuse lesions stud synovial membrane

Microscopic Pathology

- Multiple discrete nodules of hyaline cartilage
- Chondrocytes arranged in small clusters
- Cytological atypia and increased cellularity in some lesions
- Matrix usually hyaline but may be myxoid or heavily calcified
- Can undergo endochondral ossification

Top Differential Diagnoses

- Osteocartilaginous loose bodies
- Soft tissue chondroma

  - Some lesions heavily calcified
  - Nodules can undergo endochondral ossification

Predominant Pattern/Injury Type

- Neoplastic

Predominant Cell/Compartment Type

- Cartilaginous

ANCILLARY TESTS

Cytogenetics

- Clonal chromosomal changes
- Often involves 12q

DIFFERENTIAL DIAGNOSIS

Osteocartilaginous Loose Bodies

- Concentric laminations of variably calcified/ossified cartilage
- Associated with degenerative joint disease, trauma, osteochondritis dissecans

Soft Tissue Chondroma

- Lacks multinodular architecture
- Predilection for hands and feet

Juxtaarticular Chondroma

- Lacks well-defined lobular architecture
- Concentric laminations of calcified cartilage
- Often extensively ossified
- Most common in subpatellar knee

Synovial Chondrosarcoma

- Very rare
- May arise de novo or within synovial chondromatosis
- Loss of clustered growth, prominent myxoid matrix, necrosis, peripheral spindling

DIAGNOSTIC CHECKLIST

Clinically Relevant Pathologic Features

- Tissue distribution

Pathologic Interpretation Pearls

- Multinodularity
- Clustered chondrocytes

SELECTED REFERENCES

1. Campanacci DA et al: Synovial chondrosarcoma of the hip: report of two cases and literature review. Chir Organi Mov. 92(3):139-44, 2008
2. Lieger O et al: Synovial chondromatosis of the temporomandibular joint with cranial extension: a case report and literature review. J Oral Maxillofac Surg. 65(10):2073-80, 2007
3. Murphey MD et al: Imaging of synovial chondromatosis with radiologic-pathologic correlation. Radiographics. 27(5):1465-88, 2007
4. Fetsch JF et al: Tenosynovial (extraarticular) chondromatosis: an analysis of 37 cases of an underrecognized clinicopathologic entity with a strong predilection for the hands and feet and a high local recurrence rate. Am J Surg Pathol. 27(9):1260-8, 2003
5. Tallini G et al: Correlation between clinicopathological features and karyotype in 100 cartilaginous and chordoid tumours. A report from the Chromosomes and Morphology (CHAMP) Collaborative Study Group. J Pathol. 196(2):194-203, 2002
6. Sciot R et al: Synovial chondromatosis: clonal chromosome changes provide further evidence for a neoplastic disorder. Virchows Arch. 433(2):189-91, 1998
7. Sviland L et al: Synovial chondromatosis presenting as painless soft tissue mass--a report of 19 cases. Histopathology. 27(3):275-9, 1995
8. Bertoni F et al: Chondrosarcomas of the synovium. Cancer. 67(1):155-62, 1991
9. Milgram JW: Synovial osteochondromatosis: a histopathological study of thirty cases. J Bone Joint Surg Am. 59(6):792-801, 1977

SYNOVIAL CHONDROMATOSIS

Radiographic, Gross, and Microscopic Features

*(**Left**) The knee is the most common location for synovial chondromatosis and presents radiographically as diffuse periarticular punctate calcifications ➡. Other common sites are hip, elbow, shoulder, and temporomandibular joint. Synovial chondromatosis also occurs in extraarticular locations, such as tenosynovium or bursae. (**Right**) Grossly, it has a very distinctive multinodular pattern characterized by small opalescent cartilaginous nodules, which coalesce into larger conglomerates.*

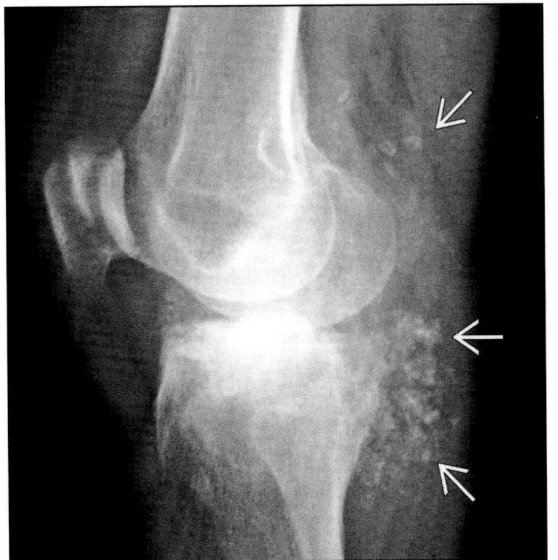

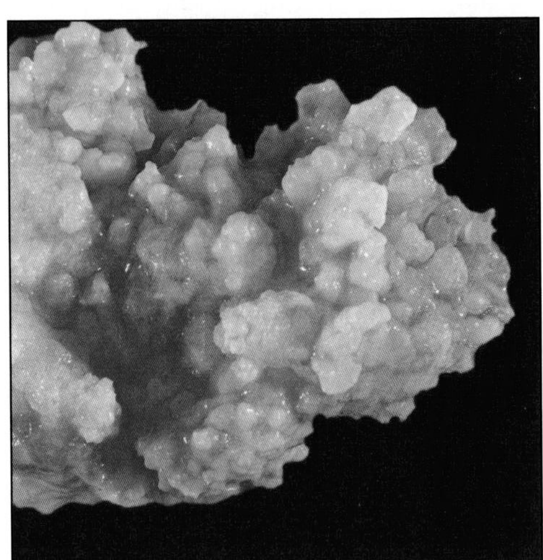

*(**Left**) This gross photograph depicts tissue removed at knee synovectomy. Note the characteristic multinodular appearance as well as how it studs the synovial membrane ➡. Detached loose bodies typically accompany such specimens. (**Right**) This low-power micrograph illustrates discrete nodules of synovial chondromatosis within subsynovial tissue. Note the sharp borders of the nodules, which are separated by fibrovascular tissue.*

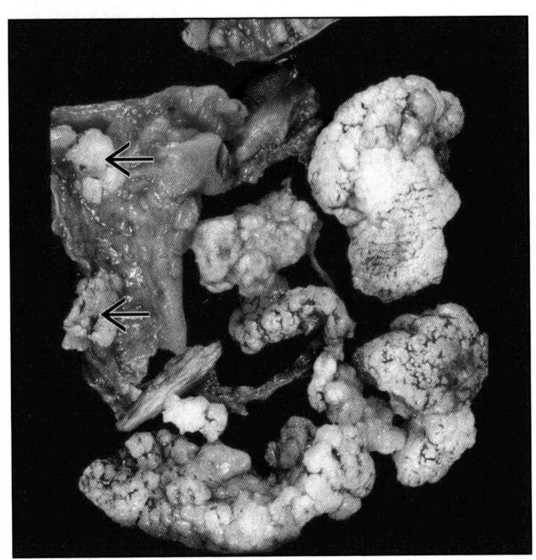

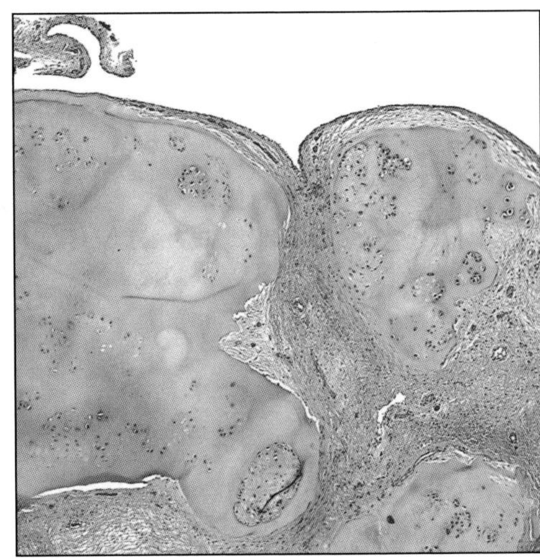

*(**Left**) In most cases of synovial chondromatosis, the matrix is pure hyaline cartilage, and the chondrocytes are arranged in small clusters. (**Right**) The chondrocytes are situated within lacunar spaces and have vacuolated eosinophilic cytoplasm and open nuclear chromatin with small nucleoli. Binucleation is common ➡. Mitoses are rare. Some cases show greater nuclear atypia that, when taken out of context, can be mistaken for chondrosarcoma.*

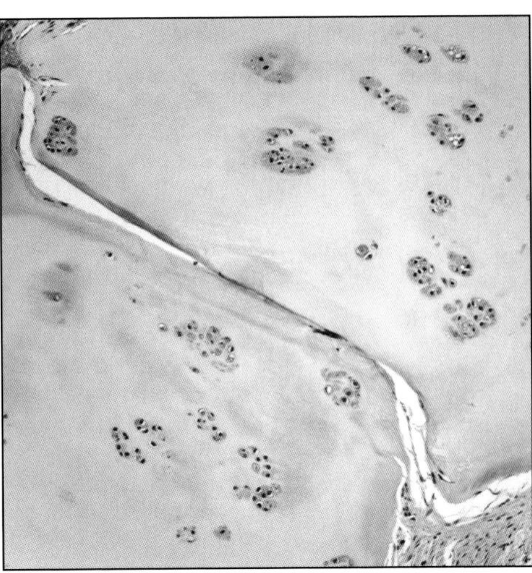

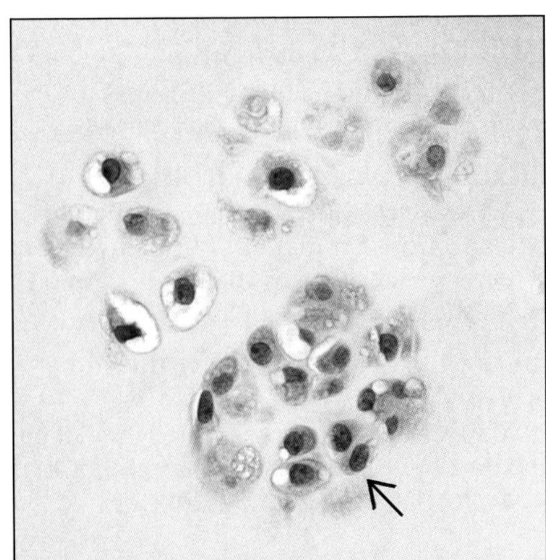

Microscopic and Radiographic Features

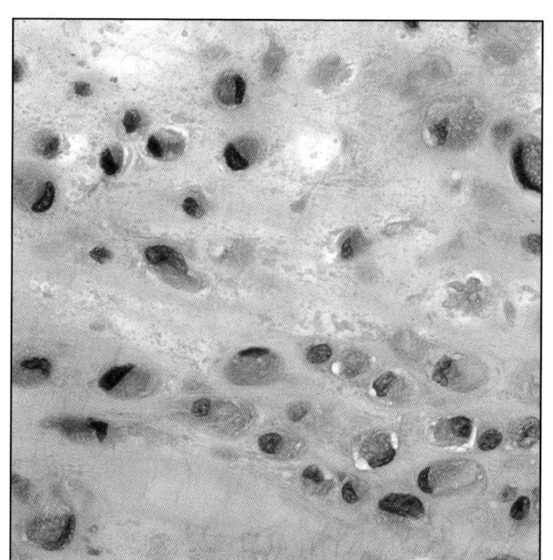

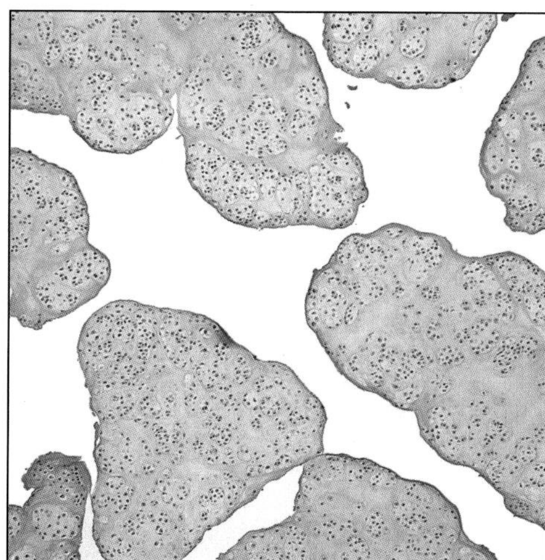

(Left) Degenerative cytological atypia can be seen in synovial chondromatosis. This high-power micrograph depicts large chondrocytes with eccentric cytoplasm and pleomorphic nuclei with smudged chromatin. **(Right)** Intraarticular loose bodies frequently occur in synovial chondromatosis. Unlike the osteocartilaginous loose bodies associated with degenerative joint disease, they lack concentric laminations and maintain the clustered arrangement of chondrocytes.

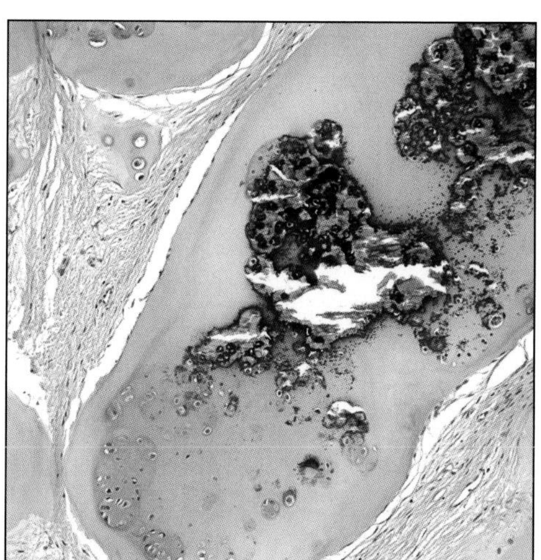

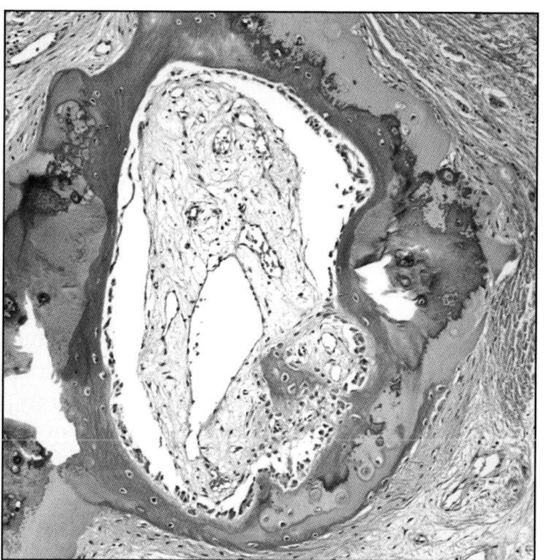

(Left) Calcification is common in synovial chondromatosis, as depicted. This pattern correlates with the punctate calcifications seen on radiographs. **(Right)** Calcified nodules can be transformed into ring-like ossified structures via endochondral ossification. Note the remnants of calcified cartilage peripheral to the bone. Such ossified nodules correspond to ring-like structures seen on radiographs.

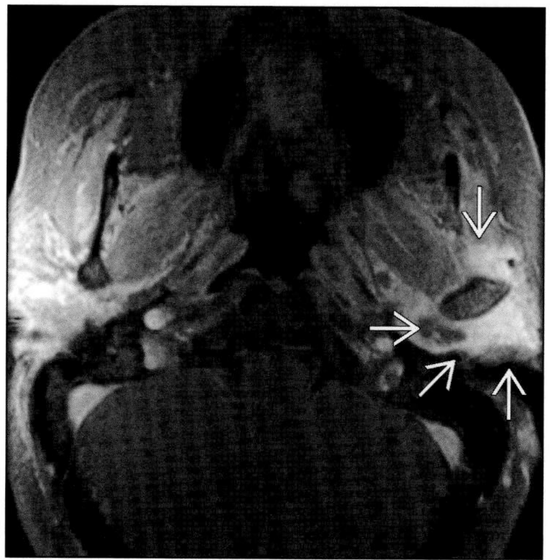

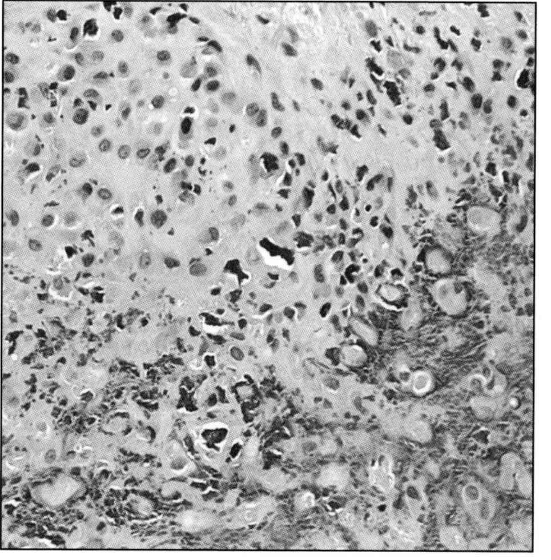

(Left) This T2-weighted MR depicts bright signaling in synovial chondromatosis ➔ of the temporomandibular joint. In this location, synovial chondromatosis presents with pain, swelling, and deviation. It frequently recurs and rarely can invade intracranially. **(Right)** Synovial chondromatosis of the temporomandibular joint can be heavily calcified, as in this example.

EXTRASKELETAL OSTEOSARCOMA

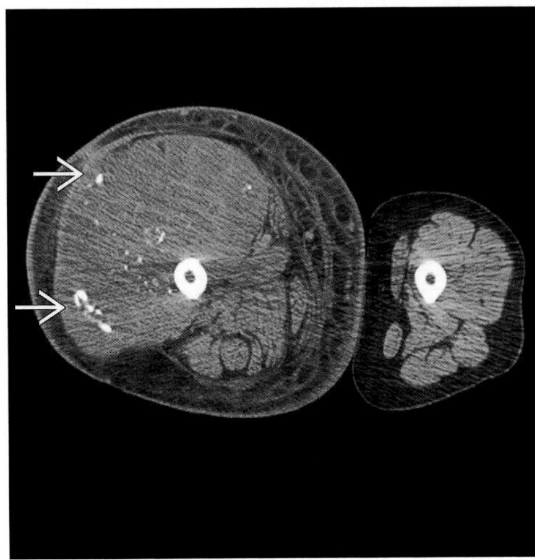

Extraskeletal osteosarcoma (ESOS) typically presents as a massive soft tissue tumor, most commonly in the thigh, as shown in this CT scan. Calcifications ➡ are common and variable in extent.

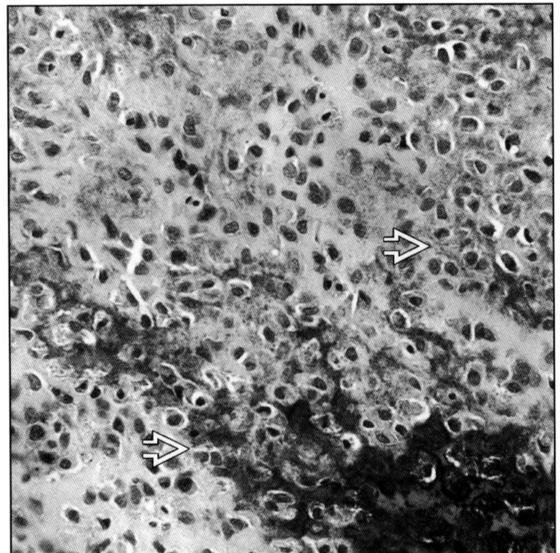

ESOSs are usually high-grade sarcomas, microscopically identical to their skeletal counterparts, characterized by malignant osteoid and bone formation. Note the lace-like pattern of ossification ⇨.

TERMINOLOGY

Abbreviations

- Extraskeletal osteosarcoma (ESOS)

Synonyms

- Soft tissue osteosarcoma
- Extraosseous osteogenic sarcoma

Definitions

- Soft tissue sarcoma in which neoplastic cells produce osteoid or bone
  - Can produce cartilage in addition to osseous matrix
  - No other lines of differentiation

ETIOLOGY/PATHOGENESIS

Environmental Exposure

- Radiation-associated (10%)
- Trauma history in some
- Rare tumors arise in myositis ossificans

CLINICAL ISSUES

Epidemiology

- Incidence
  - 1-2% of soft tissue sarcomas
  - 2-4% of osteosarcomas
- Age
  - Almost exclusively adults
  - Average: 50 years, range: 20-80 years
- Gender
  - Men outnumber women 2:1

Site

- Mostly deep-seated (70-90%)
- Lower extremity (50-70%)
  - Thigh most common site (30-50%)
  - Pelvic girdle, buttocks, leg
- Upper extremity (20%)
  - Shoulder girdle and upper arm common
- Retroperitoneum (10%)
- Rare sites: Hand, foot, larynx, tongue, spermatic cord, penis, pleura, lung, breast, colon, CNS

Presentation

- Painless mass

Natural History

- Progressive enlargement
- Local recurrence (35-50%)
- Metastasis (60%)
  - Occurs within 2-3 years
  - Lungs most common site
  - Also bone, soft tissue, lymph nodes, liver, brain

Treatment

- Surgical approaches
  - Wide local excision, resection, amputation
- Adjuvant therapy
  - Radiation
    - Local control or palliation
- Drugs
  - Chemotherapy
    - Effectiveness not proven

Prognosis

- Poor; 5-year survival (30%)
- Favorable prognostic factors: Size < 5 cm, chondroblastic histology, low MIB-1

IMAGE FINDINGS

General Features

- Large mass
- Calcifications in 50%
  - Spotty to massive
- May secondarily involve periosteum or bone

EXTRASKELETAL OSTEOSARCOMA

Key Facts

Terminology
- Soft tissue sarcoma in which neoplastic cells produce osteoid or bone

Etiology/Pathogenesis
- Radiation-associated (10%)

Clinical Issues
- 1-2% of soft tissue sarcomas
- Almost exclusively adults
- Mostly deep-seated (70-90%)
- Thigh most common (30-50%)
- Shoulder girdle and upper arm
- Retroperitoneum (10%)
- Local recurrence (35-50%)
- Metastasis (60%)
- Poor; 5-year survival (30%)

Image Findings
- Calcification in 50%
- Spotty to massive

Macroscopic Features
- Average: 8 cm, range: 1-50 cm

Microscopic Pathology
- Wide histologic variation, mixed patterns common
- Fibroblastic
- Osteoblastic
- Chondroblastic
- Giant cell rich

Top Differential Diagnoses
- Undifferentiated pleomorphic sarcoma, dedifferentiated liposarcoma, myositis ossificans

MACROSCOPIC FEATURES

General Features
- Circumscribed or infiltrative
- Firm, fleshy, gritty, or hard
  - Ossification
    - Diffuse, focal, or undetectable
    - Tends to be located in center of tumor
- Cystic hemorrhagic spaces
- Geographic necrosis
- Satellite nodules

Size
- Average: 8 cm, range: 1-50 cm

MICROSCOPIC PATHOLOGY

Histologic Features
- Identical to skeletal osteosarcoma
- Vast majority are high grade
- Striking variation in amount of osteoid
- Wide histologic variation, mixed patterns common
  - Fibroblastic
    - Resembles undifferentiated pleomorphic sarcoma or fibrosarcoma
    - Osteoid can be sparse
  - Osteoblastic
    - Polygonal cells with eccentric nuclei
    - Abundant malignant osteoid or bone
    - Fine lace-like osteoid
    - Wide osseous trabeculae
  - Chondroblastic
    - Pleomorphic chondrocytes within lobules of hyaline cartilage
    - Peripheral lobular hypercellularity
    - Often mixed with osteoblastic areas
  - Giant cell rich
    - Pleomorphic sarcoma with numerous osteoclastic giant cells
    - Osteoclasts may obscure underlying malignant histology
    - Osteoid can be sparse
  - Telangiectatic
    - Very rare in pure form
    - Telangiectatic or cystic hemorrhagic areas common in ESOS
  - Well differentiated
    - Very rare
    - Cytologically bland fibrogenic spindle cells
    - Wide seams of osteoid and woven bone
    - Resembles parosteal or low-grade central osteosarcoma
  - Small cell
    - Very rare
    - Resembles Ewing sarcoma

Cytogenetics
- Complex karyotype

DIFFERENTIAL DIAGNOSIS

Undifferentiated Pleomorphic Sarcoma
- Pleomorphic storiform sarcoma
- Stromal hyalinization can mimic osteoid
- Can have osteoclastic giant cells
- Distinguishing from fibroblastic osteosarcoma sometimes arbitrary
  - Osteocalcin immunohistochemistry may be helpful

Dedifferentiated Liposarcoma with Osteosarcomatous Differentiation
- Heterologous osteosarcomatous differentiation sometimes present
- Usually in retroperitoneal tumors
- Identification of well-differentiated liposarcomatous component rules out ESOS

Mesenchymal Chondrosarcoma
- Small round blue or spindle cell tumor
- Neoplastic cells produce cartilage that can ossify
- Pericytic vascular pattern
- Small cell ESOS very rare

EXTRASKELETAL OSTEOSARCOMA

Immunohistochemistry

Antibody	Reactivity	Staining Pattern	Comment
Actin-sm	Positive	Cytoplasmic	68%
Desmin	Positive	Cytoplasmic	25%
S100	Positive	Nuclear & cytoplasmic	25%
EMA	Positive	Cell membrane & cytoplasm	52%
Osteocalcin	Positive	Cytoplasmic	82%
CD99	Positive	Cell membrane & cytoplasm	Unknown percentage

Ewing Sarcoma
- Small round blue cell tumor
- Fibrinous matrix can mimic osteoid
- CD99(+), but can also be osteosarcoma
- Cytogenetic [t(11;22), t(7;22), t(21;22), t(2;22)] and molecular (EWS-FLI-1, EWS-ERG) confirmation

Giant Cell Tumor of Soft Tissue
- Numerous osteoclastic giant cells and mononuclear stroma cells
- Can produce bone, usually at periphery of tumor
- Lacks high-grade cytologic atypia and atypical mitotic figures
- Lacks lace-like osteoid

Myositis Ossificans
- Nonneoplastic, usually post-traumatic tumor
- Benign reactive myofibroblasts and osteoblasts
  - Can have brisk mitotic activity
  - Lacks malignant cytologic atypia
- Temporal and peripheral and bony maturation
  - Increased bone formation and maturation with time
  - More mature bone forms at periphery of tumor
  - ESOS usually ossifies centrally

Fibroosseous Pseudotumor of Digits
- Benign reactive fibroblasts and osteoblasts
- Often lack peripheral zonal maturation
- ESOS very rare in the digits

Synovial Sarcoma with Ossification
- Uniform spindle cells
- May have stromal fibrosis with heterotopic ossification
- Positive for TLE1, cytokeratin, EMA
- Cytogenetic t(x;18) and molecular (SSX-SYT) confirmation

Malignant Peripheral Nerve Sheath Tumor with Heterologous Osteosarcomatous Differentiation
- Hyperchromatic spindle cells in fascicles
- May have heterologous osseous, chondroid, or osteosarcomatous elements
- Usually S100(+) (50-60%)
- Frequent history of neurofibromatosis type 1 (50%)

Osteogenic Melanoma
- Rare melanoma with heterologous osteosarcomatous element
- S100(+)
- Often HMB-45(+) or Melan-A(+)

Ossifying Fibromyxoid Tumor
- Ovoid mesenchymal cells arranged in cords and clusters
- Fibromyxoid stroma
- Usually encased by peripheral shell of bone
- Usually bland but can show cytologic atypia

DIAGNOSTIC CHECKLIST

Clinically Relevant Pathologic Features
- Tissue distribution

Pathologic Interpretation Pearls
- Microscopically identical to skeletal osteosarcoma
- Almost always high grade

SELECTED REFERENCES

1. Yang JY et al: Small cell extraskeletal osteosarcoma. Orthopedics. 32(3):217, 2009
2. Folpe AL et al: Ossifying fibromyxoid tumor of soft parts: a clinicopathologic study of 70 cases with emphasis on atypical and malignant variants. Am J Surg Pathol. 27(4):421-31, 2003
3. Okada K et al: A low-grade extraskeletal osteosarcoma. Skeletal Radiol. 32(3):165-9, 2003
4. Konishi E et al: Extraskeletal osteosarcoma arising in myositis ossificans. Skeletal Radiol. 30(1):39-43, 2001
5. Oliveira AM et al: Primary giant cell tumor of soft tissues: a study of 22 cases. Am J Surg Pathol. 24(2):248-56, 2000
6. Fanburg-Smith JC et al: Osteocalcin and osteonectin immunoreactivity in extraskeletal osteosarcoma: a study of 28 cases. Hum Pathol. 30(1):32-8, 1999
7. Lidang Jensen M et al: Extraskeletal osteosarcomas: a clinicopathologic study of 25 cases. Am J Surg Pathol. 22(5):588-94, 1998
8. Lee JS et al: A review of 40 patients with extraskeletal osteosarcoma. Cancer. 76(11):2253-9, 1995
9. Lucas DR et al: Osteogenic melanoma. A rare variant of malignant melanoma. Am J Surg Pathol. 17(4):400-9, 1993
10. Bane BL et al: Extraskeletal osteosarcoma. A clinicopathologic review of 26 cases. Cancer. 65(12):2762-70, 1990
11. Chung EB et al: Extraskeletal osteosarcoma. Cancer. 60(5):1132-42, 1987
12. Dupree WB et al: Fibro-osseous pseudotumor of the digits. Cancer. 58(9):2103-9, 1986
13. Sordillo PP et al: Extraosseous osteogenic sarcoma. A review of 48 patients. Cancer. 51(4):727-34, 1983
14. Allan CJ et al: Osteogenic sarcoma of the somatic soft tissues. Clinicopathologic study of 26 cases and review of literature. Cancer. 27(5):1121-33, 1971

Microscopic Features

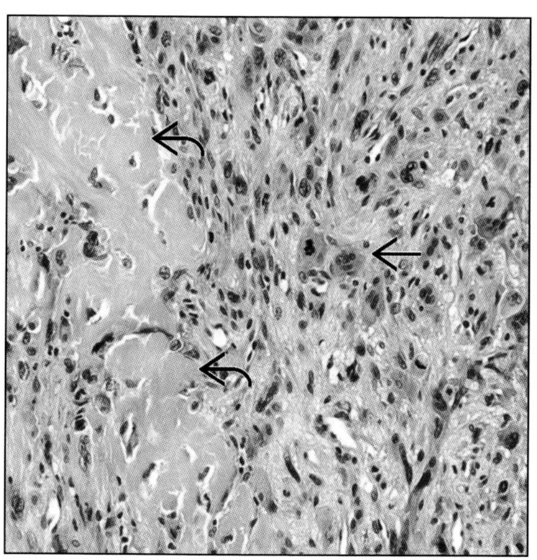

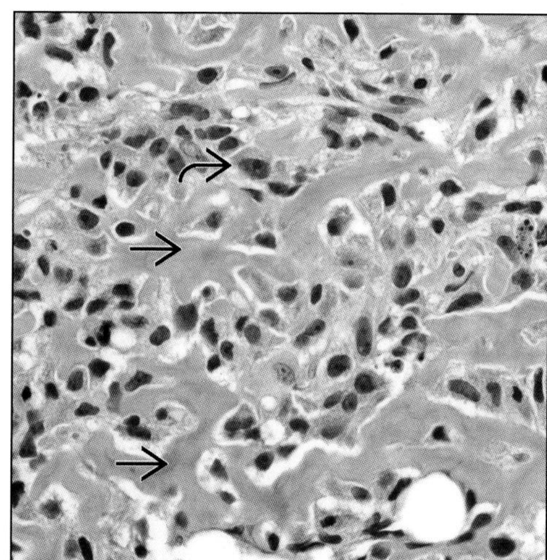

(Left) Fibroblastic ESOS resembles pleomorphic undifferentiated sarcoma (as shown) or fibrosarcoma. Identification of osteoid ⮫ is required for diagnosis. However, it can be sparse and hard to distinguish from hyalinized fibrous matrix. Osteoclastic giant cells ⇨ are often present. **(Right)** Osteoblastic osteosarcoma is characterized by polygonal osteoblastic cells with eccentric nuclei ⮫ that produce osteoid ⇨ or woven bone, often with an irregular lace-like pattern.

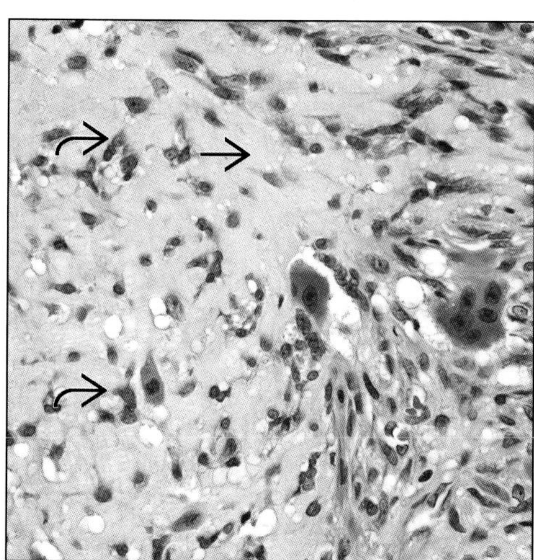

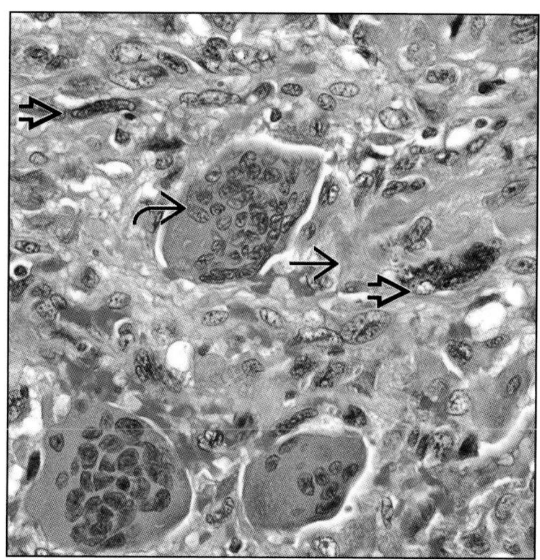

(Left) Chondroblastic osteosarcoma has pleomorphic chondrocytes ⮫ in lacunar spaces embedded within pale blue chondroid matrix ⇨. This pattern is often admixed with others, such as osteoblastic or fibroblastic patterns. **(Right)** Giant cell-rich osteosarcoma contains numerous histologically benign osteoclastic giant cells ⮫. In such tumors, one needs to search carefully for atypical cells ⇨ and osteoid ⇨ to establish the diagnosis.

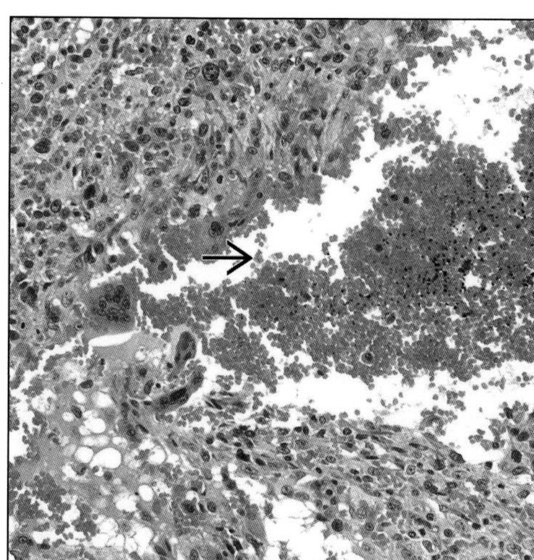

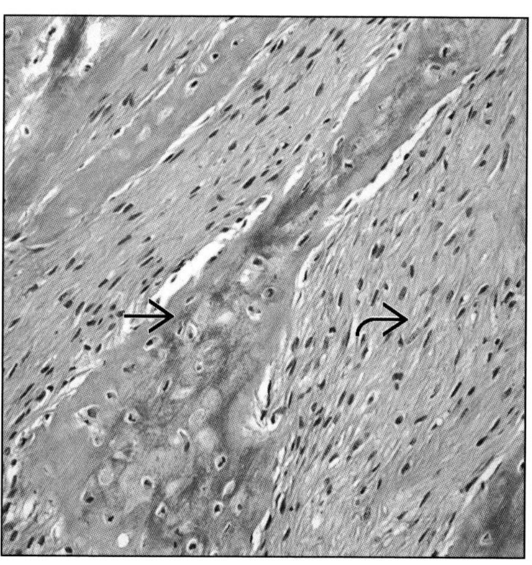

(Left) Although pure telangiectatic osteosarcoma is very rare in the soft tissue, cystic hemorrhagic spaces ⇨ (or focal telangiectatic areas) are common in ESOS. **(Right)** Only a handful of well-differentiated ESOSs have been reported. These tumors are microscopically identical to parosteal or low-grade central osteosarcoma, composed of cytologically bland fibrogenic spindle cells ⮫ in between broad trabeculae of woven bone ⇨.

EXTRASKELETAL MESENCHYMAL CHONDROSARCOMA

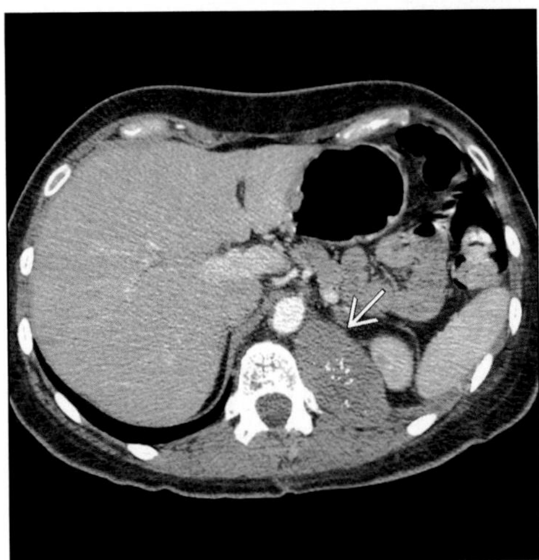

EMC typically presents as a circumscribed, calcified mass. Although most common in cranial and spinal meninges, it occurs at widely variable sites. In this case, CT shows a tumor ➔ in the retrocrural area.

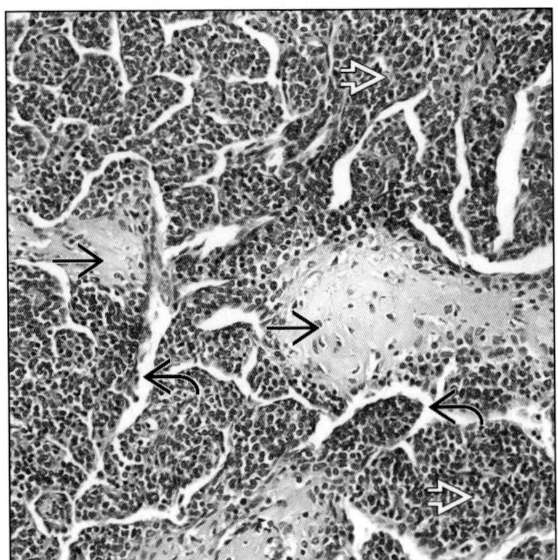

Extraskeletal mesenchymal chondrosarcoma (EMC) has a bimorphic histology consisting of small round cell areas ➔ and islands of hyaline cartilage ➔. Most have a pericytomatous vascular pattern ➔.

TERMINOLOGY

Abbreviations

- Extraskeletal mesenchymal chondrosarcoma (EMC)

Synonyms

- Hemangiopericytoma with cartilaginous differentiation

Definitions

- Bimorphic soft tissue sarcoma characterized by undifferentiated small round or spindle cells and islands of well-differentiated hyaline cartilage
  - Microscopically identical to skeletal mesenchymal chondrosarcoma

CLINICAL ISSUES

Epidemiology

- Incidence
  - < 1% of soft tissue sarcomas
  - Only 1/3 of EMCs present as primary extraskeletal tumors
    - Most are bone tumors
- Age
  - Wide age range: 0-70 years
    - Mostly 2nd and 3rd decades
    - Average age: 30 years
    - Rare congenital cases
- Gender
  - Women and men equally affected

Site

- Head and neck region
  - Cranial dura
    - Most common extraskeletal site
  - Orbit
- Lower extremities
- Reported in wide array of soft tissue and visceral locations

Presentation

- Painful or painless mass in extremity tumors
- Headache and neurological symptoms in meningeal tumors
- Proptosis and visual changes in orbital tumors

Natural History

- Fully malignant and aggressive
- Frequent metastases
  - Lungs most common
  - Can have late metastases
    - Up to 20 years following initial presentation
- Behavior regarded as unpredictable

Treatment

- Surgical approaches
  - Complete resection when possible
- Drugs
  - Role of chemotherapy poorly defined
- Radiation
  - May benefit local control

Prognosis

- Overall poor outcome
  - 50% 5-year survival
  - 25% 10-year survival
- Clinical course can be protracted

IMAGE FINDINGS

Radiographic Findings

- Well-defined soft tissue mass
- Dural-based intracranial/intraspinal tumor
- Calcifications in most
  - Stipples, rings and arcs, streaks

EXTRASKELETAL MESENCHYMAL CHONDROSARCOMA

Key Facts

Terminology
- Bimorphic soft tissue sarcoma characterized by undifferentiated small round or spindle cells and islands of well-differentiated hyaline cartilage

Clinical Issues
- < 1% of soft tissue sarcomas
- Age: Mostly 2nd and 3rd decades
- Wide range of soft tissue and visceral locations
- Common locations
  - Head and neck region
  - Cranial and spinal dura
- Clinical course can be protracted

Image Findings
- Calcifications in most

Microscopic Pathology
- Bimorphic pattern
- Small round or spindle cells
- Hyperchromatic coarse chromatin
- Thin-walled branching (pericytomatous) vascular pattern
- Hyaline cartilage islands
- Calcifications and endochondral ossification
- CD99(+) and SOX9(+)

Top Differential Diagnoses
- Ewing sarcoma
- Synovial sarcoma
- Cellular solitary fibrous tumor/hemangiopericytoma
- Osteosarcoma
- MPNST with heterologous cartilage

MACROSCOPIC FEATURES

General Features
- Multilobulated and well circumscribed
- Periphery soft and fleshy
- Center often with gritty texture or cartilaginous foci
- Necrosis and hemorrhage in some

Size
- Variable: 2-37 cm

MICROSCOPIC PATHOLOGY

Histologic Features
- Bimorphic pattern
  - Small round or spindle cells
    - Clusters or fascicles
    - Thin-walled branching (pericytomatous) vascular pattern
    - Necrosis or hemorrhage in some
  - Hyaline cartilage
    - Variable-size islands
    - Large sheets in some
    - Small hyperchromatic cells in lacunar spaces
    - Often low-grade or bland cytological features
    - Calcifications and endochondral ossification common
    - Sharp demarcation or gradual transition between cellular areas and cartilage

Cytologic Features
- Uniform round, oval, or spindle-shaped nuclei
- Hyperchromatic coarse chromatin
- Variable mitotic rate
- Scant cytoplasm
- Clear cytoplasm in some

Predominant Cell/Compartment Type
- Mesenchymal, cartilagenous

ANCILLARY TESTS

Cytogenetics
- Variable results
  - Complex numerical and structural aberrations
  - Robertsonian (13:21)(q10;q10) translocation reported in 2 cases

DIFFERENTIAL DIAGNOSIS

Ewing Sarcoma
- Uniform small round cells
- Softer, less coarse chromatin
- Lacks cartilage
- Lacks pericytomatous vascular pattern
- Glycogen-rich clear cell cytoplasm in most
- CD99(+)
- SOX9(-)
- *EWSR1* break apart by FISH
- *EWS-FLI1* or *EWS-ERG* fusion by RT-PCR

Synovial Sarcoma
- Spindle or small round cells
- Softer, less coarse chromatin
- Hyalinized and calcified stroma
- Metaplastic ossification in some
- Pericytomatous vascular pattern
- Lacks hyaline cartilage
- CD99(+)
- TLE1(+)
- Cytokeratin(+)
- *SYT* break apart by FISH
- *SSX-SYT* fusion by RT-PCR

Cellular Solitary Fibrous Tumor/ Hemangiopericytoma
- Spindle cells in haphazard or storiform arrays
- Wire-like collagen bundles
- Pericytomatous vascular pattern
- Occurs in meninges, as does EMC
- Lacks hyaline cartilage

EXTRASKELETAL MESENCHYMAL CHONDROSARCOMA

Immunohistochemistry

Antibody	Reactivity	Staining Pattern	Comment
CD99	Positive	Cell membrane & cytoplasm	Positive in cellular areas
S100	Positive	Nuclear & cytoplasmic	Positive in cartilaginous areas only
SOX9	Positive	Nuclear	Positive in cellular and cartilaginous areas
EMA	Positive	Cytoplasmic	Positive in 35%
Desmin	Positive	Cytoplasmic	Focally positive in 50%
SNF5	Positive		Staining is retained; no loss of INI1
Osteocalcin	Negative	Stromal matrix	Positive only in areas of ossification
CK-PAN	Negative		
Actin-sm	Negative		
GFAP	Negative		
Myogenin	Equivocal	Nuclear	Rare reports of positive staining
MYOD1	Equivocal	Nuclear	Rare reports of positive staining

- CD99(+)
- CD34(+)
- CD10(+)

Osteosarcoma
- Can have small cell or chondroblastic features
- Rare as a primary soft tissue tumor
- SOX9(-)
- Osteocalcin(+)

Malignant Peripheral Nerve Sheath Tumor with Heterologous Cartilage
- Rare tumors with heterologous cartilage
- Fascicular spindle cell pattern most common
- Can have small round cell pattern
- Can have pericytomatous vascular pattern
- S100 positivity in 50% of tumors

Extraskeletal Myxoid Chondrosarcoma
- Abundant myxoid matrix
- Epithelioid or spindle cells arranged in cords
- Well-formed hyaline cartilage rarely present
- SOX9(-)

Atypical Teratoid Rhabdoid Tumor
- Intracranial location
- Small round cells
- More abundant eosinophilic cytoplasm
- Lacks cartilage
- Cytokeratin(+)
- SNF5 (INI1)(-)

Sclerosing Pseudovascular Rhabdomyosarcoma
- Small round or spindle cells
- Hyalinized matrix can mimic cartilage
- Rhabdomyoblasts often sparse
- Desmin(-), MYOD1(-), and myogenin(+)
  - EMC desmin(+) in 50% of cases
  - Rare EMCs reported as positive for MYOD1 or myogenin

SELECTED REFERENCES

1. Fanburg-Smith JC et al: Immunoprofile of mesenchymal chondrosarcoma: aberrant desmin and EMA expression, retention of INI1, and negative estrogen receptor in 22 female-predominant central nervous system and musculoskeletal cases. Ann Diagn Pathol. 14(1):8-14, 2010
2. Fanburg-Smith JC et al: Reappraisal of mesenchymal chondrosarcoma: novel morphologic observations of the hyaline cartilage and endochondral ossification and beta-catenin, Sox9, and osteocalcin immunostaining of 22 cases. Hum Pathol. 41(5):653-62, 2010
3. Dantonello TM et al: Mesenchymal chondrosarcoma of soft tissues and bone in children, adolescents, and young adults: experiences of the CWS and COSS study groups. Cancer. 112(11):2424-31, 2008
4. Gengler C et al: Desmin and myogenin reactivity in mesenchymal chondrosarcoma: a potential diagnostic pitfall. Histopathology. 48(2):201-3, 2006
5. Wehrli BM et al: Sox9, a master regulator of chondrogenesis, distinguishes mesenchymal chondrosarcoma from other small blue round cell tumors. Hum Pathol. 34(3):263-9, 2003
6. Naumann S et al: Translocation der(13;21)(q10;q10) in skeletal and extraskeletal mesenchymal chondrosarcoma. Mod Pathol. 15(5):572-6, 2002
7. Granter SR et al: CD99 reactivity in mesenchymal chondrosarcoma. Hum Pathol. 27(12):1273-6, 1996
8. Shapeero LG et al: Extraskeletal mesenchymal chondrosarcoma. Radiology. 186(3):819-26, 1993
9. Nakashima Y et al: Mesenchymal chondrosarcoma of bone and soft tissue. A review of 111 cases. Cancer. 57(12):2444-53, 1986
10. Bertoni F et al: Mesenchymal chondrosarcoma of bone and soft tissues. Cancer. 52(3):533-41, 1983
11. Huvos AG et al: Mesenchymal chondrosarcoma. A clinicopathologic analysis of 35 patients with emphasis on treatment. Cancer. 51(7):1230-7, 1983
12. Guccion JG et al: Extraskeletal mesenchymal chondrosarcoma. Arch Pathol. 95(5):336-40, 1973

Microscopic Features

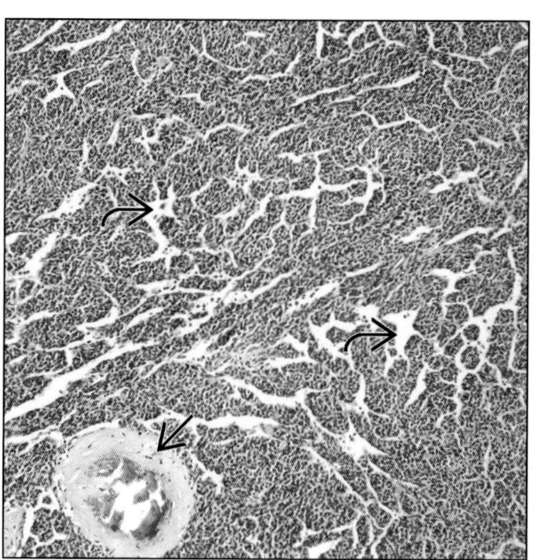

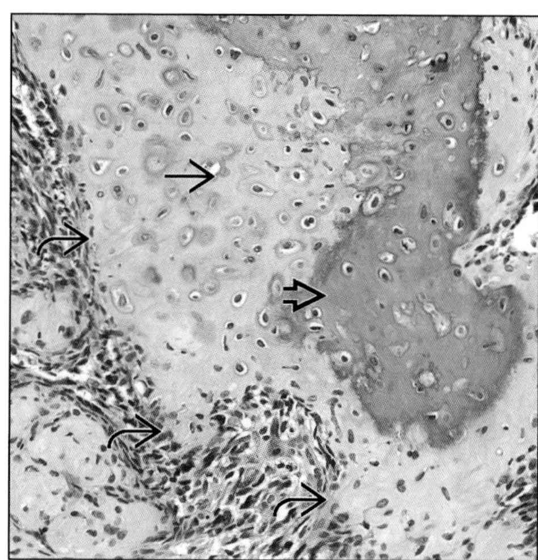

(Left) *The amount of cartilage* ➔ *is variable in EMC. In most tumors, cellular areas predominate as depicted. Note the prominent pericytomatous vascular pattern* ➔. ***(Right)*** *In some tumors, hyaline cartilage* ➔ *forms the dominant component. The interface between cellular and cartilaginous areas is usually sharply demarcated as shown* ➔ *but can be more gradual. Endochondral bone formation* ➔ *within the center of cartilage islands is common.*

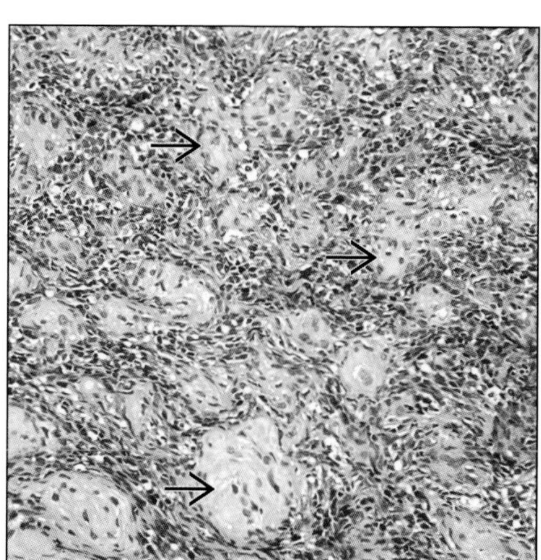

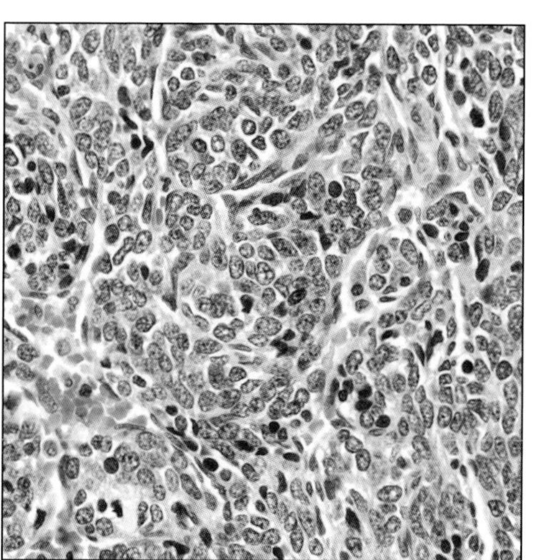

(Left) *Multiple small islands of hyaline cartilage* ➔ *blend with small round cells in this EMC, creating a multinodular pattern.* ***(Right)*** *Most EMCs are composed of closely spaced small cells with rather distinctive cytological features, consisting of round or oval nuclei with dense, coarse chromatin and very scant, indistinct cytoplasm. Note the clustered arrangement of cells within a pericytomatous vascular stroma.*

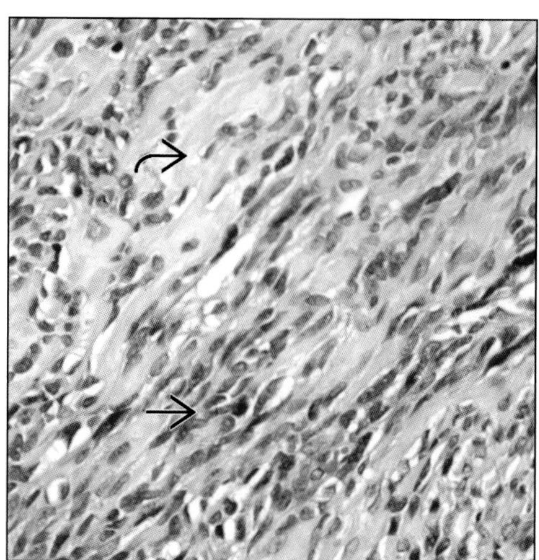

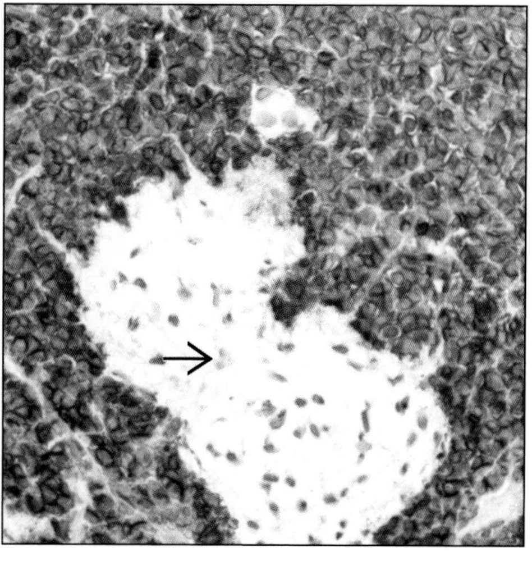

(Left) *In some tumors, the cells are spindle-shaped and arranged in fascicles* ➔. *However, spindle cell areas generally account for only a portion of a given tumor. Fibrotic stroma is occasionally present as illustrated* ➔. ***(Right)*** *Diffuse strong CD99 immunoreactivity characterizes EMC. In this example, CD99 shows a cytoplasmic membrane staining pattern, which can lead to a misdiagnosis of Ewing sarcoma. Note the cells within the cartilage island are negative* ➔.

Pericytic Lesions

Benign or Malignant

HEMANGIOPERICYTOMA

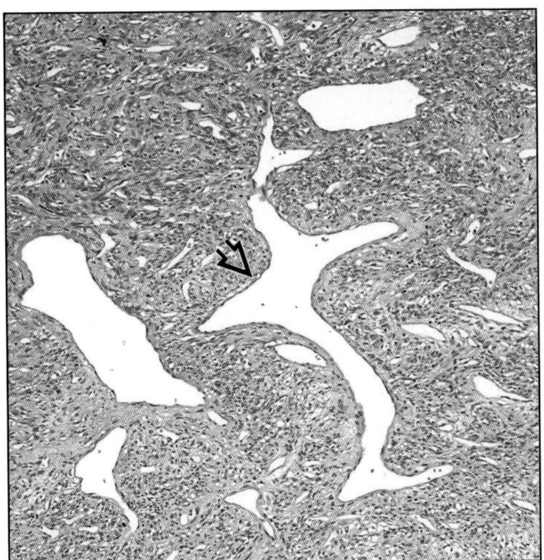

Hematoxylin & eosin shows a diffuse hemangiopericytic pattern. The vascular channels are dispersed throughout the tumor but vary in size, shape, and dilatation. Note the "staghorn" shape ⊳.

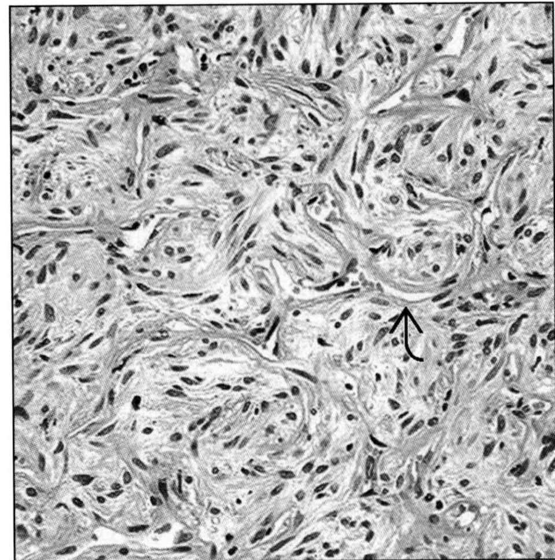

Hematoxylin & eosin shows hemangiopericytoma with myxoid change. There is a hemangiopericytic pattern, but the vessels are slit-like ⊳, not dilated.

TERMINOLOGY

Abbreviations

- Hemangiopericytoma (HPC)

Definitions

- Tumor with diffuse pattern of branching, dilated, thin-walled blood vessels composed of short spindle cells
- Diagnosis is now rarely made
  - Many different specific tumor types have hemangiopericytic vascular pattern
  - Most remaining tumors without specific differentiation are now classified as solitary fibrous tumor
- Tumors of pericytes now classified as myopericytoma

CLINICAL ISSUES

Epidemiology

- Incidence
  - Rare once other possibilities excluded
- Age
  - Adult
- Gender
  - More common in females

Site

- Deep soft tissue
  - Pelvis, retroperitoneum
  - Proximal limbs
- Subset in meninges
- Subset in sinonasal region
  - Resembles myopericytoma or glomus tumor

Presentation

- Painful or painless mass
- Hypoglycemia

Treatment

- Surgical approaches
  - Complete excision

Prognosis

- Majority benign
- Minority recur locally or metastasize

MACROSCOPIC FEATURES

General Features

- Circumscribed mass
- Tan or yellow
- Spongy cut surface

Size

- Up to 15 cm

MICROSCOPIC PATHOLOGY

Histologic Features

- Widespread hemangiopericytic pattern
- Thin-walled vessels
  - Branching "staghorn"
  - Dilated or slit-like
- Short plump spindle cells
  - Uniform nuclei
  - Scanty cytoplasm
- Malignant variant
  - Mitoses exceeding 4 per 10 HPF
  - Nuclear pleomorphism
  - Focal necrosis

Predominant Pattern/Injury Type

- Hemangiopericytic

Predominant Cell/Compartment Type

- Fibroblast

HEMANGIOPERICYTOMA

Key Facts

Terminology

- Tumor with diffuse pattern of branching, dilated, thin-walled blood vessels composed of short spindle cells
- Many tumor types have pericytomatous pattern, so diagnosis is rarely made
- Most such tumors without specific differentiation are now classified as solitary fibrous tumors

Clinical Issues

- Site: Pelvis, retroperitoneum, proximal limbs
- Subset in meninges
- Subset in sinonasal region

Microscopic Pathology

- Widespread hemangiopericytic pattern
- Thin-walled vessels
- Short plump spindle cells

ANCILLARY TESTS

Immunohistochemistry

- CD34(-) or focally positive
- CD99, Bcl-2 focally positive
- Desmin, S100 protein, CK-PAN negative

Cytogenetics

- Various nonspecific rearrangements

DIFFERENTIAL DIAGNOSIS

Solitary Fibrous Tumor

- Fibrous or hyalinized areas
- HPC pattern usually focal
- CD34(+)

Tumors with Focal Hemangiopericytic Pattern

- Benign
  - Infantile myofibroma
  - Deep benign fibrous histiocytoma
  - Myopericytoma
  - Intranodal myofibroblastoma
- Malignant
  - Synovial sarcoma
  - Mesenchymal chondrosarcoma
  - Round cell liposarcoma
  - Infantile fibrosarcoma
  - Malignant peripheral nerve sheath tumor
  - Pleomorphic sarcoma

DIAGNOSTIC CHECKLIST

Clinically Relevant Pathologic Features

- Rare cause of hypoglycemia

Pathologic Interpretation Pearls

- HPC pattern is diffuse
- Sclerosing areas usually absent

SELECTED REFERENCES

1. Gengler C et al: Solitary fibrous tumour and haemangiopericytoma: evolution of a concept. Histopathology. 48(1):63-74, 2006
2. Chan JK: Solitary fibrous tumour--everywhere, and a diagnosis in vogue. Histopathology. 31(6):568-76, 1997
3. Miettinen MM et al: Tumor size-related DNA copy number changes occur in solitary fibrous tumors but not in hemangiopericytomas. Mod Pathol. 10(12):1194-200, 1997
4. Nappi O et al: Hemangiopericytoma: histopathological pattern or clinicopathologic entity? Semin Diagn Pathol. 12(3):221-32, 1995
5. Henn W et al: Recurrent t(12;19)(q13;q13.3) in intracranial and extracranial hemangiopericytoma. Cancer Genet Cytogenet. 71(2):151-4, 1993
6. Winek RR et al: Meningioma, meningeal hemangiopericytoma (angioblastic meningioma), peripheral hemangiopericytoma, and acoustic schwannoma. A comparative immunohistochemical study. Am J Surg Pathol. 13(4):251-61, 1989

IMAGE GALLERY

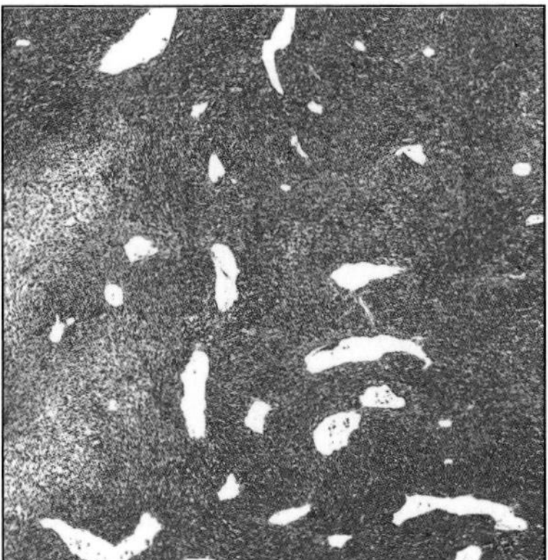

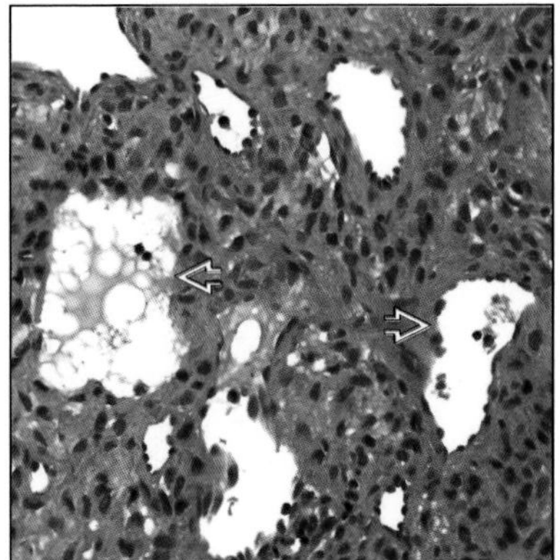

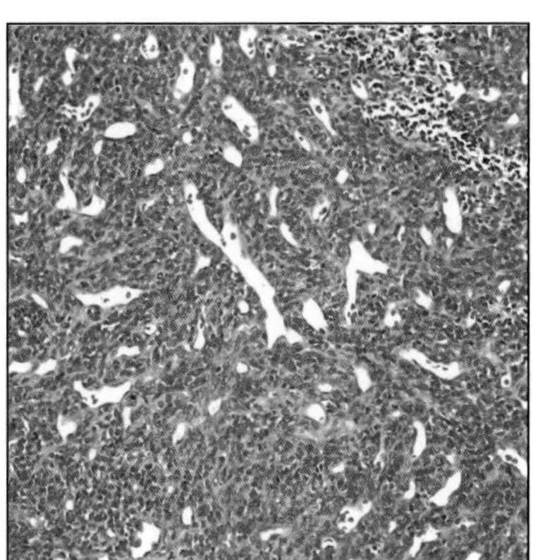

(Left) *Hematoxylin & eosin of synovial sarcoma shows focal pericytomatous vascular pattern. Many tumors previously termed malignant hemangiopericytoma are now called synovial sarcomas.* ***(Center)*** *Hematoxylin & eosin of sinonasal HPC shows spindle cells randomly lying between open thin-walled vessels ➡. Some sinonasal HPC are solitary fibrous tumors (CD34[+]); others are myopericytomas (SMA[+]).* ***(Right)*** *Hematoxylin & eosin shows a hemangiopericytic pattern in mesenchymal chondrosarcoma.*

MYOPERICYTOMA

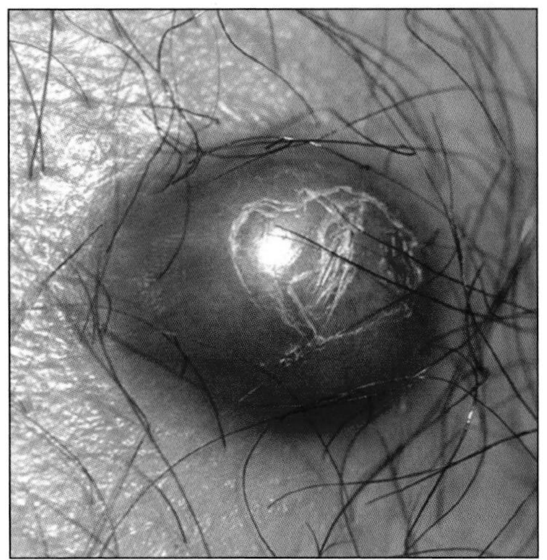

Clinical photograph shows a raised nodular lesion mimicking a vascular neoplasm arising on the lower leg of an adult male patient.

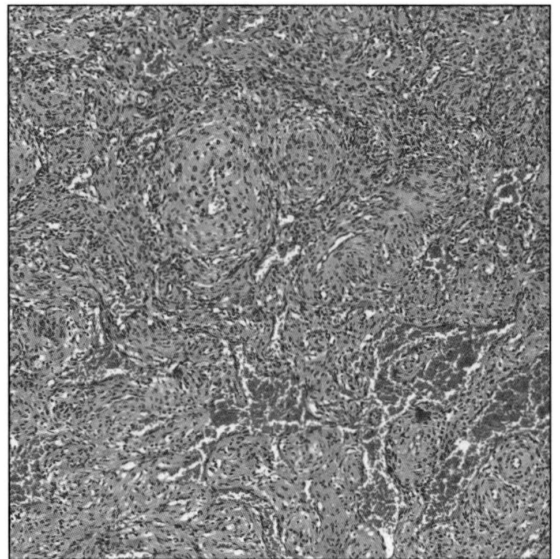

Hematoxylin & eosin shows a perivascular myoid neoplasm characterized by a concentric perivascular growth of myogenic tumor cells.

TERMINOLOGY

Synonyms

- Hemangiopericytoma

Definitions

- Benign perivascular neoplasm composed of perivascular myoid tumor cells (myopericytes)
- Myopericytoma forms morphologic spectrum with angioleiomyoma, myofibroma, and glomus tumor

CLINICAL ISSUES

Epidemiology

- Incidence
  - Rare
- Age
  - Arises most commonly in mid-adulthood
  - Children are rarely affected

Site

- Arises most commonly in dermal/subcutaneous tissues
- Arises rarely in deep soft tissues
- Distal extremities are most frequently involved
  - Proximal extremities, such as neck and trunk, more rarely involved
- Rare malignant examples usually arise in deep soft tissues

Presentation

- Painless mass
  - Usually solitary lesions
  - Multiple lesions are very rare
- Slow-growing
- Subcutaneous mass

Natural History

- Often longstanding neoplasms
- No increased number of local recurrences

Treatment

- Surgical approaches
  - Complete excision

Prognosis

- Most lesions do not recur
- Local recurrences are related to poor circumscription
- Very rare malignant myopericytomas characterized by poor clinical outcome

MACROSCOPIC FEATURES

General Features

- Nodular indurated lesions
- Variable number of vessels

MICROSCOPIC PATHOLOGY

Histologic Features

- Numerous thin-walled blood vessels
- Perivascular multilayered concentric growth
- Plump spindled &/or round myoid tumor cells
- Tumor cells with eosinophilic or amphophilic cytoplasm
- Round, plump, spindled nuclei
- Mitoses are rare
- May show focal areas similar to glomus tumor, angioleiomyoma, or myofibroma
- Areas of infarction and hemorrhage especially in deep-seated neoplasms
- Degenerative atypia may be present in longstanding neoplasms
- Prominent degenerative stromal changes in longstanding neoplasms
- May show prominent myxoid stromal changes
- Variable morphologic features
- Classic solid variant
  - Narrow, closely packed vessels

MYOPERICYTOMA

Key Facts

Terminology

- Benign perivascular neoplasm composed of perivascular myoid tumor cells (myopericytes)
- Myopericytoma forms morphologic spectrum with angioleiomyoma, myofibroma, glomus tumor, and so-called hemangiopericytoma

Clinical Issues

- Arises most commonly in mid-adulthood
- Arises most commonly in dermal/subcutaneous tissues
- Distal extremities are most frequently involved
- Usually solitary lesions
- Most lesions do not recur

Microscopic Pathology

- Numerous thin-walled blood vessels
- Perivascular multilayered concentric growth
- Plump spindled &/or round myoid tumor cells
- Round, plump, spindled nuclei
- No prominent atypia
- Homogeneous expression of actins and HCAD
- Desmin, S100 protein, CD, and epithelial markers are usually negative
- May show focal areas similar to glomus tumor, angioleiomyoma, or myofibroma
- Variable morphologic features
  - Classic solid variant
  - Hemangiopericytoma-like variant
  - Angioleiomyoma-like variant
  - Intravascular variant
  - Malignant variant

  - Vessels are concentrically surrounded by spindled &/ or round tumor cells
- Hemangiopericytoma-like variant
  - Dilated, branching, thin-walled vessels
  - Perivascular growth of myoid tumor cells
- Angioleiomyoma-like variant
  - Perivascular growth of elongated spindled cells
- Intravascular variant
  - Intravascular or intramural growth
  - Closely packed, thin-walled vessels
  - Vessels are concentrically surrounded by myoid tumor cells
- Malignant variant
  - Infiltrative growth
  - Prominent cytologic atypia
  - Numerous mitoses
  - Areas of tumor necrosis
- Rare hypocellular fibroma-like variant
- Rare immature cellular variant

Predominant Pattern/Injury Type

- Circumscribed
- Hemangiopericytic

Predominant Cell/Compartment Type

- Mesenchymal
  - Myoid tumor cells

ANCILLARY TESTS

Cytogenetics

- Characteristic t(7;12)(p21-22;q13-15)
- *ACTB-GLI* fusion

DIFFERENTIAL DIAGNOSIS

Myofibroma

- Biphasic growth
  - Undifferentiated mesenchymal tumor cells associated with numerous thin-walled vessels showing hemangiopericytoma-like growth
  - Mature, spindled, eosinophilic tumor cells
- Often multinodular growth
- Myxohyaline stromal changes
- HCAD(-): Rarely focal positivity

Angioleiomyoma

- Thick-walled vessels
- Predominance of spindled eosinophilic tumor cells
- Usually desmin(+)

Glomus Tumor

- Round tumor cells
- Sharply demarcated round nuclei

Nodular Hidradenoma

- Epithelial immunohistochemical markers are positive
- Myogenic immunohistochemical markers are negative

Leiomyoma

- Bundles and fascicles
- Spindled tumor cells
- Fibrillary eosinophilic cytoplasm
- Cigar-shaped nuclei

Dermatofibroma

- Stellate growth
- No prominent perivascular growth
- Hyalinized collagen fibers are surrounded by tumor cells
- Usually no homogeneous expression of actin and HCAD

Solitary Fibrous Tumor

- No prominent perivascular growth
- Spindled rather neuroid tumor cells
- Muscle markers are usually negative
- CD34(+)

Hemangioma

- Lobular architecture
- Predominantly proliferation of vascular structures
- No prominent concentric growth of perivascular myoid tumor cells

MYOPERICYTOMA

Immunohistochemistry

Antibody	Reactivity	Staining Pattern	Comment
Actin-sm	Positive	Cytoplasmic	Diffuse positivity
Caldesmon	Positive	Cytoplasmic	Diffuse positivity
Calponin	Positive	Cytoplasmic	Variable positivity
Desmin	Negative		Focal positivity in rare cases
S100	Negative		
CK-PAN	Negative		
EMA/MUC1	Negative		
CD34	Negative		Focal positivity in rare cases

Symplastic Hemangioma

- Lobular architecture
- Predominantly proliferation of vascular structures
- Perivascular growth of pleomorphic cells
- Perivascular cells show prominent degenerative atypia
- No homogeneous expression of actin by perivascularly proliferating cells

Pleomorphic Hyalinizing Angiectatic Tumor

- Dilated vessels with rim of fibrin
- Pleomorphic cells between vessels
- No prominent perivascular growth
- Myogenic markers are negative

Ancient Schwannoma

- Encapsulated neoplasms
- No prominent perivascular growth
- Homogeneous expression of S100 protein

DIAGNOSTIC CHECKLIST

Clinically Relevant Pathologic Features

- Gross appearance
- Organ distribution

Pathologic Interpretation Pearls

- Well-circumscribed nodular neoplasms
- Arise usually in dermal/subcutaneous tissues
- Contain numerous thin-walled blood vessels
- Characteristic perivascular, concentric growth
- Plump spindled/round myoid tumor cells
- No or only slight cytologic atypia
- Malignant cases are extremely rare and arise usually in deep soft tissues
- Expression of actins
- Expression of HCAD
- May show overlapping morphologic features with glomus tumor, myofibroma, &/or angioleiomyoma

SELECTED REFERENCES

1. Ide F et al: Perivascular myoid tumors of the oral region: a clinicopathologic re-evaluation of 35 cases. J Oral Pathol Med. 37(1):43-9, 2008
2. Matsuyama A et al: Angioleiomyoma: a clinicopathologic and immunohistochemical reappraisal with special reference to the correlation with myopericytoma. Hum Pathol. 38(4):645-51, 2007
3. Wilson T et al: Intranasal myopericytoma. A tumour with perivascular myoid differentiation: the changing nomenclature for haemangiopericytoma. J Laryngol Otol. 121(8):786-9, 2007
4. Dray MS et al: Myopericytoma: a unifying term for a spectrum of tumours that show overlapping features with myofibroma. A review of 14 cases. J Clin Pathol. 59(1):67-73, 2006
5. Gengler C et al: Solitary fibrous tumour and haemangiopericytoma: evolution of a concept. Histopathology. 48(1):63-74, 2006
6. Mentzel T et al: Myopericytoma of skin and soft tissues: clinicopathologic and immunohistochemical study of 54 cases. Am J Surg Pathol. 30(1):104-13, 2006
7. Rousseau A et al: Primary intracranial myopericytoma: report of three cases and review of the literature. Neuropathol Appl Neurobiol. 31(6):641-8, 2005
8. Dahlén A et al: Activation of the GLI oncogene through fusion with the beta-actin gene (ACTB) in a group of distinctive pericytic neoplasms: pericytoma with t(7;12). Am J Pathol. 164(5):1645-53, 2004
9. Dahlén A et al: Molecular genetic characterization of the genomic ACTB-GLI fusion in pericytoma with t(7;12). Biochem Biophys Res Commun. 325(4):1318-23, 2004
10. McMenamin ME et al: Intravascular myopericytoma. J Cutan Pathol. 29(9):557-61, 2002
11. McMenamin ME et al: Malignant myopericytoma: expanding the spectrum of tumours with myopericytic differentiation. Histopathology. 41(5):450-60, 2002
12. Mikami Y et al: Perivascular myoma: case report with immunohistochemical and ultrastructural studies. Pathol Int. 52(1):69-74, 2002
13. Granter SR et al: Myofibromatosis in adults, glomangiopericytoma, and myopericytoma: a spectrum of tumors showing perivascular myoid differentiation. Am J Surg Pathol. 22(5):513-25, 1998
14. Kutzner H: [Perivascular myoma: a new concept for "myofibroblastic" tumors with perivascular myoid differentiation] Verh Dtsch Ges Pathol. 82:301-8, 1998
15. Variend S et al: Are infantile myofibromatosis, congenital fibrosarcoma and congenital haemangiopericytoma histogenetically related? Histopathology. 26(1):57-62, 1995
16. Mentzel T et al: Infantile hemangiopericytoma versus infantile myofibromatosis. Study of a series suggesting a continuous spectrum of infantile myofibroblastic lesions. Am J Surg Pathol. 18(9):922-30, 1994

Gross and Microscopic Features

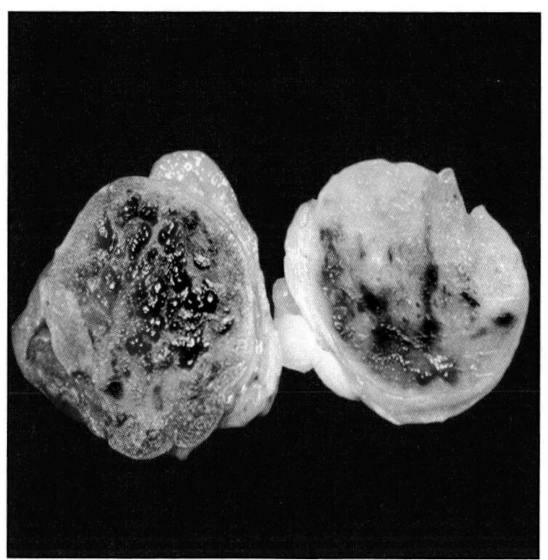

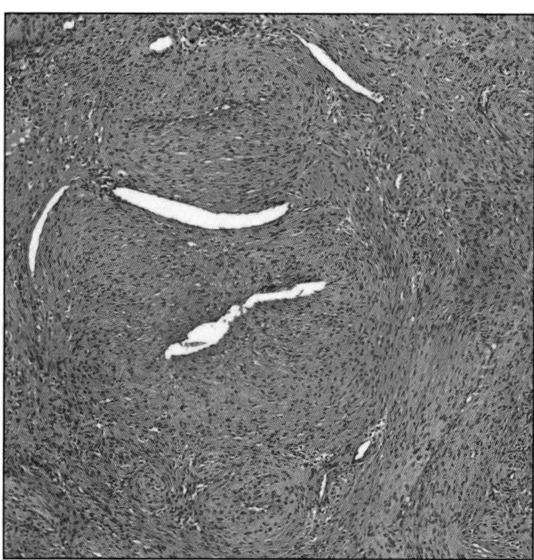

*(**Left**) Gross photograph shows a nodular, well-circumscribed neoplasm with numerous vessels and gray-white cut surfaces. (**Right**) Hematoxylin & eosin shows an example of the classic solid type of myopericytoma. Note the perivascular rims of myogenic tumor cells.*

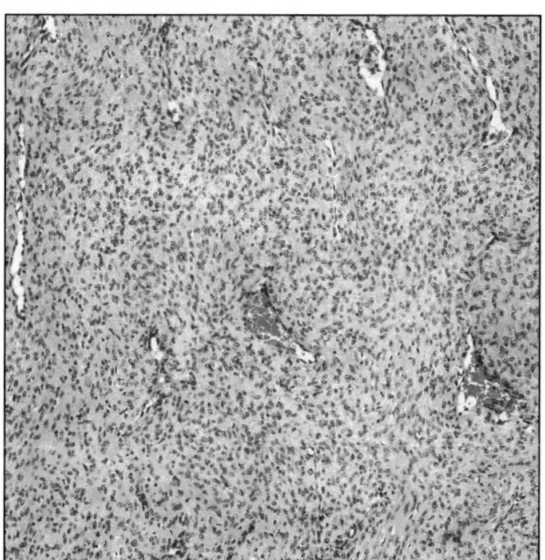

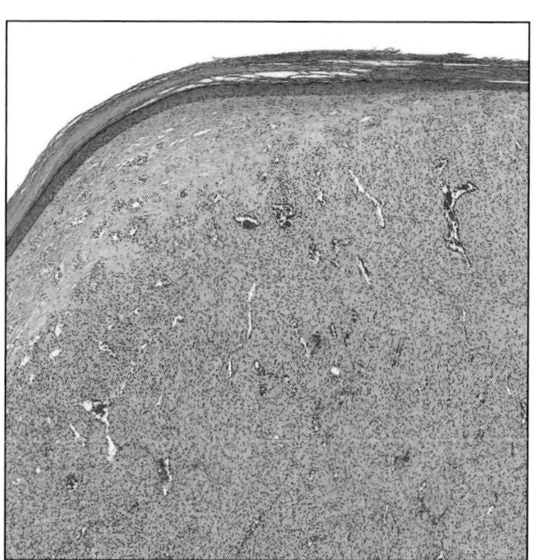

*(**Left**) Hematoxylin & eosin shows numerous narrow vessels surrounded concentrically by myogenic tumor cells. (**Right**) Hematoxylin & eosin shows a cutaneous myopericytoma.*

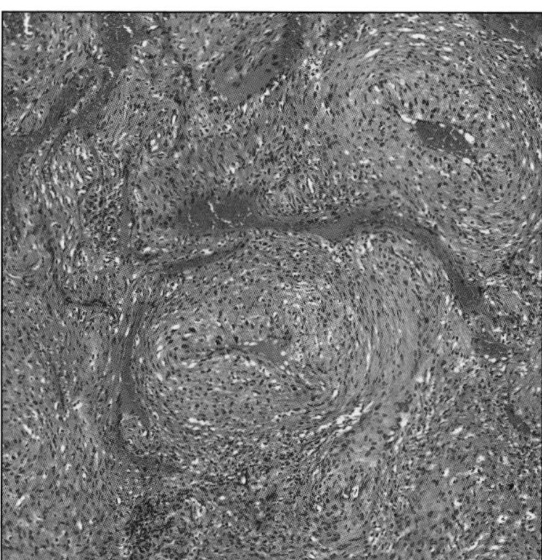

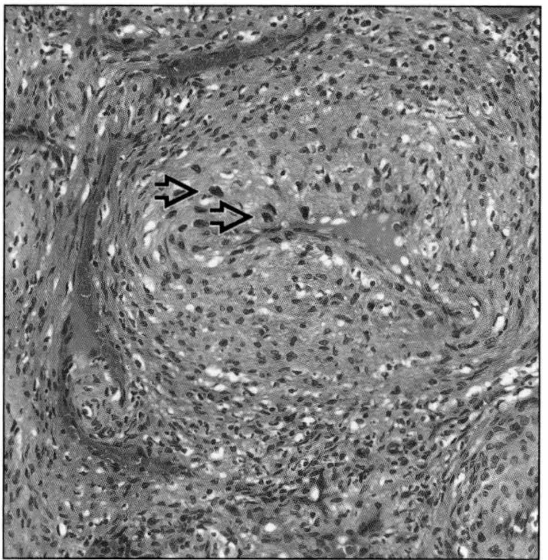

*(**Left**) Hematoxylin & eosin shows an example of the classic solid type of myopericytoma with perivascular growing eosinophilic tumor cells. (**Right**) Hematoxylin & eosin of the classic solid type of myopericytoma shows a higher power view of enlarged cells with enlarged nuclei representing cells with degenerative atypia ⇨.*

MYOPERICYTOMA

Gross and Variant Microscopic Features

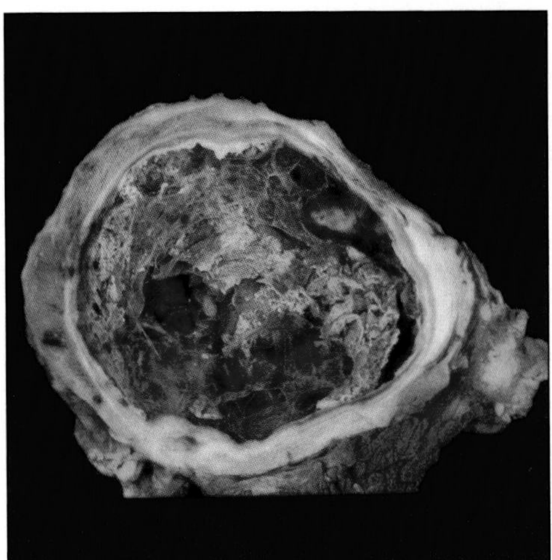

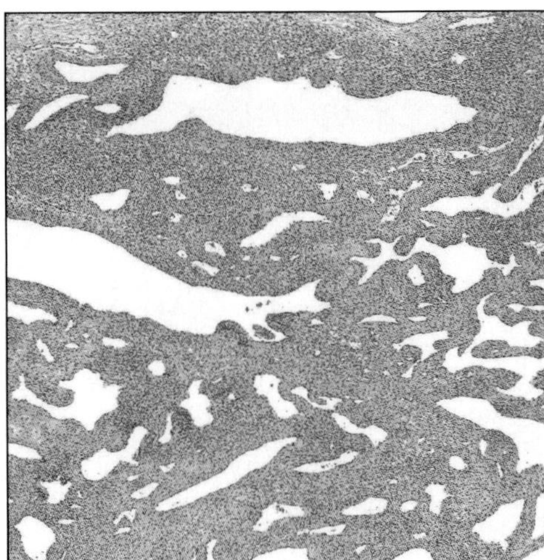

(Left) *Gross photograph shows a large myopericytoma arising on the thigh of a young female patient. Note the extensive central degenerative changes and necrosis.* ***(Right)*** *Hematoxylin & eosin shows an example of the hemangiopericytoma-like type of myopericytoma. Note the numerous dilated and branching thin-walled vessels.*

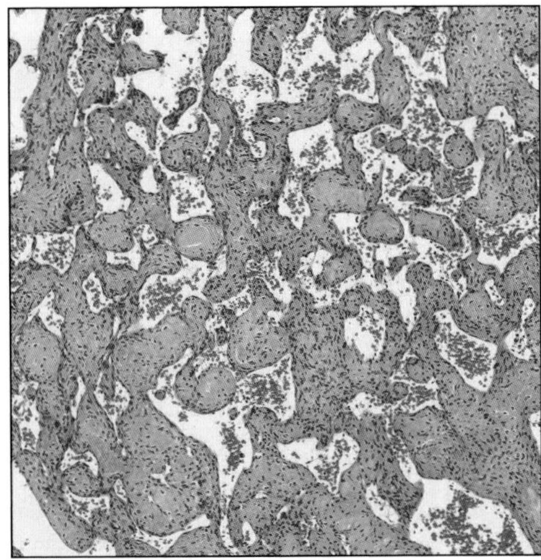

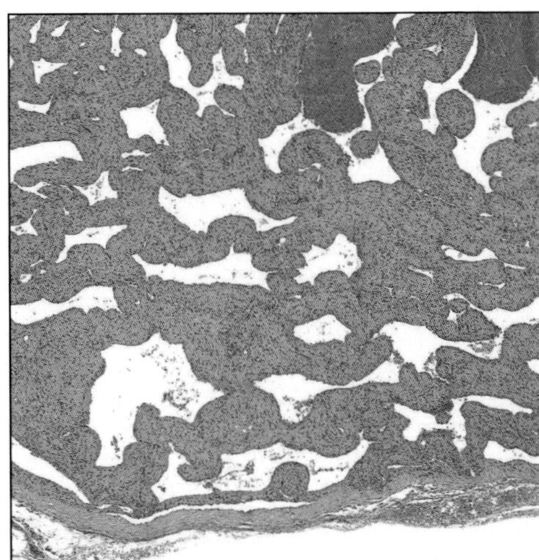

(Left) *Hematoxylin & eosin shows a myopericytoma of the hemangiopericytoma-like type with numerous branching vessels surrounded by myoid tumor cells.* ***(Right)*** *Hematoxylin & eosin shows a hemangiopericytoma-like myopericytoma. Note the perivascular growth of eosinophilic myoid tumor cells.*

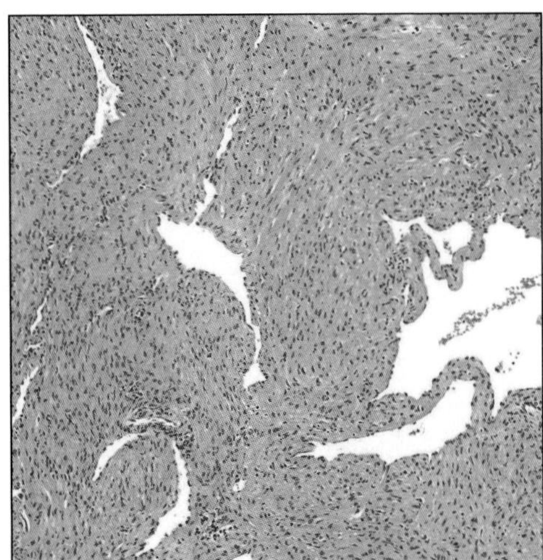

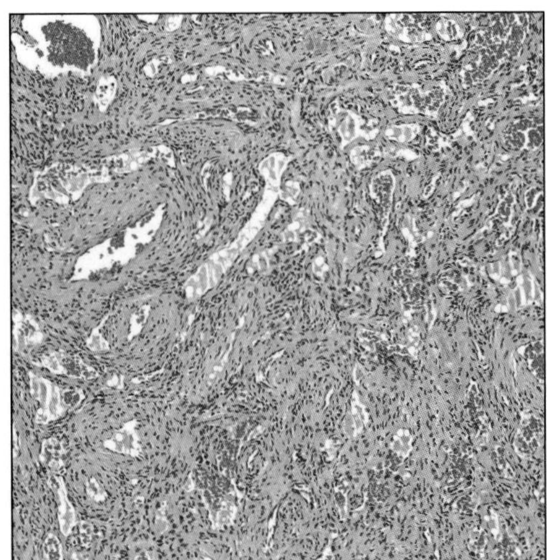

(Left) *Hematoxylin & eosin shows a myopericytoma of the angioleiomyoma-like type. Dilated and narrow vascular structures are surrounded by bundles of eosinophilic spindled tumor cells.* ***(Right)*** *Hematoxylin & eosin shows angioleiomyoma-like myopericytoma with a concentric perivascular growth of bundles of myoid tumor cells.*

Ancillary Techniques and Microscopic Features

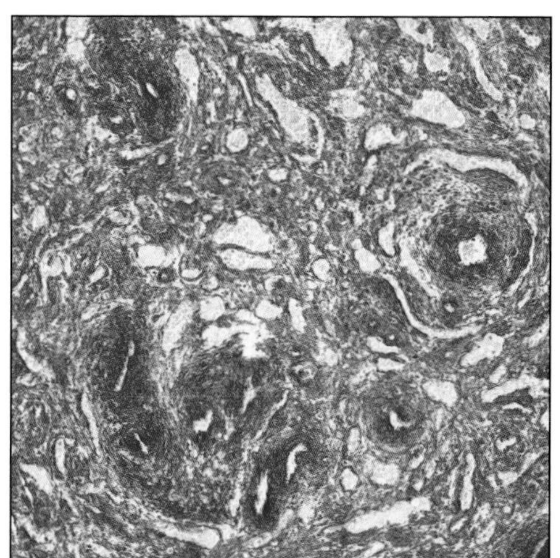

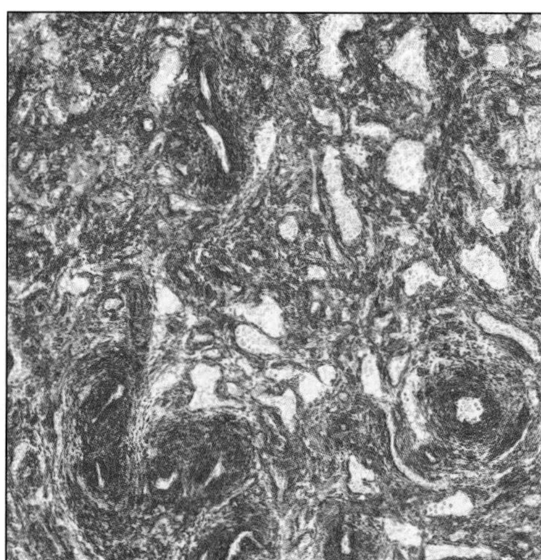

(Left) *Actin-sm shows homogeneous expression of tumor cells in myopericytoma. Note the striking perivascular growth of neoplastic cells.* ***(Right)*** *HCAD shows homogeneous positivity of neoplastic cells.*

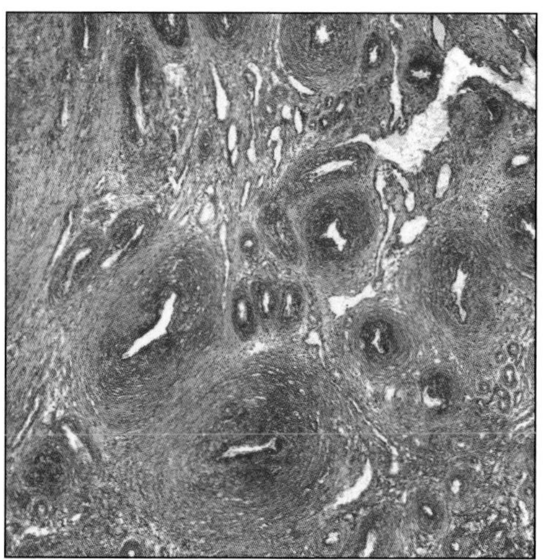

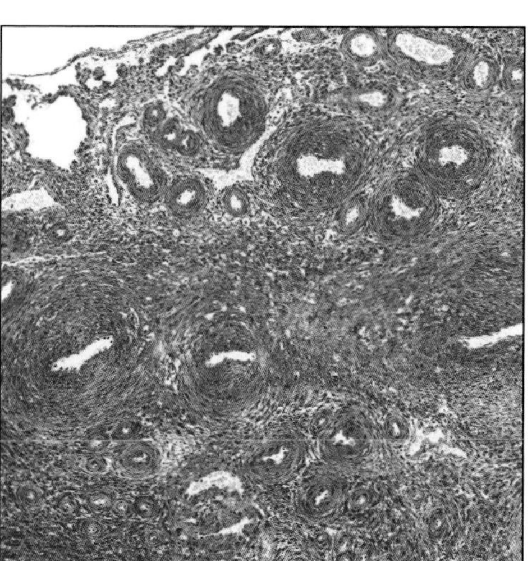

(Left) *Collagen IV shows homogeneous expression by neoplastic cells.* ***(Right)*** *Calponin shows homogeneous expression by neoplastic cells.*

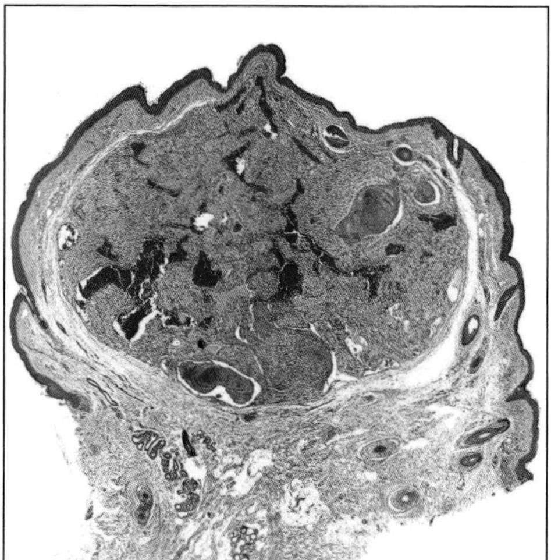

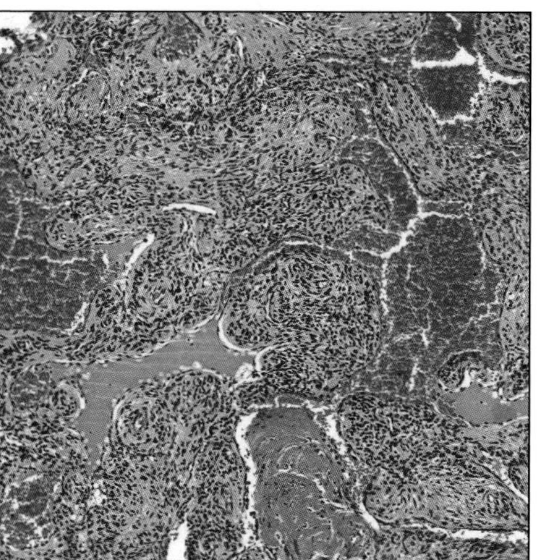

(Left) *Hematoxylin & eosin shows a cutaneous myopericytoma. Note the well-circumscribed, nodular growth.* ***(Right)*** *Hematoxylin & eosin of a cutaneous myopericytoma shows a higher power view of numerous blood vessels surrounded concentrically by myogenic tumor cells.*

MYOPERICYTOMA

Variant Microscopic Features

*(**Left**) Hematoxylin & eosin shows a case of myopericytoma with focal hemorrhages. (**Right**) Hematoxylin & eosin shows a case of myopericytoma with edema and degenerative atypia of neoplastic cells containing enlarged nuclei.*

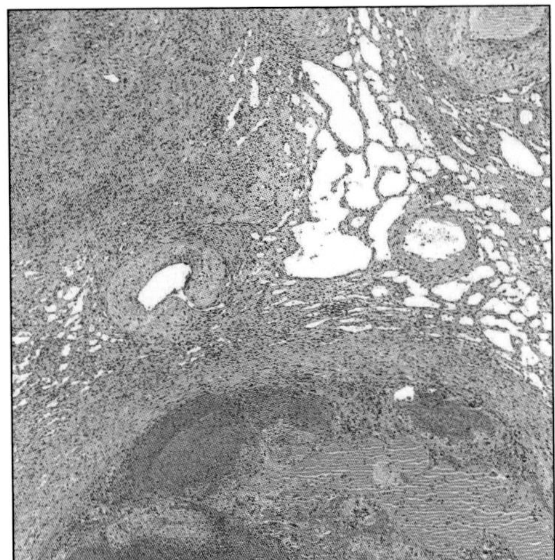

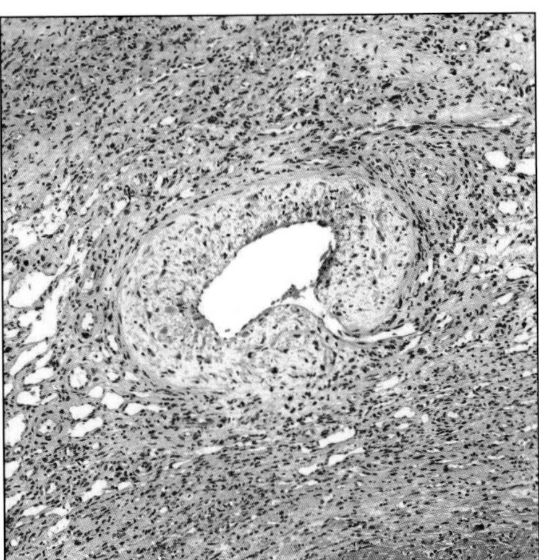

*(**Left**) Hematoxylin & eosin shows focal stromal hyalinization in this myopericytoma. (**Right**) Hematoxylin & eosin shows degenerative edema in this case of myopericytoma.*

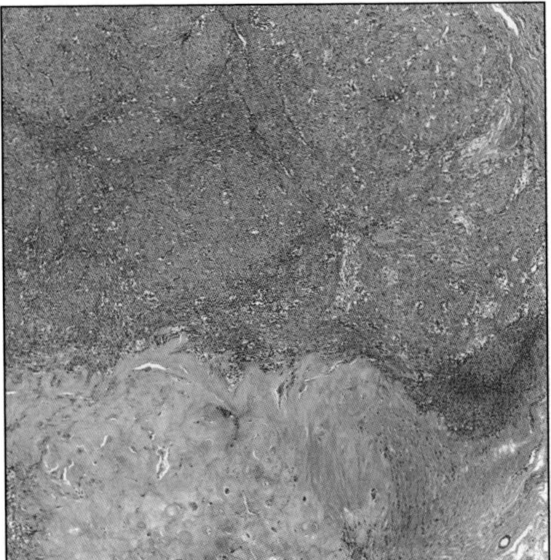

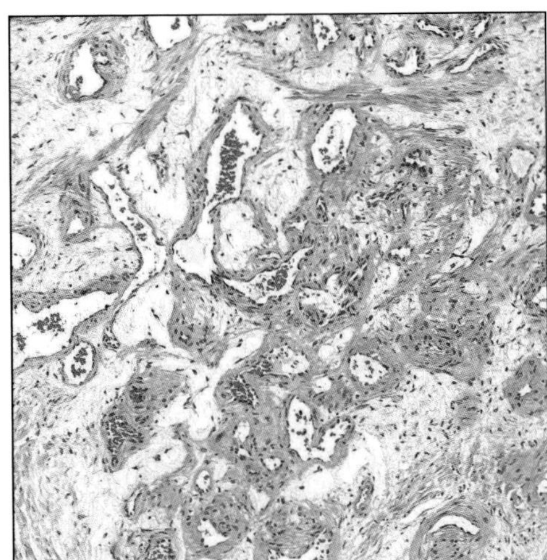

*(**Left**) Hematoxylin & eosin shows myxohyaline degeneration in this case of myopericytoma ➲. (**Right**) Hematoxylin & eosin shows an "immature" myopericytoma composed of rather undifferentiated, plump, spindled mesenchymal tumor cells showing a perivascular growth.*

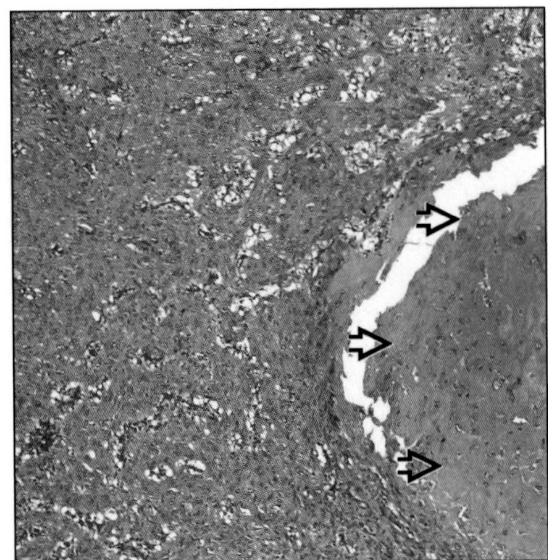

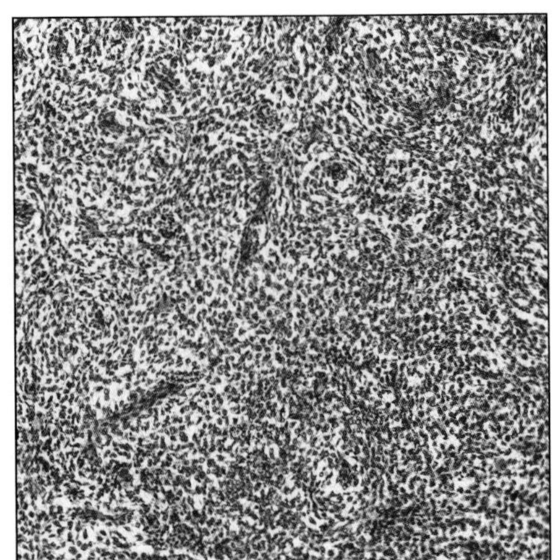

Variant Microscopic Features

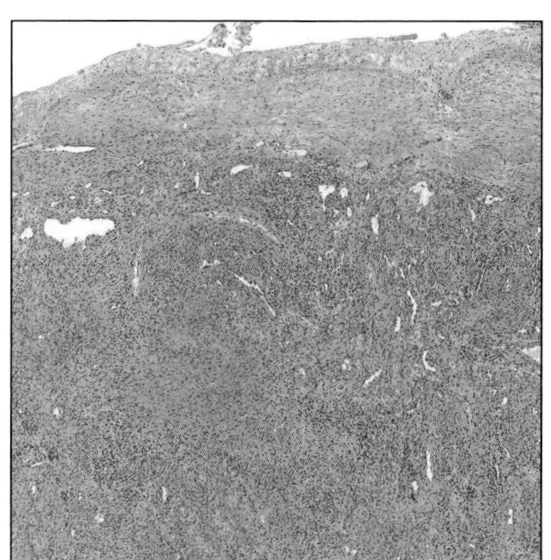

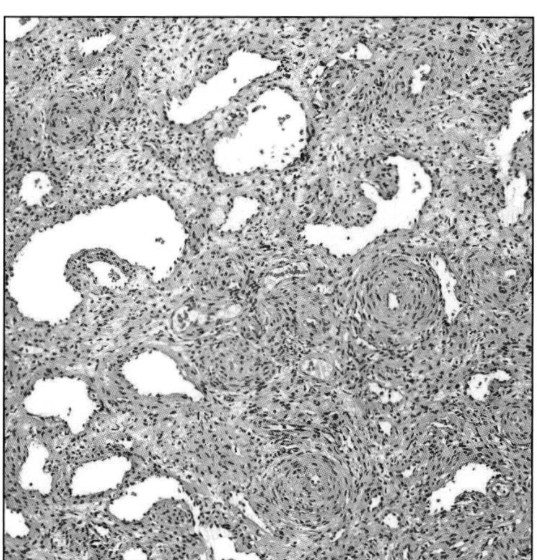

(Left) *Hematoxylin & eosin shows an intravascular myopericytoma.* ***(Right)*** *Hematoxylin & eosin shows numerous vessels and a perivascular growth of myoid tumor cells in this intravascular myopericytoma.*

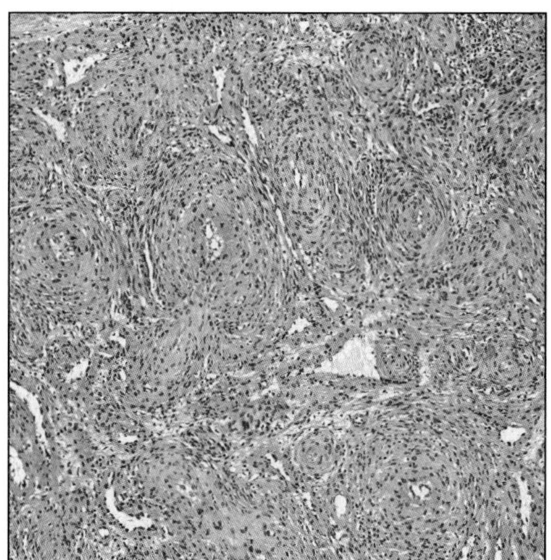

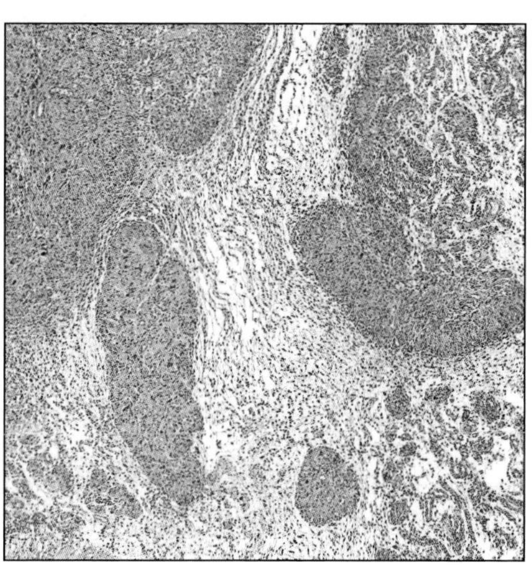

(Left) *Hematoxylin & eosin shows a higher power view of an intravascular myopericytoma. Note the concentric perivascular growth of myoid tumor cells.* ***(Right)*** *Hematoxylin & eosin shows a rare example of malignant myopericytoma. This is an ill-defined, infiltrative mesenchymal neoplasm containing numerous vascular structures. Atypical tumor cells are arranged in a perivascular fashion.*

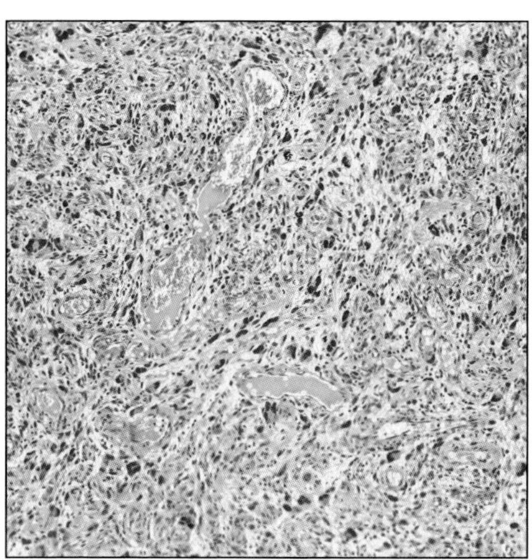

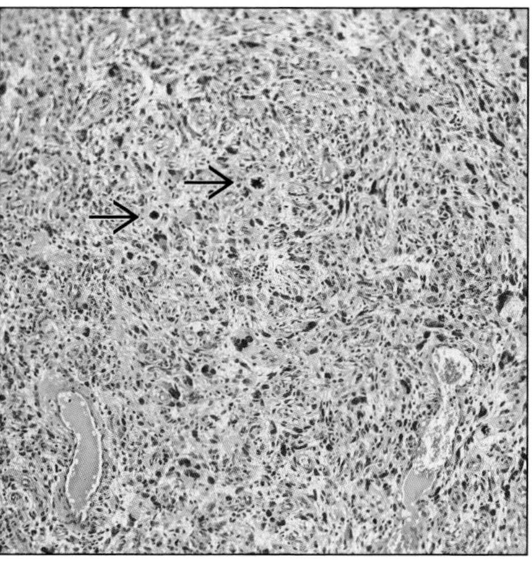

(Left) *Hematoxylin & eosin shows a malignant myopericytoma. The growing perivascular neoplastic cells contain enlarged and hyperchromatic nuclei, and multinucleated giant cells are noted.* ***(Right)*** *Hematoxylin & eosin shows atypical tumor cells with enlarged and atypical nuclei. Note the numerous atypical mitoses* →.

SINONASAL HEMANGIOPERICYTOMA

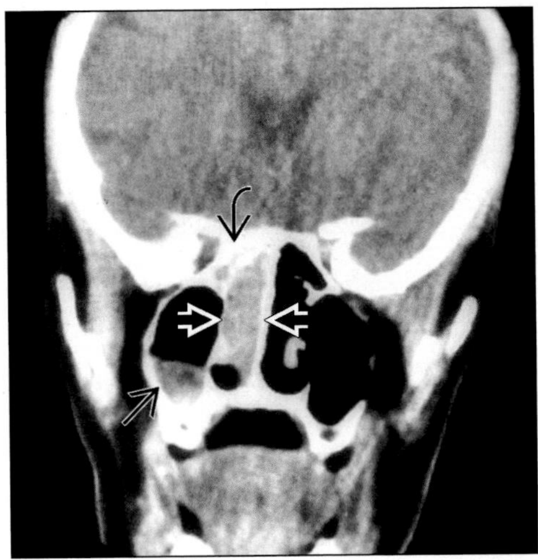

Coronal CT scan shows a sinonasal hemangiopericytoma (HPC) filling the right nasal cavity ➡ with bone erosion and extension into the adjacent ethmoid sinus ↗. The right maxillary sinus has associated sinusitis →.

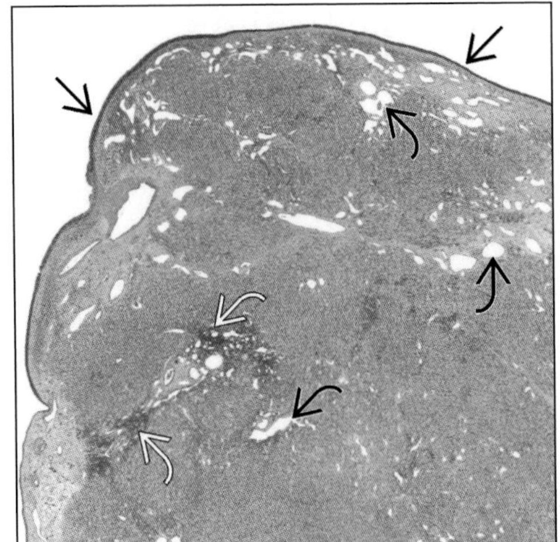

Low-power image shows sinonasal HPC with intact surface → and a subepithelial mesenchymal proliferation with prominent vascularity ↗, extravasated blood ➡, and effacing subepithelial structures.

TERMINOLOGY

Abbreviations

- Sinonasal hemangiopericytoma (HPC)

Synonyms

- Glomangiopericytoma
- Hemangiopericytoma-like tumor of sinonasal cavity
- Sinonasal glomus tumor
- Hemangiopericytoma

Definitions

- Unique sinonasal mesenchymal neoplasm demonstrating perivascular myoid phenotype

ETIOLOGY/PATHOGENESIS

Histogenesis

- Proposed cell of origin is unidentified modified perivascular glomus-like myoid cell

CLINICAL ISSUES

Epidemiology

- Incidence
  - Accounts for < 0.5% of sinonasal neoplasms
- Age
  - All age groups affected (range: 5-86 years)
    - 75% of cases occur in 6th-8th decades
    - Peak incidence in 6th-7th decades
- Gender
  - Slight female predilection

Site

- Most frequently involve nasal cavity
  - Often have concomitant paranasal sinus involvement
  - Right and left side equally effected
- Rarely arise primarily in paranasal sinuses

Presentation

- Unilateral polypoid intranasal mass
- Nasal obstruction
- Epistaxis
- Congestion &/or difficulty breathing
- Sinusitis

Treatment

- Surgical approaches
  - Complete surgical excision is treatment of choice
- Adjuvant therapy
  - Radiation therapy of unproven value

Prognosis

- Excellent overall 5-year survival (> 90%)
- Approximately 1/3 will recur/persist (range: 18-44%)
  - Recurrences can occur after many years
    - Mean interval to 1st recurrence is around 6.5 years (range: 1-17.5 years)
    - Long-term follow-up warranted
- Malignant degeneration uncommon
  - Histologic features of malignant sinonasal hemangiopericytoma similar to soft tissue "hemangiopericytoma"
    - Large size (> 5 cm)
    - Marked pleomorphism
    - Necrosis
    - Bone invasion
    - > 4 mitoses/10 high-power fields
    - Ki-67 proliferation index > 10%

IMAGE FINDINGS

Radiographic Findings

- Opacification filling nasal cavity ± adjacent sinuses
- Bone erosion or sclerosis can be seen
- Concomitant sinusitis not uncommon

SINONASAL HEMANGIOPERICYTOMA

Key Facts

Clinical Issues

- Accounts for < 0.5% of sinonasal neoplasms
- Peak incidence in 6th-7th decades
- Most frequently involve nasal cavity
- Excellent overall 5-year survival (> 90%)
- Approximately 1/3 will recur/persist (range: 18-44%)
- Often have concomitant paranasal sinus involvement

Macroscopic Features

- Mean size is 3.5 cm (range: 1.5-8 cm)

Microscopic Pathology

- Composed of uniform, cytologically bland, closely packed, round to spindle-shaped cells intimately associated with vascular component
- Prominent perivascular hyalinization is characteristic and is seen in up to 90% of cases
- Most tumors have solid or fascicular growth, but mixed growth patterns are common
- Vast majority demonstrate myoid phenotype with actin immunohistochemical positivity

Top Differential Diagnoses

- Solitary fibrous tumor
- Angiofibroma
- Lobular capillary hemangioma
- Sinonasal smooth muscle neoplasms
- Glomus tumor
- Various sarcomas with HPC-like vascular pattern

MACROSCOPIC FEATURES

General Features

- Often removed piecemeal
- If resected intact, appears as polypoid solid mass with tan hemorrhagic cut surface
- Surface mucosa typically intact

Size

- Mean size is 3.5 cm (range: 1.5-8 cm)

MICROSCOPIC PATHOLOGY

Histologic Features

- Subepithelial, well-demarcated but unencapsulated, cellular mesenchymal proliferation
  - Surface (Schneiderian) mucosa usually intact but may be eroded or show squamous metaplasia
  - Usually efface but may surround submucosal minor salivary glands
- Composed of uniform, closely packed, round to spindle-shaped cells intimately associated with vascular component
- Vascular channels are variable in size ranging from capillaries to patulous "staghorn" vessels
  - Prominent perivascular hyalinization is characteristic and seen in up to 90% of cases
- Stroma is typically scant but may be myxoid in areas
- Stromal edema may result in hypocellular zones with residual smaller cellular lobules
- Most tumors have solid or fascicular growth, but mixed growth patterns are common
  - Whorled growth patterns can be seen in up to 10% of cases
- Extravasated red blood cells are usually present
- Inflammatory cells, including eosinophils, mast cells, lymphocytes, and plasma cells, are invariably present
- Cytoplasm is lightly eosinophilic and indiscrete, resulting in syncytial appearance
  - Focal areas composed of clear cells may be seen
- Neoplastic cells have uniform oval to round nuclei
  - Nuclear chromatin is typically homogeneous or vesicular with 1 or more small nucleoli
- Rare mitoses and mild nuclear pleomorphism may be identified
- Scattered tumor giant cells (~ 5%) may be present
  - Likely represent degenerative phenomenon
  - Consist of agglomerated tumor cells
    - Giant cells have same immunophenotype as single spindle cells

ANCILLARY TESTS

Immunohistochemistry

- Vast majority demonstrate myoid phenotype with actin positivity
  - Smooth muscle actin(+) (80-100%)
  - Muscle specific actin(+) (77-100%)
- Desmin, cytokeratin, and C-kit (CD117) negative
- Factor XIIIA often positive (78%) but nonspecific
- CD34 (0-8%) occasionally positive but weak and focal
- S100 protein (0-3%) occasionally positive but weak and focal

DIFFERENTIAL DIAGNOSIS

Solitary Fibrous Tumor

- 1/3 of extrapleural solitary fibrous tumors occur in head and neck sites
  - 15% of head and neck solitary fibrous tumors occur in sinonasal sites
- Variably cellular spindle cell proliferation with stromal collagen and HPC-like vessels
- Spindle cells arranged along ropey stromal collagen in contrast to sinonasal HPCs, which typically lack collagen
- CD34 almost uniformly positive, unlike sinonasal HPC

Angiofibroma

- Majority occur in adolescent males
- Arise in posterior nasal cavity with extension into nasopharynx

- Often involve nasal cavity, sinuses, and skull base when they enlarge
- Less cellular than sinonasal HPC and composed of evenly spaced stellate fibroblasts/myofibroblasts
- Associated with abundant stromal collagen, unlike sinonasal HPC
- Cells are arranged around ectatic and capillary-sized vessels
- Stromal cells often positive for nuclear β-catenin staining
  - Some cases occur in patients with familial adenomatosis polyposis

Lobular Capillary Hemangioma

- Nasal cavity is 2nd most common head and neck site following oral cavity
- Mean size is 1.7 cm but can be up to 8 cm
- Composed of cellular lobules arranged in fibrovascular stroma
- Surface erosion is frequent
- Lobules consist of proliferation of small slit-like vascular channels emanating from larger central feeder vessels
- Cells within lobules consist of endothelial cells and pericytes
  - Mitoses can be frequent
  - Endothelial markers (CD31, CD34) will be positive, unlike sinonasal HPC

Sinonasal Smooth Muscle Neoplasms

- Uncommon
  - Leiomyomas and leiomyosarcomas occur with roughly equal frequency
- Arranged in long sweeping fascicles
- Cells have more elongated spindle cell morphology
  - Abundant fibrillary eosinophilic cytoplasm in contrast to sinonasal HPC
  - Blunt-ended oval nuclei often with paranuclear vacuole
- Usually will have desmin reactivity (in contrast to sinonasal HPC) in addition to actin reactivity

Glomus Tumor

- Extremely rare in sinonasal sites
- Histology may overlap with sinonasal HPC in some cases
  - Identical immunophenotype to sinonasal HPC
- Consists of rounded perivascular cells with central round nucleus, eosinophilic cytoplasm, and prominent cell borders
- May have spindle cell growth, but this is usually more limited than in sinonasal HPC
- Sinonasal HPC may be site-specific variant of traditional glomus tumor

Various Sarcomas with HPC-like Vascular Pattern

- Usually can be distinguished from sinonasal HPC by presence of cytologic atypica, significant mitotic activity, and necrosis

DIAGNOSTIC CHECKLIST

Clinically Relevant Pathologic Features

- Organ distribution
- Bland spindle cells with prominent vascular component
- Low mitotic rare
- Myoid phenotype (smooth muscle and muscle specific actin) immunohistochemically

Pathologic Interpretation Pearls

- Features that can lead to misdiagnosis
  - Lack of awareness of this unique sinonasal tumor
  - Bone invasion
  - Multinodularity secondary to edema or degenerative changes
  - Multinucleated tumor giant cells
  - Whorled growth pattern
  - Focal CD34 &/or S100 protein staining

SELECTED REFERENCES

1. Kuo FY et al: Sinonasal hemangiopericytoma-like tumor with true pericytic myoid differentiation: a clinicopathologic and immunohistochemical study of five cases. Head Neck. 27(2):124-9, 2005
2. Li XQ et al: Intranasal pericytic tumors (glomus tumor and sinonasal hemangiopericytoma-like tumor): report of two cases with review of the literature. Pathol Int. 53(5):303-8, 2003
3. Thompson LD et al: Sinonasal-type hemangiopericytoma: a clinicopathologic and immunophenotypic analysis of 104 cases showing perivascular myoid differentiation. Am J Surg Pathol. 27(6):737-49, 2003
4. Tse LL et al: Sinonasal haemangiopericytoma-like tumour: a sinonasal glomus tumour or a haemangiopericytoma? Histopathology. 40(6):510-7, 2002
5. Watanabe K et al: True hemangiopericytoma of the nasal cavity. Arch Pathol Lab Med. 125(5):686-90, 2001
6. Catalano PJ et al: Sinonasal hemangiopericytomas: a clinicopathologic and immunohistochemical study of seven cases. Head Neck. 18(1):42-53, 1996
7. Thiringer JK et al: Sinonasal hemangiopericytoma: case report and literature review. Skull Base Surg. 5(3):185-90, 1995
8. el-Naggar AK et al: Sinonasal hemangiopericytomas. A clinicopathologic and DNA content study. Arch Otolaryngol Head Neck Surg. 118(2):134-7, 1992
9. Eichhorn JH et al: Sinonasal hemangiopericytoma. A reassessment with electron microscopy, immunohistochemistry, and long-term follow-up. Am J Surg Pathol. 14(9):856-66, 1990
10. Batsakis JG et al: Hemangiopericytoma of the nasal cavity: electron-optic study and clinical correlations. J Laryngol Otol. 97(4):361-8, 1983
11. Compagno J: Hemangiopericytoma-like tumors of the nasal cavity: a comparison with hemangiopericytoma of soft tissues. Laryngoscope. 88(3):460-9, 1978
12. Compagno J et al: Hemangiopericytoma-like intranasal tumors. A clinicopathologic study of 23 cases. Am J Clin Pathol. 66(4):672-83, 1976

Microscopic Features

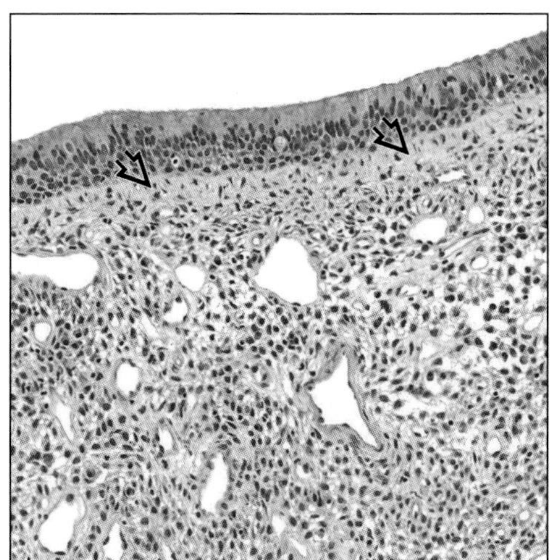

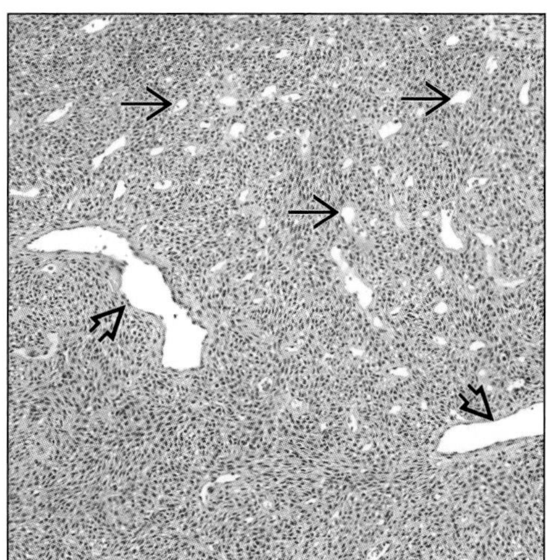

(Left) Sinonasal HPCs typically have intact surface (Schneiderian) mucosa and may or may not have a Grenz-type zone of submucosal sparing ⇨. ***(Right)*** Low-power image shows a typical sinonasal HPC with a diffuse submucosal spindle cell proliferation and extensive associated vascular component. Note the combination of numerous small capillaries → and scattered ectatic and irregular vascular spaces ⇨ (hemangiopericytoma-like).

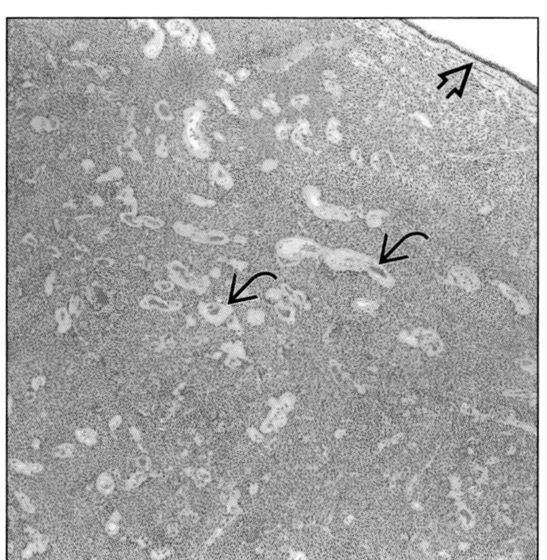

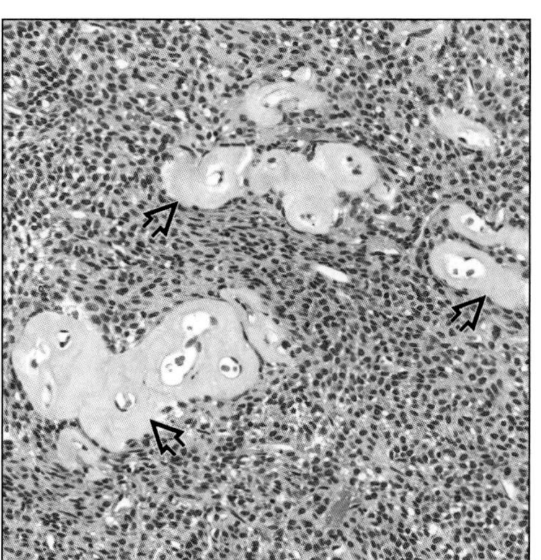

(Left) A very characteristic feature of sinonasal HPC is the presence of prominent perivascular hyalinization ↷. This histologic feature is seen in up to 90% of tumors. Note the intact Schneiderian mucosa ⇨. ***(Right)*** High-power image shows the characteristic perivascular hyalinization ⇨ consisting of a sharply demarcated zone of homogeneous and paucicellular eosinophilic collagen surrounding capillaries.

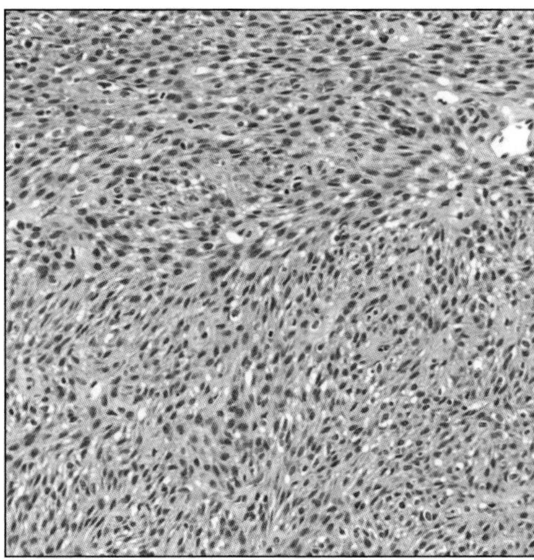

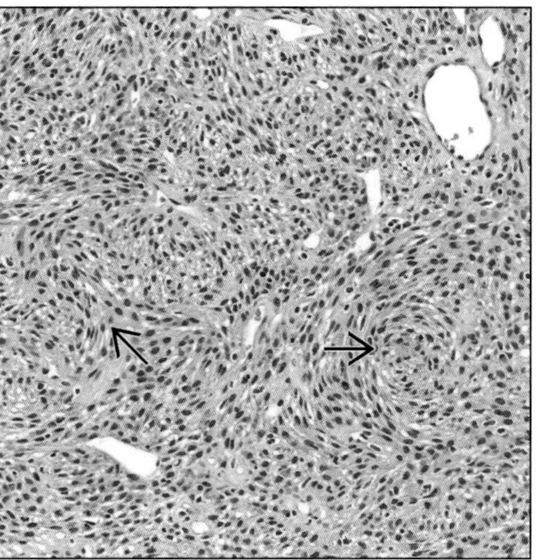

(Left) Sinonasal HPC may show a variety of growth patterns, including solid, fascicular, and whorled. Mixed patterns are not uncommon. This example demonstrates a compact fascicular growth pattern. ***(Right)*** Another example of a sinonasal HPC is shown with a prominent whorled or meningothelial-like growth pattern →. This pattern can be seen in up to 10% of sinonasal HPCs and usually is limited in extent when present.

SINONASAL HEMANGIOPERICYTOMA

Microscopic Features

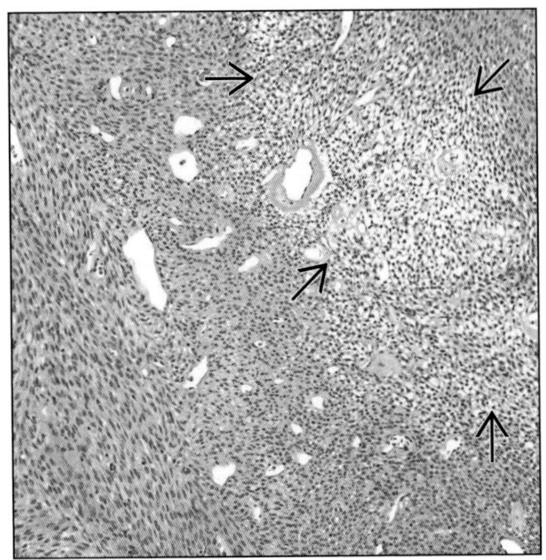
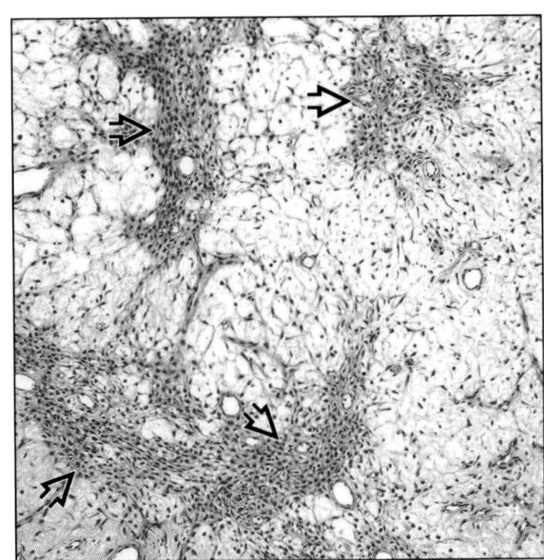

(Left) *Sinonasal HPCs have minimal stroma predominantly consisting of only mesenchymal cells and vessels. Focal areas of stromal edema* ➔ *or myxoid change can often be seen.* ***(Right)*** *Extensive stromal edema also can be seen and is usually more prominent at the periphery. The stromal edema in this example imparts a reticular appearance in the paucicellular region and multinodularity* ➔ *in the preserved cellular zones.*

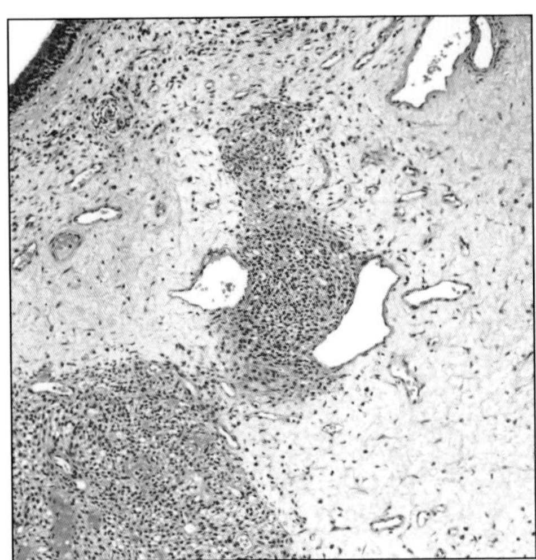
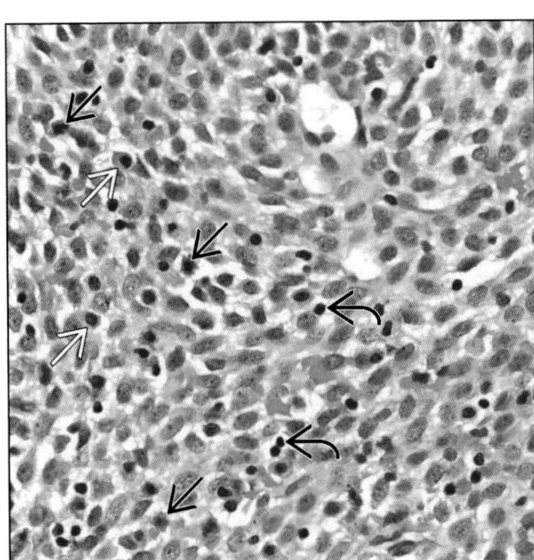

(Left) *Whereas sinonasal HPCs do not have a prominent stromal component, cellular nodules embedded within a paucicellular collagenous stroma may be present at the periphery, imparting a multinodular appearance. This is thought to result from degenerative changes.* ***(Right)*** *An inflammatory infiltrate is invariably present in sinonasal HPCs and usually consists of a mixture of eosinophils* ➔ *and mast cells, but neutrophils, plasma cells* ➔*, and lymphocytes* ➔ *may also be seen.*

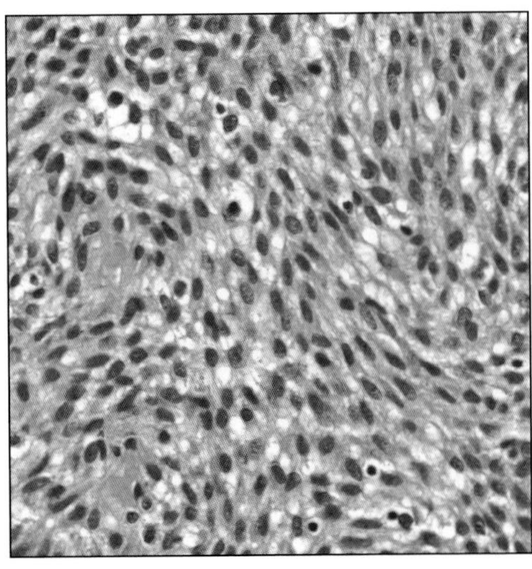
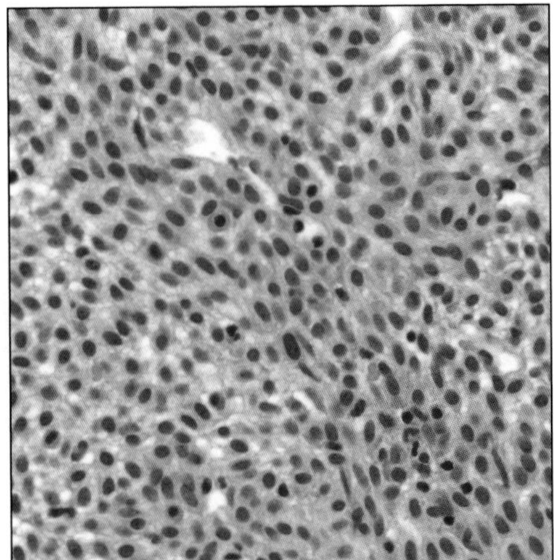

(Left) *Sinonasal HPCs are usually composed of cytologically bland spindle cells with blunt-ended oval nuclei containing even chromatin and small nucleoli. The cytoplasm is eosinophilic and finely vacuolated with indistinct cell borders imparting a syncytial growth pattern.* ***(Right)*** *In many tumors, areas with more rounded cells can be seen. These round cell areas are limited in extent and may resemble glomus tumors but lack the prominent cell borders seen in soft tissue glomus tumors.*

Variant Microscopic Features and Ancillary Techniques

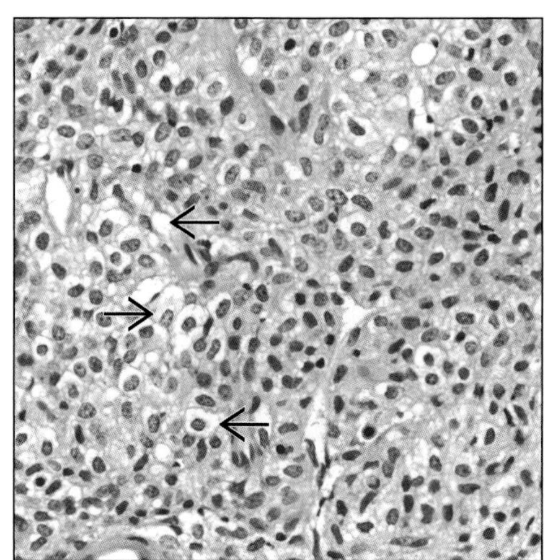

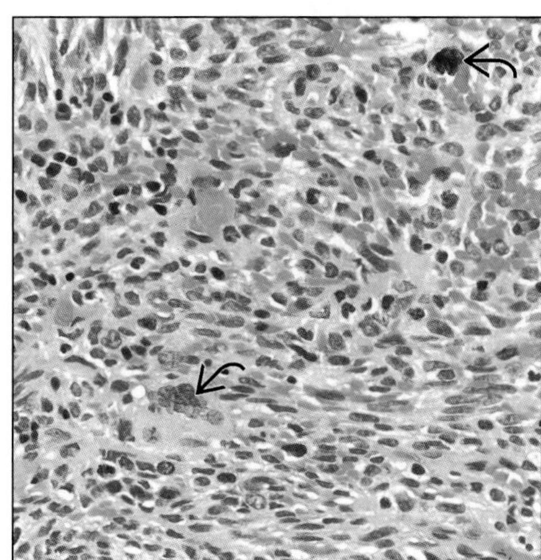

(Left) *This image is a focal area in an otherwise typical sinonasal HPC that demonstrates round cells with clear cytoplasm ⇒. Clear cytoplasm can be seen in many sinonasal HPCs, but it is usually only focal and rarely is extensive.* ***(Right)*** *Multinucleated tumor giant cells ⇒ can be seen in up to 5% of cases and likely represent a degenerative change. Note the extravasated blood, which is typical of sinonasal HPC and seen in almost all tumors.*

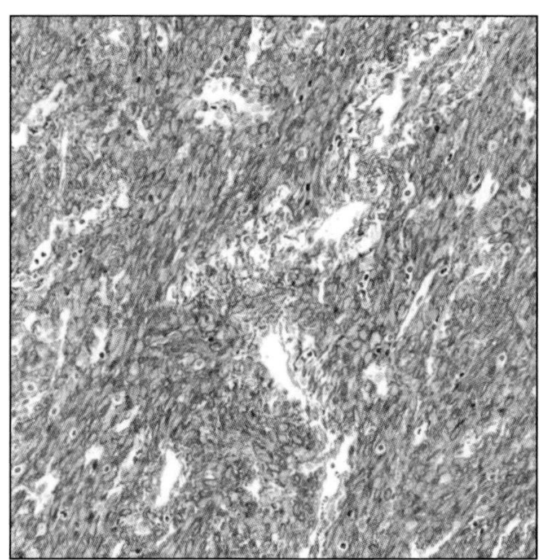

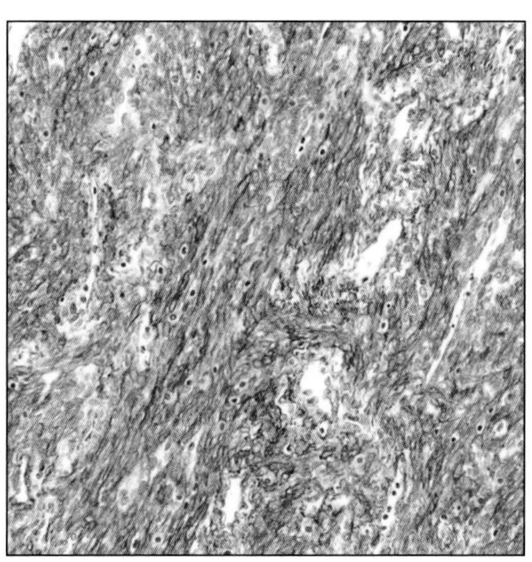

(Left) *The cells of sinonasal HPC are true pericytic cells, as they demonstrate a myoid phenotype both ultrastructurally and immunophenotypically. This example demonstrates diffuse and strong cytoplasmic staining with smooth muscle actin.* ***(Right)*** *The vast majority of sinonasal HPCs stain with actins immunohistochemically, such as this example showing diffuse and strong cytoplasmic staining with muscle specific actin.*

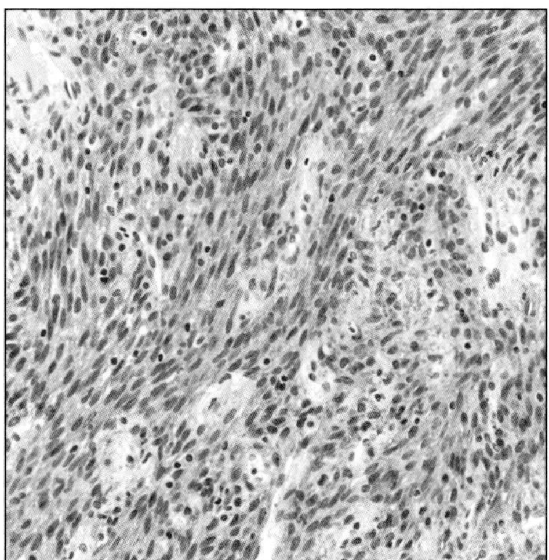

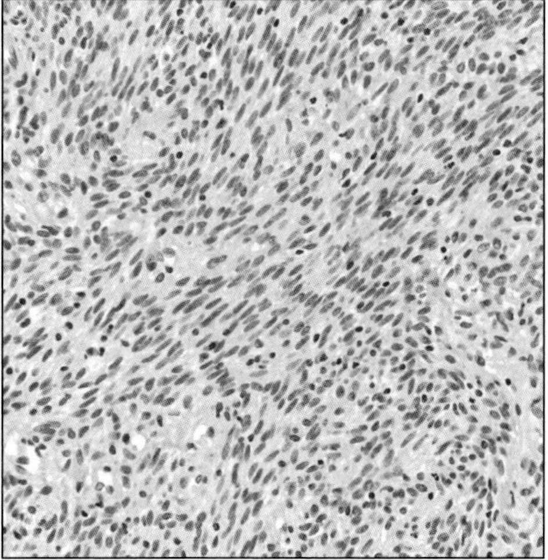

(Left) *Factor XIIIA labeling can be demonstrated in up to 80% of sinonasal HPCs; however, this is not a very specific marker, and its utility is limited in sorting out the differential diagnosis.* ***(Right)*** *While actin staining can be appreciated in most sinonasal HPCs, desmin is uniformly negative, as in this example.*

GLOMUS TUMORS

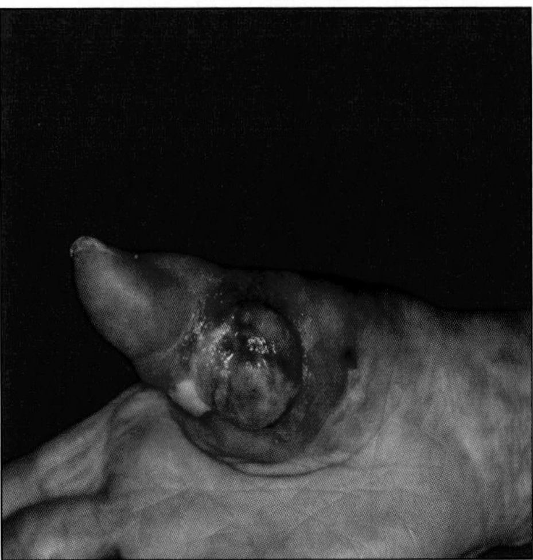

Clinical photograph shows a rare malignant glomus tumor involving the right thumb.

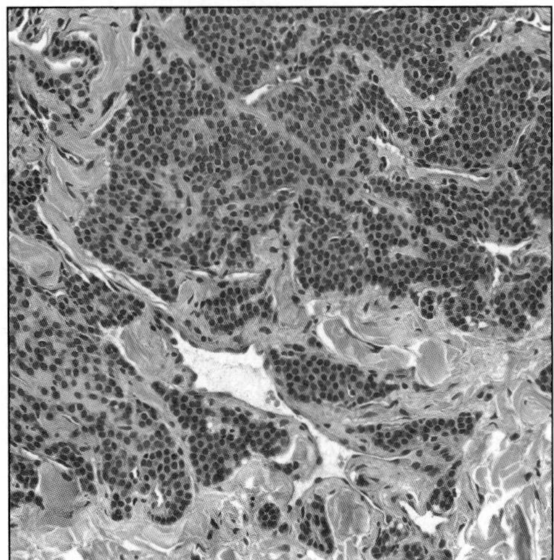

Hematoxylin & eosin shows perivascularly arranged myogenic tumor cells that contain uniform round nuclei in a benign glomus tumor.

TERMINOLOGY

Abbreviations

- Glomus tumor (GT)

Definitions

- Perivascular myogenic mesenchymal neoplasm composed of cells closely resembling smooth muscle cells of normal glomus body

CLINICAL ISSUES

Epidemiology

- Incidence
  - Rare
  - Account for < 2% of soft tissue neoplasms
- Age
  - Predominantly in young adults
  - May occur at any age
- Gender
  - No sex predilection

Site

- Distal extremities
- Often in subungual location
- Rare in other anatomic locations (e.g., visceral organs, bone, mediastinum, nerve)
- Skin, subcutis
- Rare in deep soft tissue

Presentation

- Painful mass
- Typically small red-blue nodules
- Long history of pain
- Pain with exposure to cold &/or tactile stimulation
- Usually solitary lesions
- Rare multiple neoplasms
- Multiple lesions more common in childhood

Natural History

- < 10% recur locally
- Malignant glomus tumors highly aggressive
- Metastases and death of patients in up to 40% of cases

Treatment

- Surgical approaches
  - Complete excision

Prognosis

- Benign behavior in most cases

MACROSCOPIC FEATURES

General Features

- Red-blue nodular lesions

MICROSCOPIC PATHOLOGY

Histologic Features

- Perivascular myoid tumor cells
- Small, uniform, round tumor cells
- Centrally placed, sharply punched-out, round nuclei
- Eosinophilic cytoplasm
- Each cell surrounded by basal lamina

Predominant Pattern/Injury Type

- Circumscribed

Predominant Cell/Compartment Type

- Smooth muscle

Solid Glomus Tumor

- Most common variant
- Well-circumscribed nodular neoplasm
- Contains numerous capillary-sized vessels
- Nest of tumor cells surrounding capillaries
- Stroma may show hyalinization
- Stroma may show myxoid changes
- Rare degenerative cytologic atypia

GLOMUS TUMORS

Key Facts

Terminology

- Perivascular myogenic mesenchymal neoplasm composed of cells closely resembling smooth muscle cells of normal glomus body

Clinical Issues

- Distal extremities, especially in subungual location
- Typically small, red-blue, painful nodules
- < 10% recur locally
- Malignant glomus tumors highly aggressive

Macroscopic Features

- Red-blue nodular lesions

Microscopic Pathology

- Solid glomus tumor
  - Most common variant
  - Well-circumscribed nodular neoplasm
  - Small, uniform, round tumor cells
  - Centrally placed, sharply punched-out, round nuclei
- Glomangioma
  - Comprises up to 20% of glomus tumors
- Glomangiomyoma
  - Solid glomus tumor or glomangioma and elongated, spindled smooth muscle cells
- Glomangiomatosis
  - Extremely rare variant
- Malignant glomus tumor (glomangiosarcoma)
  - Exceedingly rare neoplasms
  - Enlarged size (> 2 cm) &/or subfascial/visceral location
  - Marked nuclear atypia
  - Increased number of mitoses

- Rare vascular invasion
- Peripheral rim of collagen (fibrous pseudocapsule)
- May contain numerous hemangiopericytoma-like vessels
- Rare oncocytic changes
- Rare epithelioid variant

Glomangioma

- Comprises up to 20% of glomus tumors
- Most common type in patients with multiple lesions
- Less well circumscribed
- Dilated veins surrounded by clusters of glomus cells
- Secondary thrombosis may occur

Glomangiomyoma

- Rare subtype
- Solid glomus tumor or glomangioma and elongated, spindled smooth muscle cells

Glomangiomatosis

- Extremely rare variant
- Infiltrative growth
- Multiple nodules of solid glomus tumor
- Biologically benign lesions

Symplastic Glomus Tumor

- Cells show prominent degenerative atypia
- Multinucleated giant cells
- Enlarged nuclei
- No increased proliferative activity
- No tumor necrosis

Malignant Glomus Tumor (Glomangiosarcoma)

- Exceedingly rare neoplasms
- Criteria of malignancy
  - Enlarged size (> 2 cm)
  - Subfascial/visceral location
  - Marked nuclear atypia
  - Mitoses
  - Necrosis
  - Intravascular growth
- Preexisting benign-appearing glomus tumor may be present
- Spindle cell subtype
  - Atypical spindled tumor cells
  - Increased number of mitoses
- Round cell subtype
  - Sheets of atypical round tumor cells
  - Increased number of mitoses

Glomus Tumor of Uncertain Malignant Potential

- Nuclear pleomorphism
- 1 additional atypical feature

ANCILLARY TESTS

Cytogenetics

- Gene for inherited glomangiomas localized at 1p21-22
- Multiple familial glomus tumors may have autosomal dominant pattern of inheritance

Electron Microscopy

- Short interdigitating cytoplasmic processes
- Bundles of cytoplasmic actin-like filaments
- Dense bodies
- External lamina

DIFFERENTIAL DIAGNOSIS

Myopericytoma

- Distinction can be problematic because of overlapping morphologic features
- Perivascular onion-like growth
- Round and plump spindled tumor cells
- Nuclei usually not so sharply punched-out

Myofibroma

- Biphasic pattern
- Spindled tumor cells in more mature component
- Small undifferentiated cells associated with hemangiopericytoma-like vessels

GLOMUS TUMORS

Immunohistochemistry

Antibody	Reactivity	Staining Pattern	Comment
Actin-sm	Positive	Cytoplasmic	
HCAD	Positive	Cytoplasmic	
Collagen IV	Positive	Cell membrane	
CD34	Negative		May be positive in myxoid glomus tumor
Desmin	Negative		
CK-PAN	Negative		
S100P	Negative		

- Usually H-caldesmon(-)

Hidradenoma (Solid Form)

- Often focal stromal hyalinization
- Ductal differentiation
- Poroid and cuticular tumor cells
- Pancytokeratin(+)
- Actin(-)

Paraganglioma

- Clinical features
- Expression of neuroendocrine markers
- Sustentacular S100 protein(+) cells
- Zellballen of tumor cells

Dermal Melanocytic Nevus

- Nests of melanocytic cells
- Pigmentation of tumor cells
- Intranuclear pseudoinclusion
- Expression of S100 protein
- Expression of Melan-A

Angioleiomyoma

- Thick-walled blood vessels
- Bundles of spindled tumor cells
- Eosinophilic spindled tumor cells
- Expression of desmin

DIAGNOSTIC CHECKLIST

Clinically Relevant Pathologic Features

- Organ distribution
- Nuclear features
- Symptom complex
- Often painful neoplasms
- Biologically benign neoplasms in most cases

Pathologic Interpretation Pearls

- Perivascular myogenic mesenchymal neoplasm
- Varying number of blood vessels
- Uniform round tumor cells
- Round, sharply punched-out nuclei
- Expression of actins and H-caldesmon
- No expression of cytokeratin, desmin, S100 protein

SELECTED REFERENCES

1. Semaan MT et al: Current assessment and management of glomus tumors. Curr Opin Otolaryngol Head Neck Surg. 16(5):420-6, 2008
2. Brouillard P et al: Four common glomulin mutations cause two thirds of glomuvenous malformations ("familial glomangiomas"): evidence for a founder effect. J Med Genet. 42(2):e13, 2005
3. De Chiara A et al: Malignant Glomus Tumour: A Case Report and Review of the Literature. Sarcoma. 7(2):87-91, 2003
4. Brouillard P et al: Mutations in a novel factor, glomulin, are responsible for glomuvenous malformations ("glomangiomas"). Am J Hum Genet. 70(4):866-74, 2002
5. Mentzel T et al: CD34-positive glomus tumor: clinicopathologic and immunohistochemical analysis of six cases with myxoid stromal changes. J Cutan Pathol. 29(7):421-5, 2002
6. Calvert JT et al: Additional glomangioma families link to chromosome 1p: no evidence for genetic heterogeneity. Hum Hered. 51(3):180-2, 2001
7. Folpe AL et al: Atypical and malignant glomus tumors: analysis of 52 cases, with a proposal for the reclassification of glomus tumors. Am J Surg Pathol. 25(1):1-12, 2001
8. Takata H et al: Treatment of subungual glomus tumour. Hand Surg. 6(1):25-7, 2001
9. Boon LM et al: A gene for inherited cutaneous venous anomalies ("glomangiomas") localizes to chromosome 1p21-22. Am J Hum Genet. 65(1):125-33, 1999
10. Hiruta N et al: Malignant glomus tumor: a case report and review of the literature. Am J Surg Pathol. 21(9):1096-103, 1997
11. Van Geertruyden J et al: Glomus tumours of the hand. A retrospective study of 51 cases. J Hand Surg [Br]. 21(2):257-60, 1996
12. Pulitzer DR et al: Epithelioid glomus tumor. Hum Pathol. 26(9):1022-7, 1995
13. Haque S et al: Multiple glomus tumors of the stomach with intravascular spread. Am J Surg Pathol. 16(3):291-9, 1992
14. Gould EW et al: Locally infiltrative glomus tumors and glomangiosarcomas. A clinical, ultrastructural, and immunohistochemical study. Cancer. 65(2):310-8, 1990
15. Hulsebos TJ et al: Inheritance of glomus tumours. Lancet. 335(8690):660, 1990
16. Slater DN et al: Oncocytic glomus tumour: a new variant. Histopathology. 11(5):523-31, 1987
17. Miettinen M et al: Glomus tumor cells: evaluation of smooth muscle and endothelial cell properties. Virchows Arch B Cell Pathol Incl Mol Pathol. 43(2):139-49, 1983

Microscopic and Immunohistochemical Features

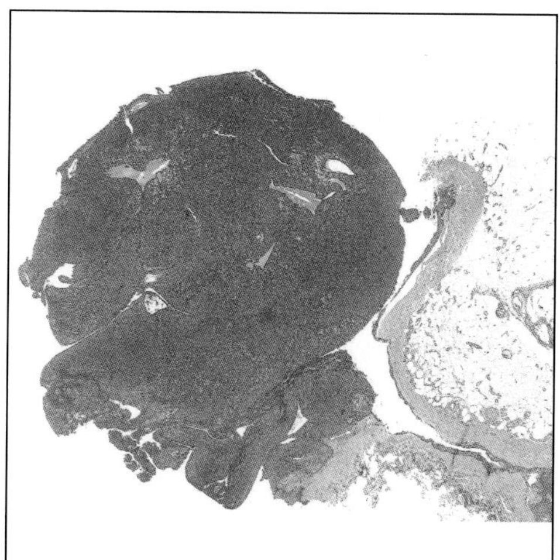

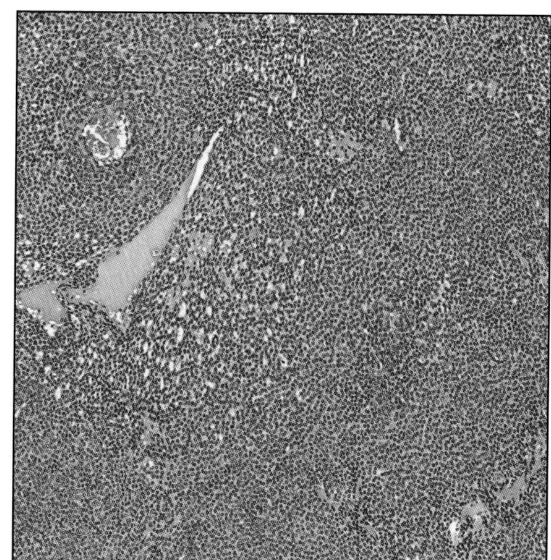

(Left) *Hematoxylin & eosin shows a solid glomus tumor. Note the nodular growth of a well-circumscribed neoplasm.* ***(Right)*** *Hematoxylin & eosin shows a solid growth of uniform round tumor cells, mimicking an adnexal cutaneous neoplasm.*

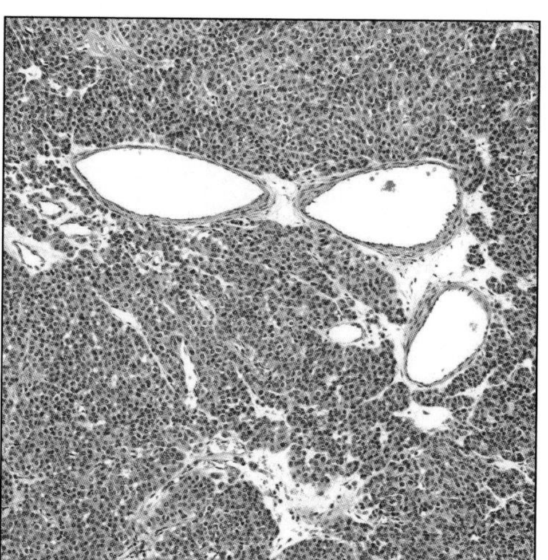

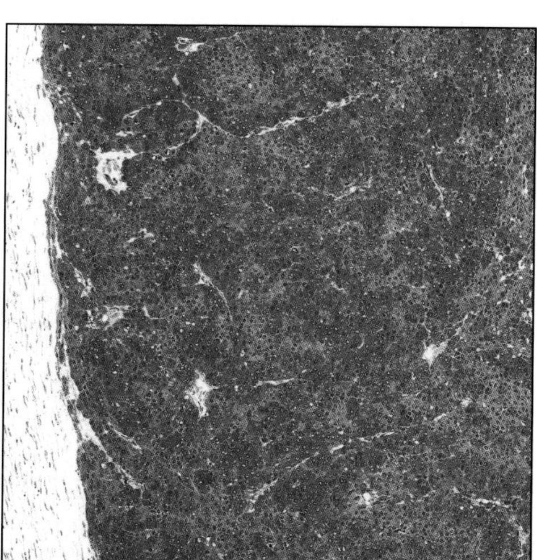

(Left) *Hematoxylin & eosin shows sheets of myogenic tumor cells with slightly enlarged nuclei.* ***(Right)*** *Actin-sm shows homogeneous expression in contrast to an adnexal neoplasm.*

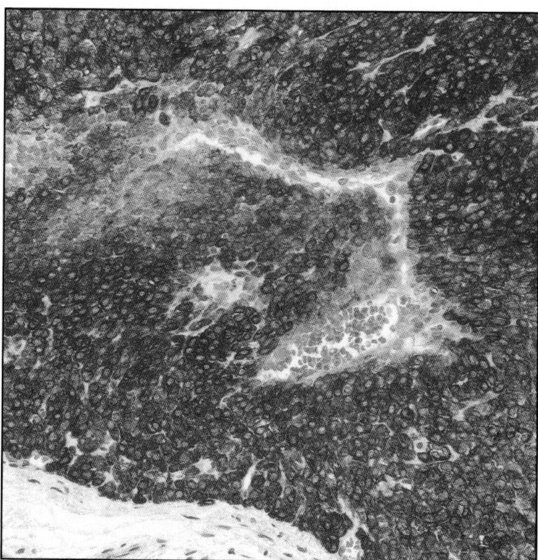

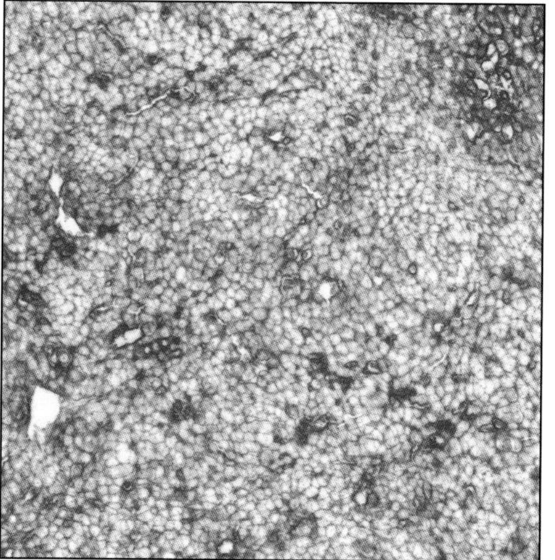

(Left) *Caldesmon shows homogeneous expression.* ***(Right)*** *Collagen IV shows the clear membranous staining of tumor cells.*

GLOMUS TUMORS

Microscopic and Immunohistochemical Features

(Left) *Hematoxylin & eosin shows a low-power view of a deep dermal-located, well-circumscribed glomangioma.* ***(Right)*** *Hematoxylin & eosin shows a perivascular arrangement of glomus cells in this example of glomangioma.*

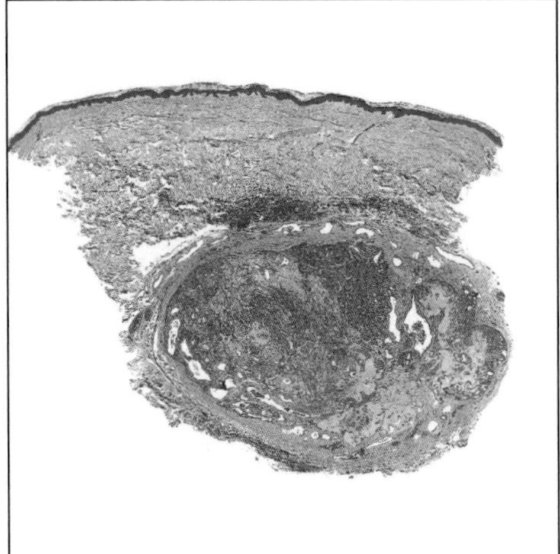

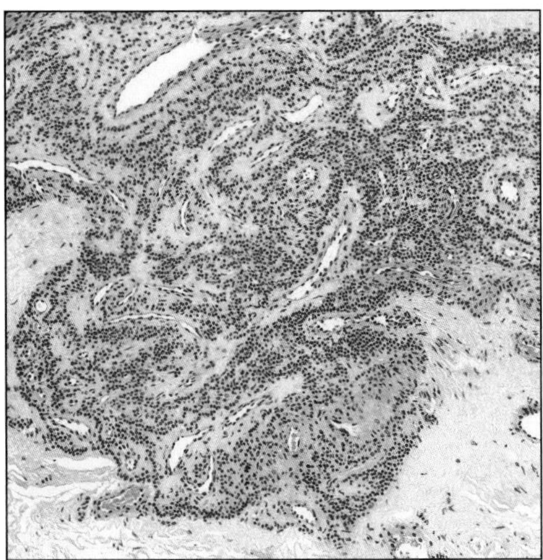

(Left) *Hematoxylin & eosin shows the bland cytology of round glomus cells containing sharply demarcated, round nuclei.* ***(Right)*** *Actin-sm shows the perivascular arrangement of round, myogenic tumor cells.*

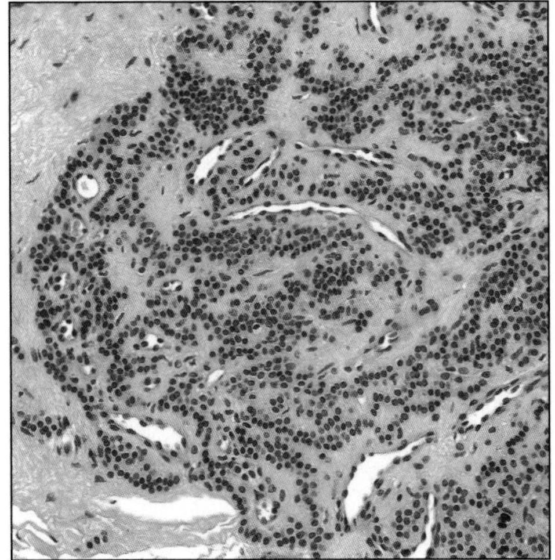

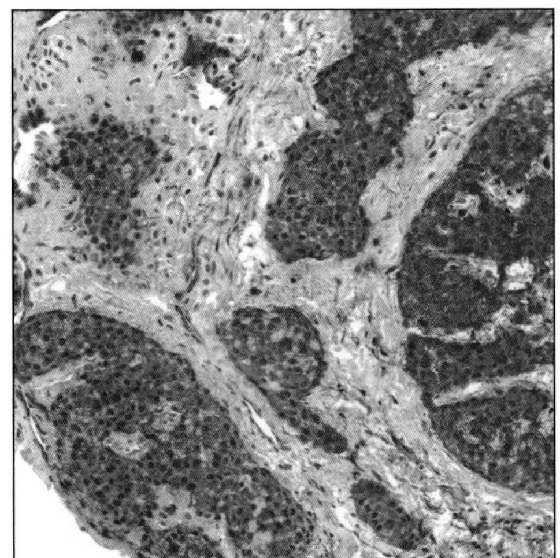

(Left) *Hematoxylin & eosin shows an example of a glomus tumor with myxoid stromal changes.* ***(Right)*** *Hematoxylin & eosin shows a "transition" of an ordinary glomus tumor (left upper corner) to a glomus tumor with myxoid stromal changes.*

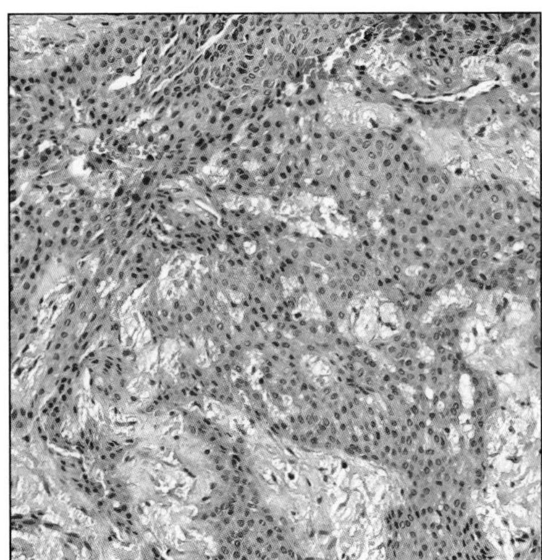

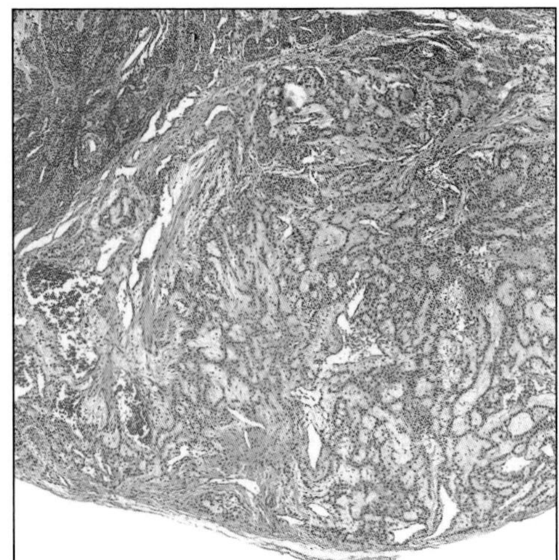

Microscopic and Immunohistochemical Features

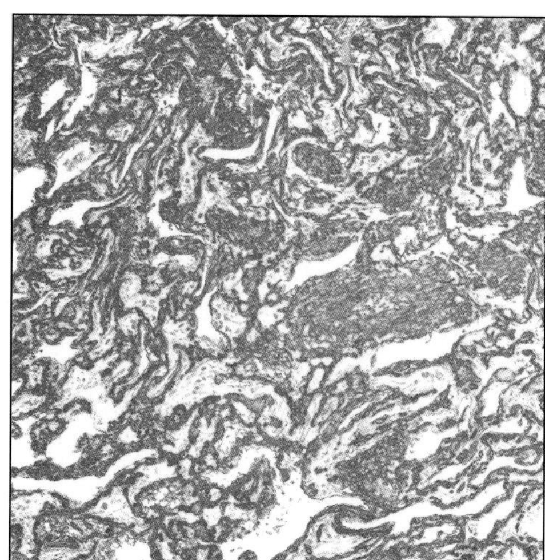

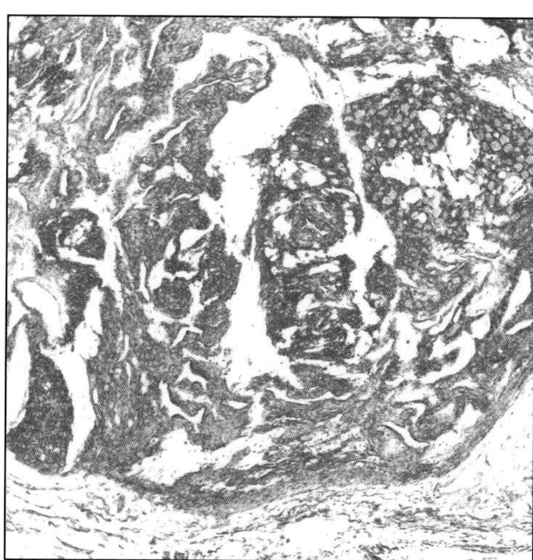

(Left) *Actin-sm shows homogeneous actin expression in this example of a rare myxoid glomus tumor.* ***(Right)*** *CD34 shows coexpression in this example of a myxoid glomus tumor. Whereas all CD34(+) glomus tumors are characterized by myxoid changes, this coexpression was not seen in all cases of glomus tumor with myxoid stromal changes.*

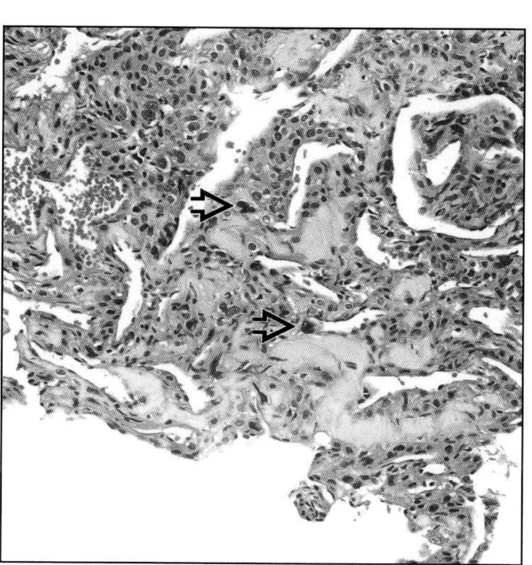

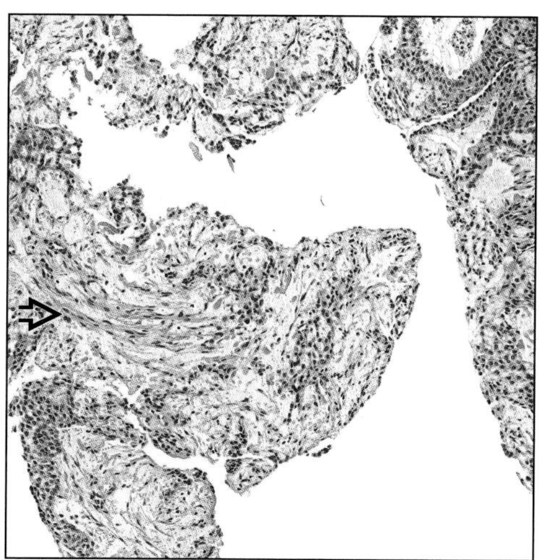

(Left) *Hematoxylin & eosin shows a rare case of symplastic glomus tumor. Note the enlarged tumor cells containing enlarged and irregular-shaped nuclei* ➩*.* ***(Right)*** *Hematoxylin & eosin shows a rare example of glomangiomyoma with myxoid stromal changes. Note the presence of elongated spindle-shaped tumor cells containing abundant eosinophilic cytoplasm and elongated nuclei* ➩*.*

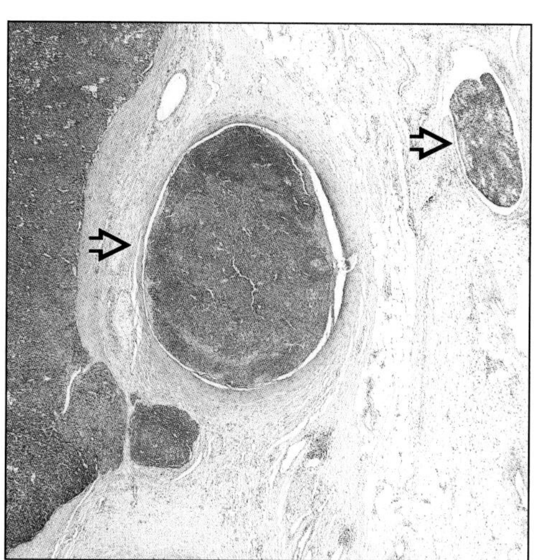

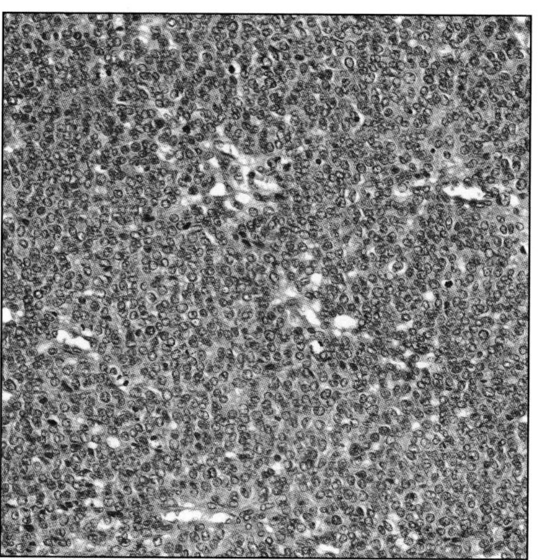

(Left) *Hematoxylin & eosin shows a very rare malignant glomus tumor with widespread vascular invasion* ➩*.* ***(Right)*** *Hematoxylin & eosin shows a high-power view of a malignant glomus tumor with prominent cytologic atypia and numerous mitoses.*

Skeletal Muscle Lesions

Inflammatory Lesions

Benign

Malignant

Examination of Rhabdomyosarcoma Specimens

FOCAL MYOSITIS

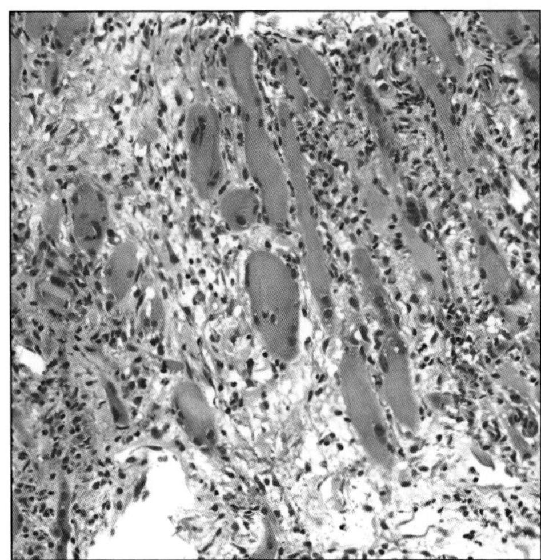

Hematoxylin & eosin shows early-stage focal myositis with interstitial edema and inflammation involving individual muscle fibers. This biopsy specimen is from the gastrocnemius muscle in a 34-year-old man.

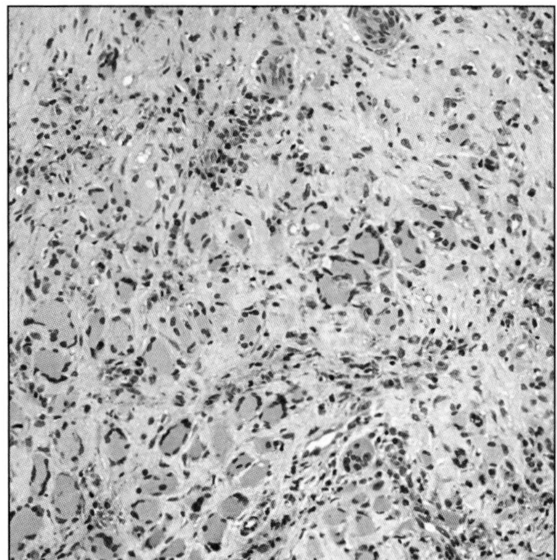

Hematoxylin & eosin shows muscle fibers separated by inflammation and fibrosis, with reduction in fiber population. The inflammatory cells are lymphocytes and plasma cells.

TERMINOLOGY

Definitions

- Benign inflammatory pseudotumor affecting single muscles

ETIOLOGY/PATHOGENESIS

Environmental Exposure

- Some cases related to trauma
- Similar changes can be seen in skeletal muscle adjacent to tumor

Idiopathic

- Not part of spectrum of sclerosing fibroinflammatory diseases
- Some cases related to denervation, but this could be secondary

CLINICAL ISSUES

Site

- Limbs, especially lower extremity
- Head and neck

Presentation

- Painful mass
- Weakness in affected part

Natural History

- Appears rapidly
- Self-limiting
- Eventual regression
- Very rare examples progress to polymyositis

Treatment

- None required
- Surgery is not indicated

Prognosis

- Residual fibrosis
- Does not usually recur

IMAGE FINDINGS

CT Findings

- Irregularity and enlargement of involved muscles
- Diffuse, poorly defined, fatty infiltration of muscle planes
- No discrete mass

MACROSCOPIC FEATURES

Size

- Between 2-10 cm in diameter

MICROSCOPIC PATHOLOGY

Histologic Features

- Inflammatory infiltrate
  - Mainly lymphocytes
- Necrosis of single muscle fibers
  - Vacuolation, fragmentation, or hyalinization
  - Phagocytosis of necrotic fibers
- Regeneration of muscle fibers
  - Basophilic cytoplasm
  - Large vesicular nuclei
- Focal denervation
  - Axonal swelling
  - Demyelination
  - Endoneurial fibrosis
- Variable fatty replacement of muscle
- Endomysial and perimysial fibrosis in older lesions
- No atypia, calcification, or ossification

Predominant Pattern/Injury Type

- Inflammatory

FOCAL MYOSITIS

Key Facts

Terminology
- Benign inflammatory pseudotumor affecting single muscle

Clinical Issues
- Children or adults
- Painful mass in limb or head and neck
- Surgery not usually required
- Can regress after incomplete excision
- Does not recur

Microscopic Pathology
- Necrosis and regeneration of muscle fibers
- Inflammation
- Variable fatty replacement of muscle and fibrosis

Top Differential Diagnoses
- Polymyositis
- Nodular fasciitis
- Proliferative myositis
- Rhabdomyosarcoma

Predominant Cell/Compartment Type
- Skeletal muscle

DIFFERENTIAL DIAGNOSIS

Polymyositis
- Involves multiple locations
- Systemic symptoms
  - Fever, malaise
  - Arthralgia, Raynaud phenomenon

Nodular Fasciitis
- Distinct mass: Circumscribed, not infiltrative
- Fascicles and storiform whorls of myofibroblasts
- Myxoid, cellular, and fibrous areas in same lesion

Proliferative Myositis
- "Checkerboard" pattern, less muscle fiber damage
- Ganglion-like fibroblasts
- Lacks fatty component

Fibromatosis
- Parallel-aligned myofibroblasts in collagen
- Infiltrates muscle with fiber damage and regeneration
- No fat, no inflammatory cells other than mast cells
- Nuclear immunoreactivity for β-catenin

Intramuscular Lipoma
- Fatty mass
- Lacks inflammation or fiber damage

Rhabdomyosarcoma
- Mass of spindled or round cells with mitoses, necrosis, rhabdomyoblastic differentiation

DIAGNOSTIC CHECKLIST

Clinically Relevant Pathologic Features
- Organ distribution

SELECTED REFERENCES

1. Georgalas C et al: Inflammatory focal myositis of the sternomastoid muscle: is there an absolute indication for biopsy? A case report and review of the literature. Eur Arch Otorhinolaryngol. 263(2):149-51, 2006
2. Dehner LP et al: Idiopathic fibrosclerotic disorders and other inflammatory pseudotumors. Semin Diagn Pathol. 15(2):161-73, 1998
3. Moskovic E et al: Benign mimics of soft tissue sarcomas. Clin Radiol. 46(4):248-52, 1992
4. Moskovic E et al: Focal myositis, a benign inflammatory pseudotumour: CT appearances. Br J Radiol. 64(762):489-93, 1991
5. Vercelli-Retta J et al: Focal myositis and its differential diagnosis. A case report and review of the literature. Ann Pathol. 8(1):54-6, 1988
6. Heffner RR Jr et al: Denervating changes in focal myositis, a benign inflammatory pseudotumor. Arch Pathol Lab Med. 104(5):261-4, 1980
7. Heffner RR Jr et al: Focal myositis. Cancer. 40(1):301-6, 1977

IMAGE GALLERY

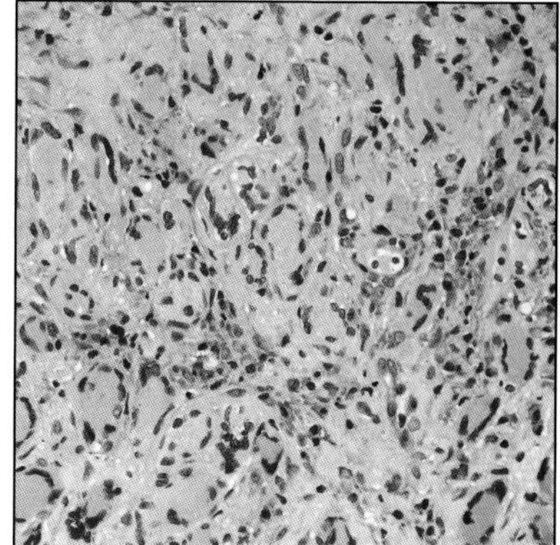

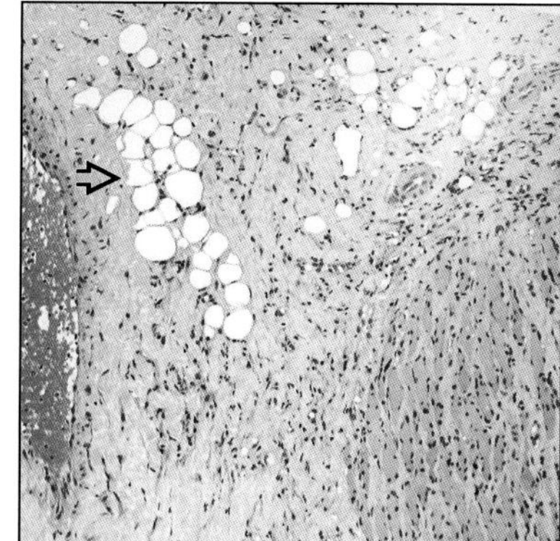

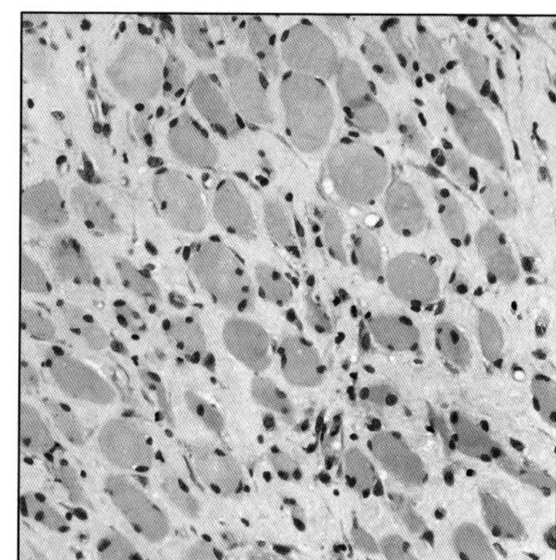

(Left) *Higher magnification demonstrates damage to and loss of muscle fibers with chronic inflammation and replacement by cellular fibrous tissue.* ***(Center)*** *Hematoxylin & eosin shows the later stage of focal myositis with less cellular fibrous tissue, inflammatory cells, and focal infiltration by adipose tissue ⊳.* ***(Right)*** *Hematoxylin & eosin shows an older lesion with interstitial fibrosis around muscle fibers, which appear to be of varying size.*

RHABDOMYOMA

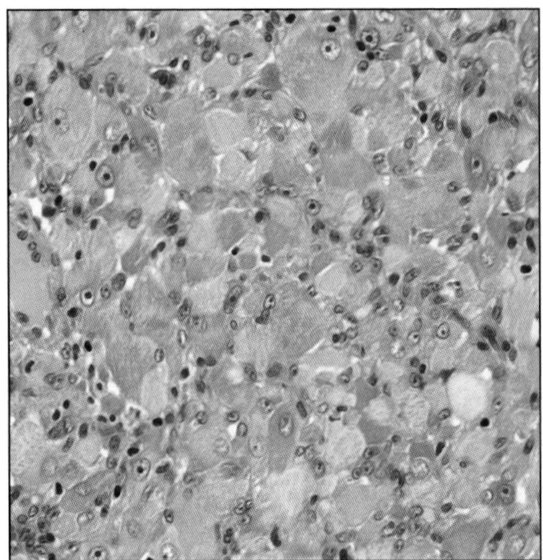

Hematoxylin & eosin shows adult rhabdomyoma composed of large polygonal cells with copious eosinophilic cytoplasm (varying in staining intensity) and small round nuclei with uniform nucleoli.

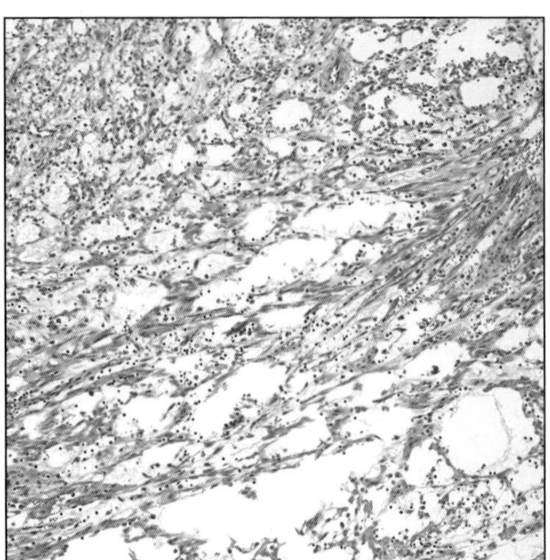

Hematoxylin & eosin shows fetal rhabdomyoma of myxoid (immature) type. Slender spindle cells form loosely organized fascicles in myxoid stroma. Note the absence of pleomorphism and necrosis.

TERMINOLOGY

Definitions

- Benign tumor with skeletal muscle differentiation
- Can arise in heart (cardiac rhabdomyoma) or extracardiac locations
- Extracardiac tumors can be of adult or fetal histologic type

ETIOLOGY/PATHOGENESIS

Developmental Anomaly

- No associations for most extracardiac lesions
- Cardiac rhabdomyoma can be associated with tuberous sclerosis
- Some fetal rhabdomyomas associated with nevoid basal cell syndrome
  - *PTCH* mutations
    - Inhibitory receptor in sonic hedgehog signaling pathway

CLINICAL ISSUES

Epidemiology

- Incidence
  - Rare
- Age
  - Adults; mean: 6th-7th decades
  - Fetal rhabdomyoma mostly in childhood; median: 4 years
    - About 1/2 in 1st year or congenital
    - Rare examples in adults up to 6th decade
- Gender
  - 75% in males
  - Genital rhabdomyoma mostly in middle-aged women
    - Rare cases in males

Site

- Most often in head and neck region, especially fetal rhabdomyoma
  - Larynx, oropharynx, mouth, neck
- Genital lesions mostly in vagina, occasionally vulva or cervix
- Rare examples in males in paratesticular region or epididymis

Presentation

- Incidental finding
- Painless mass
- Difficulty breathing

Treatment

- Surgical approaches
  - Simple complete excision

Prognosis

- Excellent after complete excision
- Can recur if incompletely excised

MACROSCOPIC FEATURES

General Features

- Usually solitary, can occasionally be multinodular or multicentric

Size

- Most lesions are small (< 10 cm diameter); median: ~ 3 cm

MICROSCOPIC PATHOLOGY

Key Microscopic Features

- Adult rhabdomyoma
  - Circumscribed
  - Large polygonal cells with abundant eosinophilic cytoplasm

RHABDOMYOMA

Key Facts

Terminology
- Benign tumor with skeletal muscle differentiation
- Extracardiac tumors can be of adult or fetal histologic type

Etiology/Pathogenesis
- Some fetal rhabdomyomas associated with nevoid basal cell syndrome

Clinical Issues
- Adults; mean: 6th-7th decades; 75% males
- Fetal rhabdomyoma mostly childhood
- Genital rhabdomyoma mostly in middle-aged women
- Most often in head and neck region, especially fetal rhabdomyoma
- Genital lesions mostly in vagina, occasionally vulva or cervix

Microscopic Pathology
- Adult rhabdomyoma
  - Circumscribed
  - Large polygonal cells with abundant eosinophilic cytoplasm
- Fetal rhabdomyoma
  - Immature (myxoid) type has long spindle cells in myxoid stroma
  - Intermediate (juvenile) type has spindled and round cells with variable skeletal muscle differentiation
- No atypia or necrosis; mitoses usually absent

Ancillary Tests
- Lesional cells are immunoreactive for desmin, myogenin, and MYOD1

  - Cross striations and crystalline cytoplasmic inclusions occasionally seen
  - Small bland nuclei, some with prominent nucleoli
  - Some vacuolated ("spider") cells
- Fetal rhabdomyoma, immature (myxoid)
  - Solitary circumscribed lesion, can be polypoid
  - Spindle cells with eosinophilic cytoplasm, occasional cross-striations
  - No atypia or necrosis, mitoses usually absent
  - Myxoid stroma
- Fetal rhabdomyoma, intermediate (juvenile)
  - More mature skeletal muscle: Strap cells, smooth muscle-like cells, and rounded rhabdomyoblasts
- Genital rhabdomyoma
  - Polypoid subepithelial lesion
  - Bundles of strap cells with eosinophilic cytoplasm, scattered rhabdomyoblast-like cells
  - Fibrous stroma

ANCILLARY TESTS

Immunohistochemistry
- Immunoreactive for desmin, myogenin, and MYOD1

Electron Microscopy
- Sarcomeric differentiation: Thick and thin filaments, Z-bands, glycogen deposits associated with filaments

DIFFERENTIAL DIAGNOSIS

DDx of Adult Rhabdomyoma
- Rhabdomyosarcoma
  - Mitoses, pleomorphism, necrosis
- Carcinoma
  - In situ changes in overlying epithelium
  - Mitoses, pleomorphism
  - Epithelial markers positive, desmin absent
- Melanoma
  - Mitoses, pleomorphism
  - S100 protein(+); HMB-45 and Melan-A in some cases
  - Desmin usually negative, myogenin(-)
- Hibernoma
  - Lobulated, cells multivacuolated, central nuclei
  - S100 protein(+), desmin(-)
- Granular cell tumor
  - Cytoplasm granular rather than fibrillary
  - S100 protein(+), CEA(+), and inhibin(+); desmin(-)

DDx of Fetal Rhabdomyoma
- Embryonal rhabdomyosarcoma
  - Mitoses, pleomorphism, necrosis

SELECTED REFERENCES

1. Walsh SN et al: Cutaneous fetal rhabdomyoma: a case report and historical review of the literature. Am J Surg Pathol. 32(3):485-91, 2008
2. Davies B et al: Paratesticular rhabdomyoma in a young adult: case study and review of the literature. J Pediatr Surg. 42(4):E5-7, 2007
3. Valdez TA et al: Recurrent fetal rhabdomyoma of the head and neck. Int J Pediatr Otorhinolaryngol. 70(6):1115-8, 2006
4. Watson J et al: Nevoid basal cell carcinoma syndrome and fetal rhabdomyoma: a case study. Ear Nose Throat J. 83(10):716-8, 2004
5. Wehner MS et al: Epididymal rhabdomyoma: report of a case, including histologic and immunohistochemical findings. Arch Pathol Lab Med. 124(10):1518-9, 2000
6. Johansen EC et al: Rhabdomyoma of the larynx: a review of the literature with a summary of previously described cases of rhabdomyoma of the larynx and a report of a new case. J Laryngol Otol. 109(2):147-53, 1995
7. Cleveland DB et al: Adult rhabdomyoma. A light microscopic, ultrastructural, virologic, and immunologic analysis. Oral Surg Oral Med Oral Pathol. 77(2):147-53, 1994
8. Kapadia SB et al: Fetal rhabdomyoma of the head and neck: a clinicopathologic and immunophenotypic study of 24 cases. Hum Pathol. 24(7):754-65, 1993
9. Metheetrairut C et al: Pharyngeal rhabdomyoma: a clinicopathological study. J Otolaryngol. 21(4):257-61, 1992
10. Gee DC et al: Benign vaginal rhabdomyoma. Pathology. 9(3):263-7, 1977

RHABDOMYOMA

Microscopic and Immunohistochemical Features

*(**Left**) Hematoxylin & eosin shows adult rhabdomyoma of larynx. The tumor is separated from the epithelium by a narrow clear zone and forms a solid sheet of cells. Laryngeal rhabdomyomas are most commonly of the adult type, although examples of fetal rhabdomyoma also occur. (**Right**) Hematoxylin & eosin shows adult rhabdomyoma. The large, rounded, uniform cells have abundant eosinophilic cytoplasm. They are arranged in confluent sheets with interspersed inflammatory cells.*

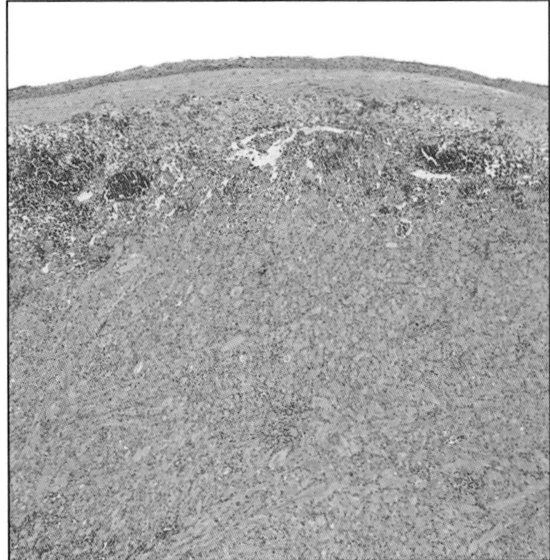

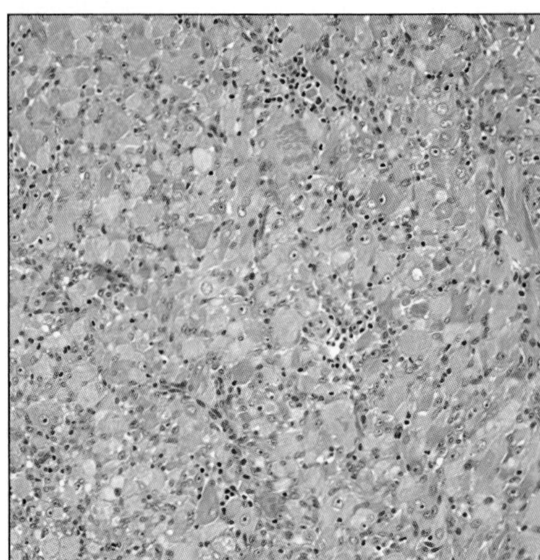

*(**Left**) Hematoxylin & eosin shows adult rhabdomyoma with vacuolated cells, some with strands of cytoplasm extending to cell's periphery ("spider" cell) ⇾. This appearance is mostly seen in cardiac rhabdomyoma. (**Right**) Hematoxylin & eosin shows adult rhabdomyoma with a large lesional cell containing crystalline rod-shaped intracytoplasmic inclusions ⇾. With electron microscopy, these are seen to be composed of hypertrophic Z-band structures.*

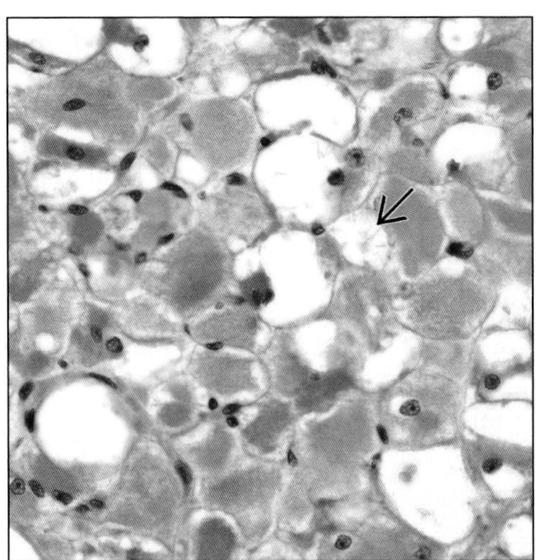

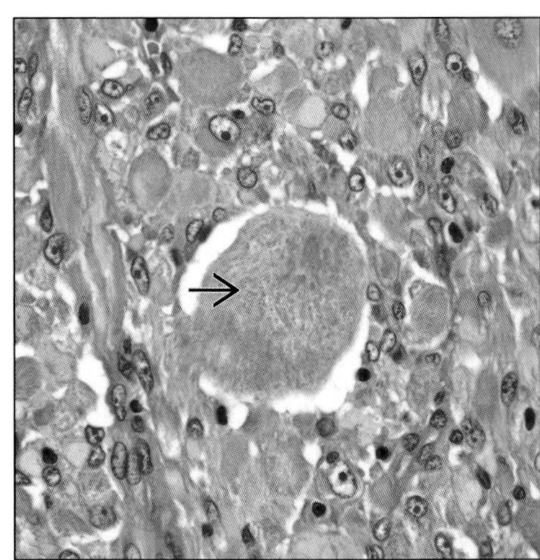

*(**Left**) Desmin stain shows adult rhabdomyoma with strong diffuse positivity throughout the lesion. This is a diagnostic finding in rhabdomyoma and can also highlight cross-striations. (**Right**) Positive myogenin shows adult rhabdomyoma with immunoreactivity in nuclei of many of the lesional cells. This is diagnostic of skeletal muscle differentiation. Cytoplasmic staining is sometimes seen but is nonspecific and should be disregarded. MYOD1 is also useful although less sensitive.*

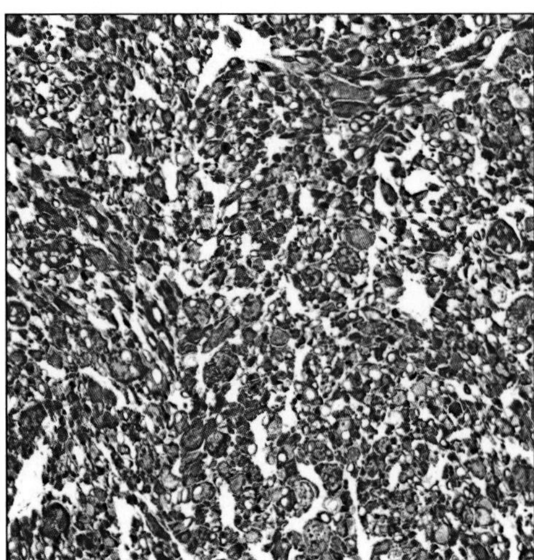

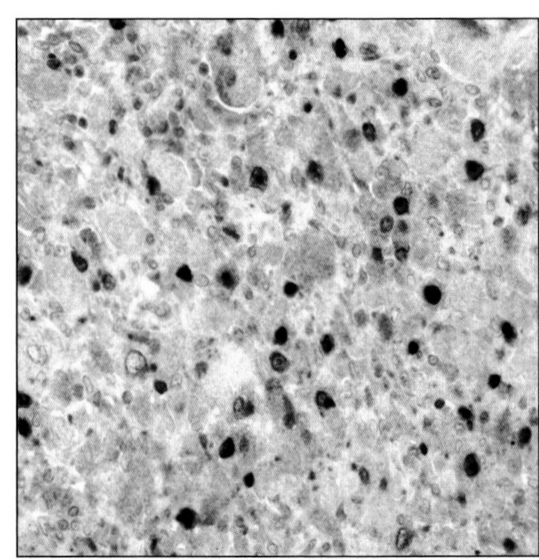

Microscopic and Immunohistochemical Features

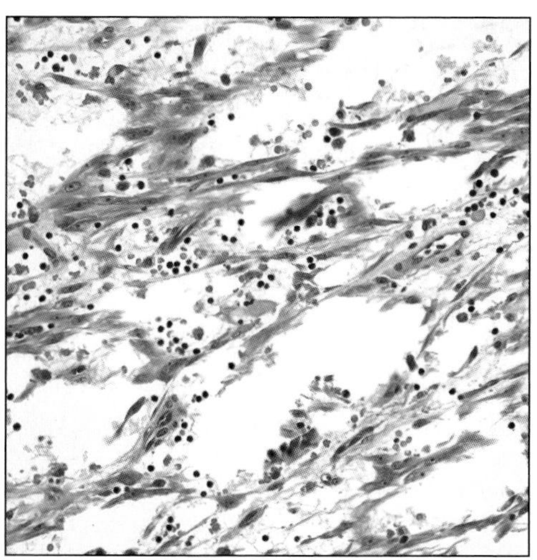

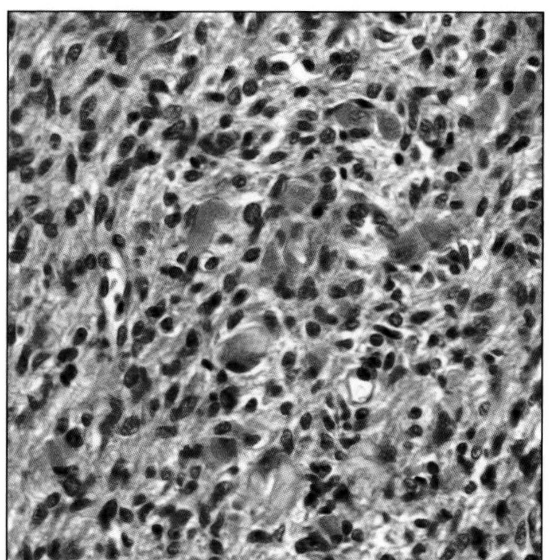

(Left) *Hematoxylin & eosin shows fetal rhabdomyoma of myxoid (immature) type, with spindle cells arranged in a vaguely fascicular pattern in myxoid stroma. Pleomorphism and necrosis are absent.* ***(Right)*** *H&E shows fetal rhabdomyoma (intermediate type). Cells show varying stages of skeletal muscle maturation, including rhabdomyoblast-like cells. As in other types of rhabdomyoma, mitotic figures, pleomorphism, and necrosis are absent, which helps to exclude embryonal rhabdomyosarcoma.*

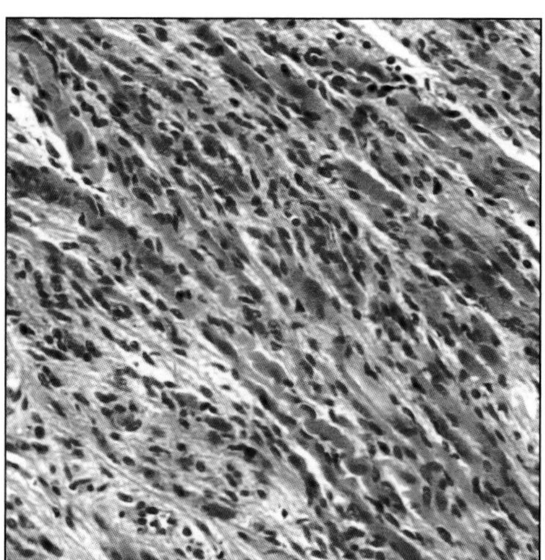

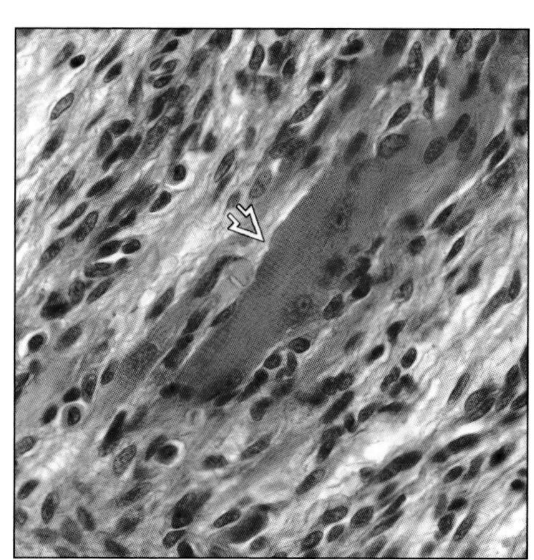

(Left) *Hematoxylin & eosin shows intermediate-type fetal rhabdomyoma manifesting relatively uniform spindle cells, with differentiation resembling late-stage embryonic skeletal muscle development. Nuclei are uniform, & no mitotic activity is seen.* ***(Right)*** *Hematoxylin & eosin shows intermediate-type fetal rhabdomyoma at higher magnification. Note variation in cell type. Typical cross-striations ➪, characteristic of skeletal muscle differentiation, are apparent in the cytoplasm.*

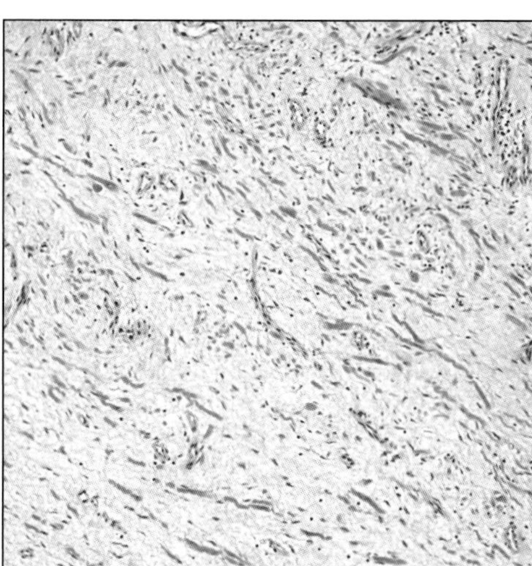

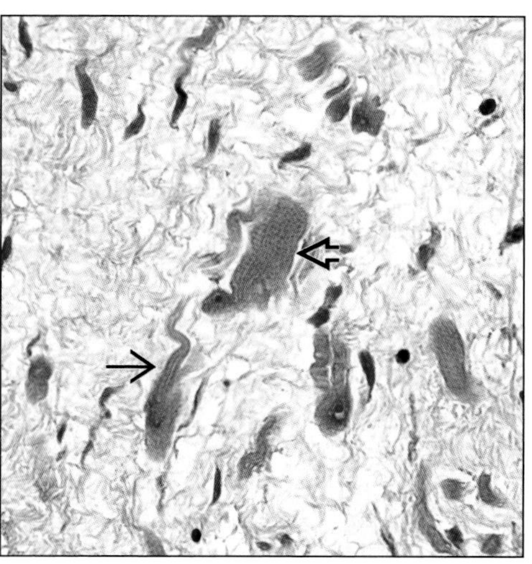

(Left) *Hematoxylin & eosin shows genital rhabdomyoma. This is a vaginal tumor with widely separated cords of cells with eosinophilic cytoplasm in a fibrous or myxoid stroma.* ***(Right)*** *Hematoxylin & eosin of the same case at higher magnification shows spindle cells that vary in shape and size. Some are slender and wavy; others are tadpole-like →, and occasional cells are strap-shaped ⇨, with cross-striations evident in this example. As with most rhabdomyomas, no mitoses are seen.*

EMBRYONAL RHABDOMYOSARCOMA

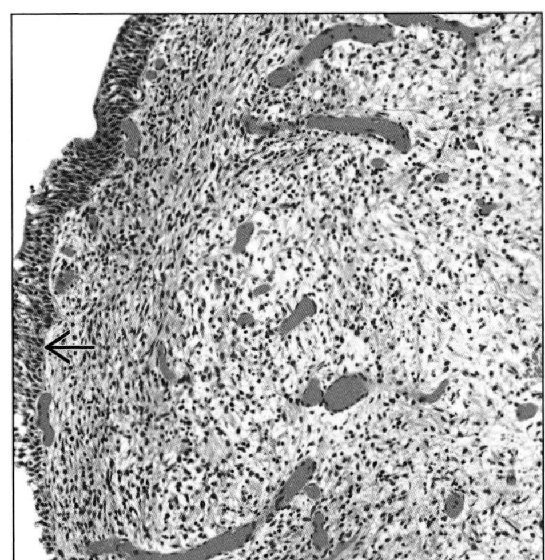

Embryonal rhabdomyosarcoma of the bladder is seen under urothelium ⇒. It is mostly of low cellularity and not easily identifiable at low power when the appearances can be mistaken for inflammation.

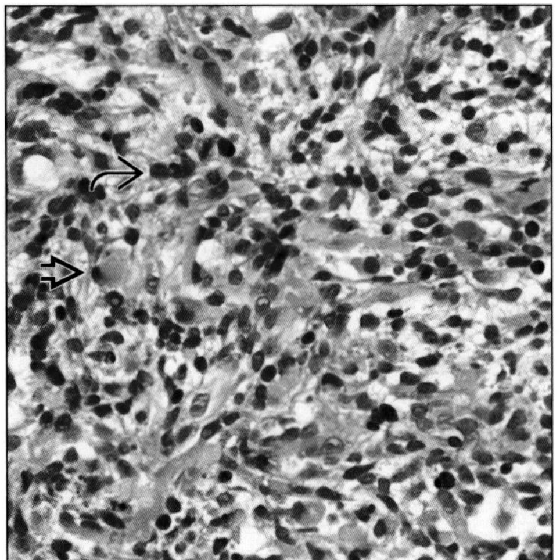

The tumor cells show a range of appearances. There are relatively undifferentiated ovoid cells ⇒ along with rhabdomyoblasts with prominent eosinophilic cytoplasm and eccentric nuclei ⇒.

TERMINOLOGY

Abbreviations

- Embryonal rhabdomyosarcoma (ERMS)

Definitions

- Malignant soft tissue tumor that shows variable differentiation toward embryonic skeletal muscle
- ERMS encompasses botryoid, spindle cell, and anaplastic variants

ETIOLOGY/PATHOGENESIS

Unknown

- Cell of origin still unknown
  - Possible candidate cells include muscle stem cells and multipotent mesenchymal stem cells
- Often occur in sites lacking skeletal muscle
  - e.g., bladder, prostate

CLINICAL ISSUES

Epidemiology

- Incidence
  - Rhabdomyosarcomas (RMS) are most frequent soft tissue sarcomas in children and young adults
  - ERMS is most common RMS subtype
    - 4.3 cases per 1,000,000 children/year in USA
    - Represent 60-70% of RMS
- Age
  - Children
  - ERMS generally affects younger population than alveolar RMS
  - Typically < 10 years of age
    - Majority in children < 5 years
    - Bimodal distribution with smaller peak in adolescence
    - Occasional cases congenital
  - Rarer in adults
    - Where pleomorphic subtype predominates
- Gender
  - Slight male preponderance
  - M:F = 1.4:1

Site

- Head and neck
  - Particularly orbital and parameningeal sites
- Genitourinary region
  - Bladder
  - Prostate
  - Paratesticular soft tissue
- Other sites
  - Retroperitoneum and pelvis
  - Biliary tract
- Much less frequent involvement of trunk and limbs than alveolar rhabdomyosarcoma (ARMS)
- Spindle cell RMS
  - Paratesticular region
- Botryoid RMS
  - Arise beneath mucosal epithelial surfaces
    - Bladder
    - Vagina
    - Extrahepatic bile ducts
    - More rarely, auditory canal or conjunctiva

Presentation

- Suddenly enlarging mass
  - Local symptoms pertaining to site of origin
    - e.g., deafness, proptosis (head and neck)
    - e.g., urinary retention (genitourinary sites)

Prognosis

- Main prognostic parameters are histologic type, disease stage, and site
- Favorable sites are head and neck (nonparameningeal), genitourinary (nonbladder, nonprostate), and bile duct
- Botryoid and spindle cell variants (excluding aggressive adult spindle cell variant) have better prognosis

EMBRYONAL RHABDOMYOSARCOMA

Key Facts

Terminology

- Malignant soft tissue tumor that shows variable differentiation toward skeletal muscle
- Encompasses botryoid, spindle cell, and anaplastic variants

Clinical Issues

- Most common rhabdomyosarcoma (RMS) subtype
  - Represents 60-70% of RMS
- Generally affects younger population than alveolar RMS
  - Majority in children < 5 years
- Head and neck
- Genitourinary region
- Other sites include retroperitoneum, pelvis, and biliary tract

Microscopic Pathology

- Loose fascicles and sheets
  - Cytology, pattern, and cellularity can vary
- Spindle, stellate, and ovoid cells
- Rhabdomyoblasts in variable numbers and stages of differentiation
- Botryoid RMS
  - Grows beneath epithelial surfaces
- Spindle cell RMS
  - Spindle cells with elongated nuclei
  - May exhibit cross-striations
- Anaplastic RMS
  - Atypical or bizarre tumor cells, present focally or more diffusely
- Complex karyotypes
- Associated with 11p15.5 loss of heterozygosity

- ERMS has significantly better prognosis than ARMS
- 5-year overall survival approximately 73%

MACROSCOPIC FEATURES

General Features

- Fleshy mass
- Margins usually infiltrative
- Tan to white
- Rubbery cut surface
- Hemorrhage
- Necrosis
- Cystic degeneration
- Botryoid RMS
  - Exophytic, polypoid tumor
  - More circumscribed margins
  - Small nodules adjacent to mucosal surface
  - Masses may fill lumen of hollow viscus
  - Gelatinous cut surface

MICROSCOPIC PATHOLOGY

Histologic Features

- Patterns variable
- Loose fascicles and sheets
- Variable cellularity
  - Can alternate between markedly cellular and looser myxoid zones
- Spindle, stellate, and ovoid cells
  - In varying stages of myogenic differentiation
  - Ovoid and elongated nuclei
    - Nuclei hyperchromatic or vesicular
- Rhabdomyoblasts
  - Cells with eccentric nuclei and variable amounts of eosinophilic cytoplasm
  - Cytoplasmic cross-striations may be visible
  - Variable numbers and stages of differentiation
  - Varying shapes
    - Strap cells
    - Tadpole cells
    - Spider cells
- Myxoid stroma
- Mitoses usually easily discernible
- Necrosis
- Tumor giant cells are rare, in contrast to alveolar RMS
- Botryoid RMS
  - Polypoid
  - Cambium layer
    - Tightly packed cellular layer of tumor cells closely abutting epithelial surface
  - Loose myxoid stroma
  - Can be of relatively low cellularity
    - May be missed or mistaken for chronic inflammation
- Spindle cell RMS
  - Spindle cells with elongated nuclei
  - May exhibit cross-striations
  - Tumors may have abundant collagenous stroma
- Anaplastic RMS
  - Pleomorphic cells
  - Atypical or bizarre tumor cells
  - Anaplasia may be present as scattered cells or as foci or large sheets of cells
    - Presence of anaplastic cells in aggregates or diffuse sheets associated with poorer survival
  - Atypical mitotic figures
  - Areas of more typical embryonal RMS present
- Mixed embryonal and alveolar RMS
  - Presence of focal alveolar pattern is associated with reduced survival
  - Tumors with any evidence of alveolar features are included among alveolar group
- Post chemotherapy
  - Cells appear more differentiated
    - Possibly residual, better differentiated component is left after selective destruction of undifferentiated tumor cells
  - Fibrosis
  - Myxoid change
  - Necrosis

EMBRYONAL RHABDOMYOSARCOMA

ANCILLARY TESTS

Immunohistochemistry

- Desmin diffusely positive
  - Can highlight cross striations
- Myogenin and MYOD1 variably positive
  - Myogenic nuclear regulatory proteins
  - Nuclear expression is specific for RMS
    - Cytoplasmic staining is nonspecific and should be disregarded
  - Myogenin is more sensitive
  - Expression of myogenin and MYOD1 usually less diffuse than in ARMS
- Variable positivity for smooth muscle actin
- H-caldesmon(-)

Cytogenetics

- Complex karyotypes
  - Often gains of chromosomes 2, 8, 12, and 13

Molecular Genetics

- Almost all RMS show regions of loss of heterozygosity (LOH)
- Most frequent LOH at chromosome 11
  - 80% of ERMS
  - Both long and short arms
  - LOH at 11p15.5 considered hallmark of ERMS
  - Genes located in 11p15.5 region include ones encoding proteins involved in growth regulation
    - These are subject to genomic imprinting (parent of origin-specific gene expression)
    - e.g., *IGF2* (paternally expressed) and *CDKN1C* (maternally expressed)
  - Genetic alterations can lead to disruption of imprinted gene expression and cause disease
- ERMS lack *PAX3/7-FOXO1* fusions

DIFFERENTIAL DIAGNOSIS

Rhabdomyoma

- Head and neck predilection, especially fetal type
- Fetal rhabdomyoma
  - No atypia or necrosis
  - Mitoses usually absent
- Adult rhabdomyoma
  - Middle-aged adults
  - Male preponderance
  - Circumscribed lesion
  - Large polygonal cells, abundant cytoplasm
- Genital rhabdomyoma
  - Mostly middle-aged women
  - Strap cells, no mitoses

Rhabdomyomatous Mesenchymal Hamartoma

- Congenital or infants
- Dermal and subcutaneous
  - Rarely in oral cavity
- Mature skeletal muscle, fat, nerves, and adnexa
- No mitoses, necrosis, or atypia

Alveolar Rhabdomyosarcoma (Including Solid Variant)

- Adolescents and young adults
- More common in extremities and trunk
- Small to medium-sized round cells
- Nests of tumor cells divided by fibrous septa
  - Resemble pulmonary alveoli
- Tumor giant cells frequent
- Myogenin expression more often diffuse and widespread than ERMS
- Characteristic translocations between *FOXO1* and *PAX3/7*

Adult-type Spindle Cell Rhabdomyosarcoma

- Most commonly in head and neck region of adults
- Predominantly spindled cells
  - Rhabdomyoblasts often scanty or rare

Pleomorphic Rhabdomyosarcoma

- Almost exclusively in adults
- Most common in extremities
- Malignant fibrous histiocytoma/pleomorphic sarcoma-like morphology
  - Marked cellular pleomorphism and cytological atypia

Sclerosing Rhabdomyosarcoma

- Abundant hyalinizing matrix
- Pronounced MYOD1 positivity
- Weaker expression of myogenin
- Desmin expression often dot-like and focal

Malignant Peripheral Nerve Sheath Tumor and Malignant Triton Tumor

- Occur mostly in adults
- May have neurofibromatosis type 1
- Focal S100 protein expression in neural component
- Desmin and myogenic marker expression is limited to rhabdomyosarcomatous portion of tumor

Leiomyosarcoma

- Adults; rare in children
- Intersecting fascicular architecture
- Cells may show typical cytological features of smooth muscle, e.g., blunt-ended nuclei
- Strong SMA and H-caldesmon expression
- Lack myogenin and MYOD1 expression

Low-Grade Myofibroblastic Sarcoma

- More common in adults
- Subset in children
  - Head and neck area
- Long fascicles of spindle tumor cells
- Ovoid nuclei with small nucleoli
- Only focal nuclear pleomorphism
- SMA(+), desmin occasionally positive
- Lack myogenin and MYOD1

Extrarenal Rhabdoid Tumor

- Infants and young children
- Larger cells
  - Eccentric nuclei
  - Hyaline inclusions

EMBRYONAL RHABDOMYOSARCOMA

Immunohistochemistry

Antibody	Reactivity	Staining Pattern	Comment
Desmin	Positive	Cytoplasmic	
CD56	Positive	Cytoplasmic	
Actin-sm	Positive	Cytoplasmic	Variable positivity
WT1	Positive	Cytoplasmic	Some tumors display cytoplasmic rather than nuclear staining
Myogenin	Positive	Nuclear	Cytoplasmic staining not diagnostic
MYOD1	Positive	Nuclear	Cytoplasmic staining not diagnostic
CD99	Positive	Cell membrane	Some tumors
AE1/AE3	Negative		
Caldesmon	Negative		
EMA	Negative		
CD34	Negative		
S100	Negative		

- Cytokeratin(+)
- Desmin(-)
- INI1(-)
  - Chromosome 22q deletions

Infantile Fibrosarcoma

- Most occur congenitally or in 1st 2 years of life
- Most common in extremities
- Intersecting fascicles of primitive ovoid and spindled tumor cells
- Often prominent hemangiopericytic vessels
- Does not express muscle markers
- Characteristic translocation with *NTRK3-ETV6* fusion

Wilms Tumor

- Occurs in kidney
- 90% occur before age 6 years
- Variable mixtures of blastemal, epithelial, and stromal elements
  - Stromal elements can show skeletal muscle differentiation but lack rhabdomyoblasts and malignant spindle or round cells
- Nuclear WT1 expression
- Keratin expression in epithelial components

Neuroblastoma

- Often in characteristic locations
  - Adrenal gland
  - Intraabdominal sympathetic chain
- Variable amount of neurofibrillary matrix
- Homer-Wright rosettes in some cases
- NB84(+)

Pleuropulmonary Blastoma

- Occur in peripheral lung and pleura
- Children in 1st decade of life
- Varying degrees of cyst formation
- Cystic foci lined by bland modified respiratory epithelium
- Small primitive cells with blastematous qualities
- Focal differentiation toward other mesenchymal lineages

Ectomesenchymoma

- Infants; very rare
- ERMS admixed with neural crest tumor
  - E.g., ganglioneuroma, neuroblastoma, malignant peripheral nerve sheath tumor

SELECTED REFERENCES

1. Williamson D et al: Fusion gene-negative alveolar rhabdomyosarcoma is clinically and molecularly indistinguishable from embryonal rhabdomyosarcoma. J Clin Oncol. 28(13):2151-8, 2010
2. Davicioni E et al: Molecular classification of rhabdomyosarcoma--genotypic and phenotypic determinants of diagnosis: a report from the Children's Oncology Group. Am J Pathol. 174(2):550-64, 2009
3. De Giovanni C et al: Molecular and cellular biology of rhabdomyosarcoma. Future Oncol. 5(9):1449-75, 2009
4. Ognjanovic S et al: Trends in childhood rhabdomyosarcoma incidence and survival in the United States, 1975-2005. Cancer. 115(18):4218-26, 2009
5. Smith AC et al: Growth regulation, imprinted genes, and chromosome 11p15.5. Pediatr Res. 61(5 Pt 2):43R-47R, 2007
6. Smith LM et al: Cytodifferentiation and clinical outcome after chemotherapy and radiation therapy for rhabdomyosarcoma (RMS). Med Pediatr Oncol. 38(6):398-404, 2002
7. Gordon T et al: Cytogenetic abnormalities in 42 rhabdomyosarcoma: a United Kingdom Cancer Cytogenetics Group Study. Med Pediatr Oncol. 36(2):259-67, 2001
8. Anderson J et al: Disruption of imprinted genes at chromosome region 11p15.5 in paediatric rhabdomyosarcoma. Neoplasia. 1(4):340-8, 1999
9. Anderson J et al: Genes, chromosomes, and rhabdomyosarcoma. Genes Chromosomes Cancer. 26(4):275-85, 1999
10. Visser M et al: Allelotype of pediatric rhabdomyosarcoma. Oncogene. 15(11):1309-14, 1997
11. Besnard-Guérin C et al: A common region of loss of heterozygosity in Wilms' tumor and embryonal rhabdomyosarcoma distal to the D11S988 locus on chromosome 11p15.5. Hum Genet. 97(2):163-70, 1996
12. d'Amore ES et al: Therapy associated differentiation in rhabdomyosarcomas. Mod Pathol. 7(1):69-75, 1994
13. Kodet R et al: Childhood rhabdomyosarcoma with anaplastic (pleomorphic) features. A report of the Intergroup Rhabdomyosarcoma Study. Am J Surg Pathol. 17(5):443-53, 1993

EMBRYONAL RHABDOMYOSARCOMA

Microscopic Features

(Left) The cells of this embryonal rhabdomyosarcoma have ovoid or spindled nuclei and moderate amounts of eosinophilic cytoplasm. Nuclear atypia is mild to moderate. The prominent myxoid stroma, a common feature, imparts a reticular or filigree pattern in this part of the tumor. ***(Right)*** The architecture of ERMS can be variable. Here, ovoid and spindle cells are present in a patternless distribution within prominent myxoid stroma. Nuclear atypia is generally minimal in this specimen.

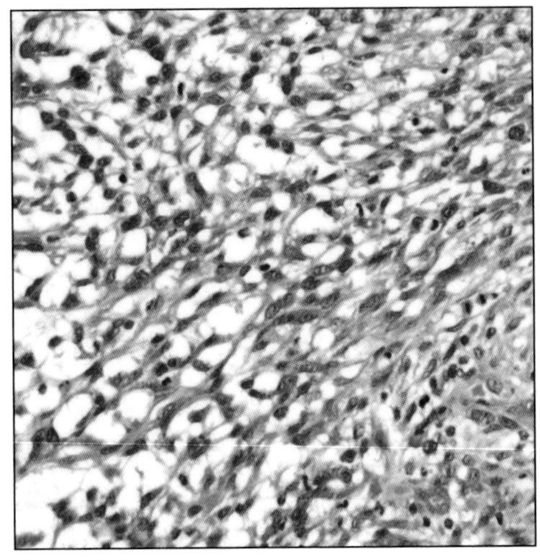

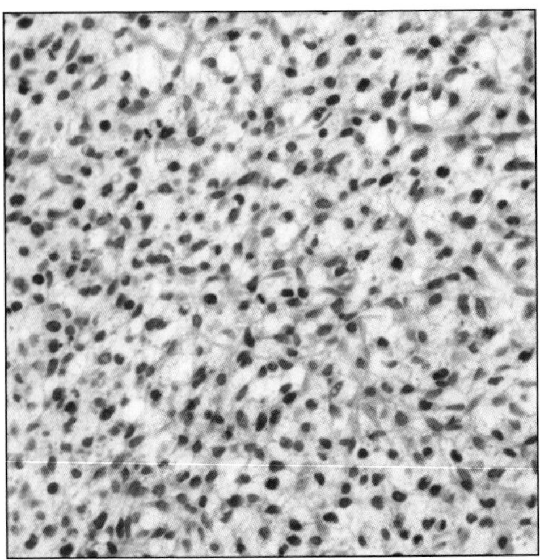

(Left) In this case of embryonal rhabdomyosarcoma, cells are in varying stages of myogenesis. Most of those in the bottom half of the field are undifferentiated. The cells at the top show skeletal muscle differentiation and are larger and polygonal with abundant eosinophilic cytoplasm. ***(Right)*** The appearances vary, and morphology can be heterogeneous between and within tumors. This case arose in the orbit of a 7-year-old girl. Cells vary from round to spindled, and there are vacuolated forms ⇨.

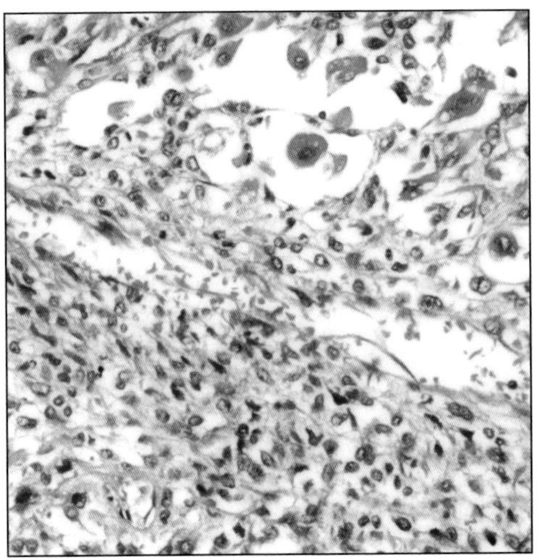

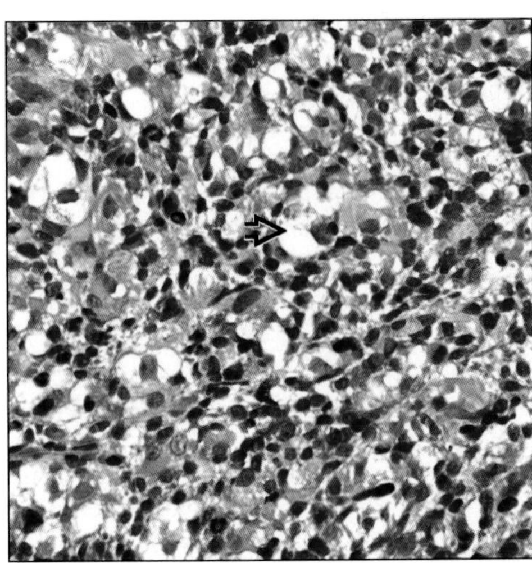

(Left) The tumor cells recapitulate embryonic skeletal muscle at varying stages of myogenesis. This example shows numerous atypical rhabdomyoblasts of varying shapes, some displaying prominent cross-striations ↷. ***(Right)*** This example of embryonal rhabdomyosarcoma of the prostate from an adolescent boy was excised post chemotherapy. There is extensive treatment-related maturation of tumor cells with remaining viable cells showing prominent rhabdomyoblastic differentiation ↷.

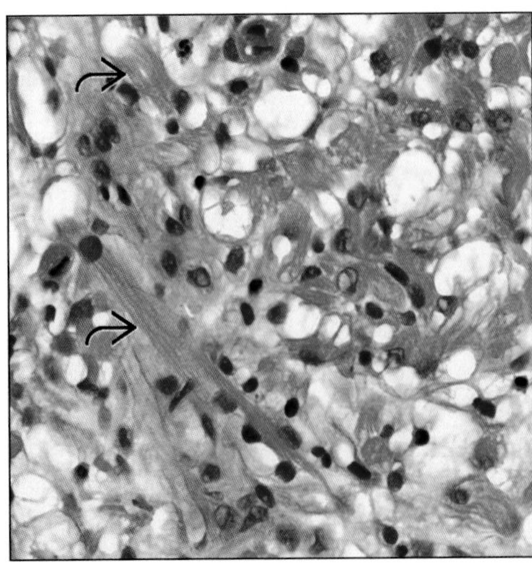

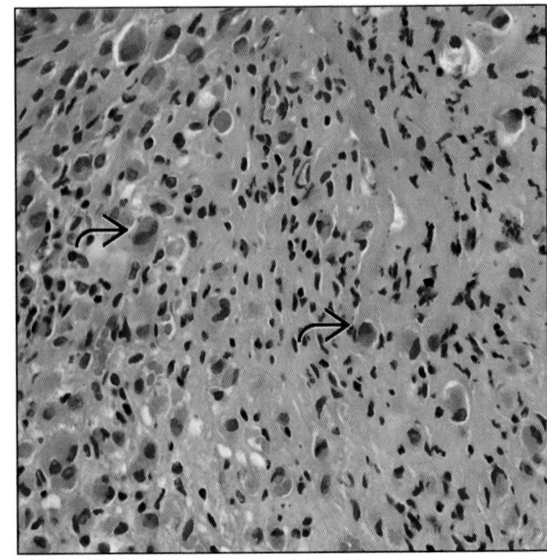

Microscopic and Immunohistochemical Features

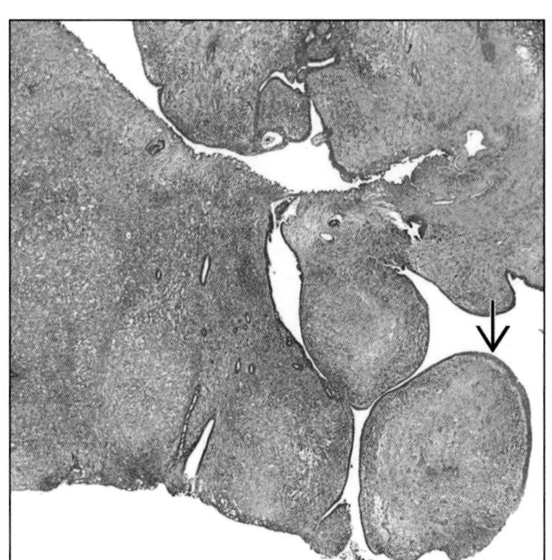

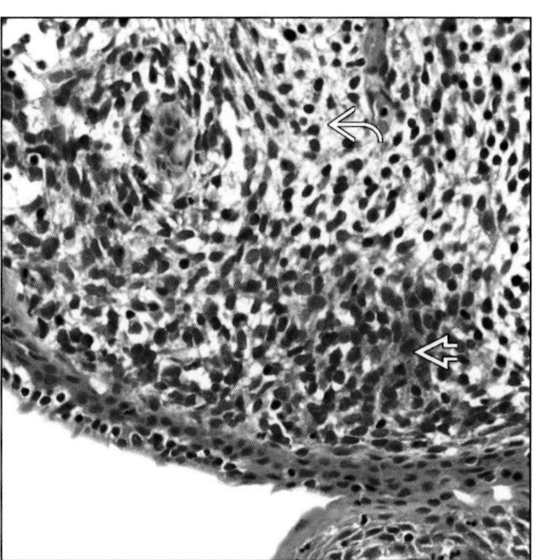

(Left) *This botryoid ERMS arose in the bladder of a 14-year-old boy. The polypoid architecture of the neoplasm is apparent. The tumor is covered by transitional epithelium ➔.* ***(Right)*** *Immediately beneath the urothelium in this botryoid variant of ERMS is a cambium layer ➔ representing a cellular condensation of tumor cells. This contrasts with the less cellular myxoid areas in deeper parts of the tumor ➔.*

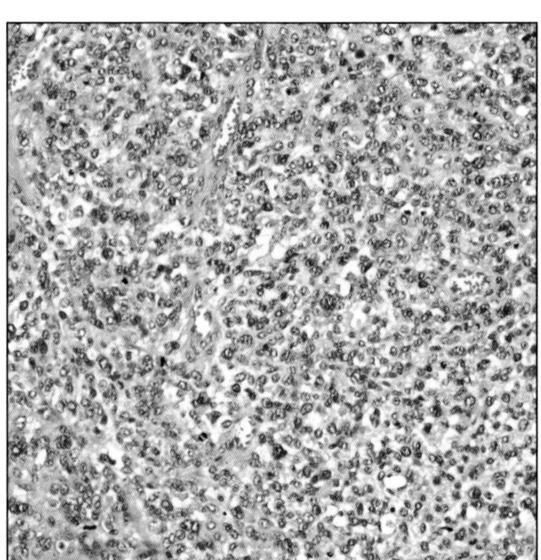

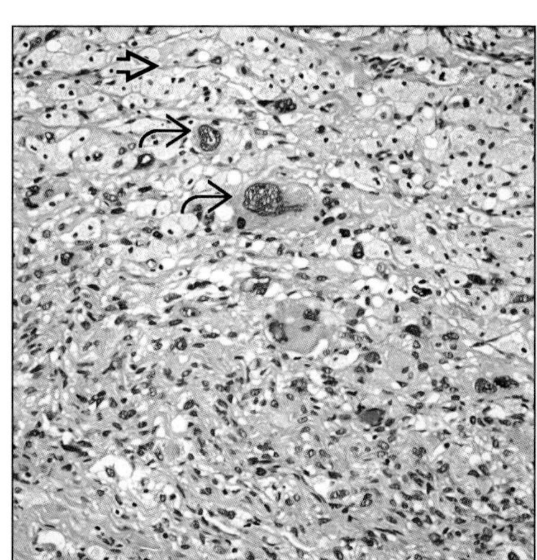

(Left) *This is an anaplastic variant of embryonal rhabdomyosarcoma that arose in the chest wall of a 4-year-old boy. The cells are relatively large and show nuclear atypia. The anaplasia can be widespread, as here, or more localized.* ***(Right)*** *This anaplastic variant of embryonal rhabdomyosarcoma shows only focal anaplasia. There are scattered, interspersed, large tumor cells with striking, bizarre nuclei ➔. Sheets of foamy histiocytes ➔ are present at the top of the field.*

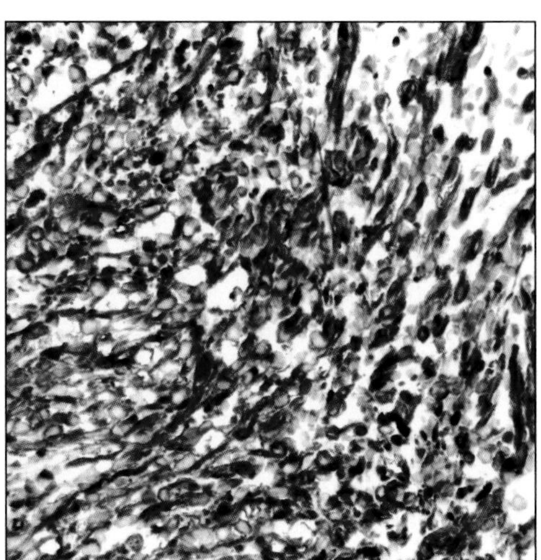

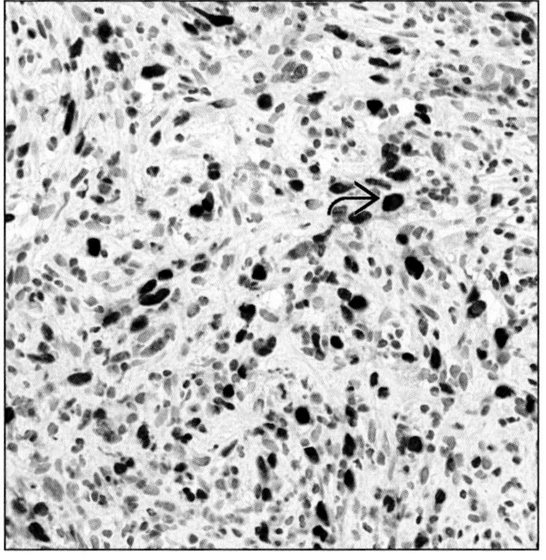

(Left) *Desmin expression is typically diffuse and strong in the cytoplasm of almost all the neoplastic cells. Sometimes cross-striations can be highlighted, especially in strap cells.* ***(Right)*** *Immunostaining for myogenin shows well-defined nuclear localization ➔. Only a proportion of tumor nuclei express this marker, and the staining is generally not as widespread as that seen in alveolar rhabdomyosarcoma. Cytoplasmic staining is nonspecific and seen in many tumor types.*

SPINDLE CELL RHABDOMYOSARCOMA

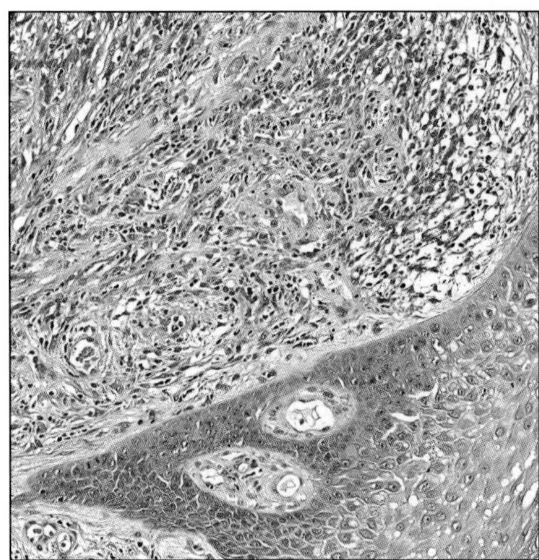

Low-power view of adult-type spindle cell rhabdomyosarcoma, in which laryngeal squamous epithelium overlies cellular tumor, shows sheets of mildly atypical cells within collagenous stroma.

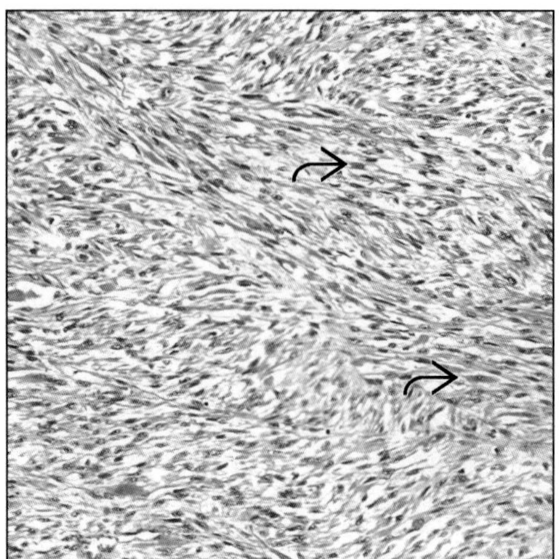

Juvenile-type spindle cell rhabdomyosarcoma shows sweeping fascicles of spindled cells present in a collagenous matrix. Focal rhabdomyoblastic differentiation is evident ➡, even at low power.

TERMINOLOGY

Abbreviations

- Spindle cell rhabdomyosarcoma (RMS)

Definitions

- Uncommon subtype of rhabdomyosarcoma occurring in both children and adults; composed of largely cellular proliferation of predominantly spindled cells
- Spindle cell RMS in children is considered variant of embryonal RMS
  - Carries good prognosis compared to other RMS subtypes
- Adult-type spindle cell rhabdomyosarcoma is aggressive neoplasm

CLINICAL ISSUES

Epidemiology

- Age
  - Children
    - < 10 years
  - Adults
    - All adult age groups (2nd-8th decades)
    - Median: Approximately 4th-5th decades
- Gender
  - Male preponderance

Site

- Children
  - Most tumors occur in paratesticular region
- Adults
  - Most common in head and neck region
    - > 50% of cases
  - Retroperitoneum
  - Extremities
  - Trunk
  - Vulva
  - Paratesticular region
- Tumors usually deeply located

Presentation

- Suddenly enlarging mass
  - Local symptoms pertaining to site of origin

Prognosis

- Behavior varies significantly between children and adults, suggesting distinct clinicopathologic subtypes
  - Good prognosis in children (when compared to other RMS subtypes)
  - Clinically aggressive in adults
    - Lymph node or blood-borne metastases

MACROSCOPIC FEATURES

General Features

- Firm white mass

Size

- Variable: 1-30 cm
  - Mean: 8 cm

MICROSCOPIC PATHOLOGY

Histologic Features

- Juvenile type
  - Fascicular architecture
    - Sweeping or loose fascicles
    - Some tumors have storiform pattern
  - Usually hypercellular
  - Spindle cells
    - Elongated nuclei
    - Nuclei can be vesicular or hyperchromatic
    - Nucleoli may be prominent
    - Pale or amphophilic fibrillary cytoplasm
    - Cross-striations
    - Prominent cell borders
  - Rhabdomyoblasts

SPINDLE CELL RHABDOMYOSARCOMA

Key Facts

Terminology

- Uncommon subtype of rhabdomyosarcoma occurring in both children and adults; composed of largely cellular proliferation of predominantly spindled cells

Clinical Issues

- Behavior appears to vary significantly between children and adults, suggesting these are distinct clinicopathological subtypes
  - Good prognosis in children (when compared to other RMS subtypes)
  - Clinically aggressive in adults
- Children
  - Most tumors occur in paratesticular region
- Adults
  - Most common in head and neck region (> 50% of cases)
  - Retroperitoneum
  - Extremities
  - Trunk
  - Vulva

Microscopic Pathology

- Long or intersecting fascicles
- Atypical spindle cells
- Elongated, vesicular nuclei
- Scattered spindle or polygonal rhabdomyoblasts

Ancillary Tests

- Desmin(+)
- Myogenin(+) and MYOD1(+)

    - Variable numbers
    - Spindle or polygonal
  - Variable amounts of intervening collagen
    - Collagen-rich type shows abundant collagen fibers, with cells in short fascicles or storiform arrangements
    - Collagen-poor type is more cellular
  - Mitotic figures usually prominent
  - Frankly pleomorphic areas absent
  - No round cell foci
- Adult type
  - Long or intersecting fascicles
  - Atypical spindle cells
    - Elongated, vesicular nuclei
    - Pale or amphophilic fibrillary cytoplasm
  - Scattered spindle or polygonal rhabdomyoblasts
    - Usually present in small numbers
    - Abundant eosinophilic cytoplasm
  - Prominent mitoses with atypical forms
  - Necrosis in some tumors
    - Sclerosing pseudovascular features in a smaller number
  - No round cell or pleomorphic areas

ANCILLARY TESTS

Immunohistochemistry

- Desmin(+)
  - Characteristically strong and diffuse cytoplasmic expression
- Myogenin(+) and MYOD1(+)
  - Myogenic nuclear regulatory proteins
  - Nuclear expression is specific for RMS
    - May be scanty or focal
  - Any cytoplasmic staining should be disregarded
- HHF-35 (muscle specific actin)(+)
- SMA frequently positive
- Occasional cases cytokeratin and epithelial membrane antigen positive
- H-caldesmon(-)
- S100 protein(-)

DIFFERENTIAL DIAGNOSIS

Rhabdomyoma

- Predilection for head and neck
  - Especially fetal type
- Fetal rhabdomyoma
  - No atypia or necrosis
  - Mitoses usually absent
- Adult rhabdomyoma
  - Male preponderance
  - Circumscribed lesion
  - Large polygonal cells, abundant cytoplasm
- Genital rhabdomyoma
  - Mostly middle-aged women
  - Mostly vagina; also vulva and cervix

Desmoid Fibromatosis

- Long fascicles of spindle and stellate myofibroblasts
- Vesicular nuclei
- Small pinpoint nucleoli
- Fibrillary cytoplasm
- No cytologic atypia
- Distinct vascular pattern
  - Small thick-walled and larger thin-walled vessels
- Prominent collagenous stroma
- Nuclear β-catenin expression
- Desmin usually negative
- Focal and weak expression of actins
- β-catenin or *APC* mutations

Nodular Fasciitis

- Short history
- Typically smaller lesions in younger adults
- Mostly superficially located
- Loose storiform rather than fascicular pattern
- Spindle and stellate cells
  - Bland nuclei
  - Fibrillary cytoplasm
- Background of lymphocytes and extravasated erythrocytes
- Sometimes osteoclast-like giant cells
- Lesional cells express actin or calponin

SPINDLE CELL RHABDOMYOSARCOMA

- Does not express desmin, myogenin, or MYOD1

Solitary Fibrous Tumor
- Typically circumscribed
- "Patternless" pattern of randomly orientated spindle to ovoid cells
- Cells usually lack atypia
- Hemangiopericytic vascular pattern
- Diffuse or focal collagenization
- Diffuse CD34 expression

Cellular Schwannoma
- Location
  - Retroperitoneum
  - Pelvis
  - Posterior mediastinum
- Background may contain lymphocytes and sheets of foamy histiocytes
- Strong and diffuse S100 protein expression
- Does not express desmin, myogenin, or MYOD1

Embryonal Rhabdomyosarcoma
- Usually pediatric
- Location
  - Head and neck
  - Genitourinary region
  - Retroperitoneum, pelvis, biliary tract
- Often show increased proliferation in subepithelial zone (cambium layer)
- Less fascicular organization than adult-type spindle cell rhabdomyosarcoma
- Myxoid stroma common
- Associated with 11p15.5 loss of heterozygosity (LOH)

Sclerosing Rhabdomyosarcoma
- Abundant hyalinizing matrix
- Pronounced MYOD1 expression
- Weaker myogenin expression
- Desmin expression often dot-like and focal

Pleomorphic Rhabdomyosarcoma
- Older adults
- Most common in extremities
- Pleomorphic sarcoma/malignant fibrous histiocytoma-like morphology
- Diffuse cellular pleomorphism
- Marked nuclear atypia, often with bizarre or giant tumor cells

Pleomorphic Undifferentiated Sarcoma
- Often storiform pattern
- Markedly atypical cells
  - Spindle and polygonal
  - Bizarre and multinucleate forms
- Abundant and atypical mitoses
- No discernible microscopic differentiation
- No specific differentiation by immunohistochemistry

Malignant Peripheral Nerve Sheath Tumor and Malignant Triton Tumor
- Usually occur in older adults
- May have history of neurofibromatosis type 1
- May be seen to arise from large nerves
- Can have areas of alternating high and lower cellularity
  - "Marbled" pattern
- Buckled or bullet-shaped nuclei
- Amphophilic to basophilic cytoplasm
- Can show extensive necrosis with perivascular preservation
- S100 protein expression in small numbers of nuclei
- Desmin and myogenin/MYOD1 expression focal in Triton tumor
  - Limited to rhabdomyosarcomatous portion of tumor

Synovial Sarcoma
- Majority in young adults
- Tumor may have focal biphasic morphology with epithelial-like elements
- Cellular fascicles of spindle cells
  - Uniform nuclei that lack atypia
  - Prominent nuclear overlapping
  - Cells have elongated nuclei with darkly amphophilic to basophilic cytoplasm
- Focal expression of cytokeratin and EMA
- Nuclear expression of TLE1
- Often express CD99 and Bcl-2
- Typically lack actin and desmin
- No expression of myogenic markers
- Nested reticulin pattern
- Characteristic translocation: t(X;18)
  - Fusion genes *SYT-SSX1* and *SSX2*

Leiomyosarcoma
- Tumors may show focal features characteristic of smooth muscle
  - e.g., blunt-ended nuclei
  - Paranuclear vacuolation
- Intersecting fascicular architecture
- Strong SMA and H-caldesmon expression
- Lack myogenin and MYOD1 expression

Low-Grade Myofibroblastic Sarcoma
- Long fascicles of spindle tumor cells
- Elongated nuclei with vesicular chromatin
- Small nucleoli
- Can express actin
- Less likely to express desmin
- Lack myogenin and MYOD1 expression

Fibrosarcoma
- Diagnosis of exclusion
- Herringbone fascicular pattern
- Negative for desmin and myogenic markers

Dermatofibrosarcoma Protuberans
- Young adults
- Location
  - Trunk
  - Proximal and distal extremities
  - Head and neck
  - Dermis and subcutis
- Storiform pattern
- Uniform spindle cells
  - Lack atypia
- Diffuse CD34 expression
- Negative for desmin and myogenic markers

SPINDLE CELL RHABDOMYOSARCOMA

Immunohistochemistry

Antibody	Reactivity	Staining Pattern	Comment
Desmin	Positive	Cytoplasmic	
Myogenin	Positive	Nuclear	
MYOD1	Positive	Nuclear	
Actin-sm	Positive	Cytoplasmic	Positive in less than 1/4 of tumors
CD56	Positive	Cytoplasmic	
CD34	Positive	Cytoplasmic	Positive in small number of tumors
WT1	Positive	Cytoplasmic	Some tumors display cytoplasmic rather than nuclear staining
EMA	Positive	Cell membrane	Positive in rare tumors
Caldesmon	Negative		
S100	Negative		
GFAP	Negative		
TLE1	Negative		
β-catenin	Negative		
AE1/AE3	Equivocal	Cytoplasmic	Positive in rare tumors

Spindle Cell/Sarcomatoid Carcinoma

- Older adults
- History of carcinoma at primary site
- Epithelium may show dysplastic or in situ changes
- Eosinophilic spindle cells lacking organized fascicular pattern
- At least focal expression of cytokeratins or EMA
- Desmin(-)
- Myogenin(-) and MYOD1(-)

Spindle Cell Melanoma

- Junctional activity may be present in epidermis
- Cells often have nested architecture
- Diffuse S100 protein expression
- HMB-45 and Melan-A expression
- Desmin usually negative
- Myogenin and MYOD1 negative
- Melanin pigment may be identifiable
- Nested reticulin pattern

Dedifferentiated Liposarcoma

- Usually in retroperitoneum and intraabdominal cavity
- May have adjacent well-differentiated liposarcomatous component
  - Atypical adipocytes, spindle cells, and sometimes lipoblasts
- Nuclear expression of CDK4 and MDM2
- No expression of myogenic markers
- MDM2 amplification

Gastrointestinal Stromal Tumor

- Uniform spindle or epithelioid cells
- Lobulated or short fascicular architecture
- Nuclear pleomorphism rare
- Cytoplasmic vacuoles common
- Typically CD117(+) and CD34(+)
- Subset express H-caldesmon
- Scant actin and desmin
- Myogenin(-) and MYOD1(-)
- *KIT* or *PDGFRA* mutations

Inflammatory Myofibroblastic Tumor

- Often in children and young adults
- May present with B symptoms
  - e.g., fever, anemia, weight loss
- Spindled to stellate myofibroblastic cells
- Variable fibrosis and keloid-like collagen
- Lymphoplasmacytic inflammatory cell infiltrate
- *ALK* gene rearrangements in approximately 50% of cases
  - ALK(+) by immunohistochemistry

SELECTED REFERENCES

1. Stock N et al: Adult-type rhabdomyosarcoma: analysis of 57 cases with clinicopathologic description, identification of 3 morphologic patterns and prognosis. Am J Surg Pathol. 33(12):1850-9, 2009
2. Mentzel T et al: Spindle cell rhabdomyosarcoma in adults: clinicopathological and immunohistochemical analysis of seven new cases. Virchows Arch. 449(5):554-60, 2006
3. Parham DM et al: Rhabdomyosarcomas in adults and children: an update. Arch Pathol Lab Med. 130(10):1454-65, 2006
4. Nascimento AF et al: Spindle cell rhabdomyosarcoma in adults. Am J Surg Pathol. 29(8):1106-13, 2005
5. Rubin BP et al: Spindle cell rhabdomyosarcoma (so-called) in adults: report of two cases with emphasis on differential diagnosis. Am J Surg Pathol. 22(4):459-64, 1998
6. Leuschner I: Spindle cell rhabdomyosarcoma: histologic variant of embryonal rhabdomyosarcoma with association to favorable prognosis. Curr Top Pathol. 89:261-72, 1995
7. d'Amore ES et al: Therapy associated differentiation in rhabdomyosarcomas. Mod Pathol. 7(1):69-75, 1994
8. Edel G et al: Spindle cell (leiomyomatous) rhabdomyosarcoma, a rare variant of embryonal rhabdomyosarcoma. Pathol Res Pract. 189(1):102-7; discussion 107-10, 1993
9. Leuschner I et al: Spindle cell variants of embryonal rhabdomyosarcoma in the paratesticular region. A report of the Intergroup Rhabdomyosarcoma Study. Am J Surg Pathol. 17(3):221-30, 1993
10. Miettinen M: Rhabdomyosarcoma in patients older than 40 years of age. Cancer. 62(9):2060-5, 1988

SPINDLE CELL RHABDOMYOSARCOMA

Microscopic Features

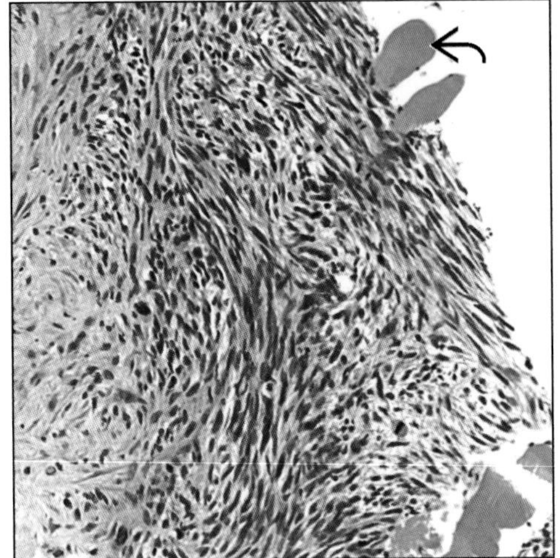

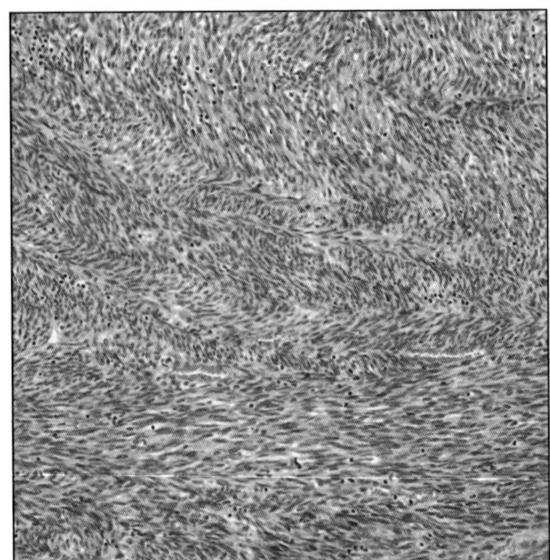

(Left) *Needle core biopsy of adult-type spindle cell rhabdomyosarcoma shows cellular tumor composed of cells with elongated hyperchromatic nuclei, arranged in long sweeping fascicles, adjacent to skeletal muscle fibers* ↪*.* ***(Right)*** *Adult-type spindle cell rhabdomyosarcoma shows a prominent "herringbone" fascicular architecture, reminiscent of fibrosarcoma. This tumor was strongly desmin and myogenin positive, but this morphology can overlap with many spindle cell sarcomas.*

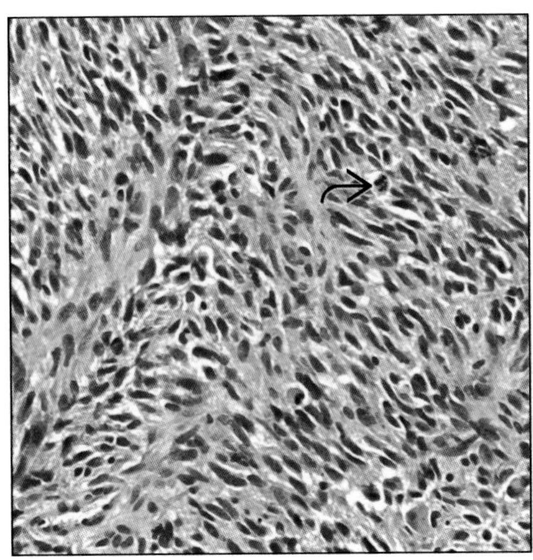

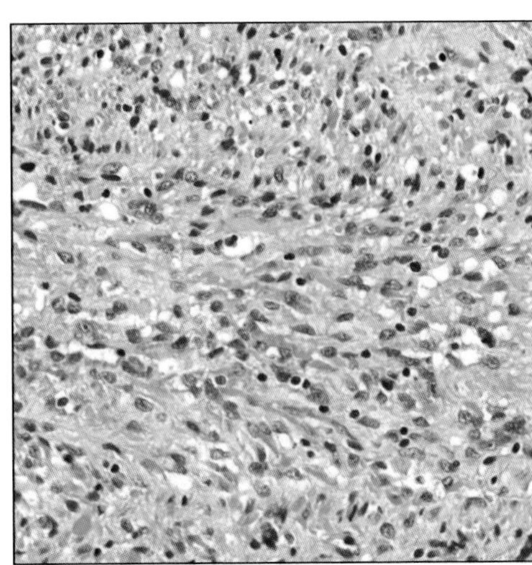

(Left) *This tumor is markedly cellular, composed of tightly packed fascicles of spindle cells with hyperchromatic, mildly to moderately atypical nuclei. A mitotic figure is prominent* ↪*.* ***(Right)*** *The tumor is composed of fascicles of cells with elongated nuclei and small amounts of fibrillary cytoplasm. The morphology can be fairly nonspecific, resembling different types of spindle cell sarcoma. Here, the fascicular pattern and eosinophilic cytoplasm are reminiscent of leiomyosarcoma.*

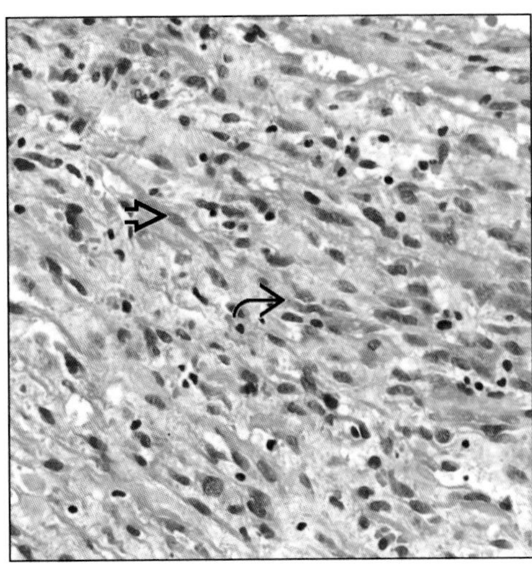

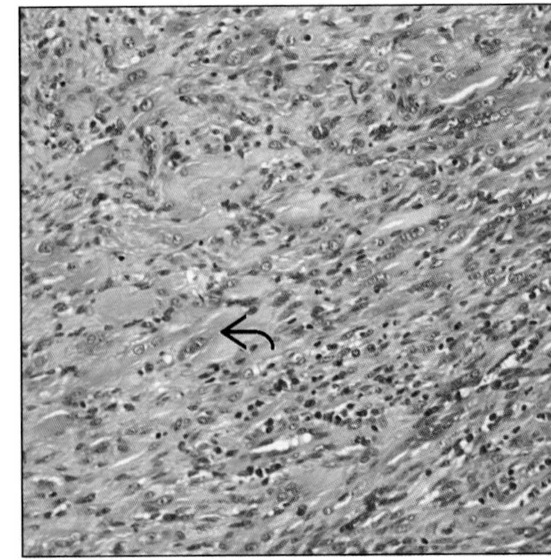

(Left) *Higher power view of adult-type spindle cell rhabdomyosarcoma shows that the spindle cells can appear heterogeneous within a given tumor. The nuclei in this case display a mixture of forms, varying from ovoid* ⇨ *to wavy or buckled* ↪*.* ***(Right)*** *Juvenile-type spindle cell rhabdomyosarcoma shows atypical spindle cells and prominent rhabdomyoblasts* ↪ *against a collagenous background. There is also a moderate mixed chronic inflammatory cell infiltrate in this example.*

Microscopic Features and Ancillary Techniques

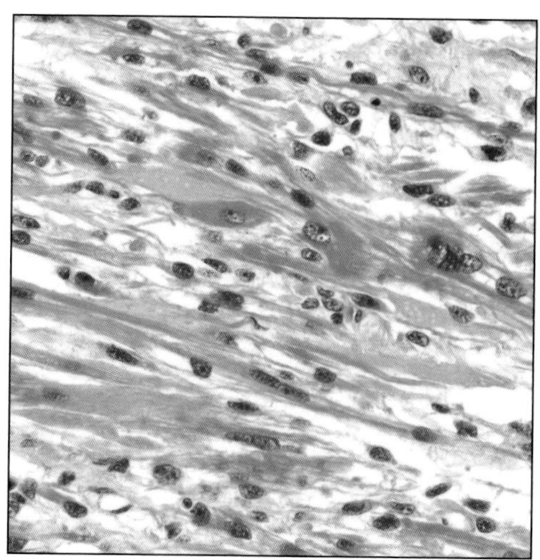

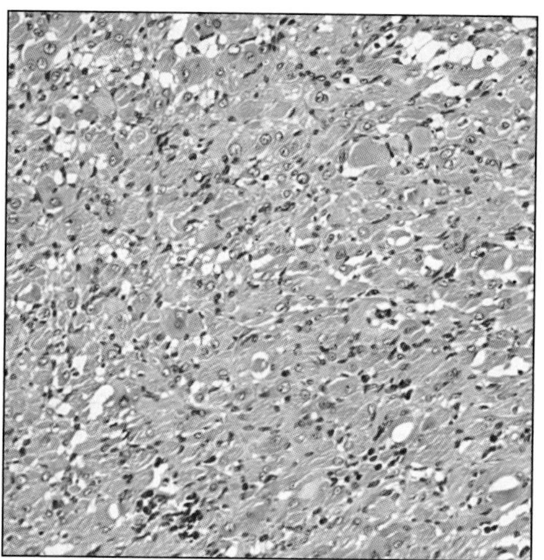

(Left) *Juvenile-type spindle cell rhabdomyosarcoma shows prominent rhabdomyoblastic differentiation. These cells vary in shape and size, and they have pleomorphic nuclei with coarse chromatin and abundant eosinophilic cytoplasm.* ***(Right)*** *Adult-type spindle cell rhabdomyosarcoma shows a high degree of differentiation. This case from a middle-aged woman shows fascicular areas, as well as large areas in which the tumor cells display rhabdomyoblastic features.*

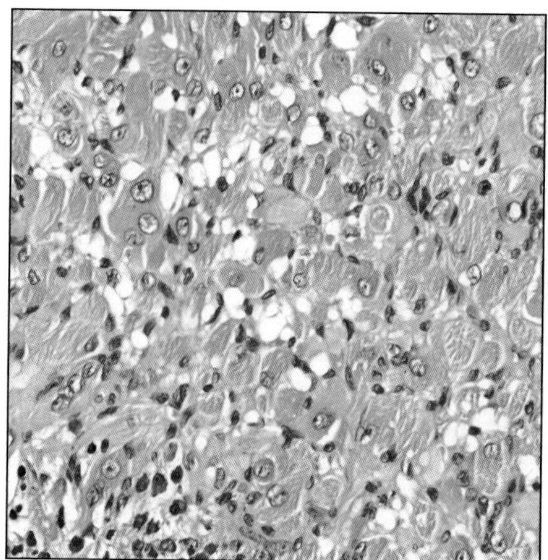

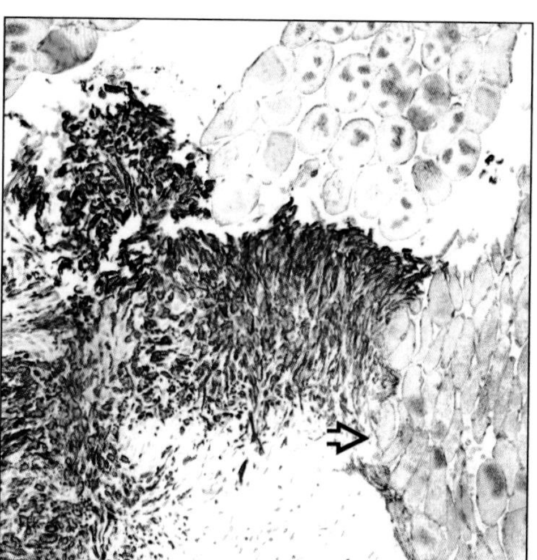

(Left) *Adult-type spindle cell rhabdomyosarcoma at high power shows marked rhabdomyoblastic differentiation. Spindled areas are not present in this field, which is composed entirely of sheets of polygonal rhabdomyoblasts with abundant eosinophilic cytoplasm.* ***(Right)*** *Spindle cell rhabdomyosarcoma displays widespread, strong cytoplasmic desmin expression, contrasting with the weaker positivity seen in the fascicles of normal skeletal muscle ⮚ that the tumor is seen to infiltrate.*

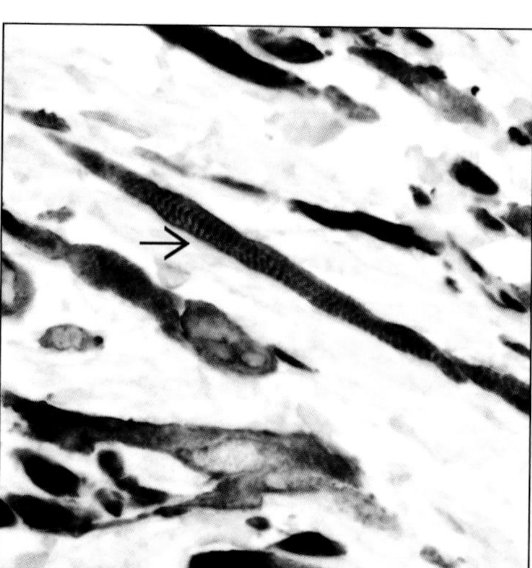

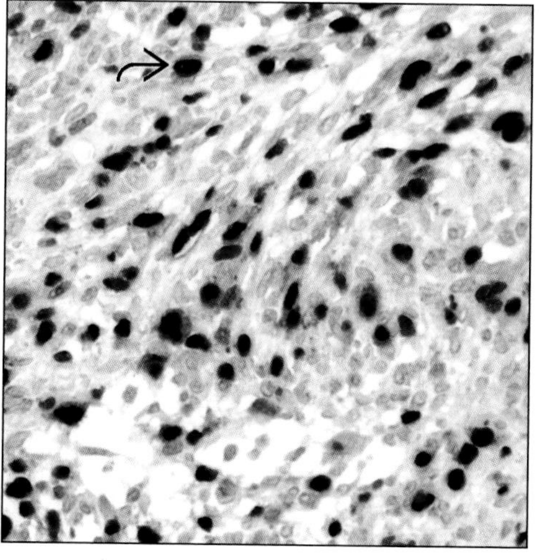

(Left) *Desmin expression in spindle cell rhabdomyosarcoma is typically strong. Atypical elongated rhabdomyoblasts show intense cytoplasmic staining, and cross-striations → are easily visible here.* ***(Right)*** *Many tumor nuclei show strong expression of myogenin ↷. In general, expression is patchy within some nuclei, rather than diffuse and widespread. Cytoplasmic staining of myogenin or MYOD1 should be disregarded.*

ALVEOLAR RHABDOMYOSARCOMA

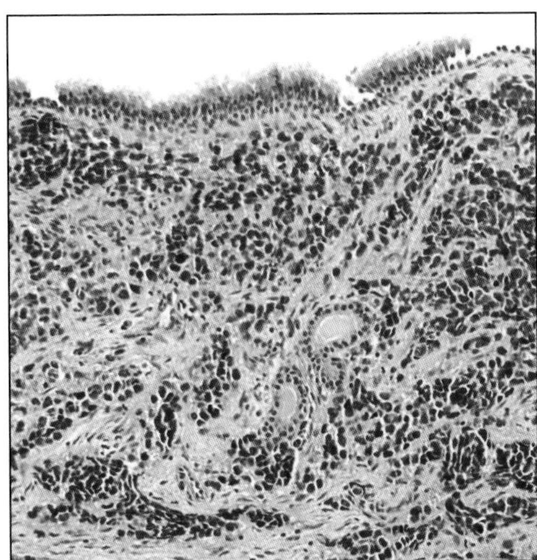

Alveolar rhabdomyosarcoma from the postnasal space is seen. Respiratory-type epithelium overlies fibrous tissue extensively infiltrated by sheets and nests of monomorphic round cell tumor.

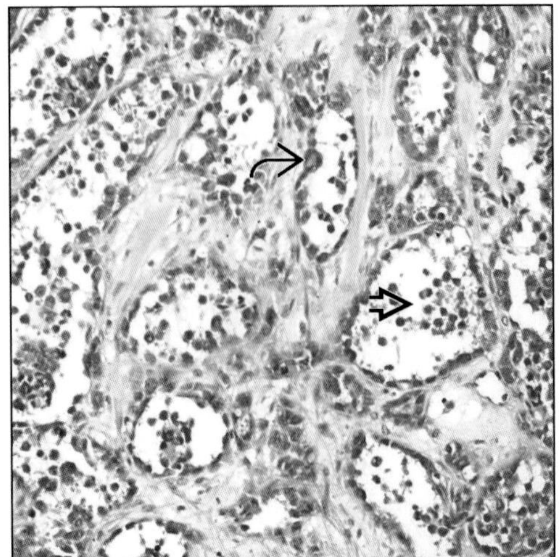

The tumor is composed of round cells with peripheral cellular preservation [curved arrow], but central discohesion and necrosis [open arrow] as well, somewhat resembling the appearance of pulmonary alveoli.

TERMINOLOGY

Abbreviations

- Alveolar rhabdomyosarcoma (ARMS)

Definitions

- High-grade malignant round cell neoplasm characterized by recurrent chromosomal translocations showing variable differentiation toward skeletal muscle

ETIOLOGY/PATHOGENESIS

Genetic Events

- Characteristic balanced translocations
  - Produce chimeric fusion proteins
    - These act as aberrant transcription factors
    - Regulate expression of specific target genes
- Target cell/cell of origin still unknown

CLINICAL ISSUES

Epidemiology

- Incidence
  - Accounts for approximately 30% of rhabdomyosarcomas
  - 2nd most common rhabdomyosarcoma
    - After embryonal RMS
- Age
  - Predominantly adolescents and young adults
  - Peak incidence: 10-25 years
  - Rare in adults > 45 years
  - Congenital in small number of cases
- Gender
  - M = F
- Ethnicity
  - No ethnic or geographical predilections

Site

- Deep soft tissue
- Most common in extremities
- Head and neck
- Trunk
- Pelvis
- Retroperitoneum
- Perineum

Presentation

- Suddenly enlarging mass
  - Local symptoms pertaining to site of origin
    - Proptosis or cranial nerve deficits (head and neck)
    - Paresthesia or paresis (paraspinal areas of trunk)
  - Can present with widespread dissemination
    - Lymphadenopathy or marrow infiltration
    - Rarely may present without obvious primary
- Deep mass

Treatment

- Multimodality approach
- RMS is sensitive to both chemotherapy and radiation therapy
- Systemic chemotherapy
  - In conjunction with surgery, radiation therapy, or both modalities
- Radiotherapy
  - To maximize local control
- Surgery
  - Excise primary tumor when possible, without major functional or cosmetic defects
  - Complete resection often difficult or impossible

Prognosis

- Tend to be high-stage lesions at presentation
- Prognosis of ARMS significantly worse than for embryonal RMS
  - Accurate distinction between RMS subtypes is therefore crucial for appropriate management

ALVEOLAR RHABDOMYOSARCOMA

Key Facts

Terminology

- High-grade malignant round cell neoplasm showing partial differentiation towards skeletal muscle

Etiology/Pathogenesis

- Characteristic *PAX-FOXO1* balanced translocations in most
  - t(2;13)(q35;q14) (majority)
  - t(1;13)(p36;q14) in 10-15%

Clinical Issues

- Accounts for approximately 30% of rhabdomyosarcomas
- Predominantly adolescents and young adults
- Sites: Deep soft tissue of extremities, head and neck, and trunk
- Can present with widespread dissemination
- Tend to be high-stage lesions at presentation

Microscopic Pathology

- Poorly differentiated round cells
- Hyperchromatic nuclei, scanty cytoplasm
- Alveolar-like spaces formed by central loss of cohesion
- Multinucleate giant tumor cells in some cases
- Fibrovascular septa separate nests
- Rhabdomyoblasts can be present
- Solid variant
  - Lacks alveolar architecture
- Mixed alveolar and embryonal rhabdomyosarcoma
  - Behavior and classification as ARMS
- Desmin usually strong and diffuse
- Myogenin and MYOD1 are sensitive and specific for skeletal muscle differentiation

MACROSCOPIC FEATURES

General Features

- Fleshy mass
- Infiltrative margins
- Tan cut surface
- Hemorrhage
- Necrosis

MICROSCOPIC PATHOLOGY

Histologic Features

- Poorly differentiated round cells
  - Medium size
  - Hyperchromatic nuclei
  - Scanty cytoplasm
- Sheets and nests
  - Alveolar-like spaces formed by central loss of cohesion
  - Central cells poorly preserved and necrotic
  - Many appear freely floating
- Fibrovascular septa separate nests
- Rare clear cell appearance
  - Due to cytoplasmic glycogen
  - Vacuolated cells may be confused with lipoblasts
- Rhabdomyoblasts can be present
  - Less frequent than in embryonal RMS
- Multinucleate giant tumor cells in some cases
  - Peripheral or wreath-like nuclei
- Very rarely atypical cells, similar to anaplastic variant of embryonal RMS
- Tumor metastases often show alveolar pattern
- **Solid variant**
  - Sheets and islands of densely packed tumor cells
    - Cytomorphology of typical ARMS
    - Lack alveolar pattern
  - Occasional small nests may be present
  - Foci of more typical ARMS may be seen on careful examination
  - More likely to be fusion(-) for *PAX3/7-FOXO1*
  - Very rarely atypical cells, similar to anaplastic variant of embryonal RMS
- **Mixed alveolar and embryonal rhabdomyosarcoma**
  - Foci of embryonal morphology
    - Spindle cells or myxoid stroma
  - Behavior and classification as ARMS

Lymph Nodes

- Nodal metastases may be presenting factor

Predominant Pattern/Injury Type

- Neoplastic

Predominant Cell/Compartment Type

- Mesenchymal, muscle, skeletal

Genetics

- Characteristic balanced recurrent translocations
  - Majority of cases (80-85%) of ARMS
  - Translocations are not feature of other RMS subtypes
- Fusion of 2 genes, each encoding transcription factors
  - *FOXO1*
    - Chromosome 13
    - Member of forkhead transcription factor family
  - *PAX3* or *PAX7*
    - Chromosomes 2 and 1, respectively
    - Members of paired box family of transcription factors
    - High degree of homology
- Fusion genes lead to formation of chimeric proteins that act as aberrant transcription factors
- Mechanism by which fusion protein causes sarcomagenesis is not established
  - Hypothesized to generate novel transcription program in unknown target cell
  - Downstream targets are tumorigenic and myogenic factors that are still being characterized
- t(2;13)(q35;q14)
  - Majority (60%) of ARMS cases
- t(1;13)(p36;q14)
  - 10-15% of ARMS cases
- Patients with metastatic disease

 - Those with *PAX7-FOXO1* appear to have better prognosis than those with *PAX3-FOXO1*
- Patients with locoregional ARMS
  - Fusion status not associated with outcome differences
- Approximately 20% of cases of ARMS are fusion(-) by routine RT-PCR
  - Fusion(-) ARMS are genetically heterogeneous
    - May have alternate fusions with other genes
    - Some may be truly fusion(-)
- Histological appearances of ARMS do not predict presence or type of gene fusion
- However, solid architecture with absence of typical alveolar pattern predicts high possibility of fusion negativity

ANCILLARY TESTS

Immunohistochemistry

- Desmin
  - Intermediate filament protein
  - Positive in both skeletal and smooth muscle neoplasms
  - Diffuse positivity typical in ARMS
- Myogenin and MYOD1
  - Myogenic nuclear regulatory proteins
  - Members of MYOD family of transcription factors
    - Initiate myogenesis in vivo and in vitro
    - Act on other myogenic genes, inducing transcription and those causing skeletal muscle differentiation
  - Most sensitive and specific markers for skeletal muscle differentiation
  - Nuclear expression is specific for RMS
    - Cytoplasmic staining is nonspecific and should be disregarded
- Variable positivity for actins, including actin-sm
- Variable expression of neuroendocrine markers
  - CD56 often positive

In Situ Hybridization

- Detects *FOXO1* breakpoint

PCR

- Detects *FOXO1-PAX3/PAX7* fusion transcripts

DIFFERENTIAL DIAGNOSIS

Embryonal Rhabdomyosarcoma

- Often in urogenital or head and neck sites
- Younger age group
- Unusual in limbs
- Sheets and fascicles of cells
- Lack alveolar architecture
- At least focal spindle cell areas
- Stroma often myxoid
- Rhabdomyoblastic differentiation usually more pronounced
- Desmin and myogenin expression less diffuse
- Absence of *PAX-FOXO1* fusions

Sclerosing Rhabdomyosarcoma

- Abundant hyalinizing matrix
- Pronounced MYOD1 positivity
- Weaker expression of myogenin
- Desmin expression often dot-like and focal
- Lack *PAX-FOXO1* fusions

Pleomorphic Rhabdomyosarcoma

- Almost exclusively in adults
- Most common in extremities
- Solid sheets of cells
- Lack alveolar architecture
- Marked cytological atypia
- Desmin and myogenin expression often more focal
- Lack *PAX-FOXO1* fusions

Lymphoma/Leukemia

- Often systemic involvement by disease
- Usually sites of lymphadenopathy
- Architecture dispersed and sheet-like rather than nested
- Expression of broad spectrum of hematolymphoid markers
- Desmin(-)
- Lack *PAX-FOXO1* fusions

Ewing Sarcoma/PNET

- Cells more uniform and smaller than in ARMS
- Can show rosette formation
- Many cases CD99(+)
- May rarely express desmin
  - Negative for myogenic markers
- Expression of neural/neuroectodermal markers in PNET
- Usually CD56(-)
- Absence of intercellular reticulin
- Characteristic translocations involving *EWSR1*

Desmoplastic Small Round Cell Tumor

- Intraabdominal location
- Prominent stromal fibroplasia
- Polyphenotypic immunoprofile
  - Myogenin(-) and MYOD1(-)
- Characteristic translocation t(11;22(p13;q12)
  - *EWSR1-WT1* fusion gene

Neuroblastoma

- Younger age group
- Often in characteristic locations
  - Adrenal gland
  - Intraabdominal sympathetic chain
- Variable amount of neurofibrillary matrix
- Homer-Wright rosettes in some cases
- NB84(+)
- *MYCN* amplification in subset of tumors
- Absence of *PAX-FOXO1* fusions

Small Cell/Neuroendocrine Carcinoma

- Older adults
- Primary tumor site may be identifiable
- Cells show crush artifact
- Nuclear molding
- CK-PAN expression
  - Cytoplasmic dot positivity in Merkel cell carcinoma

Immunohistochemistry

Antibody	Reactivity	Staining Pattern	Comment
Desmin	Positive	Cytoplasmic	Diffuse and strong
Myogenin	Positive	Nuclear	Strong
MYOD1	Positive	Nuclear	Strong
CD56	Positive	Cytoplasmic	Helps distinguish from Ewing sarcoma
Actin-sm	Positive	Cytoplasmic	Occasional focal positivity
Synaptophysin	Positive	Cytoplasmic	Occasional focal expression
AE1/AE3	Positive		Occasional focal expression
CD99	Positive		May occasionally show positivity
Chromogranin-A	Positive	Cytoplasmic	Occasional focal expression
Caldesmon	Negative		
S100	Negative		
CD34	Negative		
CD45	Negative		
FLI-1	Negative		Helps distinguish from Ewing sarcoma
Neuroblastoma	Negative		Helps distinguish from neuroblastoma
WT1	Negative		Helps distinguish from desmoplastic small round cell tumor

- Desmin(-)
- Absence of *PAX-FOXO1* fusions

Olfactory Neuroblastoma

- Specific sites
  - Sinonasal tract
- Wider age range
  - Bimodal peak
    - 2nd and 6th decades
- Lobulated architecture
- Variable amount of neurofibrillary material
- Positive for neuroendocrine markers
- S100(+) sustentacular-like cells
- Desmin(-)
- Absence of *PAX-FOXO1* fusions

Extrarenal Rhabdoid Tumor

- Often infants and very young children
- Larger cells
  - Eccentric nuclei
  - Abundant cytoplasm
  - Hyaline inclusions
- Keratin(+)
- Desmin(-)
- SNF5(-)
  - Chromosome 22q deletions
- Absence of *PAX-FOXO1* fusions

GRADING

High Grade

- ARMS are classified as high-grade sarcomas

SELECTED REFERENCES

1. Parham DM et al: Correlation between histology and PAX/FKHR fusion status in alveolar rhabdomyosarcoma: a report from the Children's Oncology Group. Am J Surg Pathol. 31(6):895-901, 2007
2. Walterhouse D et al: Optimal management strategies for rhabdomyosarcoma in children. Paediatr Drugs. 9(6):391-400, 2007
3. Tomescu O et al: Inducible short-term and stable long-term cell culture systems reveal that the PAX3-FKHR fusion oncoprotein regulates CXCR4, PAX3, and PAX7 expression. Lab Invest. 84(8):1060-70, 2004
4. Barr FG et al: Genetic heterogeneity in the alveolar rhabdomyosarcoma subset without typical gene fusions. Cancer Res. 62(16):4704-10, 2002
5. Sorensen PH et al: PAX3-FKHR and PAX7-FKHR gene fusions are prognostic indicators in alveolar rhabdomyosarcoma: a report from the children's oncology group. J Clin Oncol. 20(11):2672-9, 2002
6. Dias P et al: Strong immunostaining for myogenin in rhabdomyosarcoma is significantly associated with tumors of the alveolar subclass. Am J Pathol. 156(2):399-408, 2000
7. Bennicelli JL et al: PAX3 and PAX7 exhibit conserved cis-acting transcription repression domains and utilize a common gain of function mechanism in alveolar rhabdomyosarcoma. Oncogene. 18(30):4348-56, 1999
8. Merlino G et al: Rhabdomyosarcoma--working out the pathways. Oncogene. 18(38):5340-8, 1999
9. Kelly KM et al: Common and variant gene fusions predict distinct clinical phenotypes in rhabdomyosarcoma. J Clin Oncol. 15(5):1831-6, 1997
10. Bennicelli JL et al: Mechanism for transcriptional gain of function resulting from chromosomal translocation in alveolar rhabdomyosarcoma. Proc Natl Acad Sci U S A. 93(11):5455-9, 1996
11. Boman F et al: Clear cell rhabdomyosarcoma. Pediatr Pathol Lab Med. 16(6):951-9, 1996
12. Etcubanas E et al: Rhabdomyosarcoma, presenting as disseminated malignancy from an unknown primary site: a retrospective study of ten pediatric cases. Med Pediatr Oncol. 17(1):39-44, 1989
13. Douglass EC et al: A specific chromosomal abnormality in rhabdomyosarcoma. Cytogenet Cell Genet. 45(3-4):148-55, 1987
14. Turc-Carel C et al: Consistent chromosomal translocation in alveolar rhabdomyosarcoma. Cancer Genet Cytogenet. 19(3-4):361-2, 1986
15. Enzinger FM et al: Alveolar rhabdomyosarcoma. An analysis of 110 cases. Cancer. 24(1):18-31, 1969

ALVEOLAR RHABDOMYOSARCOMA

Microscopic Features

*(**Left**) The alveolar architecture is often inapparent, as in this case. It may not be present in all sections or might not be represented due to sampling error. Here, the tumor is present as solid sheets of monomorphic cells with scant cytoplasm, intersected by thick fibrous septa. (**Right**) At a slightly higher power, the cells show a degree of nuclear atypia and are of intermediate size with round to ovoid nuclei displaying an uneven chromatin pattern.*

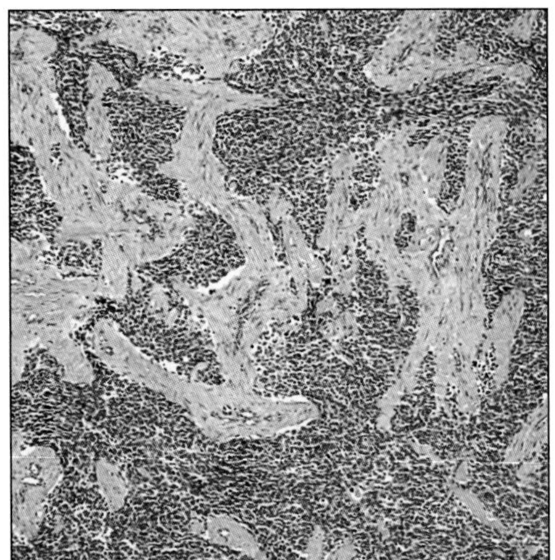

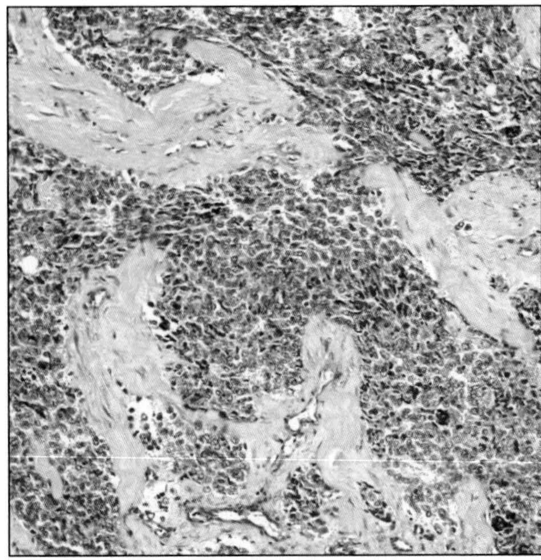

*(**Left**) Note the metastatic tumor deposit within a lymph node. Even at sites of metastasis, the distinct alveolar architecture is frequently maintained. The peripheral cells are well preserved, but central cells are discohesive ⇨, poorly preserved, and often necrotic. (**Right**) Formation of tumor giant cells is a frequent feature. Several giant cells of varying sizes are present in this field, with nuclei in peripherally distributed, wreath-like formations →.*

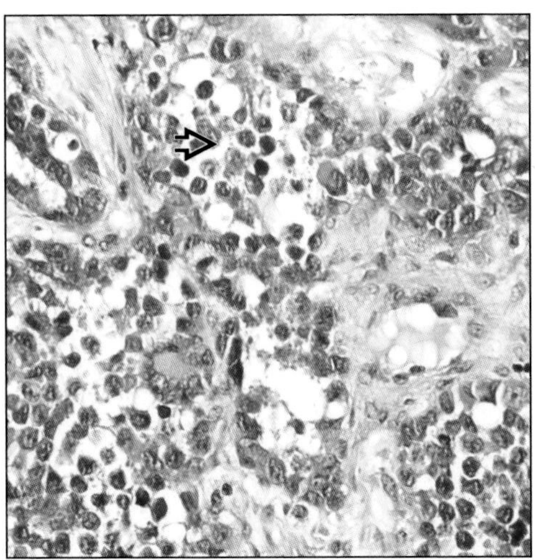

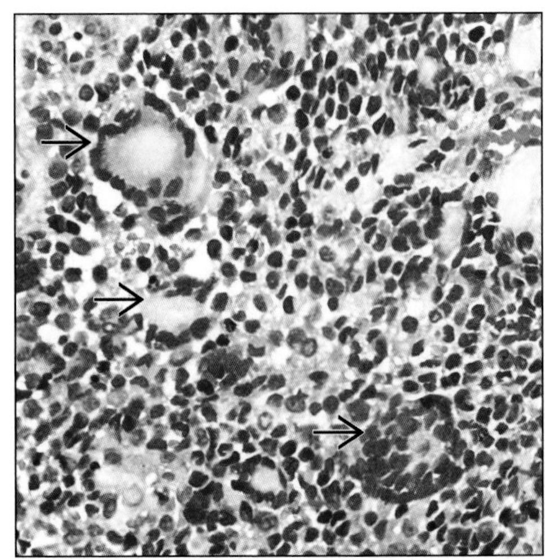

*(**Left**) Rarely, the tumor cells exhibit prominent cytoplasmic clearing in ARMS, such as in this case →. These cytoplasmic vacuolations can occasionally be mistaken for lipoblasts, but nuclear indentation is not seen here. (**Right**) Tumors can show a variable degree of rhabdomyoblastic differentiation, prominent in this specimen. Many cells within the alveolar structures are large and polygonal, with abundant eosinophilic cytoplasm →. Cross-striations may be discernible at higher power.*

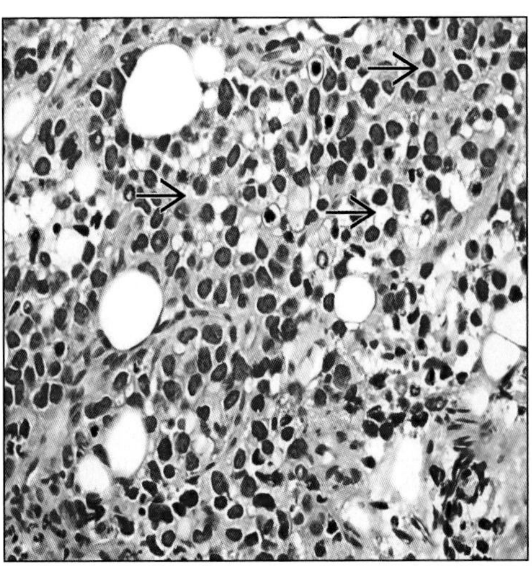

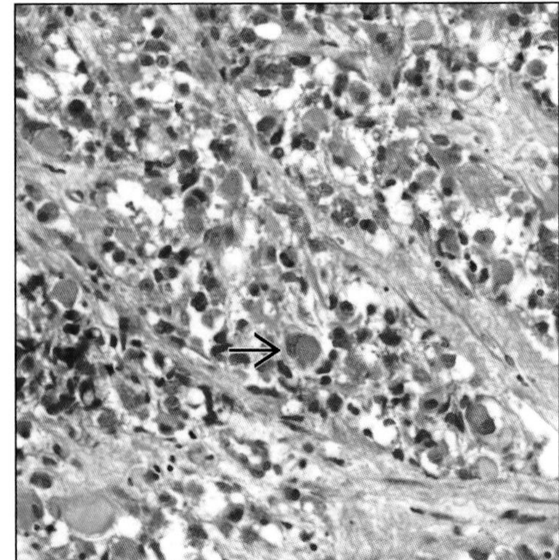

Microscopic Features and Ancillary Techniques

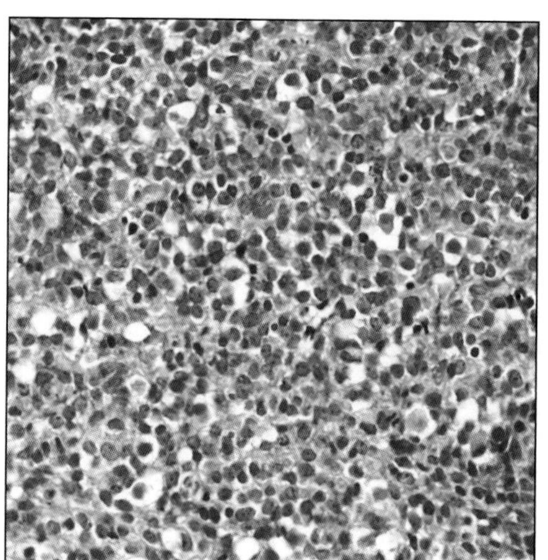

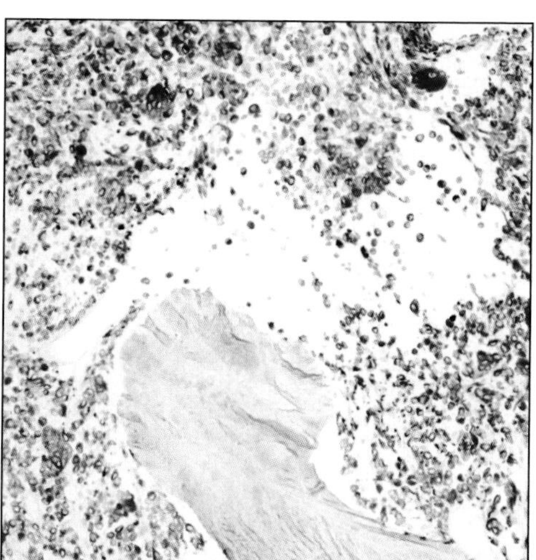

(Left) *ARMS, solid variant, is shown. Alveolar architecture is entirely absent in this tumor, showing solid sheets of medium-sized cells with round or ovoid nuclei. Careful sampling of the specimen may identify small areas of alveolar architecture, but this was not present in this specimen.* ***(Right)*** *Some patients present with disseminated metastases. This bone marrow biopsy specimen shows marked infiltration of the marrow space by tumor, which shows diffuse desmin expression.*

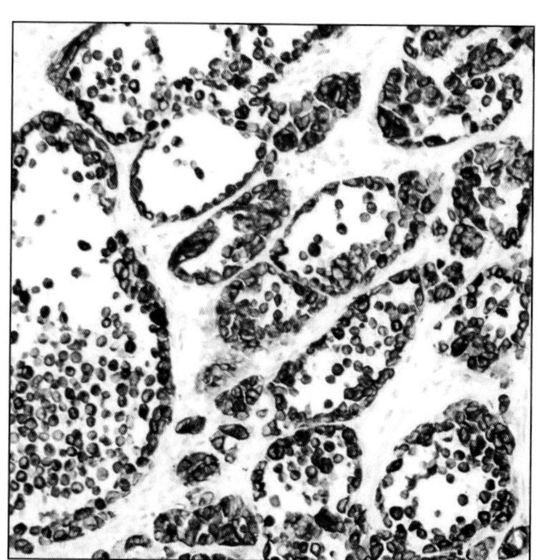

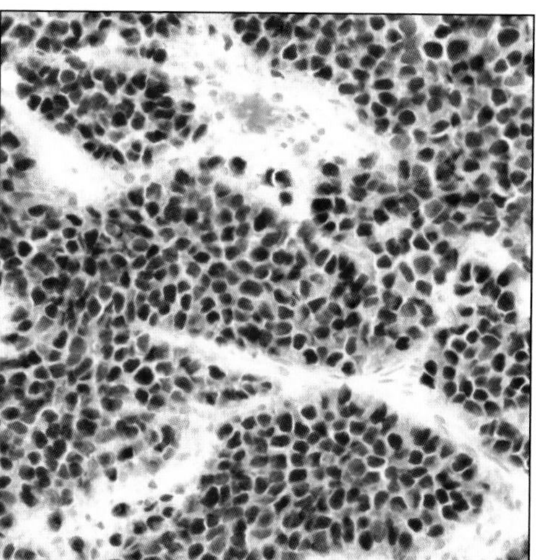

(Left) *Cytoplasmic desmin expression is typically strong and diffuse, and the alveolar pattern is clearly highlighted in this example.* ***(Right)*** *There is diffuse strong nuclear expression of myogenin. This diffuse level of positivity for myogenin is rarely seen in embryonal or pleomorphic rhabdomyosarcoma. Myogenin is a nuclear transcription factor, and any aberrant cytoplasmic staining should be disregarded.*

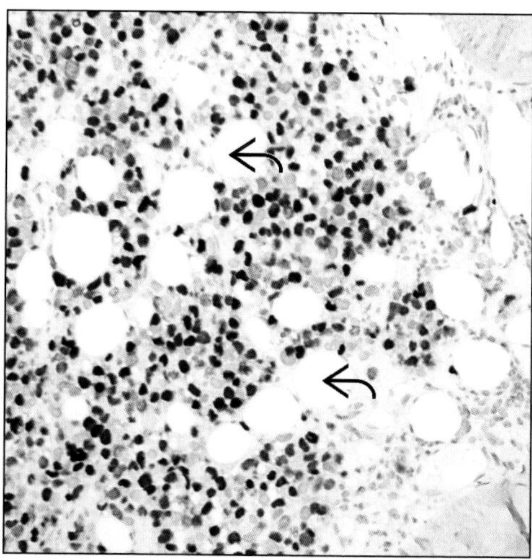

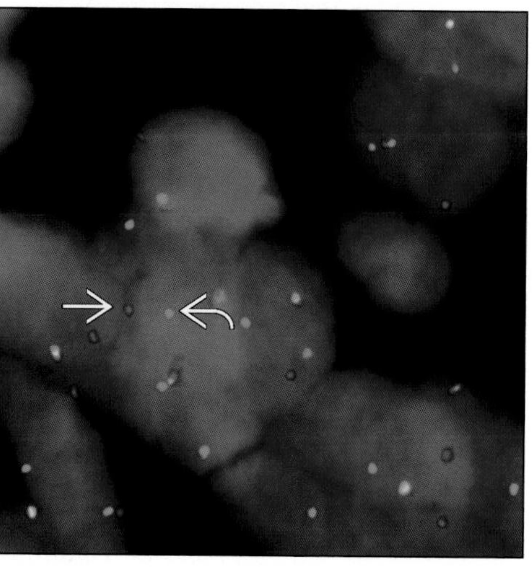

(Left) *Nuclear myogenin expression of metastatic ARMS is shown in a bone marrow biopsy specimen of a patient presenting with thrombocytopenia. Almost all the marrow space ⮫ is infiltrated by the tumor.* ***(Right)*** *In this fluorescence in situ hybridization in ARMS, dual color break-apart probes are used for the FOXO1 gene on chromosome 13q14 and show split red ➔ & green ➔ signals, indicating an abnormal clone with a translocation involving FOXO1.*

SCLEROSING PSEUDOVASCULAR RHABDOMYOSARCOMA

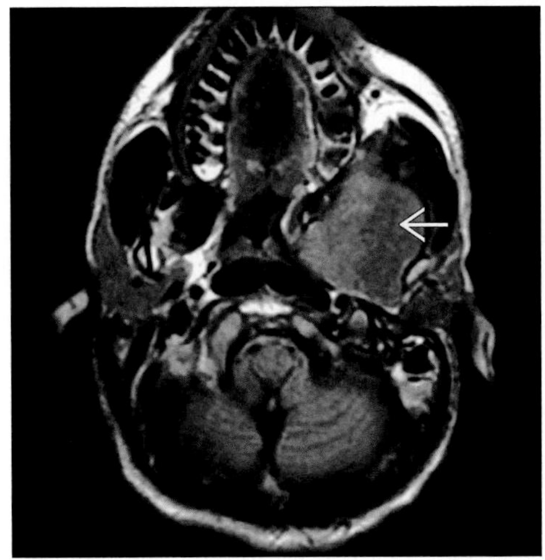

Sclerosing pseudovascular rhabdomyosarcoma most often affects the extremities and the head and neck. This MR image depicts a destructive mass ➔ involving the maxillary sinus of a 26-year-old man.

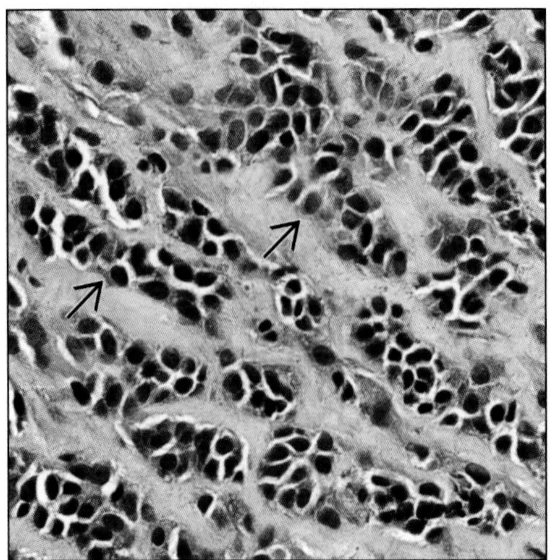

Sclerosing RMS is characterized by cords and clusters of small round cells or spindle cells and extensive hyalinizing fibrosis. Poorly cohesive cell clusters resemble vascular structures ➔.

TERMINOLOGY

Abbreviations

- Rhabdomyosarcoma (RMS)

Synonyms

- Sclerosing RMS, carcinoma-like RMS, microalveolar RMS, desmoplastic RMS

Definitions

- Variant of RMS characterized by extensive stromal fibrosis and pseudovascular, microalveolar, or cord-like architecture

CLINICAL ISSUES

Epidemiology

- Incidence
  - Rare; only 34 reports
- Age
  - Adults and children
  - Median age: 30 years; range: 0.3-79 years

Site

- Extremities and head and neck most common

Presentation

- Painless mass in extremity
- Obstructive symptoms in head and neck

Treatment

- Surgical approaches
  - Wide excision
- Adjuvant therapy
  - Chemotherapy &/or radiotherapy

Prognosis

- Poor
- Often unresectable
- Local recurrence: 25%
- Metastasis: 20%

MACROSCOPIC FEATURES

General Features

- White to tan, firm to fleshy, hemorrhagic areas

Size

- Median: 6 cm; range: 0.3-12 cm

MICROSCOPIC PATHOLOGY

Histologic Features

- Hyalinizing stromal fibrosis
  - Can mimic osteoid or chondroid matrix
- Pseudovascular, microalveolar, cord-like, single cell strand patterns
- Solid cellular areas in some
- Spindle cell fascicular areas in some

Cytologic Features

- Small round blue cells and spindle cells
- Scant eosinophilic or clear cytoplasm
- Rare rhabdomyoblasts

DIFFERENTIAL DIAGNOSIS

Alveolar Rhabdomyosarcoma

- Larger alveolar spaces
- More cohesive growth pattern
- Wreath-like giant cells in most
- Lacks spindle cells
- Very diffuse myogenin staining
- t(2:13) or t(1:13) rearrangement in majority

Sclerosing Epithelioid Fibrosarcoma

- Cords and single cell strands
- Epithelioid cytology
- Desmin(-)
- MYOD1(-), myogenin(-)
- Some have t(7;16) with *FUS-CREB3L2* fusion

SCLEROSING PSEUDOVASCULAR RHABDOMYOSARCOMA

Key Facts

Terminology

- Variant of RMS characterized by extensive stromal fibrosis and pseudovascular, microalveolar, or cord-like architecture

Clinical Issues

- Rare; only 34 reports
- Adults and children
- Median age: 30 years; range: 0.3-79 years
- Extremities and head and neck most common
- Poor prognosis

Microscopic Pathology

- Hyalinizing stromal fibrosis
  - Can mimic osteoid or chondroid matrix
- Small round blue cells or spindle cells
- Pseudovascular, microalveolar, cord-like, single cell strand patterns
- Solid cellular areas in some
- Spindle cell fascicular areas in some
- Rare rhabdomyoblasts
- Only focal myogenin staining

Top Differential Diagnoses

- Alveolar RMS
- Sclerosing epithelioid fibrosarcoma
- Angiosarcoma
- Osteosarcoma
- Infiltrating carcinoma
- Mesenchymal chondrosarcoma
- Extraskeletal myxoid chondrosarcoma

Immunohistochemistry

Antibody	Reactivity	Staining Pattern	Comment
MYOD1	Positive	Nuclear	Diffuse, strong staining
Desmin	Positive	Cytoplasmic	Focal or diffuse, sometimes dot-like
Myogenin	Positive	Nuclear	Focal, sometimes negative
S100	Negative		
CD31	Negative		
CK-PAN	Negative		
Actin-sm	Equivocal	Cytoplasmic	Sometimes positive
CD99	Equivocal	Cell membrane & cytoplasm	Sometimes positive

Angiosarcoma

- More complex branching architecture
- Often with epithelioid cytology
- CD31(-) and CD34(+)
- Desmin(-), MYOD1(-), myogenin(-)

Osteosarcoma

- Rare as soft tissue primary tumor
- Larger, more pleomorphic cells
- Lace-like osteoid
- Desmin(-), MYOD1(-), myogenin(-)

Chondrosarcoma

- Mesenchymal chondrosarcoma
  - Small round blue cells or spindle cells
  - Islands of well-formed cartilage
  - Pericytomatous vascular pattern
  - CD99(+)
  - Desmin(-), MYOD1(-), myogenin(-)
- Extraskeletal myxoid chondrosarcoma
  - Cords and clusters of epithelioid or spindle cells
  - Abundant myxoid matrix
  - Desmin(-), MYOD1(-), myogenin(-)
  - t(9:22) or t(9:17)

Infiltrating Carcinoma

- Epithelioid cytology
- Cytokeratin(+)
- Desmin(-), MYOD1(-), myogenin(-)

SELECTED REFERENCES

1. Stock N et al: Adult-type rhabdomyosarcoma: analysis of 57 cases with clinicopathologic description, identification of 3 morphologic patterns and prognosis. Am J Surg Pathol. 33(12):1850-9, 2009
2. Wang J et al: Sclerosing rhabdomyosarcoma: a clinicopathologic and immunohistochemical study of five cases. Am J Clin Pathol. 129(3):410-5, 2008
3. Kuhnen C et al: Sclerosing pseudovascular rhabdomyosarcoma-immunohistochemical, ultrastructural, and genetic findings indicating a distinct subtype of rhabdomyosarcoma. Virchows Arch. 449(5):572-8, 2006
4. Chiles MC et al: Sclerosing rhabdomyosarcomas in children and adolescents: a clinicopathologic review of 13 cases from the Intergroup Rhabdomyosarcoma Study Group and Children's Oncology Group. Pediatr Dev Pathol. 8(1):141, 2005
5. Croes R et al: Adult sclerosing rhabdomyosarcoma: cytogenetic link with embryonal rhabdomyosarcoma. Virchows Arch. 446(1):64-7, 2005
6. Nascimento AF et al: Spindle cell rhabdomyosarcoma in adults. Am J Surg Pathol. 29(8):1106-13, 2005
7. Folpe AL et al: Sclerosing rhabdomyosarcoma in adults: report of four cases of a hyalinizing, matrix-rich variant of rhabdomyosarcoma that may be confused with osteosarcoma, chondrosarcoma, or angiosarcoma. Am J Surg Pathol. 26(9):1175-83, 2002
8. Mentzel T et al: Sclerosing, pseudovascular rhabdomyosarcoma in adults. Clinicopathological and immunohistochemical analysis of three cases. Virchows Arch. 436(4):305-11, 2000

SCLEROSING PSEUDOVASCULAR RHABDOMYOSARCOMA

Gross and Microscopic Features

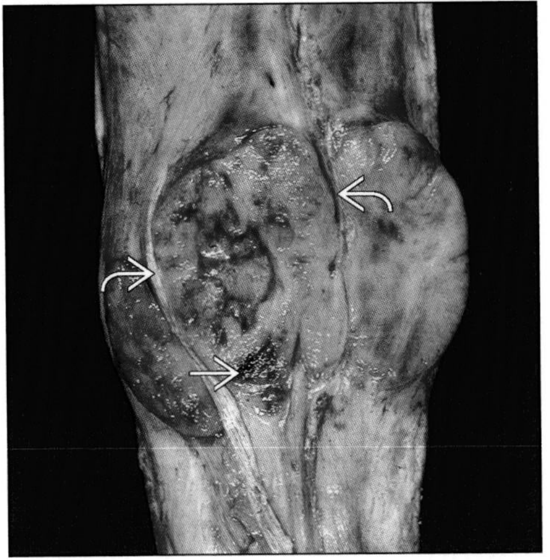

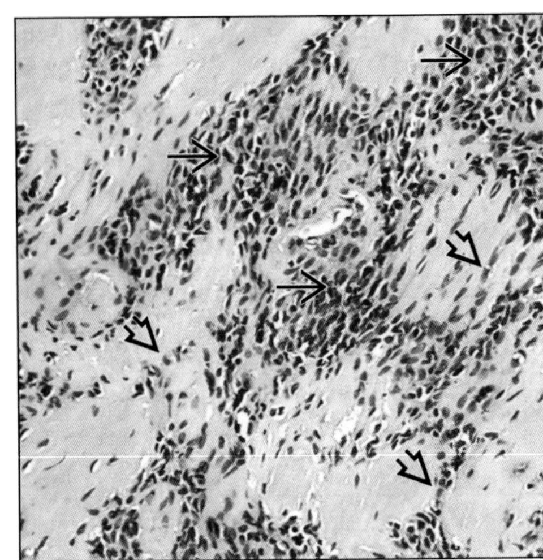

*(**Left**) This gross specimen depicts recurrent sclerosing pseudovascular RMS in the calf of a 60-year-old-man who had an amputation. The tumor is fleshy and lobulated with areas of hemorrhage ➡ and extends through the intermuscular fascia ↪ to involve multiple compartments. (**Right**) Hyalinizing stromal fibrosis is a defining feature of this entity. This low-power micrograph depicts sheets → and cords ⇨ of hyperchromatic small round and spindle cells within a fibrotic milieu.*

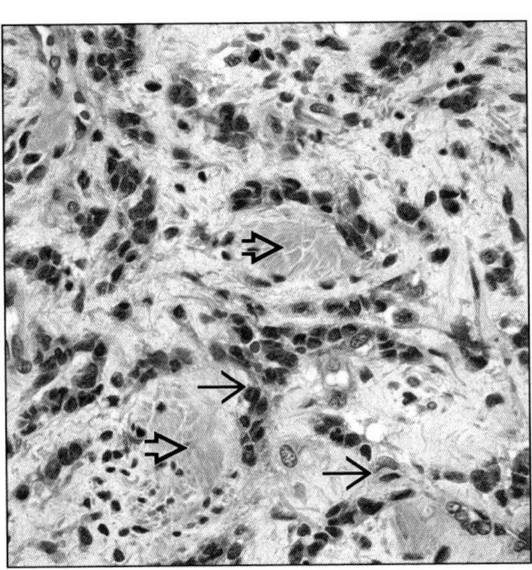

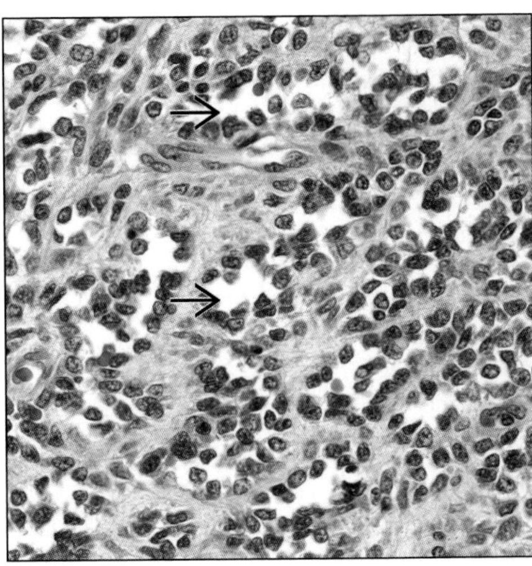

*(**Left**) Branching cords of neoplastic cells form pseudovascular structures → in this tumor. Note the collagen bundles ⇨ within the stroma. (**Right**) This micrograph depicts a microalveolar pattern characterized by clusters of loosely cohesive small round cells → separated by fibrous stroma. Compared to alveolar RMS, the alveolar spaces in sclerosing pseudovascular RMS are smaller and more cohesive. Unlike alveolar RMS, sclerosing pseudovascular RMS lacks wreath-like giant cells.*

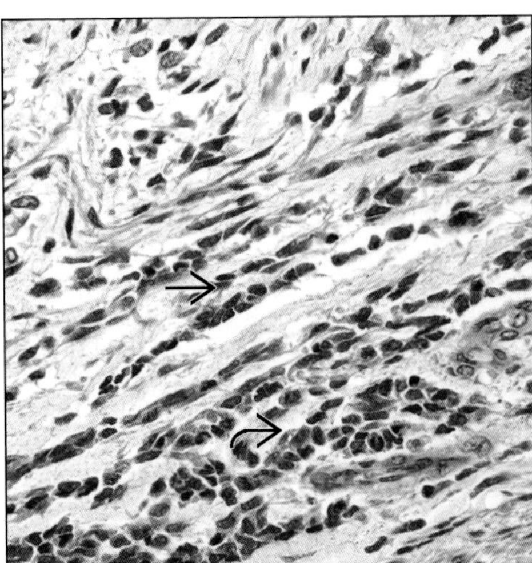

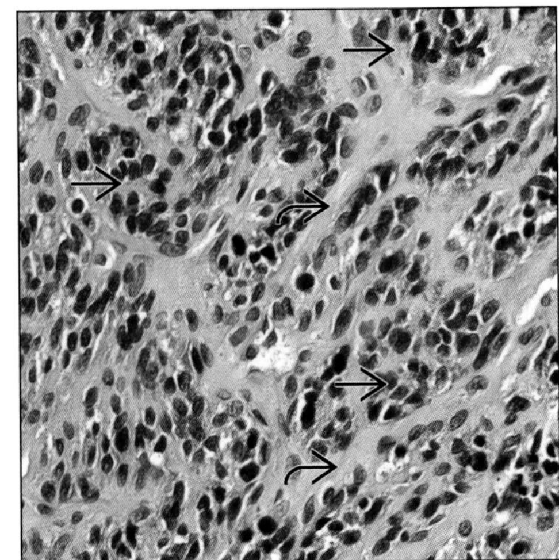

*(**Left**) In some tumors, the neoplastic cells are arranged in single cell strands → and elongated cords ↪, which can mimic infiltrating carcinoma. Immunohistochemistry readily distinguishes sclerosing pseudovascular RMS from carcinoma. (**Right**) The cells can also be arranged in a nested pattern consisting of small cell clusters → separated by fibrous septa ↪.*

Microscopic and Immunohistochemical Features

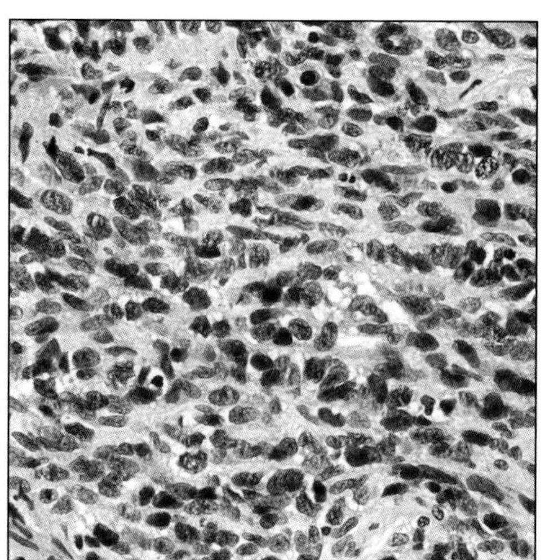

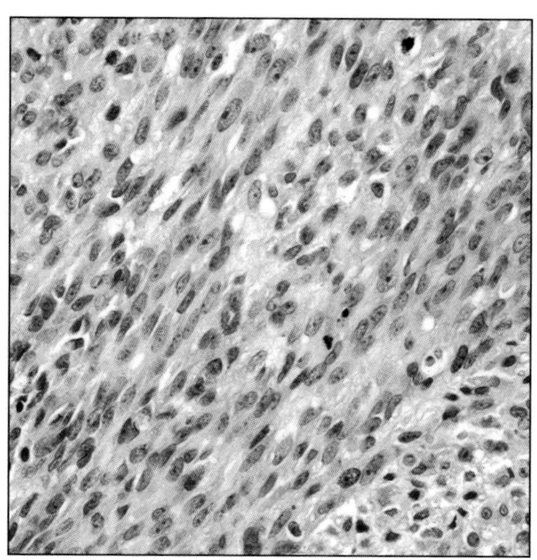

(Left) *Solid sheets of malignant cells are often present in sclerosing pseudovascular RMS. The cells are closely spaced and have round to oval hyperchromatic nuclei with scant eosinophilic cytoplasm.* ***(Right)*** *Some tumors have prominent fascicular spindle cell areas. In such cases the distinction between sclerosing pseudovascular RMS and adult-type spindle cell RMS with sclerotic areas becomes arbitrary.*

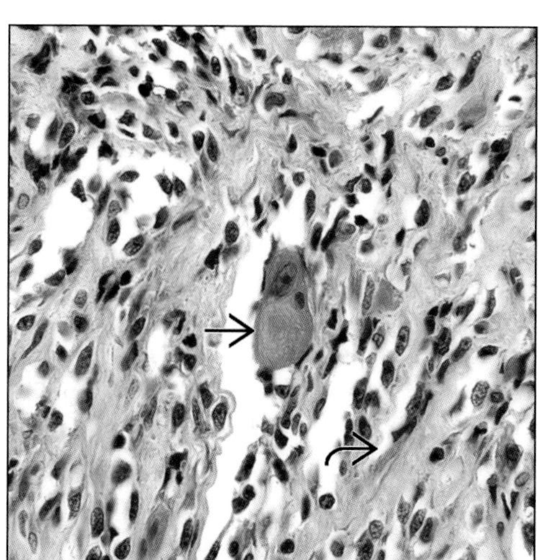

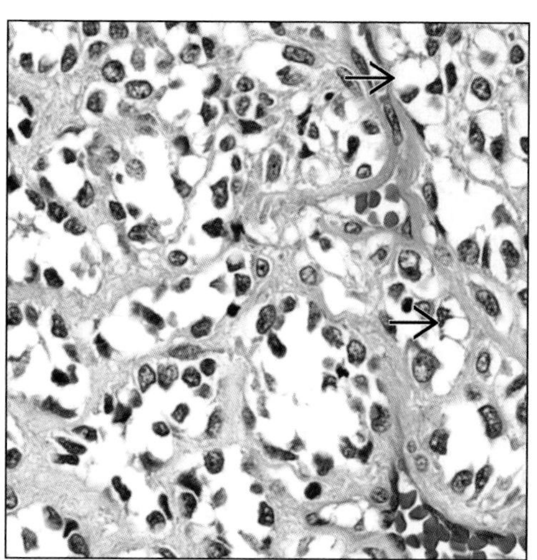

(Left) *Although often sparse and hard to find in sclerosing pseudovascular RMS, rhabdomyoblasts were readily identified in this tumor. Rhabdomyoblasts have abundant deeply eosinophilic cytoplasm and are polygonal ⇒ or fusiform-shaped ⇗.* ***(Right)*** *Clear cell change is present in some tumors evidenced here by neoplastic cells with cytoplasmic vacuolization ⇒.*

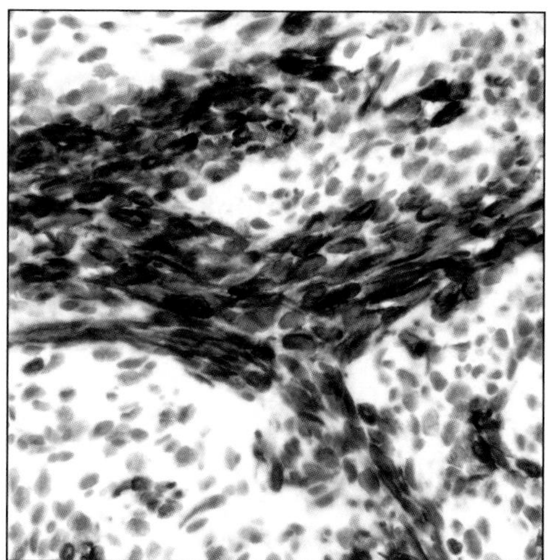

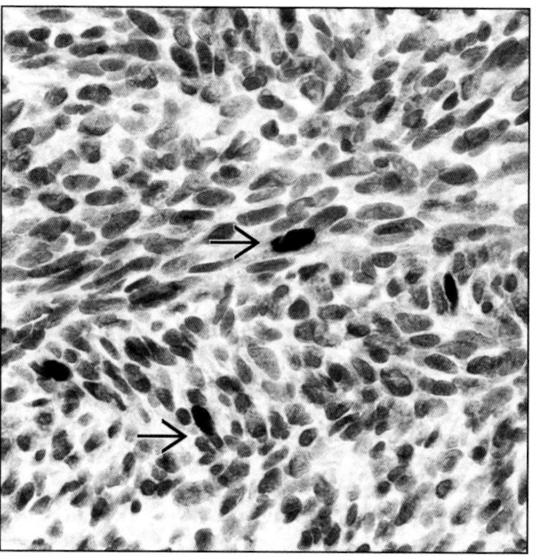

(Left) *Sclerosing pseudovascular RMS is usually strongly positive for desmin as shown. However, the degree of staining varies from focal to diffuse.* ***(Right)*** *Although most tumors are myogenin(+), staining is often very focal, involving only scattered nuclei ⇒. This finding distinguishes it from alveolar RMS, which typically shows very diffuse myogenin staining. MYOD1 (not shown) is reported to be more diffusely positive than myogenin in sclerosing pseudovascular RMS.*

PLEOMORPHIC RHABDOMYOSARCOMA

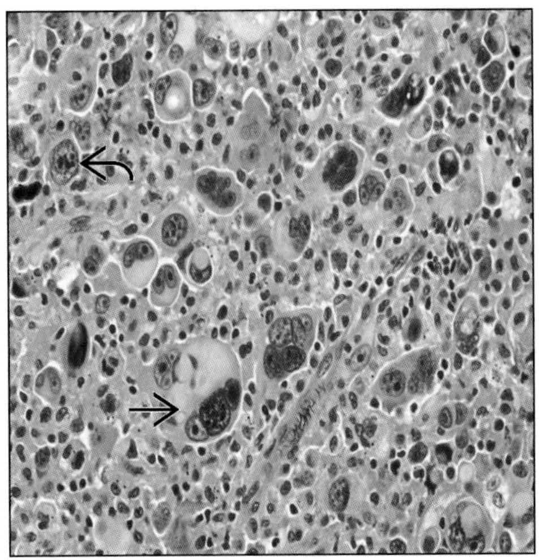

Pleomorphic rhabdomyosarcoma is shown with sheets of markedly anaplastic, frequently bizarre ⇗ or multinucleate ⇒ polygonal cells. The morphology is indistinguishable from other pleomorphic tumors.

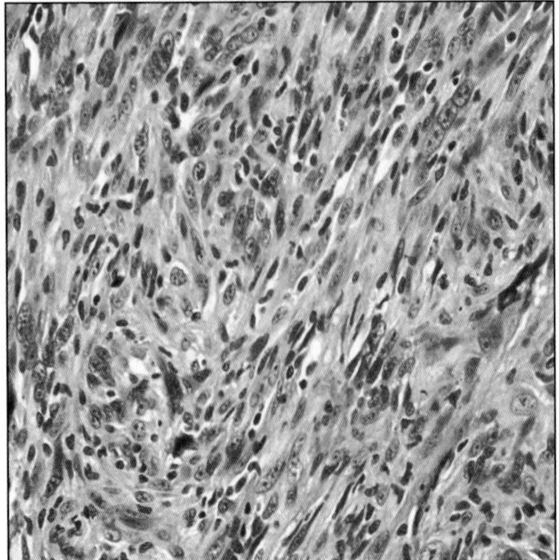

In this specimen, the tumor shows a fascicular architecture with bundles of atypical spindle cells with vesicular or hyperchromatic nuclei.

TERMINOLOGY

Definitions

- High-grade sarcoma occurring almost exclusively in adults and displaying evidence of skeletal muscle differentiation
- Diagnosis requires identification of pleomorphic rhabdomyoblasts and expression of skeletal muscle specific immunohistochemical markers

CLINICAL ISSUES

Epidemiology

- Age
  - Older adults
    - Median: 6th decade
  - Very rare cases reported in children and adolescents
- Gender
  - M > F

Site

- Deep soft tissues of lower extremity, particularly thigh
- Abdomen/retroperitoneum
- Spermatic cord and testes
- Upper extremity
- Mouth and orbit

Presentation

- Suddenly enlarging mass
- Painful mass

Prognosis

- Aggressive clinical course
  - Frequent early metastasis

MACROSCOPIC FEATURES

General Features

- Usually large (> 10 cm)
- Fairly circumscribed
- Firm, white to tan cut surface
- Variable hemorrhage
- Necrosis often extensive

MICROSCOPIC PATHOLOGY

Histologic Features

- Densely cellular
- Morphology of undifferentiated pleomorphic sarcoma
  - Markedly atypical spindle to polygonal cells
  - Sheet-like, fascicular, or storiform arrangements
  - Large hyperchromatic or vesicular, often bizarre nuclei
  - Eosinophilic cytoplasm
- Pleomorphic rhabdomyoblasts may be present
  - Polygonal
  - Spindled
  - Strap- or racquet-like shapes
  - Cross-striations rare
- Classified into "classic," "round cell," and "spindle cell" patterns by some authors

Predominant Pattern/Injury Type

- Neoplastic

Predominant Cell/Compartment Type

- Mesenchymal, muscle, skeletal

ANCILLARY TESTS

Immunohistochemistry

- Strong, sometimes focal, desmin positivity
- Strong focal nuclear myogenin and MYOD1
  - Usually less pronounced than in pediatric RMS
- Variable, focal expression of smooth muscle markers
  - Muscle specific actin, actin-sm
- Negative for CD45, S100, and cytokeratin

PLEOMORPHIC RHABDOMYOSARCOMA

Key Facts

Terminology

- High-grade sarcoma occurring almost exclusively in adults and displaying evidence of skeletal muscle differentiation
- Diagnosis requires identification of pleomorphic rhabdomyoblasts and expression of skeletal muscle specific immunohistochemical markers

Clinical Issues

- Older adults
- Deep soft tissues of lower extremity
  - Multiple other sites

Microscopic Pathology

- Morphology of pleomorphic sarcoma
- Markedly atypical spindle to polygonal cells
- Pleomorphic polygonal rhabdomyoblasts may be present
- Expression of desmin and myogenic markers

Cytogenetics

- No consistent chromosomal abnormalities identified
- Most tumors have complex karyotypes

Electron Microscopy

- Rudimentary sarcomeres

DIFFERENTIAL DIAGNOSIS

Other Pleomorphic Sarcomas

- Pleomorphic leiomyosarcoma
  - Lower grade areas with intersecting fascicles
  - Myogenin(-) and MYOD1(-)
- Pleomorphic liposarcoma
  - Pleomorphic lipoblasts
- Undifferentiated pleomorphic sarcoma
  - Absence of skeletal muscle markers

Alveolar or Embryonal Rhabdomyosarcoma

- Children and adolescents
- May have focally atypical areas
  - Diffuse, marked pleomorphism absent
- Areas of more typical alveolar or embryonal RMS
- Characteristic translocation in alveolar RMS

Anaplastic Large Cell Lymphoma

- Expresses broad spectrum of leucocyte markers

Undifferentiated or Metastatic Carcinoma

- Dysplastic changes in overlying epithelium
- History of carcinoma at primary site
- At least focally positive for cytokeratin or EMA
- Desmin(-)

Melanoma

- In situ changes in overlying epithelium
- Positive for S100
- Often HMB-45(+) and Melan-A(+)
- Desmin usually negative
- Myogenin(-) and MYOD1(-)
- Melanin pigment may be identifiable

SELECTED REFERENCES

1. Li G et al: Cytogenetic and real-time quantitative reverse-transcriptase polymerase chain reaction analyses in pleomorphic rhabdomyosarcoma. Cancer Genet Cytogenet. 192(1):1-9, 2009
2. Furlong MA et al: Pleomorphic rhabdomyosarcoma in adults: a clinicopathologic study of 38 cases with emphasis on morphologic variants and recent skeletal muscle-specific markers. Mod Pathol. 14(6):595-603, 2001
3. Furlong MA et al: Pleomorphic rhabdomyosarcoma in children: four cases in the pediatric age group. Ann Diagn Pathol. 5(4):199-206, 2001
4. Schürch W et al: Pleomorphic soft tissue myogenic sarcomas of adulthood. A reappraisal in the mid-1990s. Am J Surg Pathol. 20(2):131-47, 1996
5. Hollowood K et al: Rhabdomyosarcoma in adults. Semin Diagn Pathol. 11(1):47-57, 1994
6. Gaffney EF et al: Pleomorphic rhabdomyosarcoma in adulthood. Analysis of 11 cases with definition of diagnostic criteria. Am J Surg Pathol. 17(6):601-9, 1993

IMAGE GALLERY

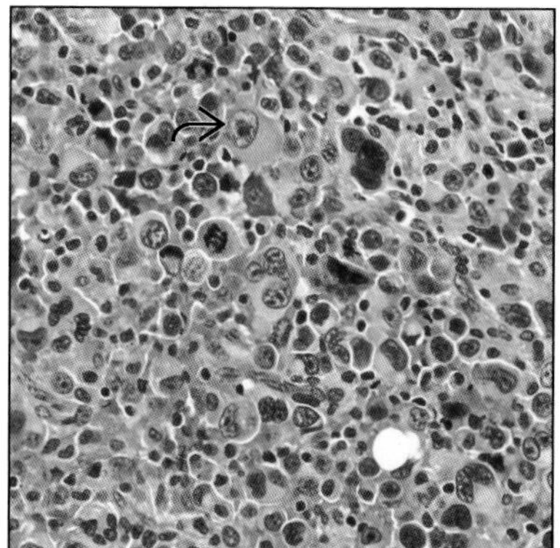

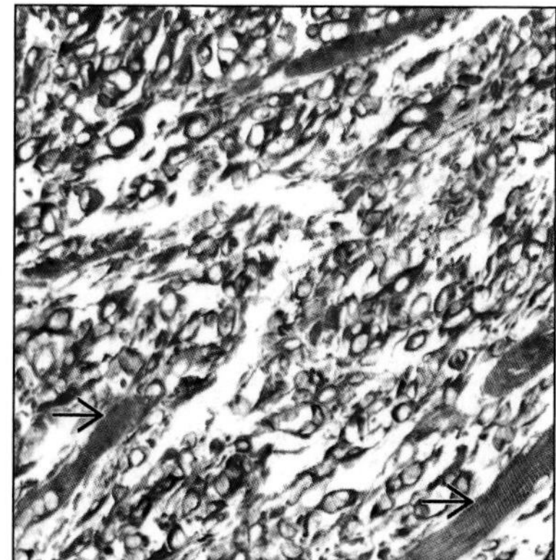

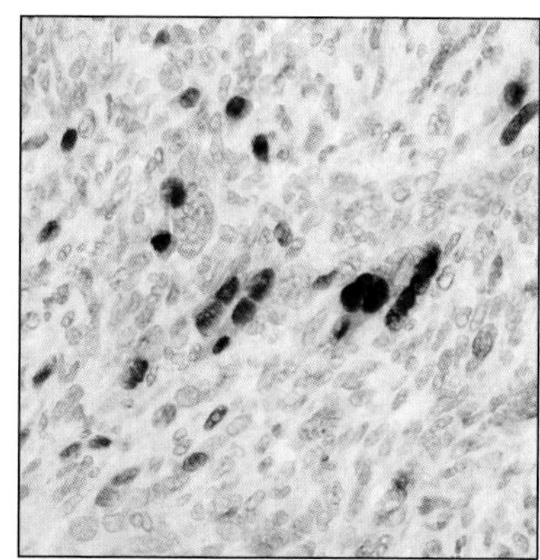

(Left) *Tumor cells are frequently large and polygonal ⮫ with abundant eosinophilic cytoplasm and resemble pleomorphic rhabdomyoblasts.* ***(Center)*** *There is diffuse, strong positivity for desmin within this tumor. Note also the intervening normal skeletal muscle fibers ⮕.* ***(Right)*** *Myogenin expression confirms skeletal muscle differentiation. Staining should be nuclear and is often patchy.*

PROTOCOL FOR THE EXAMINATION OF RHABDOMYOSARCOMA SPECIMENS

Rhabdomyosarcoma and Related Neoplasms: Resection or Biopsy

Surgical Pathology Cancer Case Summary (Checklist)

Procedure

___ Biopsy
___ Excision, local
___ Excision, radical
___ Excision, compartmentectomy
___ Amputation (specify type): ___________________________
___ Other (specify): ___________________________
___ Not specified

Specimen Laterality

___ Right
___ Left
___ Midline
___ Indeterminate
___ Not specified

Tumor Site

___ Bladder/prostate
___ Cranial parameningeal
___ Extremity
___ Genitourinary (not bladder/prostate)
___ Head and neck (excluding parameningeal)
___ Orbit
___ Other(s) (includes trunk, retroperitoneum, etc.)
(Specify): ___________________________
___ Not specified

Tumor Size

Greatest dimension: _________ cm
*Additional dimensions: _________ x _________ cm
___ Cannot be determined

**Tumor Depth for Soft Tissue-based Tumors*

*___ Dermal
*___ Subcutaneous
*___ Subfascial
*___ Intramuscular
*___ Intraabdominal
*___ Retroperitoneal
*___ Intracranial
*___ Organ based
*___ Other (specify): ___________________________
*___ Cannot be assessed

Histologic Type

___ Embryonal, botryoid
___ Embryonal, spindle cell
___ Embryonal, not otherwise specified (NOS)
___ Alveolar
___ Mixed embryonal and alveolar rhabdomyosarcoma
(Specify percentage of each type): ___________________________
___ Rhabdoid rhabdomyosarcoma
___ Sclerosing rhabdomyosarcoma
___ Undifferentiated sarcoma
___ Ectomesenchymoma

PROTOCOL FOR THE EXAMINATION OF RHABDOMYOSARCOMA SPECIMENS

____ Other (specify): ____________________________

____ Rhabdomyosarcoma, subtype indeterminate

Anaplasia

____ Not identified

____ Focal (single or few scattered anaplastic cells)

____ Diffuse (clusters or sheets of anaplastic cells)

____ Indeterminate

____ Cannot be assessed

Margins

____ Cannot be assessed

____ Sarcoma involvement of margins not identified

Distance of sarcoma from closest margin: _________ mm OR _________ cm

Specify margin: ____________________________

____ Indeterminate

Lymph Nodes

____ No regional lymph nodes sampled

____ Metastatic involvement of regional lymph nodes not identified

____ Regional lymph node metastasis present

Specify: Number examined: _________

Number involved: ________

Distant Metastasis

____ Not applicable

____ Distant metastasis present

*Specify site(s), if known: ____________________________

The Intergroup Rhabdomyosarcoma Study Postsurgical Clinical Grouping System

Note: Clinical information required to definitively assign stage group (e.g., gross residual disease or distant metastatic disease) may not be available to the pathologist. Alternatively, this protocol may not be applicable to some situations (e.g., group IIIA). If applicable, the appropriate stage group may be assigned by the pathologist.

____ Not applicable

____ Cannot be assessed

Group I

____ A) Localized tumor, confined to site of origin, completely resected

____ B) Localized tumor, infiltrating beyond site of origin, completely resected

Group II

____ A) Localized tumor, gross total resection, but with microscopic residual disease

____ B) Locally extensive tumor (spread to regional lymph nodes), completely resected

____ C) Locally extensive tumor (spread to regional lymph nodes), gross total resection, but microscopic residual disease

Group III

____ A) Localized or locally extensive tumor, gross residual disease after biopsy only

____ B) Localized or locally extensive tumor, gross residual disease after major resection (> 50% debulking)

Group IV

____ Any size tumor, ± regional lymph node involvement, with distant metastases, with respect to surgical approach to primary tumor

**Modified Site, Size, Metastasis Staging for Rhabdomyosarcoma (for relevant stage) (select all that apply)*

Note: Clinical information required to definitively assign stage (e.g., nodal status or distant metastatic disease) may not be available to the pathologist.

*____ Not applicable

*____ Cannot be assessed

*____ Stage I (requires all of the following to be true)

*____ Tumor involves orbit, head and neck, or genitourinary site (excluding bladder, prostate, and cranial parameningeal)

*____ Tumor metastatic to distant site not identified

*____ Stage II (requires all of the following to be true)

*____ Tumor does not involve orbit, nonparameningeal head and neck, or nonbladder/nonprostate genitourinary tract

*____ Tumor size ≤ 5 cm

*____ Tumor involvement of lymph nodes not identified

PROTOCOL FOR THE EXAMINATION OF RHABDOMYOSARCOMA SPECIMENS

*____ Tumor metastatic to distant site not identified

*____ Stage III (select one if applicable)

*____ Tumor involves bladder or prostate and is metastatic to regional lymph nodes but distant metastases are not identified

*____ Tumor involves site other than orbit, nonparameningeal head and neck, or nonbladder/nonprostate genitourinary tract and is > 5 cm, but distant metastases are not identified

*____ Stage IV

*____ Distant metastases present

*Additional Pathologic Findings

*Specify: ____________________________

**Data elements with asterisks are not required. However, these elements may be clinically important but are not yet validated or regularly used in patient management. Adapted with permission from College of American Pathologists, "Protocol for the Examination of Specimens from Patients with Rhabdomyosarcoma." Web posting date October 2009, www.cap.org.*

Smooth Muscle Lesions

Benign

Malignant

CONGENITAL SMOOTH MUSCLE HAMARTOMA

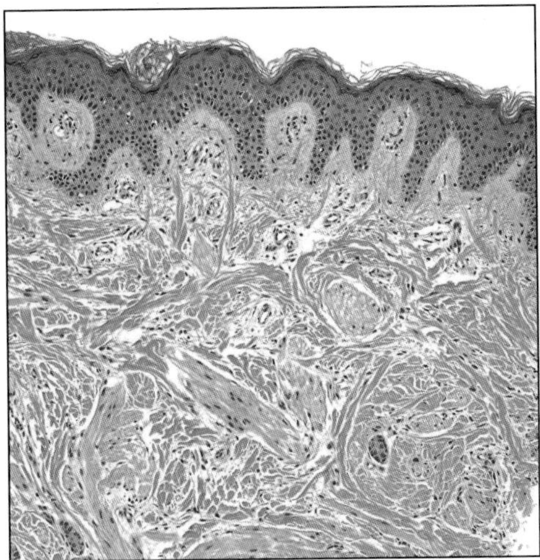

Hematoxylin & eosin shows a haphazard arrangement of smooth muscle bundles in the dermis.

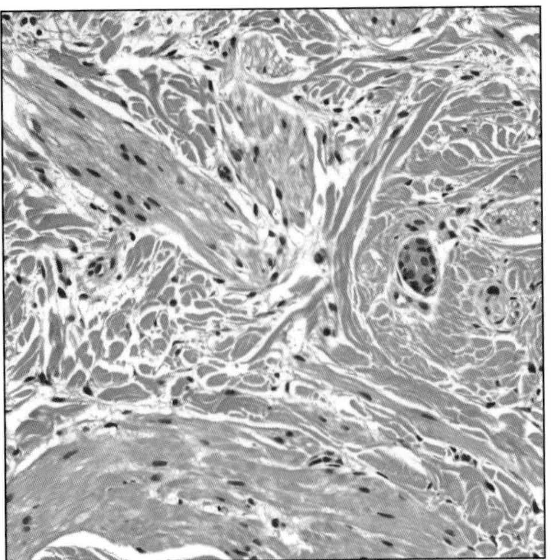

Hematoxylin & eosin shows a fascicular arrangement of smooth muscle with characteristic elongated blunt-ended nuclei.

TERMINOLOGY

Synonyms

- Smooth muscle hamartoma

Definitions

- Rare benign smooth muscle tumor presenting in infants
- Characterized by disorganized proliferation of smooth muscle bundles

CLINICAL ISSUES

Epidemiology

- Age
  - Infants

Site

- Lumbosacral area and proximal extremities

Presentation

- Macule or plaque
  - Indurated
  - Often hyperpigmented
  - May have coarse hairs
- Pseudo-Darier sign
  - Piloerection induced by mechanical stimulation
- Occasionally presents as multiple lesions
- Occasional familial cases

Treatment

- Surgical approaches
  - Simple excision

Prognosis

- Excellent

MACROSCOPIC FEATURES

General Features

- Ill-defined dermal thickening

Size

- Usually < 2 cm diameter

MICROSCOPIC PATHOLOGY

Histologic Features

- Haphazard arrangement of benign smooth muscle bundles
  - Resembles arrector pili muscle
  - Spindled cells arranged in fascicles
  - Elongated, blunt-ended nuclei
  - Eosinophilic cytoplasm
  - No pleomorphism
  - No mitotic activity
  - No necrosis

Predominant Pattern/Injury Type

- Fascicular

Predominant Cell/Compartment Type

- Mesenchymal, muscle, smooth

DIFFERENTIAL DIAGNOSIS

Cutaneous Leiomyoma (Pilar Leiomyoma)

- Presents in young adults
- Usually multiple
- Solid rather than haphazard fascicles

Leiomyosarcoma

- Diffuse or nodular
- Mitotic activity
- Nuclear atypia

CONGENITAL SMOOTH MUSCLE HAMARTOMA

Key Facts

Terminology
- Rare lesion presenting in infants, characterized by disorganized proliferation of benign smooth muscle bundles in dermis, often involving subcutis

Clinical Issues
- Infants
- Most common in lumbosacral area
- Macule or plaque
- Often hyperpigmented, may have coarse hairs

Microscopic Pathology
- Benign smooth muscle bundles
  - Haphazard arrangement
  - Thin fascicles rather than solid growth pattern
  - No atypia
  - No mitoses
  - No necrosis

Immunohistochemistry

Antibody	Reactivity	Staining Pattern	Comment
Actin-sm	Positive	Cytoplasmic	Diffuse
Desmin	Positive	Cytoplasmic	Diffuse
HCAD	Positive	Cytoplasmic	Diffuse
S100P	Negative		
AE1/AE3	Negative		
EMA/MUC1	Negative		
Myogenin	Negative		

Schwannoma
- Circumscribed
- Often encapsulated
- S100(+)
- EMA(+) rim of perineurial cells

Neurofibroma
- Wavy spindle cell
- S100(+)
- Meissner bodies in diffuse neurofibroma

Fetal Rhabdomyoma
- Skeletal muscle differentiation
  - Striations
  - Myogenin(+), MYOD1(+)

Normal Skin from Special Sites
- Skin from nipple, vulva, or scrotum has high concentration of normal smooth muscle bundles

DIAGNOSTIC CHECKLIST

Pathologic Interpretation Pearls
- Confined to dermis
- No atypical features

SELECTED REFERENCES

1. Gualandri L et al: Multiple familial smooth muscle hamartomas. Pediatr Dermatol. 18(1):17-20, 2001
2. Gagné EJ et al: Congenital smooth muscle hamartoma of the skin. Pediatr Dermatol. 10(2):142-5, 1993
3. Zvulunov A et al: Congenital smooth muscle hamartoma. Prevalence, clinical findings, and follow-up in 15 patients. Am J Dis Child. 144(7):782-4, 1990
4. Johnson MD et al: Congenital smooth muscle hamartoma. A report of six cases and a review of the literature. Arch Dermatol. 125(6):820-2, 1989

IMAGE GALLERY

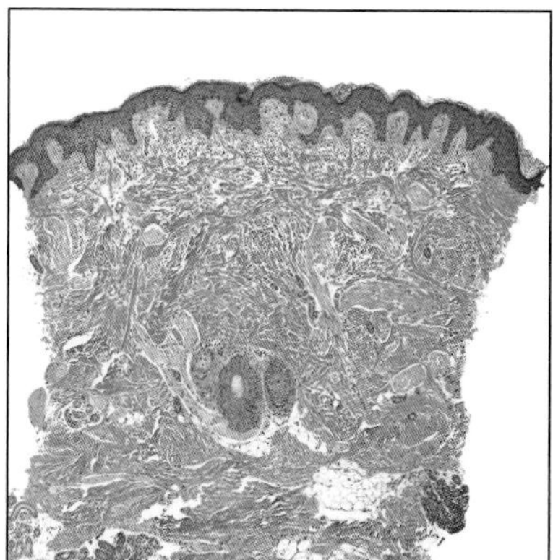

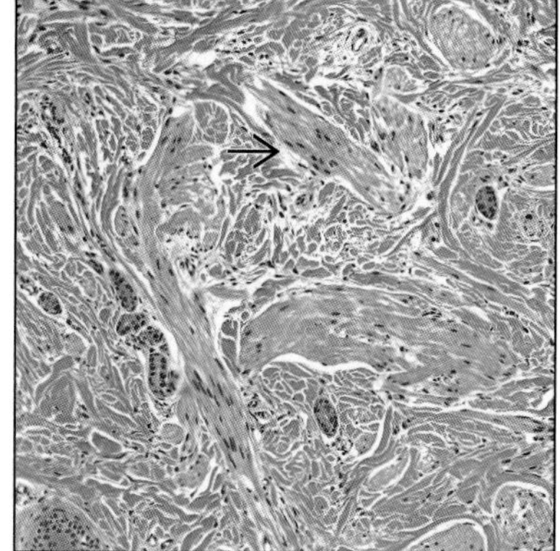

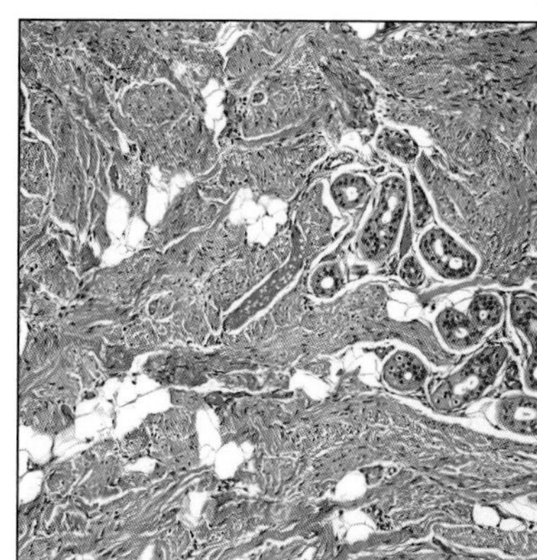

(Left) *Hematoxylin & eosin shows low-power view with disorganized proliferation of smooth muscle bundles throughout the dermis.* ***(Center)*** *Hematoxylin & eosin shows haphazard pattern of smooth muscle bundles ⇒. The smooth muscle bundles resemble arrector pili muscles but are present in a greater density than normal arrector pili muscles.* ***(Right)*** *Hematoxylin & eosin shows the proliferation of smooth muscle extending into the deep reticular dermis/subcutis.*

SUPERFICIAL LEIOMYOMA

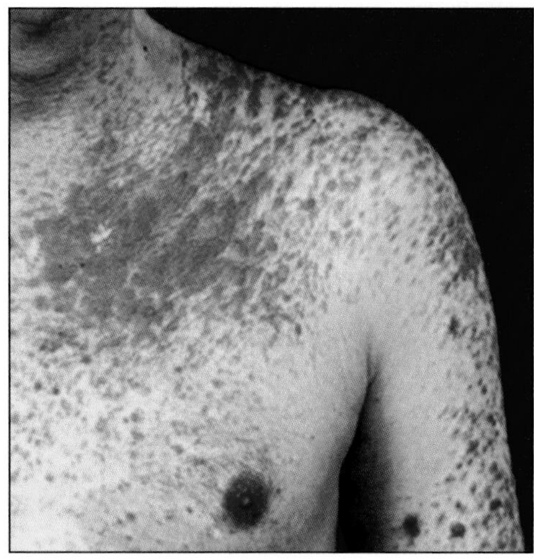

Multiple cutaneous leiomyomas are seen involving the chest, lower neck, shoulder, and upper arm. Typical of superficial leiomyomas, these lesions tend to involve more than 1 body site and involve extensor surfaces.

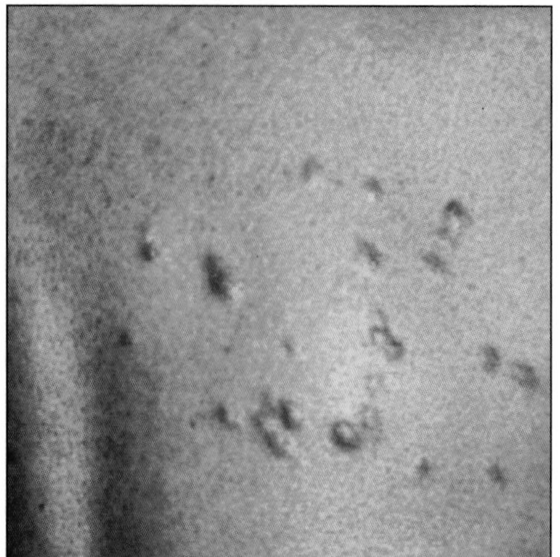

Superficial leiomyomas are usually under 2 cm and appear as multiple pink or brown papules or nodules. Clinically they tend to elicit pain and are often distributed in a dermatomal fashion.

TERMINOLOGY

Synonyms

- Cutaneous leiomyoma, pilar leiomyoma, piloleiomyoma, leiomyoma cutis

Definitions

- Uncommon benign cutaneous smooth muscle neoplasm originating from arrector pili muscles

ETIOLOGY/PATHOGENESIS

Genetics

- Some cases are familial
  - Autosomal dominant inheritance pattern with incomplete penetrance
- Most patients are shown to have germline fumarate hydratase gene mutations
  - Gene on 1q43 and enzyme involved with tricarboxylic acid (Krebs) cycle
- May be associated with uterine leiomyomas (98%) and renal cell carcinoma (10-15%)
  - Syndrome known as hereditary leiomyomatosis and renal cell cancer, multiple cutaneous and uterine leiomyomatosis syndrome, or Reed syndrome
    - Renal cell carcinomas are usually papillary, tubulopapillary, or collecting duct type

CLINICAL ISSUES

Epidemiology

- Age
  - Most develop in adolescence or early adulthood
  - Some are congential or develop in childhood

Site

- Predilection for extensor surfaces of extremities, trunk, and head & neck
  - 2 or more body sites are often affected

Presentation

- Most often multiple painful pink or brown papules
  - Papules may coalesce into nodules
  - Lesions tend to follow dermatomal distribution
- Pain can be induced by cold exposure, pressure, or in states of emotion
- Rare cases are solitary and painless

Treatment

- Options, risks, complications
  - Depends on number of lesions and symptomatology
  - Medical management with follow-up is option for those with extensive lesions
  - Imaging to rule out renal mass or large atypical uterine lesions is warranted
  - Cryotherapy and laser ablation have been used with mixed results
- Surgical approaches
  - For localized and symptomatic lesions

Prognosis

- Do not undergo malignant degeneration
- Surgically treated lesions often develop recurrence (more likely representing new lesions)

MACROSCOPIC FEATURES

Size

- Most are less than 2 cm

MICROSCOPIC PATHOLOGY

Histologic Features

- Bundles and fascicles of differentiated smooth muscle cells
  - Cells have abundant fibrillary pink cytoplasm and oval, blunt-ended (cigar-shaped) nuclei
- Unencapsulated, haphazardly arranged, with irregular borders, and confined to dermis

SUPERFICIAL LEIOMYOMA

Key Facts

Terminology
- Benign cutaneous smooth muscle neoplasm arising from arrector pili muscles

Etiology/Pathogenesis
- Many are shown to have germline fumarate hydratase gene mutations
- May be associated with uterine leiomyomas and renal cell carcinoma

Clinical Issues
- Most develop in adolescence or early adulthood
- Predilection for extensor surfaces of extremities as well as trunk
- Most often present with multiple painful pink or brown papules

Microscopic Pathology
- Bundles and fascicles of differentiated smooth muscle cells
- Proliferation is unencapsulated, haphazardly arranged, with irregular borders, and confined to dermis
- Degenerative atypia and occasional mitotic figures (up to 1 per 10 HPF) are acceptable

Top Differential Diagnoses
- Genital leiomyoma
- Smooth muscle hamartoma
- Dermatomyofibroma
- Myofibroma
- Angiomyoma (angioleiomyoma, vascular leiomyoma)
- Superficial leiomyosarcoma

  - Often intimately associated with hair follicles
  - Fascicles often dissect between dermal collagen
- Rare cases are circumscribed
- Overlying epidermal hyperplasia is frequently present
- Degenerative atypia and occasional mitotic figures (up to 1 per 10 HPF) are acceptable
  - Higher mitotic activity, diffuse (nondegenerative) atypia, necrosis, and subcutaneous extension are more suggestive of leiomyosarcoma

Immunohistochemistry
- Tumor cells are strongly positive for desmin, smooth muscle actin, and muscle specific actin

DIFFERENTIAL DIAGNOSIS

Genital Leiomyoma
- Usually solitary and painless and arise from specialized dermal smooth muscle (e.g., dartos in scrotum)
- Common sites include scrotum, penis, nipple, areola, and vulva
- Tend to be more circumscribed, cellular, and histologically heterogeneous than pilar leiomyomas
  - Histologic heterogeneity can include myxoid change and epithelioid cells

Smooth Muscle Hamartoma
- Usually solitary, larger, and located in lumbar region
- May be associated with increased hair &/or pigment (Becker nevus)
- Smooth muscle bundles tend to be more well defined than in leiomyoma, but there is significant histologic overlap

Dermatomyofibroma
- Solitary plaque lesion usually located on shoulder or trunk
- Fascicular spindle cell proliferation parallel to epidermis without effacement of dermal structures
- Cells have myofibroblastic appearance and are typically negative for desmin

Myofibroma
- Circumscribed and often nodular with biphasic histology
  - Fascicles and whorls of myofibroblasts alternating with primitive round cells associated with hemangiopericytomatous vascular pattern
  - Necrosis and mitotic figures can be seen; spindle cells are typically negative for desmin

Angiomyoma
- Solitary subcutaneous nodule that may be painful; usually occur in lower extremity (wide distribution though)
- Circumscribed with less fascicular arrangement and intimately associated with evenly distributed, thick-walled to cavernous vascular spaces

Superficial Leiomyosarcoma
- Larger lesions that are usually solitary and often extend into subcutis
- Atypia and mitotic activity (and necrosis) beyond that acceptable in leiomyoma

SELECTED REFERENCES

1. Badeloe S et al: Clinical and molecular genetic aspects of hereditary multiple cutaneous leiomyomatosis. Eur J Dermatol. 19(6):545-51, 2009
2. Holst VA et al: Cutaneous smooth muscle neoplasms: clinical features, histologic findings, and treatment options. J Am Acad Dermatol. 46(4):477-90; quiz, 491-4, 2002
3. Yokoyama R et al: Superficial leiomyomas. A clinicopathologic study of 34 cases. Acta Pathol Jpn. 37(9):1415-22, 1987
4. Tavassoli FA et al: Smooth muscle tumors of the vulva. Obstet Gynecol. 53(2):213-7, 1979
5. Fox SR Jr: Leiomyomatosis cutis. N Engl J Med. 263:1248-50, 1960

SUPERFICIAL LEIOMYOMA

Microscopic Features

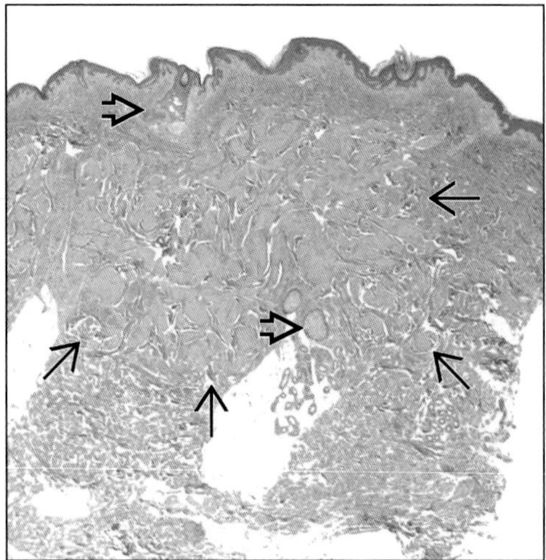

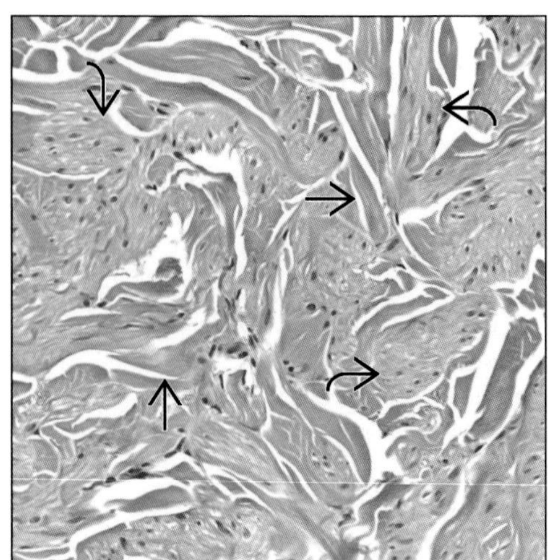

(Left) *Low-power image shows a superficial (pilar) leiomyoma involving the majority of the dermis. The lesion is unencapsulated and vaguely circumscribed but does have an irregular border* ➔ *with displacement of dermal appendages* ⇨. ***(Right)*** *At higher power, superficial leiomyomas consist of short fascicles or bundles of smooth muscle* ↱ *haphazardly arranged within the dermis and tend to dissect between dermal collagen bundles* ➔.

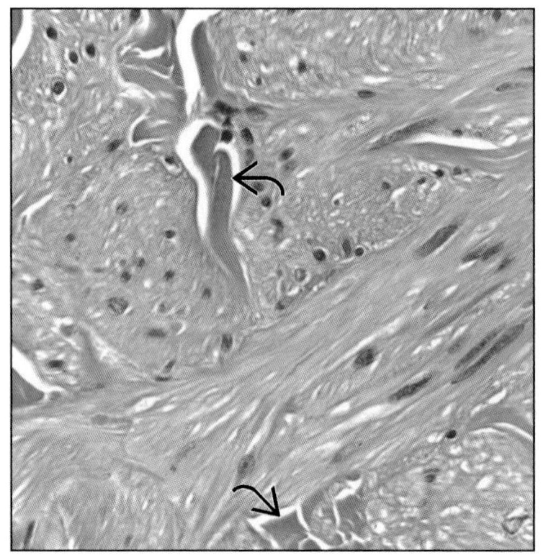

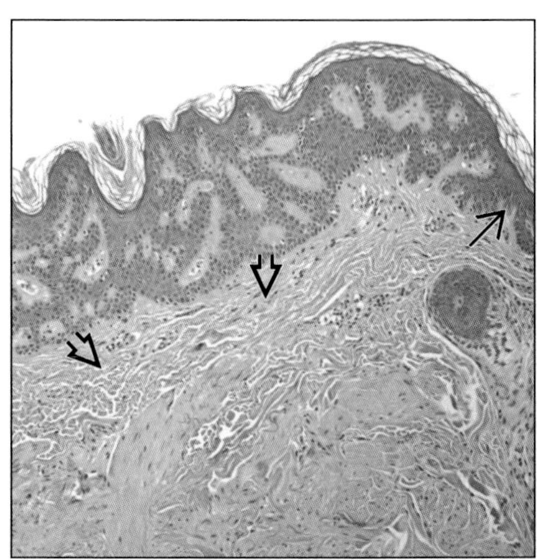

(Left) *The smooth muscle fascicles/bundles consist of elongated spindled cells with abundant fibrillary eosinophilic cytoplasm. Nuclei are oval with blunt ends (cigar-shaped) and show little cytologic atypia or mitotic activity. Note the characteristic pattern of fascicles dissecting between dermal collagen bundles* ↱. ***(Right)*** *Many superficial leiomyomas have a Grenz zone* ⇨ *and epidermal hyperplasia, such as this case with elongated rete pegs adjacent to normal epidermis* ➔.

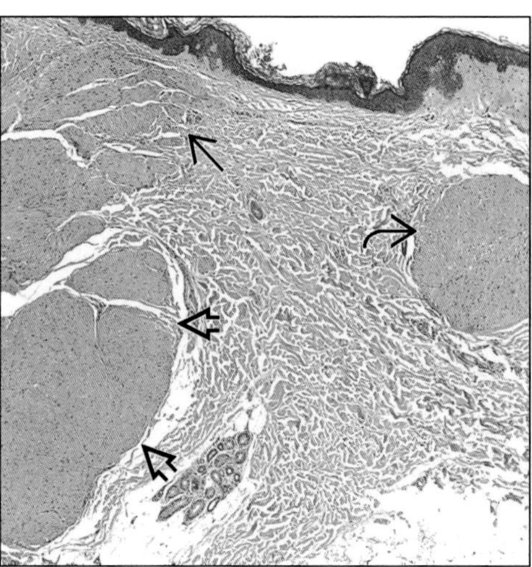

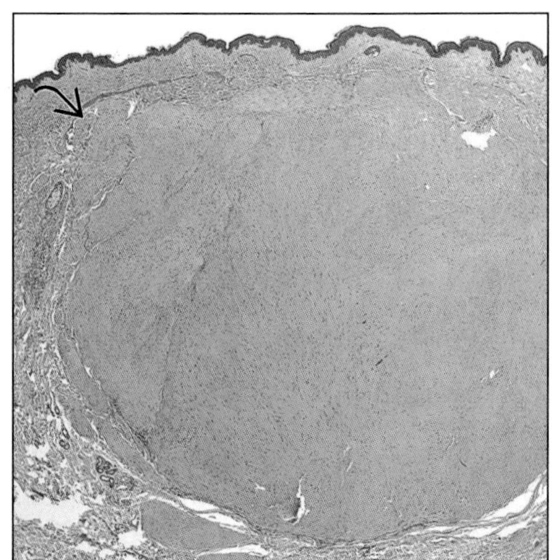

(Left) *Surgical specimens often reveal incipient pilar leiomyomas* ↱ *adjacent to the primary tumor. The primary tumor in this example does show areas of circumscription* ⇨, *but other areas have the more typical infiltrative pattern* ➔. ***(Right)*** *Rare examples of superficial leiomyoma are well circumscribed, such as this solitary lesion, which shows only focal areas with an irregular border* ↱. *Solitary lesions such as this 1, more often present without pain symptoms.*

Microscopic Features and Differential Diagnosis

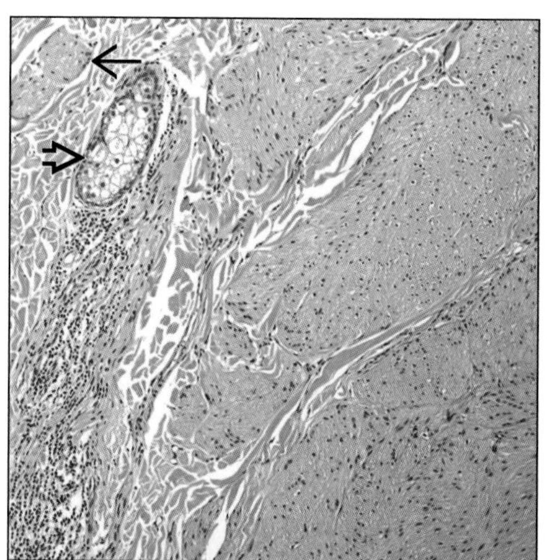

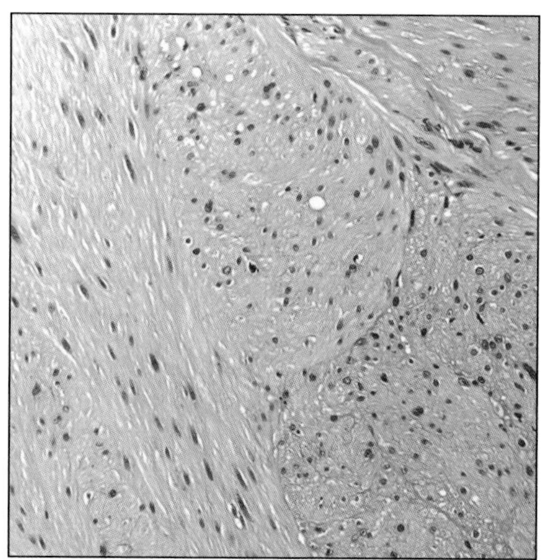

*(**Left**) Similar to typical superficial leiomyomas, solitary and circumscribed cutaneous leiomyomas can arise from the pilar smooth muscle. This solitary and circumscribed tumor was located adjacent to a sebaceous gland ⇨ and pilar smooth muscle bundle →, indicating likely origin from this pilosebaceous unit. (**Right**) Solitary superficial leiomyomas are less often characterized by small smooth muscle fascicles intersecting between dermal collagen and are more often solid tumors.*

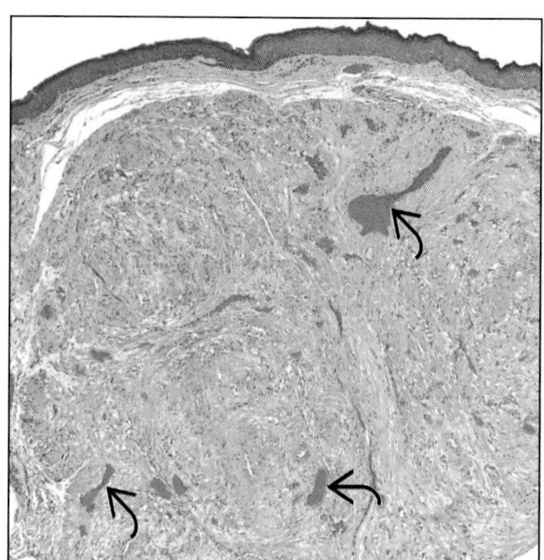

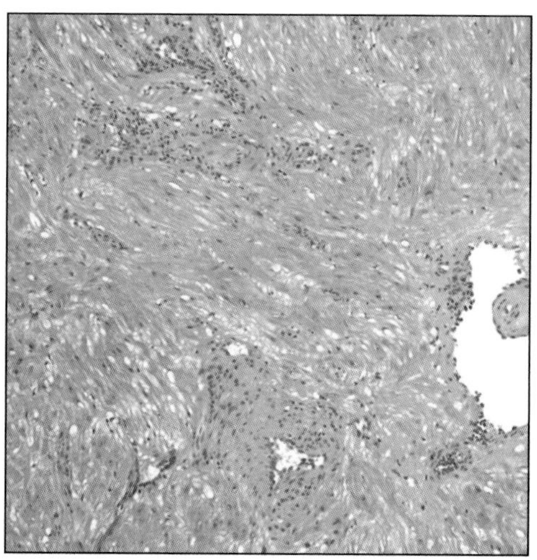

*(**Left**) In contrast to superficial leiomyomas, angiomyomas are usually circumscribed and contain numerous variably sized slit-like vascular channels that stand out at low power ↶. In addition, they are usually solitary and located in the lower extremity. (**Right**) Sheets of smooth muscle cells with abundant fibrillary eosinophilic cytoplasm intimately associated with thick-walled, often slit-like vascular channels characterize angiomyomas at higher power.*

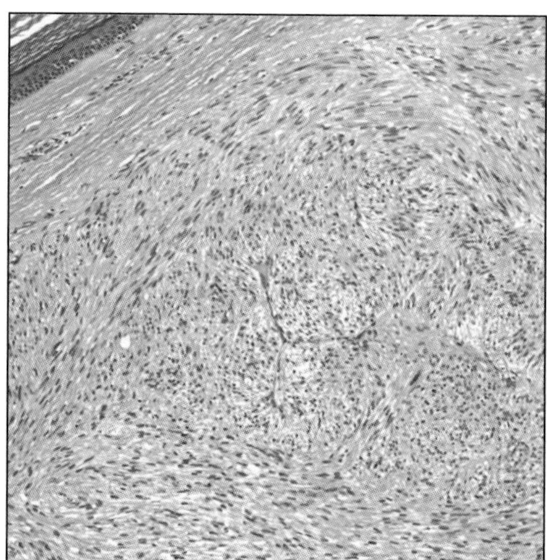

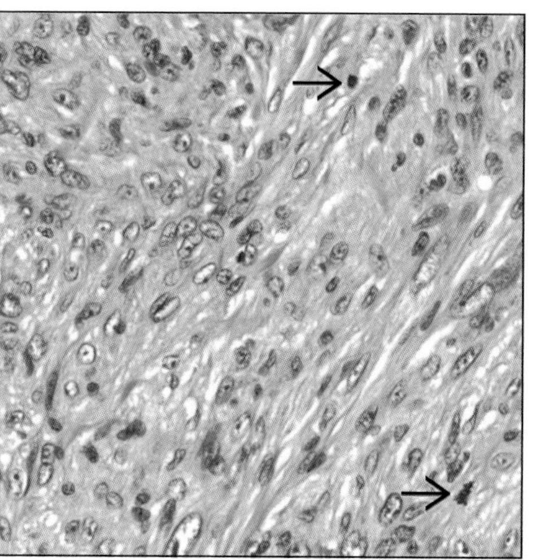

*(**Left**) Superficial leiomyosarcomas also consist of fascicles of cells with abundant fibrillary eosinophilic cytoplasm with blunt-ended oval nuclei. However, these are more cellular and demonstrate less dissection of dermal collagen. They are usually solitary and larger as compared to superficial leiomyomas. (**Right**) At higher power, superficial leiomyosarcomas will show moderate to marked nuclear atypia with higher nuclear-to-cytoplasmic ratios and frequent mitotic figures →.*

DEEP LEIOMYOMA

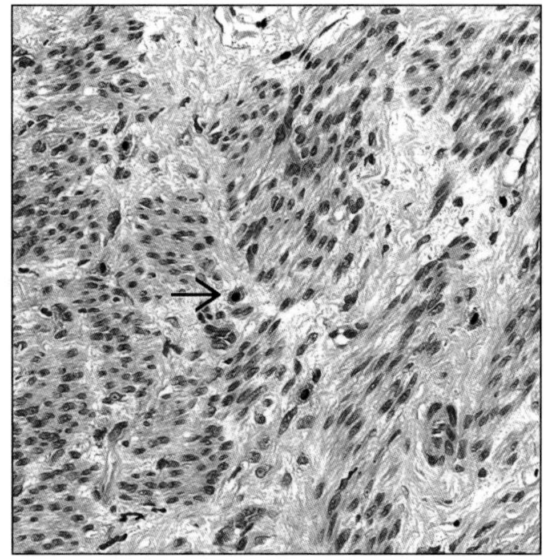

Hematoxylin & eosin shows short fascicles of uniform spindle cells with blunt- or round-ended nuclei and eosinophilic cytoplasm. There is a fibrous stroma with scattered mast cells ➔.

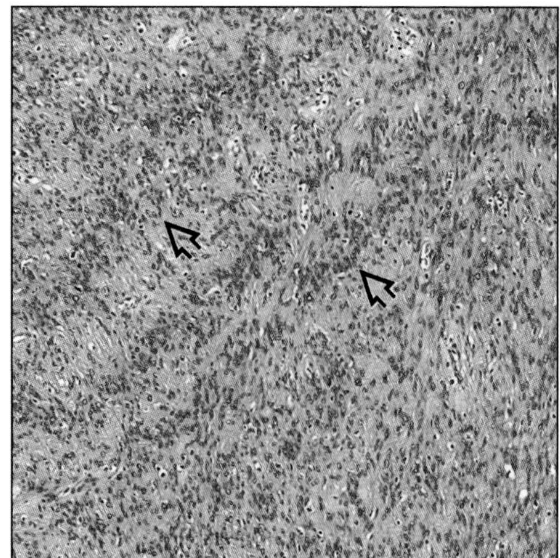

Hematoxylin & eosin shows nuclear palisading ➢. This is more common in retroperitoneal leiomyomas in females, which resemble those of the uterus. This should not be misinterpreted as a schwannoma.

TERMINOLOGY

Definitions

- Benign smooth muscle tumor involving deep soft tissue of limbs or retroperitoneum

CLINICAL ISSUES

Epidemiology

- Incidence
  - Rare: 4% of benign soft tissue tumors
- Age
  - 4th-6th decade of life
- Gender
  - M < F

Site

- Deep subcutis or subfascial in limbs
- Retroperitoneum, especially in females
  - Resemble uterine leiomyomas

Presentation

- Painless mass
- Slow growing

Treatment

- Simple excision

Prognosis

- Benign tumor
- Correctly diagnosed cases do not recur or metastasize

MACROSCOPIC FEATURES

General Features

- Well circumscribed
- Gray-white cut surface
- Myxoid areas
- Foci of calcification
- Rare cystic change
- Necrosis absent

Size

- 5-20 cm
- Retroperitoneal tumors can reach very large size

MICROSCOPIC PATHOLOGY

Predominant Pattern/Injury Type

- Sheets

Predominant Cell/Compartment Type

- Smooth muscle

Key Microscopic Features

- Short fascicles or nests of uniform spindle-shaped smooth muscle cells
  - Nontapered nuclei
  - Abundant eosinophilic cytoplasm
- Focal epithelioid cell morphology
- No nuclear pleomorphism
  - Occasional degenerative atypia seen; no nucleoli
- No necrosis
- No mitoses except in retroperitoneal tumors in females
  - Not exceeding 5 per 50 high-power fields (HPF)
    - 5-10 per 50 HPF = uncertain malignant potential
- Variable fibrosis, myxoid change, calcification
- Occasional foci of fat (lipoleiomyoma)

ANCILLARY TESTS

Electron Microscopy

- Transmission
  - Shows typical smooth muscle differentiation
    - Myofilament bundles with dense bodies throughout cytoplasm
    - Pinocytic vesicles, external lamina

DEEP LEIOMYOMA

Key Facts

Clinical Issues
- Rare: 4% of benign soft tissue tumors
- Slow-growing mass
- Usually painless
- Deep subcutis or subfascial in limbs in either sex
- Retroperitoneum, especially in females
  - Range of appearances like uterine leiomyoma

Macroscopic Features
- Well circumscribed
- Retroperitoneal tumors can reach very large size
- No necrosis
- No hemorrhage
- Focal myxoid change and cyst formation
- Foci of calcification

Microscopic Pathology
- Short fascicles of benign smooth muscle cells
- Focal epithelioid cell morphology
- No nuclear pleomorphism
- No necrosis
- No mitoses except in female retroperitoneum

Ancillary Tests
- Positive for actin-sm, desmin, HCAD
- ER, PR diffusely in female retroperitoneum

Top Differential Diagnoses
- Leiomyosarcoma
  - Any necrosis or pleomorphism
  - Any mitoses in deep somatic soft tissue leiomyomas

Immunohistochemistry

Antibody	Reactivity	Staining Pattern	Comment
Desmin	Positive	Cytoplasmic	Strong diffuse staining
Actin-sm	Positive	Cytoplasmic	Strong diffuse staining
Caldesmon	Positive	Cytoplasmic	Strong diffuse staining
ER	Positive	Nuclear	Diffuse staining in females; negative in males
PR	Positive	Nuclear	Diffuse staining in females; negative in males
CD34	Equivocal	Cell membrane	In occasional cases

DIFFERENTIAL DIAGNOSIS

Gastrointestinal Stromal Tumor
- Can have mitotic activity and necrosis
- Relation to bowel in most cases
- Immunoreactive for CD117, DOG1

Leiomyosarcoma
- Atypia, necrosis
- Presence of any mitoses in deep tumors in males
- > 10 mitoses per 50 HPF in retroperitoneal tumors in females
- Weak, focal, or absent staining for ER, PR

Cellular Schwannoma
- Encapsulated
- S100 protein diffusely positive
- Absence of smooth muscle antigens

PEComa
- Cells in nests separated by slender connective tissue septa
- Clear or finely granular cytoplasm
- Ovoid uniform nuclei
- HMB-45, Melan-A ,and actin-sm expressed
  - HCAD, desmin in some

DIAGNOSTIC CHECKLIST

Clinically Relevant Pathologic Features
- Organ distribution
  - Retroperitoneal in females

Pathologic Interpretation Pearls
- No necrosis or pleomorphism
- Mitoses absent except in retroperitoneal tumors in females
  - Diffuse nuclear immunoreactivity for ER, PR

SELECTED REFERENCES

1. Miettinen M et al: Evaluation of biological potential of smooth muscle tumours. Histopathology. 48(1):97-105, 2006
2. Hornick JL et al: Criteria for malignancy in nonvisceral smooth muscle tumors. Ann Diagn Pathol. 7(1):60-6, 2003
3. Weiss SW: Smooth muscle tumors of soft tissue. Adv Anat Pathol. 9(6):351-9, 2002
4. Billings SD et al: Do leiomyomas of deep soft tissue exist? An analysis of highly differentiated smooth muscle tumors of deep soft tissue supporting two distinct subtypes. Am J Surg Pathol. 25(9):1134-42, 2001
5. Paal E et al: Retroperitoneal leiomyomas: a clinicopathologic and immunohistochemical study of 56 cases with a comparison to retroperitoneal leiomyosarcomas. Am J Surg Pathol. 25(11):1355-63, 2001
6. Horiuchi K et al: Multiple smooth muscle tumors arising in deep soft tissue of lower limbs with uterine leiomyomas. Am J Surg Pathol. 22(7):897-901, 1998
7. Fletcher CD et al: The difficulty in predicting behavior of smooth-muscle tumors in deep soft tissue. Am J Surg Pathol. 19(1):116-7, 1995
8. Kilpatrick SE et al: Leiomyoma of deep soft tissue. Clinicopathologic analysis of a series. Am J Surg Pathol. 18(6):576-82, 1994

DEEP LEIOMYOMA

Microscopic Features

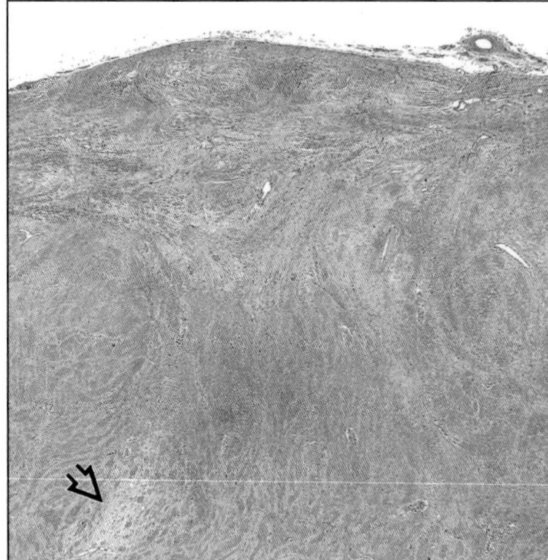

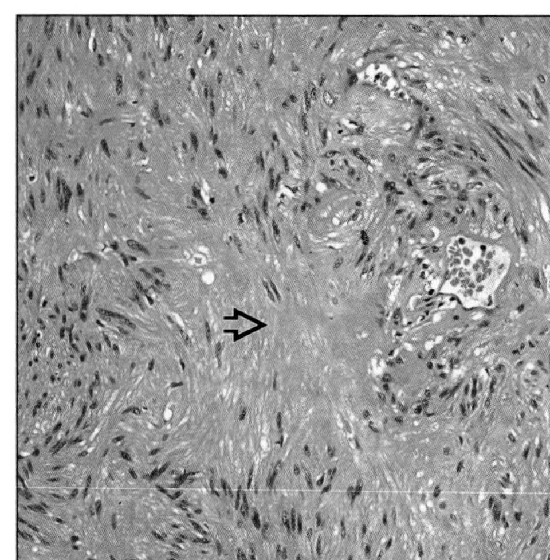

(Left) *A deep leiomyoma with a circumscribed (but nonencapsulated) margin is apparent. The tumor shows variable cellularity and focal myxoid change ⇨. This differs from a schwannoma, which is usually encapsulated.* ***(Right)*** *A deep leiomyoma with focus of stromal collagenization ⇨ is seen. This appearance can resemble that of schwannoma, especially when there are hyalinized or thrombotic vessels nearby. Such areas can also undergo hyalinization or calcification.*

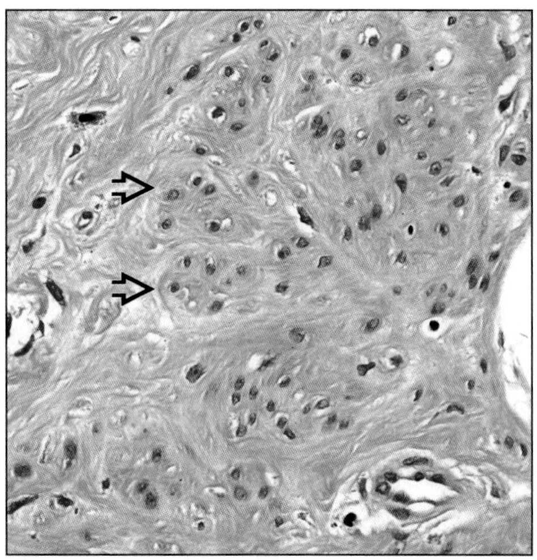

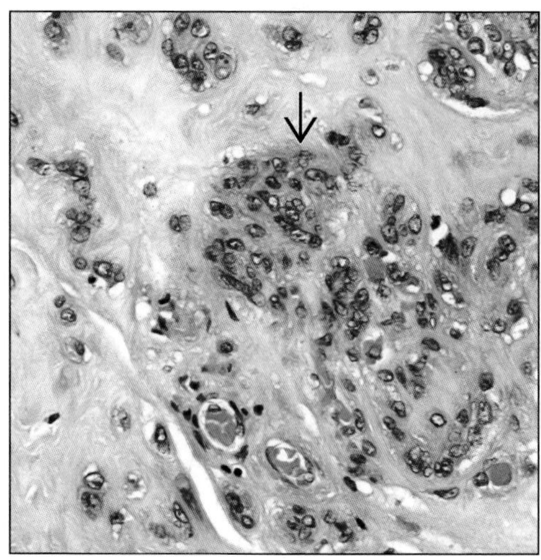

(Left) *Hematoxylin & eosin shows small nests of cells with epithelioid change ⇨. The cells are rounded with uniform nuclei and eosinophilic cytoplasm. The cell margins are focally distinct.* ***(Right)*** *Clusters and short cords of epithelioid smooth muscle cells → are visible in hyalinized stroma. The nuclei are rounded, focally vesicular, and lack atypia or mitotic activity. This is usually a focal finding in deep leiomyoma, with other areas showing more typical spindle cells.*

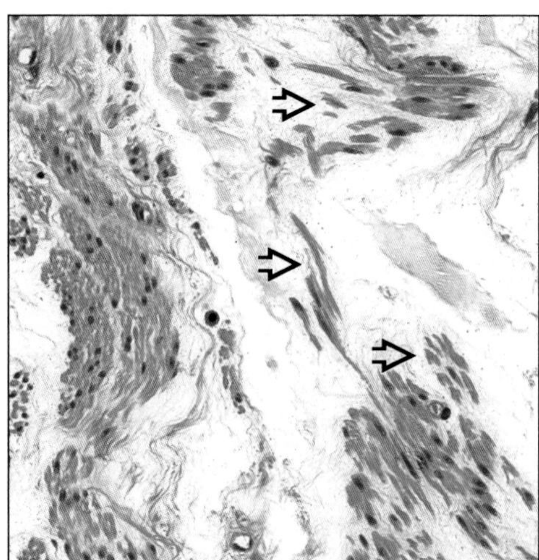

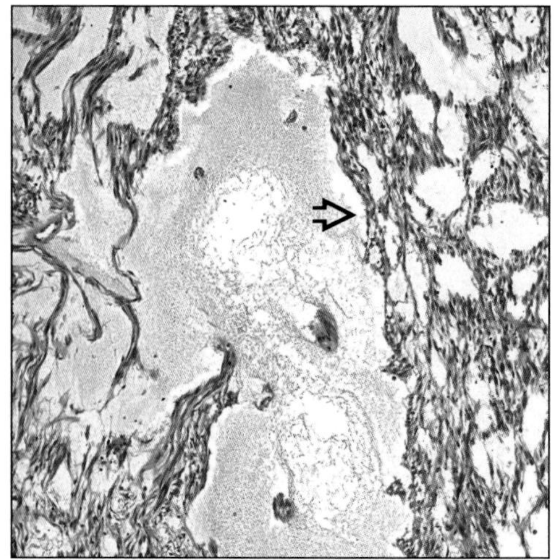

(Left) *Hematoxylin & eosin shows stromal myxoid change. The muscle bundles are separated by variable amounts of myxoid stroma, which in places dissects between single cells ⇨. Cell morphology is often more distinct in the single cells.* ***(Right)*** *Hematoxylin & eosin shows increased myxoid stromal change resulting in microcysts of varying size. Note the complex reticular pattern ⇨ in which cords of tumor cells are separated by accumulations of myxoid stroma.*

Microscopic and Immunohistochemical Features

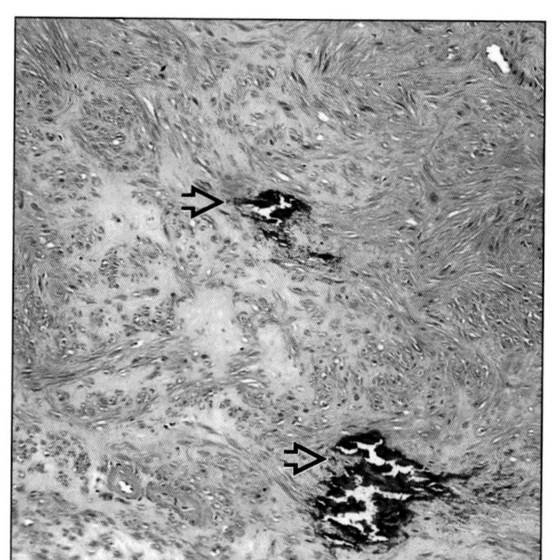

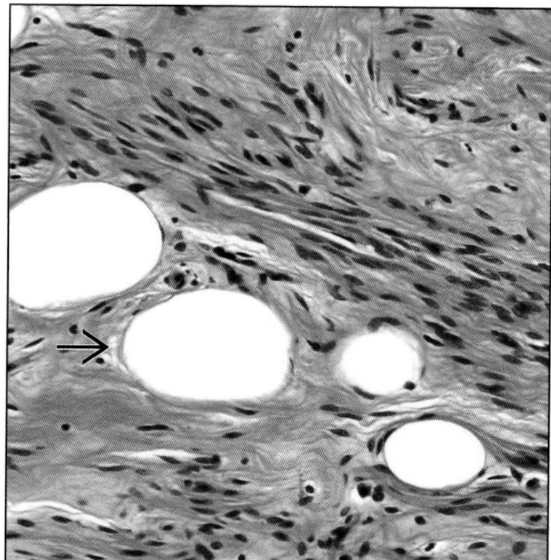

(Left) *Hematoxylin & eosin shows focal stromal calcification ⊳. This is a relatively common finding in a deep leiomyoma, especially in retroperitoneal examples, and can be detected by various imaging techniques. It is not associated with tumor necrosis.* ***(Right)*** *In this lipoleiomyoma, small islands of adipose tissue → are present within a benign smooth muscle tumor. This example arose in the retroperitoneum, but such tumors can also be found in the deep subcutis.*

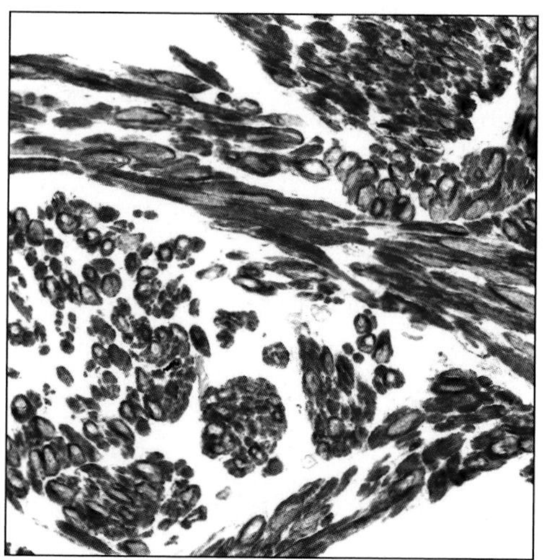

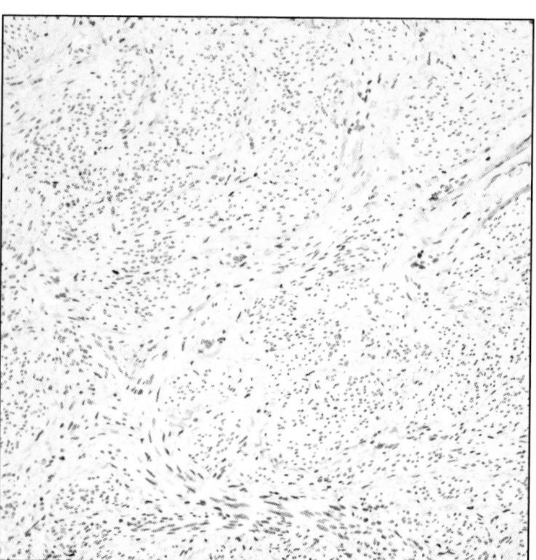

(Left) *Positive desmin shows strong diffuse immunoreactivity in tumor cell cytoplasm. Other smooth muscle markers, such as actin-sm and HCAD are also positive. Occasional examples are focally cytokeratin(+) also.* ***(Right)*** *This is a marker of cell proliferation and is usually found in very few nuclei in deep leiomyoma. In this example, Ki-67 staining is entirely negative, indicating a lack of cell proliferation. This is in parallel with an absence of mitotic activity.*

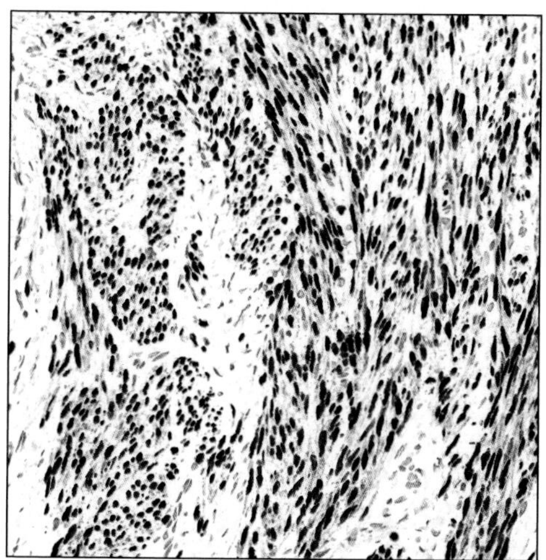

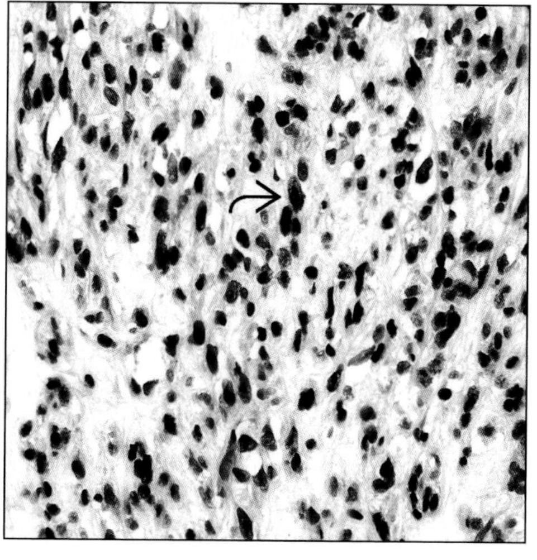

(Left) *The nuclei are diffusely and strongly reactive for hormone receptors in a deep leiomyoma of the female retroperitoneum. Such positivity is found in both spindled and epithelioid cells. Leiomyomas in males are negative. This contrasts with leiomyosarcoma, in which staining is focal, weak, or absent.* ***(Right)*** *Positive PR shows uniform staining confined to nuclei of lesional cells ⇗. This is a typical finding in deep leiomyoma. PR is negative in deep leiomyoma of the extremities.*

LEIOMYOMATOSIS PERITONEALIS DISSEMINATA

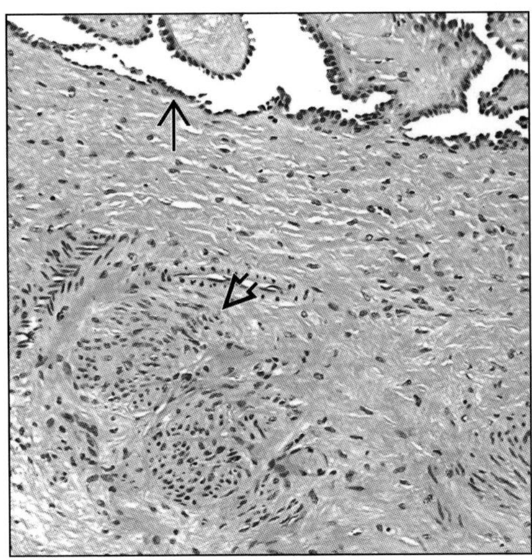

Hematoxylin & eosin shows ill-defined, variably sized nodules of spindled or ovoid cells ⇨ in a sparsely cellular fibrous stroma. Note relationship to peritoneal surface →.

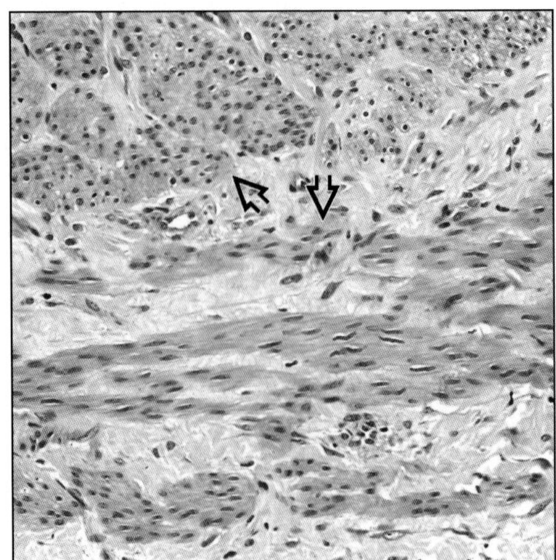

Hematoxylin & eosin shows smooth muscle bundles in transverse section with epithelioid-like cellular morphology ⇨.

TERMINOLOGY

Abbreviations

- Leiomyomatosis peritonealis disseminata (LPD)

Definitions

- Multiple smooth muscle-like deposits
  - In abdomen or pelvis
  - Beneath peritoneal surfaces

ETIOLOGY/PATHOGENESIS

Associated with

- Pregnancy
- Hormonal therapy
- Hormone-secreting tumors
- Rarely in patients with concomitant endometriosis
- Rarely familial

Genetic Analysis

- Clonality shown in multiple lesions

CLINICAL ISSUES

Epidemiology

- Incidence
  - Relatively uncommon
- Age
  - Fertile period
    - Especially in 4th decade
  - Very rarely postmenopausal
- Gender
  - Females
  - Very rarely in males
- Ethnicity
  - More common in African-Americans

Presentation

- Incidental finding
- Abdominal pain

Natural History

- Lesions regress if hormonal stimulus removed
- Can recur in subsequent pregnancy

Treatment

- Surgical approaches
  - Excision occasionally needed
- Drugs
  - Gonadotrophin-releasing hormone antagonists
  - Progestogens

Prognosis

- Excellent

MACROSCOPIC FEATURES

General Features

- Large number of separate nodules
  - Widespread over parietal and visceral surfaces
  - Varying sizes
    - 0.5-5 cm diameter
  - Circumscribed or infiltrative

MICROSCOPIC PATHOLOGY

Histologic Features

- Subperitoneal nodules: 3 cell types
  - Majority composed of smooth muscle cells: Nontapered, round-ended nuclei, eosinophilic cytoplasm
  - Some composed of myofibroblasts: Tapered cells, ovoid pale nuclei, less cytoplasm
  - A few mainly fibroblastic: Tapered, pointed nuclei, inconspicuous cytoplasm
- No atypia or necrosis
- Mitoses rare: No abnormal forms
- Can be decidualized

LEIOMYOMATOSIS PERITONEALIS DISSEMINATA

Key Facts

Etiology/Pathogenesis
- Associated with
  - Pregnancy
  - Hormonal therapy
  - Hormone-secreting tumors

Clinical Issues
- Females
- Fertile period
  - Especially in 4th decade
- Throughout abdomen and pelvis

Microscopic Pathology
- Subperitoneal nodules
- Mature smooth muscle or myofibroblastic cells
- No atypia or necrosis

Ancillary Tests
- Smooth muscle: SMA, desmin, H-caldesmon, ER, and PR positive

- Stromal hyalinization in regressing lesions
- Rare component of endometriosis

Predominant Pattern/Injury Type
- Multinodular
- Fascicular

Predominant Cell/Compartment Type
- Spindle

ANCILLARY TESTS

Immunohistochemistry
- Smooth muscle type
  - SMA, desmin, H-caldesmon, ER, PR positive
- Myofibroblastic type
  - SMA, calponin positive

DIFFERENTIAL DIAGNOSIS

Metastatic Leiomyosarcoma
- Atypia, mitoses, necrosis
- Previous primary sarcoma

DIAGNOSTIC CHECKLIST

Clinically Relevant Pathologic Features
- Age distribution
- Organ distribution

Pathologic Interpretation Pearls
- Multiple subperitoneal foci
- Normal-looking smooth muscle

SELECTED REFERENCES

1. Halama N et al: Familial clustering of Leiomyomatosis peritonealis disseminata: an unknown genetic syndrome? BMC Gastroenterol. 5:33, 2005
2. Bristow RE et al: Leiomyomatosis peritonealis disseminata and ovarian Brenner tumor associated with tamoxifen use. Int J Gynecol Cancer. 11(4):312-5, 2001
3. Strinić T et al: Leiomyomatosis peritonealis disseminata in a postmenopausal woman. Arch Gynecol Obstet. 264(2):97-8, 2000
4. Quade BJ et al: Disseminated peritoneal leiomyomatosis. Clonality analysis by X chromosome inactivation and cytogenetics of a clinically benign smooth muscle proliferation. Am J Pathol. 150(6):2153-66, 1997
5. Tavassoli FA et al: Peritoneal leiomyomatosis (leiomyomatosis peritonealis disseminata): a clinicopathologic study of 20 cases with ultrastructural observations. Int J Gynecol Pathol. 1(1):59-74, 1982
6. Kaplan C et al: Leiomyomatosis peritonealis disseminata with endometrium. Obstet Gynecol. 55(1):119-22, 1980
7. Pieslor PC et al: Ultrastructure of myofibroblasts and decidualized cells in leiomyomatosis peritonealis disseminata. Am J Clin Pathol. 72(5):875-82, 1979
8. Parmley TH et al: Histogenesis of leiomyomatosis peritonealis disseminata (disseminated fibrosing deciduosis). Obstet Gynecol. 46(5):511-6, 1975
9. Crosland DB: Leiomyomatosis peritonealis disseminata: a case report. Am J Obstet Gynecol. 117(2):179-81, 1973

IMAGE GALLERY

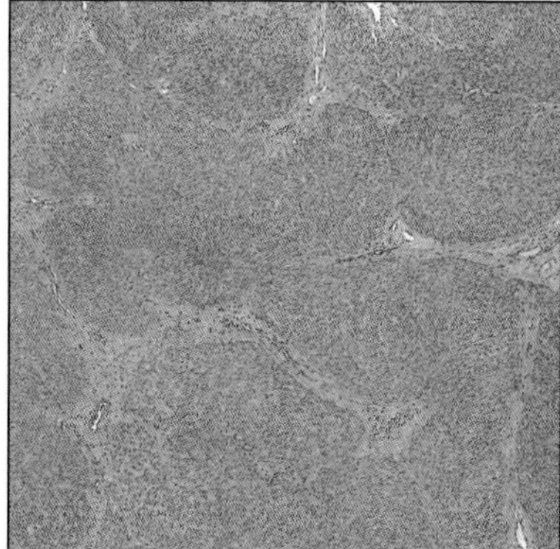

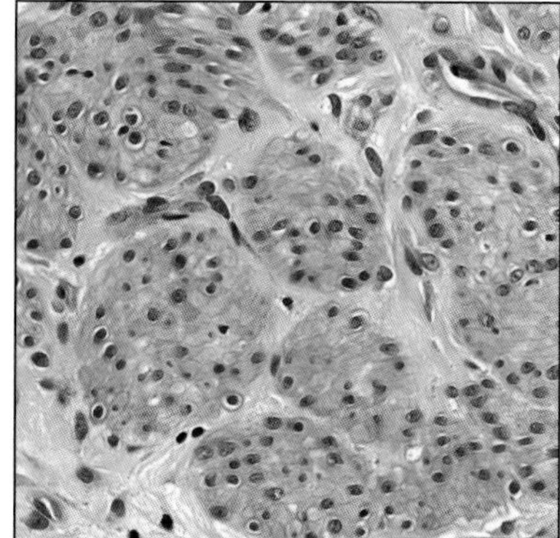

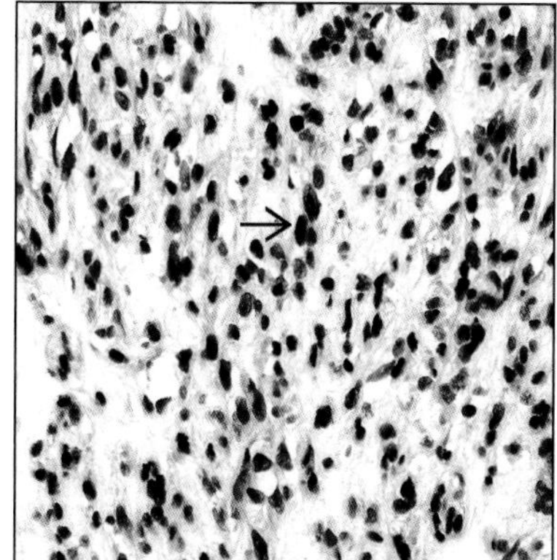

(Left) Hematoxylin & eosin shows multiple cellular nodules of varying size. (Center) Hematoxylin & eosin shows smooth muscle bundles in transverse section with epithelioid-like cellular morphology. (Right) ER shows diffuse nuclear immunoreactivity ⇒. Leiomyomatosis peritonealis disseminata can resemble normal uterine smooth muscle and display hormone receptor positivity.

INTRAVASCULAR LEIOMYOMATOSIS

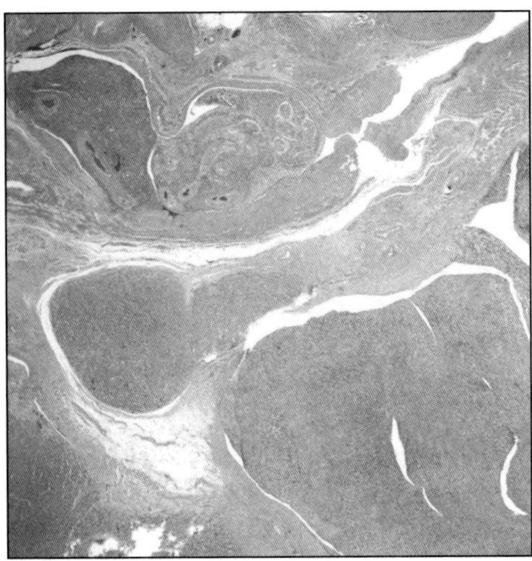

Hematoxylin & eosin from a hysterectomy specimen shows intravascular growth of the lesion, which is more cellular than the investing vessels.

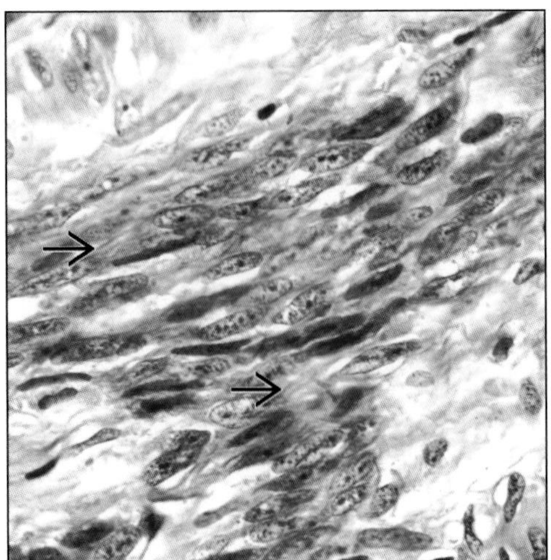

Hematoxylin & eosin shows the intravascular process at high magnification. Note the delicate longitudinal striations of the spindle cells →.

TERMINOLOGY

Synonyms

- Intravenous leiomyomatosis

Definitions

- Rare condition featuring growth of nodules of benign smooth muscle in veins of myometrium, some with extension into extrauterine veins

CLINICAL ISSUES

Presentation

- Not applicable
- Usually premenopausal women
  - Median age: Early 40s
- Abnormal vaginal bleeding
- Pelvic pain
- Enlarged uterus
- Some patients (10-20%) have tumor extending into vena cava or heart
  - Present with cardiac symptoms

Prognosis

- Overall good
- Most patients cured by hysterectomy
- About 30% experience persistence of disease
  - Occasional cases fatal
    - Extension into hepatic veins, heart, or lungs
  - Can result in presentation as "benign metastasizing leiomyomas"

MACROSCOPIC FEATURES

General Features

- Coiled myometrial masses
- Some lesions extend grossly into uterine veins in broad ligament

MICROSCOPIC PATHOLOGY

Histologic Features

- Intravascular proliferation of lesion, showing features of gynecologic leiomyoma
  - Nodules of intravascular lesion can be richly vascular themselves
  - Some cases believed to arise in vessels whereas others may be associated with extravascular leiomyoma
- Spindle cells with eosinophilic cytoplasm
  - Delicate longitudinal striations can be seen
- Blunt-ended to tapered nuclei
  - Bipolar configuration
  - Smooth nuclear membranes
  - Inconspicuous nucleoli
- Minimal mitotic activity

DIFFERENTIAL DIAGNOSIS

Plexiform Nerve Sheath Tumors

- Extravascular lesions
- Plexiform neurofibroma essentially diagnostic of neurofibromatosis type 1 (NF1)
- Plexiform schwannomas can be associated with neurofibromatosis type 2 (NF2)
- Strong S100 protein expression

Leiomyoma

- Extravascular lesions
- Brightly eosinophilic cells arranged in perpendicular arrays
- Blunt-ended pale nuclei
- Paranuclear vacuoles
- Minimal mitotic activity
- Expresses actin, desmin, calponin, caldesmon
  - Usually S100 protein(-)
- Female genital tract leiomyomas express hormone receptors

INTRAVASCULAR LEIOMYOMATOSIS

Key Facts

Terminology

- Rare condition featuring growth of nodules of benign smooth muscle in veins of myometrium, some with extension into extrauterine veins

Clinical Issues

- Most patients cured by hysterectomy
  - Overall good prognosis
- About 30% experience persistence of disease
- Occasional cases fatal
  - Extension into hepatic veins, heart, or lungs
- Can result in presentation as "benign metastasizing leiomyomas"

Microscopic Pathology

- Intravascular proliferation of lesion, showing features of a gynecologic leiomyoma
- No atypia or necrosis
- ER(+) and PR(+)

Immunohistochemistry

Antibody	Reactivity	Staining Pattern	Comment
Desmin	Positive	Cytoplasmic	Immunohistochemical profile is essentially identical to that of uterine leiomyomas
Actin-sm	Positive	Cytoplasmic	
Calponin	Positive	Cytoplasmic	
Caldesmon	Positive	Cytoplasmic	
ER	Positive	Nuclear	
PR	Positive	Nuclear	

- Estrogen receptor and progesterone receptor

Leiomyosarcoma

- Criteria for malignancy differ between gynecologic sites and somatic soft tissues
  - In soft tissue sites, minimal mitotic activity sufficient for sarcoma diagnosis
  - In gynecologic sites, > 5 mitoses/high-power field suggested cutoff for sarcoma diagnosis
- Brightly eosinophilic fascicles arranged in perpendicular arrays
- Blunt-ended hyperchromatic nuclei
- Paranuclear vacuoles
- Expresses actin, desmin, calponin, caldesmon
  - ER and PR staining usually lost in female genital tract leiomyosarcomas

SELECTED REFERENCES

1. Kir G et al: Immunohistochemical profile of intravenous leiomyomatosis. Eur J Gynaecol Oncol. 25(4):481-3, 2004
2. Dal Cin P et al: Intravenous leiomyomatosis is characterized by a der(14)t(12;14)(q15;q24). Genes Chromosomes Cancer. 36(2):205-6, 2003
3. Quade BJ et al: Intravenous leiomyomatosis: molecular and cytogenetic analysis of a case. Mod Pathol. 15(3):351-6, 2002
4. Clement PB et al: Intravenous leiomyomatosis of the uterus. A clinicopathological analysis of 16 cases with unusual histologic features. Am J Surg Pathol. 12(12):932-45, 1988
5. Clement PB: Intravenous leiomyomatosis of the uterus. Pathol Annu. 23 Pt 2:153-83, 1988
6. Norris HJ et al: Mesenchymal tumors of the uterus. V. Intravenous leiomyomatosis. A clinical and pathologic study of 14 cases. Cancer. 36(6):2164-78, 1975

IMAGE GALLERY

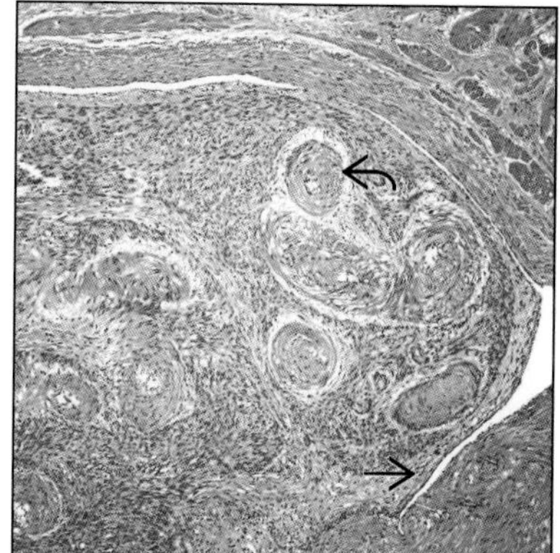

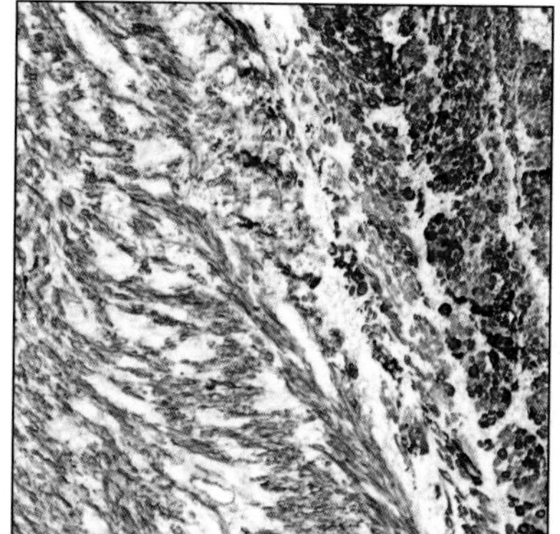

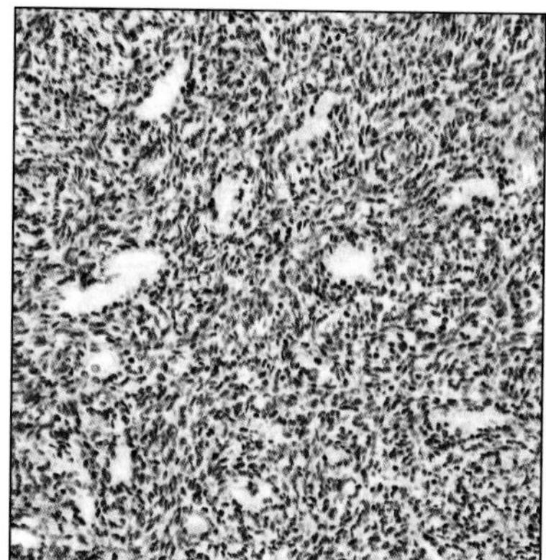

*(**Left**) Hematoxylin & eosin shows a vein containing the lesion. An endothelial-lined space is seen at the lower right ⇒. Note that the intravenous leiomyomatosis itself has prominent vessels ⇗. (**Center**) Actin-sm shows labeling of the lesional cells, as well as the investing vein seen on the right side of the field. Desmin shows a similar pattern. (**Right**) PR shows strong nuclear labeling in intravascular leiomyomatosis, a feature in common with other gynecologic leiomyomas. Similar labeling would be expected with ER.*

BENIGN METASTASIZING LEIOMYOMA

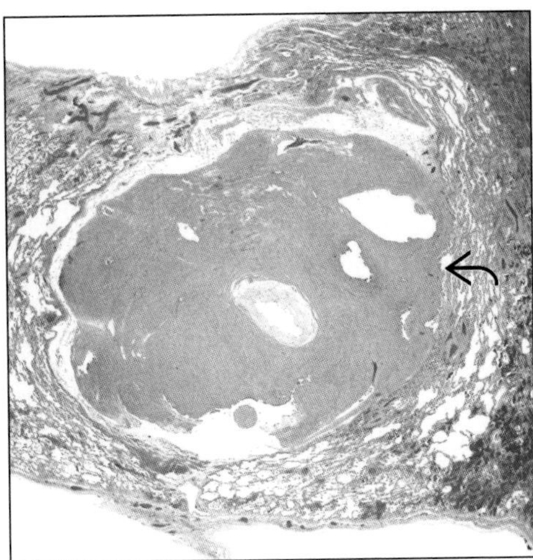

Hematoxylin & eosin show a well-marginated lung nodule detected in a woman with a remote history of a uterine leiomyoma. A vascular wall ➔ can be seen.

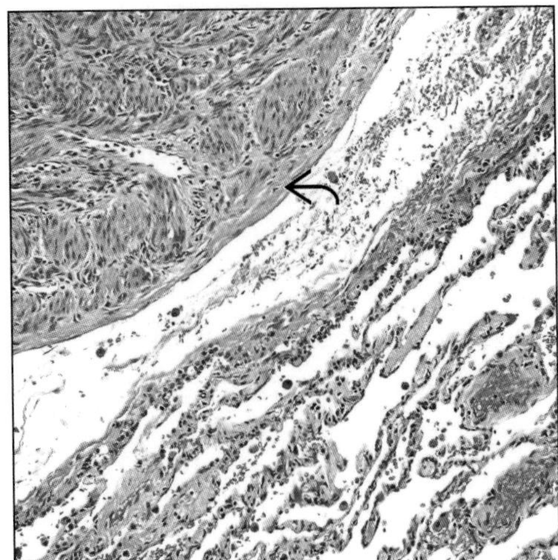

Hematoxylin & eosin shows the margin between this bland smooth muscle lesion and the surrounding lung. A compressed vessel wall surrounds the lesion ➔.

TERMINOLOGY

Abbreviations

- Benign metastasizing leiomyoma (BML)

Definitions

- Rare lesion usually typified by multiple benign-appearing smooth muscle neoplasms of lung in women with coexisting or past uterine leiomyoma
  - Subset associated with intravenous leiomyomatosis

CLINICAL ISSUES

Epidemiology

- Incidence
  - Rare
- Age
  - Late reproductive years
- Gender
  - Exclusively female

Presentation

- Many patients are asymptomatic
  - Occasional patients have respiratory or cardiac symptoms
    - Subset associated with cor pulmonale
    - Progressive dyspnea typical
  - Most cases involve lungs
    - Abdomen, lymph nodes, deep soft tissues, bone, heart, nervous system all reported sites
  - Typically long latency between hysterectomy for uterine leiomyoma and detection of extrauterine lesions
    - Median interval in largest series: 16 years

Natural History

- Disease may remain stable for many years

Treatment

- Surgical excision of metastases
- Hormonal manipulation
  - LHRH agonists
  - Antiestrogens
  - Aromatase inhibitors

Prognosis

- Overall good
- Reports of deaths from respiratory failure

MACROSCOPIC FEATURES

General Features

- Well-marginated nodules
- Typically involves 1 or both lungs

MICROSCOPIC PATHOLOGY

Histologic Features

- Lung lesions are identical to those of uterine leiomyomas
- Brightly eosinophilic cytoplasm
- Blunt-ended nuclei
- Essentially no mitotic activity
- Perpendicularly oriented hypocellular fascicles

ANCILLARY TESTS

Immunohistochemistry

- Identical to that of uterine leiomyomas
  - Desmin
  - Actin
  - Calponin
  - Caldesmon
  - ER
  - PR
  - Low Ki-67 labeling index (2-3%) as per uterine leiomyomas

BENIGN METASTASIZING LEIOMYOMA

Key Facts

Terminology
- Rare lesion usually typified by multiple benign-appearing smooth muscle neoplasms of lung in women with coexisting or past uterine leiomyoma

Clinical Issues
- Rare
- Late reproductive years
- Exclusively female
- Surgical excision of metastases
- Hormonal manipulation
- Overall good
- Reports of deaths from respiratory failure

Microscopic Pathology
- Lung lesions identical to those of uterine leiomyomas

Ancillary Tests
- Smooth muscle antigens positive
- ER(+) and PR(+)

DIFFERENTIAL DIAGNOSIS

Metastatic Leiomyosarcoma
- Features of malignancy
  - Atypia
  - Mitoses
  - Necrosis
- Different molecular and immunohistochemical profile from BML, same as uterine leiomyoma
  - Higher Ki-67 labeling index
  - Weak or absent immunolabeling for hormone receptors (ER and PR)
  - Shorter telomere length
  - Different micro-RNA pattern

Lymphangiomyomatosis (LAM)
- Typical in women in late reproductive years and multifocal
- Part of perivascular epithelioid cell family of tumors ("PEComa family")
  - Renal and extrarenal angiomyolipoma, clear cell myomelanocytic tumor
  - Clear cell tumor of lung (sugar tumor)
  - Clear cell myomelanocytic tumor
- "PEComa family" members co-label with smooth muscle markers and HMB-45
- Like BML, LAM often expresses hormone receptors ER and PR
  - Differs from leiomyoma by labeling with HMB-45

SELECTED REFERENCES

1. Nuovo GJ et al: Benign metastasizing leiomyoma of the lung: clinicopathologic, immunohistochemical, and micro-RNA analyses. Diagn Mol Pathol. 17(3):145-50, 2008
2. Patton KT et al: Benign metastasizing leiomyoma: clonality, telomere length and clinicopathologic analysis. Mod Pathol. 19(1):130-40, 2006
3. Rivera JA et al: Hormonal manipulation of benign metastasizing leiomyomas: report of two cases and review of the literature. J Clin Endocrinol Metab. 89(7):3183-8, 2004
4. Kayser K et al: Benign metastasizing leiomyoma of the uterus: documentation of clinical, immunohistochemical and lectin-histochemical data of ten cases. Virchows Arch. 437(3):284-92, 2000
5. Tietze L et al: Benign metastasizing leiomyoma: a cytogenetically balanced but clonal disease. Hum Pathol. 31(1):126-8, 2000
6. Esteban JM et al: Benign metastasizing leiomyoma of the uterus: histologic and immunohistochemical characterization of primary and metastatic lesions. Arch Pathol Lab Med. 123(10):960-2, 1999
7. Jautzke G et al: Immunohistological detection of estrogen and progesterone receptors in multiple and well differentiated leiomyomatous lung tumors in women with uterine leiomyomas (so-called benign metastasizing leiomyomas). A report on 5 cases. Pathol Res Pract. 192(3):215-23, 1996
8. Gal AA et al: Leiomyomatous neoplasms of the lung: a clinical, histologic, and immunohistochemical study. Mod Pathol. 2(3):209-16, 1989

IMAGE GALLERY

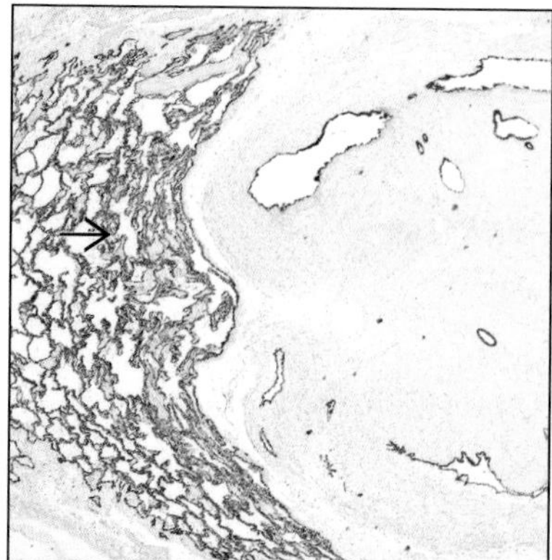

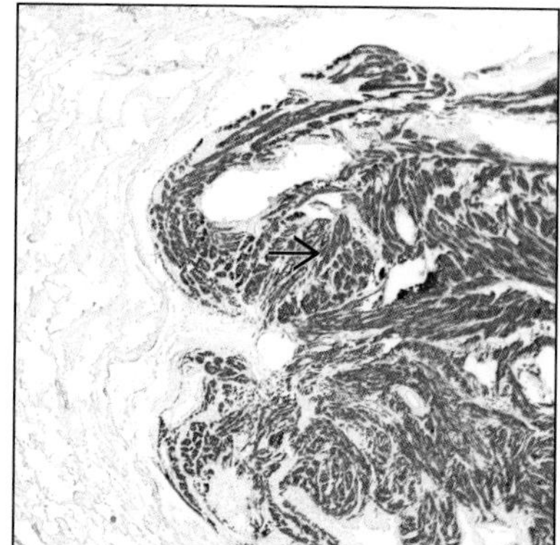

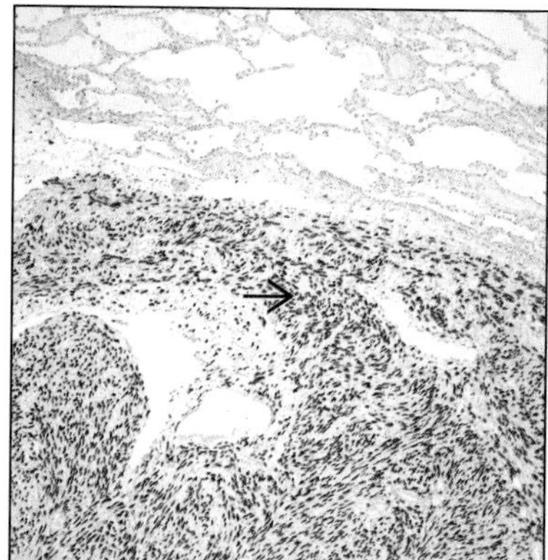

(Left) *Negative CK-PAN shows labeling in the surrounding ⇒ lung tissue but not in the lesion.* ***(Center)*** *Positive desmin shows strong immunolabeling in the lesional cells ⇒.* ***(Right)*** *Positive ER strongly labels the nuclei ⇒. As a general rule, benign smooth muscle neoplasms of the female genital tract express hormone receptors, which are often lost in leiomyosarcomas.*

MAMMARY-TYPE MYOFIBROBLASTOMA

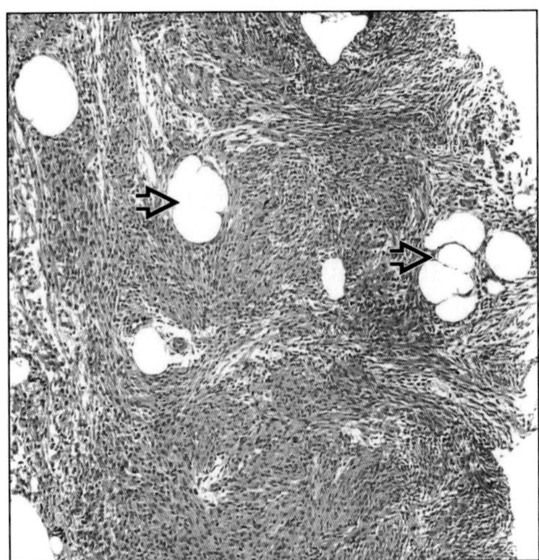

Hematoxylin & eosin shows a cellular spindle cell proliferation incorporating subcutaneous fat ⇨.

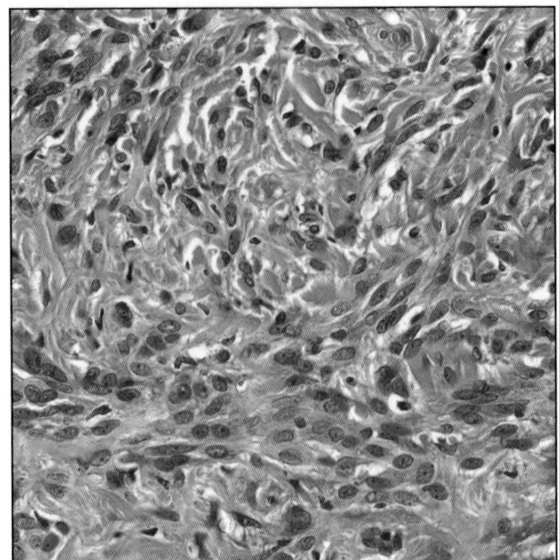

Hematoxylin & eosin shows short uniform spindle cells arranged in fascicles and cords, infiltrating between collagen bundles.

TERMINOLOGY

Synonyms

- Mammary myofibroblastoma
- Extramammary myofibroblastoma

Definitions

- Benign spindle cell lesion of modified smooth muscle cells in fibrous and fatty stroma
- Originally described in breast
- Also occurs in soft tissue locations including in "milk-line"
  - Subcutis
    - Inguinal region most common

CLINICAL ISSUES

Epidemiology

- Incidence
  - Rare
  - Mainly inguinal region
- Age
  - 4th-7th decades (mean age: 55)
- Gender
  - Predominantly males

Presentation

- Painless mass

Treatment

- Surgical approaches
  - Simple excision is usually curative

Prognosis

- Excellent: Reported cases have not recurred or metastasized

MACROSCOPIC FEATURES

General Features

- Circumscribed, nonencapsulated
- Firm to hard, whorled cut surface
- Tan, yellow, or white

Size

- Between 2-13 cm diameter (median: 6 cm)

MICROSCOPIC PATHOLOGY

Histologic Features

- Bland spindle cells, rare focal atypia
- Rarely epithelioid
- Tapered or ovoid nuclei, moderate eosinophilic cytoplasm
- Mitoses up to 6 per 10 HPF
- Irregular collagen bands, mast cells
- Mature adipose tissue, variable amount
- Rare chondroid metaplasia
- Rare hemangiopericytic pattern

Predominant Pattern/Injury Type

- Spindled

Predominant Cell/Compartment Type

- Smooth muscle cell
- Myofibroblast

ANCILLARY TESTS

Cytogenetics

- Monosomy of 13q, 16q
- Loss at RB/13q14 and FKHR/13q14 loci

Electron Microscopy

- Transmission
  - Suggests modified smooth muscle differentiation

MAMMARY-TYPE MYOFIBROBLASTOMA

Key Facts

Terminology
- Benign spindle cell lesion of modified smooth muscle cells in fibrous and fatty stroma

Clinical Issues
- Identical to mammary myofibroblastoma
- Rare, mainly inguinal region
- 4th-7th decades (mean age: 55), mostly in males
- Simple excision is usually curative

Microscopic Pathology
- Bland spindle cells
- Rare focal atypia or epithelioid appearance
- Mitoses up to 6 per 10 HPF
- Adipose tissue component
- Coexpression of desmin and CD34

Top Differential Diagnoses
- Spindle cell lipoma
- Solitary fibrous tumor

Immunohistochemistry

Antibody	Reactivity	Staining Pattern	Comment
CD34	Positive	Cell membrane & cytoplasm	90% of cases
Desmin	Positive	Cytoplasmic	75% of cases
Actin-sm	Positive	Cytoplasmic	25% of cases
HCAD	Positive	Cytoplasmic	50% of mammary myofibroblastomas, 2-10% of cells

DIFFERENTIAL DIAGNOSIS

Spindle Cell Lipoma
- Different location: Neck or back
- Myxoid areas
- Rarely desmin(+)
- Similar cytogenetic findings

Solitary Fibrous Tumor
- Variable cellularity: Fibrous and cellular areas
- Hemangiopericytic pattern
- CD34(+), desmin(-)
- Lacks the genetic features

Cellular Angiofibroma
- In genital and inguinal areas
- Approximately equal sex distribution
- More prominent vascular pattern
- Desmin(-)
- Similar cytogenetic findings

SELECTED REFERENCES

1. Maggiani F et al: Cellular angiofibroma: another mesenchymal tumour with 13q14 involvement, suggesting a link with spindle cell lipoma and (extra)-mammary myofibroblastoma. Histopathology. 51(3):410-2, 2007
2. Mukonoweshuro P et al: Paratesticular mammary-type myofibroblastoma. Histopathology. 50(3):396-7, 2007
3. Maggiani F et al: Extramammary myofibroblastoma is genetically related to spindle cell lipoma. Virchows Arch. 449(2):244-7, 2006
4. Magro G et al: H-caldesmon expression in myofibroblastoma of the breast: evidence supporting the distinction from leiomyoma. Histopathology. 42(3):233-8, 2003
5. McMenamin ME et al: Mammary-type myofibroblastoma of soft tissue: a tumor closely related to spindle cell lipoma. Am J Surg Pathol. 25(8):1022-9, 2001
6. Wargotz ES et al: Myofibroblastoma of the breast. Sixteen cases of a distinctive benign mesenchymal tumor. Am J Surg Pathol. 11(7):493-502, 1987

IMAGE GALLERY

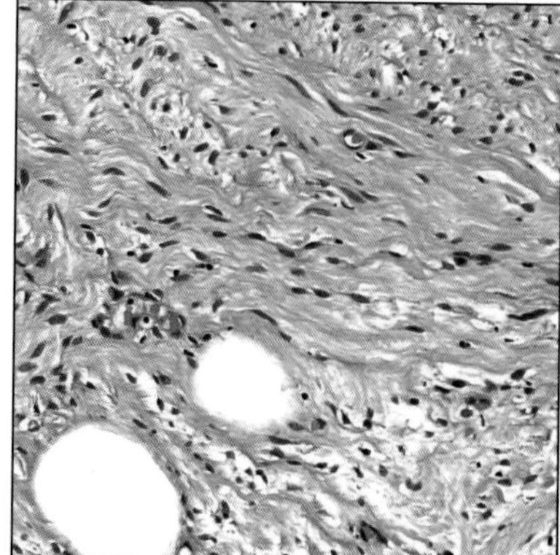

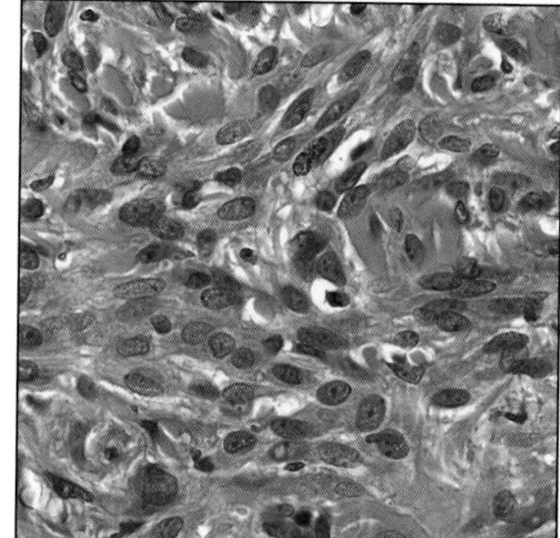

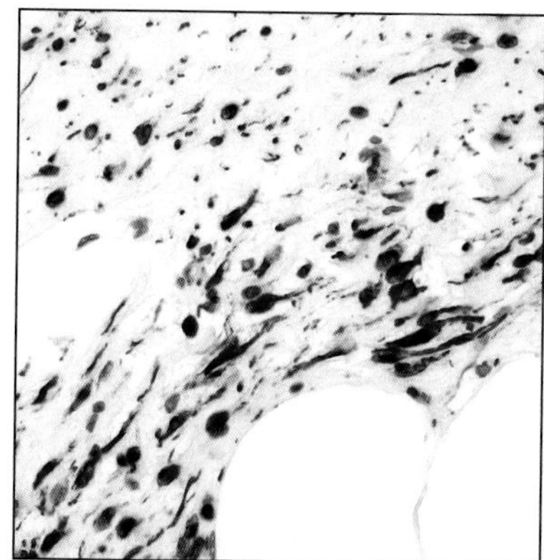

*(**Left**) Hematoxylin & eosin shows an area of low cellularity with slender spindle cells dispersed between collagen fibers. (**Center**) Hematoxylin & eosin shows more cellular area. The cells have ovoid nuclei with punctate nucleoli, without pleomorphism, and with scanty eosinophilic cytoplasm. Note relationship to collagen bundles. (**Right**) Positive desmin shows focal cytoplasmic immunoreactivity in lesional cells.*

PALISADED MYOFIBROBLASTOMA

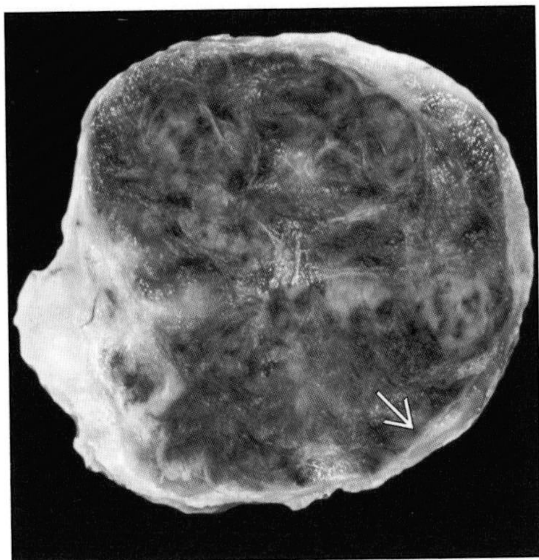

Gross pathology photograph shows a hemorrhagic tumor extensively replacing the lymph node. Residual nodal tissue is seen at the periphery ➡.

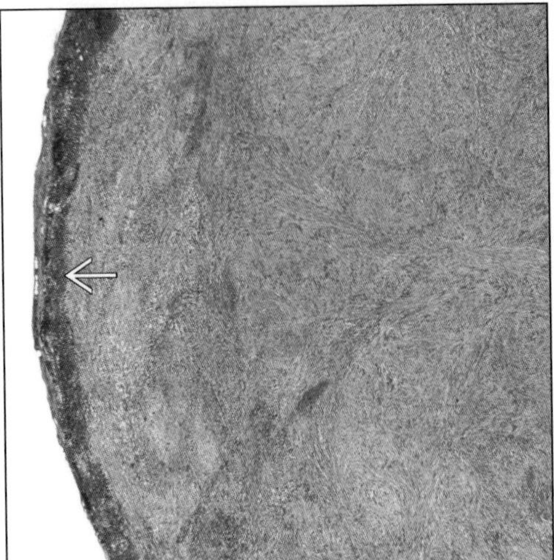

Hematoxylin & eosin shows a cellular tumor with irregular fascicles and vague palisades of uniform spindle cells. Note rim of compressed lymph node ➡.

TERMINOLOGY

Synonyms

- Intranodal hemorrhagic spindle cell tumor with amianthoid fibers
- Solitary spindle cell tumor with myoid differentiation of lymph node

Definitions

- Benign spindle cell tumor of modified smooth muscle cells in lymph node

CLINICAL ISSUES

Epidemiology

- Incidence
  - Rare
  - Mainly inguinal region
  - Occasionally in submandibular lymph node
  - Rarely multicentric
- Age
  - 5th and 6th decades
- Gender
  - Mostly in males

Presentation

- Painless mass

Treatment

- Surgical approaches
  - Lymphadenectomy is usually curative

Prognosis

- Excellent: Rarely recurs, no metastases reported

MACROSCOPIC FEATURES

General Features

- Circumscribed, replaces node to variable extent
- Solid
- Cut surface often dark red or black due to hemorrhage
- Paler firm areas

Size

- Up to 5 cm in diameter

MICROSCOPIC PATHOLOGY

Histologic Features

- Rim of lymph node tissue
- Uniform long spindle cells, rarely epithelioid change
- Focal palisading, often around hyalinized blood vessels
- Microhemorrhages with occasional sieve-like architecture
- Hemosiderin pigment
- Amianthoid fibers
  - Thick collagen fibers (280-1000 nm); normal: 8-150 nm in diameter
  - Radially disposed
  - Irregular rounded or stellate eosinophilic masses
  - Occasionally calcified

Predominant Pattern/Injury Type

- Spindled

Predominant Cell/Compartment Type

- Myofibroblast
- Smooth muscle cell

ANCILLARY TESTS

Immunohistochemistry

- Positive for actins and calponin
- Negative for
  - Desmin, H-caldesmon
  - S100 protein
  - CD31, CD34, HHV8
- Cyclin-D1 overexpressed

PALISADED MYOFIBROBLASTOMA

Key Facts

Terminology
- Benign spindle cell tumor of modified smooth muscle cells in lymph node

Clinical Issues
- Mainly inguinal region
- Mostly in males

Macroscopic Features
- Cut surface often dark red or black

Microscopic Pathology
- Rim of lymph node tissue
- Focal palisading, amianthoid fibers

Ancillary Tests
- Actin(+), desmin(-), and CD34(-)

Top Differential Diagnoses
- Kaposi sarcoma
- Schwannoma

Electron Microscopy
- Transmission
  - Features of smooth muscle or myofibroblastic differentiation
    - Moderate rough endoplasmic reticulum
    - Peripheral bundles of myofilaments
    - Fragments of external lamina

DIFFERENTIAL DIAGNOSIS

Kaposi Sarcoma
- Nuclear atypia
- Mitotic activity
- HHV8, CD34, CD31, D2-40 positive
- SMA(-)

Cellular Schwannoma
- Rare in lymph node
- S100 protein(+)

Leiomyoma
- Nuclei are blunt ended
- Cells arranged in rectilinear fascicles
- SMA, desmin, H-caldesmon positive

Solitary Fibrous Tumor
- Variable fibrosis and cellularity
- Hemangiopericytic pattern
- CD34(+)

DIAGNOSTIC CHECKLIST

Clinically Relevant Pathologic Features
- Tissue distribution
  - Located within lymph node

SELECTED REFERENCES

1. Nguyen T et al: Intranodal palisaded myofibroblastoma. Arch Pathol Lab Med. 131(2):306-10, 2007
2. Kleist B et al: Intranodal palisaded myofibroblastoma with overexpression of cyclin D1. Arch Pathol Lab Med. 127(8):1040-3, 2003
3. Eyden B et al: Intranodal myofibroblastoma: study of a case suggesting smooth-muscle differentiation. J Submicrosc Cytol Pathol. 33(1-2):157-63, 2001
4. Creager AJ et al: Recurrent intranodal palisaded myofibroblastoma with metaplastic bone formation. Arch Pathol Lab Med. 123(5):433-6, 1999
5. White JE et al: Intranodal leiomyoma or myofibroblastoma: an identical lesion? Histopathology. 26(2):188-90, 1995
6. Lee JY et al: Solitary spindle cell tumor with myoid differentiation of the lymph node. Arch Pathol Lab Med. 113(5):547-50, 1989
7. Suster S et al: Intranodal hemorrhagic spindle-cell tumor with "amianthoid" fibers. Report of six cases of a distinctive mesenchymal neoplasm of the inguinal region that simulates Kaposi's sarcoma. Am J Surg Pathol. 13(5):347-57, 1989
8. Weiss SW et al: Palisaded myofibroblastoma. A benign mesenchymal tumor of lymph node. Am J Surg Pathol. 13(5):341-6, 1989

IMAGE GALLERY

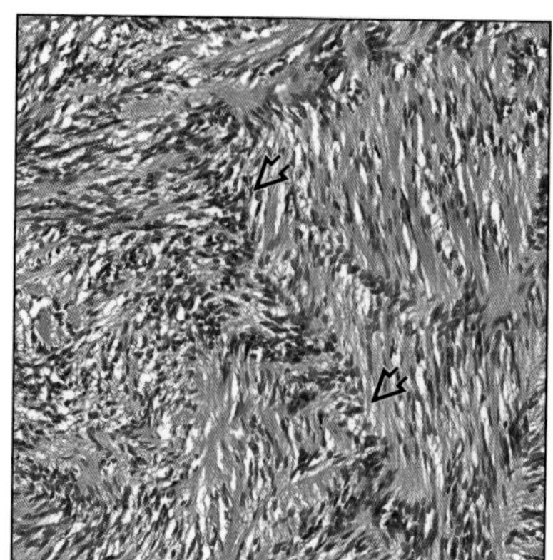

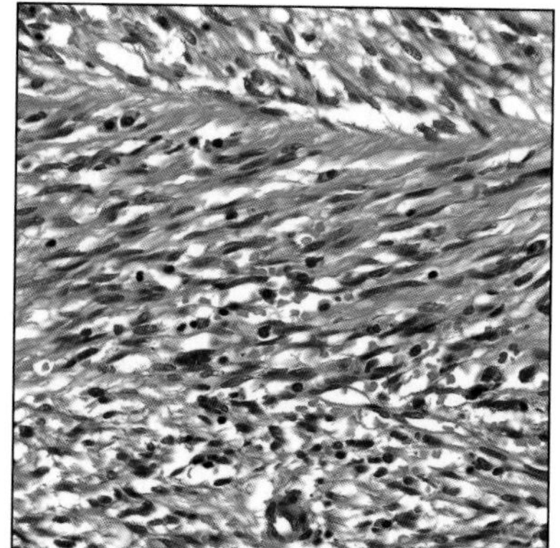

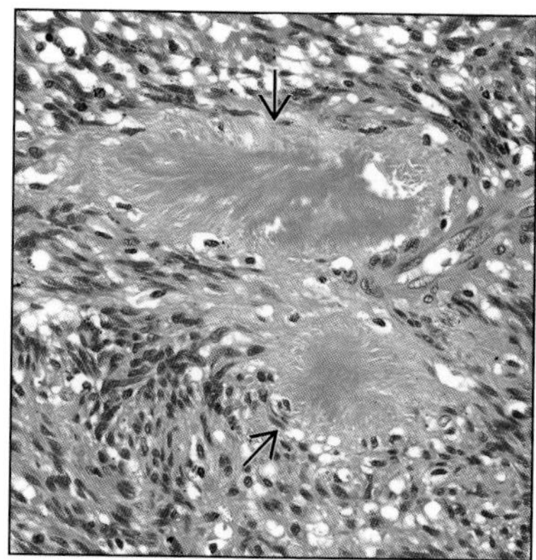

(Left) *Hematoxylin & eosin shows spindle cells with eosinophilic cytoplasm and elongated nuclei with focal palisading ⇨. The cells lack pleomorphism.* ***(Center)*** *Hematoxylin & eosin shows lesional cells with elongated nuclei. There is intercellular old and recent hemorrhage with extravasated red blood cells, hemosiderin pigment, and lymphocytes.* ***(Right)*** *Hematoxylin & eosin shows foci of amianthoid fibers composed of eosinophilic collagen bundles → among spindle cells. Note collagenous foci with a characteristic lighter peripheral zone.*

LEIOMYOSARCOMA

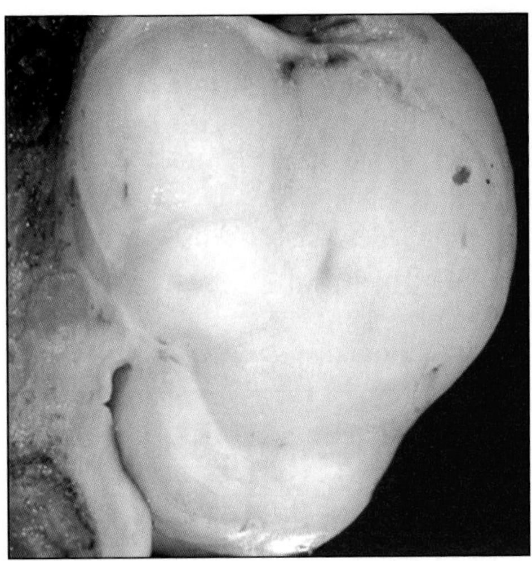

Gross pathology photograph shows a leiomyosarcoma arising in association with a large deep vessel. This is a common presentation of leiomyosarcomas.

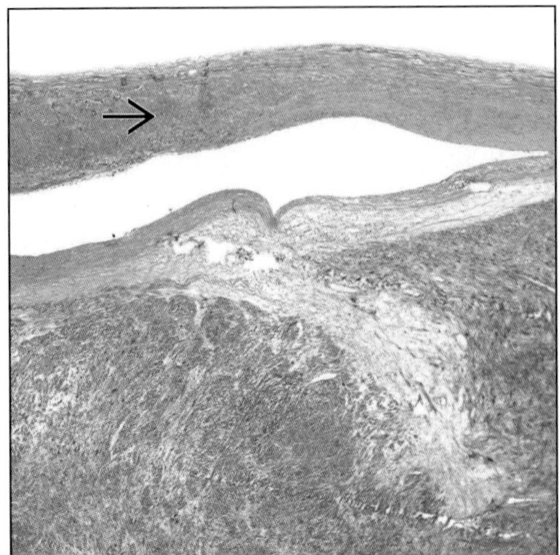

Hematoxylin & eosin shows a leiomyosarcoma associated with a large vein ⇒. Note that the cytoplasm of the lesional cells is brightly eosinophilic, identical to that of the vein.

TERMINOLOGY

Abbreviations

- Leiomyosarcoma (LMS)

Definitions

- Malignant neoplasm composed of cells exhibiting smooth muscle differentiation

ETIOLOGY/PATHOGENESIS

Infectious Agents

- Epstein-Barr virus associated in immunosuppressed patients
- Occasional examples associated with radiation

CLINICAL ISSUES

Epidemiology

- Incidence
  - Rare: 10-15% of extremity sarcomas
  - Most common overall sarcoma type if uterine and visceral examples are included
- Age
  - Middle-aged adults
- Gender
  - No gender preference overall
    - Retroperitoneal and inferior vena cava lesions more common in women

Presentation

- Deep soft tissue mass, often asymptomatic in extremities
  - Retroperitoneum most common site
    - Retroperitoneal lesions can be associated with abdominal pain
  - Vena cava examples often symptomatic
    - Upper portion: Budd-Chiari syndrome (hepatomegaly, jaundice, ascites)
    - Mid-portion: Renal obstruction
    - Lower portion: Lower extremity edema
- Uterine examples considered separately with unique diagnostic criteria

Treatment

- Surgical excision
  - Radiation
  - Chemotherapy

Prognosis

- Outcome depends on site and stage as per other sarcoma types
  - Lesions restricted to cutis essentially never metastasize
    - Some observers have advocated diagnosing them as "atypical smooth muscle tumors"
  - Subcutaneous lesions
    - Up to 1/3 of tumors metastasize
    - 10-20% of patients with subcutaneous lesion die of leiomyosarcoma
  - Retroperitoneum: About 80% of patients die of disease, typically with metastases
  - Bone: Metastases in up to 1/2 of patients
    - 5-year survival: 65%
  - Vena cava: 5- and 10-year survival: 50% and 30%, respectively
  - Head and neck
    - Few data available
    - Over 1/2 metastasize

MICROSCOPIC PATHOLOGY

Histologic Features

- Perpendicularly oriented fascicles of spindle cells
- Brightly eosinophilic cytoplasm
- Blunt-ended nuclei
- Nuclear atypia
- Some examples are epithelioid

LEIOMYOSARCOMA

Key Facts

Terminology

- Malignant neoplasm composed of cells exhibiting smooth muscle differentiation

Etiology/Pathogenesis

- Epstein-Barr virus-associated in immunosuppressed patients

Clinical Issues

- Retroperitoneal and inferior vena cava lesions more common in women
- Deep soft tissue mass, often asymptomatic in extremities
- Retroperitoneum most common site
- Site and stage dependent as per other sarcoma types
- Surgical excision
- Rare: 10-15% of extremity sarcomas
- Most common sarcoma type if uterine examples are included

Microscopic Pathology

- Perpendicularly oriented fascicles of spindle cells
- Brightly eosinophilic cytoplasm
- Blunt-ended nuclei
- Nuclear atypia

Ancillary Tests

- Labels as per smooth muscle: Desmin, actin, calponin, caldesmon
  - Some cases label with keratins

Top Differential Diagnoses

- Gastrointestinal stromal tumor (in gastrointestinal tract)
- Fibromatosis (in most sites)

- Any number of mitoses sufficient in subcutis, scrotal lesions, or deep soft tissue if nuclear atypia is present
- In vulva, some observers offered > 5 mitosis per 10 HPF as "cutoff," but recurrences reported in lesions with any mitotic activity
- In uterus
  - Diffuse moderate to marked cytologic atypia **and**
  - Mitotic rate 10 or more mitoses per 10 HPFs **and**
  - Tumor cell necrosis

Predominant Pattern/Injury Type

- Fascicular

Predominant Cell/Compartment Type

- Mesenchymal, muscle, smooth

Variant and Special Forms

- **Myxoid leiomyosarcoma**
  - Grossly gelatinous
  - Extensive myxoid change, but zones of typical leiomyosarcoma allow diagnosis
    - Express desmin and actin
    - Subset labels with keratin antibodies
  - Tends to be low grade
  - Clinicopathologic features otherwise as per typical leiomyosarcoma
- **Inflammatory leiomyosarcoma**
  - Characterized by dense inflammation that masks underlying lesion
    - Histiocytes, xanthoma cells, lymphocytes, neutrophils
  - Areas of more typical morphology must be sought
  - Clinicopathologic features otherwise as per typical leiomyosarcoma
- **Pleomorphic leiomyosarcoma**
  - Defined as pleomorphic areas in > 2/3 of tumor
    - Ordinary leiomyosarcomatous fascicular area covers < 1/3
  - More aggressive since higher grade
    - In 1 series, 65% of patients died of disease
  - Subset features osteoclast-like giant cells
- **Epstein-Barr-virus-associated leiomyosarcoma**
  - a.k.a. Epstein-Barr-virus-associated smooth muscle tumors (EBV-SMT)
    - Regarded as "leiomyoma" and "leiomyosarcoma," but term EBV-SMT may be more appropriate
    - Appearances are somewhat unique
    - Found in immunosuppressed patients
    - Frequently multifocal
    - Each tumor is unique molecular event; no clear-cut metastases reported
  - Histologic features
    - Monomorphic, spindled, smooth muscle cells arranged in short intersecting fascicles
    - Subpopulation of more primitive round cells are either admixed with spindled cells or form discrete nodules
    - Variable lymphocytic infiltrate composed primarily of T cells
    - Mitotic activity variable (0-18 per 10 HPF)
    - Necrosis and myxoid change in some cases
    - All are EBV-encoded RNA (EBER) positive
    - All express SMA, desmin in ~ 1/2
  - Reducing immunosuppression in transplant patients should be key treatment
    - Rapid tumor reduction following reduced immunosuppression reported, but some lesions persist
    - About 5% die of disease
  - Treatment is primarily surgical
  - Sirolimus (inhibitor of mTOR-associated protein pathway) effective in some lesions
- **Leiomyosarcoma with osteoclast-like giant cells**
  - Same demographics as per typical leiomyosarcoma
  - Areas with same histology as per typical leiomyosarcoma
    - Reactive with smooth muscle markers: Actins and desmin
  - Areas with osteoclast-like giant cells
    - Some giant cells appear bland (like histiocytes), but others cytologically malignant
    - Benign-appearing osteoclast-like giant cells label with CD68 but not muscle markers

- Cytologically malignant giant cells label with smooth muscle markers
  - No osteoid/matrix formation seen
- **Epithelioid leiomyosarcoma**
  - Literature confounded because many epithelioid gastrointestinal stromal tumors (GIST) were termed epithelioid leiomyosarcoma in past
  - Found anywhere in body
  - Distinct epithelioid morphology but more nuclear atypia than gastrointestinal stromal tumors
  - Older studies reported actin(+), desmin(-) immunophenotype, but desmin labels most lesions using modern immunohistochemistry
    - Possible reflection of misdiagnosed GISTs
    - Less sensitive desmin antibodies in past

ANCILLARY TESTS

Immunohistochemistry

- Label as per smooth muscle: Desmin, actin, calponin, caldesmon
  - Some cases label with keratins

Cytogenetics

- Complex variable karyotypes
- No characteristic translocation, mutation, or fusion product known

DIFFERENTIAL DIAGNOSIS

Skin and Subcutaneous Fat/Fascia

- Sarcomatoid squamous cell carcinoma
  - Can have epithelial in situ component
  - Expresses CK5/6 and p63, in contrast to leiomyosarcoma
- Dermatofibroma/fibrous histiocytoma
  - Storiform pattern
  - Collagen trapping pattern at periphery
  - Often has secondary inflammatory constituents (lymphoplasmacytic cells, foamy histiocytes, hemosiderin)
  - Typically lacks desmin, is factor XIIIa positive
  - Uniform cells
  - Characteristic genetic alteration; fusion gene *COL1A1-PDGFB*
- Leiomyoma
  - Bland cytology
  - Mitoses infrequent
- Nodular fasciitis
  - Loose storiform rather than fascicular pattern
  - Backdrop of lymphocytes and extravasated erythrocytes, often osteoclast-like giant cells
  - Bland nuclei
  - Immunoreactive for actin or calponin but not desmin or caldesmon

Gastrointestinal Tract

- Gastrointestinal stromal tumor
  - Uniform nuclei, less developed perpendicular fascicular pattern
  - Typically immunoreactive for CD117 and CD34, scant actin and desmin
  - *KIT* mutations common: Not observed in LMS
  - Some lesions have *PDGFRA* mutations
- Leiomyoma
  - Usually involves esophagus
  - Some cases associated with muscularis mucosae (colon)
  - Hypocellular with bland cytology and no mitotic activity
  - Smooth muscle immunophenotype
- Inflammatory fibroid polyp
  - Most common in submucosa of gastric antrum
  - Bland stellate cells, often arranged in "onion-skin" pattern around small submucosal vessels
  - Inflammatory backdrop rich in eosinophils
  - Labels for CD34 and cyclin-D1, not for CD117, desmin, or actin
  - *PDGFRA* mutations
- Fibromatosis
  - Sweeping fascicles of bland cells, gaping vessels, focal loose storiform pattern
  - Generally less cellular than leiomyosarcomas
  - Involves mesentery more than muscularis propria
  - Usually actin(+), desmin(-)
  - β-catenin nuclear labeling on immunohistochemistry
  - β-catenin or *APC* mutations
- Schwannoma
  - Most common in stomach
  - Striking lymphoid cuff surrounds lesion
  - Strong S100 protein labeling, negative desmin
- Inflammatory myofibroblastic tumor
  - Stellate to spindle cells with abundant background lymphoplasmacytic cells
  - More likely in mesentery than in muscularis propria
  - Variable actin and desmin
  - Subset labels for ALK protein
  - Subset with *ALK* gene rearrangements

Genital Tract

- Embryonal rhabdomyosarcoma (RMS)
  - Often pediatric
  - Tendency to proliferate in subepithelial zone (Cambium layer)
  - Less fascicular organization than LMS
  - Nuclear labeling for myogenin and MYOD1
- Angiomyofibroblastoma
  - Epithelioid nests of cells and prominent vessels; perivascular accentuation of cells, few mitoses
  - Variable labeling with actin, desmin labeling common, variable CD34
  - Immunolabeling for ER, PR common
- Cellular angiofibroma
  - Spindle cells and thick-walled vessels, few mitoses
  - Variable labeling with actin, desmin; CD34 labeling common
  - Immunolabeling for ER, PR common
- Aggressive angiomyxoma
  - Infiltrative growth pattern, hypocellular, lesional cells "spin off" vessels, few mitoses
  - Variable labeling with actin, desmin labeling common, variable CD34
  - Immunolabeling for ER, PR common

- Leiomyoma
  - Female genital tract: Variable patterns but brightly eosinophilic cells, uniform bland nuclei, infrequent mitoses (vulva)
  - Male genital tract: Eosinophilic cells, uniform bland nuclei; mitoses should be very rare or absent if there is cytologic atypia
  - Desmin and actin reactive
  - Immunolabeling for ER, PR common

Head and Neck

- Sarcomatoid carcinoma
  - In this site, majority of spindle cell malignant neoplasms are sarcomatoid carcinomas
  - Eosinophilic spindle cells lacking organized fascicular pattern
  - In situ component should be sought
  - Some cases label with keratins; p63 can also be useful
  - Lack smooth muscle markers
- Myofibrosarcoma
  - More likely to present in children than leiomyosarcoma
  - Tend to be low grade
  - Storiform pattern
  - Stellate cytoplasm
  - Shows myofibroblastic differentiation on immunohistochemistry
  - Can express α-actin, less likely to express desmin
- Rhabdomyosarcoma
  - Embryonal rhabdomyosarcoma similar to genital rhabdomyosarcoma; often pediatric
  - Spindle cell examples known in adults, often sclerotic
  - Less organized fascicles than those of leiomyosarcoma
  - Immunolabeling with specific skeletal muscle markers
  - MYOD1 and myogenin helpful
- Fibromatosis
  - As per gastrointestinal tract above
- Nodular fasciitis
  - Typically small lesions in younger patients than LMS
  - As per section above (skin)
- Myofibroma
  - Commonly pediatric
  - Biphasic pattern: Lobulated myoid zones and cellular zones enriched with hemangiopericytomatous vessels
  - Usually actin(+) but desmin(-)
- Cellular schwannoma
  - Adults
  - Often in nasal cavity
  - Bone destruction common
  - Infiltrative pattern: Lesions unencapsulated
  - Mitotic activity not commensurate with cellularity
  - Usually foci with foam cells, hemosiderin, and thick-walled vessels can be found
  - Strong diffuse S100 protein labeling

Bone

- Fibrosarcoma
  - Appears similar to leiomyosarcoma but lacks smooth muscle differentiation
  - Lacks expression of myoid markers
- Myofibrosarcoma
  - As per head and neck above
- Undifferentiated pleomorphic sarcoma (malignant fibrous histiocytoma)
  - Pleomorphic nuclei, storiform pattern rather than organized fascicles
  - No specific differentiation by immunolabeling
  - Complex karyotypes with no specific genetic alteration

Deep Soft Tissues

- Monophasic synovial sarcoma
  - Spindled cells with prominent nuclear overlapping
  - Cells have scant dark amphophilic to lightly basophilic cytoplasm
  - Uniform nuclei
  - Focal keratin and epithelial membrane antigen labeling
  - Often CD99 reactive
  - Can have calponin
  - Typically lack actin and desmin
  - CD34(-)
  - Usually Bcl-2 reactive
  - Characteristic translocation: t(X;18) and fusion genes: *SYT-SSX1/SSX2*
- Malignant peripheral nerve sheath tumor
  - Sometimes associated with large nerve trunk, especially in patients with neurofibromatosis type 1
  - Areas of low and high cellularity
  - Tendency for subendothelial proliferation
  - Nuclear pleomorphism; bullet-shaped nuclei
  - Rare examples with zones of skeletal muscle differentiation (Triton tumor)
  - Focal S100 protein
  - Smooth muscle markers usually negative
  - No characteristic translocation; early reports of fusion genes (*SYT-SSX*) presumably result of poor PCR technique
- Myofibrosarcoma
  - As per head and neck above
- Smooth muscle differentiation is component of well-differentiated and dedifferentiated liposarcoma
  - Fat-forming component must be sought
- Deep leiomyoma
  - Typically in females during fertile years
  - Often no connection to female genital tract itself
  - Variant patterns unified by bland brightly eosinophilic cells
  - Scattered mitoses may be encountered but no nuclear atypia
  - ER/PR expression common
  - Label with typical smooth muscle markers (desmin, actin, calponin, caldesmon)
- Solitary fibrous tumor
  - Most examples behave indolently
  - Spindle cell tumor with so-called "patternless pattern"
  - Prominent staghorn-shaped vascular channels
  - Negative S100 protein, actin, desmin
  - CD34, CD99, and Bcl-2 expression

LEIOMYOSARCOMA

Immunohistochemistry

Antibody	Reactivity	Staining Pattern	Comment
Desmin	Positive	Cytoplasmic	
Actin-sm	Positive	Cytoplasmic	
Calponin	Positive	Cytoplasmic	
Caldesmon	Positive	Cytoplasmic	
CK-PAN	Positive	Cytoplasmic	Reactive in ~ 1/3 of cases; usually focal
ER	Negative	Not applicable	Occasional gynecologic examples focally reactive
CD34	Negative	Cytoplasmic	Usually negative
PR	Negative	Not applicable	Occasional gynecologic examples focally reactive
S100	Negative	Not applicable	Occasional cases focally reactive
HMB-45	Negative	Not applicable	Occasional cases focally reactive

- Fibromatosis
  - As per gastrointestinal tract tumors above

DIAGNOSTIC CHECKLIST

Pathologic Interpretation Pearls

- Attention to gender and anatomic site important in evaluating smooth muscle tumors
  - Old tenet "all retroperitoneal smooth muscle tumors are malignant" can be wrong in female pelvis

SELECTED REFERENCES

1. Toledo G et al: Smooth muscle tumors of the uterus: a practical approach. Arch Pathol Lab Med. 132(4):595-605, 2008
2. Deyrup AT et al: Leiomyosarcoma of the kidney: a clinicopathologic study. Am J Surg Pathol. 28(2):178-82, 2004
3. Montgomery E et al: Leiomyosarcoma of the head and neck: a clinicopathological study. Histopathology. 40(6):518-25, 2002
4. Billings SD et al: Do leiomyomas of deep soft tissue exist? An analysis of highly differentiated smooth muscle tumors of deep soft tissue supporting two distinct subtypes. Am J Surg Pathol. 25(9):1134-42, 2001
5. Fisher C et al: Leiomyosarcoma of the paratesticular region: a clinicopathologic study. Am J Surg Pathol. 25(9):1143-9, 2001
6. Oda Y et al: Pleomorphic leiomyosarcoma: clinicopathologic and immunohistochemical study with special emphasis on its distinction from ordinary leiomyosarcoma and malignant fibrous histiocytoma. Am J Surg Pathol. 25(8):1030-8, 2001
7. Sigel JE et al: The utility of cytokeratin 5/6 in the recognition of cutaneous spindle cell squamous cell carcinoma. J Cutan Pathol. 28(10):520-4, 2001
8. Iwata J et al: Immunohistochemical detection of cytokeratin and epithelial membrane antigen in leiomyosarcoma: a systematic study of 100 cases. Pathol Int. 50(1):7-14, 2000
9. Miettinen M et al: Gastrointestinal stromal tumors and leiomyosarcomas in the colon: a clinicopathologic, immunohistochemical, and molecular genetic study of 44 cases. Am J Surg Pathol. 24(10):1339-52, 2000
10. Rubin BP et al: Myxoid leiomyosarcoma of soft tissue, an underrecognized variant. Am J Surg Pathol. 24(7):927-36, 2000
11. de Saint Aubain Somerhausen N et al: Leiomyosarcoma of soft tissue in children: clinicopathologic analysis of 20 cases. Am J Surg Pathol. 23(7):755-63, 1999
12. Antonescu CR et al: Primary leiomyosarcoma of bone: a clinicopathologic, immunohistochemical, and ultrastructural study of 33 patients and a literature review. Am J Surg Pathol. 21(11):1281-94, 1997
13. Kaddu S et al: Cutaneous leiomyosarcoma. Am J Surg Pathol. 21(9):979-87, 1997
14. Moran CA et al: Primary leiomyosarcomas of the lung: a clinicopathologic and immunohistochemical study of 18 cases. Mod Pathol. 10(2):121-8, 1997
15. Merchant W et al: Inflammatory leiomyosarcoma: a morphological subgroup within the heterogeneous family of so-called inflammatory malignant fibrous histiocytoma. Histopathology. 27(6):525-32, 1995
16. Mentzel T et al: Leiomyosarcoma with prominent osteoclast-like giant cells. Analysis of eight cases closely mimicking the so-called giant cell variant of malignant fibrous histiocytoma. Am J Surg Pathol. 18(3):258-65, 1994
17. Suster S: Epithelioid leiomyosarcoma of the skin and subcutaneous tissue. Clinicopathologic, immunohistochemical, and ultrastructural study of five cases. Am J Surg Pathol. 18(3):232-40, 1994
18. Miettinen M: Keratin subsets in spindle cell sarcomas. Keratins are widespread but synovial sarcoma contains a distinctive keratin polypeptide pattern and desmoplakins. Am J Pathol. 138(2):505-13, 1991
19. Hashimoto H et al: Leiomyosarcoma of the external soft tissues. A clinicopathologic, immunohistochemical, and electron microscopic study. Cancer. 57(10):2077-88, 1986
20. Shmookler BM et al: Retroperitoneal leiomyosarcoma. A clinicopathologic analysis of 36 cases. Am J Surg Pathol. 7(3):269-80, 1983
21. Fields JP et al: Leiomyosarcoma of the skin and subcutaneous tissue. Cancer. 47(1):156-69, 1981
22. Wile AG et al: Leiomyosarcoma of soft tissue: a clinicopathologic study. Cancer. 48(4):1022-32, 1981

Microscopic Features

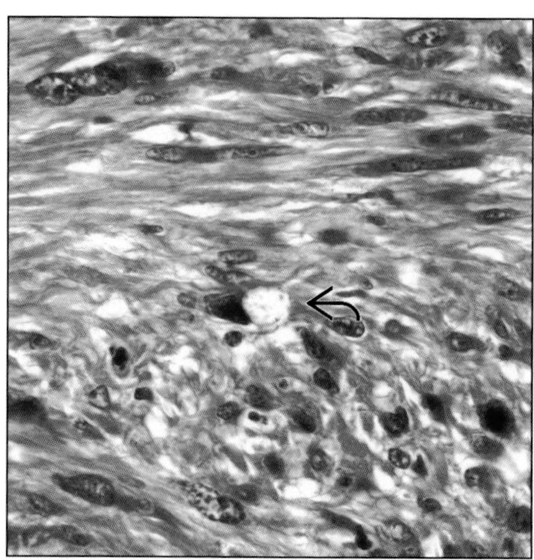

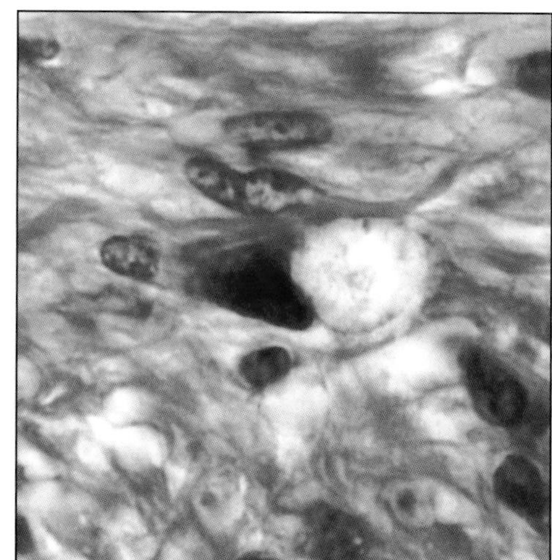

(Left) *Hematoxylin & eosin shows a classic appearance of a leiomyosarcoma. The proliferating cells contain blunt-ended nuclei and fibrillary eosinophilic cytoplasm. A paranuclear vacuole is in the center of the field ⮳.* ***(Right)*** *Hematoxylin & eosin shows high magnification of a paranuclear vacuole depicted in a leiomyosarcoma. The cells above the vacuolated one have blunt-ended nuclei.*

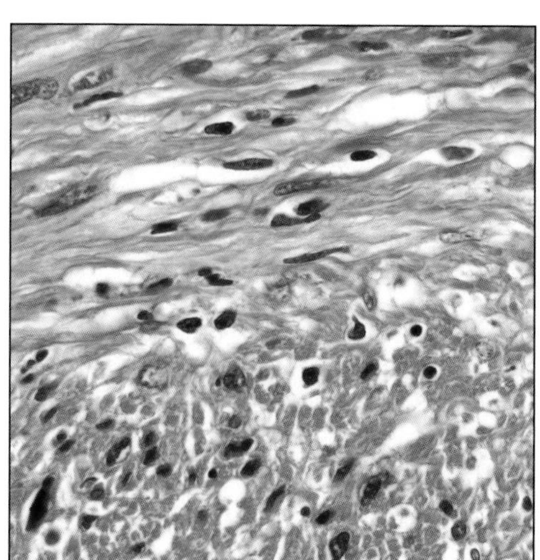

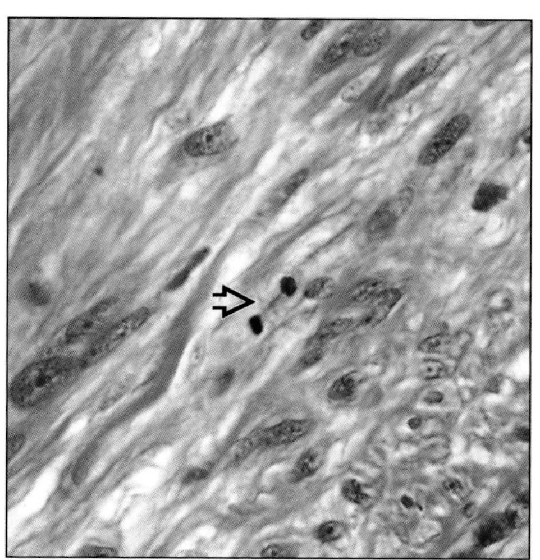

(Left) *Hematoxylin & eosin shows perpendicularly oriented fascicles. The cells in the upper part of the field are in a fascicular arrangement, whereas the ones at the bottom of the field are aligned perfectly en face.* ***(Right)*** *This image shows an anaphase bridge ⇨ in the center of the field, an indication that this neoplasm has chromosome instability rather than a characteristic translocation or gene rearrangement.*

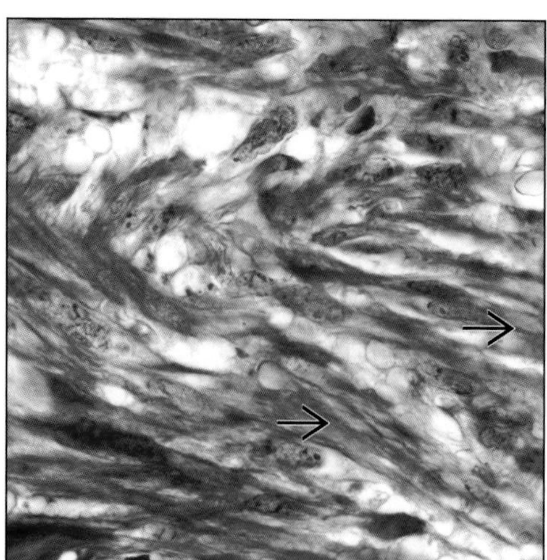

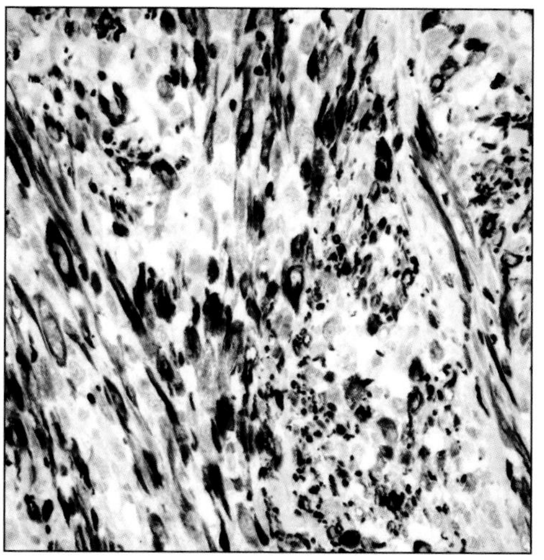

(Left) *Masson trichrome stain highlights delicate red cytoplasmic filaments → in this well-differentiated leiomyosarcoma.* ***(Right)*** *Desmin immunostain shows striking cytoplasmic labeling in this leiomyosarcoma. This lesion was in the colonic wall. In the gastrointestinal tract, leiomyosarcomas are rare and often confused with gastrointestinal stromal tumors, which usually have weaker, more focal expression of desmin (if any).*

LEIOMYOSARCOMA

Microscopic Features

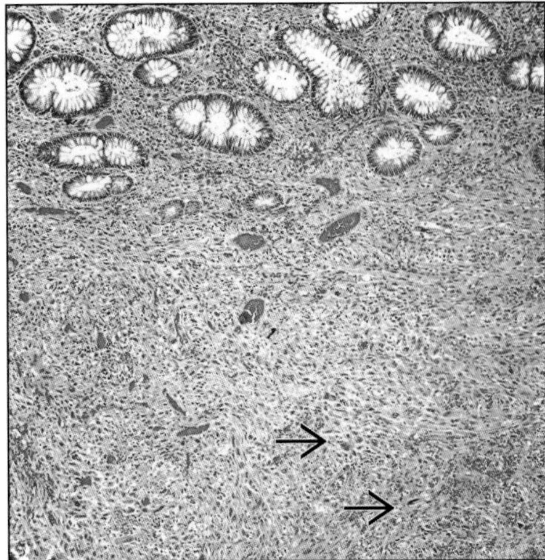

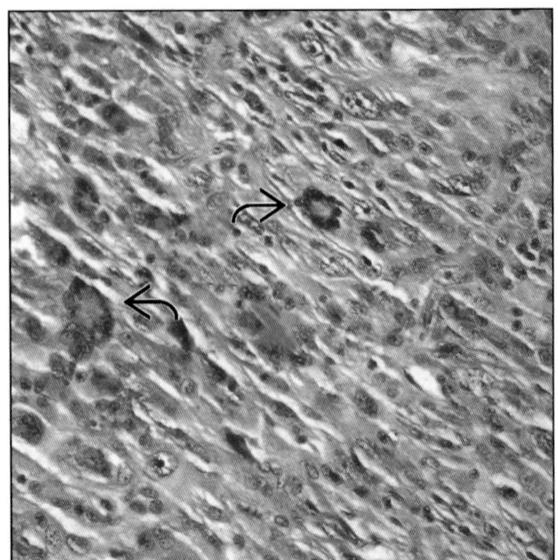

(Left) *Hematoxylin and eosin shows a leiomyosarcoma of the colon extending from the muscularis propria into the mucosa. Even at this magnification pleomorphic nuclei are evident ⇒, a feature that is against a diagnosis of gastrointestinal stromal tumor.* ***(Right)*** *This leiomyosarcoma displays prominent osteoclast-like giant cells ⇗. In the past, such lesions were sometimes mistaken for undifferentiated pleomorphic sarcomas (malignant fibrous histiocytomas).*

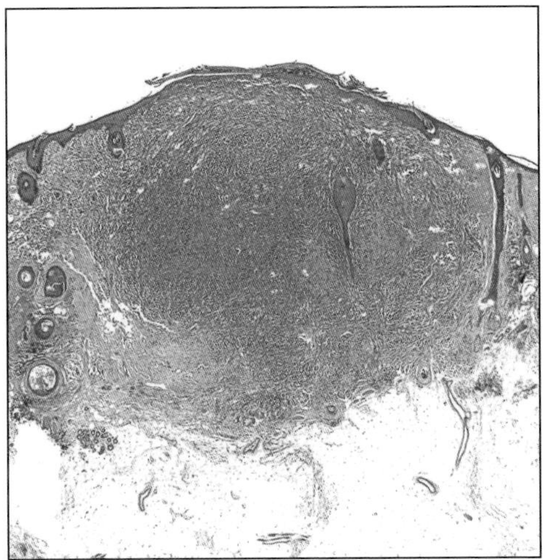

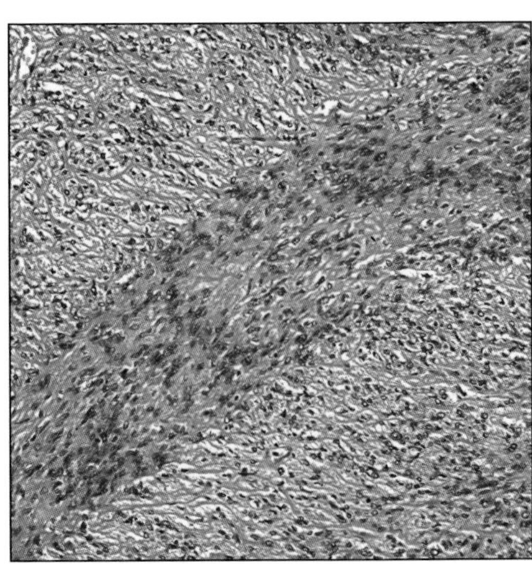

(Left) *Based on the lack of involvement of the subcutaneous adipose tissue, a favorable prognosis would be anticipated for this lesion. In fact, some observers have suggested diagnosing such superficial lesions as "atypical smooth muscle tumors."* ***(Right)*** *Note the nuclear palisading in this cutaneous leiomyosarcoma in the same case. Although this pattern suggests a nerve sheath tumor, the perpendicular arrangement of the fascicles supports an interpretation of leiomyosarcoma.*

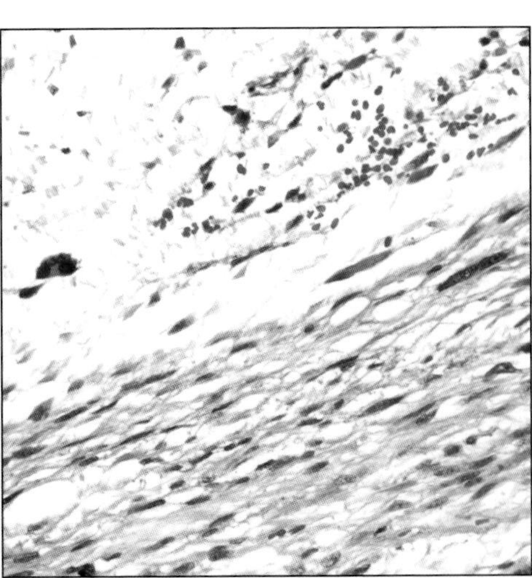

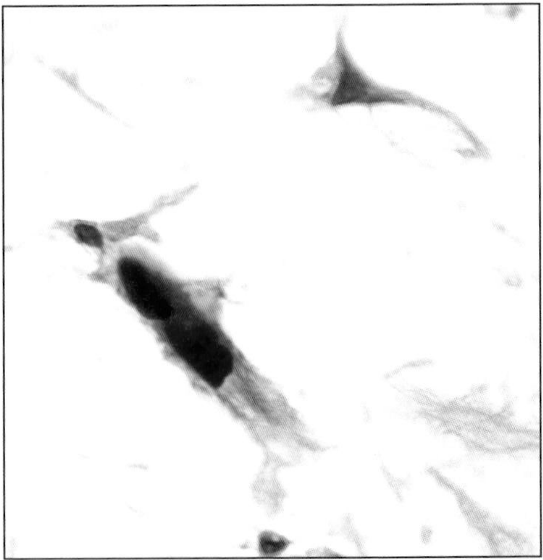

(Left) *Hematoxylin and eosin shows a myxoid leiomyosarcoma. The bottom of the field shows typical leiomyosarcoma features, whereas the top is myxoid with a pleomorphic cell. A predominance in pleomorphic zones would qualify a tumor as a "pleomorphic leiomyosarcoma."* ***(Right)*** *This cell, found in the myxoid zone of the lesion depicted in the previous image, shows blunt-ended nuclear contours. Note the delicate eosinophilic filaments in the cytoplasm.*

Microscopic Features

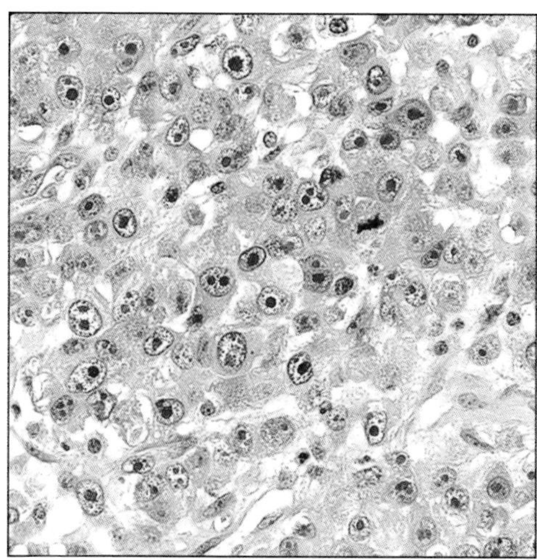

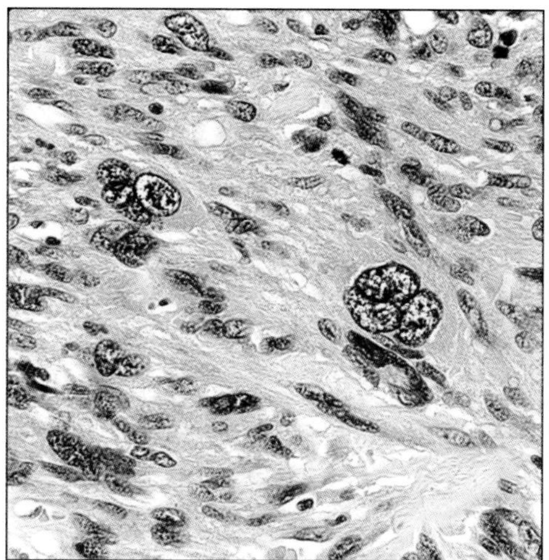

(Left) *Epithelioid leiomyosarcoma shows abundant eosinophilic cytoplasm and cytologically malignant nuclei. A diagnosis of such cases often requires use of immunohistochemistry to exclude melanoma and carcinomas.* ***(Right)*** *This leiomyosarcoma displays striking nuclear pleomorphism. When this feature is the overriding one, such tumors behave more aggressively and have been classified as "pleomorphic leiomyosarcoma."*

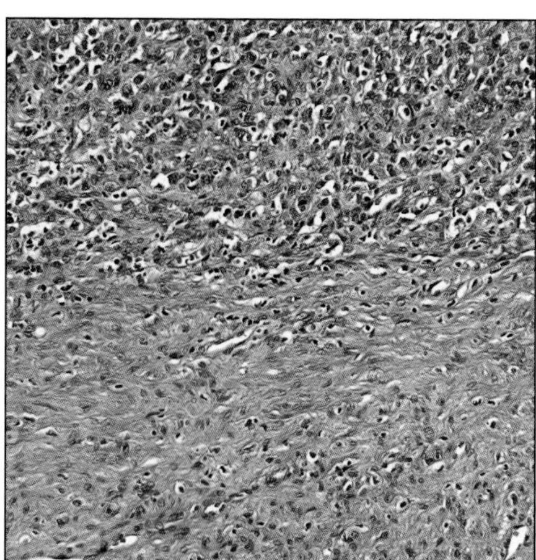

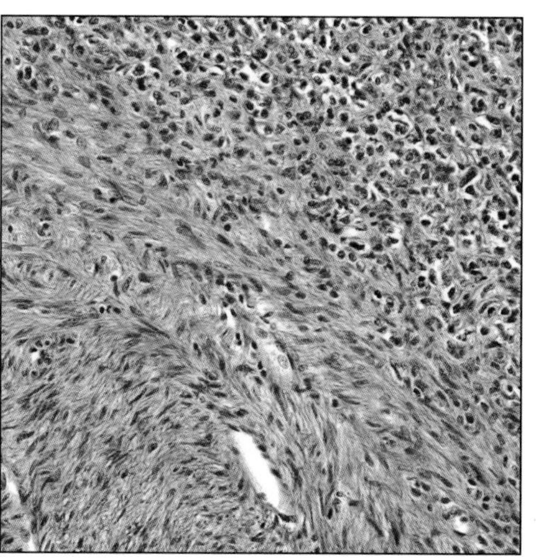

(Left) *Epstein-Barr-virus-associated smooth muscle tumor manifests a dual population of fascicular eosinophilic cells and smaller darker cells at the top of the field. (Courtesy A. Deyrup, MD.)* ***(Right)*** *Higher magnification of the Epstein-Barr-virus-associated smooth muscle tumor. These tumors have EBV-encoded RNA (EBER) and express SMA, but only 54% are desmin positive. (Courtesy A. Deyrup, MD.)*

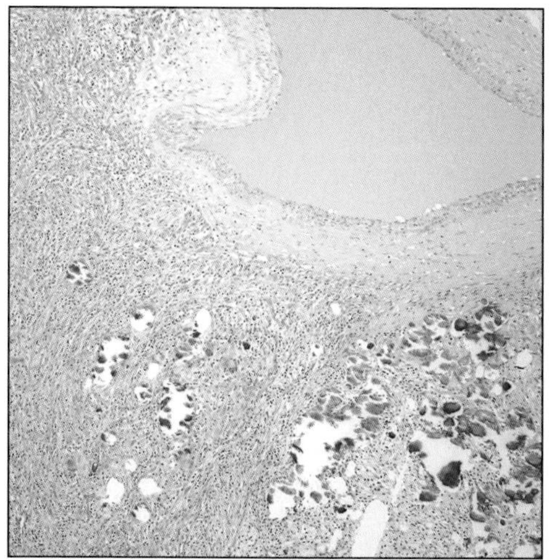

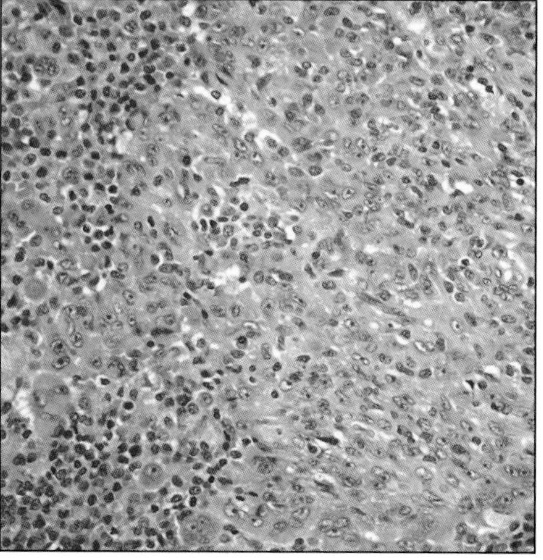

(Left) *An inflammatory leiomyosarcoma associated with a large vein is seen.* ***(Right)*** *At a higher magnification the proliferating cells are seen as epithelioid in this example. The inflammatory component is primarily lymphoplasmacytic.*

Vascular Lesions

Benign

Intermediate

Malignant

BACILLARY ANGIOMATOSIS

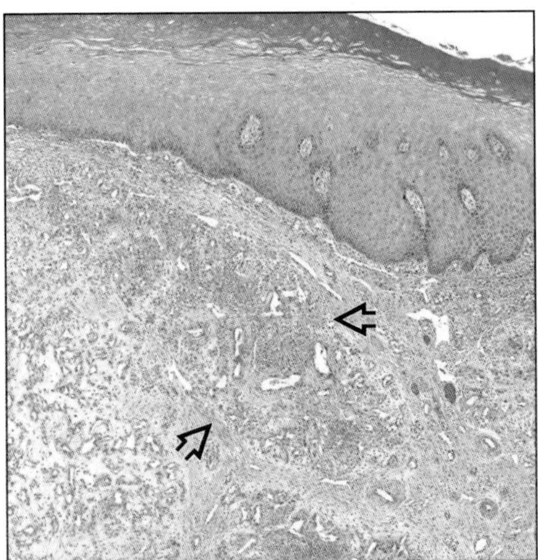

Low-power examination of bacillary angiomatosis demonstrates a superficial dermal proliferation of blood vessels in a lobular configuration ⇨ associated with edema and inflammation.

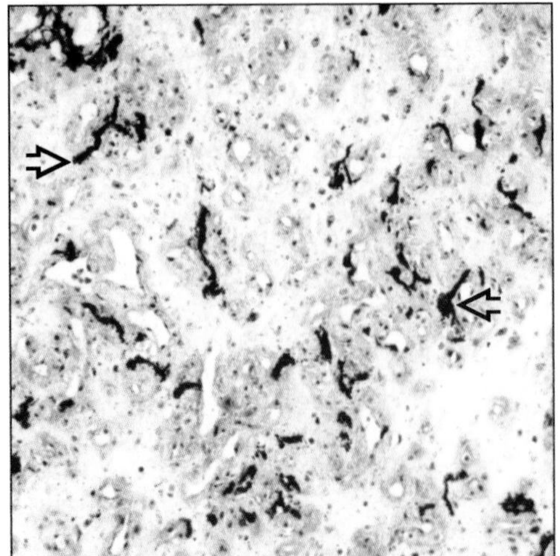

Warthin-Starry silver stain preparation shows numerous clusters of bacterial organisms ⇨ around blood vessels.

TERMINOLOGY

Abbreviations

- Bacillary angiomatosis (BA)

Synonyms

- Epithelioid angiomatosis

Definitions

- Reactive vascular proliferation associated with *Bartonella* bacterial infection

ETIOLOGY/PATHOGENESIS

Infectious Agents

- Caused by infection with *Bartonella* (gram-negative coccobacilli) species, usually *B. henselae* or *B. quintana*
  - Most patients have a history of cat exposure (and may have preceding scratch or bite)
- Most patients are immunocompromised, especially due to HIV/AIDS
  - Also has been associated with organ transplantation, systemic steroids, and leukemia

CLINICAL ISSUES

Epidemiology

- Age
  - May occur in adults and children

Site

- Can involve any cutaneous site; uncommonly may involve mucosal sites and deep soft tissues
  - Internal organ involvement rare but may affect liver (peliosis hepatis)

Presentation

- Skin nodules or, less likely, plaques
  - Typically present with multiple lesions, often pyogenic granuloma-like

Treatment

- Drugs
  - Antibiotics typically lead to resolution of lesions

Prognosis

- Typically good, but depends on patient's immune status and sites involved

MACROSCOPIC FEATURES

General Features

- Reddish-brown, dermal-based, nodular, hemorrhagic lesion

MICROSCOPIC PATHOLOGY

Histologic Features

- Typically nodular to dome-shaped/polypoid dermal-based vascular proliferation
  - May have overlying epidermal ulceration and collarette (similar to pyogenic granuloma)
- Vessels are arranged in loose lobular configuration
  - Endothelial cells show mild enlargement and oval to epithelioid shape
  - Deeper parts of lesion may show greater cellularity and crowding of vessels
  - No significant cytologic atypia or atypical mitotic activity
- Background stroma shows fibrosis, edema, and mixed inflammatory infiltrate
  - Infiltrate is rich in neutrophils with nuclear dust, macrophages, and may show focal collections of basophilic granular material (clumps of bacteria)
    - Neutrophils are more plentiful in deeper lesions

BACILLARY ANGIOMATOSIS

Key Facts

Terminology
- Reactive vascular proliferation associated with *Bartonella* (gram-negative coccobacilli) bacterial infection

Etiology/Pathogenesis
- Most patients are immunocompromised, especially HIV/AIDS
- Also associated with organ transplantation, systemic steroids, and leukemia

Clinical Issues
- Can involve any cutaneous site, uncommonly involves mucosal sites, deep soft tissues

Microscopic Pathology
- Nodular to dome-shaped/polypoid dermal-based vascular proliferation
- Infiltrate of neutrophils with nuclear dust, macrophages, focal clumps of basophilic granular material (bacteria)

ANCILLARY TESTS

Histochemistry
- Warthin-Starry
  - Reactivity: Positive
  - Staining pattern
    - Granular (coccobacillary organisms)
- GMS (Gomori methenamine silver)
  - Reactivity: Positive
  - Staining pattern
    - Granular (coccobacillary organisms)

PCR
- PCR for *Bartonella* species may be ordered if organisms are not identified on histochemical stains

DIFFERENTIAL DIAGNOSIS

Pyogenic Granuloma
- Polypoid dermal-based lesion composed of lobular collection of capillary-type vessels
- Overlying ulceration and peripheral epidermal collarette are typically present, similar to BA
- No evidence of organisms identified on H&E or special stains

Kaposi Sarcoma
- Plaque-like or nodular collection of slit-like vessels lined by atypical spindle cells
- Inflammatory infiltrate is typically composed of lymphocytes and plasma cells, not neutrophils
- No bacterial organisms identified
- HHV8(+) is diagnostic

DIAGNOSTIC CHECKLIST

Clinically Relevant Pathologic Features
- Organ distribution

Pathologic Interpretation Pearls
- Proliferation of vessels associated with neutrophils and clumps of bacterial organisms

SELECTED REFERENCES

1. Amsbaugh S et al: Bacillary angiomatosis associated with pseudoepitheliomatous hyperplasia. Am J Dermatopathol. 28(1):32-5, 2006
2. Tucci E et al: Localized bacillary angiomatosis in the oral cavity: observations about a neoplasm with atypical behavior. Description of a case and review of the literature. Minerva Stomatol. 55(1-2):67-75, 2006
3. Maurin M et al: Bartonella infections: diagnostic and management issues. Curr Opin Infect Dis. 11(2):189-93, 1998
4. LeBoit PE et al: Bacillary angiomatosis. The histopathology and differential diagnosis of a pseudoneoplastic infection in patients with human immunodeficiency virus disease. Am J Surg Pathol. 13(11):909-20, 1989

IMAGE GALLERY

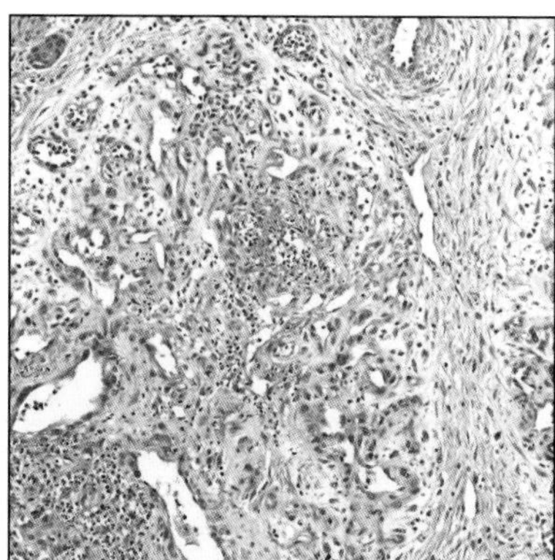

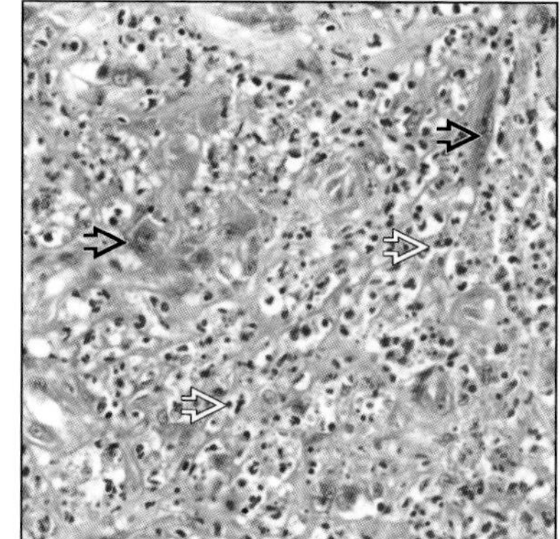

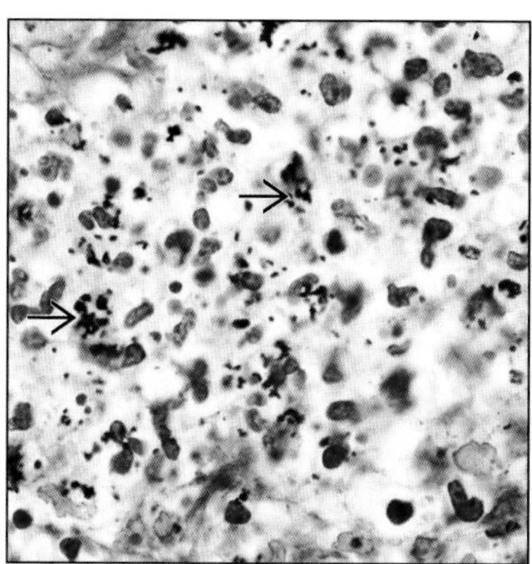

(Left) *Intermediate magnification shows a proliferation of small blood vessels arranged in a vaguely lobular configuration with prominent stromal edema, mild fibrosis, and mixed inflammatory infiltrate.* ***(Center)*** *High magnification of bacillary angiomatosis demonstrates a proliferation of small blood vessels with swollen endothelial cells ⇨ surrounded by edema and inflammation ➡.* ***(Right)*** *Warthin-Starry stain demonstrates positive staining of numerous clusters ⇒ and single bacterial organisms.*

PAPILLARY ENDOTHELIAL HYPERPLASIA

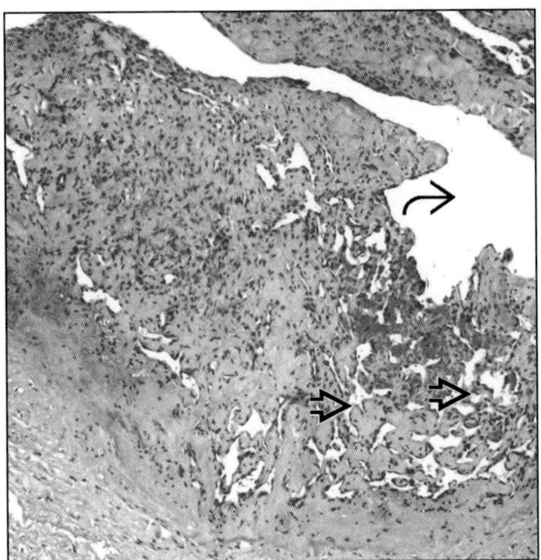

Papillary endothelial hyperplasia (PEH) is a well-circumscribed reactive lesion in which papillary fronds ➡ lined by a single layer of endothelial cells proliferate within a vascular lumen ↗.

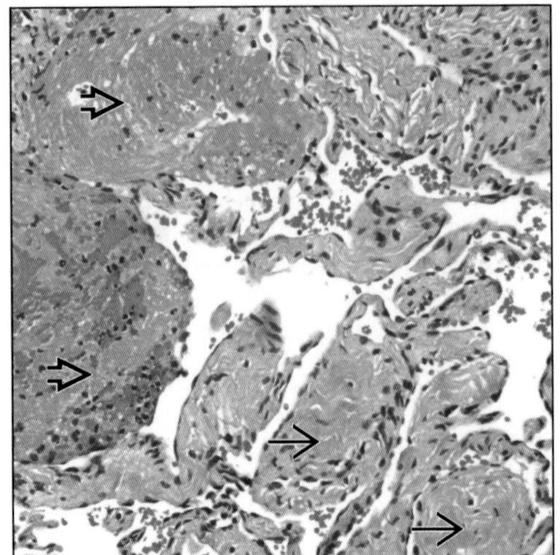

Fibrin thrombi ➡ are apparent in early stages and with time are replaced by papillary fronds with a fibrous core → characteristic of PEH.

TERMINOLOGY

Abbreviations

- Papillary endothelial hyperplasia (PEH)

Synonyms

- Masson tumor
- Vegetant intravascular hemangioendothelioma
- Intravascular angiomatosis

Definitions

- Benign, reactive, intravascular papillary endothelial proliferation

ETIOLOGY/PATHOGENESIS

Reactive Vascular Proliferation

- Manifestation of organizing intravascular thrombus
- PEH-like changes may be present in preexisting hemangiomas or vascular malformations

CLINICAL ISSUES

Site

- Wide distribution
- Common sites include
  - Head & neck, fingers, trunk

Presentation

- Painless mass
- Located in deep dermis or subcutaneous tissue

Treatment

- Excision is curative

Prognosis

- Excellent
- Cases with underlying hemangioma or vascular malformation may recur

MACROSCOPIC FEATURES

General Features

- Cystic mass with red-purple discoloration
- Often surrounded by pseudocapsule

Size

- Mostly small in size (< 2 cm)

MICROSCOPIC PATHOLOGY

Histologic Features

- Circumscribed lesion with pseudocapsule
  - Residual smooth muscle or elastic lamina of preexisting vessel may be apparent
- Fibrin thrombus
- Papillary structures lined by endothelial cells
  - Endothelial cells in single layer
  - Papillae form anastomosing network
- Papillary cores may consist of fibrin or fibrous connective tissue
- Vessel rupture may lead to extension of papillary endothelial proliferation into adjacent soft tissue
- Rare examples of extravascular variant in soft tissue have been reported
  - Represent reactive endothelial proliferation in organizing hematoma

Cytologic Features

- Nuclei lining papillae may appear plump or hobnail in appearance
- Significant nuclear pleomorphism is absent

ANCILLARY TESTS

Electron Microscopy

- Transmission
  - Differentiated endothelial cells line papillae
    - Luminal micropinocytotic vesicles

PAPILLARY ENDOTHELIAL HYPERPLASIA

Key Facts

Terminology
- Benign, reactive, intravascular papillary endothelial proliferation

Clinical Issues
- Wide site distribution; located in deep dermis or subcutaneous tissue

Macroscopic Features
- Small, cystic lesions with red-purple discoloration

Microscopic Pathology
- Circumscribed lesion with pseudocapsule
- Papillary structures lined by endothelial cells
- Significant nuclear pleomorphism is absent

Top Differential Diagnoses
- Angiosarcoma
  - PEH lacks nuclear atypia, tumor cell necrosis, and mitotic activity present in angiosarcoma

---

    - Tight junctions and basal lamina
    - Weibel-Palade bodies
  - Undifferentiated &/or pericytic cells present within papillary cores

DIFFERENTIAL DIAGNOSIS

Angiosarcoma
- Angiosarcoma is infiltrative process, unlike PEH, which is intraluminal
- Even PEH cases with soft tissue extension have bulk of the lesion confined to vascular lumen
- PEH lacks nuclear atypia, tumor cell necrosis, and mitotic activity present in angiosarcoma

Vascular Neoplasm
- PEH-like changes may occur in hemangiomas complicated by thrombosis

Arteriovenous Malformation (AVM)
- PEH-like changes may occur in background of AVM
- Important to recognize since these may recur

Hematoma
- Soft tissue hematomas may have foci of PEH
- May be mistaken for angiosarcoma

DIAGNOSTIC CHECKLIST

Clinically Relevant Pathologic Features
- Tissue distribution
  - Intravascular process

Pathologic Interpretation Pearls
- Intravascular papillary proliferation lined by endothelial cells without significant nuclear atypia

SELECTED REFERENCES

1. Pins MR et al: Florid extravascular papillary endothelial hyperplasia (Masson's pseudoangiosarcoma) presenting as a soft-tissue sarcoma. Arch Pathol Lab Med. 117(3):259-63, 1993
2. Hashimoto H et al: Intravascular papillary endothelial hyperplasia. A clinicopathologic study of 91 cases. Am J Dermatopathol. 5(6):539-46, 1983
3. Barr RJ et al: Intravascular papillary endothelial hyperplasia. A benign lesion mimicking angiosarcoma. Arch Dermatol. 114(5):723-6, 1978
4. Clearkin KP et al: Intravascular papillary endothelial hyperplasia. Arch Pathol Lab Med. 100(8):441-4, 1976
5. Kuo T et al: Masson's "vegetant intravascular hemangioendothelioma:" a lesion often mistaken for angiosarcoma: study of seventeen cases located in the skin and soft tissues. Cancer. 38(3):1227-36, 1976
6. Salyer WR et al: Intravascular angiomatosis: development and distinction from angiosarcoma. Cancer. 36(3):995-1001, 1975

IMAGE GALLERY

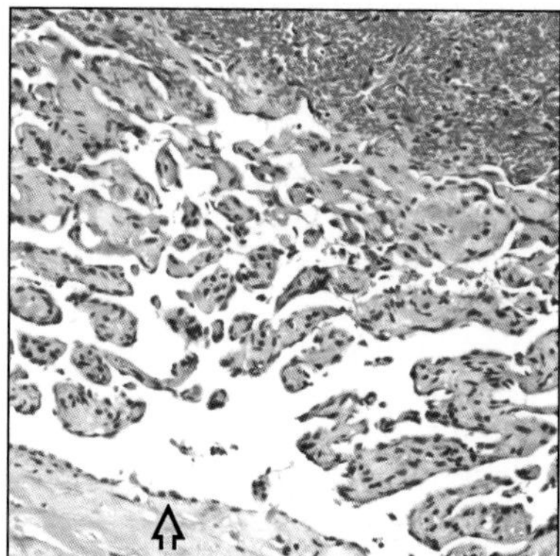
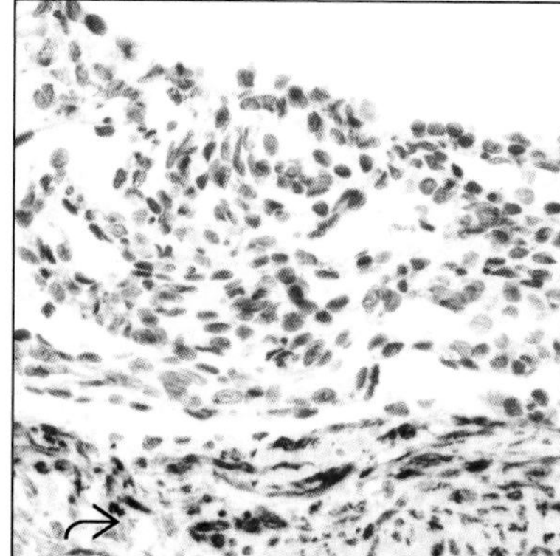
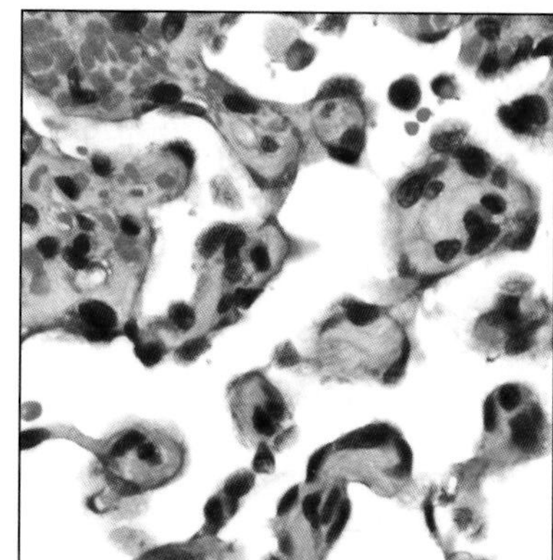

*(**Left**) PEH can be mistaken for the dissecting vascular spaces seen in low-grade angiosarcoma. Note the endothelium lining ⇨ of the blood vessel lumen. (**Center**) A desmin immunostain highlights remnants of smooth muscle in the blood vessel wall ↗ and confirms the intravascular location of PEH. (**Right**) A single layer of endothelial cells line the papillary fronds in PEH. The endothelial cells may be plump and swollen but do not show significant nuclear atypia.*

CAPILLARY, VENOUS, AND CAVERNOUS HEMANGIOMAS

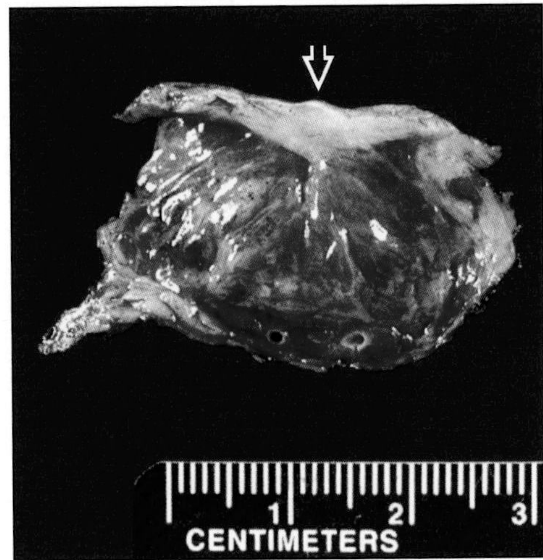

Capillary hemangiomas present as small, superficial, well-circumscribed, red-purple nodules. The overlying skin is intact in this example ⇒ but may be ulcerated ("pyogenic granuloma").

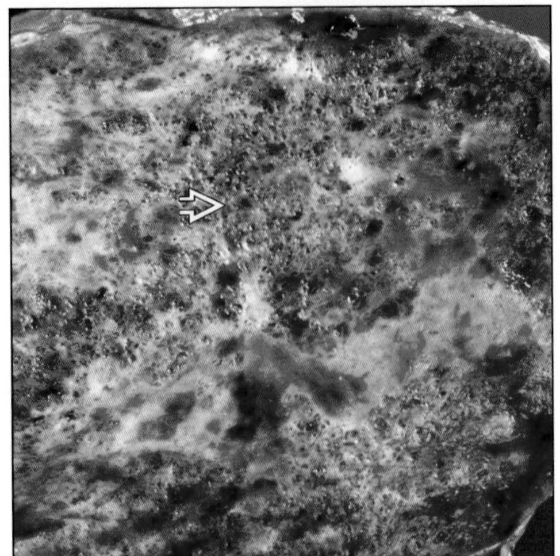

The cut surface of cavernous hemangiomas is typically spongy in appearance ⇒ with cystic spaces of variable size filled with blood.

TERMINOLOGY

Abbreviations

- Pyogenic granuloma (PG)

Synonyms

- Capillary hemangioma = lobular hemangioma

Definitions

- Benign vascular tumors composed of blood vessels of various size lined by plump to flattened endothelial cells with no atypia

ETIOLOGY/PATHOGENESIS

Developmental Anomaly

- Juvenile capillary hemangiomas may be congenital
- Venous hemangiomas may represent vascular malformations

CLINICAL ISSUES

Epidemiology

- Age
  - Depends on subtype
- Gender
  - Capillary and cavernous hemangiomas in adults occur more commonly in women

Site

- Depends on subtype

Presentation

- Painless mass
- Red elevated papule(s)

Natural History

- Juvenile capillary hemangiomas regress spontaneously with time

Treatment

- Surgical approaches
  - Surgical excision is curative
- Drugs
  - Glucocorticoids or interferon-α therapy for large or symptomatic juvenile hemangiomas
- Watchful waiting for juvenile hemangiomas that regress with time

Prognosis

- Recurrences are rare; occur in incompletely excised lesion

MACROSCOPIC FEATURES

General Features

- Elevated nodular red-purple lesions
- Usually involve skin or subcutaneous tissue
- Discoloration may not be obvious in deep-seated lesions
- Recurrences may be sessile

Size

- Variable size

Capillary (Lobular) Hemangioma

- Most common type of hemangioma
- Variants
  - **Juvenile hemangioma**
    - Occurs in infancy; 1:200 births
    - About 1/5 multiple; rarely familial
    - Flat red lesion in early stage
  - **Pyogenic granuloma (PG)**
    - Occurs on skin and mucosal surfaces
    - Gingiva, fingers, lips, face, and tongue are most common sites of involvement
    - Polypoid friable lesions that bleed easily and are often ulcerated
  - **Intravenous pyogenic granuloma**
    - Neck and upper extremity are common sites

CAPILLARY, VENOUS, AND CAVERNOUS HEMANGIOMAS

Key Facts

Terminology

- Benign vascular tumors composed of blood vessels lined by plump to flattened endothelial cells with no atypia

Etiology/Pathogenesis

- May be congenital

Clinical Issues

- Capillary and cavernous hemangiomas in adults occur more commonly in women

Macroscopic Features

- Capillary hemangioma is commonest subtype of hemangioma
- Juvenile hemangioma occurs in infancy
- Pyogenic granuloma occurs on skin and mucosal surfaces
- Cavernous hemangiomas present as birthmarks
- Venous hemangiomas are rare and present in adulthood

Microscopic Pathology

- Nodules of small capillary sized vessels in lobular pattern in capillary hemangioma
- Large, cystically dilated blood vessels filled with blood in cavernous hemangioma
- Large, thick-walled veins in venous hemangioma
- Lining endothelium in all lesions does not show atypia
- Thrombosis, hemorrhage, and calcification may be present

    - Red-brown intravascular polyp
    - May be mistaken for organizing thrombus
  - **Pregnancy-related pyogenic granuloma**
    - Gingiva commonest site
    - Regress after delivery
  - **Senile angioma (cherry angioma)**
    - Trunk and extremity
    - Ruby red papule with halo around it

Venous Hemangioma

- Rare, presents in adulthood, predilection for limbs

Cavernous Hemangioma

- Common symptomatic birthmark
- Soft, compressible, purple lesions

MICROSCOPIC PATHOLOGY

Key Descriptors

- Histologic Features
  - **Capillary hemangioma**
    - Nodules of small capillaries arranged in lobular architecture
    - Large "feeder" vessel supplies each lobule
    - Vascular lumen may be inconspicuous in early lesions
    - Flat to plump endothelial cells with no atypia
    - Mitotic figures may be present
    - Surface epithelium may be atrophic or ulcerated in PG
    - Marked acute and chronic inflammation present in PG
  - **Venous hemangioma**
    - Large, thick-walled blood vessels
    - Dilated lumen with thrombi or phleboliths
    - Cystically dilated vessels may mimic cavernous hemangioma
  - **Cavernous hemangioma**
    - Large, cystically dilated blood vessels filled with blood
    - Lined by flat endothelium without atypia
    - Organizing thrombi and Masson tumor-like change may be present
    - Recanalizing thrombi may create sinusoidal pattern ("sinusoidal hemangioma")

DIFFERENTIAL DIAGNOSIS

Arteriovenous Malformation (AVM)

- May mimic venous hemangioma
- Unlike AVMs, elastic stain shows absence of internal elastic lamina in venous hemangioma

Kaposi Sarcoma (KS)

- Angiomatous form of KS may be mistaken for PG
  - PG is well circumscribed and shows lobular arrangement
- KS shows spindle cell areas with slit-like spaces
- KS shows nuclear immunoreactivity for HHV8

Reactive Granulation Tissue

- Lacks lobular architecture of capillaries seen in PG

DIAGNOSTIC CHECKLIST

Pathologic Interpretation Pearls

- Lobular architecture of blood vessels is typical of capillary hemangiomas
- Cavernous hemangiomas may show Masson tumor-like changes

SELECTED REFERENCES

1. Jackson R: The natural history of strawberry naevi. J Cutan Med Surg. 2(3):187-9, 1998
2. Coffin CM et al: Vascular tumors in children and adolescents: a clinicopathologic study of 228 tumors in 222 patients. Pathol Annu. 28 Pt 1:97-120, 1993
3. Mills SE et al: Lobular capillary hemangioma: the underlying lesion of pyogenic granuloma. A study of 73 cases from the oral and nasal mucous membranes. Am J Surg Pathol. 4(5):470-9, 1980

CAPILLARY, VENOUS, AND CAVERNOUS HEMANGIOMAS

Microscopic Features

(Left) *Capillary hemangiomas are well-circumscribed lesions composed of nodules of capillary-sized vessels with variable luminal size.* ***(Right)*** *Each lobule in lobular capillary hemangioma is supplied by a large "feeder vessel" ➔. The capillary lumen may be inconspicuous in early lesions but becomes more apparent as the lesion matures.*

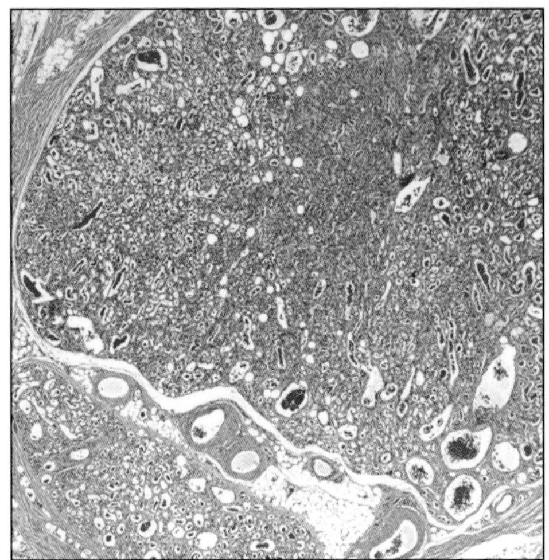

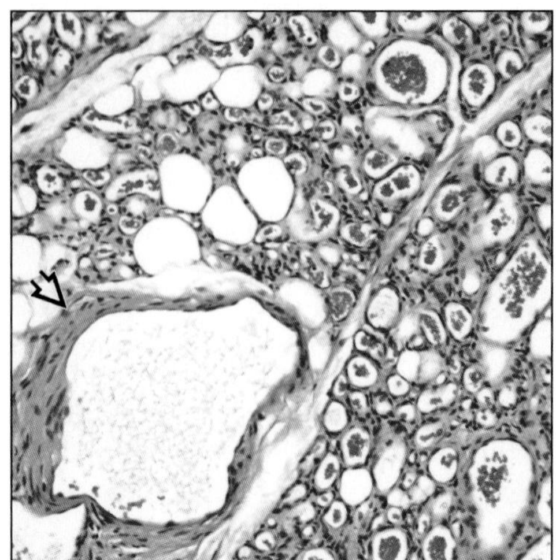

(Left) *The lobular configuration of capillary hemangiomas is apparent at low-power examination ➔. Lobules of capillaries are centered in dermis and subcutaneous tissue in this example, and the overlying skin is intact ➚.* ***(Right)*** *The skin overlying capillary hemangiomas may ulcerate ➔ and mimic inflamed granulation tissue, often referred to as "pyogenic granulomas." The sharp separation ➚ between the 2 nodules of proliferating capillaries is a useful diagnostic clue.*

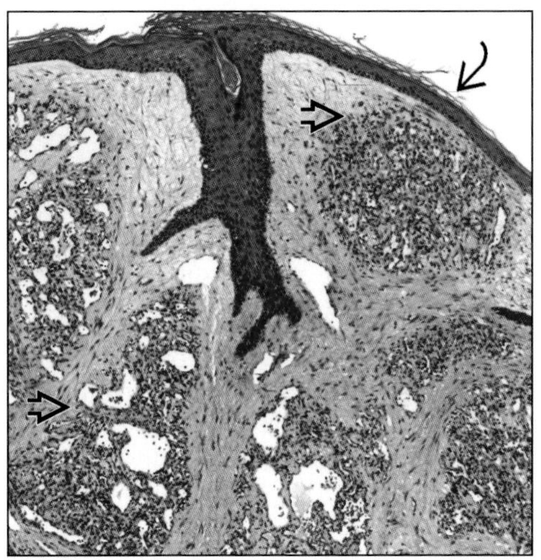

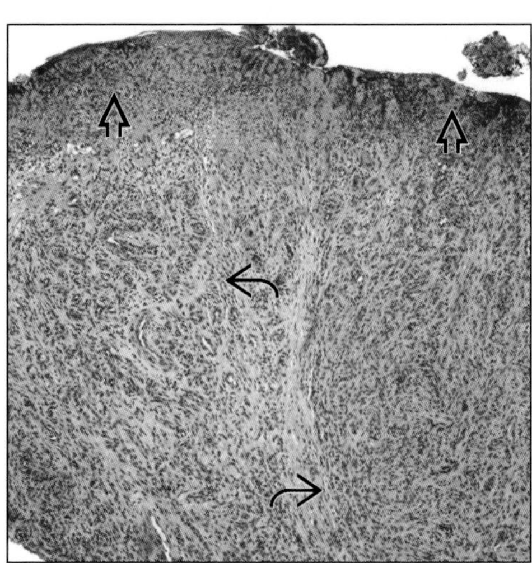

(Left) *At the cellular level, capillary hemangiomas are composed of proliferating endothelial cells, pericytes, and a component of inflammatory cells. Endothelial cells lining the capillaries may be flat ➚ or plump ➔ in appearance.* ***(Right)*** *Mitotic figures may be present ➔ in capillary hemangiomas. The well-circumscribed, lobular architecture at low power as well as the lack of nuclear hyperchromasia and atypia in the lining endothelial cells are helpful in ruling out malignancy.*

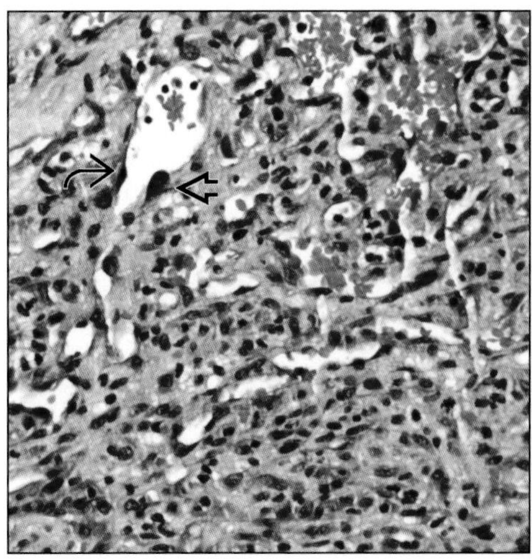

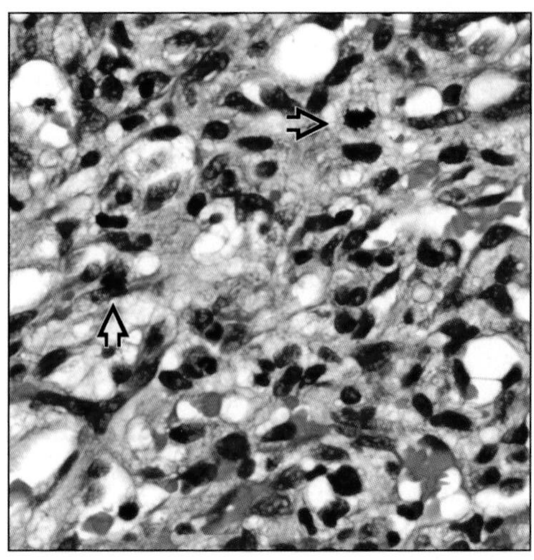

Microscopic Features

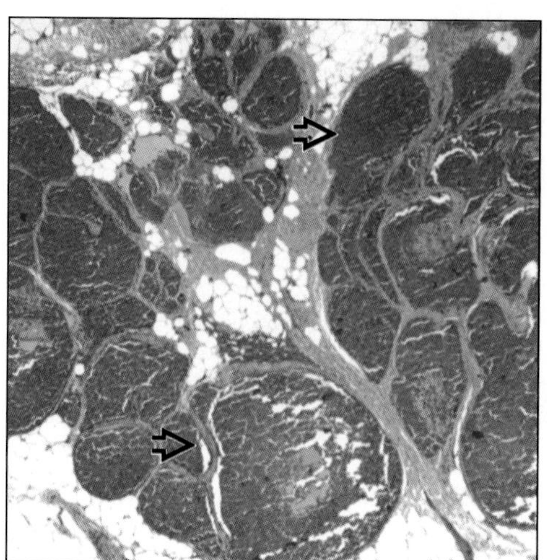

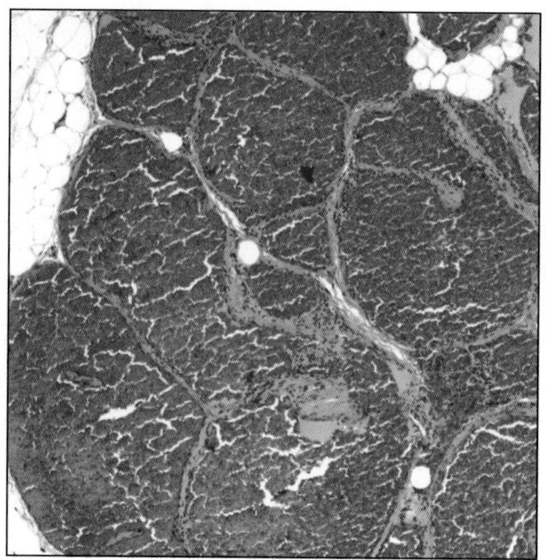

(Left) *Cavernous hemangiomas are also well-circumscribed nodular lesions composed of lobules of cystically dilated ➾ vascular spaces filled with blood.* ***(Right)*** *The endothelial cells lining the cystically dilated blood vessels are flat and attenuated in appearance and show no nuclear atypia.*

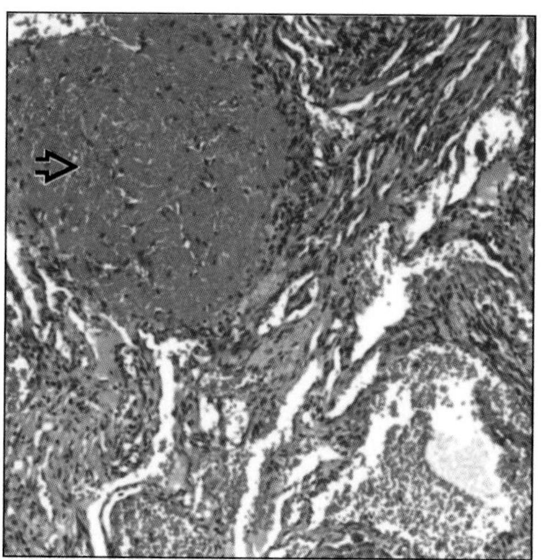

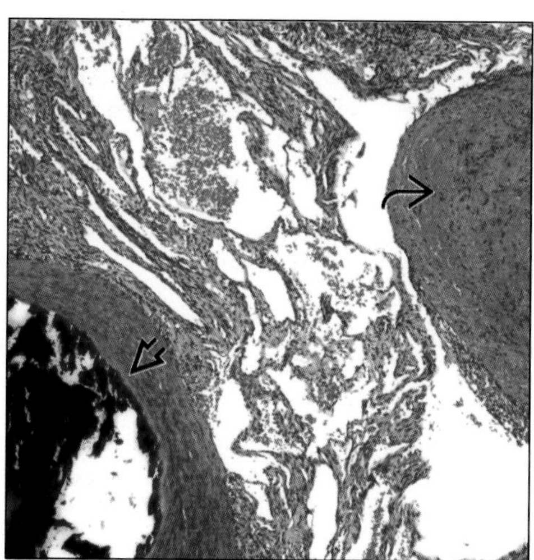

(Left) *Large collections of blood within these cavernous spaces increases predisposition to thrombus formation ➾, which may undergo reorganization to Masson tumor (intravascular papillary endothelial hyperplasia)-like changes.* ***(Right)*** *Large intralesional thrombi may also undergo calcification ➾ and be apparent on imaging studies as phleboliths. A noncalcified thrombus ➚ is also present in this example of cavernous hemangioma.*

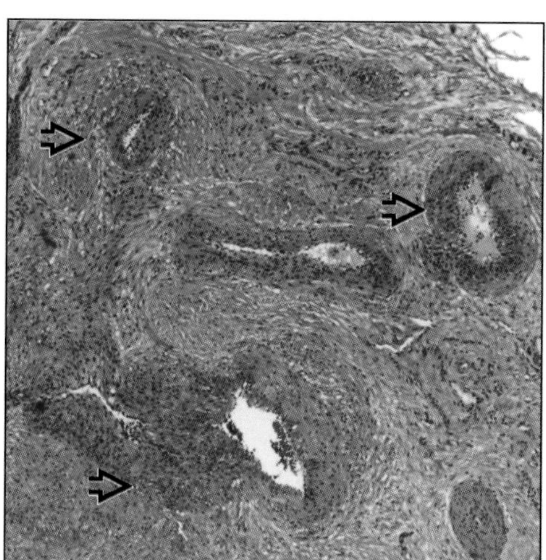

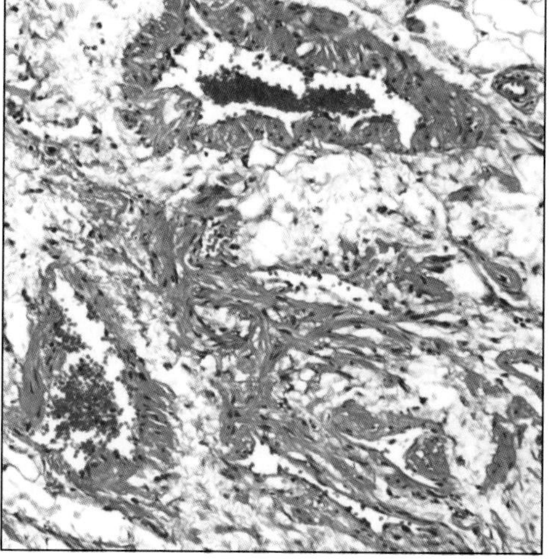

(Left) *Venous hemangiomas are composed of circumscribed, nodular collections of thick-walled blood vessels ➾. The lack of an internal elastic lamina in these proliferating vessels is helpful in distinguishing venous hemangiomas from arteriovenous malformations.* ***(Right)*** *The smooth muscle layer surrounding the veins in venous hemangioma may be variable in thickness and not well formed. Cystically dilated veins in venous hemangiomas may mimic a cavernous hemangioma.*

INTRAMUSCULAR HEMANGIOMA

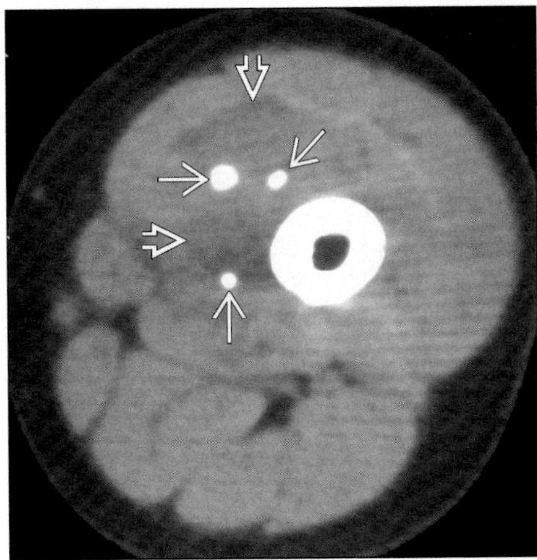

Axial CT through the mid-thigh shows phleboliths ➡ within an intramuscular hemangioma. The low-density areas ⇨ represent fat within the lesion.

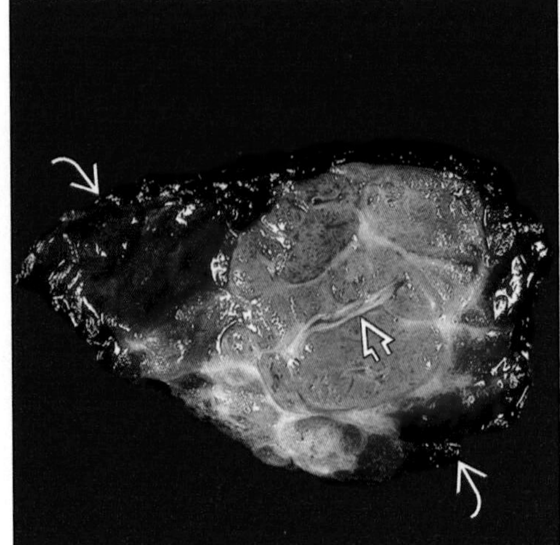

Gross photograph demonstrates a solid tan mass involving skeletal muscle ➡. The lesion has an irregular border with the muscle, and there are grossly evident large vascular structures ⇨.

TERMINOLOGY

Synonyms

- Intramuscular angioma
- Intramuscular angiolipoma

Definitions

- Benign vascular proliferation located within skeletal muscle with varying amounts of mature adipose tissue

ETIOLOGY/PATHOGENESIS

Developmental Anomaly

- Likely represents vascular malformation
- No relation to trauma

CLINICAL ISSUES

Epidemiology

- Incidence
  - Uncommon
    - < 0.8% of benign vascular lesions
    - Relatively common among deep-seated soft tissue tumors
- Age
  - All ages affected
  - Most occur in young adults
    - 85% diagnosed prior to age 30
- Gender
  - Women and men equally affected

Site

- Most frequent in lower extremities
  - Thigh is most common site
- Other common anatomic sites: Head and neck, upper extremities, trunk
- Can occur in any skeletal muscle site as well as in cardiac muscle

Presentation

- Deep-seated, slow-growing mass
- Frequently associated with pain
  - Pain often occurs during exercise
  - Pain more often occurs in long narrow muscles (e.g., thigh muscles)

Treatment

- Surgical approaches
  - Complete excision

Prognosis

- 30-50% recurrence rate
  - Often secondary to incomplete excision
  - Histologic parameters (e.g., vessel type) not predictive of recurrence risk

IMAGE FINDINGS

Radiographic Findings

- Intramuscular soft tissue mass
  - Fatty areas will appear low density on CT
- Frequently show foci of calcification
  - Phleboliths
  - Metaplastic ossification

MACROSCOPIC FEATURES

General Features

- Ill-defined mass within skeletal muscle
- Color varies depending on cellularity, vessel type, and amount of adipose tissue

Size

- Wide size range: 1-29 cm; mean size: 6.5 cm

INTRAMUSCULAR HEMANGIOMA

Key Facts

Terminology
- Benign vascular proliferation located within skeletal muscle with varying amounts of mature adipose tissue

Etiology/Pathogenesis
- Likely represents vascular malformation
- No relation to trauma

Clinical Issues
- 85% diagnosed prior to age 30
- Most frequent in lower extremity muscles
- 30-50% recurrence rate
- Deep-seated, slow-growing mass
- Frequently associated with pain
- < 0.8% of benign vascular lesions

Microscopic Pathology
- Typically consist of mixture of thick-walled veins, arteries, capillaries, and ectatic thin-walled vascular spaces
- Vacular and adipose elements infiltrate among skeletal muscle fibers
- Historically classified into capillary, cavernous, and mixed types

Top Differential Diagnoses
- Angiosarcoma
- Intramuscular lipoma
- Well-differentiated liposarcoma
- Angiomatosis

MICROSCOPIC PATHOLOGY

Histologic Features
- Vary greatly in histologic appearance
  - Typically consist of mixture of thick-walled veins, arteries, capillaries, and ectatic thin-walled vascular spaces
  - Associated with varying amounts of mature adipose tissue
  - Vacular and adipose elements infiltrate among skeletal muscle fibers
    - Muscle atrophy and degenerative sarcolemmal changes may be seen
- Historically classified into capillary, cavernous, and mixed types
  - Majority are of mixed type, limiting use of this classification system
  - May have lymphatic component, too
- Capillary type
  - More frequent in head and neck sites
  - Composed of numerous small (capillary-sized) vessels
  - Lumen formation typically apparent
  - Solid growth akin to juvenile hemangiomas may be seen
  - Endothelial cells are plump and cytologically bland with rare mitoses
- Cavernous type
  - More common in trunk locations
  - Endothelial cells are attenuated and cytologically bland
- Presurgical embolization may result in secondary changes and presence of embolization material

DIFFERENTIAL DIAGNOSIS

Angiosarcoma
- Very uncommon in deep-seated locations
- Complex anastomosing vascular channels
- Multilayered endothelial cells
- Pleomorphic and hyperchromatic nuclei

Intramuscular Lipoma
- Similar site predilection to intramuscular hemangioma
- Does not have a prominent vascular component
- Less recurrence risk (15%) than intramuscular hemangioma

Well-Differentiated Liposarcoma
- May have vascular stroma but lacks mixed vessel component with ectatic and large venous channels
- Will have atypical hyperchromatic stromal cells
  - May have lipoblasts

Angiomatosis
- Histologically identical in many cases, so distinction is clinical
  - Usually congenital
  - Involves large region of body and multiple tissues (e.g., skin, muscle, and bone)

DIAGNOSTIC CHECKLIST

Pathologic Interpretation Pearls
- Features that can lead to misdiagnosis
  - Abundant adipose and relative paucity of vascular proliferation
  - Entrapped muscle fibers with degenerative sarcolemmal nuclei
  - Extensive post-embolization degenerative changes
  - Markedly cellular capillary-type intramuscular hemangioma

SELECTED REFERENCES

1. Beham A et al: Intramuscular angioma: a clinicopathological analysis of 74 cases. Histopathology. 18(1):53-9, 1991
2. Cohen AJ et al: Intramuscular hemangioma. JAMA. 249(19):2680-2, 1983
3. Lin JJ et al: Two entities in angiolipoma. A study of 459 cases of lipoma with review of literature on infiltrating angiolipoma. Cancer. 34(3):720-7, 1974

INTRAMUSCULAR HEMANGIOMA

Microscopic Features

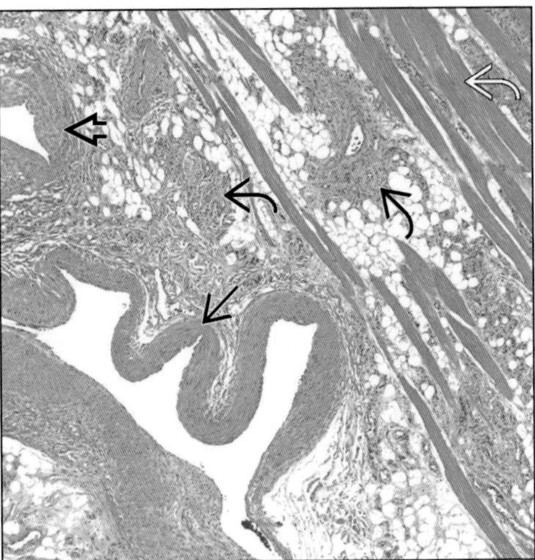

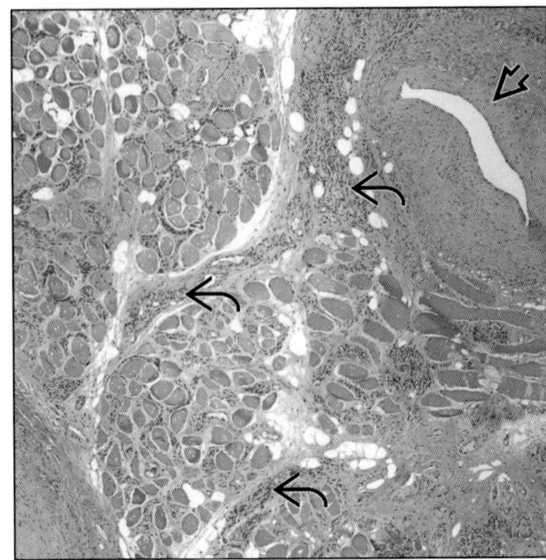

*(**Left**) Typical appearance of intramuscular hemangioma is a complex mixture of vessels, including ectatic vessels ➔, capillaries ➙, arteries ➪, and adipose tissue that appears to infiltrate skeletal muscle ➙. (**Right**) Another mixed-type intramuscular hemangioma composed of a proliferation of capillaries ➙ appears to infiltrate skeletal muscle, imparting a checkerboard-like appearance. Arteries ➪ and a small amount of adipose tissue are present as well.*

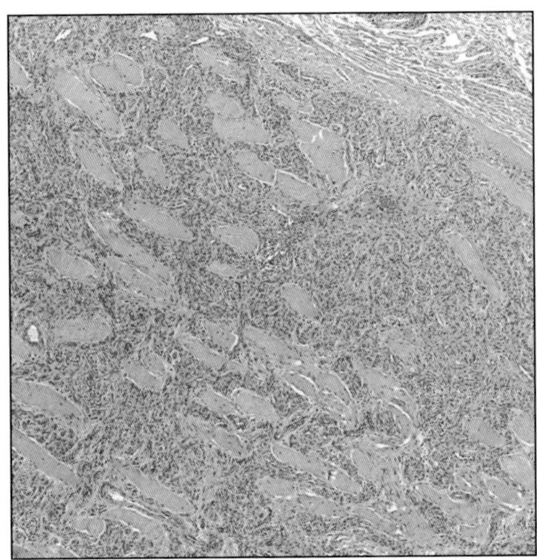

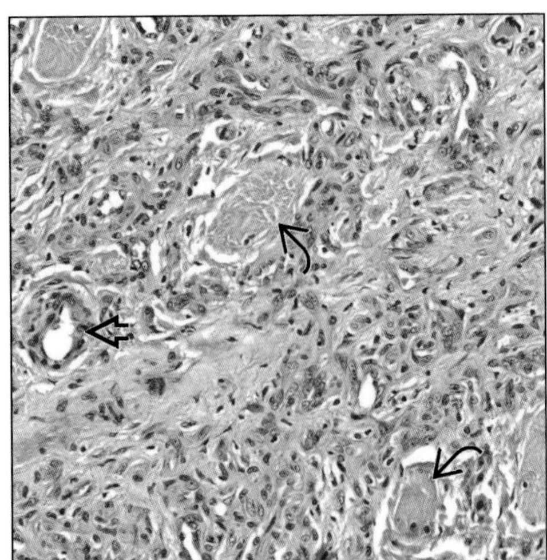

*(**Left**) Low-power view shows a capillary-type intramuscular hemangioma composed of a cellular proliferation of capillary-sized vessels arranged around skeletal muscle fibers. (**Right**) High-power view shows capillary-type intramuscular hemangioma composed of capillary-sized vessels with small to inconspicuous lumens. Scattered arterioles ➪ and degenerating muscle fibers ➙ are present. The endothelial nuclei are cytologically bland, helping to differentiate this from an angiosarcoma.*

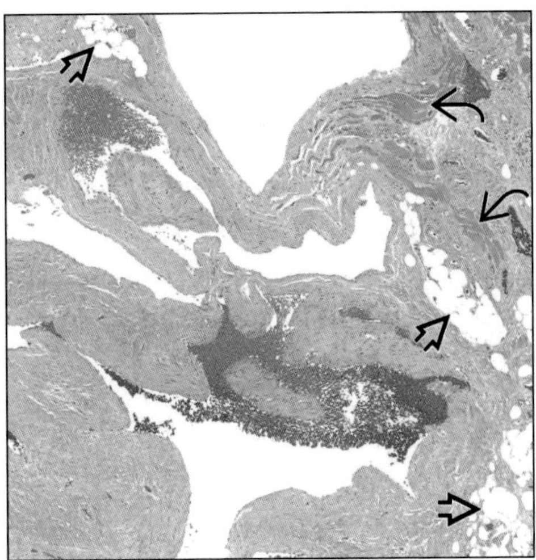

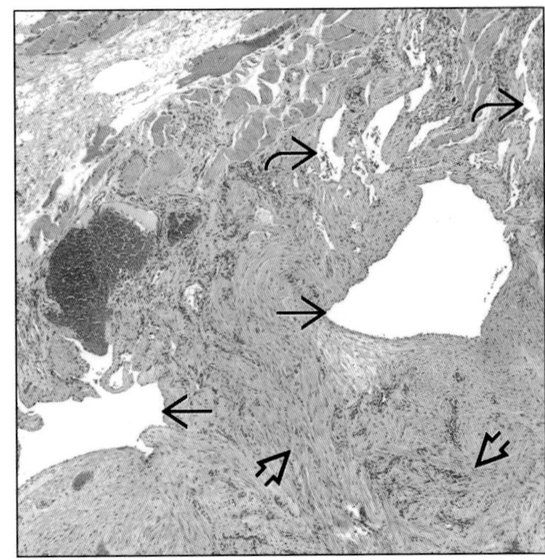

*(**Left**) Cavernous intramuscular hemangioma is characterized by ectatic thin-walled vascular spaces with associated adipose tissue ➪ and infiltrating degenerating skeletal muscle ➙. (**Right**) Cavernous intramuscular hemangiomas are frequently associated with an irregular proliferation of smooth muscle bundles ➪ and smaller slit-like vascular channels ➙ at the periphery of the larger ectatic vessels ➔.*

Microscopic Features

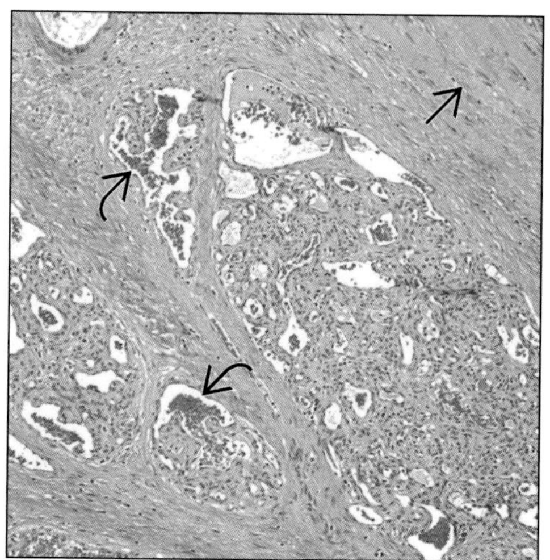

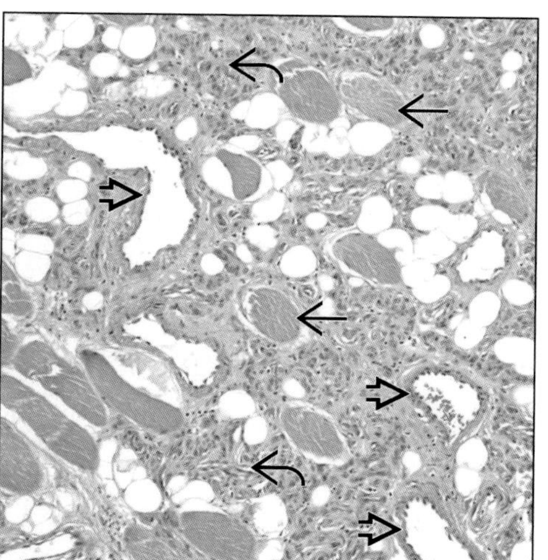

(Left) *Some intramuscular hemangiomas have a lobulated appearance, imparting a resemblance to lobular capillary hemangioma. The lobules in this example are composed of numerous small capillaries with larger feeder-type vascular channels* ⮫*. Note the compressed zone of skeletal muscle* →. **(Right)** *High-power view of a typical intramuscular hemangioma shows capillaries* ⮫ *and arterioles* ⇨ *associated with mature adipose and insinuating among skeletal muscle fibers* →.

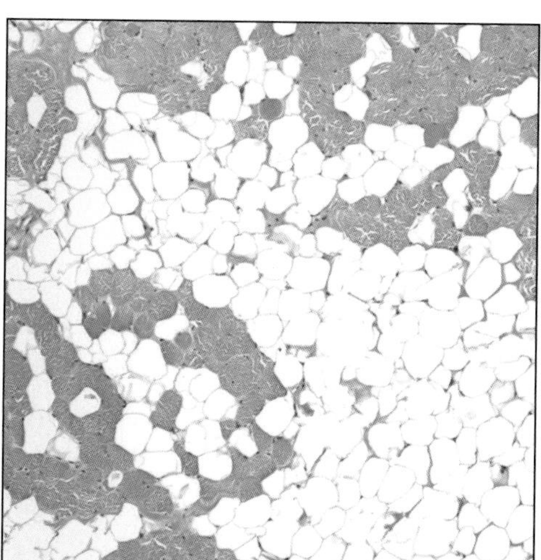

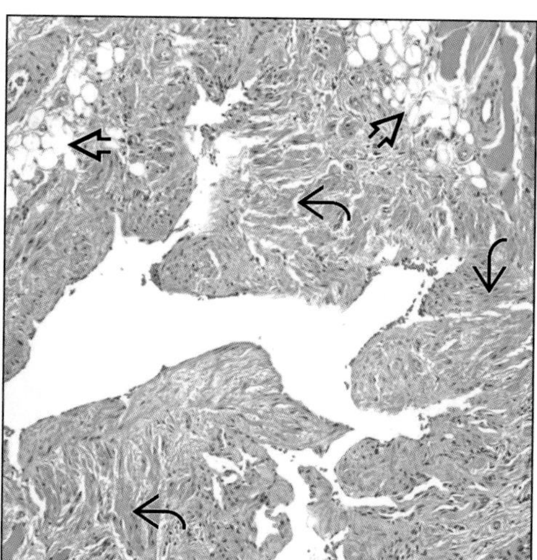

(Left) *Some intramuscular hemangiomas, such as this example, can easily be confused with intramuscular lipomas due to abundant adipose tissue and relative paucity of vascular elements.* **(Right)** *Extensive adipose tissue is often seen in cavernous types of intramuscular hemangioma, such as this tumor, which had extensive adipose tissue and only focal vascular areas. Note the adipose tissue* ⇨*, ectatic vascular channels, and irregular smooth muscle proliferation around the lumen* ⮫.

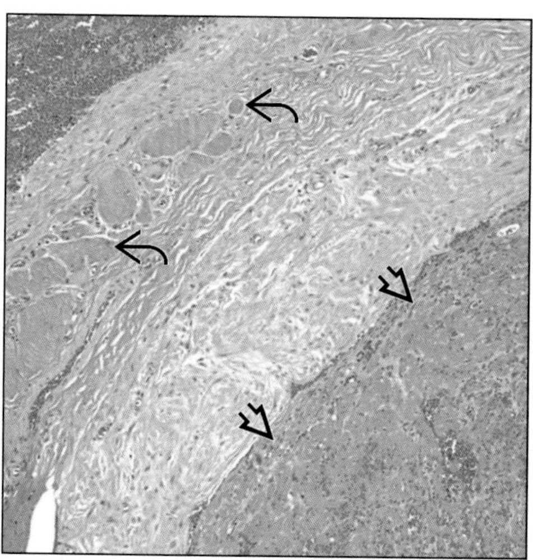

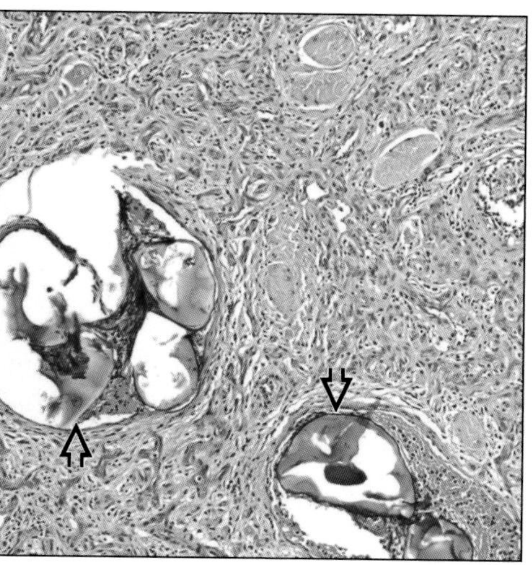

(Left) *Secondary changes are common in intramuscular hemangioma. Note the compressed and atrophic skeletal muscle bundles* ⮫ *in this cavernous intramuscular hemangioma. Cavernous examples frequently develop thrombi* ⇨ *that may calcify and become phleboliths, which suggest the diagnosis on imaging studies.* **(Right)** *Many tumors are embolized prior to resection and show embolization material and thrombus in vessels* ⇨ *with secondary inflammation &/or necrosis.*

SINUSOIDAL HEMANGIOMA

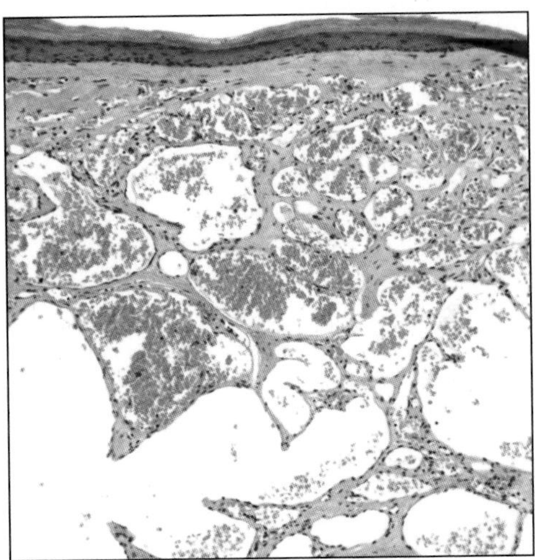

Histologic section shows the superficial portion of a cutaneous sinusoidal hemangioma with large dilated vascular spaces.

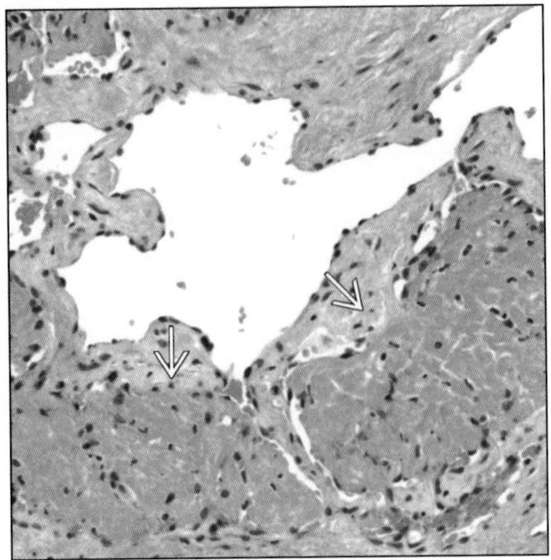

Histologic section shows sinusoidal vascular spaces with thrombosis ➡, a finding often seen in sinusoidal hemangioma.

TERMINOLOGY

Abbreviations
- Sinusoidal hemangioma (SH)

Synonyms
- Cavernous hemangioma (variant of)

Definitions
- Acquired vascular lesion in adults; features similar to cavernous hemangioma/venous malformation

ETIOLOGY/PATHOGENESIS

Unknown
- May represent reactive vascular proliferation rather than true neoplastic process

CLINICAL ISSUES

Epidemiology
- Incidence
    - Rare tumors
- Age
    - Typically occurs in adults
- Gender
    - More common in females

Site
- Often occurs on extremities, trunk, or breast

Presentation
- Subcutaneous or dermal mass
    - Solitary, painless, bluish (deep) or red (superficial) nodule
        - Freely movable

Treatment
- Surgical approaches
    - Complete excision is curative but not necessary given benign nature of lesions

Prognosis
- Excellent, no malignant potential

MACROSCOPIC FEATURES

Size
- Typically < 2.0 cm

MICROSCOPIC PATHOLOGY

Histologic Features
- Proliferation of numerous thin-walled anastomosing vessels
    - Well-circumscribed proliferation of vessels in sinusoidal pattern
    - Vessels are thin walled and closely packed, with little intervening stroma
        - Occasional cases may show smooth muscle in vessel walls
        - Pseudopapillary pattern may be seen (due to tangential sectioning)
        - Thrombosis may occur and be associated with intravascular papillary endothelial hyperplasia (Masson tumor)
    - Lining cells are small endothelial cells with nuclear hyperchromasia
    - Mitotic figures typically not seen
    - Calcifications may rarely be present

Cytologic Features
- Nuclei are hyperchromatic but show regular borders and uniform chromatin

Predominant Pattern/Injury Type
- Vascular proliferation

SINUSOIDAL HEMANGIOMA

Key Facts

Terminology

- Acquired vascular lesion in adults; features similar to venous malformation

Clinical Issues

- Painless bluish or red nodule
- Complete excision is curative, but not necessary given benign nature of lesions
- Excellent, no malignant potential

Microscopic Pathology

- Well-circumscribed vascular proliferation
- Vessels are thin walled and closely packed, with little intervening stroma
- Lining cells are small endothelial cells with nuclear hyperchromasia
- Pseudopapillary pattern may be seen (due to tangential sectioning)

Predominant Cell/Compartment Type

- Endothelial

DIFFERENTIAL DIAGNOSIS

Venous Malformation (Cavernous Hemangioma)

- Typically occurs in children
- Often larger and more poorly circumscribed than sinusoidal hemangioma
- Does not show as closely packed vessels or ramified pattern

Cherry Angioma

- Very common small papular lesions occurring in adults
- Superficial papillary dermal lesions, as opposed to sinusoidal hemangioma (which is typically deep dermal or subcutaneous)

Arteriovenous Hemangioma (Malformation)

- Typically occurs on lips, perioral skin, or nose of older men
- Proliferation of large, thick-walled blood vessels with smooth muscle in their walls, which mostly represent veins
- Feeder vessel (ascending muscular artery) may be present in some cases

Glomeruloid Hemangioma

- Associated with Castleman syndrome and **p**olyneuropathy, **o**rganomegaly, **e**ndocrinopathy, **m**onoclonal paraproteinemia, and **s**kin lesions (POEMS) syndrome
- Typically presents as multiple eruptive lesions on trunk and limbs
- Dilated vascular spaces filled by grape-like clusters of capillaries, reminiscent of renal glomeruli

DIAGNOSTIC CHECKLIST

Pathologic Interpretation Pearls

- Closely packed lobular proliferation of vessels in deep dermis or subcutis

SELECTED REFERENCES

1. Nakamura M et al: Calcifying sinusoidal haemangioma on the back. Br J Dermatol. 141(2):377-8, 1999
2. Ruck P et al: Diffuse sinusoidal hemangiomatosis of the spleen. A case report with enzyme-histochemical, immunohistochemical, and electron-microscopic findings. Pathol Res Pract. 190(7):708-14; discussion 715-7, 1994
3. Calonje E et al: New entities in cutaneous soft tissue tumours. Pathologica. 85(1095):1-15, 1993
4. Calonje E et al: Sinusoidal hemangioma. A distinctive benign vascular neoplasm within the group of cavernous hemangiomas. Am J Surg Pathol. 15(12):1130-5, 1991

IMAGE GALLERY

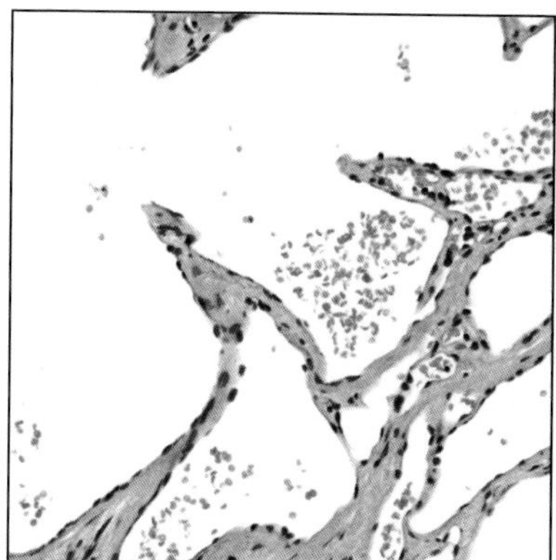

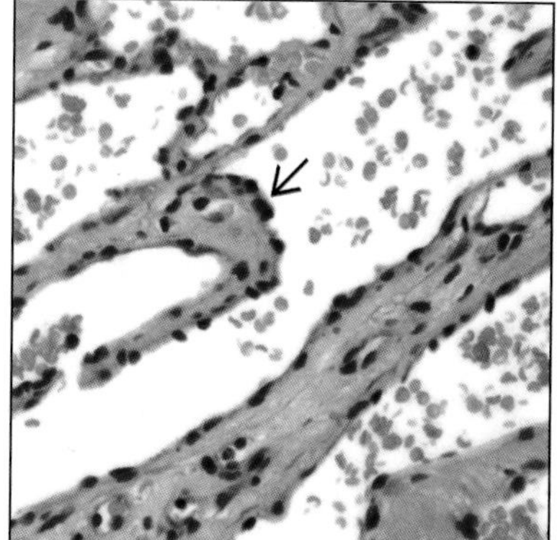

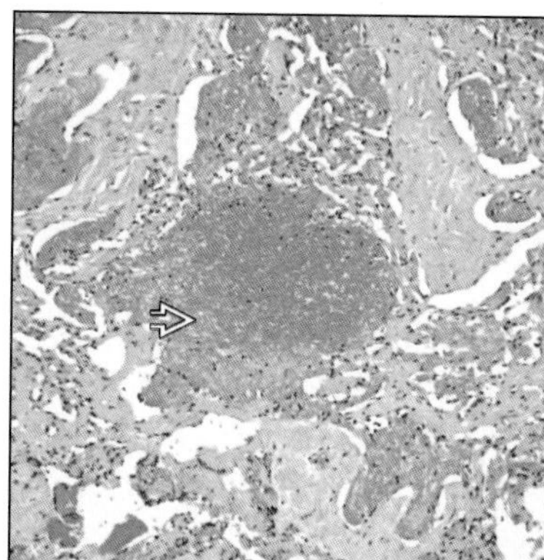

(Left) *Histologic section shows pseudopapillary areas with thin, endothelial-lined stroma projecting into dilated vascular spaces.* ***(Center)*** *Histologic section shows the cytologic features of the endothelial cells, which show small, uniform nuclei with hyperchromasia ➔.* ***(Right)*** *Another example of a sinusoidal hemangioma shows hemorrhage and thrombosis (Masson change) ➔.*

MICROVENULAR HEMANGIOMA

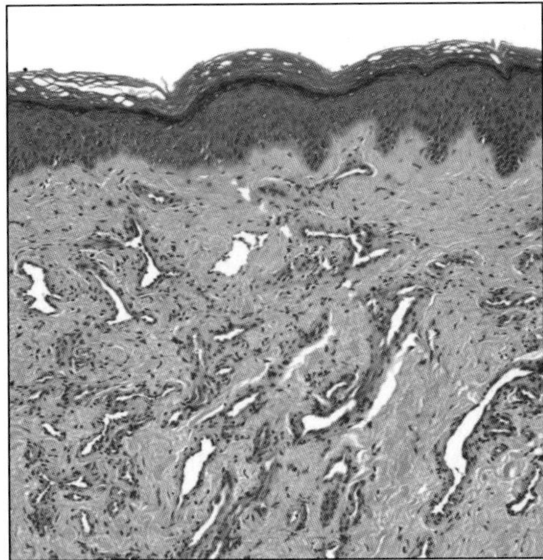

Histologic section shows increased numbers of small blood vessels in the superficial dermis with irregular branching and narrow lumina.

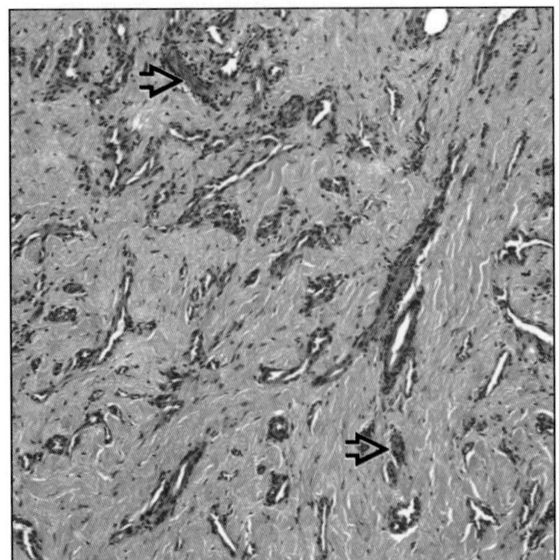

Higher magnification of the histologic section shows a proliferation of small blood vessels with thin walls and small to collapsed lumina ➡ associated with a sclerotic stroma.

TERMINOLOGY

Abbreviations

- Microvenular hemangioma (MVH)

Synonyms

- Microcapillary angioma

Definitions

- Slowly growing benign vascular proliferation composed of small, collapsed vessels

ETIOLOGY/PATHOGENESIS

Unknown

- In most cases

Hormonal Influence

- Some cases reportedly related to pregnancy or contraceptives

CLINICAL ISSUES

Epidemiology

- Age
  - Young to middle-aged adults
- Gender
  - Occurs in both males and females about equally

Site

- Typically occurs on upper extremities, especially forearms

Presentation

- Slow-growing papule or nodule

Natural History

- Often present for only a few weeks to months at presentation

Treatment

- Surgical approaches
  - Simple excision is curative but not necessary, as these are benign lesions

Prognosis

- Excellent

MACROSCOPIC FEATURES

Size

- Small, typically < 1 cm

MICROSCOPIC PATHOLOGY

Histologic Features

- Poorly circumscribed dermal proliferation of small blood vessels that diffusely involve reticular dermis
  - Branching vessels typically present
  - Most vessels show narrow or collapsed lumina
    - A few erythrocytes may be present with lumina
  - Endothelial cells may be slightly enlarged, but lack significant cytologic atypia
  - Some cases may show large epithelioid cells resembling those seen in epithelioid (histiocytoid) hemangiomas
- Tufted groups of vessels may be seen in deep dermis
- Background of mild dermal sclerosis
- Inflammation and hemosiderin deposition typically lacking

Cytologic Features

- Endothelial cells may be enlarged, but they show bland nuclei without significant atypia or pleomorphism

MICROVENULAR HEMANGIOMA

Key Facts

Terminology

- Microvenular hemangioma (MVH)
- Synonym: Microcapillary angioma
- Slowly growing, benign vascular proliferation composed of small, collapsed vessels

Clinical Issues

- Young to middle-aged adults
- Typically occur on upper extremities, especially forearms

Microscopic Pathology

- Poorly circumscribed dermal proliferation of small blood vessels that diffusely involve reticular dermis
- Most vessels show narrow or collapsed lumina
- Endothelial cells may be slightly enlarged but lack significant cytologic atypia
- Tufted groups of vessels may be seen in deep dermis

DIFFERENTIAL DIAGNOSIS

Kaposi Sarcoma

- May show thin-walled vessels but typically also has irregular anastomosing spaces lined by atypical spindle cells
- Plasma cells and hyaline globules are lacking in MVH
- HHV8(+) by immunohistochemistry

Stasis Changes/Stasis Dermatitis

- Superficial proliferation of small, thick-walled blood vessels
- Shows prominent hemosiderin deposition throughout dermis (lacking in MVH)
- Often shows more inflammation and overlying spongiosis (stasis dermatitis)
- Clinical presentation distinctive: Lower extremities of elderly adults

Early Scar

- Angiogenesis in early scars may mimic MVH
- Typically greater fibrosis, inflammation, extravasated red blood cells, and hemosiderin deposition in scars

Targetoid Hemosiderotic Hemangioma (Hobnail Hemangioma)

- While deeper small vessels are similar to those in MVH, superficial vessels are larger and dilated
- Hobnailed endothelial cells project into vascular lumina
- Hemosiderin deposition is typically very prominent

DIAGNOSTIC CHECKLIST

Pathologic Interpretation Pearls

- Benign vascular proliferation composed of small, collapsed vessels
- Branching vessels typically present
- Endothelial cells may be enlarged but lack cytologic atypia
- Background of mild dermal sclerosis

SELECTED REFERENCES

1. Chang SE et al: Microvenular hemangioma in a boy with acute myelogenous leukemia. Pediatr Dermatol. 20(3):266-7, 2003
2. Kim YC et al: Microvenular hemangioma. Dermatology. 206(2):161-4, 2003
3. Rikihisa W et al: Microvenular haemangioma in a patient with Wiskott-Aldrich syndrome. Br J Dermatol. 141(4):752-4, 1999
4. Hunt SJ et al: Acquired benign and "borderline" vascular lesions. Dermatol Clin. 10(1):97-115, 1992
5. Hunt SJ et al: Microvenular hemangioma. J Cutan Pathol. 18(4):235-40, 1991
6. Bantel E et al: [Understanding microcapillary angioma, observations in pregnant patients and in females treated with hormonal contraceptives.] Z Hautkr. 64(12):1071-4, 1989

IMAGE GALLERY

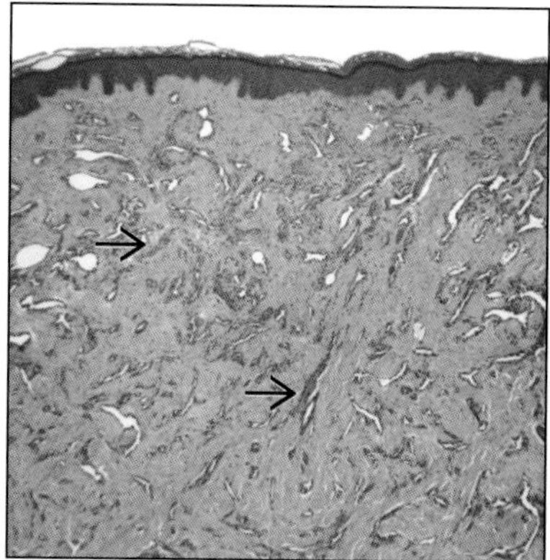

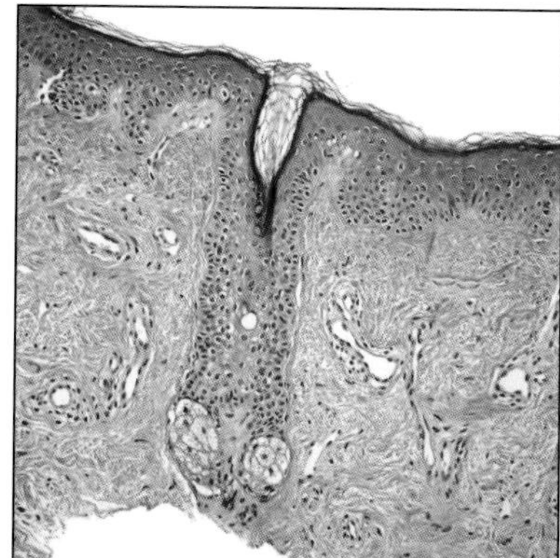

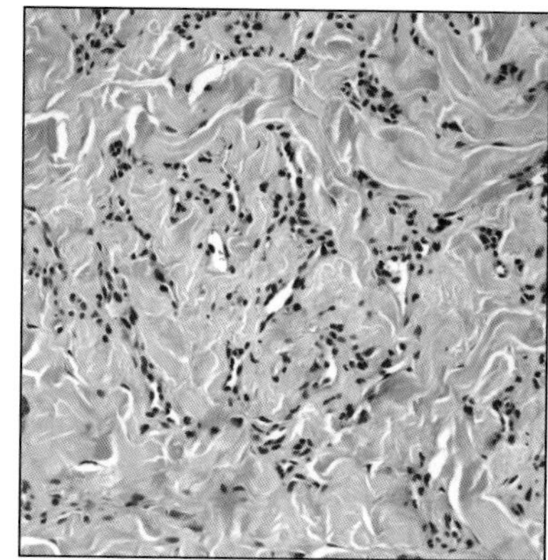

(Left) Scanning magnification of skin shows a diffuse dermal proliferation of small, elongated blood vessels with narrow to collapsed ⇒ lumina and a background of dermal sclerosis. (Center) Superficial portion of a subtle lesion of microvenular hemangioma shows scattered small blood vessels in the superficial dermis. (Right) High-power examination shows bland cytologic features of the endothelial cells, with small, hyperchromatic-staining nuclei. No mitoses or necrosis are present.

HOBNAIL HEMANGIOMA

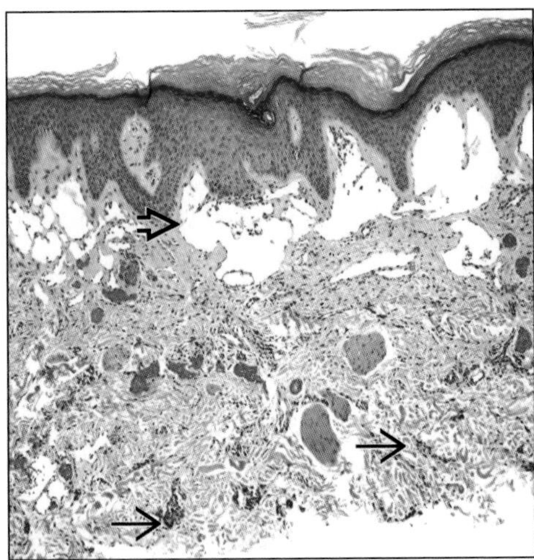

Low magnification of a hobnail hemangioma shows superficial dilated vascular spaces ⇨ in the papillary dermis with deeper small blood vessels and stromal hemosiderin deposits →.

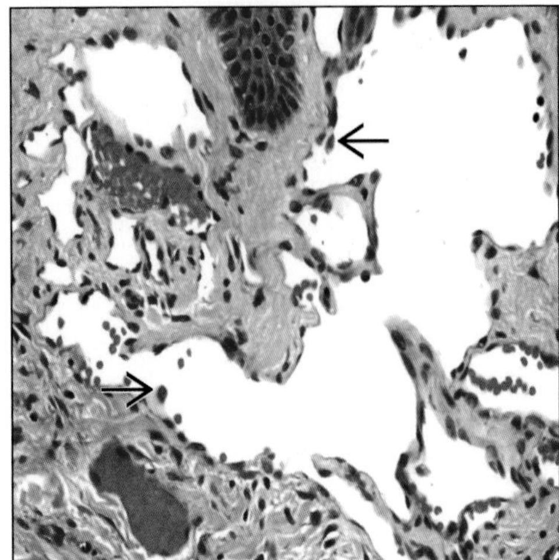

Higher power examination demonstrates a hobnail hemangioma with superficial dilated vessels lined by small endothelial cells protruding into the lumina → and showing nuclear hyperchromasia.

TERMINOLOGY

Abbreviations

- Hobnail hemangioma (HH)

Synonyms

- Targetoid hemosiderotic hemangioma (clinical term)

Definitions

- Benign vascular proliferation, typically wedge-shaped, showing intravascular papillae and hobnailed endothelial cells

ETIOLOGY/PATHOGENESIS

Unknown

- Trauma has been implicated in some cases
  - Postulated to represent traumatized lymphangioma or hemangioma

CLINICAL ISSUES

Epidemiology

- Age
  - Young to middle-aged adults
- Gender
  - More common in males

Site

- Typically presents on lower extremities; also may occur on upper extremities, rarely in oral cavity

Presentation

- Skin papule or nodule
  - Often pigmented due to hemosiderin deposition
  - May show a halo ("targetoid" appearance) in minority of cases

Treatment

- Surgical approaches
  - Complete excision is curative but not necessary given lesions' benign nature

Prognosis

- Excellent, with no tendency for local recurrence

MACROSCOPIC FEATURES

General Features

- Dermal-based reddish brown lesion with hemorrhage

Size

- Small, usually < 2 cm

MICROSCOPIC PATHOLOGY

Histologic Features

- Vascular proliferation with wedge-shaped appearance
- Superficial vessels are dilated and thin walled
  - Some vessels may resemble lymphatics
  - Focal papillary projections with fibrous cores may be present
  - Vessels are lined by small, bland-appearing endothelial cells with hobnail appearance (nuclei project into lumina)
  - Mitoses should not be present
- Deeper vessels are progressively smaller and show narrow lumina
- Hemorrhage and hemosiderin deposition are typically prominent
- Inflammation is usually minimal

Cytologic Features

- Bland, plump endothelial cells with uniform-appearing nuclei

Predominant Pattern/Injury Type

- Vascular

HOBNAIL HEMANGIOMA

Key Facts

Terminology
- Targetoid hemosiderotic hemangioma
- Benign vascular proliferation, typically wedge-shaped, showing intravascular papillae and hobnail endothelial cells

Etiology/Pathogenesis
- Postulated to represent traumatized lymphangioma or hemangioma

Clinical Issues
- Typically presents on lower extremities; also may occur on upper extremities, rarely in oral cavity

Microscopic Pathology
- Superficial vessels are dilated and thin walled
- Deeper vessels are progressively smaller
- Vessels are lined by small, bland-appearing endothelial cells with hobnail appearance

Predominant Cell/Compartment Type
- Endothelial

DIFFERENTIAL DIAGNOSIS

Progressive Lymphangioma
- Thin-walled, dilated superficial vascular spaces with narrower deeper vessels
- Lacks hobnail endothelial cell morphology and hemosiderin deposition of HH

Kaposi Sarcoma
- Shows proliferation of slit-like spaces lined by atypical spindle cells
- Typically lacks superficial dilated vascular spaces and hobnail cells
- HHV8(+) by immunohistochemistry

Microvenular Hemangioma
- Proliferation of small, round to slit-like, thin-walled vessels involving reticular dermis
- Lacks superficial dilated vascular spaces, hobnail cells, and hemosiderin deposition

Retiform Hemangioendothelioma
- Dermal and subcutaneous tumor characterized by proliferation of arborizing vessels lined by hobnail endothelial cells
- Typically prominent lymphoid infiltrate, which is lacking in HH
- HH is typically more superficial, and deeper vessels are smaller and compact

DIAGNOSTIC CHECKLIST

Pathologic Interpretation Pearls
- Wedge-shaped vascular proliferation
- Dilated superficial vessels, deeper small/collapsed vessels
- Intravascular papillae and hobnail endothelial cells
- Prominent hemosiderin deposition

SELECTED REFERENCES

1. Fernandez-Flores A et al: Clinical changes in "true" hobnail hemangioma during menstruation. Bratisl Lek Listy. 109(3):141-3, 2008
2. Franke FE et al: Hobnail hemangiomas (targetoid hemosiderotic hemangiomas) are true lymphangiomas. J Cutan Pathol. 31(5):362-7, 2004
3. Pabuccuoğlu U et al: Hobnail haemangioma occurring on the nasal dorsum. Br J Dermatol. 146(1):162-4, 2002
4. Guillou L et al: Hobnail hemangioma: a pseudomalignant vascular lesion with a reappraisal of targetoid hemosiderotic hemangioma. Am J Surg Pathol. 23(1):97-105, 1999
5. Santonja C et al: Hobnail hemangioma. Dermatology. 191(2):154-6, 1995

IMAGE GALLERY

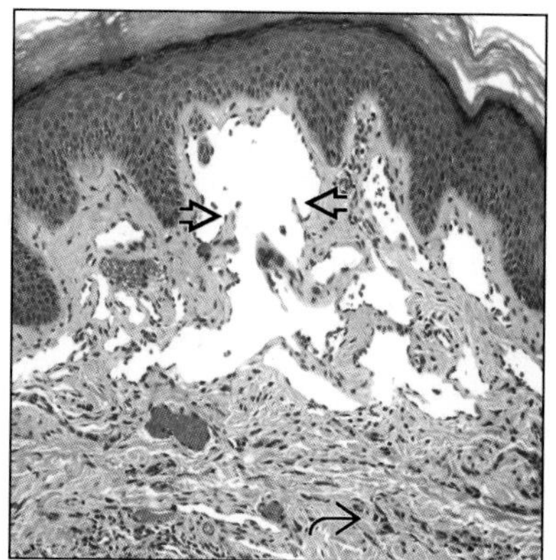

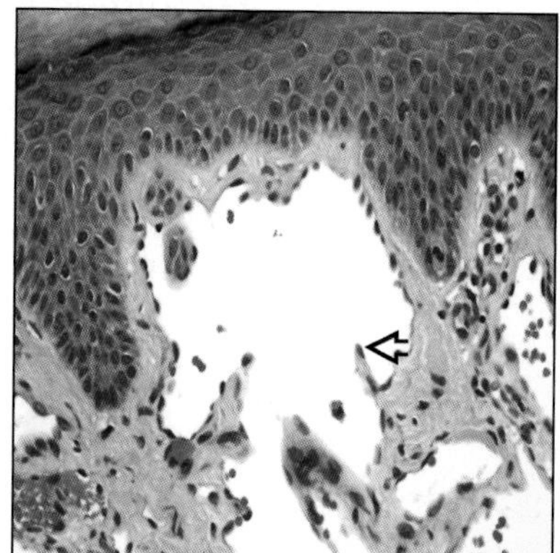

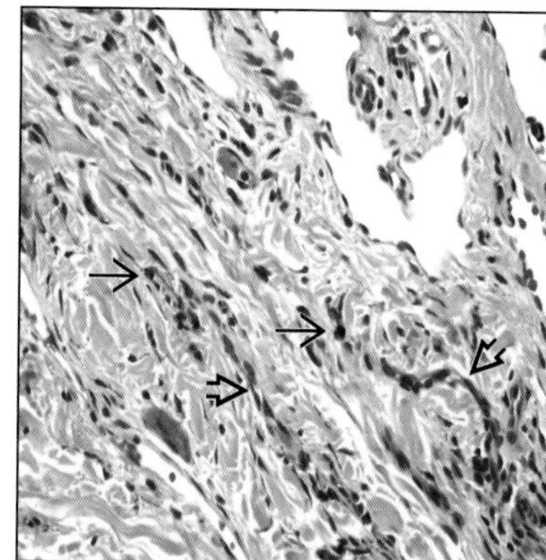

*(**Left**) Low magnification shows the superficial portion of a hobnail hemangioma with dilated vascular spaces, papillary endothelial structures ⇨, and stromal hemosiderin deposits ➔. (**Center**) Higher magnification of the tumor shows the bland cytologic features of the endothelial cells protruding into the vascular spaces ⇨. (**Right**) Histologic examination of the deeper aspect of the lesion shows smaller blood vessels ⇨ and prominent hemosiderin deposition in the stroma ➔.*

GLOMERULOID HEMANGIOMA

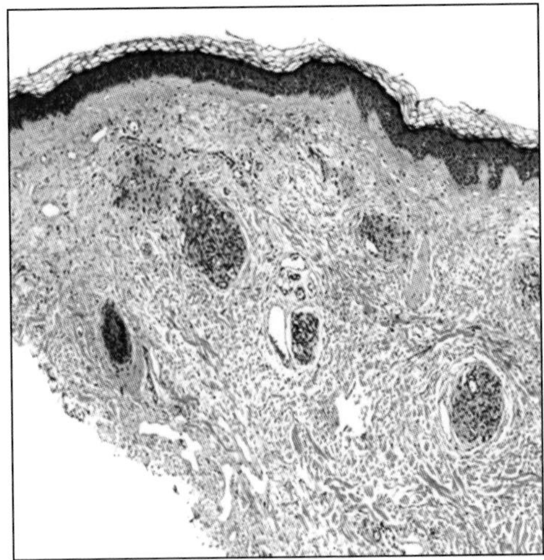

Low magnification shows a superficial dermal proliferation of small clusters of vessels with a glomeruloid pattern.

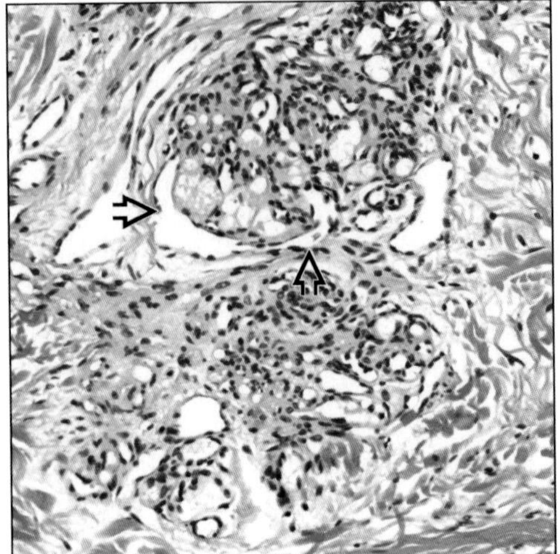

High-power view of a glomeruloid hemangioma shows small, grape-like clusters of vessels projecting into vascular lumens (with peripheral crescentic spaces ⇨).

TERMINOLOGY

Abbreviations

- Glomeruloid hemangioma (GH)

Synonyms

- Glomeruloid angioma

Definitions

- Benign proliferation of small vessels mimicking renal glomeruli

ETIOLOGY/PATHOGENESIS

Paraneoplastic Syndromes

- Association with **p**olyneuropathy, **o**rganomegaly, **e**ndocrinopathy, **M**-protein, **s**kin changes (POEMS syndrome) or multicentric Castleman disease in almost all cases

Unknown

- Rare cases not associated with POEMS syndrome

CLINICAL ISSUES

Epidemiology

- Incidence
  - Rare tumors
- Gender
  - More common in females
- Ethnicity
  - More common in Asians (Japanese)

Site

- Trunk and extremities

Presentation

- Multiple red to purple eruptive papules (POEMS syndrome)
  - Most patients also have diffuse skin hyperpigmentation
- Single lesions reported in patients without POEMS

Treatment

- Surgical approaches
  - Excision is curative but not necessary in most cases
- Adjuvant therapy
  - Treatment of underlying plasma cell disorder may lead to regression of lesions

Prognosis

- Excellent, no malignant potential

MACROSCOPIC FEATURES

General Features

- Dermal-based, well-circumscribed, unencapsulated lesions

Size

- Small, typically only a few millimeters

MICROSCOPIC PATHOLOGY

Histologic Features

- Dermal-based proliferation of dilated spaces containing small capillary-type vessels
- Vessels show distinctive grape-like clusters projecting into lumina, mimicking renal glomeruli
- Endothelial cells are mildly enlarged, and many show cytoplasmic eosinophilic globules
  - Cytoplasmic globules (secondary lysosomes containing immunoglobulins) are PAS(+)
- Endothelial cells may show nuclear hyperchromasia but do not show significant cytologic atypia
- Few mitoses, no necrosis or infiltrative features

GLOMERULOID HEMANGIOMA

Key Facts

Terminology
- Glomeruloid angioma

Etiology/Pathogenesis
- Association with polyneuropathy, organomegaly, endocrinopathy, M-protein, skin changes (POEMS) or multicentric Castleman syndrome in most cases

Clinical Issues
- More common in Asians (especially Japanese)
- Multiple red to purple eruptive papules (POEMS syndrome)

Microscopic Pathology
- Vessels show distinctive grape-like clusters mimicking renal glomeruli
- Endothelial cells are mildly enlarged and many show cytoplasmic eosinophilic globules
- Cytoplasmic globules (immunoglobulins) are PAS(+)

DIFFERENTIAL DIAGNOSIS

Acquired Tufted Hemangioma (Angioblastoma)
- Slowly spreading macules and plaques in young children and adults
- Multiple dermal and subcutaneous vascular lobules composed of spindled and polygonal-shaped cells
- Some cases may show overlapping features with glomeruloid hemangioma

Lobular Capillary Hemangioma (Pyogenic Granuloma)
- Often shows polypoid configuration with epidermal collarette
- Lobular proliferation typically associated with ulceration, edema, and acute inflammation

Targetoid Hemosiderotic Hemangioma (Hobnail Hemangioma)
- Superficial dilated vessels and smaller, narrow deeper vessels lined by plump (hobnailed) cells
- Extravasated red blood cells and prominent stromal hemosiderin deposition

Kaposi Sarcoma
- Clinical history distinctive
  - HIV(+) with multiple lesions, or lower extremity lesion in elderly Mediterranean male
- Cords or fascicles of spindled cells with slit-like lumina associated with hemosiderin deposition and plasma cells
- HHV8(+) (not reported in glomeruloid hemangioma)

DIAGNOSTIC CHECKLIST

Pathologic Interpretation Pearls
- Dermal proliferation of vessels showing distinctive glomeruloid groups or clusters mimicking renal glomeruli

SELECTED REFERENCES

1. Forman SB et al: Glomeruloid hemangiomas without POEMS syndrome: series of three cases. J Cutan Pathol. 34(12):956-7, 2007
2. Perdaens C et al: POEMS syndrome characterized by glomeruloid angioma, osteosclerosis and multicentric Castleman disease. J Eur Acad Dermatol Venereol. 20(4):480-1, 2006
3. Uthup S et al: Renal involvement in multicentric Castleman disease with glomeruloid hemangioma of skin and plasmacytoma. Am J Kidney Dis. 48(2):e17-24, 2006
4. Rongioletti F et al: Glomeruloid hemangioma. A cutaneous marker of POEMS syndrome. Am J Dermatopathol. 16(2):175-8, 1994
5. Chan JK et al: Glomeruloid hemangioma. A distinctive cutaneous lesion of multicentric Castleman's disease associated with POEMS syndrome. Am J Surg Pathol. 14(11):1036-46, 1990

IMAGE GALLERY

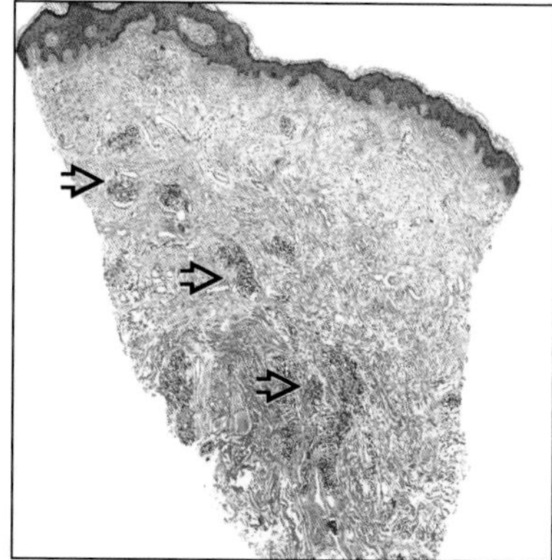

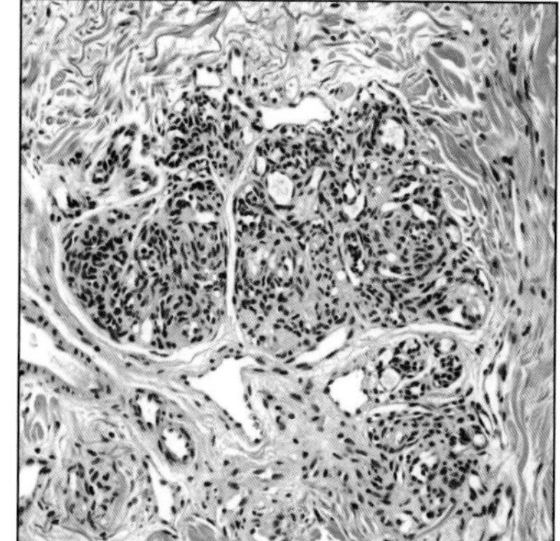

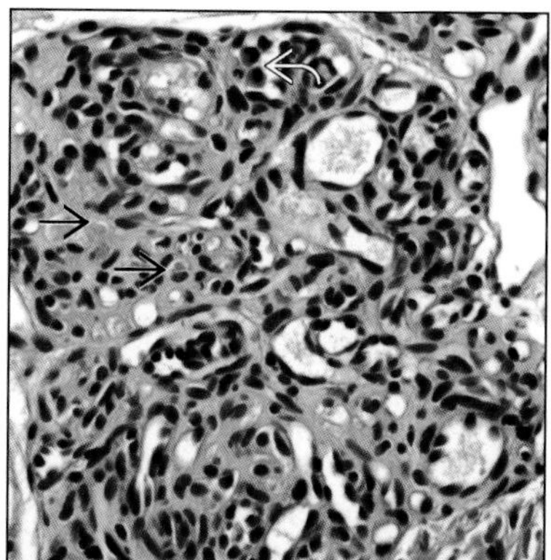

(Left) *Scanning magnification view of a glomeruloid hemangioma shows small clusters of vessels ⇨ in the mid to deep dermis.* *(Center)* *Higher magnification shows the grape-like pattern of clustered small vessels, mimicking renal glomeruli.* *(Right)* *High magnification of the vessels in a glomeruloid hemangioma shows endothelial cells with oval- to spindle-shaped nuclei. Cytoplasmic eosinophilic globules are present focally →. A few intraluminal eosinophils are also seen ➨.*

ACQUIRED TUFTED ANGIOMA

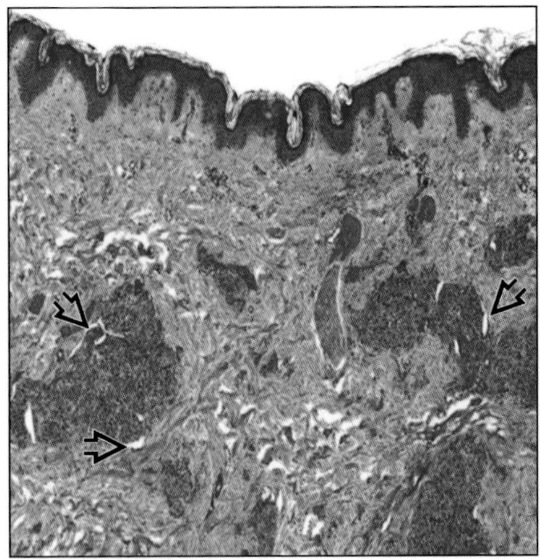

Scanning magnification of a tufted angioma shows scattered dermal lobular collections of vessels. The lobules bulge into dilated vessels, with a few peripheral semilunar spaces identified ➲.

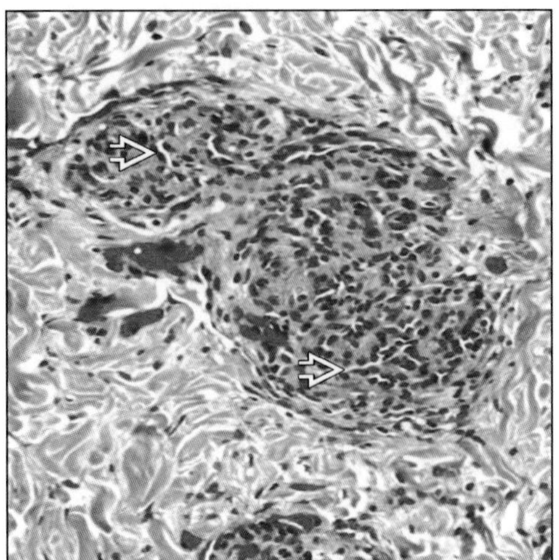

Higher magnification of 1 lobule shows a proliferation of small, slit-like vascular spaces ➲ lined by bland oval to spindle-shaped endothelial cells.

TERMINOLOGY

Abbreviations

- Acquired tufted angioma (ATA)

Synonyms

- Tufted angioma
- Angioblastoma (of Nakagawa)
- Progressive capillary hemangioma

Definitions

- Multiple scattered cannonball-like cellular collections of small vessels in dermis

ETIOLOGY/PATHOGENESIS

Unknown

- Most cases sporadic, rare familial case described
- Some cases associated with pregnancy or liver transplantation

CLINICAL ISSUES

Epidemiology

- Incidence
  - Rare tumors
- Age
  - Children and young adults

Site

- Neck, shoulders, and upper trunk most common

Presentation

- Slow growing
  - Erythematous macules and plaques

Prognosis

- Excellent, completely benign behavior
- May be associated with Kasabach-Merritt syndrome (consumptive coagulopathy)

MACROSCOPIC FEATURES

General Features

- Reddish brown nonencapsulated dermal lesion

Size

- Typically small papules but may be large plaque

MICROSCOPIC PATHOLOGY

Histologic Features

- Multiple scattered lobular collections of small capillary-type vessels throughout the dermis
  - Have typical cannonball appearance at low-power examination
  - Collections are larger in middle and lower dermis
  - Cleft-like lumina often present around capillary tufts, may impart glomerular-like appearance
  - Capillaries may be so closely packed that lumina may be inconspicuous
  - Cells are oval to spindled-shaped
  - May show nuclear hyperchromasia but lack significant cytologic atypia
  - A few mitoses may be present
- Hemosiderin deposition may be seen
- Inflammation typically not present
- Subcutaneous tissue typically not involved

DIFFERENTIAL DIAGNOSIS

Lobular Capillary Hemangioma

- Shows exophytic appearance and epidermal collarette, often ulcerated and acutely inflamed
- Proliferation of small capillary-type blood vessels typically arranged in a few larger nodular collections, rather than multiple smaller dispersed collections seen in ATA

ACQUIRED TUFTED ANGIOMA

Key Facts

Terminology
- Acquired tufted angioma (ATA)
- Angioblastoma (of Nakagawa)
- Multiple cannonball-like cellular collections of small vessels in dermis

Clinical Issues
- Children and young adults
- Rare tumors
- Slowly growing erythematous macules and plaques

Microscopic Pathology
- Scattered lobular collections of small capillary-type vessels throughout dermis, may involve subcutis
- Cleft-like lumina often present around capillary tufts, may impart glomerular-like appearance
- Cells are oval to spindled-shaped
- Mitoses may be present, but cells lack significant cytologic atypia

Glomeruloid Hemangioma
- Usually associated with Castleman disease or polyoneuropathy, organomegaly, endocrinopathy, M-protein, skin changes (POEMS syndrome)
- Smaller capillary-like collections inside vascular spaces with clefts around them
- Cytoplasmic globules, which are PAS(+) (immunoglobulin aggregates)

Infantile (Juvenile) Hemangioma
- Cellular dermal nodules composed of lobular collections of oval endothelial cells
- Vascular lumina often small and slit-like, become larger later-stage lesions

Targetoid Hemosiderotic Hemangioma (Hobnail Hemangioma)
- Superficial dilated vessels and smaller, narrow deeper vessels lined by plump (hobnailed) cells
- Extravasated red blood cells and prominent stromal hemosiderin deposition

Kaposi Sarcoma
- Proliferation of interlacing bundles of spindle cells forming slit-like vascular spaces
- Cytoplasmic hyalinized globules, plasma cells, and hemosiderin deposits typically present
- HHV8(+) by immunohistochemistry

DIAGNOSTIC CHECKLIST

Pathologic Interpretation Pearls
- Multiple scattered cannonball-like lobular collections of small capillary-type vessels throughout dermis

SELECTED REFERENCES

1. Arai E et al: Usefulness of D2-40 immunohistochemistry for differentiation between kaposiform hemangioendothelioma and tufted angioma. J Cutan Pathol. 33(7):492-7, 2006
2. Lee B et al: Adult-onset tufted angioma: a case report and review of the literature. Cutis. 78(5):341-5, 2006
3. Ishikawa K et al: The spontaneous regression of tufted angioma. A case of regression after two recurrences and a review of 27 cases reported in the literature. Dermatology. 210(4):346-8, 2005
4. Wong SN et al: Tufted angioma: a report of five cases. Pediatr Dermatol. 19(5):388-93, 2002
5. Igarashi M et al: The relationship between angioblastoma (Nakagawa) and tufted angioma: report of four cases with angioblastoma and a literature-based comparison of the two conditions. J Dermatol. 27(8):537-42, 2000
6. Padilla RS et al: Acquired "tufted" angioma (progressive capillary hemangioma). A distinctive clinicopathologic entity related to lobular capillary hemangioma. Am J Dermatopathol. 9(4):292-300, 1987
7. Scott OL: Tufted Haemangioma. Proc R Soc Med. 70(4):283, 1977

IMAGE GALLERY

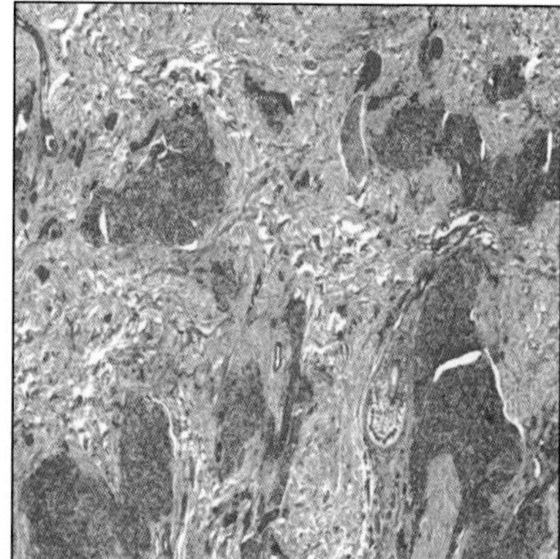

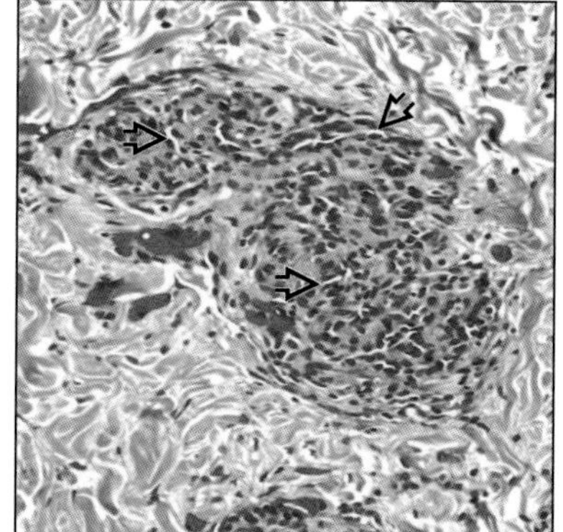

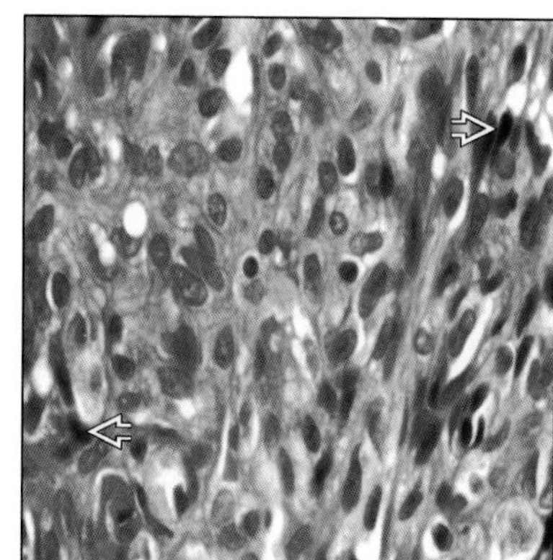

(Left) *Low-magnification view shows diffuse dermal proliferation of clustered blood vessels.* ***(Center)*** *Higher magnification shows a lobular cluster of blood vessels lined by small, oval to spindle-shaped cells. Lumina are collapsed and slit-like ⇨.* ***(Right)*** *High-power view shows bland cytologic features of the tufted angioma endothelial cells. Some of the cells show mild nuclear hyperchromasia ➡, but no significant cytologic atypia is identified.*

SPINDLE CELL HEMANGIOMA

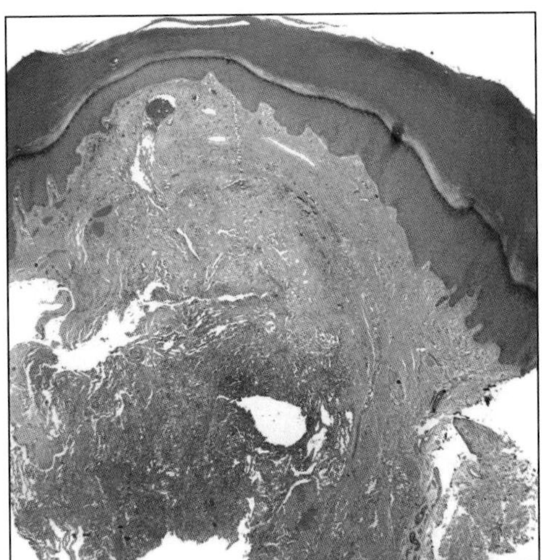

Hematoxylin & eosin shows a noncircumscribed lesion in the dermis and subcutis composed of an admixture of thin-walled dilated blood vessels and sheets of spindle cells.

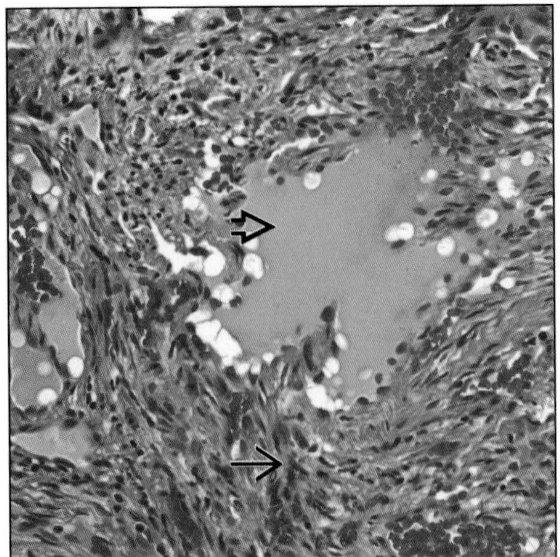

Hematoxylin & eosin shows straight/curved fascicles of uniform spindle cells ➙ with irregularly shaped vascular spaces ➲ and small areas of hemorrhage.

TERMINOLOGY

Synonyms

- Formerly called spindle cell hemangioendothelioma

Definitions

- Benign vascular tumor characterized by cavernous and spindled areas

CLINICAL ISSUES

Epidemiology

- Age
  - Young adults

Site

- Distal extremities
  - Acral location most common

Presentation

- Subcutaneous mass
  - Sometimes multifocal
- Associated with Mafucci syndrome, Klippel-Trenaunay syndrome, varicosities, and congenital lymphedema

Treatment

- Surgical approaches
  - Excision

Prognosis

- Local recurrence in 50-60%
- No metastatic potential

MICROSCOPIC PATHOLOGY

Histologic Features

- Dilated vessels often with focal thrombi
- Solid spindled cell areas
- Vacuolated endothelial cells, so-called "blister cells"
- ~ 50% of cases are at least partially intravascular

Predominant Pattern/Injury Type

- Circumscribed
  - Cavernous thin-walled vascular spaces
  - Solid spindled cell areas resembling Kaposi sarcoma

Predominant Cell/Compartment Type

- Vascular

DIFFERENTIAL DIAGNOSIS

Kaposi Sarcoma

- Patch stage
  - Irregular vessels dissecting through collagen
- Plaque/tumor stage
  - Areas with fascicles of spindled cells with slit-like vascular lumens
- Immunoreactive for HHV8 latent nuclear antigen

Kaposiform Hemangioendothelioma

- Almost exclusively in children
- Dilated vessels
- Solid spindled cell areas
- Glomeruloid nests of rounded endothelial cells
- Associated with Kasabach-Merritt phenomenon

Epithelioid Hemangioendothelioma

- Cords of epithelioid endothelial cells
- Vacuolated endothelial cells
- Myxohyaline-hyaline stroma
- Lacks cavernous vascular spaces

Organizing Thrombus/Intravascular Papillary Endothelial Hyperplasia

- Less prominent spindle cell proliferation
- Lacks so-called "blister cells"
- Papillary architecture of endothelial cells overlying fibrin cores

SPINDLE CELL HEMANGIOMA

Key Facts

Terminology

- Formerly called spindle cell hemangioendothelioma

Clinical Issues

- Subcutaneous mass
- Usually acral location
- Sometimes multifocal
- Associated with Mafucci syndrome in some cases
- Local recurrence in 50-60%
- No metastatic potential

Microscopic Pathology

- Dilated vessels often with focal thrombi
- Solid spindled cell areas
- Vacuolated endothelial cells, so-called "blister cells"
- Negative for HHV8 latent nuclear antigen

Top Differential Diagnoses

- Kaposi sarcoma
- Kaposiform hemangioendothelioma
- Epithelioid hemangioendothelioma

Immunohistochemistry

Antibody	Reactivity	Staining Pattern	Comment
CD31	Positive	Cell membrane & cytoplasm	In endothelial cells
CD34	Positive	Cell membrane & cytoplasm	In endothelial cells
FVIIIRAg	Positive	Cell membrane & cytoplasm	In endothelial cells (of historical interest only)
Actin-sm	Positive	Cytoplasmic	In spindle cells focally
S100	Negative		
HHV8	Negative		

DIAGNOSTIC CHECKLIST

Pathologic Interpretation Pearls

- Combination of ectatic vessels, spindled cells, and vacuolated endothelial cells ("blister cells") is key feature
- At least partially intravascular in ~ 1/2 of cases

SELECTED REFERENCES

1. Lyons LL et al: Kaposiform hemangioendothelioma: a study of 33 cases emphasizing its pathologic, immunophenotypic, and biologic uniqueness from juvenile hemangioma. Am J Surg Pathol. 28(5):559-68, 2004
2. Perkins P et al: Spindle cell hemangioendothelioma. An analysis of 78 cases with reassessment of its pathogenesis and biologic behavior. Am J Surg Pathol. 20(10):1196-204, 1996
3. Fanburg JC et al: Multiple enchondromas associated with spindle-cell hemangioendotheliomas. An overlooked variant of Maffucci's syndrome. Am J Surg Pathol. 19(9):1029-38, 1995
4. Imayama S et al: Spindle cell hemangioendothelioma exhibits the ultrastructural features of reactive vascular proliferation rather than of angiosarcoma. Am J Clin Pathol. 97(2):279-87, 1992
5. Fletcher CD et al: Spindle cell haemangioendothelioma: a clinicopathological and immunohistochemical study indicative of a non-neoplastic lesion. Histopathology. 18(4):291-301, 1991
6. Scott GA et al: Spindle cell hemangioendothelioma. Report of seven additional cases of a recently described vascular neoplasm. Am J Dermatopathol. 10(4):281-8, 1988
7. Weiss SW et al: Spindle cell hemangioendothelioma. A low-grade angiosarcoma resembling a cavernous hemangioma and Kaposi's sarcoma. Am J Surg Pathol. 10(8):521-30, 1986
8. Weiss SW et al: Epithelioid hemangioendothelioma: a vascular tumor often mistaken for a carcinoma. Cancer. 50(5):970-81, 1982

IMAGE GALLERY

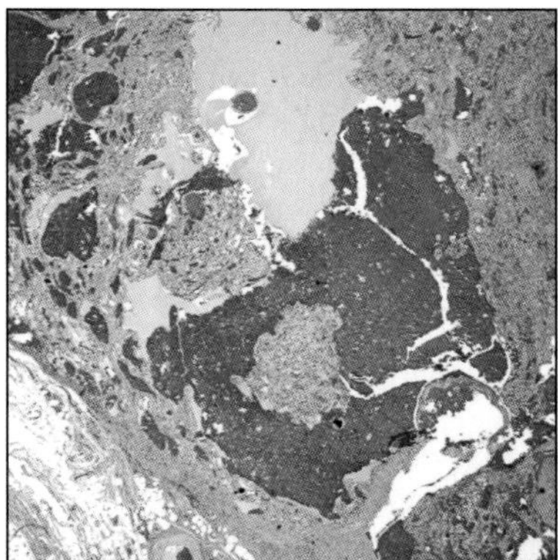

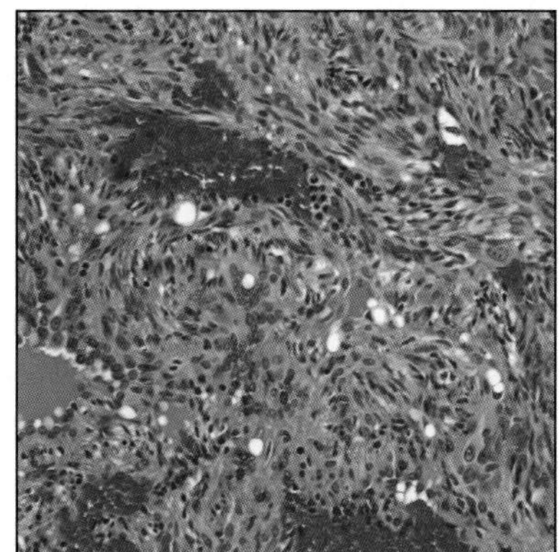

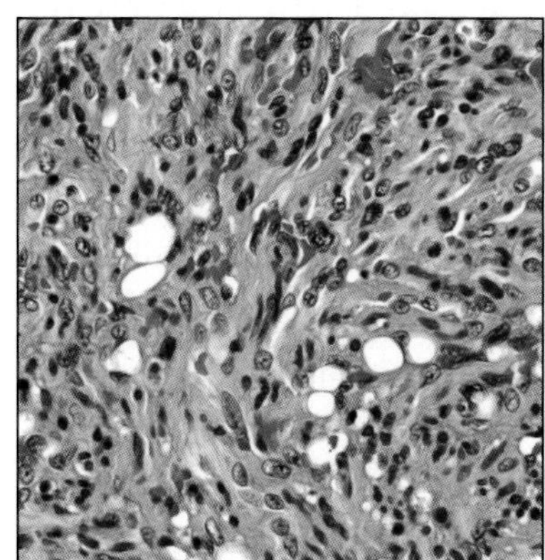

(Left) *Hematoxylin & eosin shows a well-circumscribed intravascular tumor with ectatic vascular spaces and a cellular spindle cell proliferation.* ***(Center)*** *Hematoxylin & eosin shows a more solid area of the spindled cell proliferation that mimics Kaposi sarcoma. However, nuclear atypia and significant mitotic activity are lacking.* ***(Right)*** *Hematoxylin & eosin shows a high-power view of the spindled cells and the characteristic vacuolated endothelial cells (so-called "blister cells").*

EPITHELIOID HEMANGIOMA

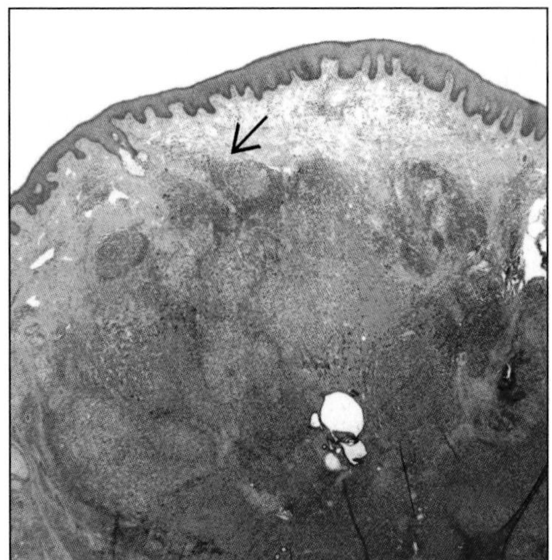

Hematoxylin & eosin shows a low-power view of epithelioid hemangioma demonstrating vascular proliferation in association with lymphoid aggregates ➔.

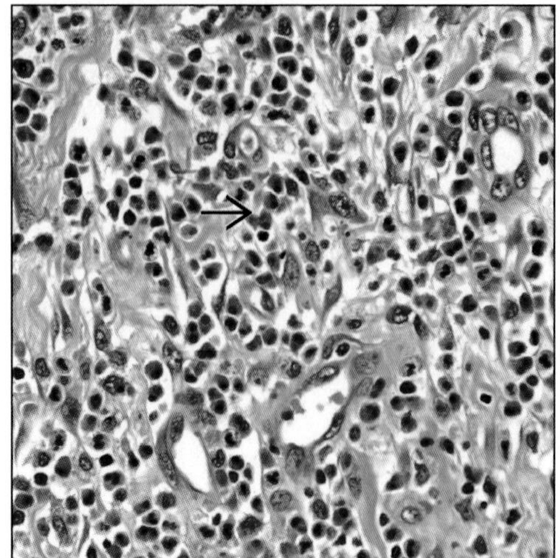

Hematoxylin & eosin shows capillaries lined with epithelioid endothelial cells admixed with numerous eosinophils ➔.

TERMINOLOGY

Synonyms

- Angiolymphoid hyperplasia with eosinophilia, histiocytoid hemangioma

Definitions

- Benign vascular tumor with epithelioid endothelial cells, usually accompanied by lymphoid aggregates and eosinophils

CLINICAL ISSUES

Presentation

- Dermal or subcutaneous nodules
- Most commonly involves head and neck, especially around ear
- Usually solitary but may be multiple in same region

Prognosis

- Benign
  - Local recurrence in up to 1/3
  - No metastasis

MICROSCOPIC PATHOLOGY

Histologic Features

- Lobular proliferation of capillaries usually surrounding central vessel
  - Capillaries lined by epithelioid endothelial cells
  - Epithelioid endothelial cells with abundant eosinophilic cytoplasm
  - Not all vessels necessarily have epithelioid endothelial cells
- Lymphoid aggregates
  - May show germinal center formation
- Abundant eosinophils
- Usually superficial dermal tumors
- Rare deep or intravascular tumors
- Endothelial cells positive for CD31 and CD34
  - Immunohistochemical stains can bring out hard-to-see vascular component in cases with obscuring lymphoid aggregates

Predominant Cell/Compartment Type

- Vascular

DIFFERENTIAL DIAGNOSIS

Epithelioid Hemangioendothelioma

- Cords of tumor cells in myxohyaline matrix
- Vessels not well formed
- Lacks inflammatory component

Epithelioid Angiosarcoma

- Complex interanastomosing vascular pattern
- Nuclear atypia and mitotic activity
- Lacks characteristic inflammatory component

Kimura Disease

- Endemic in Asian population
- Lymphadenopathy
- Lacks epithelioid endothelial cells

Cutaneous Follicle Center Cell B-Cell Lymphoma

- Irregular germinal centers without polarization
- Often with sheets of neoplastic B cells
- Lacks vascular proliferation
- Lacks eosinophils

Angiomatoid (Malignant) Fibrous Histiocytoma

- Fibrous pseudocapsule with lymphoid aggregates; eosinophils rare
- Sheet-like proliferation of histiocyte-like cells
- Blood-filled cystic spaces
- ~ 50% positive for CD68, desmin, &/or EMA
- Negative for vascular markers

EPITHELIOID HEMANGIOMA

Key Facts

Terminology

- Angiolymphoid hyperplasia with eosinophilia, histiocytoid hemangioma
- Benign vascular tumor with epithelioid endothelial cells, usually accompanied by lymphoid aggregates and eosinophils

Clinical Issues

- Most commonly involves head and neck, especially around ear

Microscopic Pathology

- Lobular proliferation of capillaries usually surrounding central vessel
  - Capillaries lined by epithelioid endothelial cells
- Lymphoid aggregates
  - Density of lymphoid aggregates can obscure underlying vascular proliferation on low-power examination
- Abundant eosinophils
- Lacks complex vasculature of angiosarcoma
- Lacks nuclear pleomorphism of epithelioid angiosarcoma
- Not all tumor vessels are necessarily lined by epithelioid endothelial cells
- Usually superficial dermal tumors
- Endothelial cells positive for CD31 and CD34
  - Immunohistochemical stains can bring out hard-to-see vascular component in cases with obscuring lymphoid aggregates

Immunohistochemistry

Antibody	Reactivity	Staining Pattern	Comment
CD34	Positive	Cell membrane	
CD31	Positive	Cell membrane	
Actin-sm	Positive	Cytoplasmic	In pericytes around vessels
Desmin	Negative		
S100	Negative		
AE1/AE3	Negative	Cytoplasmic	Very occasionally positive

Epithelioid Sarcoma

- Epithelioid hemangioma with more solid areas sometimes confused with epithelioid sarcoma
- Epithelioid sarcoma composed of nodules of tumor cells without vascular lumen formation
- Central necrosis often seen in tumor nodules
- Immunoreactive for cytokeratin and EMA; ~ 50-60% immunoreactive for CD34
- CD31(-)

Epithelioid Sarcoma-like Hemangioendothelioma

- Sheet-like proliferation of epithelioid tumor cells
- Lacks obvious vessel formation
- Rare intracytoplasmic lumens
- Immunoreactive for cytokeratin, CD31
- CD34(-)
- Lacks significant inflammatory component

Arthropod Bite Reaction

- Numerous eosinophils
- Lymphoid aggregates common
- Lacks vascular proliferation

DIAGNOSTIC CHECKLIST

Pathologic Interpretation Pearls

- Vascular proliferation with associated inflammatory infiltrate containing eosinophils: Consider epithelioid hemangioma
- Some tumor vessels may lack epithelioid endothelial cells

SELECTED REFERENCES

1. Macarenco RS et al: Angiolymphoid hyperplasia with eosinophilia showing prominent granulomatous and fibrotic reaction: a morphological and immunohistochemical study. Am J Dermatopathol. 28(6):514-7, 2006
2. Suzuki H et al: A case of angiolymphoid hyperplasia with eosinophilia (ALHE) of the upper lip. J Dermatol. 32(12):991-5, 2005
3. Zarrin-Khameh N et al: Angiolymphoid hyperplasia with eosinophilia associated with pregnancy: a case report and review of the literature. Arch Pathol Lab Med. 129(9):1168-71, 2005
4. Fetsch JF et al: Observations concerning the pathogenesis of epithelioid hemangioma (angiolymphoid hyperplasia). Mod Pathol. 4(4):449-55, 1991
5. Haas AF et al: Angiolymphoid hyperplasia with eosinophilia of the hand. A case report. J Dermatol Surg Oncol. 17(9):731-4, 1991
6. Urabe A et al: Epithelioid hemangioma versus Kimura's disease. A comparative clinicopathologic study. Am J Surg Pathol. 11(10):758-66, 1987

EPITHELIOID HEMANGIOMA

Microscopic Features

*(**Left**) Hematoxylin & eosin shows a low-power view of epithelioid hemangioma. There are prominent lymphoid aggregates, some with germinal center formation, in association with the vascular proliferation. (**Right**) Hematoxylin & eosin shows germinal center formation ➡ within associated lymphoid aggregates. The germinal centers have a normal polarized architecture.*

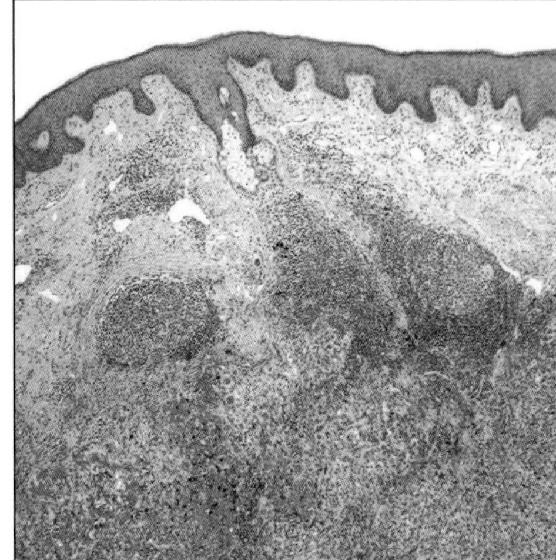

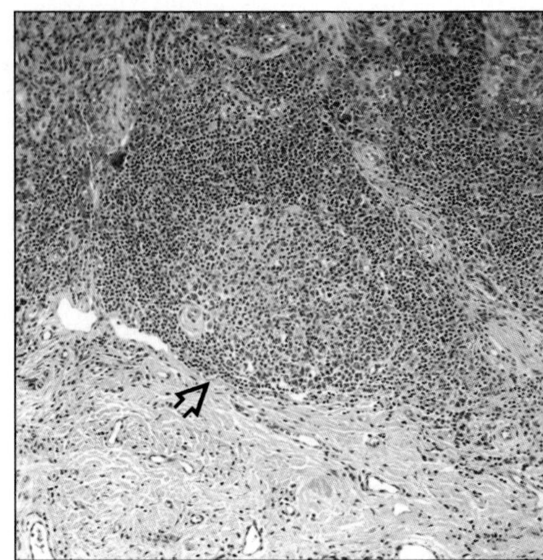

*(**Left**) Hematoxylin & eosin shows larger central vessels surrounded by capillaries with epithelioid endothelial cells that have relatively abundant eosinophilic cytoplasm. (**Right**) Hematoxylin & eosin shows a medium-power view of epithelioid hemangioma. The capillaries are well formed without architectural complexity. Although the majority are lined by epithelioid endothelial cells, some of the vessels are not.*

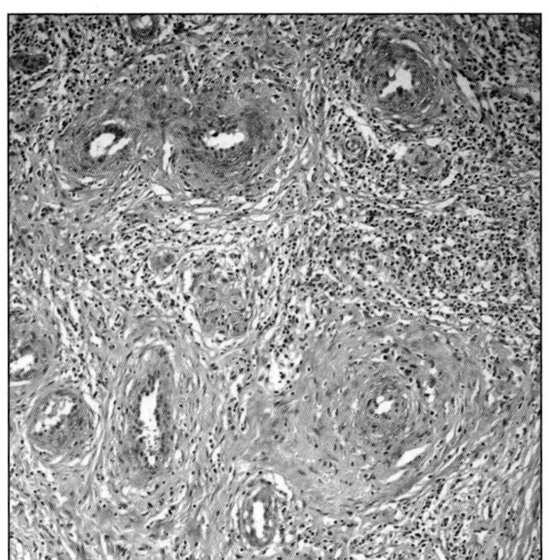

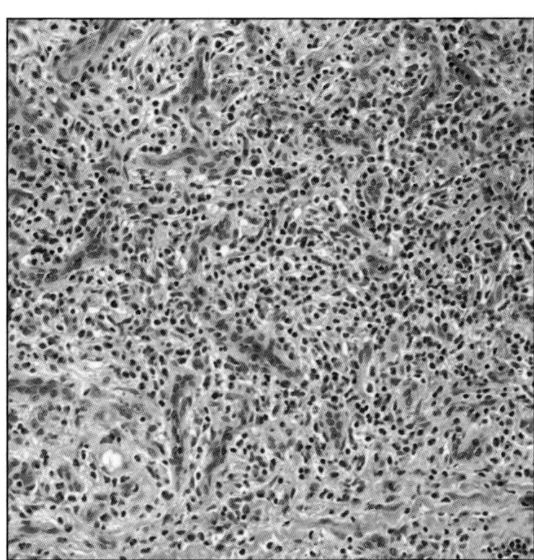

*(**Left**) Hematoxylin & eosin shows capillaries lined by epithelioid endothelial cells with abundant eosinophilic cytoplasm. The nuclei are enlarged with an open chromatin pattern. The nuclei lack hyperchromasia or pleomorphism. There are abundant admixed eosinophils. (**Right**) Hematoxylin & eosin shows the lobular architecture of the vascular proliferation. This is sometimes difficult to appreciate because of the lymphoid aggregates and background inflammation.*

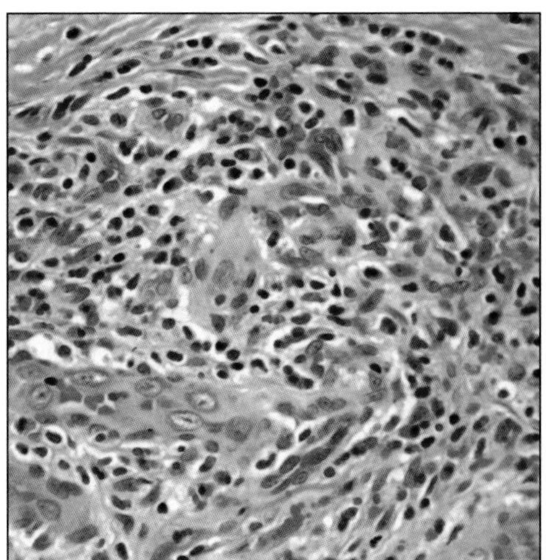

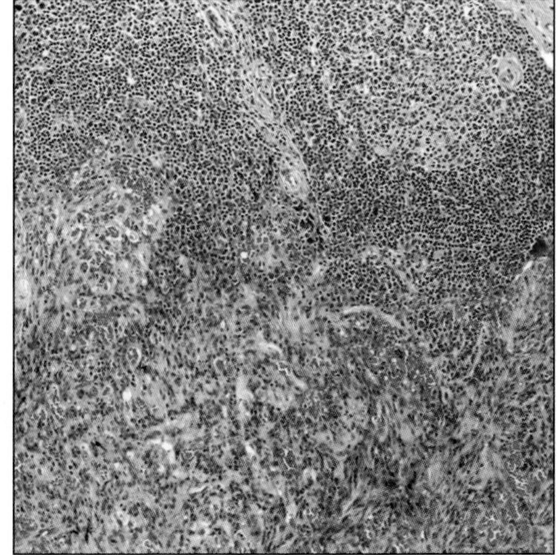

Variant Microscopic Features

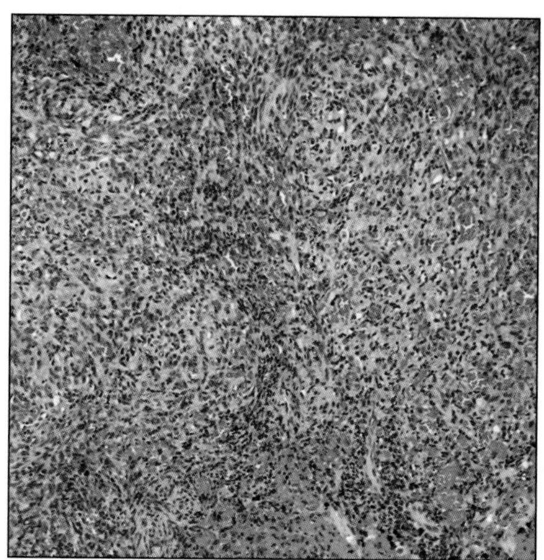

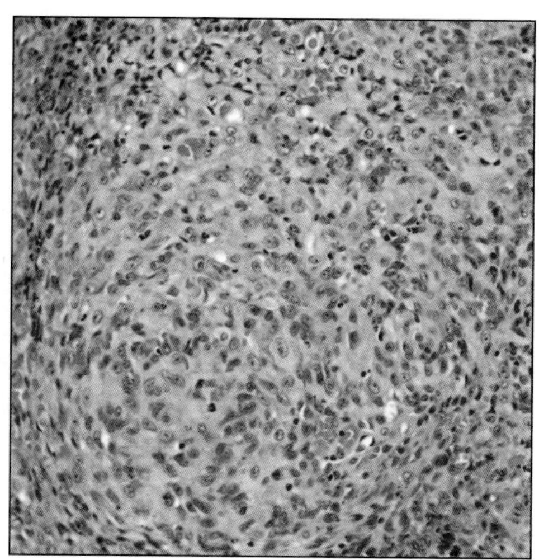

(Left) *Hematoxylin & eosin shows an epithelioid hemangioma with a more solid growth pattern. The solid areas still have a vaguely lobular appearance.* ***(Right)*** *Hematoxylin & eosin shows a high-power view of a sheet-like area within an epithelioid hemangioma. Note that the nuclei, though enlarged, do not have hyperchromasia or pleomorphism.*

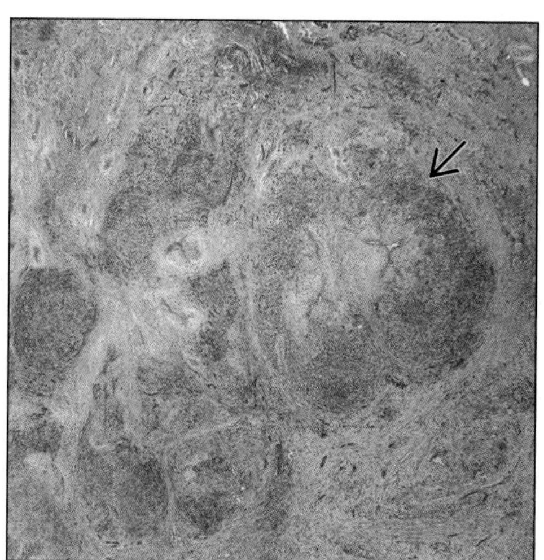

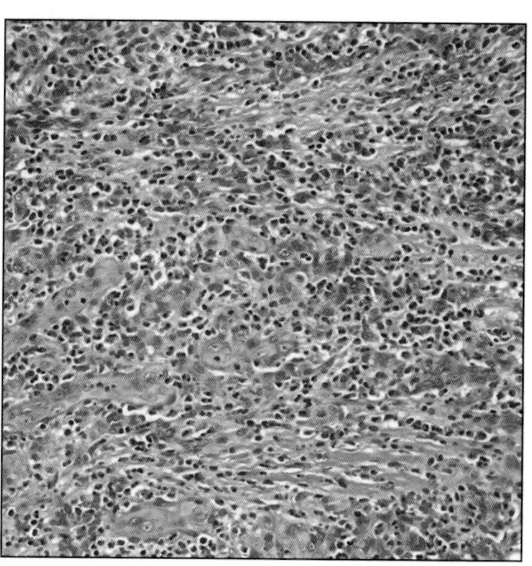

(Left) *Hematoxylin & eosin shows prominent lymphoid aggregates* ⇨ *within an epithelioid hemangioma. In some cases the lymphoid aggregates can obscure the underlying vascular proliferation at low power.* ***(Right)*** *Hematoxylin & eosin shows compressed vessels with epithelioid endothelial cells in an epithelioid hemangioma. This should not be confused with the cord-like proliferation of epithelioid hemangioendothelioma.*

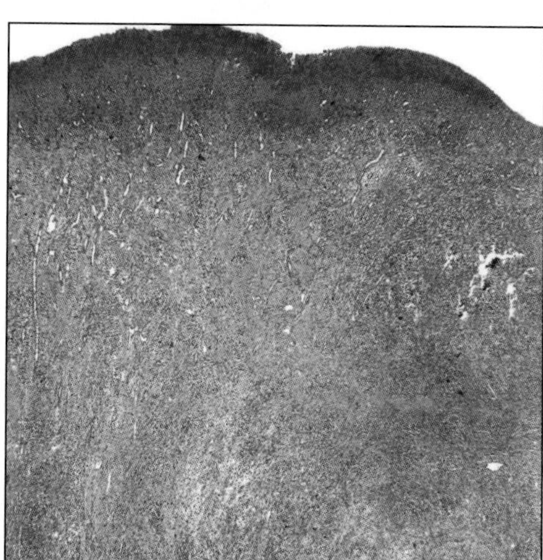

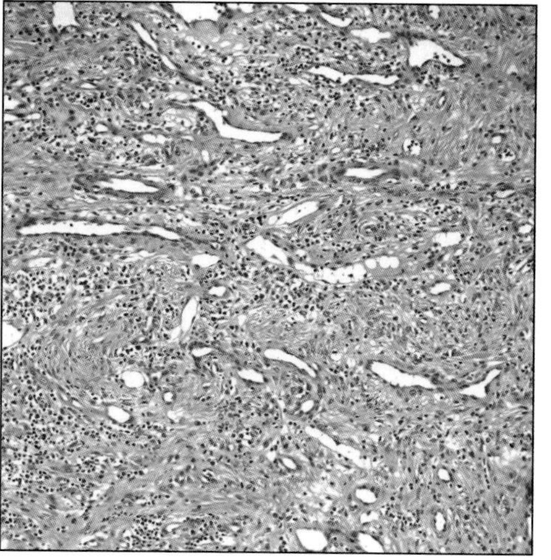

(Left) *Hematoxylin & eosin demonstrates an epithelioid hemangioma with an ulcerated epidermis. Occasional cases of epithelioid hemangioma may be ulcerated, and this finding is not indicative of malignancy.* ***(Right)*** *Hematoxylin & eosin highlights that the vessels in epithelioid hemangioma are well formed and lack architectural complexity. Although the defining feature is epithelioid endothelial cells lining capillaries, not all of the tumor vessels have this feature.*

ANGIOMATOSIS

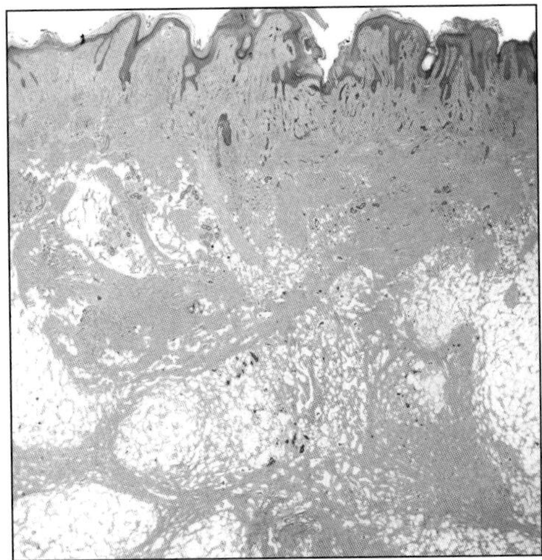

This example of angiomatosis shows a diffuse vascular proliferation involving the upper dermis and extending down into the subcutaneous adipose tissue.

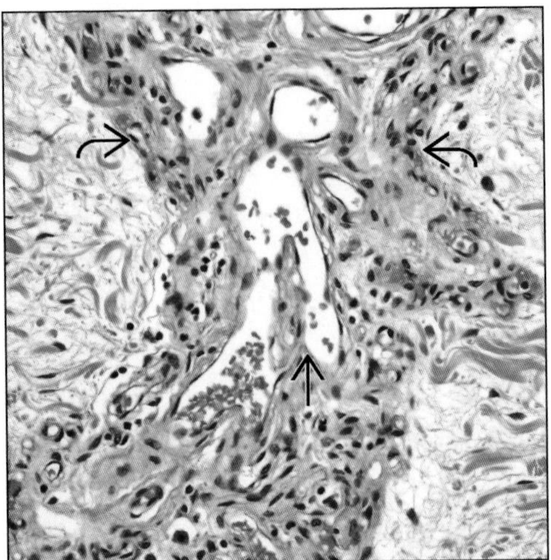

A large cavernous vessel with an irregular wall ➔ is surrounded by numerous small to medium-sized capillaries ➔.

TERMINOLOGY

Synonyms

- Diffuse hemangioma
- Vascular malformation
- Infiltrating angiolipoma

Definitions

- Diffuse, benign, vascular lesion of soft tissue affecting large segments of body or multiple tissue planes in contiguous fashion

ETIOLOGY/PATHOGENESIS

Developmental Anomaly

- Likely represents congenital malformation
  - Thought to arise in early intrauterine life during limb-bud formation

CLINICAL ISSUES

Epidemiology

- Age
  - Most present in early childhood
  - 2/3 develop by 2nd decade of life
- Gender
  - Females affected slightly more than males

Site

- Lower extremities (> 50%)
- Chest wall, abdomen, and upper extremities may also be affected

Presentation

- Diffuse and persistent swelling
- Pain and discoloration
- Swelling worsened by strenuous exercise

Treatment

- Conservative but complete excision

Prognosis

- Benign lesion with frequent recurrences and persistent disease
  - Majority will develop recurrences (60-90%)
  - Multiple recurrences (40%)
  - Likely reflects incomplete excision
- Metastases or malignant transformation not reported

IMAGE FINDINGS

CT Findings

- Ill-defined, nonhomogeneous mass
- Serpiginous densities in low-density areas
  - Correspond to tortuous vessels

MACROSCOPIC FEATURES

General Features

- Ill-defined mass

Size

- 3-26 cm

Gross Features

- Variable coloration
- Most have predominantly fatty appearance

MICROSCOPIC PATHOLOGY

Predominant Pattern/Injury Type

- Vascular malformation

Predominant Cell/Compartment Type

- Vascular
- Adipose

ANGIOMATOSIS

Key Facts

Terminology
- Diffuse, benign, vascular lesion of soft tissue affecting large segments of body or multiple tissue planes in contiguous fashion

Clinical Issues
- Most present in early childhood
- Lower extremities (> 50%)
- Benign lesion with frequent recurrences and persistent disease

Macroscopic Features
- Predominantly fatty appearance

Microscopic Pathology
- Haphazard arrangement of venous-, cavernous-, and capillary-sized vessels
  - Most common and most characteristic pattern

Diagnostic Checklist
- Clinicopathologic diagnosis

Microscopic Features
- 2 common patterns
  - Haphazard arrangement of venous-, cavernous-, and capillary-sized vessels
    - Irregular and thick to attenuated walls with herniations and intimal redundancies
    - Clusters of capillary vessels within or adjacent to vein walls
    - Large amounts of mature adipose tissue
    - Most common and most characteristic pattern
  - Infiltrating capillary hemangioma
    - Nodules of tumor infiltrate into soft tissue
    - Large amounts of mature adipose tissue
    - Previously referred to as infiltrating angiolipoma
- May involve multiple tissue planes (vertical involvement)
  - Skin, subcutis, muscle, and bone
- May involve only single tissue type
  - Multiple muscles
- Lacks distinct lobular pattern
- Osseous involvement can occur

DIFFERENTIAL DIAGNOSIS

Glomangiomatosis
- Diffusely infiltrating
- Well-formed vessels of varying size surrounded by clusters of glomus cells
- Often accompanied by mature adipose tissue
- May be associated with pain

Infantile Hemangioma (Capillary Hemangioma)
- Distinct lobular pattern
- Lacks extensive involvement

Intramuscular Hemangioma
- Homogeneous groups of capillary-sized vessels
- Lacks mixture of vessel sizes
- Lacks soft tissue involvement
- May require clinical correlation to make distinction

DIAGNOSTIC CHECKLIST

Clinically Relevant Pathologic Features
- Clinicopathologic diagnosis
  - Requires the above benign microscopic features
  - Must affect large segments of body in contiguous fashion

SELECTED REFERENCES

1. Rao VK et al: Angiomatosis of soft tissue. An analysis of the histologic features and clinical outcome in 51 cases. Am J Surg Pathol. 16(8):764-71, 1992
2. Howat AJ et al: Angiomatosis: a vascular malformation of infancy and childhood. Report of 17 cases. Pathology. 19(4):377-82, 1987
3. Koblenzer PJ et al: Angiomatosis (hamartomatous hem-lymphangiomatosis). Report of a case with diffuse involvement. Pediatrics. 28:65-76, 1961

IMAGE GALLERY

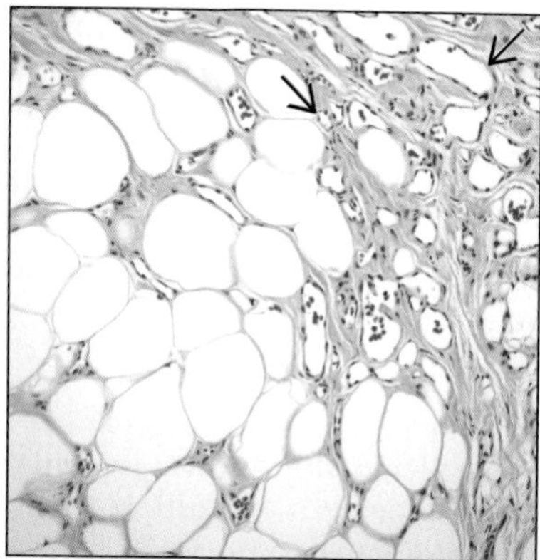

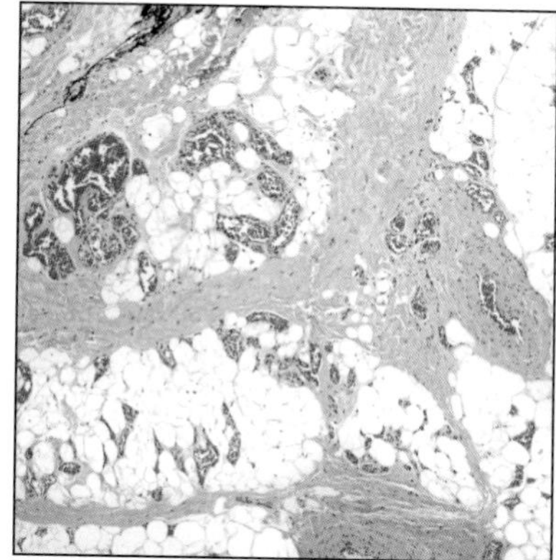

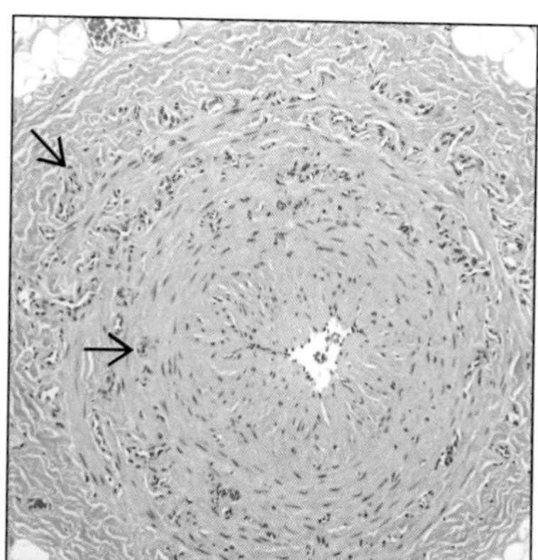

*(**Left**) Numerous small and dilated capillaries ⇒ are shown infiltrating the fibrous connective tissue and extending down into the adjacent adipose tissue. (**Center**) Scattered vessels of varying size and wall thickness are seen within the fibrous connective tissue and lobules of mature adipose tissue. (**Right**) Numerous small capillaries ⇒ are distributed within and adjacent to this thick-walled artery.*

LYMPHANGIOMA AND LYMPHANGIOMATOSIS

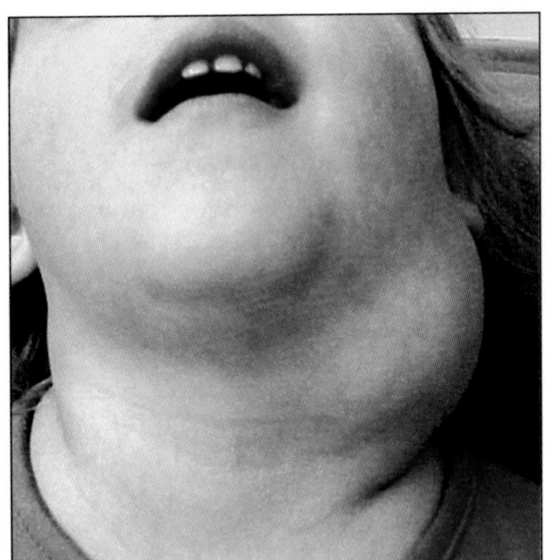

Clinical photograph shows a large deep lymphangioma (cystic hygroma) on the lateral neck of a child.

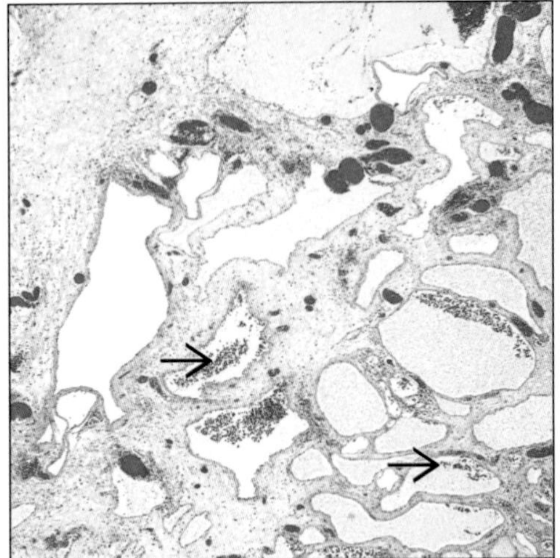

Histologic examination shows multiple dilated endothelial-lined channels. There are small collections of lymphocytes ➔ within the lumens, along with fluid and erythrocytes. (Courtesy B. Nelson, DDS.)

TERMINOLOGY

Synonyms

- Lymphangioma circumscriptum (superficial cutaneous lymphangioma) (LAC)
- Lymphangiomatosis (generalized lymphangioma, systemic angiomatosis) (LAS)
- Cystic lymphangioma (cystic hygroma)
- Deep lymphangioma (cavernous lymphangioma)
- Lymphatic malformation

Definitions

- Proliferation of lymphatic vessels; may be
  - Superficial (lymphangioma circumscription)
  - Deep (cavernous lymphangioma)
  - Diffusely involve most organ systems (lymphangiomatosis)

ETIOLOGY/PATHOGENESIS

Developmental Anomaly

- Most cases of lymphangioma considered developmental or congenital malformations/ hamartomas, **not** true neoplasms
  - Maldevelopment of embryonic lymphangiogenesis most likely etiology
    - Leads to sequestered lymphatics that fail to communicate with normal lymphovascular system
  - May be due to maternal infections or substance abuse
  - LAS considered congenital in most cases

Genetics

- Associated with genetic syndromes including Turner syndrome (cystic hygroma), Noonan syndrome, Maffucci syndrome, trisomies 13, 18, 21
- Mutations in *VEGFR-C*, *VEGFR3*, *PROX1*, *FOXC2*, and *SOX18* genes implicated

Acquired

- Rare acquired cases occur in adults
  - Likely associated with infection or trauma

CLINICAL ISSUES

Epidemiology

- Incidence
  - More common in children: Estimated 6% of benign childhood tumors
- Age
  - Often present at birth or within 1st 2 years of life (approximately 90% of cases)
  - LAS usually presents within 1st 2 decades of life
- Gender
  - Intraabdominal lymphangiomas have slight male predominance
  - LAS has no gender predilection

Site

- Head and neck most common site for cystic lymphangiomas
  - Usually posterior triangle but can occur in anterior triangle
  - Also occur in axillae, abdomen, and internal organs
- Cavernous type more frequent in oral cavity, upper trunk, limbs, and abdominal sites
  - Intraabdominal lymphangiomas occur in mesentery, omentum, and retroperitoneum
- LAC: Axillary folds, neck, and trunk are most common sites
- LAS: Can affect any organ system, but often involves bones, soft tissues, and skin

Presentation

- Cystic mass lesion; may be superfical or deep
  - Typically presents as large, slow-growing, painless mass (deep lymphangioma) or as multiple small, grouped, superficial vesicular lesions (LAC)

LYMPHANGIOMA AND LYMPHANGIOMATOSIS

Key Facts

Terminology
- Lymphangioma circumscriptum (superficial lymphangioma) (LAC)
- Lymphangiomatosis (systemic angiomatosis) (LAS)
- Cystic lymphangioma (cystic hygroma)
- Deep lymphangioma (cavernous lymphangioma)

Etiology/Pathogenesis
- Most cases considered developmental malformations/ hamartomas, **not** true neoplasms
- Associated with trisomies and other genetic syndromes, including Turner (cystic hygroma), Noonan, and Maffucci

Clinical Issues
- More common in children (6% of benign childhood tumors); present at birth or within 1st 2 years of life
- Typically presents as large, slow-growing, painless mass (deep lymphangioma) or as multiple small, grouped, superficial vesicular lesions (LAC)
- Excellent prognosis in most cases, although may be fatal if involving mediastinum or internal organs
- Recurrence rate high if removal incomplete

Microscopic Pathology
- Variably sized anastomosing vascular spaces lined by small, bland endothelial cells
- Often contain abundant proteinaceous debris, scattered lymphocytes, and erythrocytes
- Walls show stromal fibrosis (older lesions) and may contain smooth muscle
- Endothelial cells are small with uniform, bland-appearing, oval to flattened, hyperchromatic nuclei

- Lymphangiomatosis presents with numerous cystic lesions, both superficial and deep
- Soft and fluctuant swellings on palpation
- Intraabdominal cases may present with abdominal distension, mass on palpation
  - May also develop abdominal obstruction, volvulus, and infarction
- Generalized lymphangiomatosis: Depends on affected site
  - Bone: Pathologic fractures
  - Lungs: Dyspnea, wheezing due to chylothorax, chylous ascites
  - Spleen: Splenomegaly, left upper quadrant pain

Treatment
- Surgical approaches
  - May be indicated in large deep lesions, especially if symptomatic
  - LAS not amenable to surgical excision
- Drugs
  - Intralesional injection of sclerosing agents, including bleomycin and OK-432

Prognosis
- Excellent in most cases, although lymphangiomatosis may be fatal if involving mediastinum or internal organs, especially lungs
- Recurrence rate high with incomplete removal
- No malignant transformation reported

IMAGE FINDINGS

Ultrasonographic Findings
- Unilocular or multilocular anechoic mass
- Can be used in utero to detect cystic lymphangioma (associated with hydrops fetalis, Turner syndrome, and high death rate)

CT Findings
- Nonenhancing cystic lesions with homogeneous attenuation
- Visceral and osseous lesions often show contrast enhancement
- May displace surrounding organs

MACROSCOPIC FEATURES

General Features
- Multiple cystic spaces with clear to whitish fluid

MICROSCOPIC PATHOLOGY

Histologic Features
- Variably-sized anastomosing vascular spaces lined by small, bland endothelial cells
- Dilated lumens
  - Often contain abundant proteinaceous debris, scattered lymphocytes, and erythrocytes
- Walls show stromal fibrosis (older lesions) and occasional myxoid change
  - Often contain lymphoid infiltrates
    - May show occasional reactive germinal centers
  - Mast cells are common
  - Hemosiderin deposition in stroma may be seen
- Large vessels may contain smooth muscle in their walls
- Cavernous hemangiomas have infiltrative margins and often extend into surrounding tissues

Cytologic Features
- Endothelial cells are small with uniform, bland-appearing, oval to flattened, hyperchromatic nuclei

Predominant Pattern/Injury Type
- Cystic, macroscopic

Predominant Cell/Compartment Type
- Lymphatics

LYMPHANGIOMA AND LYMPHANGIOMATOSIS

ANCILLARY TESTS

Immunohistochemistry

- Endothelial lining cells show variable positivity with vascular markers CD31, CD34, and FVIIIRAg
- Newer lymphatic markers, including podoplanin (D2-40), VEGFR-3, and LYVE-1, typically positive

DIFFERENTIAL DIAGNOSIS

Hemangiomas

- Most cases show smaller vascular spaces with more red blood cells, less proteinaceous material, and fewer lymphocytes
- Often well-circumscribed, noninfiltrative borders

Progressive Lymphangioma

- Form of cutaneous lymphangioma with distinct clinical findings
  - Typically presents on lower extremities of adults as slow-growing patches or plaques
- Histologic findings very similar to other forms of lymphangioma
  - Superficially dilated spaces that become progressively smaller with deep extension

Secondary Lymphangiectasia

- May be due to local factors, such as obstruction (e.g., due to tumor), scarring, or previous radiation therapy
- Identical histologic findings; can only be distinguished by clinical history or other findings (if present)

Atypical Vascular Proliferation

- Radiation induced; most frequent in breast
- Clinically, presents as multiple small vesicles in radiation field
- Irregularly dilated vascular spaces lined by atypical endothelial cells

Lymphangioma-like Kaposi Sarcoma

- Usually shows at least focal areas of more typical Kaposi sarcoma
  - Infiltrative slit-like spaces lined by hyperchromatic spindle-shaped cells
  - Stromal hemosiderin deposition and inflammatory infiltrate containing plasma cells
- HHV8(+) is diagnostic

Angiosarcoma/Lymphangiosarcoma

- Highly atypical vascular proliferation showing irregular, anastomosing vascular spaces
- Poorly circumscribed, infiltrative neoplasm
- Endothelial cells typically show epithelioid or spindle cell features, prominent nuclear enlargement, and atypia with enlarged nucleoli
  - Endothelial multilayering often present
  - Mitotic figures easily identified

DIAGNOSTIC CHECKLIST

Clinically Relevant Pathologic Features

- Margins
  - High recurrence rate with positive margins

Pathologic Interpretation Pearls

- Proliferation of superficial &/or deep dilated vascular spaces lined by bland oval or flattened endothelial cells

SELECTED REFERENCES

1. Ji RC et al: Multiple expressions of lymphatic markers and morphological evolution of newly formed lymphatics in lymphangioma and lymph node lymphangiogenesis. Microvasc Res. Epub ahead of print, 2010
2. Kim DH et al: Lymphangiomatosis involving the inferior vena cava, heart, pulmonary artery and pelvic cavity. Korean J Radiol. 11(1):115-8, 2010
3. Chen EY et al: Similar histologic features and immunohistochemical staining in microcystic and macrocystic lymphatic malformations. Lymphat Res Biol. 7(2):75-80, 2009
4. Gedikbasi A et al: Multidisciplinary approach in cystic hygroma: prenatal diagnosis, outcome, and postnatal follow up. Pediatr Int. 51(5):670-7, 2009
5. Patel GA et al: Cutaneous lymphangioma circumscriptum: frog spawn on the skin. Int J Dermatol. 48(12):1290-5, 2009
6. Patel GA et al: Zosteriform lymphangioma circumscriptum. Acta Dermatovenerol Alp Panonica Adriat. 18(4):179-82, 2009
7. Rattan KN et al: Pediatric chylolymphatic mesenteric cyst - a separate entity from cystic lymphangioma: a case series. J Med Case Reports. 3:111, 2009
8. Richmond B et al: Adult presentation of giant retroperitoneal cystic lymphangioma: case report. Int J Surg. 7(6):559-60, 2009
9. Edwards JR et al: Lymphatics and bone. Hum Pathol. 39(1):49-55, 2008
10. François M et al: Sox18 induces development of the lymphatic vasculature in mice. Nature. 456(7222):643-7, 2008
11. Santo S et al: Prenatal ultrasonographic diagnosis of abdominal cystic lymphangioma: a case report. J Matern Fetal Neonatal Med. 21(8):565-6, 2008
12. Norgall S et al: Elevated expression of VEGFR-3 in lymphatic endothelial cells from lymphangiomas. BMC Cancer. 7:105, 2007
13. Wilting J et al: Embryonic development and malformation of lymphatic vessels. Novartis Found Symp. 283:220-7; discussion 227-9, 238-41, 2007
14. Wilting J et al: The transcription factor Prox1 is a marker for lymphatic endothelial cells in normal and diseased human tissues. FASEB J. 16(10):1271-3, 2002
15. Prevo R et al: Mouse LYVE-1 is an endocytic receptor for hyaluronan in lymphatic endothelium. J Biol Chem. 276(22):19420-30, 2001

Gross and Microscopic Features

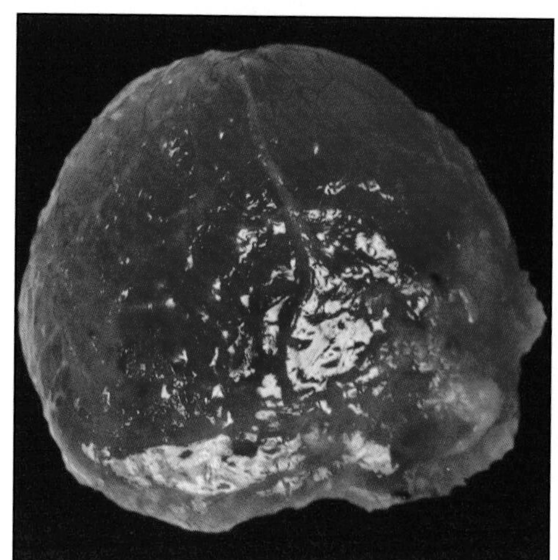

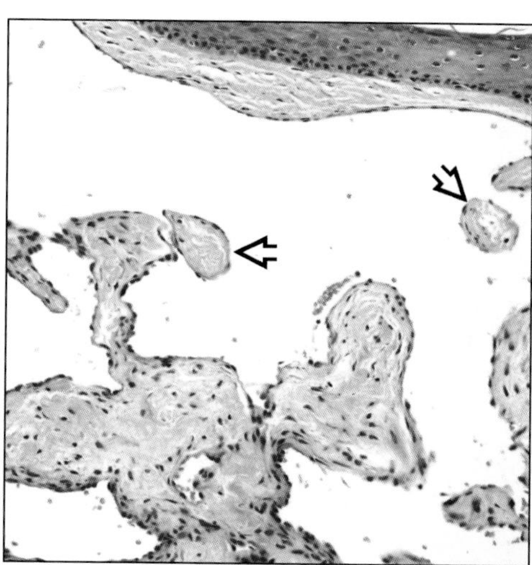

(Left) *Macroscopic view of a lymphangioma shows a reddish brown translucent cystic mass. Small vessels are noted within the lining; the cyst was filled with clear, watery fluid. (Courtesy B. Nelson, DDS.)* ***(Right)*** *Low-magnification examination of a superficial lymphangioma shows widely dilated spaces in the superficial dermis. The lumens show several papillary projections ⇨ with slightly fibrinous cores lined by small, hyperchromatic-staining endothelial cells.*

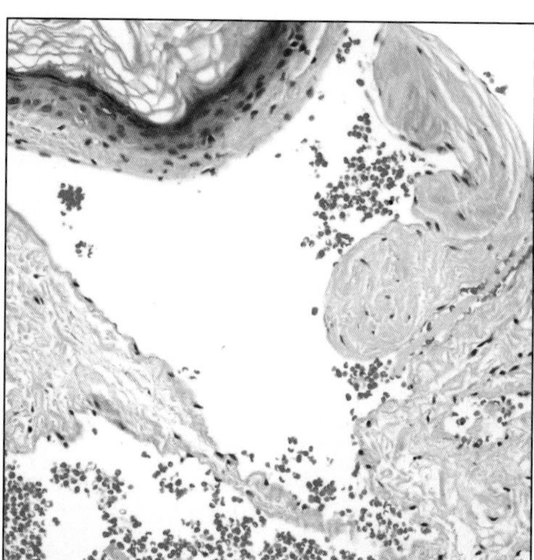

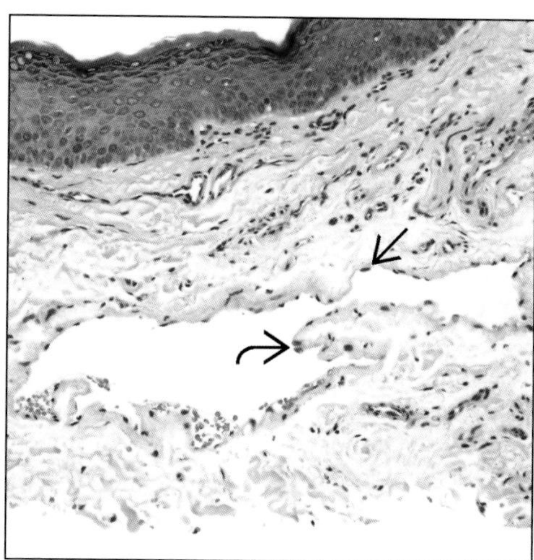

(Left) *Examination of a superficial lymphangioma shows a large, irregularly dilated space lined by thin endothelial cells containing scattered red blood cells in the superficial dermis.* ***(Right)*** *Higher magnification examination of a superficial lymphangioma shows the dilated spaces lined by small, bland endothelial cells with uniform, hyperchromatic-staining oval ↷ to flattened → nuclei.*

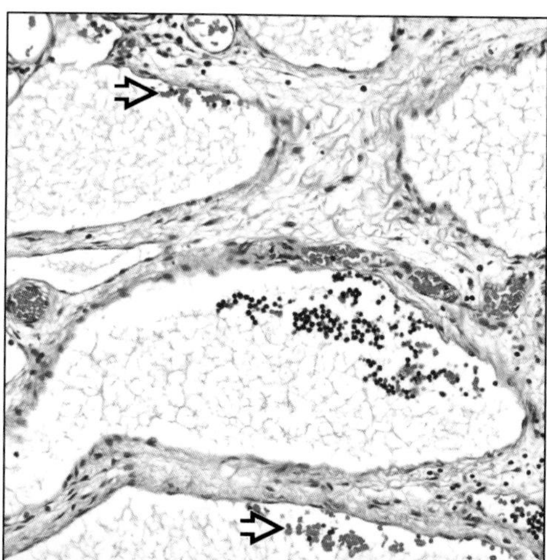

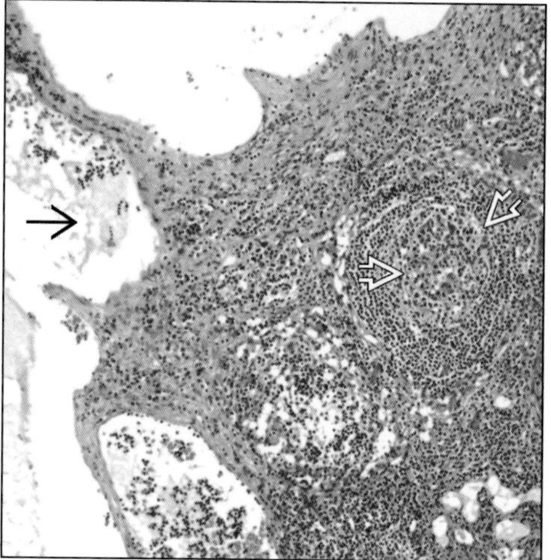

(Left) *Deep lymphangioma shows large vascular channels filled with proteinaceous material, a few lymphocytes, and scattered erythrocytes ⇨. (Courtesy B. Nelson, DDS.)* ***(Right)*** *Another deep lymphangioma shows a lumen lined by flattened endothelium and containing proteinaceous fluid →. There is a lymphocytic aggregate with a germinal center ➡ in the surrounding connective tissue. (Courtesy B. Nelson, DDS.)*

PROGRESSIVE LYMPHANGIOMA

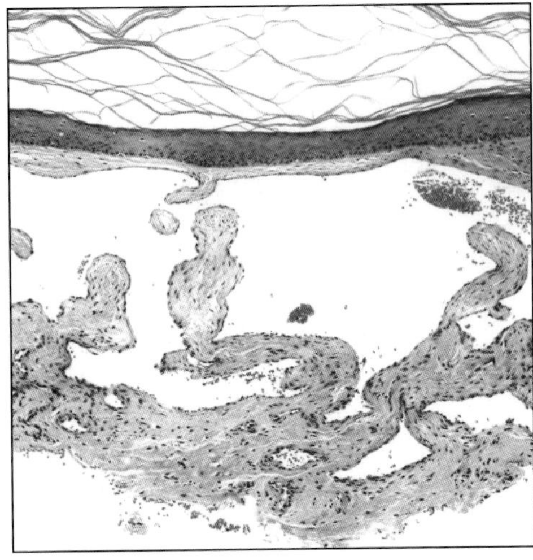

Low-magnification histologic examination of a progressive lymphangioma shows widely dilated lymphatic spaces in the superficial dermis.

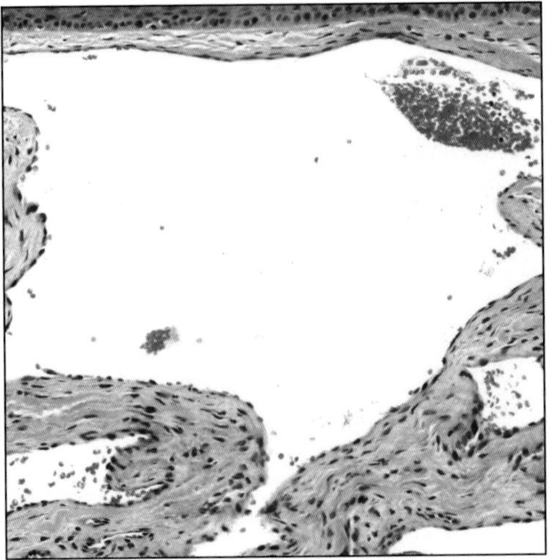

Higher magnification shows the widely dilated lymphatic spaces lined by a single layer of small, flattened, bland endothelial cells.

TERMINOLOGY

Synonyms

- Acquired progressive lymphangioma
- Benign lymphangioendothelioma

Definitions

- Benign localized proliferation of lymphatic vessels

ETIOLOGY/PATHOGENESIS

Unknown

- May be related to trauma in some cases

CLINICAL ISSUES

Epidemiology

- Age
  - Middle-aged or older adults
- Gender
  - No predilection

Site

- Usually presents on lower extremities but may occur anywhere

Presentation

- Slow-growing lesion
- Patches or plaques

Treatment

- Surgical approaches
  - Complete surgical excision is curative
- Drugs
  - Corticosteroids have been reported to induce complete regression in some cases

Prognosis

- Excellent; local recurrences are rare, metastases do not occur

MACROSCOPIC FEATURES

General Features

- Dermal-based mass lesion with cystic spaces and hemorrhage

Size

- May measure up to several centimeters

MICROSCOPIC PATHOLOGY

Histologic Features

- Dermal and subcutaneous proliferation of dilated vascular channels
- Spaces are often widely dilated superficially but become narrower with deep extension
- Vascular channels are lined by monomorphous, bland-appearing endothelial cells
- Endothelial-lined papillary projections may be present
- Endothelial cells may show mild hyperchromasia, but no significant atypia is present

Predominant Pattern/Injury Type

- Vascular proliferation

Predominant Cell/Compartment Type

- Endothelial

ANCILLARY TESTS

Immunohistochemistry

- Usually not necessary for diagnosis
- Endothelial cells positive for CD31, CD34, and D2-40

PROGRESSIVE LYMPHANGIOMA

Key Facts

Terminology
- Benign localized proliferation of lymphatic vessels

Clinical Issues
- Usually presents on lower extremities but may occur anywhere
- Prognosis excellent; local recurrences rare, and metastases do not occur

Microscopic Pathology
- Dermal and subcutaneous proliferation of dilated vascular channels
- Spaces are often widely dilated superficially but become narrower with deep extension
- Endothelial cells may show mild hyperchromasia, but no significant atypia is present

DIFFERENTIAL DIAGNOSIS

Lymphangioma Circumscriptum
- Presents at birth or in early childhood as multiple small lesions grouped together
- Superficial dermis is involved; deep dilated lymphatics possible as well

Lymphangioma-like Kaposi Sarcoma (KS)
- Usually shows more typical areas of KS and inflammatory infiltrate, including plasma cells
- HHV8 immunohistochemistry positive

Atypical Vascular Proliferation (Radiotherapy-related)
- Clinically, presents as multiple tiny vesicles in radiation field
- Histologically, lymphatic spaces are more widely dilated

Lymphangiomatosis
- Clinically very distinctive, with diffuse involvement of many organ systems

Angiosarcoma
- Highly atypical vascular proliferation with dissection throughout dermis and subcutis in most cases
- Significant cytologic atypia, endothelial multilayering, and mitoses are present

DIAGNOSTIC CHECKLIST

Pathologic Interpretation Pearls
- Proliferation of dilated lymphatic channels lined by bland endothelial cells
- Widely dilated spaces superficially; narrower spaces with deep extension

SELECTED REFERENCES

1. Paik AS et al: Acquired progressive lymphangioma in an HIV-positive patient. J Cutan Pathol. 34(11):882-5, 2007
2. Hwang LY et al: Acquired progressive lymphangioma. J Am Acad Dermatol. 49(5 Suppl):S250-1, 2003
3. Guillou L et al: Benign lymphangioendothelioma (acquired progressive lymphangioma): a lesion not to be confused with well-differentiated angiosarcoma and patch stage Kaposi's sarcoma: clinicopathologic analysis of a series. Am J Surg Pathol. 24(8):1047-57, 2000
4. Cossu S et al: Lymphangioma-like variant of Kaposi's sarcoma: clinicopathologic study of seven cases with review of the literature. Am J Dermatopathol. 19(1):16-22, 1997
5. Rosso R et al: Acquired progressive lymphangioma of the skin following radiotherapy for breast carcinoma. J Cutan Pathol. 22(2):164-7, 1995
6. Meunier L et al: Acquired progressive lymphangioma. Br J Dermatol. 131(5):706-8, 1994

IMAGE GALLERY

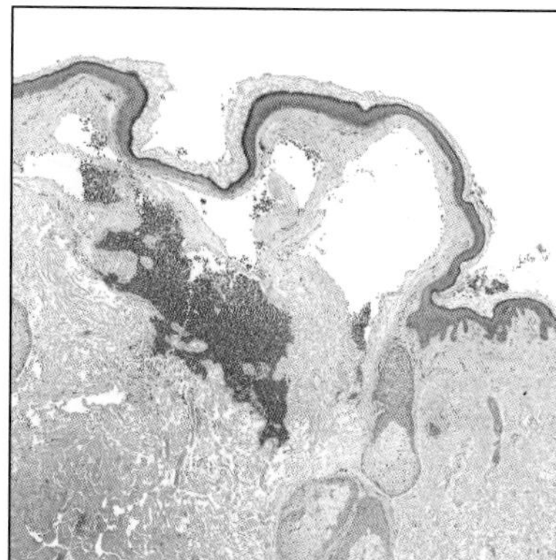

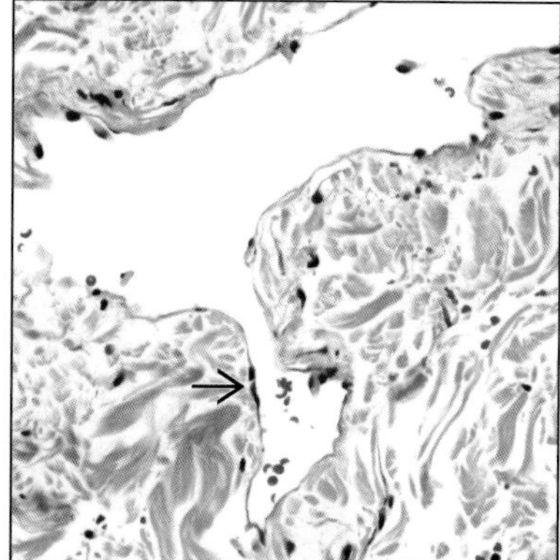

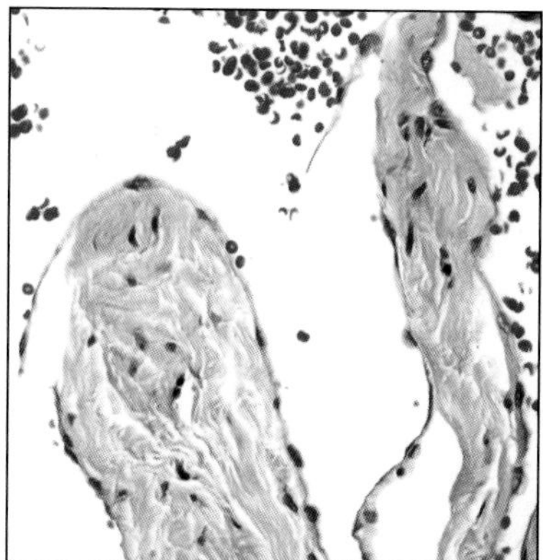

(Left) *Low-power examination shows superficial dermal dilated lymphatic spaces, some of which contain numerous red blood cells.* ***(Center)*** *High-power examination shows the irregular contours of the lymphatic spaces and the small, bland lining endothelial cells →.* ***(Right)*** *High-power examination shows a papillary projection protruding into the lymphatic space.*

MASSIVE LOCALIZED LYMPHEDEMA IN MORBID OBESITY

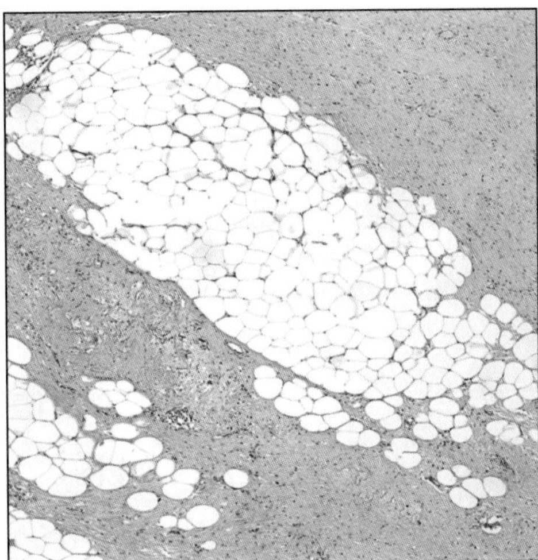

Hematoxylin & eosin shows cellular fibrous septa of variable width within the subcutaneous adipose tissue. No nuclear pleomorphism is seen in either the fibrous septa or fat.

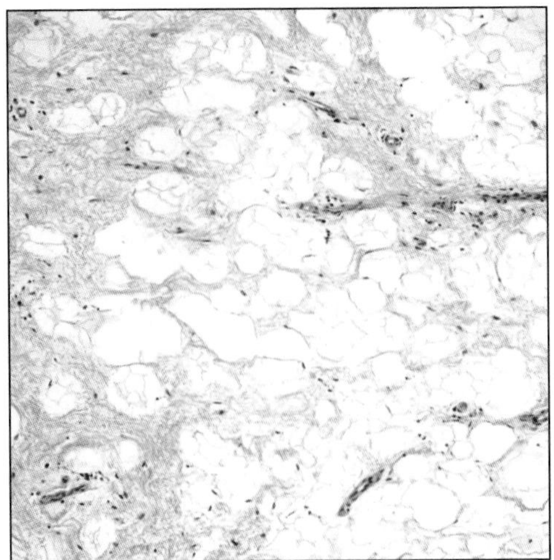

Hematoxylin & eosin shows scattered fibroblasts within fibrous trabeculae and mature adipocytes. The adipocytes are of uniform size, and no atypical cells or lipoblasts are seen.

TERMINOLOGY

Definitions

- Pseudoneoplastic process related to localized lymphatic obstruction

CLINICAL ISSUES

Presentation

- Painless mass
  - Seen in morbidly obese patients (> 300 lbs)
  - Most common on medial thigh
    - Can occur in other locations such as abdomen and axilla

Prognosis

- Benign
  - Recurrence or persistence common

IMAGE FINDINGS

CT Findings

- Soft tissue streaking due to expanded subcutaneous septa
- Cysts
- No discrete mass

MACROSCOPIC FEATURES

Gross Pathologic Examination

- Overlying skin has "peau d'orange" appearance
- Pronounced fibrous tissue septa in subcutaneous fat
- Cyst formation common
- Cut section weeps serous fluid

MICROSCOPIC PATHOLOGY

Histologic Features

- Expanded subcutaneous septa
  - Prominent edema
  - Increased mildly atypical fibroblasts
  - Preserved lobular architecture of subcutaneous fat
  - Pseudocyst formation in adipose tissue common
- Mild perivascular lymphocytic infiltrate
- Reactive capillary vascular proliferation sometimes present at interface of subcutaneous septa and lobules
- Absence of pleomorphic hyperchromatic cells of well-differentiated liposarcoma/atypical lipomatous tumor
- Overlying dermis often sclerotic

Predominant Pattern/Injury Type

- Fibrous

Predominant Cell/Compartment Type

- Adipose

DIFFERENTIAL DIAGNOSIS

Sclerosing Variant of Well-Differentiated Liposarcoma/Atypical Lipomatous Tumor

- Fibrous bands with atypical hyperchromatic cells
- Irregular adipocytes
- *MDM2* amplification

Myxofibrosarcoma

- Hyperchromatic spindled cells
- Variable pleomorphism
- Well-developed arcing vasculature
- Myxoid stroma

Myxoid Liposarcoma

- Hyperchromatic small spindled cells and lipoblasts
- Delicate plexiform vasculature
- Abundant myxoid stroma
- t(12;16) translocation

MASSIVE LOCALIZED LYMPHEDEMA IN MORBID OBESITY

Key Facts

Clinical Issues

- Seen in morbidly obese patients (> 300 lbs)

Macroscopic Features

- Overlying skin has "peau d'orange" appearance
- Pronounced fibrous tissue septa in subcutaneous fat
- Cyst formation common
- Cut section weeps serous fluid

Microscopic Pathology

- Expanded subcutaneous septa
- Prominent edema fluid
- No pleomorphic hyperchromatic cells
- Absence of plexiform vasculature, prominent myxoid stroma, and lipoblasts of myxoid liposarcoma
- Preserved lobular architecture of subcutaneous fat
- Reactive capillary vascular proliferation often present at interface of subcutaneous septa and lobules

DIAGNOSTIC CHECKLIST

Clinically Relevant Pathologic Features

- Symptom complex
  - Morbidly obese patients
  - Ill-defined mass
  - Medial thigh most common location
- Gross appearance
  - Widened subcutaneous septae
  - Cystic degeneration common
  - Cut surface weeps serous fluid
  - "Peau d'orange" appearance of overlying skin

Pathologic Interpretation Pearls

- Preservation of lobular architecture
  - Fibrosis along subcutaneous septa rather than irregular fibrosis of well-differentiated liposarcoma
- Mildly atypical fibroblasts in areas of fibrosis but no pleomorphic cells as typically seen in well-differentiated liposarcoma
- Proliferation of reactive capillaries often present at interface of fibrous septa and adipose tissue
- Overlying dermis shows evidence of stasis change
  - Dilated lymphatics in reticular dermis
  - Lobular proliferation of relatively thick-walled vessels in superficial dermis

SELECTED REFERENCES

1. Asch S et al: Massive localized lymphedema: an emerging dermatologic complication of obesity. J Am Acad Dermatol. 59(5 Suppl):S109-10, 2008
2. Bogusz AM et al: Massive localized lymphedema with unusual presentations: report of two cases and review of the literature. Int J Surg Pathol. Epub ahead of print, 2008
3. Fife CE et al: Lymphedema in the morbidly obese patient: unique challenges in a unique population. Ostomy Wound Manage. 54(1):44-56, 2008
4. Rosenberg AE: Pseudosarcomas of soft tissue. Arch Pathol Lab Med. 132(4):579-86, 2008
5. Goshtasby P et al: Pseudosarcoma: massive localized lymphedema of the morbidly obese. Obes Surg. 16(1):88-93, 2006
6. Jensen V et al: Massive localized lipolymphedema pseudotumor in a morbidly obese patient. Lymphology. 39(4):181-4, 2006
7. Brooks JS et al: Not so massive localized lymphedema. Hum Pathol. 32(1):139, 2001
8. Barr J: Massive localized lymphedema of suprapubic origin. Plast Reconstr Surg. 106(7):1663-4, 2000
9. Wu D et al: Massive localized lymphedema: additional locations and association with hypothyroidism. Hum Pathol. 31(9):1162-8, 2000
10. Farshid G et al: Massive localized lymphedema in the morbidly obese: a histologically distinct reactive lesion simulating liposarcoma. Am J Surg Pathol. 22(10):1277-83, 1998

IMAGE GALLERY

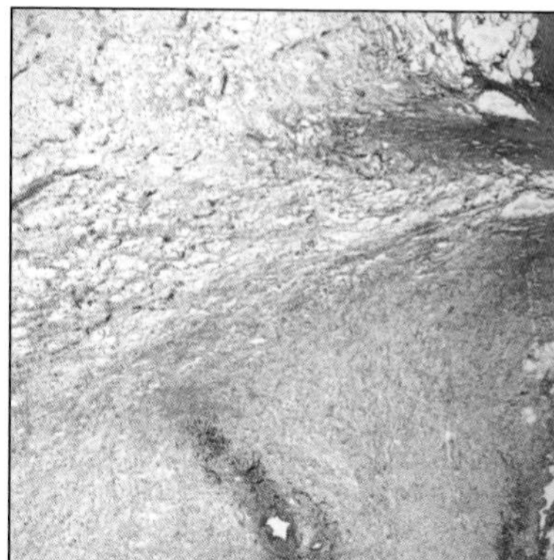

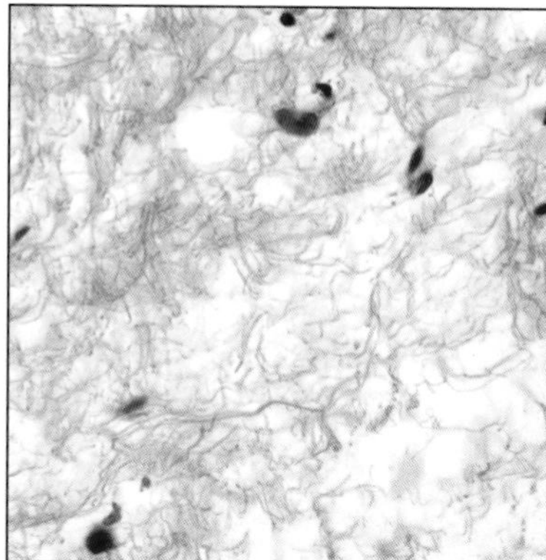

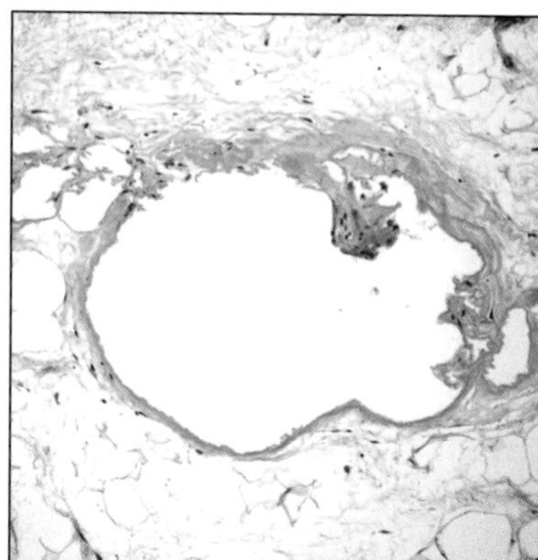

(Left) *Hematoxylin & eosin at low power shows markedly widened fibrous septa with a loose edematous appearance and remnants of subcutaneous fat lobule.* ***(Center)*** *Hematoxylin & eosin shows mildly atypical fibroblasts in areas of fibrosis. These fibroblasts lack the pleomorphism of the atypical cells of well-differentiated liposarcoma. Note how the delicate collagen fibers are separated by edema.* ***(Right)*** *Hematoxylin & eosin shows pseudocyst formation within subcutaneous fat.*

ATYPICAL VASCULAR PROLIFERATION

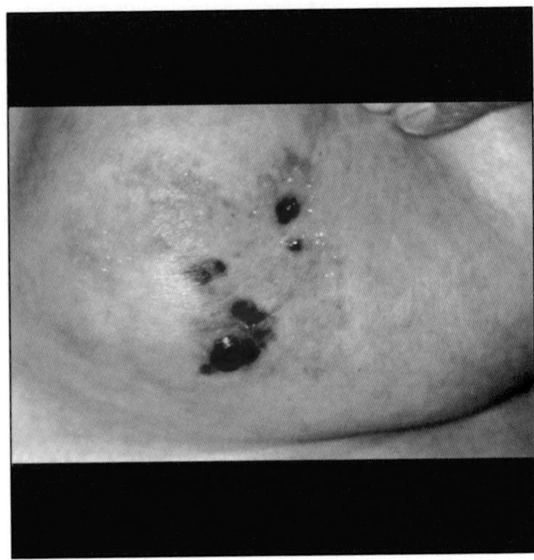

Multiple red papules and nodules are seen in a patient with an atypical vascular proliferation after radiotherapy.

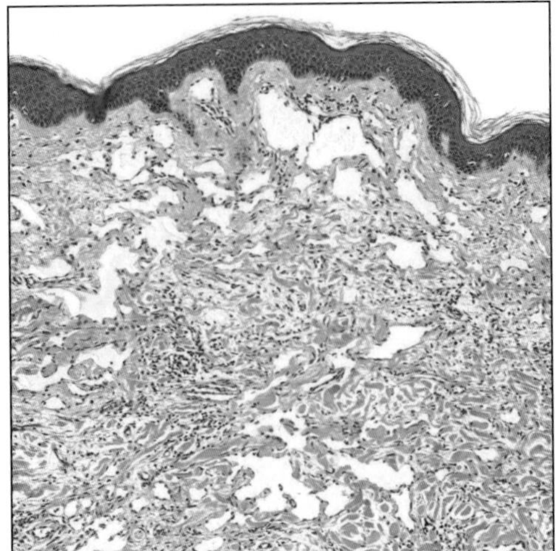

Low-power view shows a superficially located, lymphangioma-like vascular lesion composed of dilated vascular structures lined by cytologically bland endothelial cells.

TERMINOLOGY

Abbreviations

- (Post-irradiation) atypical vascular proliferation (AVP)

Synonyms

- Atypical vascular lesion (AVL)
- Benign lymphangiomatous papulae (BLAP)

Definitions

- Vascular proliferation after radiotherapy excluding obvious post-irradiation angiosarcoma, arising predominantly in breast

ETIOLOGY/PATHOGENESIS

Environmental Exposure

- Occurs after radiotherapy (40-60 Gy)
- Develops after a median of 3 years after radiotherapy

CLINICAL ISSUES

Epidemiology

- Incidence
  - Exact incidence difficult to establish
  - Relative risk is increased about 10x following radiation therapy
  - Incidence for post-irradiation AVP is equal after mastectomy or breast-conserving therapy
- Age
  - Wide age range; median in late 50s
  - Usually 1 decade earlier than radiation-induced cutaneous angiosarcoma

Site

- Occurs most frequently after radiation therapy for breast cancer
- Seen in skin of breast &/or chest wall
- Develops less frequently after radiation for gynecological or other malignancies

Presentation

- Small, red to brown papules (usually less than 5 mm)
- Often multifocal
- Presents only rarely as large plaques

Treatment

- Surgical approaches
  - All lesions must be excised completely

Prognosis

- Very difficult to estimate exact prognosis
- Presence of significant cytologic atypia worsens prognosis
- Presence of increased proliferative activity (Ki-67) worsens prognosis
- Presence of increased p53 expression worsens prognosis

MICROSCOPIC PATHOLOGY

Histologic Features

- Rather well-circumscribed, superficially located, dermal lesions
- Extension into subcutaneous tissue usually not seen
- Rather small, symmetrical, and often wedge-shaped lesions
- Dilated &/or narrow vascular structures
- Dissection of preexisting dermal collagen may be present
- Anastomosing vascular structures may be present
- Single layer of slightly enlarged endothelial cells
- Neither endothelial multilayering nor prominent cytologic atypia
- No increased endothelial mitoses
- Neither confluent hemorrhages nor necrosis

ATYPICAL VASCULAR PROLIFERATION

Key Facts

Terminology
- Vascular proliferation after radiotherapy excluding obvious post-irradiation angiosarcoma, arising predominantly in breast

Clinical Issues
- Exact incidence is difficult to establish
- Occurs most frequently after radiation therapy of breast cancer
- Small papules, usually less than 5 mm
- Papules are red to brown colored
- Often multifocal
- All lesions must be excised completely
- Wide age range; median in late 50s

Microscopic Pathology
- Rather well-circumscribed, superficially located, dermal lesions
- Rather small, symmetrical, and wedge-shaped lesions
- Dilated &/or narrow vascular structures
- Sometimes anastomosing vessels are seen
- Sometimes dissecting vascular structures are seen
- Single layer of slightly enlarged endothelial cells
- Expression of CD31 and podoplanin
- No endothelial multilayering
- No prominent cytologic atypia
- No increased endothelial mitoses
- No increased expression of Ki-67
- No increased expression of p63
- No amplification of *c-myc*

Cytologic Features
- Slightly enlarged endothelial cells
- Slightly enlarged but uniform nuclei

DIFFERENTIAL DIAGNOSIS

Hobnail Hemangioma
- Solitary papules or nodules
- Biphasic growth (superficial dilated vessels; in deeper areas, narrow vessels)
- Hobnail endothelial cells
- Stromal fibrosis, hemosiderin deposits

Lymphangioma Circumscriptum
- Represents developmental malformation (infants, adults)
- Clinically, groups of small vesicles containing clear fluid are present
- Small and superficially located lesions

Progressive Lymphangioma (Benign Lymphangioendothelioma)
- Presents clinically as large, slowly increasing, pink to reddish brown plaques
- Infiltrating and dissecting lymphatics
- Lymphatics orientated horizontally in dermis

Well-Differentiated Angiosarcoma
- Tends to involve deeper structures
- Anastomosing and infiltrating vascular structures
- Endothelial multilayering and endothelial atypia
- Increased number of endothelial mitoses
- Increased Ki-67 and p53 expression
- Evidence of *c-myc* amplification
- Post-irradiation atypical vascular proliferations and obvious angiosarcomas are best regarded as points of morphologic spectrum
- Post-irradiation atypical vascular proliferation most likely represents potential precursor of cutaneous angiosarcoma

DIAGNOSTIC CHECKLIST

Clinically Relevant Pathologic Features
- Symptom time frame
- Gross appearance
- Invasive pattern
- Nuclear features

Pathologic Interpretation Pearls
- AVP and post-irradiation well-differentiated cutaneous angiosarcoma represent morphologic spectrum
- All lesions showing features of AVP have to be excised completely

SELECTED REFERENCES

1. Manner J et al: MYC high level gene amplification is a distinctive feature of angiosarcomas after irradiation or chronic lymphedema. Am J Pathol. 176(1):34-9, 2010
2. Patton KT et al: Atypical vascular lesions after surgery and radiation of the breast: a clinicopathologic study of 32 cases analyzing histologic heterogeneity and association with angiosarcoma. Am J Surg Pathol. 32(6):943-50, 2008
3. Gengler C et al: Vascular proliferations of the skin after radiation therapy for breast cancer: clinicopathologic analysis of a series in favor of a benign process: a study from the French Sarcoma Group. Cancer. 109(8):1584-98, 2007
4. Brenn T et al: Radiation-associated cutaneous atypical vascular lesions and angiosarcoma: clinicopathologic analysis of 42 cases. Am J Surg Pathol. 29(8):983-96, 2005
5. Di Tommaso L et al: The capillary lobule: a deceptively benign feature of post-radiation angiosarcoma of the skin: report of three cases. Am J Dermatopathol. 27(4):301-5, 2005
6. Requena L et al: Benign vascular proliferations in irradiated skin. Am J Surg Pathol. 26(3):328-37, 2002
7. Fineberg S et al: Cutaneous angiosarcoma and atypical vascular lesions of the skin and breast after radiation therapy for breast carcinoma. Am J Clin Pathol. 102(6):757-63, 1994

ATYPICAL VASCULAR PROLIFERATION

Microscopic Features

*(**Left**) A benign lymphangiomatous papule that represents the "benign" end of the spectrum of atypical vascular proliferations after radiotherapy is characterized by rather circumscribed superficial dermal vascular lesions composed of lymphatic vascular structures. (**Right**) High-power view shows dilated vascular structures lined by uniform endothelial cells. Neither back-to-back arrangement of neoplastic vascular structures nor endothelial multilayering is noted.*

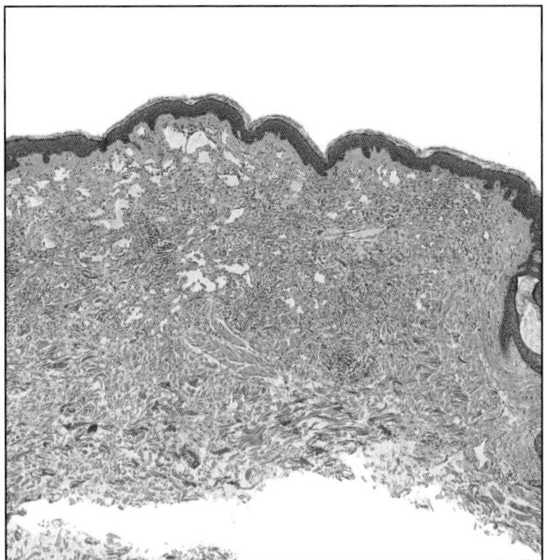

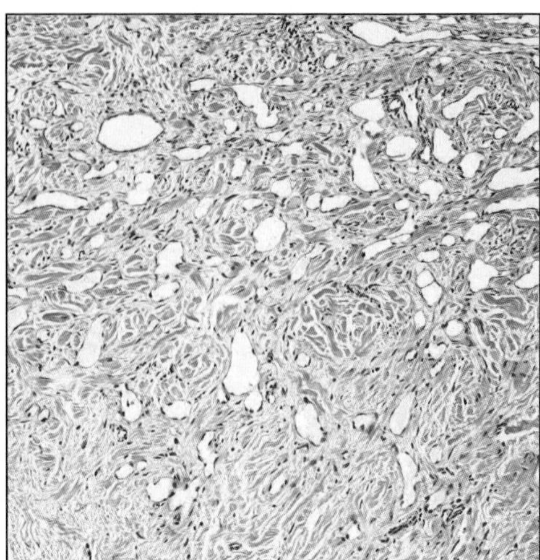

*(**Left**) The lining endothelial cells are only slightly enlarged and contain uniform nuclei with a finely dispersed chromatin. Note the endothelial bridges ⇨ in the absence of endothelial multilayering. Scattered lymphocytes are present →, a frequent finding in these lesions. (**Right**) A plaque-like atypical vascular proliferation after radiotherapy with a prominent lymphocytic infiltration demonstrates focally dilated, lymphangioma-like vascular structures ⇨.*

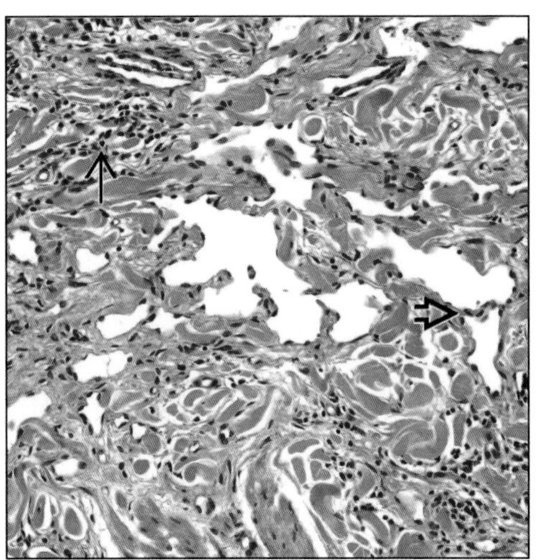

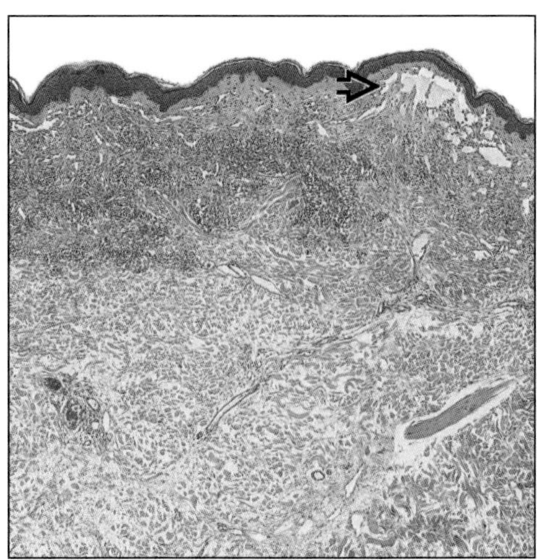

*(**Left**) This case of an atypical vascular proliferation after radiotherapy is composed of dilated and narrow vascular structures set in a collagenous stroma. Even at low power, scattered endothelial cells with enlarged and hyperchromatic nuclei are noted, a suspicious finding in these neoplasms ⇨. (**Right**) Narrow vascular structures are lined by slightly atypical endothelial cells. Note the dissecting infiltrating growth of neoplastic vascular structures.*

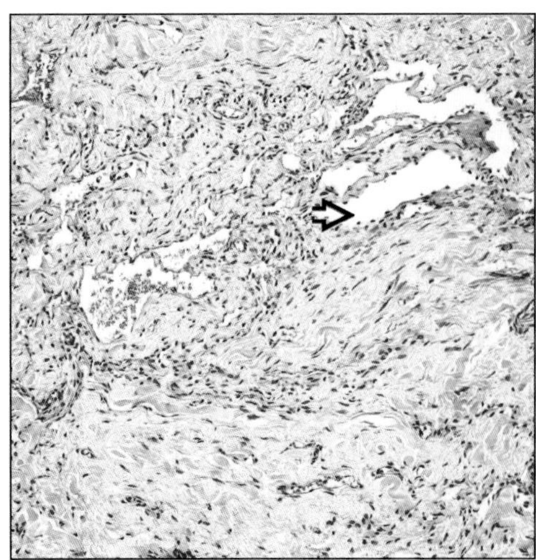

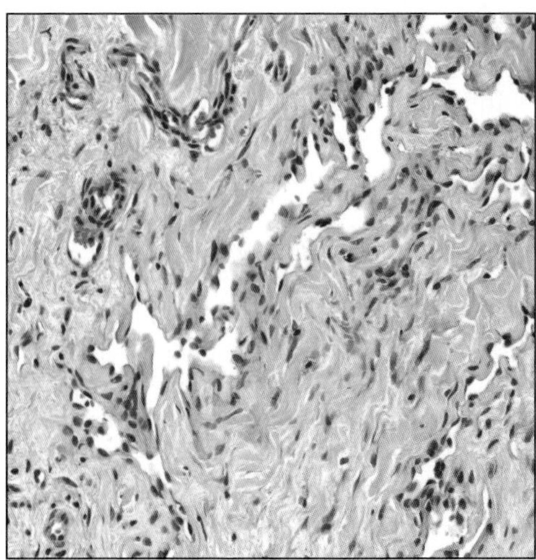

Microscopic and Immunohistochemical Features

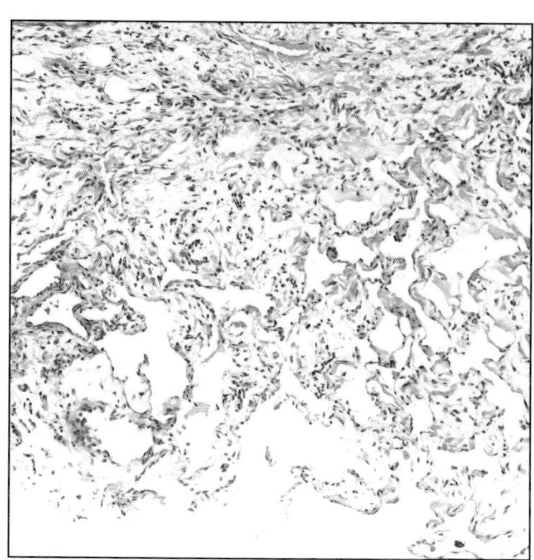

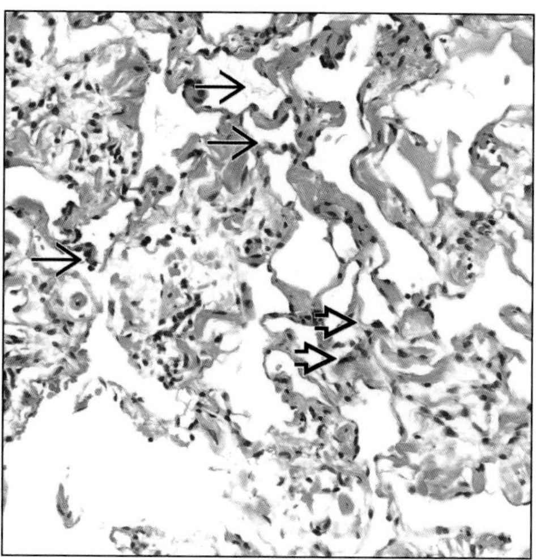

(Left) *In this cellular example of an atypical vascular proliferation after radiotherapy, numerous dilated vascular structures with slight variations of the vessel wall thickness are present.* ***(Right)*** *At higher power, numerous endothelial bridges ➔ and scattered endothelial cells with enlarged and hyperchromatic nuclei ➲ are present.*

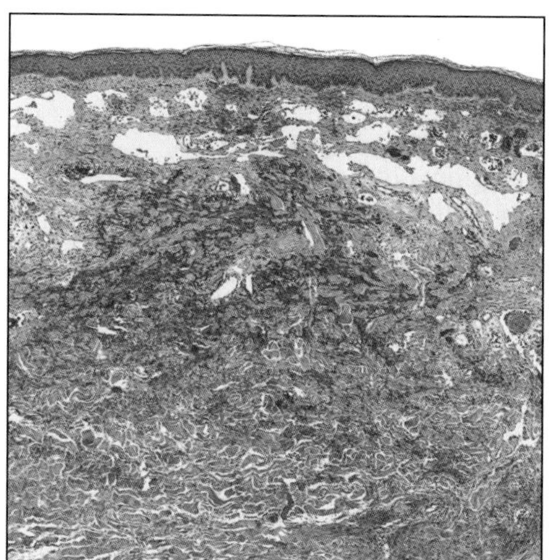

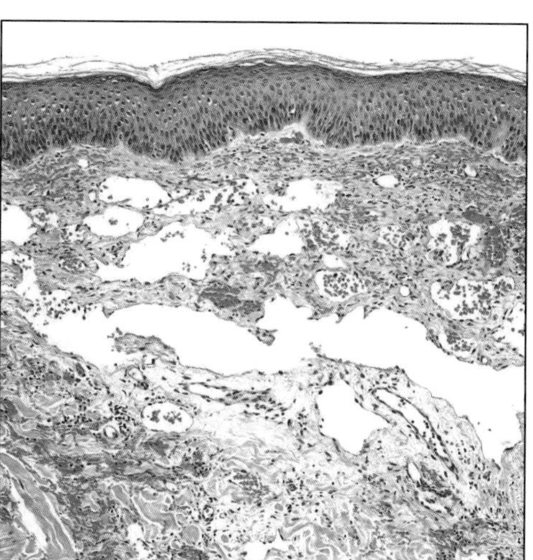

(Left) *This is a case of an atypical vascular proliferation with confluent areas of hemorrhage that represent a further suspicious morphologic finding in these neoplasms.* ***(Right)*** *This lesion is composed of mainly dilated vascular structures lined by slightly enlarged endothelial cells.*

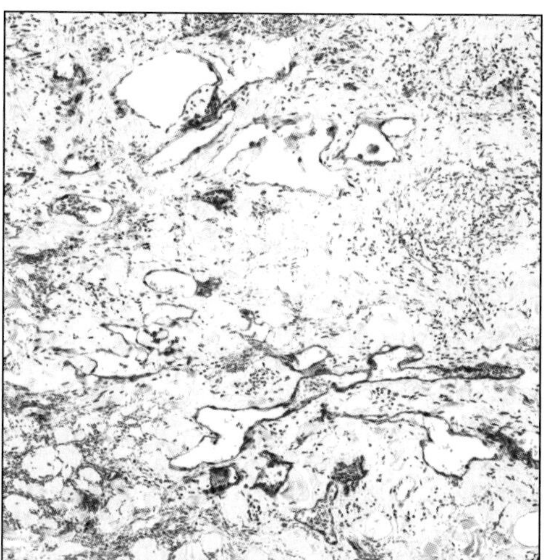

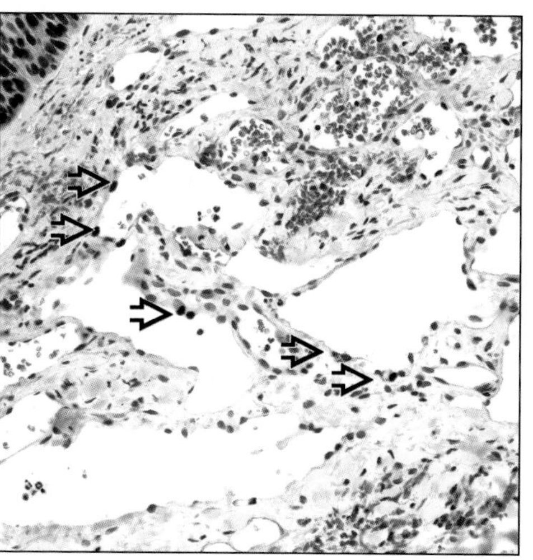

(Left) *Podoplanin antibodies highlight the lining endothelial cells. Despite slightly nuclear atypica, no endothelial multilayering nor anastomosing vascular structures are present.* ***(Right)*** *The presence of scattered Ki-67(+) endothelial cells ➲ represents a suspicious finding in cases of atypical vascular proliferation after radiotherapy.*

KAPOSIFORM HEMANGIOENDOTHELIOMA

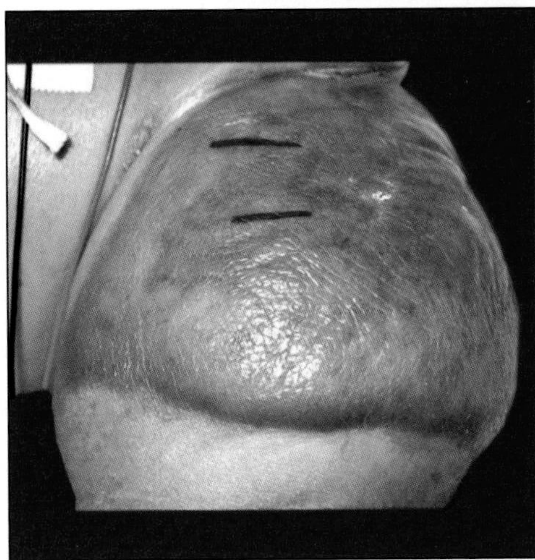

Clinical photograph shows a large inguinal tumor in an infant. More superficial tumors typically present as an erythematous or violaceous mass.

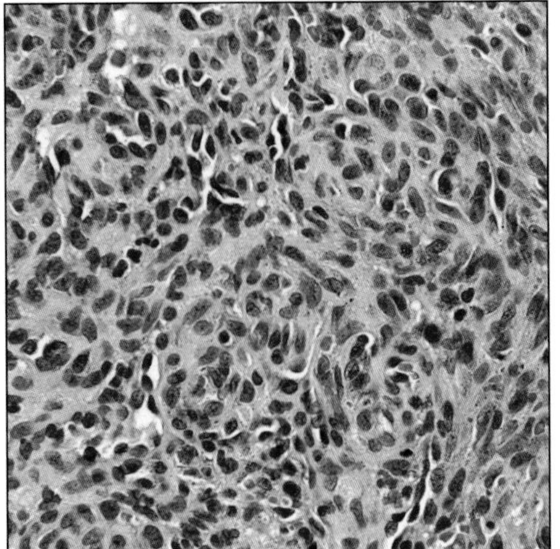

Hematoxylin & eosin shows proliferation of spindled endothelial cells. The spindled cells are arranged in short fascicles and form slit-like vascular lumens similar to Kaposi sarcoma.

CLINICAL ISSUES

Epidemiology

- Age
  - Majority present in childhood to teen years
  - Approximately 1/2 of kaposiform hemangioendothelioma cases present in 1st year of life

Presentation

- Painful or painless mass
  - Presents as superficial or deep mass
  - Cutaneous lesions present as violaceous plaques
  - Deep tumors often multiple nodules
  - Associated with Kasabach-Merritt syndrome (especially retroperitoneal tumors)
    - Consumptive coagulopathy
    - Thrombocytopenia
    - Majority of all cases of Kasabach-Merritt syndrome associated with kaposiform hemangioendothelioma

Treatment

- Surgical approaches
  - Wide excision
- Drugs
  - Vincristine
  - Cyclophosphamide
  - Methotrexate
  - Actinomycin D
  - α-interferon

Prognosis

- Rare regional lymph node metastasis
- No distant metastasis
- Mortality approximately 10%, related to local effects of tumor or Kasabach-Merritt syndrome

MICROSCOPIC PATHOLOGY

Histologic Features

- Multinodular growth pattern
- Spindled areas resembling Kaposi sarcoma
- Capillary hemangioma-like areas
- Mitoses but minimal atypia
- Immunohistochemistry
  - Positive for CD31, CD34, FLI-1, and podoplanin (especially in peripheral lymphatic component)
  - Negative for GLUT1

Predominant Cell/Compartment Type

- Endothelial

DIFFERENTIAL DIAGNOSIS

Kaposi Sarcoma

- Clinical features
  - Immunocompromised and older patients
- Microscopic features
  - Early Kaposi sarcoma shows neoplastic vessels dissecting through dermal collagen
  - Later lesions with solid spindle cell areas
  - Lacks capillary hemangioma-like areas
  - Positive for HHV8 latent nuclear antigen on immunohistochemistry

Acquired Tufted Angioma

- Clinical features
  - Similar demographics as kaposiform hemangioendothelioma
    - Most cases present in children
    - Occasional cases in adults
  - Also associated with Kasabach-Merritt syndrome
- Microscopic features
  - Nodular proliferation of closely packed capillaries in dermis ("cannonball" pattern)
  - Bland oval to spindled endothelial cells

Key Facts

Clinical Issues

- Presents in infants and young children
- Associated with Kasabach-Merritt syndrome (especially retroperitoneal tumors)
  - Consumptive coagulopathy
  - Thrombocytopenia
- Rare regional lymph node metastasis
- No distant metastasis
- Mortality approximately 10%, related to local effects of tumor or Kasabach-Merritt syndrome

Microscopic Pathology

- Spindled areas resembling Kaposi sarcoma
- Areas resembling capillary hemangiomas
- Minimal atypia
- Positive for CD31, CD34, FLI-1, and podoplanin
- Negative for HHV8

- Essentially indistinguishable from kaposiform hemangioendothelioma
- May represent part of kaposiform hemangioendothelioma spectrum

Spindle Cell Hemangioma

- Clinical features
  - Occurs in adults
  - Distal extremities
- Microscopic features
  - Often partially intravascular
  - Ectatic vessels
  - Spindled cells
  - Vacuolated endothelial cells
    - So-called "blister" cells
  - May have areas of thrombosis or phleboliths

DIAGNOSTIC CHECKLIST

Clinically Relevant Pathologic Features

- Age distribution
  - Vast majority occur in children
- Symptom complex
  - Kasabach-Merritt syndrome

Pathologic Interpretation Pearls

- Vascular tumor in children composed predominantly of spindled endothelial cells: Consider kaposiform hemangioendothelioma

SELECTED REFERENCES

1. Debelenko LV et al: D2-40 immunohistochemical analysis of pediatric vascular tumors reveals positivity in kaposiform hemangioendothelioma. Mod Pathol. 18(11):1454-60, 2005
2. Cheuk W et al: Immunostaining for human herpesvirus 8 latent nuclear antigen-1 helps distinguish Kaposi sarcoma from its mimickers. Am J Clin Pathol. 121(3):335-42, 2004
3. Lyons LL et al: Kaposiform hemangioendothelioma: a study of 33 cases emphasizing its pathologic, immunophenotypic, and biologic uniqueness from juvenile hemangioma. Am J Surg Pathol. 28(5):559-68, 2004
4. Brasanac D et al: Retroperitoneal kaposiform hemangioendothelioma with tufted angioma-like features in an infant with Kasabach-Merritt syndrome. Pathol Int. 53(9):627-31, 2003
5. Chu CY et al: Transformation between Kaposiform hemangioendothelioma and tufted angioma. Dermatology. 206(4):334-7, 2003
6. Mac-Moune Lai F et al: Kaposiform hemangioendothelioma: five patients with cutaneous lesion and long follow-up. Mod Pathol. 14(11):1087-92, 2001
7. Mentzel T et al: Kaposiform hemangioendothelioma in adults. Clinicopathologic and immunohistochemical analysis of three cases. Am J Clin Pathol. 108(4):450-5, 1997
8. Zukerberg LR et al: Kaposiform hemangioendothelioma of infancy and childhood. An aggressive neoplasm associated with Kasabach-Merritt syndrome and lymphangiomatosis. Am J Surg Pathol. 17(4):321-8, 1993

IMAGE GALLERY

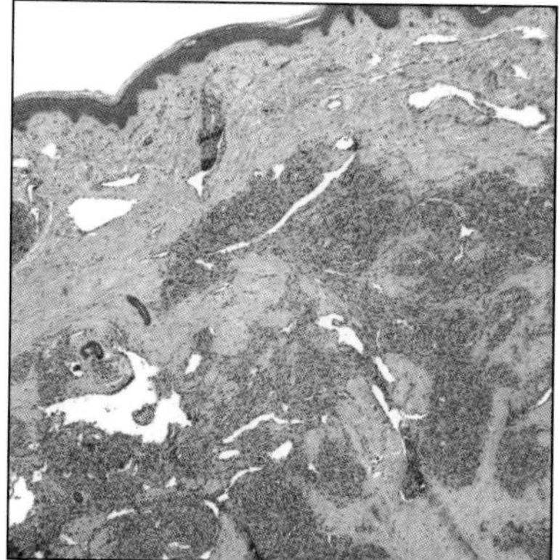

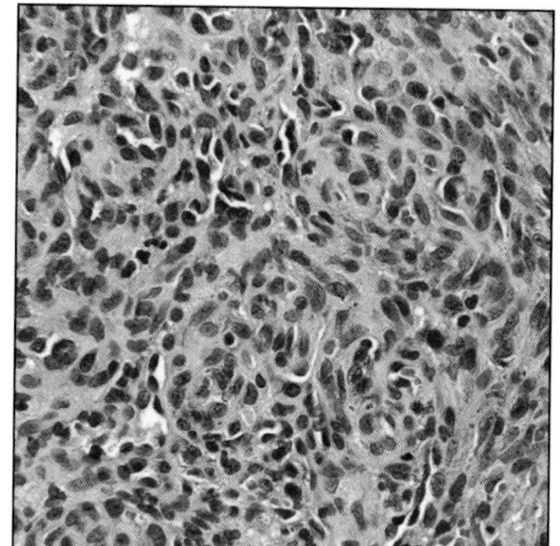

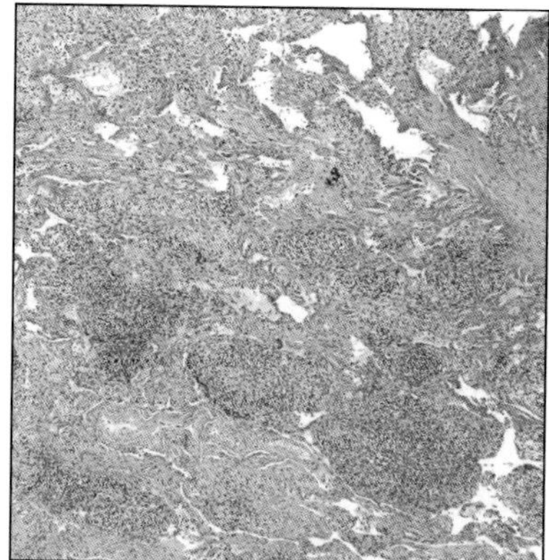

(Left) *Hematoxylin & eosin shows a low-power view of kaposiform hemangioendothelioma demonstrating irregular nodules of spindled cells in the dermis as well as ectatic vessels.* ***(Center)*** *Hematoxylin & eosin shows proliferation of spindled endothelial cells. The spindled cells are arranged in short fascicles and form slit-like vascular lumens similar to Kaposi sarcoma.* ***(Right)*** *Hematoxylin & eosin shows hemangioma-like area within kaposiform hemangioendothelioma.*

RETIFORM HEMANGIOENDOTHELIOMA

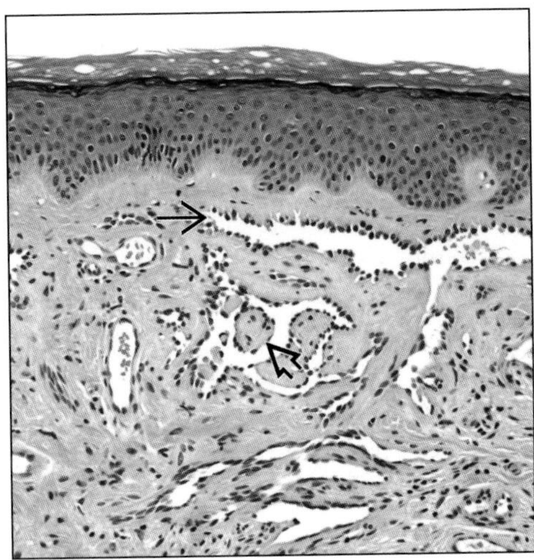

Low-magnification view of a retiform hemangioendothelioma shows superficial dermal involvement by elongated vascular spaces ➔. Focal papillary structures are present ➢.

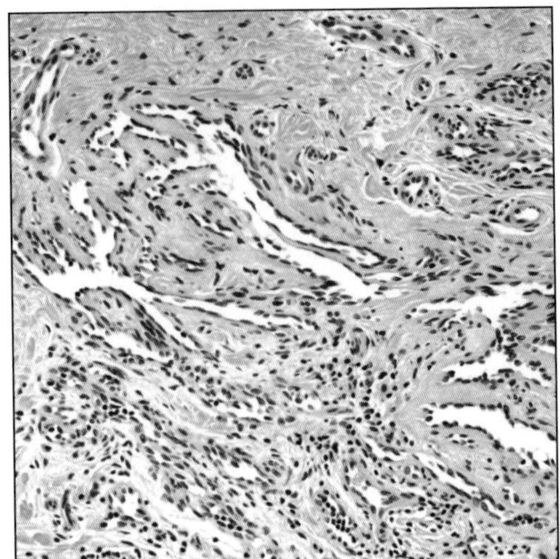

Higher magnification view shows a proliferation of elongated vessels lined by hyperchromatic hobnailed endothelial cells. The surrounding stroma shows fibrosis and scattered lymphocytes.

TERMINOLOGY

Abbreviations

- Retiform hemangioendothelioma (RHE)
- Hemangioendothelioma (HE)

Synonyms

- Hobnail hemangioendothelioma

Definitions

- Low-grade malignant vascular tumor composed of elongated vessels resembling rete testes

ETIOLOGY/PATHOGENESIS

Unknown

- Rare cases associated with lymphedema or preceding radiation
- 1 case reported to be positive for HHV8

CLINICAL ISSUES

Epidemiology

- Incidence
  - Rare vascular tumor
- Age
  - Typically middle-aged adults but may occur in children
- Gender
  - More common in females

Site

- Trunk or extremities

Presentation

- Large nodular to plaque-like lesion

Treatment

- Surgical approaches
  - Complete excision is necessary to prevent recurrence

Prognosis

- Locally aggressive, rarely metastasizing (although lymph node metastases reported in several cases)

MACROSCOPIC FEATURES

General Features

- Typically poorly circumscribed dermal &/or subcutaneous tumor

Size

- May be large tumors (up to 12 cm)

MICROSCOPIC PATHOLOGY

Histologic Features

- Dermal-based infiltrative proliferation of distinctive, elongated, arborizing blood vessels resembling rete testis
- Vascular spaces are lined by endothelial cells with characteristic hobnail morphology
  - Endothelial cells show hyperchromasia but typically do not show prominent cytologic atypia
  - Mitotic figures may be present but are usually rare
- Very prominent lymphocytic infiltrate reported in most cases
- May show invasion of subcutaneous tissues
- Some cases show significant overlap with Dabska tumor (both have hobnailed cells), with prominent papillary structures and hyaline cores

Cytologic Features

- Hobnail cells with oval nuclei with mild hyperchromasia

RETIFORM HEMANGIOENDOTHELIOMA

Key Facts

Terminology
- Retiform hemangioendothelioma (RHE)
- Low-grade malignant vascular tumor composed of elongated vessels resembling rete testes

Clinical Issues
- Typically middle-aged adults, but may occur in children
- Locally aggressive, very rarely metastasizing (although lymph node metastases reported)

Microscopic Pathology
- Distinctive, elongated, arborizing blood vessels resembling rete testis
- Often show papillary-like intraluminal projections, some of which may have a hyaline core
- Vascular spaces are lined by endothelial cells with characteristic hobnail morphology
- Some cases show significant overlap with Dabska tumor

ANCILLARY TESTS

Immunohistochemistry
- Tumor cells react with vascular endothelial markers CD31, CD34, and FVIIIRAg
- Most cases negative with lymphatic markers D2-40 and VEGFR-3, but rare positive cases

DIFFERENTIAL DIAGNOSIS

Papillary Intralymphatic Angioendothelioma (Dabska Tumor)
- More common in children, but some cases in young adults reported
- Papillary structures more common
- Typically do not show prominent rete-like elongated vessels of RHE
- Some cases show significant overlap with RHE (both have hobnailed cells)

Composite Hemangioendothelioma
- By definition, composed of at least 2 distinct HE types
  - Predominant histologic components usually are epithelioid HE and RHE

Kaposi Sarcoma
- Much more common, associated with HIV/AIDS
- Proliferation of small, slit-like vascular spaces lined by spindle cells, lacking rete-like pattern of RHE
- HHV8(+) (only 1 case of RHE reported to be positive)

Angiosarcoma
- Typically occurs in older adults or post-mastectomy
- Proliferation of atypical spindled or epithelioid endothelial cells, often forming anastomosing vascular spaces and showing infiltrative features

DIAGNOSTIC CHECKLIST

Pathologic Interpretation Pearls
- Proliferation of distinctive elongated blood vessels (lined by hobnail cells) resembling rete testis

SELECTED REFERENCES

1. Emberger M et al: Retiform hemangioendothelioma: presentation of a case expressing D2-40. J Cutan Pathol. 36(9):987-90, 2009
2. Parsons A et al: Retiform hemangioendotheliomas usually do not express D2-40 and VEGFR-3. Am J Dermatopathol. 30(1):31-3, 2008
3. Tan D et al: Retiform hemangioendothelioma: a case report and review of the literature. J Cutan Pathol. 32(9):634-7, 2005
4. Schommer M et al: Retiform hemangioendothelioma: another tumor associated with human herpesvirus type 8? J Am Acad Dermatol. 42(2 Pt 1):290-2, 2000
5. Calonje E et al: Retiform hemangioendothelioma. A distinctive form of low-grade angiosarcoma delineated in a series of 15 cases. Am J Surg Pathol. 18(2):115-25, 1994

IMAGE GALLERY

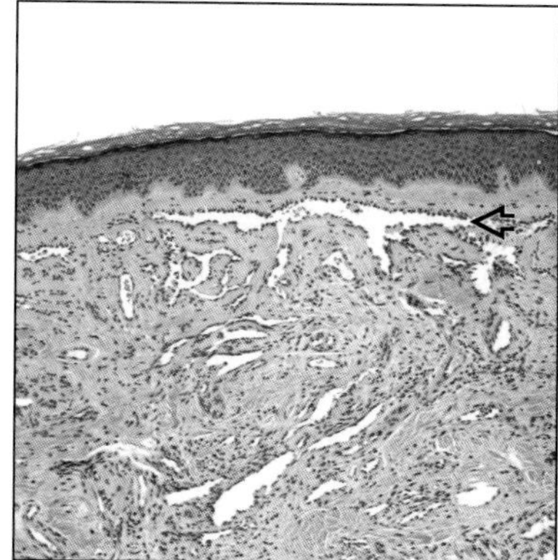

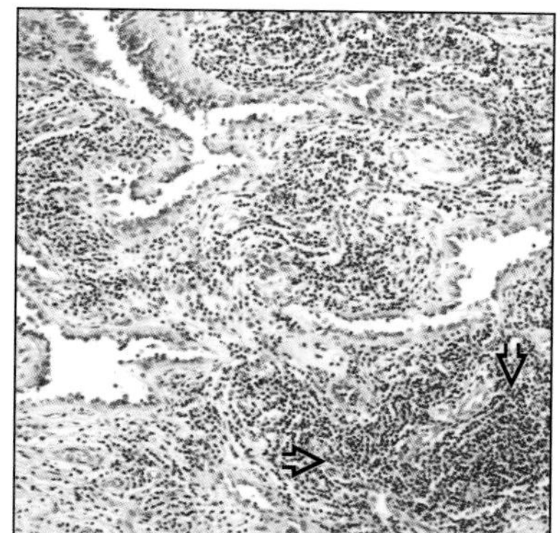

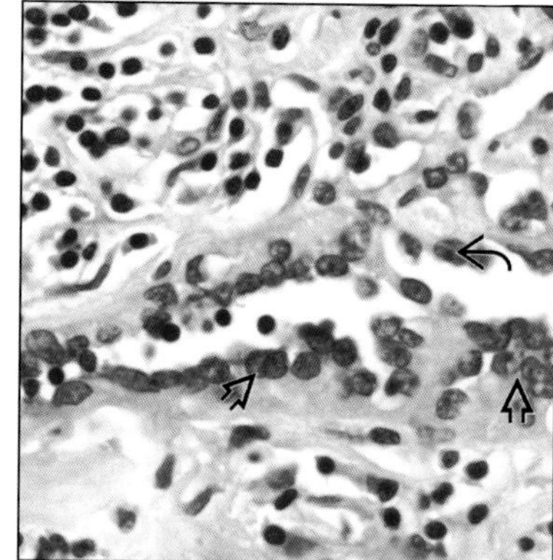

(Left) *Low-magnification examination of a RHE shows superficial dermal involvement by irregular, elongated, branching vascular spaces* ⊳. ***(Center)*** *Deep area of a retiform HE shows elongated vascular spaces surrounded by prominent lymphoid aggregates* ⊳. ***(Right)*** *High-magnification view shows hyperchromatic endothelial cells with hobnail features, nuclear crowding* ⊳*, and focally enlarged nucleoli* ⊳*.*

PAPILLARY INTRALYMPHATIC ANGIOENDOTHELIOMA (DABSKA)

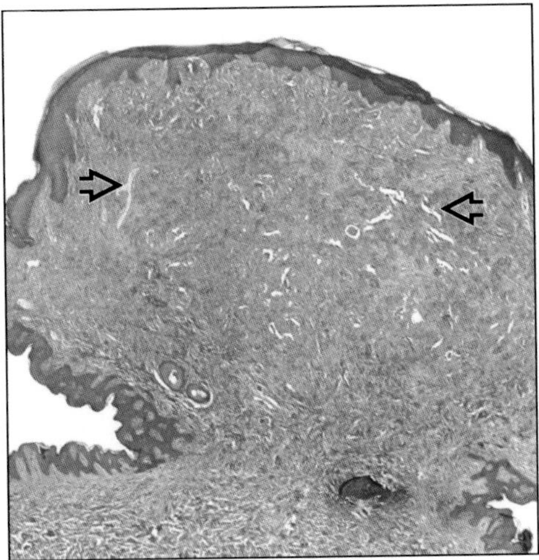

Scanning magnification view of a papillary intralymphatic angioendothelioma (Dabska tumor) shows a polypoid lesion in the skin with irregular dilated vascular spaces.

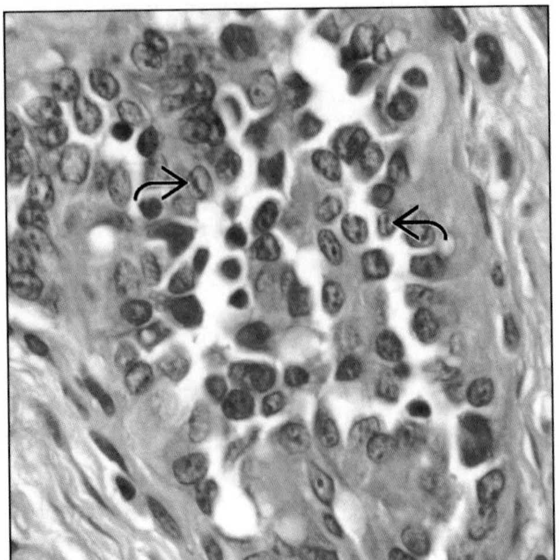

High-power examination shows papillae lined by mildly enlarged hobnailed cells projecting into the vascular lumens. The cells show vesicular chromatin, small nucleoli, and occasional grooves.

TERMINOLOGY

Abbreviations

- Papillary intralymphatic angioendothelioma (PILA)

Synonyms

- Dabska tumor
- Endovascular papillary angioendothelioma

Definitions

- Low-grade malignant vascular tumor composed of hobnailed endothelial cells

ETIOLOGY/PATHOGENESIS

Unknown

- May be associated with vascular or lymphatic tumor/ malformation

CLINICAL ISSUES

Epidemiology

- Incidence
  - Rare tumors
- Age
  - Typically occur in children (minority in adults)
- Gender
  - Slight female predominance

Site

- Distal extremities most common but may occur in other sites

Presentation

- Plaque-like lesion of dermis + subcutis
  - May show overlying violaceous skin discoloration

Treatment

- Surgical approaches
  - Complete surgical excision recommended to prevent metastasis (rare) or recurrence

Prognosis

- High rate of local recurrence, rare metastasis (to lymph nodes)

MACROSCOPIC FEATURES

General Features

- Dermal-based infiltrative tumor with extension into subcutis

Size

- Can be quite large (average: 7 cm)

MICROSCOPIC PATHOLOGY

Histologic Features

- Dermal proliferation of vessels lined by enlarged, cuboidal endothelial cells
  - Intravascular papillary projections with hyaline cores
  - Endothelial cells show prominent hobnail features with plump, rounded profiles protruding into lumens
  - Cytoplasmic vacuolation may be seen
  - Mitotic figures absent or rare
- Typically associated with surrounding lymphoid infiltrate and sclerotic collagen
- Vessels often extend into subcutaneous tissues
- Associated lymphatic or vascular tumor or malformation in some cases

Cytologic Features

- Hobnail cells show high nuclear to cytoplasmic ratio, nuclei may show grooves

PAPILLARY INTRALYMPHATIC ANGIOENDOTHELIOMA (DABSKA)

Key Facts

Terminology

- Dabska tumor
- Endovascular papillary angioendothelioma

Clinical Issues

- Typically occur in children (minority in adults)
- Distal extremities most common, but may occur in other sites
- High rate of local recurrence, rare metastasis

Microscopic Pathology

- Dermal proliferation of vessels with papillary projections lined by enlarged, cuboidal endothelial cells
- Endothelial cells show prominent hobnail features with plump, rounded profiles protruding into lumens
- Typically associated with surrounding lymphoid infiltrate and sclerotic collagen

ANCILLARY TESTS

Immunohistochemistry

- Typically positive for vascular markers including FVIIIRAg, CD31, and CD34
- Most cases also positive for lymphatic markers D2-40 and VEGFR-3

DIFFERENTIAL DIAGNOSIS

Retiform Hemangioendothelioma (RHE)

- Most cases occur in adults, but some present in children
- Proliferation of vessels forming distinct elongated rete-like structures lined by hobnail cells
- Some cases of RHE show significant overlap with Dabska tumor, with prominent papillary structures

Composite Hemangioendothelioma (HE)

- By definition, composed of at least 2 distinct HE types
  - Predominant histologic components usually are epithelioid HE and RHE

Kaposi Sarcoma

- Much more common, associated with HIV infection and AIDS in most cases
- Proliferation of small, slit-like vascular spaces lined by spindle cells, lacking papillary pattern of Dabska
- HHV8(+)

Angiosarcoma

- Typically occurs in older adults or post-mastectomy
- Proliferation of atypical spindled or epithelioid endothelial cells, forming anastomosing vascular spaces and showing infiltrative features

DIAGNOSTIC CHECKLIST

Pathologic Interpretation Pearls

- Dermal proliferation of vessels with papillary projections lined by enlarged, cuboidal endothelial cells

SELECTED REFERENCES

1. Emanuel PO et al: Dabska tumor arising in lymphangioma circumscriptum. J Cutan Pathol. 35(1):65-9, 2008
2. Fukunaga M: Expression of D2-40 in lymphatic endothelium of normal tissues and in vascular tumours. Histopathology. 46(4):396-402, 2005
3. Fanburg-Smith JC et al: Papillary intralymphatic angioendothelioma (PILA): a report of twelve cases of a distinctive vascular tumor with phenotypic features of lymphatic vessels. Am J Surg Pathol. 23(9):1004-10, 1999
4. Dabska M: Malignant endovascular papillary angioendothelioma of the skin in childhood. Clinicopathologic study of 6 cases. Cancer. 24(3):503-10, 1969

IMAGE GALLERY

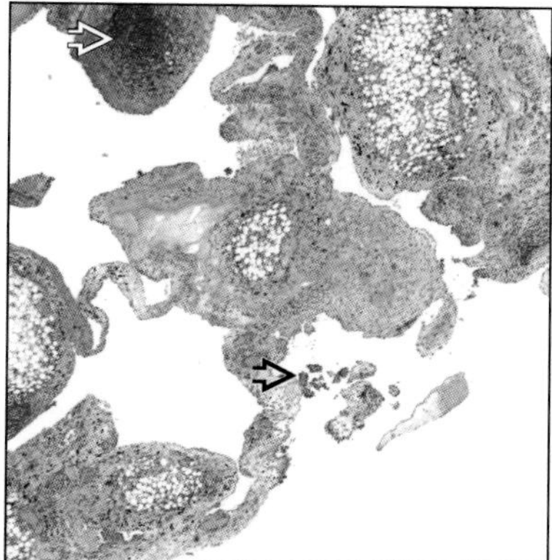

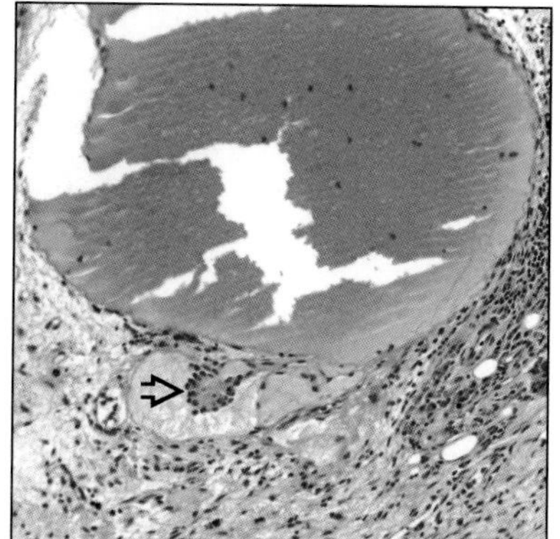

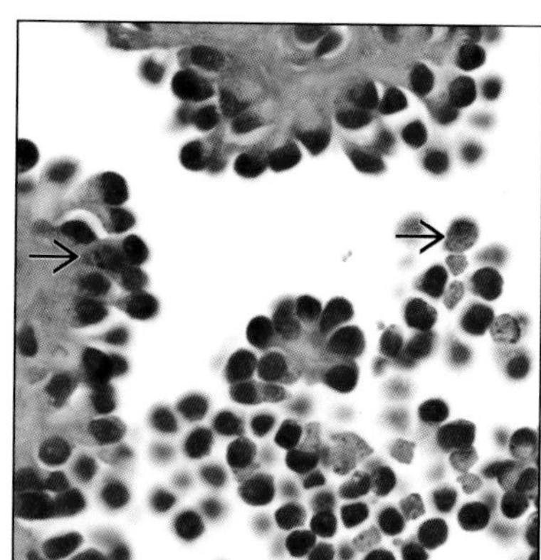

(Left) *Low magnification of a PILA shows a background of lymphangioma-like areas with scattered lymphoid aggregates ⇨. Note focal intraluminal papillary projections ⇨.* ***(Center)*** *Dilated vascular space filled with red blood cells overlying a smaller space with a prominent papillary intralymphatic projection is lined by hobnailed cells ⇨.* ***(Right)*** *Multiple prominent intralymphatic projections of papillary structures with hyaline cores are lined by plump hyperchromatic-staining endothelial cells, some of which contain cytoplasmic hemosiderin pigment →.*

COMPOSITE HEMANGIOENDOTHELIOMA

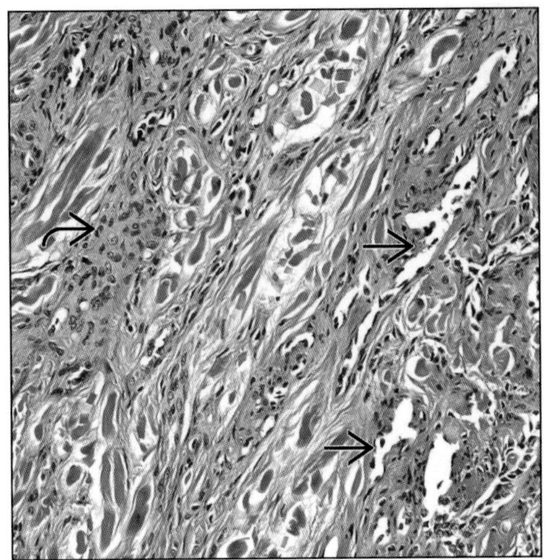

Composite hemangioendothelioma usually presents as a dermal/subcutaneous tumor on an acral extremity. It has complex histology with admixtures of various elements, most often retiform ➔ and epithelioid HE ➔.

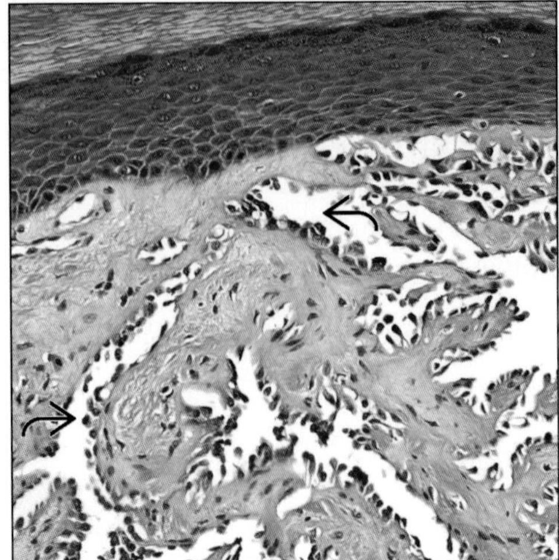

Retiform HE is the most common component of composite HE, composed of elongated, thin-walled channels lined by endothelial cells that protrude into the lumen, forming a "hobnail" pattern ➔.

TERMINOLOGY

Abbreviations

- Hemangioendothelioma (HE)

Definitions

- Endothelial neoplasm of low malignant potential composed of admixture of histologically benign, intermediate, and malignant components

ETIOLOGY/PATHOGENESIS

Developmental Anomaly

- Can arise from preexisting or congenital vascular malformation

CLINICAL ISSUES

Epidemiology

- Incidence
  - Rare: Only 25 reported cases

Site

- Dermis and subcutis
  - Acral extremities
    - Foot/ankle region (50%)
    - Hand/forearm (25%)
- Oral mucosa (12%)
- Other sites: Thigh, upper arm, back, inguinal lymph nodes, mediastinum

Presentation

- Enlarging nodular or multinodular erythematous or violaceous mass
  - Satellite nodules
  - Ulceration
- Bleeding
- Edema

Natural History

- High local recurrence rate (50%)
  - Often many years after primary excision
- Metastases (15%)
  - Usually to regional lymph nodes

Treatment

- Surgical approaches
  - Wide local excision

Prognosis

- No reports of death from disease to date

MACROSCOPIC FEATURES

General Features

- Nodular or multinodular mass
- Red to purple
- Infiltrative border

Size

- Average: 5 cm; range: 1-30 cm

MICROSCOPIC PATHOLOGY

Histologic Features

- Complex admixture of variety of vasoformative patterns
- Retiform HE pattern
  - Most common and usually dominant
  - Long, branching, thin-walled vessels
  - Single layer of bland endothelial cells that protrude intraluminally (hobnail pattern)
  - Intraluminal papillary structures in some
- Epithelioid HE pattern
  - 2nd most common
  - Cords, strands, or sheets of epithelioid endothelial cells
    - Abundant eosinophilic cytoplasm

COMPOSITE HEMANGIOENDOTHELIOMA

Key Facts

Terminology

- Endothelial neoplasm of low malignant potential composed of admixture of histologically benign, intermediate, and malignant components

Clinical Issues

- Acral extremities
- Enlarging nodular erythematous or violaceous mass
- Local recurrence (50%)
- Metastases (15%)
- No reports of death from disease to date

Microscopic Pathology

- Complex admixture of variety of vasoformative patterns
- Retiform and epithelioid HE patterns most common

Top Differential Diagnoses

- Retiform hemangioendothelioma
- Epithelioid hemangioendothelioma
- Well-differentiated angiosarcoma

    - Intracytoplasmic vacuoles
    - Myoxhyaline stroma
  - Well-differentiated angiosarcoma pattern
    - Anastomosing spaces lined by atypical cells, often multilayered
    - Dissecting growth pattern
    - Minor component when present
  - Spindle cell hemangioma pattern
    - Sheets and fascicles of spindle-shaped endothelial cells
    - Slit-like vascular spaces
    - Cavernous spaces, often with organizing thrombi and phleboliths
  - Other patterns
    - Arteriovenous malformation
    - Lymphangioma
    - Epithelioid hemangioma
    - Kaposiform HE
    - Poorly differentiated angiosarcoma

DIFFERENTIAL DIAGNOSIS

Retiform Hemangioendothelioma

- Skin and soft tissue of acral extremities
- Pure pattern, lacks other vascular components

Epithelioid Hemangioendothelioma

- Various skin, soft tissue, osseous, and visceral sites
- Pure pattern, lacks other vascular components

Well-Differentiated Angiosarcoma

- Most often cutaneous tumor on scalp/face of elderly patient
- Dissecting channels lined by atypical, multilayered endothelial cells
- High-grade or epithelioid components in many tumors

Spindle Cell Hemangioma

- Skin and soft tissue of acral extremities
- Spindle cell and cavernous patterns
- Thrombi and phleboliths

Kaposi Sarcoma

- Fascicles of atypical spindle cells
- Slit-like, blood-filled spaces
- HHV8(+)

SELECTED REFERENCES

1. Aydingöz IE et al: Composite haemangioendothelioma with lymph-node metastasis: an unusual presentation at an uncommon site. Clin Exp Dermatol. 34(8):e802-6, 2009
2. Requena L et al: Cutaneous composite hemangioendothelioma with satellitosis and lymph node metastases. J Cutan Pathol. 35(2):225-30, 2008
3. Fukunaga M et al: Composite hemangioendothelioma: report of 5 cases including one with associated Maffucci syndrome. Am J Surg Pathol. 31(10):1567-72, 2007
4. Nayler SJ et al: Composite hemangioendothelioma: a complex, low-grade vascular lesion mimicking angiosarcoma. Am J Surg Pathol. 24(3):352-61, 2000

IMAGE GALLERY

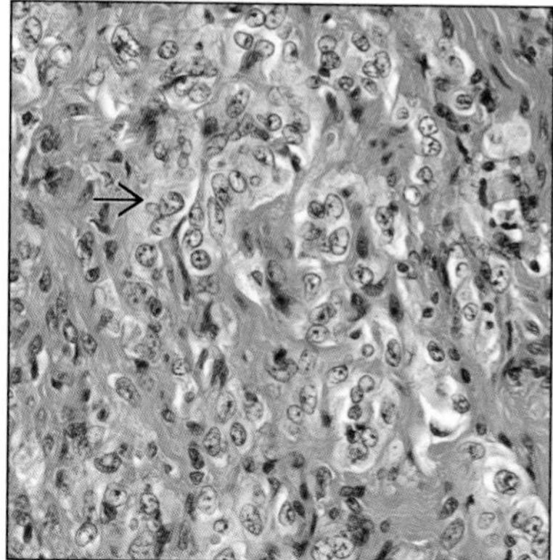

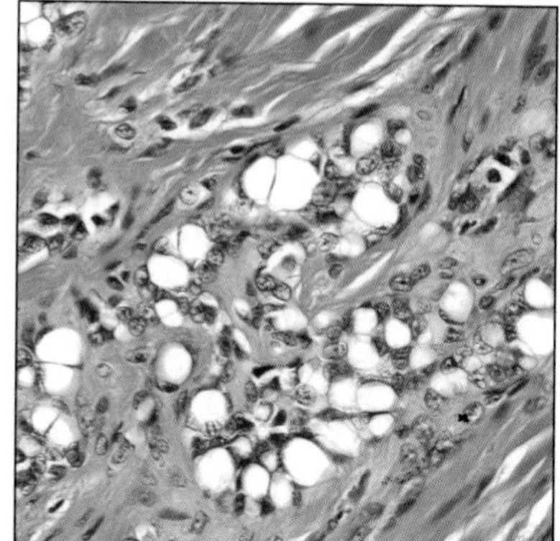

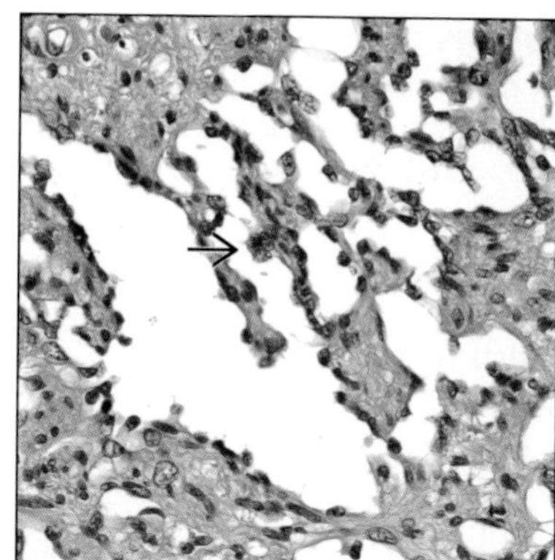

(Left) *An epithelioid HE component, present in most composite HEs, consists of cords ⇒, strands, or sheets of cells with abundant eosinophilic cytoplasm within a hyalinized or myxohyaline stroma.* ***(Center)*** *Epithelioid cells with intracytoplasmic vacuoles can mimic lipoblasts.* ***(Right)*** *Angiosarcoma-like areas are present in some tumors characterized by irregular anastomosing channels lined by atypical endothelial cells ⇒. It is not associated with worse prognosis.*

EPITHELIOID SARCOMA-LIKE HEMANGIOENDOTHELIOMA

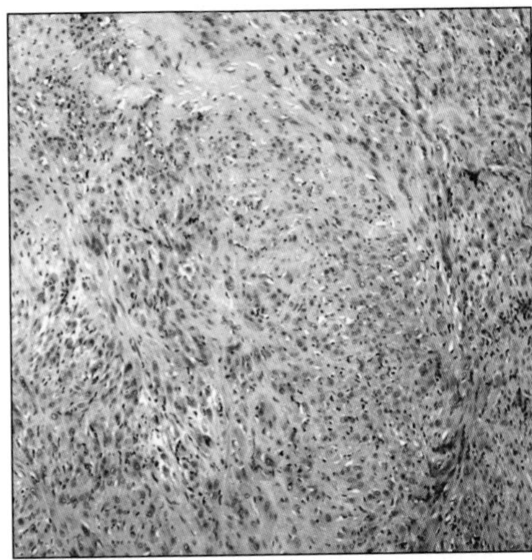

Hematoxylin & eosin demonstrates ill-defined nodular growth pattern of epithelioid sarcoma-like hemangioendothelioma.

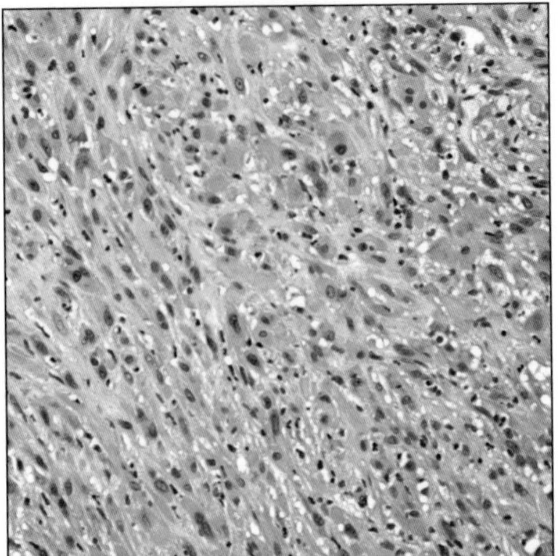

Hematoxylin & eosin shows epithelioid tumor cells with relatively abundant eosinophilic cytoplasm. The tumor transitions from epithelioid areas to more spindled areas in the left side of the image.

TERMINOLOGY

Definitions

- Vascular tumor of apparent intermediate malignancy that histologically closely resembles epithelioid sarcoma

CLINICAL ISSUES

Epidemiology

- Age
  - Most common in young adults (range: 17-70 years)

Site

- Most common in lower extremity

Presentation

- May present in superficial or deep soft tissue
  - Cutaneous lesions may be ulcerated

Treatment

- Surgical approaches
  - Wide excision
- Adjuvant therapy
  - No known role for adjuvant therapy

Prognosis

- Risk of local recurrence
- Risk of regional metastasis
- No reported case of distant metastasis to date

MICROSCOPIC PATHOLOGY

Histologic Features

- Ill-defined nodules, sheets, or short fascicles
- Predominantly epithelioid morphology
  - Round nuclei with relatively abundant eosinophilic cytoplasm
- Usually transitions to more spindled cells arranged in fascicles
- No multicellular vascular channels present
- Only rare intracytoplasmic lumen formation in approximately 1/2 of cases
- Mitotic rate low
  - < 5 mitotic figures/50 HPF

ANCILLARY TESTS

Immunohistochemistry

- CD31(+), cytokeratin(+), FLI-1(+)(nuclear stain), vimentin (+), CD34(-)
  - CD31 staining is strong with membranous pattern
  - Be careful of overinterpreting entrapped CD31(+) histiocytes

DIFFERENTIAL DIAGNOSIS

Epithelioid Sarcoma

- Nodules of epithelioid cells
  - Nodules often more defined and granuloma like
  - Nodules may have central necrosis (not seen in epithelioid sarcoma-like hemangioendothelioma)
  - Nuclei enlarged but otherwise relatively bland
- Sometimes predominantly spindled
- Low mitotic rate
- Immunophenotype: Cytokeratin(+), EMA(+), CD34(+) (~ 50-60%), vimentin(+), CD31(-), FLI-1(-), SNF5(-)

Epithelioid Hemangioendothelioma

- Cord-like arrangement of epithelioid cells
  - Sometimes arranged as small nests/groups of tumor cells
- Myxohyaline stroma
- Intracytoplasmic lumens common
- ~ 50% arise within preexisting vessel
- Nuclear features usually bland
  - Significant atypia seen in ~ 25% of cases

EPITHELIOID SARCOMA-LIKE HEMANGIOENDOTHELIOMA

Key Facts

Terminology

- Vascular tumor of apparent intermediate malignancy that histologically closely resembles epithelioid sarcoma

Clinical Issues

- Presents most commonly in young adults

Microscopic Pathology

- Ill-defined nodules, sheets, or short fascicles
- Predominantly epithelioid morphology
- Immunophenotype: CD31(+), cytokeratin(+), FLI-1(+), vimentin(+), CD34(-)
- No multicellular vascular channels present
- Only rare intracytoplasmic lumen formation in approximately 1/2 of cases

Top Differential Diagnoses

- Epithelioid sarcoma
- Epithelioid hemangioendothelioma

- Associated with more aggressive behavior
- Immunophenotype: CD31(+), CD34(+), FLI-1(+) (nuclear stain), vimentin(+), cytokeratin(+) (~ 25% of cases)

Epithelioid Angiosarcoma

- May be predominantly solid sheets
- Multicellular vascular channels usually present at least focally
- More prominent nuclear atypia
- High mitotic rate

Granulomatous Inflammatory Conditions

- Granuloma annulare
  - Histiocytic proliferation palisading around altered collagen fibers
  - Histiocytes with smaller nuclei than tumor cells of epithelioid sarcoma-like hemangioendothelioma
  - No transitions to spindled, fascicular areas
- Sarcoidosis
  - Discrete nodules of histiocytes (epithelioid granulomas)

Epithelioid Hemangioma

- Capillaries lined by epithelioid endothelial cells
- May have more solid areas
- Prominent inflammatory component
  - Lymphoid aggregates
  - Eosinophils

DIAGNOSTIC CHECKLIST

Clinically Relevant Pathologic Features

- Rare tumor
- Limited collective experience with this entity

Pathologic Interpretation Pearls

- High index of suspicion required
- Distinction from epithelioid sarcoma requires immunohistochemistry
  - Strong membranous CD31 expression
    - Beware of entrapped CD31(+) histiocytes, which have more granular membranous staining pattern
  - Nuclear staining for FLI-1 helpful
  - Negative for CD34 to date

SELECTED REFERENCES

1. Watabe A et al: Epithelioid sarcoma-like haemangioendothelioma: a case report. Acta Derm Venereol. 89(2):208-9, 2009
2. Tokyol C et al: Epithelioid sarcoma-like hemangioendothelioma: a case report. Tumori. 91(5):436-9, 2005
3. Billings SD et al: Epithelioid sarcoma-like hemangioendothelioma. Am J Surg Pathol. 27(1):48-57, 2003
4. Mentzel T et al: Epithelioid hemangioendothelioma of skin and soft tissues: clinicopathologic and immunohistochemical study of 30 cases. Am J Surg Pathol. 21(4):363-74, 1997

IMAGE GALLERY

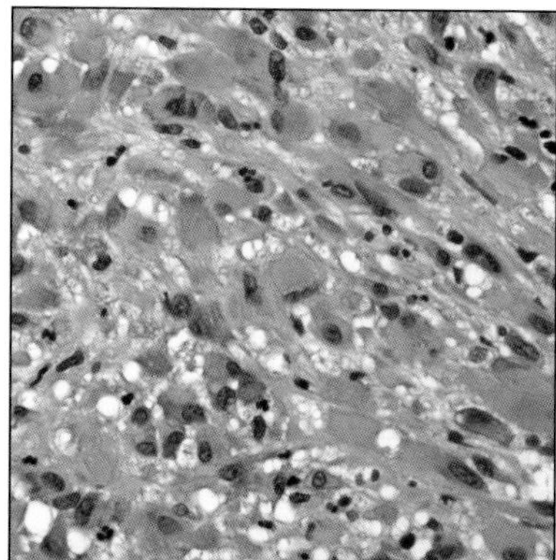

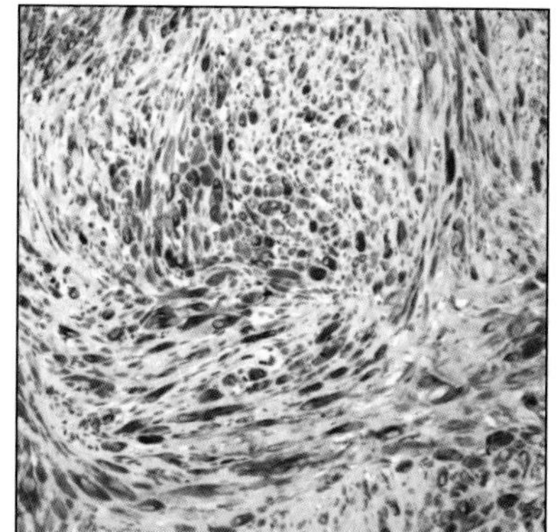

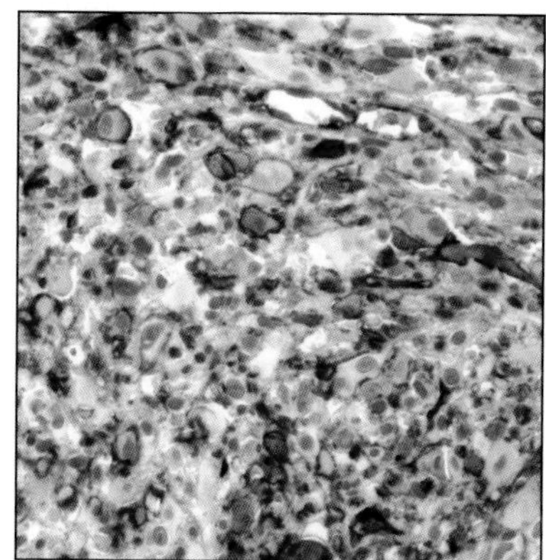

*(**Left**) Hematoxylin & eosin shows a high-power view of epithelioid tumor cells. The nuclei are large but not pleomorphic. (**Center**) Cytokeratin AE1/AE3 stain demonstrates diffuse staining throughout the tumor. (**Right**) CD31 stain demonstrates strong, linear membranous staining in the tumor cells.*

KAPOSI SARCOMA

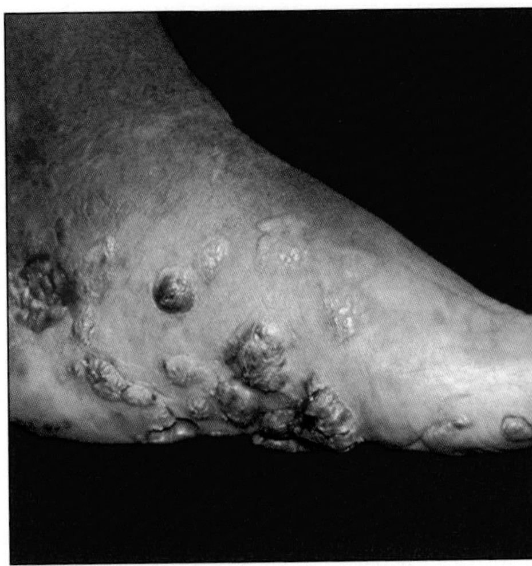

Clinical photograph shows a case of classical Kaposi sarcoma arising in an elderly man who presented with multiple nodular lesions.

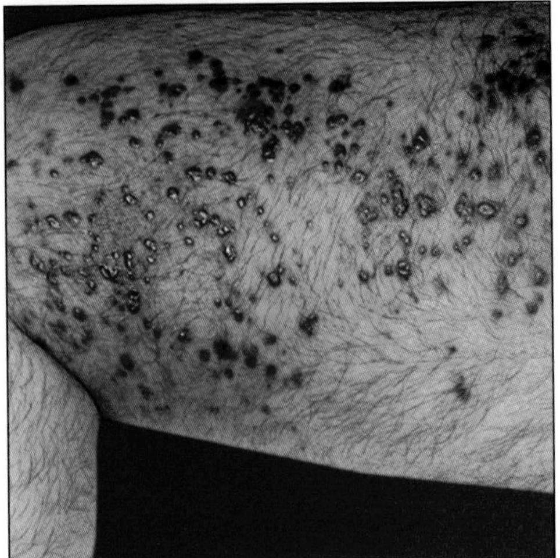

Clinical photograph shows an HIV-positive patient who developed multiple small lesions on the trunk and lower extremities.

TERMINOLOGY

Abbreviations

- Kaposi sarcoma (KS)

Definitions

- Locally aggressive endothelial neoplasm associated with human herpes virus 8 (HHV8)

ETIOLOGY/PATHOGENESIS

Infectious Agents

- Associated with HHV8
  - HHV8 is found in all forms of disease
  - HHV8 is detected in peripheral blood

CLINICAL ISSUES

Site

- Most typical site of involvement is skin
- Mucosal membranes, lymph nodes, and visceral organs may be affected

Natural History

- 4 main different clinical and epidemiologic forms are recognized
  - **Classical indolent form**
    - Occur predominantly in elderly men of Mediterranean/East European descent
    - Purplish, reddish-blue, dark brown plaques and nodules
    - Usually in distal extremities
  - **Endemic African form**
    - Occurs in middle-aged adults and children in equatorial Africa
    - Patients are not infected by HIV
  - **Iatrogenic form**
    - Occurs in patients treated by immunosuppressive agents
  - **AIDS-associated form**
    - Occurs in patients infected by HIV-1
    - Most aggressive form
    - Lesions are seen on face, genitals, lower extremities
    - Mucosal membranes, lymph nodes, and visceral organs are frequently involved

Treatment

- Options, risks, complications
  - Chemo- &/or radiotherapy
  - Cryotherapy may be useful
- Surgical approaches
  - Surgical treatment of single lesions only

Prognosis

- Classical indolent form
  - Indolent clinical course
  - Lymph node and visceral organ involvement occurs only infrequently
- Endemic African form
  - Protracted clinical course
  - Lymphadenopathic form is progressive and highly lethal
- Iatrogenic form
  - May resolve entirely after withdrawal of immunosuppressive treatment
- AIDS-associated form
  - Most aggressive type of KS
- Prognosis depends on epidemiological-clinical type of KS
- Prognosis is strongly related to stage of disease
- Prognosis is strongly related to additional infectious diseases

MACROSCOPIC FEATURES

General Features

- Skin lesions range in size from very small to several centimeters

KAPOSI SARCOMA

Key Facts

Terminology
- Locally aggressive endothelial neoplasm associated with human herpes virus 8

Clinical Issues
- Most typical site of involvement is skin
- Mucosal membranes, lymph nodes, and visceral organs may be affected
- 4 main different clinical and epidemiologic forms are recognized
  - Classical indolent form
  - Endemic African form
  - Iatrogenic form
  - AIDS-associated form
- Prognosis depends on epidemiological-clinical type

Macroscopic Features
- Skin lesions range in size from very small to several centimeters

Microscopic Pathology
- Histologic features of all forms of KS do not differ
- KS shows different stages of disease
- Patch stage of KS
  - Increased vascular spaces in reticular dermis
  - Scattered lymphocytes and plasma cells
- Plaque stage of KS
  - More extensive vascular proliferation
- Nodular stage of KS
  - Well-circumscribed, cellular nodules
  - Intersecting cellular fascicles of spindled tumor cells

- Hemorrhagic nodules of variable size in visceral organs and lymph nodes

MICROSCOPIC PATHOLOGY

Histologic Features
- Histologic features of all forms of KS do not differ
- KS shows different stages of disease
- **Patch stage of KS**
  - Increased vascular spaces in reticular dermis
    - Papillary dermis is not involved in early stages
  - Vascular spaces dissect collagen bundles
  - Perivascular and periadnexal growth of vascular spaces
  - Vascular spaces are lined by flat, uniform endothelial cells
  - Scattered lymphocytes and plasma cells
  - Extravasated erythrocytes and hemosiderin deposits
- **Plaque stage of KS**
  - More extensive vascular proliferation
  - Denser inflammatory infiltrate
  - Hyaline globules representing destroyed erythrocytes may be found
- **Nodular stage of KS**
  - Well-circumscribed, cellular nodules
  - Intersecting cellular fascicles of spindled tumor cells
  - Slit- and sieve-like spaces containing erythrocytes
  - Mild cytologic atypia
  - Numerous mitoses
- Some patients develop lymphangiomatous lesions &/ or hemangiomatous lesions

Cytologic Features
- Bland flat and spindled endothelial tumor cells

DIFFERENTIAL DIAGNOSIS

Hobnail Hemangioma
- Solitary vascular lesions
- Biphasic growth
  - Dilated vessels in superficial parts, narrow vascular spaces in deeper parts of dermis
- Hobnail endothelial cells
- HHV8(-)

Capillary Hemangioma
- Different clinical findings
- Lobular growth of narrow capillaries
- HHV8(-)

Lymphangioma
- Common pediatric lesions
- Rather well-circumscribed lesions
- Dilated vascular spaces
- Usually no inflammatory infiltrate
- HHV8(-)

Progressive Lymphangioma (Benign Lymphangioendothelioma)
- Slowly growing, solitary, plaque-like lesions
- No spindled tumor cells
- No prominent inflammatory infiltrate
- HHV8(-)

Spindle Cell Hemangioma
- Combination of KS-like features with cavernous hemangioma-like features
- No increased mitoses in spindled tumor cells
- Scattered epithelioid tumor cells
- HHV8(-)

Kaposiform Hemangioendothelioma
- Occurs usually in infants and young children
- Often in retroperitoneal and abdominal location
- Only rarely in skin of adult patients
- Infiltrative, cellular lobules
- No increased number of mitoses
- HHV8(-)

Cutaneous Angiosarcoma
- Different clinical findings
- Anastomosing vascular structures
- Prominent nuclear atypia

KAPOSI SARCOMA

Immunohistochemistry

Antibody	Reactivity	Staining Pattern	Comment
CD31	Positive	Cell membrane & cytoplasm	
CD34	Positive	Cell membrane & cytoplasm	
HHV8	Positive	Nuclear	
FLI-1	Positive	Nuclear	
Actin-sm	Negative		Only around larger, preexisting vessels

- Endothelial multilayering
- HHV8(-)

Microvenular Hemangioma

- Usually solitary vascular lesions
- Narrow vascular structures
- Dermal fibrosis
- Complete rim of actin(+) myopericytes
- HHV8(-)

Lymphangiomatosis (of the Limbs)

- Solitary, large, plaque-like lesions
- No increased number of mitoses
- No prominent inflammatory infiltrate
- HHV8(-)

Tufted Hemangioma

- Cannonball distribution of vascular tufts
- CD31(+) endothelial cells are completely surrounded by actin(+) myopericytes
- Crescent-shaped clefts
- HHV8(-)

DIAGNOSTIC CHECKLIST

Clinically Relevant Pathologic Features

- Age distribution
- Gross appearance
- Organ distribution

Pathologic Interpretation Pearls

- All clinical forms of KS follow similar morphologic stages
- Dissecting narrow vascular spaces, inflammatory cells, and hemosiderin deposits are useful findings in early stages of KS
- HHV8 immunohistochemical antibodies represent specific and sensitive marker for KS

SELECTED REFERENCES

1. Sharma-Walia N et al: Kaposi's sarcoma associated herpes virus (KSHV) induced COX-2: a key factor in latency, inflammation, angiogenesis, cell survival and invasion. PLoS Pathog. 6(2):e1000777, 2010
2. O'Hara CD et al: Endothelial lesions of soft tissues: a review of reactive and neoplastic entities with emphasis on low-grade malignant ("borderline") vascular tumors. Adv Anat Pathol. 10(2):69-87, 2003
3. Folpe AL et al: Expression of Fli-1, a nuclear transcription factor, distinguishes vascular neoplasms from potential mimics. Am J Surg Pathol. 25(8):1061-6, 2001
4. Goedert JJ: The epidemiology of acquired immunodeficiency syndrome malignancies. Semin Oncol. 27(4):390-401, 2000
5. Guillou L et al: Benign lymphangioendothelioma (acquired progressive lymphangioma): a lesion not to be confused with well-differentiated angiosarcoma and patch stage Kaposi's sarcoma: clinicopathologic analysis of a series. Am J Surg Pathol. 24(8):1047-57, 2000
6. Reed JA et al: Demonstration of Kaposi's sarcoma-associated herpes virus cyclin D homolog in cutaneous Kaposi's sarcoma by colorimetric in situ hybridization using a catalyzed signal amplification system. Blood. 91(10):3825-32, 1998
7. Borroni G et al: Bullous lesions in Kaposi's sarcoma: case report. Am J Dermatopathol. 19(4):379-83, 1997
8. Cossu S et al: Lymphangioma-like variant of Kaposi's sarcoma: clinicopathologic study of seven cases with review of the literature. Am J Dermatopathol. 19(1):16-22, 1997
9. Perniciaro C et al: Familial Kaposi's sarcoma. Cutis. 57(4):220-2, 1996
10. Ioachim HL et al: Kaposi's sarcoma of internal organs. A multiparameter study of 86 cases. Cancer. 75(6):1376-85, 1995
11. Ioachim HL et al: Kaposi's sarcoma of internal organs. A multiparameter study of 86 cases. Cancer. 75(6):1376-85, 1995
12. Chang Y et al: Identification of herpesvirus-like DNA sequences in AIDS-associated Kaposi's sarcoma. Science. 266(5192):1865-9, 1994
13. Tappero JW et al: Kaposi's sarcoma. Epidemiology, pathogenesis, histology, clinical spectrum, staging criteria and therapy. J Am Acad Dermatol. 28(3):371-95, 1993
14. Nickoloff BJ: The human progenitor cell antigen (CD34) is localized on endothelial cells, dermal dendritic cells, and perifollicular cells in formalin-fixed normal skin, and on proliferating endothelial cells and stromal spindle-shaped cells in Kaposi's sarcoma. Arch Dermatol. 127(4):523-9, 1991
15. Kao GF et al: The nature of hyaline (eosinophilic) globules and vascular slits of Kaposi's sarcoma. Am J Dermatopathol. 12(3):256-67, 1990
16. Dictor M: Kaposi's sarcoma. Origin and significance of lymphaticovenous connections. Virchows Arch A Pathol Anat Histopathol. 409(1):23-35, 1986

KAPOSI SARCOMA

Clinical and Microscopic Features

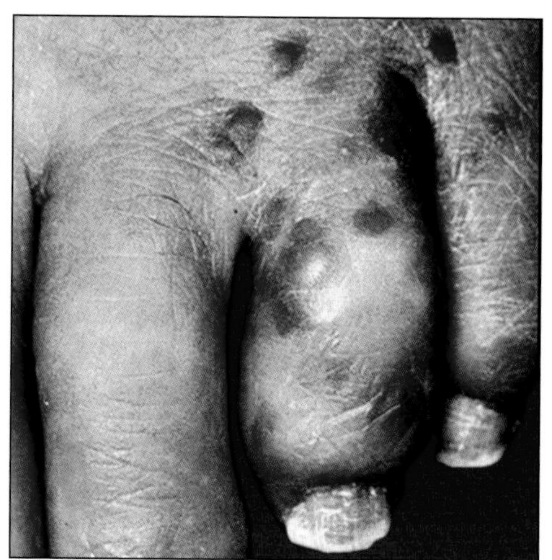

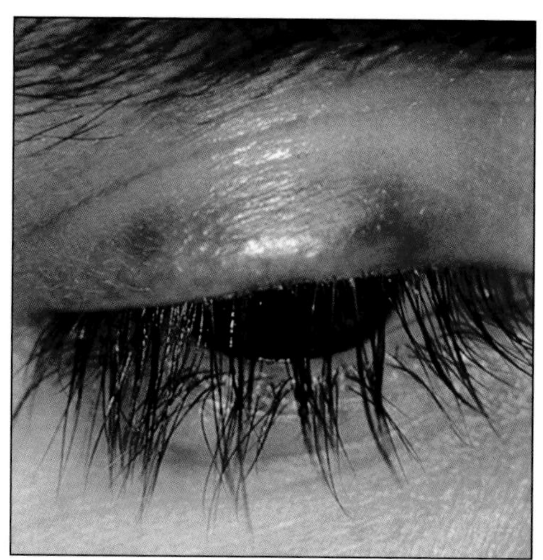

(Left) *Early forms of Kaposi sarcoma may cause diagnostic problems. This elderly patient developed multiple small lesions on the toe. Small, slightly elevated, relatively circumscribed brown papules are noted.* ***(Right)*** *Patients with AIDS-related Kaposi sarcoma may present with lesions at unusual anatomic sites, as did this young patient who developed small reddish lesions on his upper eyelid.*

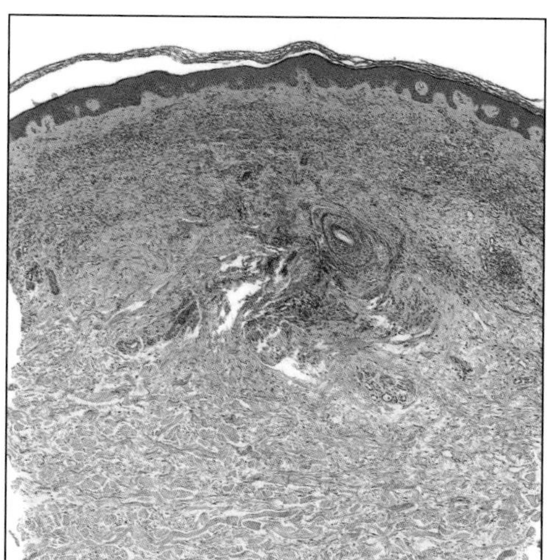

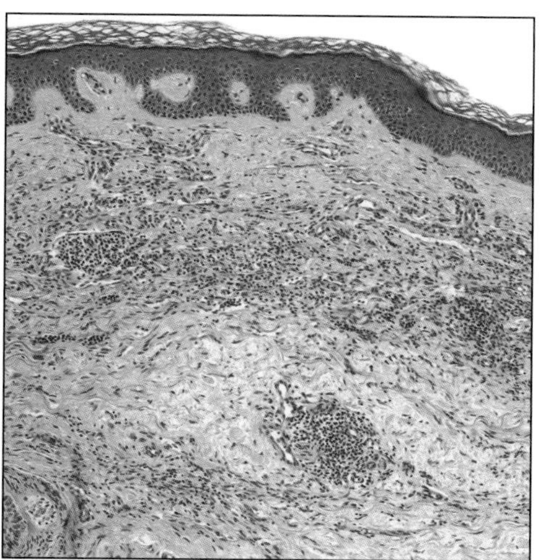

(Left) *In early lesions of Kaposi sarcoma flat, plaque-like lesions are seen. Note that the upper part of the papillary dermis is not involved, which represents an important finding to differentiate from other vascular lesions.* ***(Right)*** *Early lesions of Kaposi sarcoma show a proliferation of thin-walled vessels associated with scattered spindle cell and numerous inflammatory cells.*

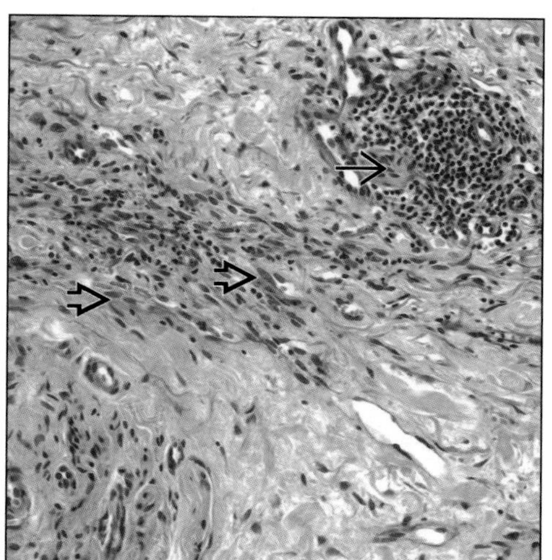

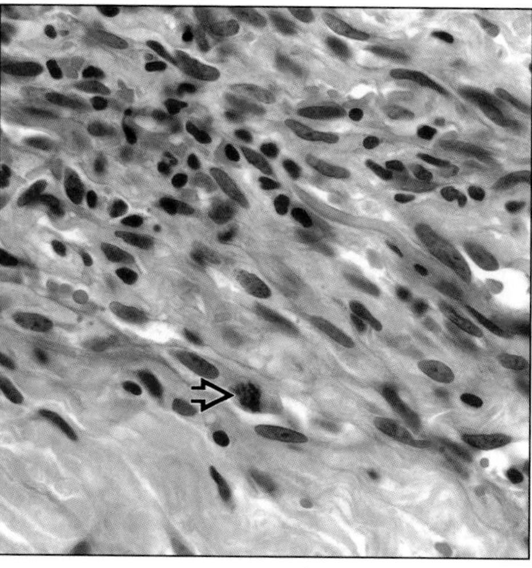

(Left) *Dissecting spindle cells ⇨ are associated with numerous inflammatory cells that are arranged in small clusters → or diffusely between the proliferating spindled cells.* ***(Right)*** *At higher power, narrow vascular spaces and cytologically bland spindled cells are seen. Note the presence of inflammatory cells and scattered mitoses ⇨ of the spindled tumor cells.*

KAPOSI SARCOMA

Microscopic Features and Ancillary Techniques

*(**Left**) The inflammatory infiltrate in Kaposi sarcoma usually contains a number of plasma cells ⇨. In addition, narrow vascular spaces and scattered spindled cells are present. (**Right**) Especially in early lesions of Kaposi sarcoma, the nuclear staining of endothelial cells for HHV8 is very helpful for making the correct diagnosis.*

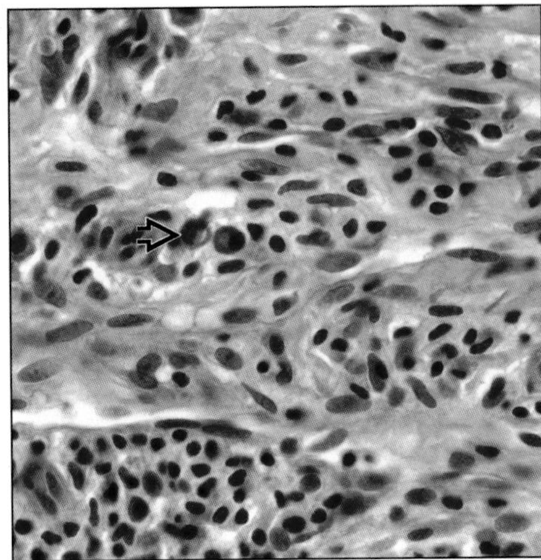

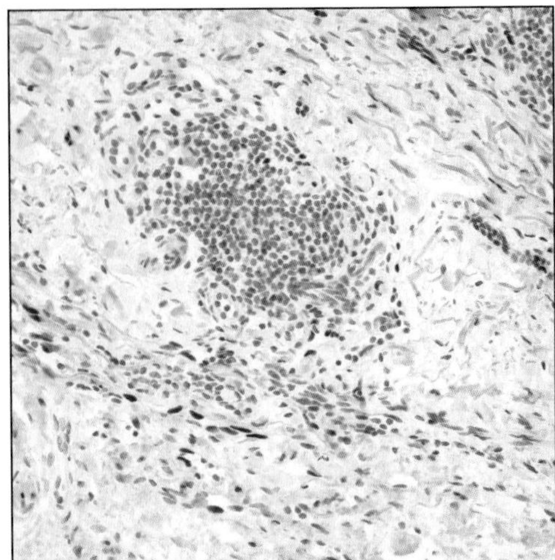

*(**Left**) A very early form of Kaposi sarcoma shows scattered spindled cells, dilated and narrow vascular spaces, as well as few inflammatory cells set in a slightly fibrosed dermal tissue. (**Right**) Iron stainings reveal abundant hemosiderin deposits, which represents an important finding in early forms of Kaposi sarcoma.*

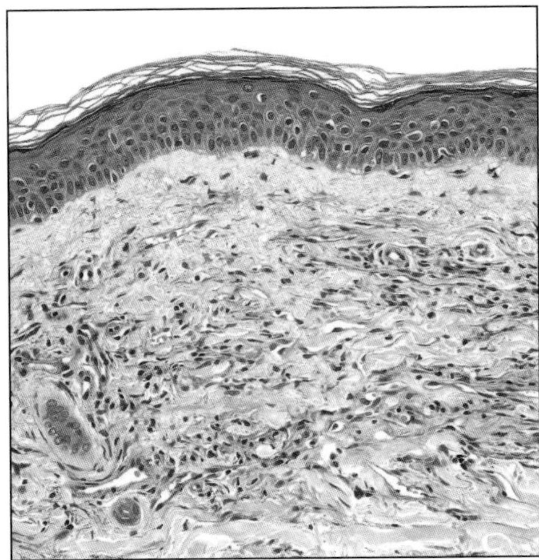

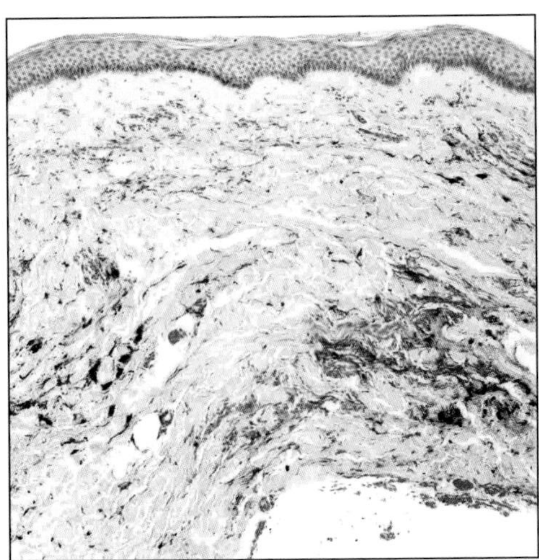

*(**Left**) An exophytic, ulcerated, and cellular lesion arising in the foot of an elderly male patient is noted in this nodular stage Kaposi sarcoma. (**Right**) Higher power views reveals cellular bundles and fascicles of spindle cells, as well as slit- and sieve-like vascular spaces containing numerous erythrocytes.*

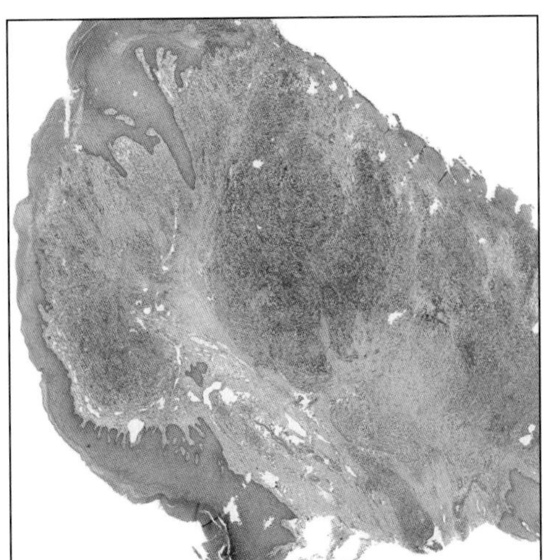

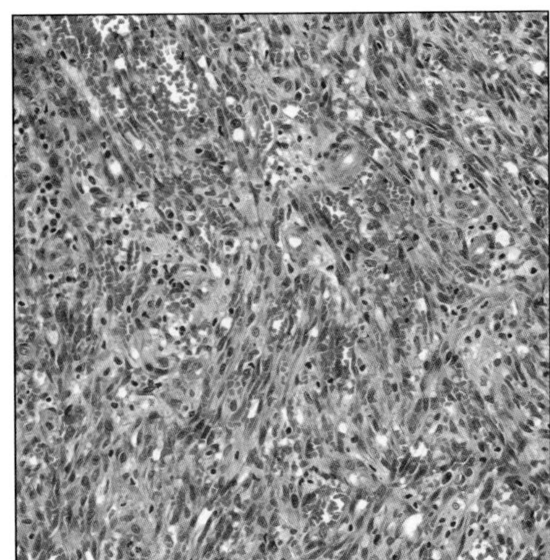

Microscopic and Immunohistochemical Features

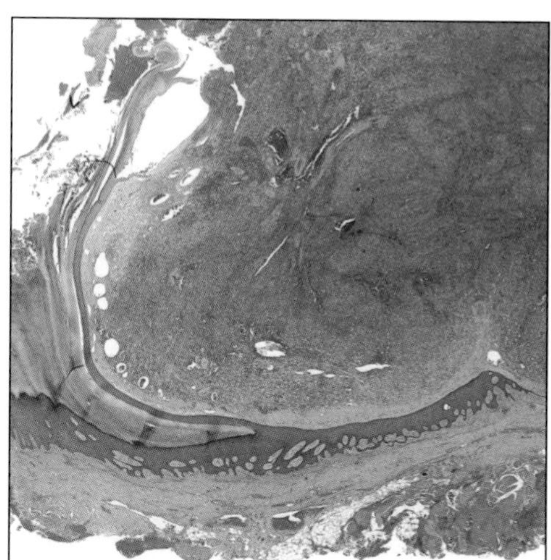

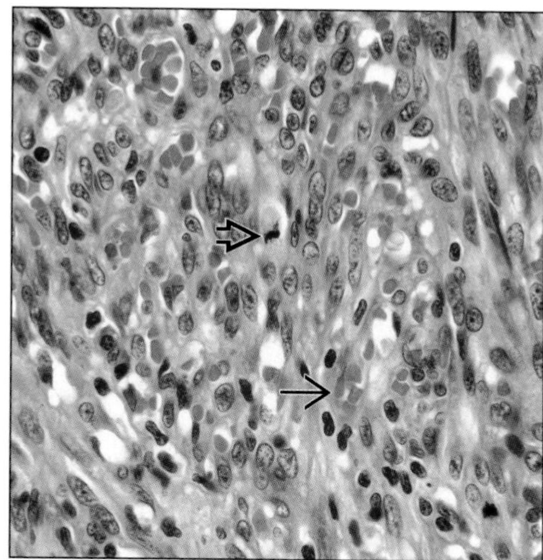

(Left) *Low-power view of nodular stage of Kaposi sarcoma shows a well-circumscribed exophytic nodular lesion with ulceration of the epidermis.* ***(Right)*** *High-power view shows cytologically bland spindled tumor cells containing uniform spindled nuclei. Despite the lack of atypia, mitoses are easily found ⇨. Small sieve-like spaces that contain erythrocytes → are seen between the spindled cells.*

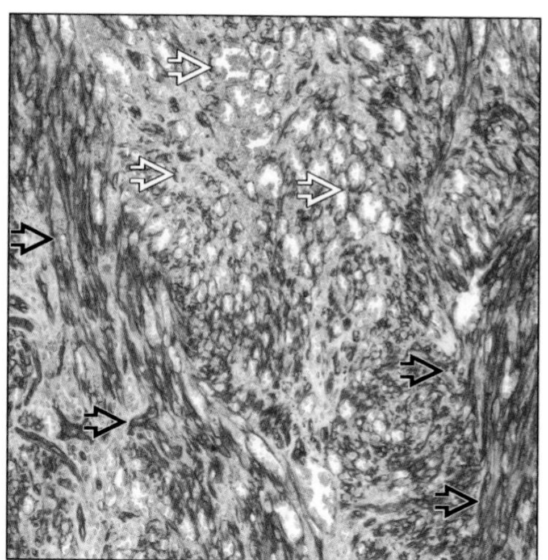

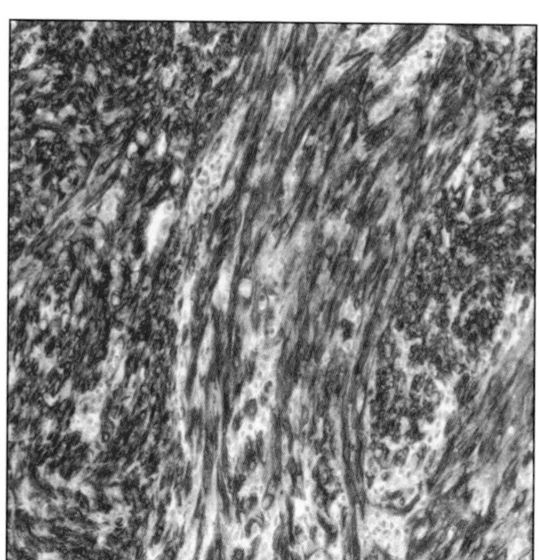

(Left) *Tumor cells stain positively for the endothelial marker CD31. In addition to cellular spindle cell fascicles ⇨, small vascular spaces lined by CD31(+) endothelial cells are noted ⇨.* ***(Right)*** *A homogeneous expression of CD34 by neoplastic cells is seen in this example of nodular Kaposi sarcoma.*

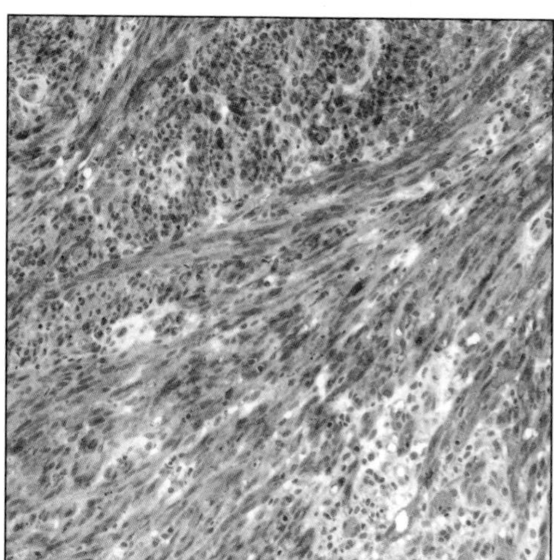

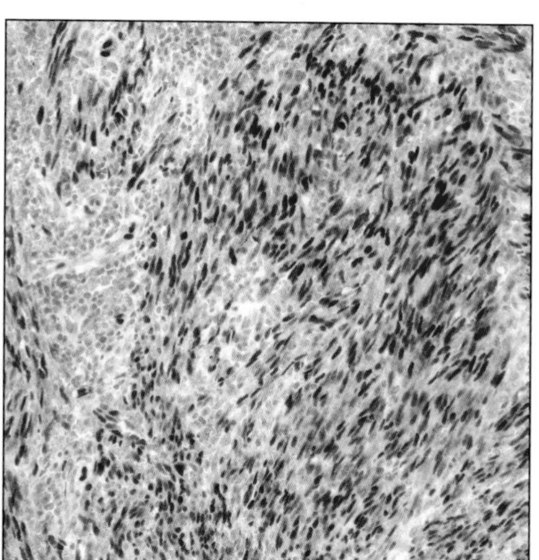

(Left) *Expression of podoplanin by neoplastic cells is usually seen in cases of Kaposi sarcoma and can be shown by immunohistochemistry using antibody D2-40.* ***(Right)*** *The nuclear staining of tumor cells for HHV8 as shown here is diagnostic for Kaposi sarcoma.*

KAPOSI SARCOMA

Microscopic and Immunohistochemical Features

*(**Left**) Low-power view shows an inguinal lymph node infiltrated by a cellular spindle cell neoplasm in this 65-year-old male patient with known Kaposi sarcoma who developed a nodular lesion in his groin. (**Right**) The neoplasm is composed of cellular fascicles of spindled cells, and numerous erythrocytes are seen.*

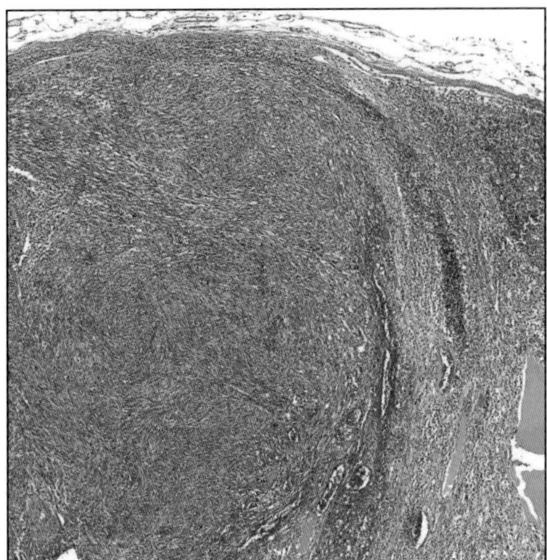

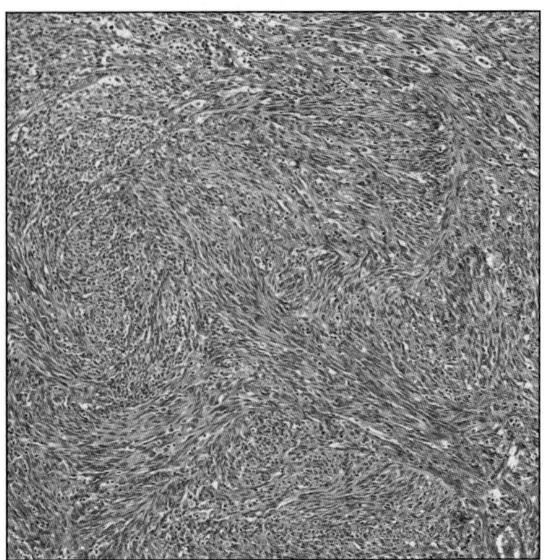

*(**Left**) High-power view shows cytologically bland spindled cells and scattered inflammatory cells. Note the focal deposits of hemosiderin pigment ➡. (**Right**) Ki-67 immunostaining reveals increased proliferative activity of the spindled cells in this intranodal neoplasm.*

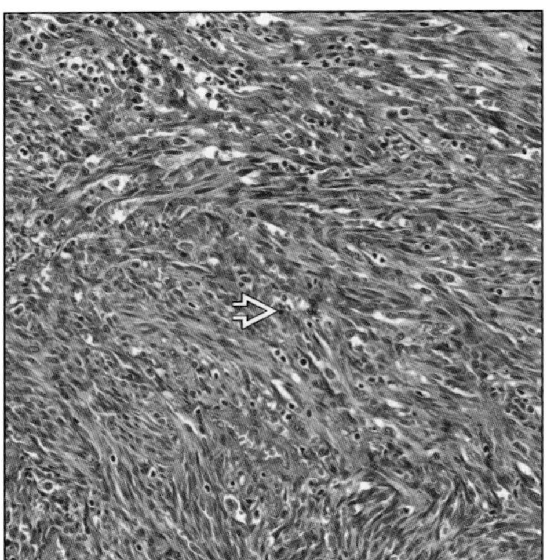

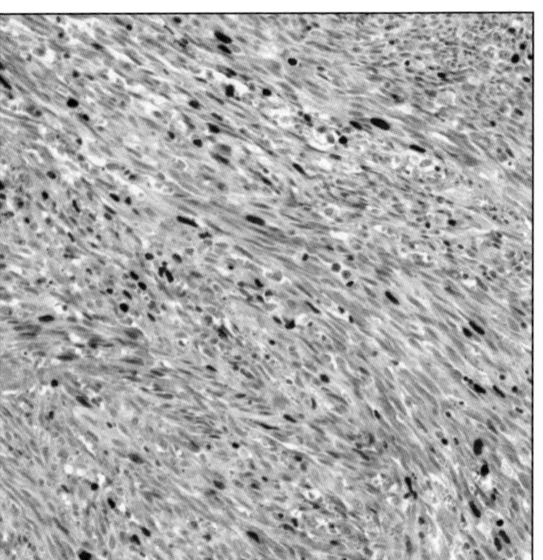

*(**Left**) Neoplastic spindled cells stain positively for CD34. (**Right**) A homogeneous expression of HHV8 by neoplastic spindled cells is diagnostic in this case of intranodal Kaposi sarcoma.*

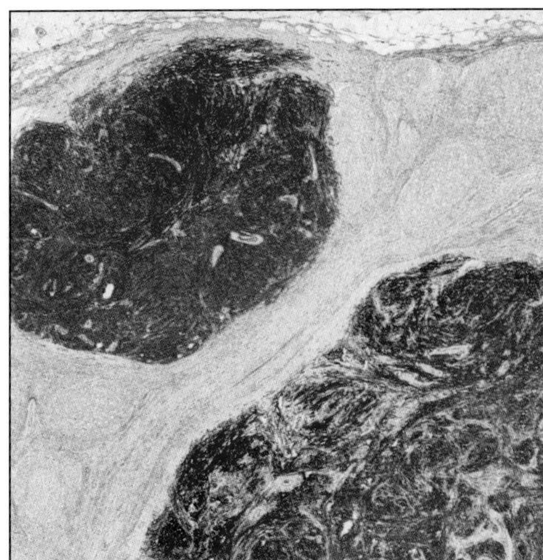

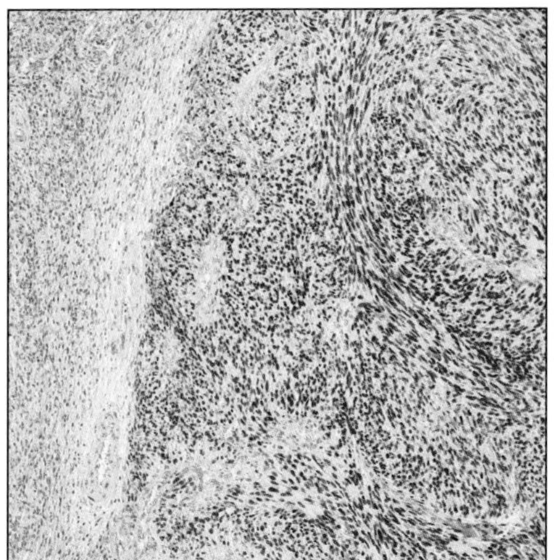

Clinical and Variant Microscopic Features

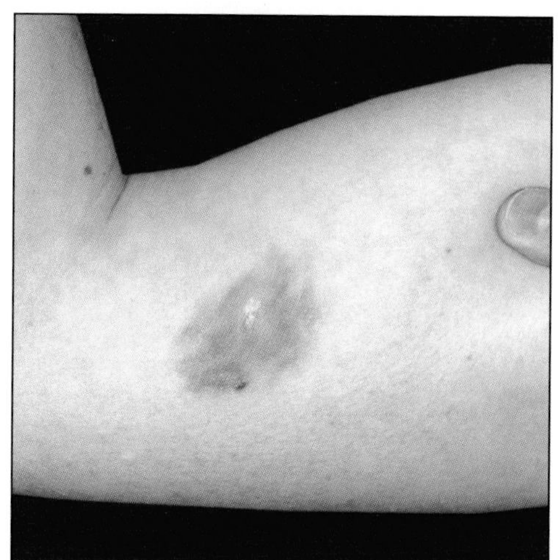

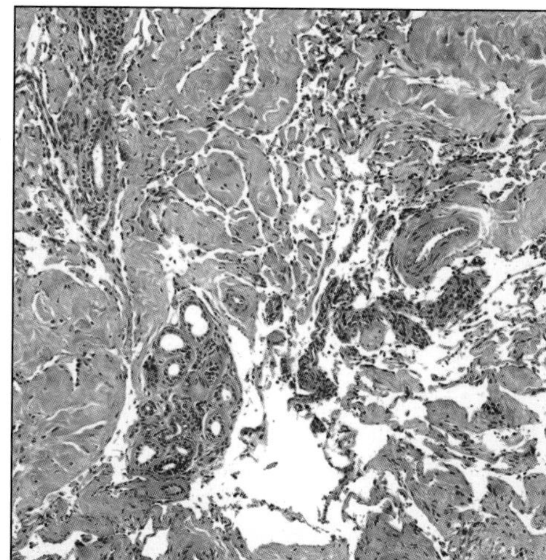

(Left) *A 30-year-old male patient presented with an irregularly shaped, slightly painful lesion on his right upper arm.* ***(Right)*** *Histologically, a lymphangioendothelioma-like lesion composed of narrow and dilated lymphatic-like vascular structures growing around adnexal structures was seen.*

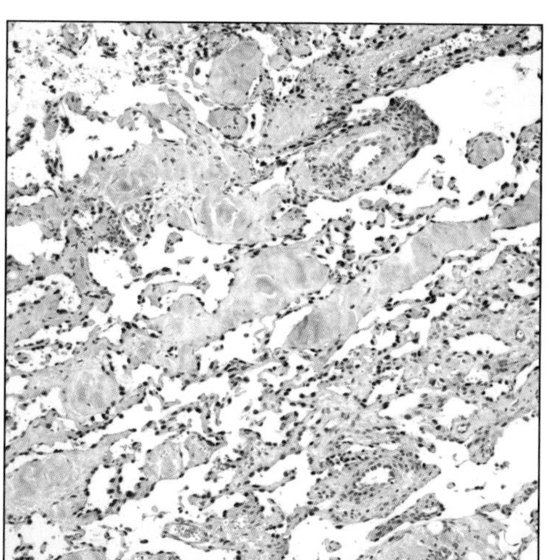

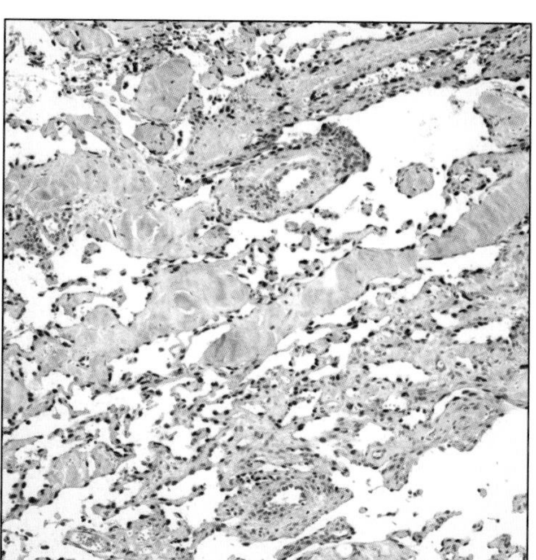

(Left) *The endothelial cells of this lymphangioendothelioma-like lesion stained positively with the lymphatic marker podoplanin.* ***(Right)*** *In addition, a homogeneous and diagnostic nuclear expression of HHV8 by endothelial cells was noted, and the final diagnosis of a lymphangioendothelioma-like Kaposi sarcoma was established.*

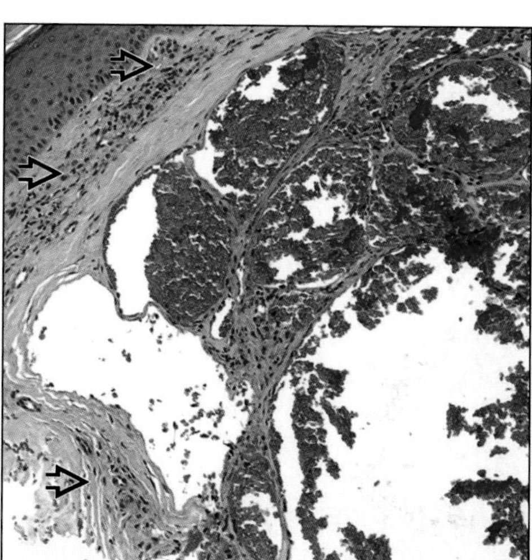

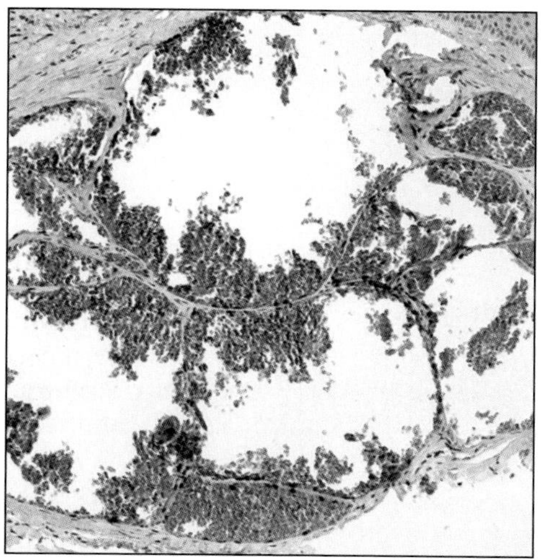

(Left) *An elderly male patient presented with a bluish dermal nodule. Histologically, a cavernous hemangioma-like vascular lesion was seen. Note the scattered inflammatory cells ➲.* ***(Right)*** *With immunohistochemistry, the endothelial cells stained positively for HHV8, and the lesion was diagnosed as a rare hemangioma-like Kaposi sarcoma.*

EPITHELIOID HEMANGIOENDOTHELIOMA

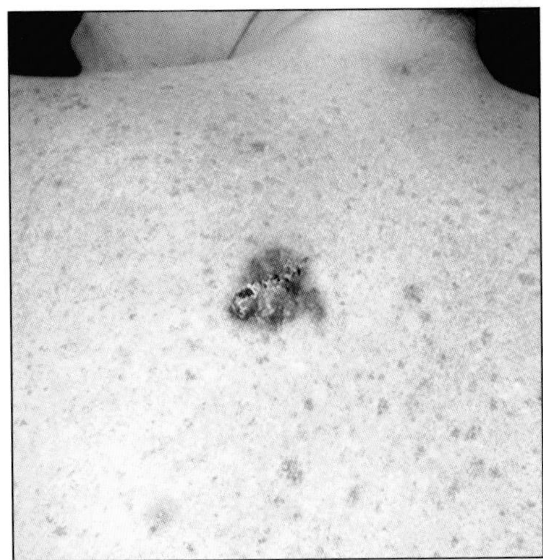

Clinical photograph shows a rare cutaneous epithelioid hemangioendothelioma presenting as an exophytic lesion.

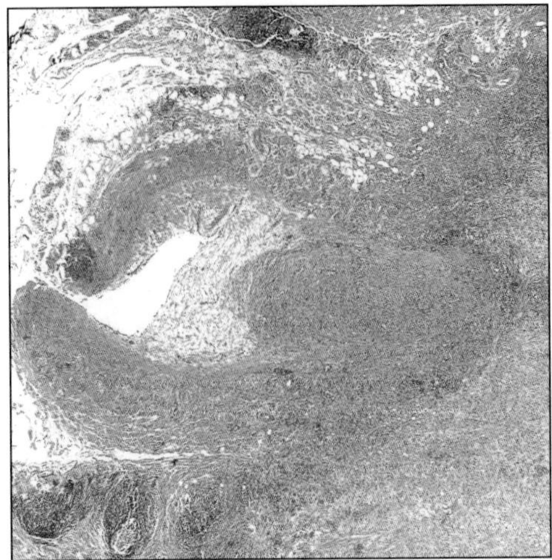

Hematoxylin & eosin shows an epithelioid hemangioendothelioma arising in deep soft tissue as an ill-defined angiocentric neoplasm.

TERMINOLOGY

Abbreviations

- Epithelioid hemangioendothelioma (EHE)

Synonyms

- Intravascular bronchioloalveolar tumor
- Angioglomoid tumor

Definitions

- Angiocentric vascular neoplasm with metastatic potential composed of epithelioid endothelial cells

CLINICAL ISSUES

Epidemiology

- Incidence
  - Rare vascular tumor
- Age
  - All age groups
  - Rare in childhood
- Gender
  - M = F

Site

- Superficial or deep soft tissue
- Extremities
- Head & neck region
- Rare in skin
- Visceral organs (often multicentric)

Presentation

- Painful mass
- Solitary mass
- Multicentric in a number of cases
- Edema
  - May be present
- Occlusion of vessels
  - 1/2 of cases arise in/are associated with preexisting vessels
  - May cause more profound symptoms

Treatment

- Surgical approaches
  - Wide local excision with clear margins
- Adjuvant therapy
  - No adjuvant chemo-/radiotherapy

Prognosis

- Intermediate behavior between hemangioma and angiosarcoma
- Local recurrence rate (10-15%)
- Metastatic rate (20-30%)
- Mortality (10-20%)
- Better prognosis in superficial cases
- Adverse prognostic factors
  - > 3 mitoses per 50 high-power fields
  - Tumor size > 3 cm

IMAGE FINDINGS

General Features

- Best diagnostic clue
  - May show calcifications
- Location
  - Soft tissue of extremities

MACROSCOPIC FEATURES

General Features

- Well-circumscribed nodular lesion
- Fusiform intravascular mass resembling organizing thrombus

MICROSCOPIC PATHOLOGY

Histologic Features

- Expansion of vessels in angiocentric cases
- Centrifugal extension into soft tissues

EPITHELIOID HEMANGIOENDOTHELIOMA

Key Facts

Terminology

- Vascular neoplasm with metastatic potential composed of epithelioid endothelial cells

Clinical Issues

- Rare vascular tumor
- Superficial or deep soft tissue
  - Rare in skin
- ~ 50% associated with preexisting vessel
- Behavior intermediate between hemangioma and angiosarcoma
  - Metastatic rate (20-30%)
  - Mortality (10-20%)
- Painful mass
- All age groups
- Wide local excision with clear margins
- Adverse prognostic factors
  - > 3 mitoses per 50 high-power fields
  - Tumor size > 3 cm

Macroscopic Features

- Well-circumscribed nodular lesion

Microscopic Pathology

- Rare obvious vascular channels
- Short strands, cords, solid nests, or single cells
- Bland, epithelioid, round or slightly spindled endothelial cells
- Intracytoplasmic lumina
- Myxohyaline, chondroid-like stroma
- Expression of endothelial markers
  - CD31, CD34, FLI-1

- Rare obvious vascular channels
- Short strands, cords, solid nests, single cells
- Round to slightly spindled endothelial tumor cells
- Eosinophilic cytoplasm
- Vesicular nuclei
- Small nucleoli
- Intracytoplasmic vacuoles
  - Represent miniature endothelial lumina
  - May contain erythrocytes
- Bland epithelioid tumor cells
- Rare mitoses
- Myxohyaline stroma
- Chondroid stroma
- Metaplastic calcification &/or ossification in ~ 10% of cases
- Stroma contains sulfated acid mucopolysaccharides
- Atypical features in ~ 1/3 of cases
  - Increased cellularity
  - Solid nests
  - Marked nuclear atypia
  - Enlarged nuclei
  - Prominent nucleoli
  - Mitoses
  - Spindling of tumor cells
  - Necrosis

Predominant Pattern/Injury Type

- Angiocentric
- Ill defined

Predominant Cell/Compartment Type

- Epithelioid

ANCILLARY TESTS

Cytogenetics

- Translocation t(1;3)(p36.3;q25) in some

Electron Microscopy

- Immature cell junctions, abundant intermediate filaments
- Weibel-Palade bodies, intracytoplasmic lumen formation

DIFFERENTIAL DIAGNOSIS

Epithelioid Hemangioma

- Lobular architecture
- Well-formed vascular channels
- Complete rim of actin(+) (myo)pericytes
- Mixed inflammatory infiltrate with eosinophils

Chondroid Lipoma

- Lobular lesion
- Often encapsulated
- Lipogenic component (adipocytes, lipoblasts)
- Eosinophilic tumor cells
- No expression of endothelial immunohistochemical markers

Myoepithelioma

- Epithelial differentiation (ducts, cysts, squamous differentiation, apocrine differentiation)
- No angiocentric growth
- S100 protein expression in most cases
- No expression of endothelial immunohistochemical markers

Metastatic Carcinoma

- Clinical findings
- Higher degree of atypia
- Homogeneous expression of epithelial immunohistochemical markers
- Endothelial immunohistochemical markers negative

Epithelioid Sarcoma

- Distal extremities
- Young patients
- May show granuloma-like growth pattern
- Nodules of round eosinophilic tumor cells surrounding necrotic debris
- Homogeneous expression of pancytokeratin and EMA
- No expression of CD31

EPITHELIOID HEMANGIOENDOTHELIOMA

Immunohistochemistry

Antibody	Reactivity	Staining Pattern	Comment
CD31	Positive	Cell membrane & cytoplasm	
CD34	Positive	Cell membrane & cytoplasm	Not specific
FLI-1	Positive	Nuclear	
Podoplanin	Positive	Cytoplasmic	In ~ 20%
CK-PAN	Positive	Cytoplasmic	In ~ 20-25%
Actin-sm	Positive	Cytoplasmic	In ~ 20-25%
S100P	Negative		
Desmin	Negative		
CD117	Negative		
EMA	Equivocal	Cell membrane & cytoplasm	In ~ 10%

- Loss of expression of INI1

Extraskeletal Myxoid Chondrosarcoma

- Well-demarcated neoplasm
- Often presence of a fibrous pseudocapsule
- Gelatinous nodules separated by fibrous septa
- Eosinophilic tumor cells with uniform nuclei
- Hypovascular stroma
- No expression of endothelial immunohistochemical markers
- Translocations (9;22)(q22;q12) or (9;17)(q22;q11) in most cases

Myxoid/Round Cell Liposarcoma

- Small undifferentiated mesenchymal tumor cells
- Univacuolated lipoblasts
- Characteristic thin-walled, branching vessels
- Mucin pooling
- Translocation (12;16)(q13;p11) in > 90%

Epithelioid Angiosarcoma

- Sheets of atypical endothelial tumor cells
- Irregular infiltrating vascular channels
- Increasing cellularity
- Increasing atypia
- Increasing mitoses
- Frequent tumor necrosis

DIAGNOSTIC CHECKLIST

Clinically Relevant Pathologic Features

- Painful mass

Pathologic Interpretation Pearls

- Often arises from preexisting vessel
- Bland epithelioid endothelial cells
- Intracytoplasmic vacuoles
- Myxohyaline, chondroid stroma
- Expression of endothelial immunohistochemical markers

SELECTED REFERENCES

1. Clarke LE et al: Cutaneous epithelioid hemangioendothelioma. J Cutan Pathol. 35(2):236-40, 2008
2. Deyrup AT et al: Epithelioid hemangioendothelioma of soft tissue: a proposal for risk stratification based on 49 cases. Am J Surg Pathol. 32(6):924-7, 2008
3. Egberts F et al: Metastasizing epithelioid hemangioendothelioma of the nose in childhood. J Cutan Pathol. 35 Suppl 1:80-2, 2008
4. Celikel C et al: Epithelioid hemangioendothelioma with multiple organ involvement. APMIS. 115(7):881-8, 2007
5. Bagan P et al: Prognostic factors and surgical indications of pulmonary epithelioid hemangioendothelioma: a review of the literature. Ann Thorac Surg. 82(6):2010-3, 2006
6. Tsarouha H et al: Chromosome analysis and molecular cytogenetic investigations of an epithelioid hemangioendothelioma. Cancer Genet Cytogenet. 169(2):164-8, 2006
7. Leowardi C et al: Malignant vascular tumors: clinical presentation, surgical therapy, and long-term prognosis. Ann Surg Oncol. 12(12):1090-101, 2005
8. Tsuji M et al: Epithelioid hemangioendothelioma with osteoclast-like giant cells. Pathol Res Pract. 198(7):501-5, 2002
9. Mendlick MR et al: Translocation t(1;3)(p36.3;q25) is a nonrandom aberration in epithelioid hemangioendothelioma. Am J Surg Pathol. 25(5):684-7, 2001
10. Quante M et al: Epithelioid hemangioendothelioma presenting in the skin: a clinicopathologic study of eight cases. Am J Dermatopathol. 20(6):541-6, 1998
11. Mentzel T et al: Epithelioid hemangioendothelioma of skin and soft tissues: clinicopathologic and immunohistochemical study of 30 cases. Am J Surg Pathol. 21(4):363-74, 1997
12. Tsang WY et al: The family of epithelioid vascular tumors. Histol Histopathol. 8(1):187-212, 1993
13. Gray MH et al: Cytokeratin expression in epithelioid vascular neoplasms. Hum Pathol. 21(2):212-7, 1990
14. Ellis GL et al: Epithelioid hemangioendothelioma of the head and neck: a clinicopathologic report of twelve cases. Oral Surg Oral Med Oral Pathol. 61(1):61-8, 1986
15. Weiss SW et al: Epithelioid hemangioendothelioma: a vascular tumor often mistaken for a carcinoma. Cancer. 50(5):970-81, 1982

Microscopic Features

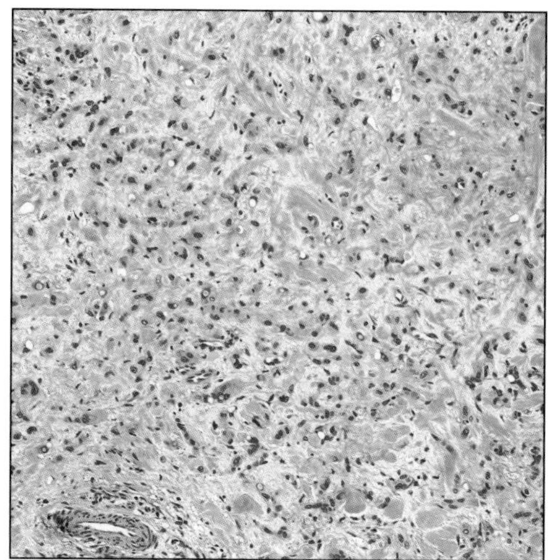

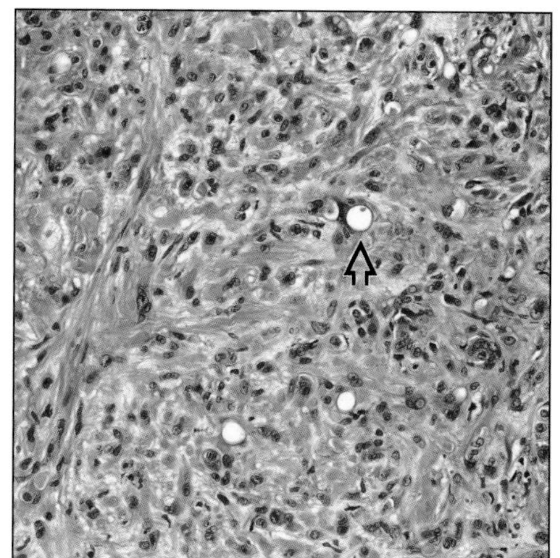

(Left) *Hematoxylin & eosin shows strands, clusters, and single epithelioid tumor cells.* ***(Right)*** *Hematoxylin & eosin shows relatively bland epithelioid tumor cells. Note the scattered cells containing cytoplasmic vacuoles* ➩.

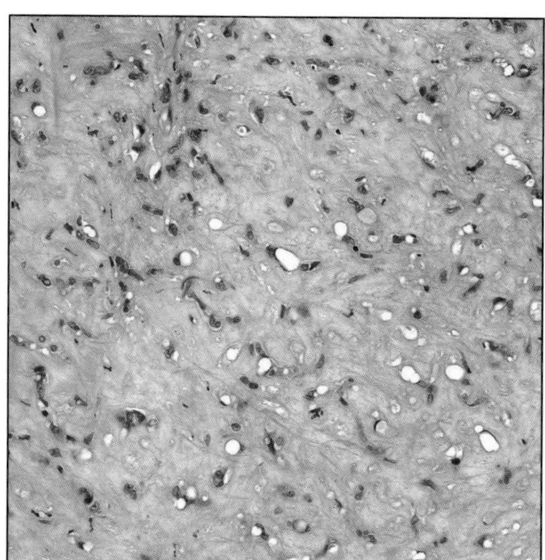

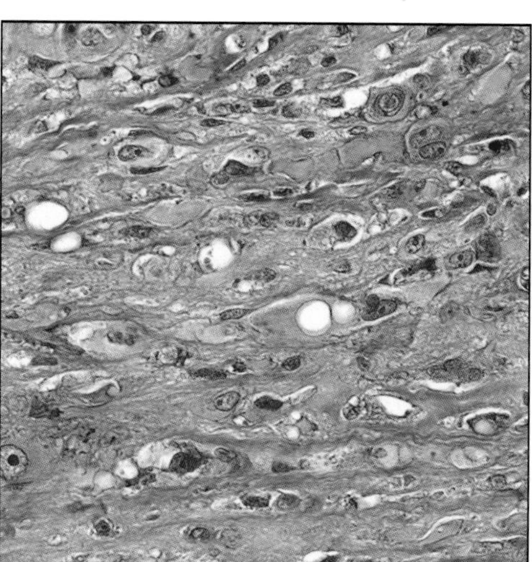

(Left) *Hematoxylin & eosin shows vacuolated epithelioid tumor cells dispersed within a myxohyaline stroma.* ***(Right)*** *Alcian blue staining highlights the prominent myxoid stroma. Note tumor cells with cytoplasmic vacuoles, a typical finding in epithelioid hemangioendothelioma.*

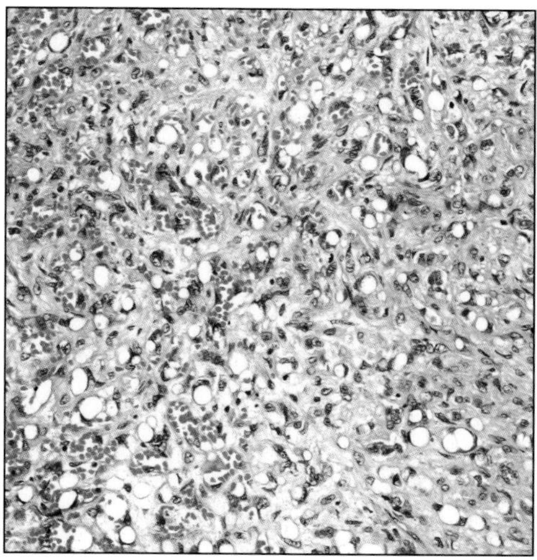

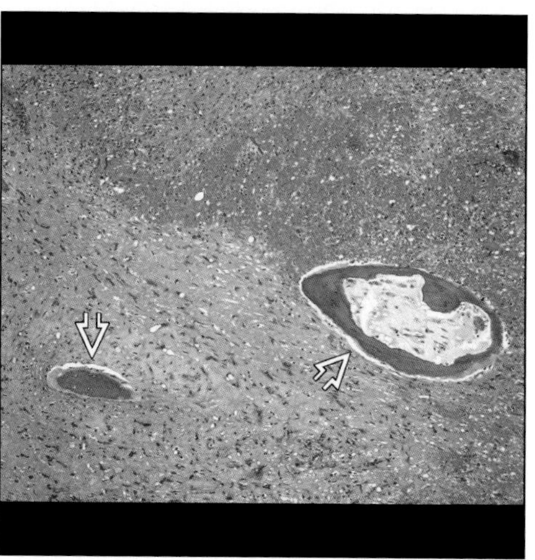

(Left) *Hematoxylin & eosin shows numerous vacuolated tumor cells mimicking lipoblasts.* ***(Right)*** *Hematoxylin & eosin shows focal metaplastic ossification* ➩.

EPITHELIOID HEMANGIOENDOTHELIOMA

Clinical and Microscopic Features

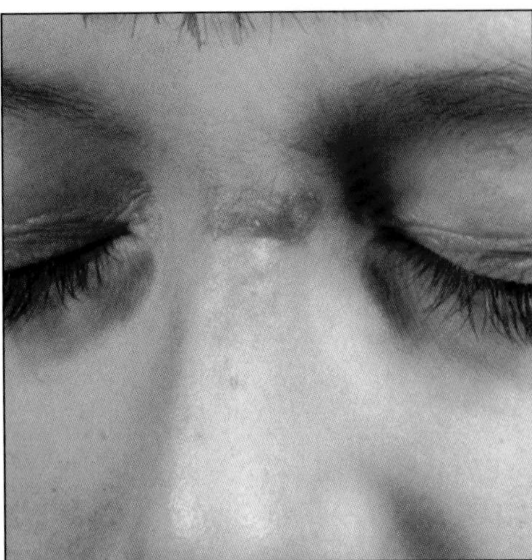

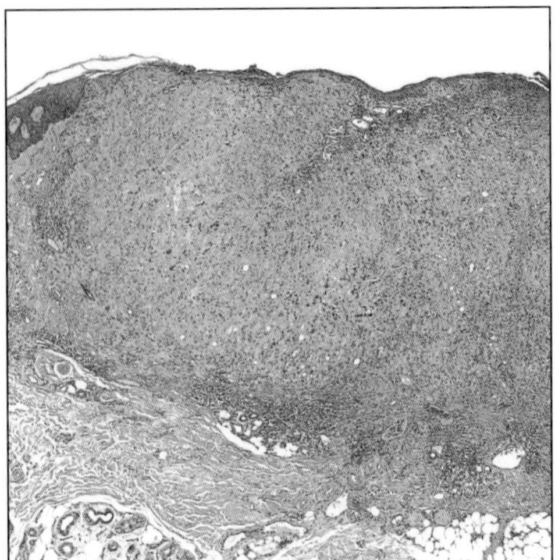

(Left) *Clinical photograph shows a flat dermal/ subcutaneous neoplasm that represents a metastasizing epithelioid hemangioendothelioma arising in a young boy.* ***(Right)*** *Hematoxylin & eosin shows epithelioid hemangioendothelioma in the dermis. Note the surface ulceration and inflammatory infiltrate at demarcated lower border.*

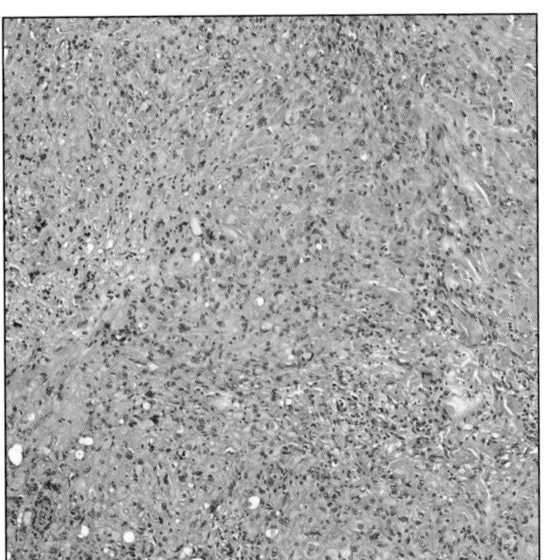

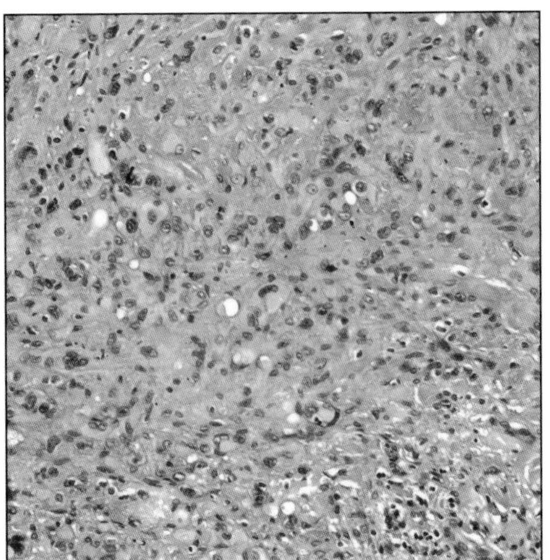

(Left) *Hematoxylin & eosin shows a sheet of epithelioid tumor cells in the dermis.* ***(Right)*** *Hematoxylin & eosin shows focal myxohyaline stroma in this dermal lesion. Note the scattered cytoplasmic vacuoles, imparting a characteristic low-power appearance.*

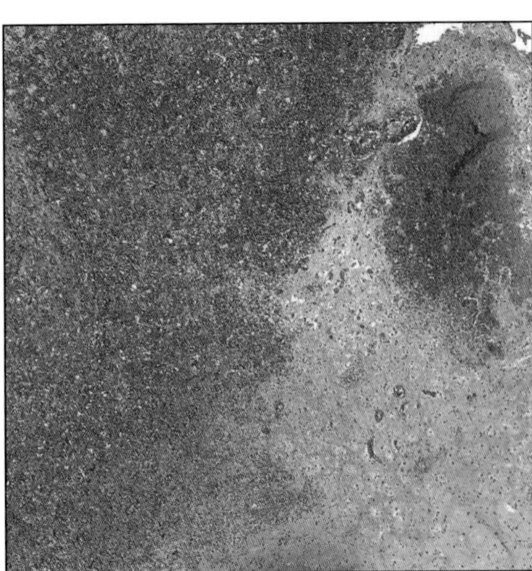

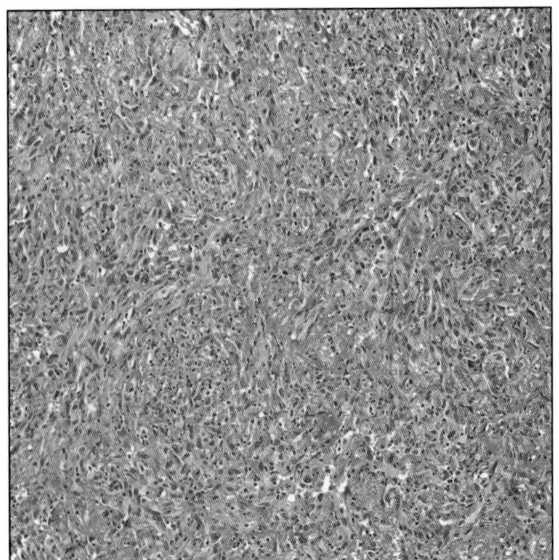

(Left) *Hematoxylin & eosin shows a case of epithelioid hemangioendothelioma arising in the brain. Note the presence of hemorrhage.* ***(Right)*** *Hematoxylin & eosin shows higher magnification of intracerebral epithelioid hemangioendothelioma. Note the marked cellularity.*

Microscopic and Immunohistochemical Features

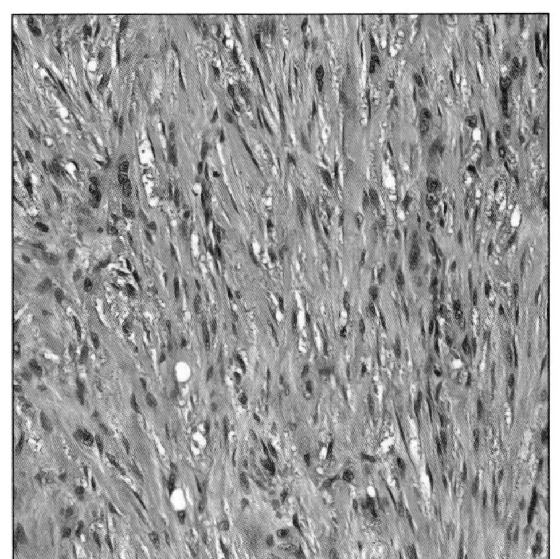

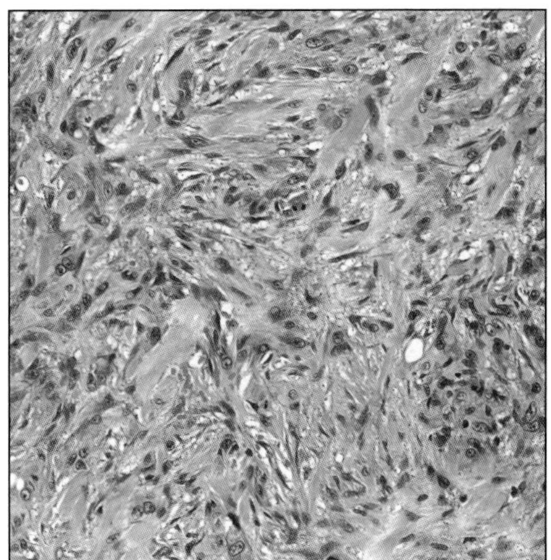

(Left) *Hematoxylin & eosin shows an example of epithelioid hemangioendothelioma with a prominent spindle cell component.* ***(Right)*** *Hematoxylin & eosin shows epithelioid hemangioendothelioma with increased cytologic atypia and scattered mitoses.*

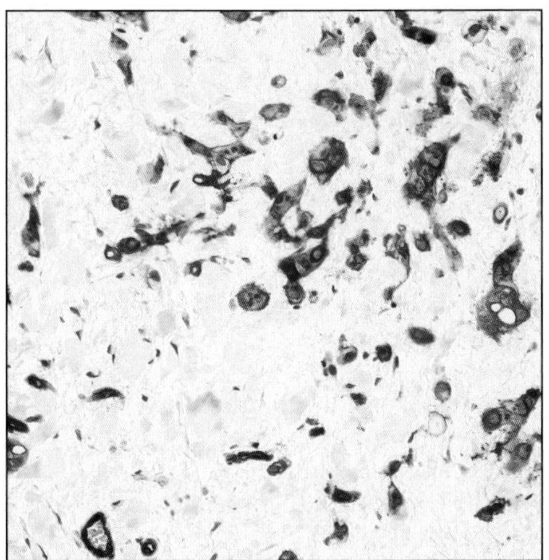

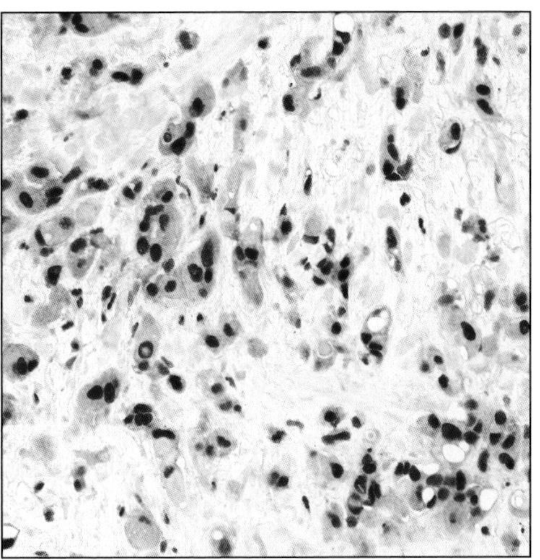

(Left) *CD31 shows membranous/cytoplasmic expression. Note scattered vacuolated tumor cells.* ***(Right)*** *FLI-1 shows diffuse immunostaining in tumor cell nuclei. Although not specific, this is a useful marker to confirm endothelial differentiation.*

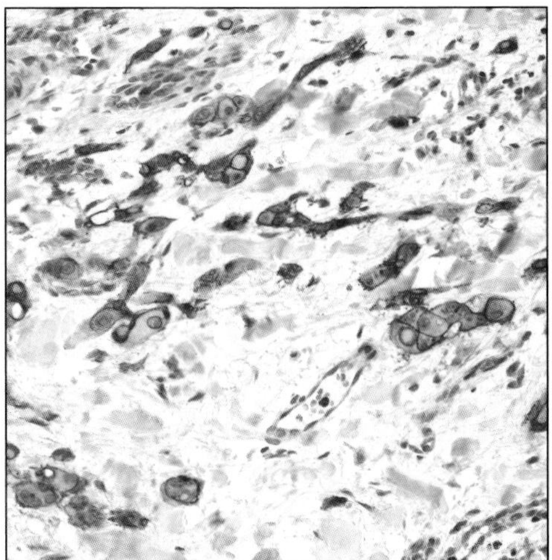

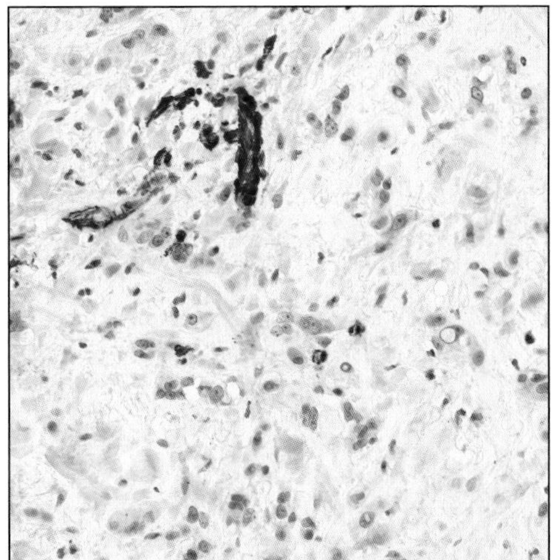

(Left) *Podoplanin shows well-defined positivity on tumor cell membranes.* ***(Right)*** *Actin-sm shows no immunoreactivity in tumor cells and the absence of pericytic layer.*

CUTANEOUS ANGIOSARCOMA

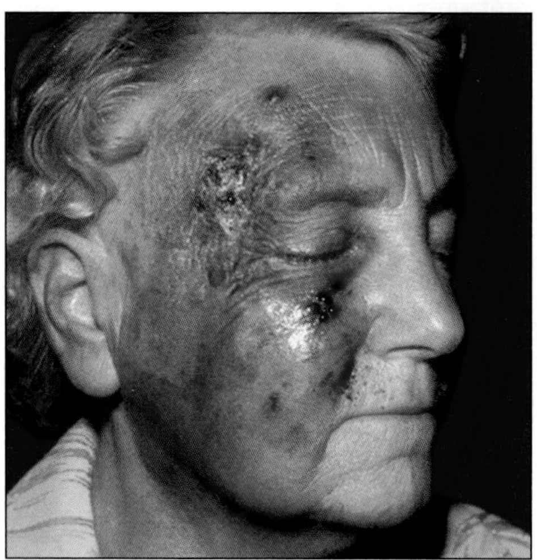

Clinical photograph shows an ill-defined, erythematous and plaque-like, hemorrhagic, cutaneous neoplasm in this male patient.

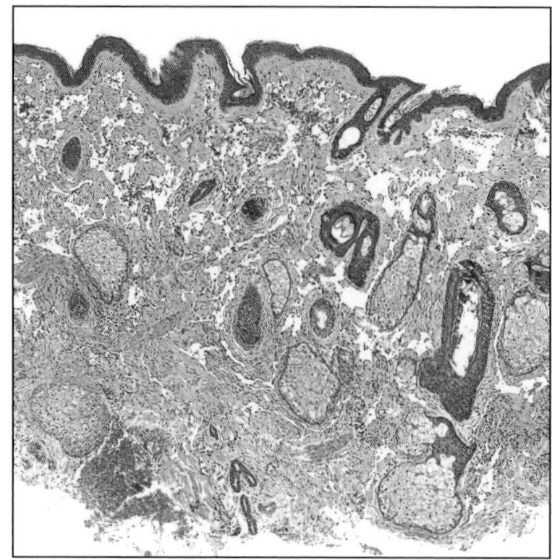

Hematoxylin & eosin shows a well-differentiated cutaneous angiosarcoma arising in sun-damaged skin.

TERMINOLOGY

Abbreviations

- Angiosarcoma (AS)

Synonyms

- Hemangiosarcoma
- Lymphangiosarcoma
- Malignant hemangioendothelioma

Definitions

- Malignant mesenchymal neoplasm of cells recapitulating variably morphologic and functional features composed of endothelial cells
- Clear differentiation between lymphangiosarcoma and sarcoma with blood vessel differentiation remains problematic

ETIOLOGY/PATHOGENESIS

Developmental Anomaly

- Congenital lymphedema

Environmental Exposure

- Chronic lymphedema, i.e., after mastectomy (Stewart-Treves syndrome)
- Radiotherapy
- Sun exposure

CLINICAL ISSUES

Epidemiology

- Incidence
  - Rare
  - Increasing rate due to use of radiotherapy and prolonged actinic damage
- Age
  - More frequent in elderly patients
  - Very rare in children
- Gender
  - M > F

Site

- Relatively frequent in head and neck area
- Radiation fields
- Areas of acquired or congenital lymphedema

Presentation

- Idiopathic (actinic) angiosarcoma
  - Arises predominantly in actinically damaged skin
  - Scalp, upper forehead, face
  - Elderly patients
  - Often initially mistaken for inflammatory lesion or cutaneous lymphoma/pseudolymphoma
- Radiation-induced angiosarcoma
  - Arises at variable times after therapeutic irradiation (e.g., for breast cancer)
- Angiosarcoma associated with chronic lymphedema
  - Congenital lymphedema
  - Acquired lymphedema (Stewart-Treves syndrome)
- Ill-defined lesions
- Plaque-like, red, indurated lesions
- Bruise-like lesions
- Nodular or multinodular appearance of older lesions
- Often multifocal

Treatment

- Surgical approaches
  - Wide excision with clear margins
- Adjuvant therapy
  - Benefit of adjuvant/neoadjuvant chemotherapy unclear

Prognosis

- Poor prognosis
  - Repeated local recurrences
  - Metastases occur often after repeated recurrences
    - Lymph node
    - Lung
  - 5-year survival (15-20%)

CUTANEOUS ANGIOSARCOMA

Key Facts

Terminology
- Malignant mesenchymal neoplasm of cells variably recapitulating morphologic and functional features composed of endothelial cells

Etiology/Pathogenesis
- Idiopathic (actinic) angiosarcoma
  - Predominantly in actinically damaged skin
  - Often initially mistaken for inflammatory lesion or cutaneous lymphoma/pseudolymphoma
- Radiation-induced angiosarcoma
- Angiosarcoma associated with chronic lymphedema

Clinical Issues
- Needs wide excision with clear margins
- Poor prognosis
- Necrosis and epithelioid cytomorphology are adverse prognostic factors

Image Findings
- Ill-defined, plaque- or bruise-like, often red lesions

Macroscopic Features
- Ill-defined, hemorrhagic lesions

Microscopic Pathology
- Vascular spaces of irregular size and shape
- Anastomosing vascular channels
- Multilayering, heaping up, and papillary formation of endothelial cells
- Enlarged, hyperchromatic, irregular-shaped nuclei
- No complete rim of actin(+) (myo)pericytes
- Increased Ki-67 expression

  - Necrosis and epithelioid cytomorphology represent adverse prognostic factors

IMAGE FINDINGS

General Features
- Best diagnostic clue
  - Ill-defined, plaque-like lesions
- Location
  - Actinically damaged skin of scalp and face

Specimen Radiographic Findings
- Diagnostic pathologic vascular structures may be present

MACROSCOPIC FEATURES

General Features
- Ill-defined, hemorrhagic lesions
- Flat or ulcerated epidermis
- Often sponge-like appearance

MICROSCOPIC PATHOLOGY

Histologic Features
- Vascular spaces of irregular size and shape
- Anastomosing vascular channels
  - Infiltrate and dissect preexisting structures
- Multilayering, heaping up, and papillary formation of endothelial cells
- Solid tumor areas in poorly differentiated neoplasms
- Enlarged endothelial cells
- Enlarged, hyperchromatic, and irregular-shaped nuclei
- Epithelioid cytomorphology seen only rarely in superficial location
- Increased number of mitoses
- Increased Ki-67 expression
- Tumor necrosis in poorly differentiated neoplasms
- Prominent inflammatory infiltrate often seen
- No complete rim of actin(+) (myo)pericytes
- Associated lymphangiomatosis in angiosarcoma associated with chronic lymphedema

Predominant Pattern/Injury Type
- Diffuse
- Hemorrhagic
- Ill-defined
- Infiltrative

Predominant Cell/Compartment Type
- Endothelial

DIFFERENTIAL DIAGNOSIS

Hemangioma
- Lobular growth
- Well-formed vascular structures
- No endothelial multilayering
- No prominent cytologic atypia
- Complete rim of actin(+) (myo)pericytes

Acquired Elastotic Hemangioma
- Plaque-like superficial vascular proliferation
- Well-formed vascular structures
- No endothelial multilayering
- No prominent cytologic atypia
- Complete rim of actin(+) (myo)pericytes

Epithelioid Angiomatous Nodule
- Small, well-circumscribed lesions
- Well-formed vessels in periphery
- No prominent cytologic atypia

Atypical Vascular Proliferation after Radiotherapy
- Circumscribed, solitary lesions
- No endothelial multilayering
- No prominent cytologic atypia

Acantholytic Carcinoma
- Homogeneous expression of epithelial immunohistochemical markers

CUTANEOUS ANGIOSARCOMA

Immunohistochemistry			
Antibody	**Reactivity**	**Staining Pattern**	**Comment**
CD31	Positive	Cell membrane & cytoplasm	
CD34	Positive	Cell membrane & cytoplasm	Not sensitive, not specific
FLI-1	Positive	Nuclear	Not specific
Podoplanin	Positive	Cell membrane & cytoplasm	Not specific
VEGF	Positive	Cell membrane & cytoplasm	
CK-PAN	Negative		
S100	Negative		
Actin-sm	Equivocal		Only rarely positive

- No expression of endothelial immunohistochemical markers

Retiform Hemangioendothelioma

- Young adults
- Distal extremities
- Rete testis-like growth pattern
- Hobnail cytomorphology
- No prominent cytologic atypia

Cutaneous Lymphoma/Pseudolymphoma

- Neoplastic vascular structures not present

DIAGNOSTIC CHECKLIST

Clinically Relevant Pathologic Features

- Invasive pattern
- Organ distribution

Pathologic Interpretation Pearls

- Ill-defined, irregular, infiltrating, anastomosing vessels
- Enlarged endothelial cells with multilayering, piling up, and papillary formation
- Nuclear atypia
- Expression of CD31, podoplanin
- Lack of complete rim of actin(+) (myo)pericytes
- Increased expression of Ki-67

SELECTED REFERENCES

1. DeMartelaere SL et al: Neoadjuvant chemotherapy-specific and overall treatment outcomes in patients with cutaneous angiosarcoma of the face with periorbital involvement. Head Neck. 30(5):639-46, 2008
2. Deyrup AT et al: Sporadic cutaneous angiosarcomas: a proposal for risk stratification based on 69 cases. Am J Surg Pathol. 32(1):72-7, 2008
3. Rouhani P et al: Cutaneous soft tissue sarcoma incidence patterns in the U.S. : an analysis of 12,114 cases. Cancer. 113(3):616-27, 2008
4. Abraham JA et al: Treatment and outcome of 82 patients with angiosarcoma. Ann Surg Oncol. 14(6):1953-67, 2007
5. Nagano T et al: Docetaxel: a therapeutic option in the treatment of cutaneous angiosarcoma: report of 9 patients. Cancer. 110(3):648-51, 2007
6. Requena L et al: Pseudolymphomatous cutaneous angiosarcoma: a rare variant of cutaneous angiosarcoma readily mistaken for cutaneous lymphoma. Am J Dermatopathol. 29(4):342-50, 2007
7. Mendenhall WM et al: Cutaneous angiosarcoma. Am J Clin Oncol. 29(5):524-8, 2006
8. Brenn T et al: Radiation-associated cutaneous atypical vascular lesions and angiosarcoma: clinicopathologic analysis of 42 cases. Am J Surg Pathol. 29(8):983-96, 2005
9. Billings SD et al: Cutaneous angiosarcoma following breast-conserving surgery and radiation: an analysis of 27 cases. Am J Surg Pathol. 28(6):781-8, 2004
10. Brenn T et al: Cutaneous epithelioid angiomatous nodule: a distinct lesion in the morphologic spectrum of epithelioid vascular tumors. Am J Dermatopathol. 26(1):14-21, 2004
11. Morgan MB et al: Cutaneous angiosarcoma: a case series with prognostic correlation. J Am Acad Dermatol. 50(6):867-74, 2004
12. Rossi S et al: Utility of the immunohistochemical detection of FLI-1 expression in round cell and vascular neoplasm using a monoclonal antibody. Mod Pathol. 17(5):547-52, 2004
13. Kahn HJ et al: Monoclonal antibody D2-40, a new marker of lymphatic endothelium, reacts with Kaposi's sarcoma and a subset of angiosarcomas. Mod Pathol. 15(4):434-40, 2002
14. Requena L et al: Benign vascular proliferations in irradiated skin. Am J Surg Pathol. 26(3):328-37, 2002
15. Folpe AL et al: Vascular endothelial growth factor receptor-3 (VEGFR-3): a marker of vascular tumors with presumed lymphatic differentiation, including Kaposi's sarcoma, kaposiform and Dabska-type hemangioendotheliomas, and a subset of angiosarcomas. Mod Pathol. 13(2):180-5, 2000
16. Orchard GE et al: An immunocytochemical assessment of 19 cases of cutaneous angiosarcoma. Histopathology. 28(3):235-40, 1996
17. Morrison WH et al: Cutaneous angiosarcoma of the head and neck. A therapeutic dilemma. Cancer. 76(2):319-27, 1995
18. Calonje E et al: Retiform hemangioendothelioma. A distinctive form of low-grade angiosarcoma delineated in a series of 15 cases. Am J Surg Pathol. 18(2):115-25, 1994
19. Fineberg S et al: Cutaneous angiosarcoma and atypical vascular lesions of the skin and breast after radiation therapy for breast carcinoma. Am J Clin Pathol. 102(6):757-63, 1994
20. Prescott RJ et al: Cutaneous epithelioid angiosarcoma: a clinicopathological study of four cases. Histopathology. 25(5):421-9, 1994

Clinical and Microscopic Features

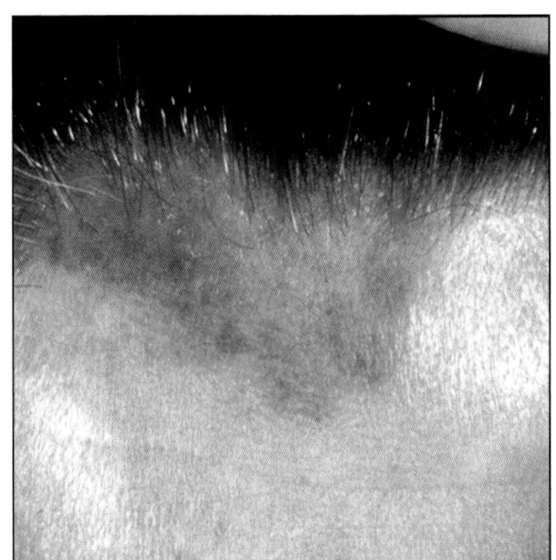

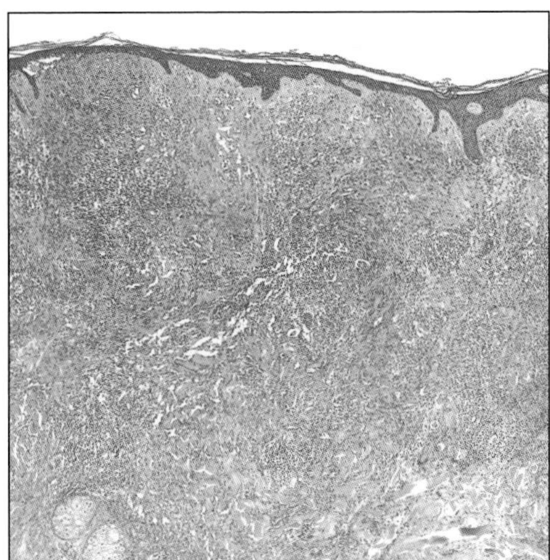

(Left) *Clinical photograph shows a plaque-like, brown cutaneous lesion mimicking an inflammatory disorder.* ***(Right)*** *Hematoxylin & eosin shows a skin specimen containing numerous inflammatory cells. In addition, the irregular and anastomosing vascular spaces are lined and surrounded by atypical endothelial cells.*

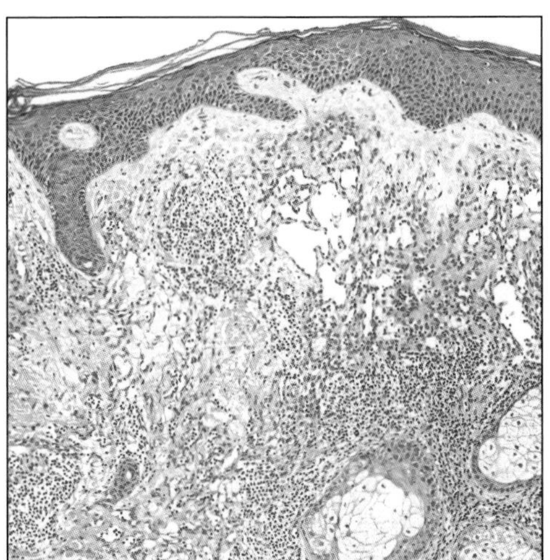

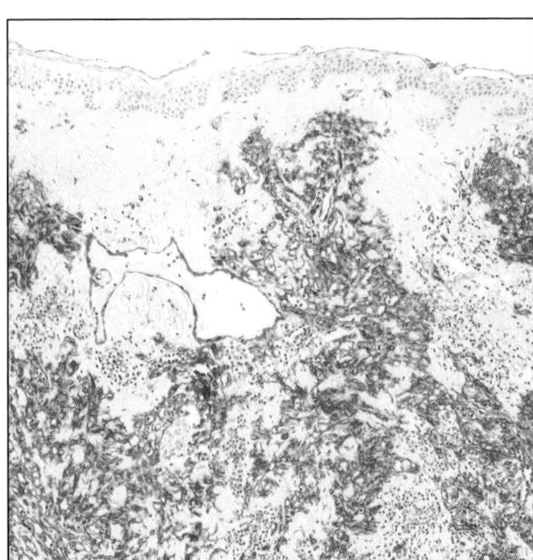

(Left) *Hematoxylin & eosin shows dilated vascular spaces lined by atypical endothelial tumor cells with enlarged nuclei.* ***(Right)*** *CD31 shows a diffuse network of neoplastic vascular spaces.*

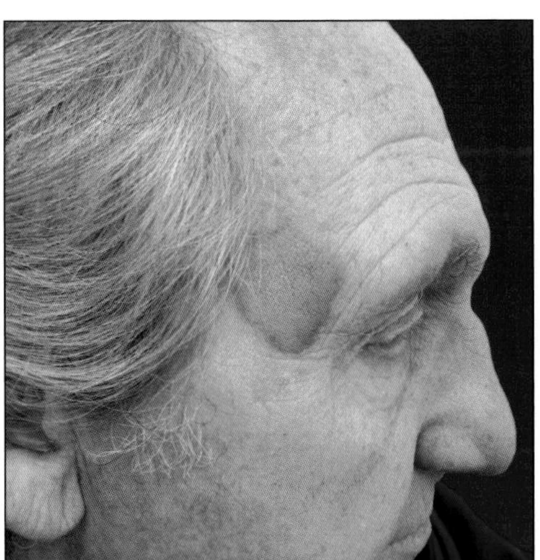

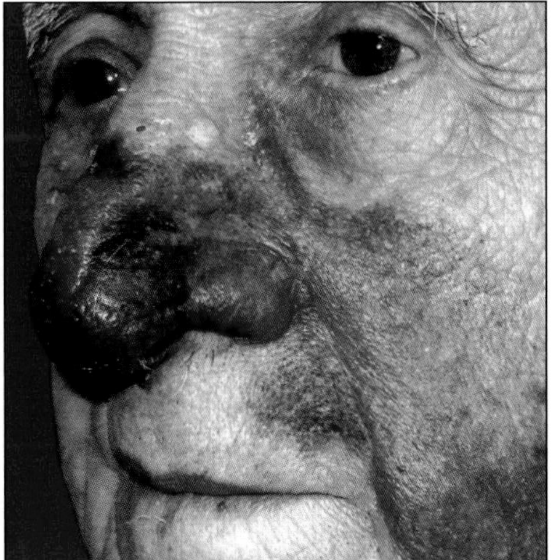

(Left) *Clinical photograph shows a relatively well-circumscribed example of cutaneous angiosarcoma.* ***(Right)*** *Clinical photograph shows an extensive cutaneous angiosarcoma with ill-defined red and bluish areas.*

CUTANEOUS ANGIOSARCOMA

Microscopic Features and Ancillary Techniques

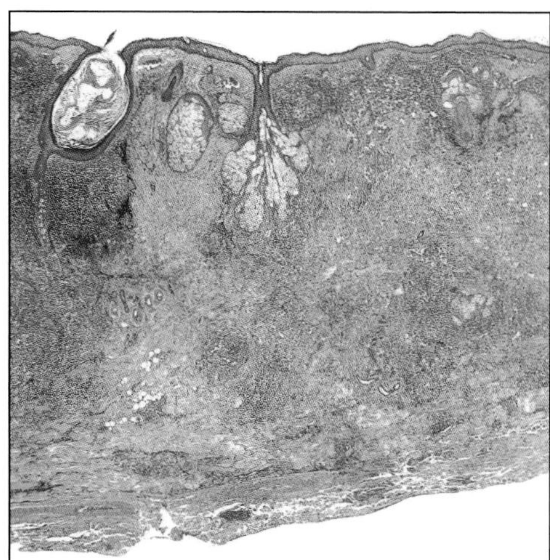

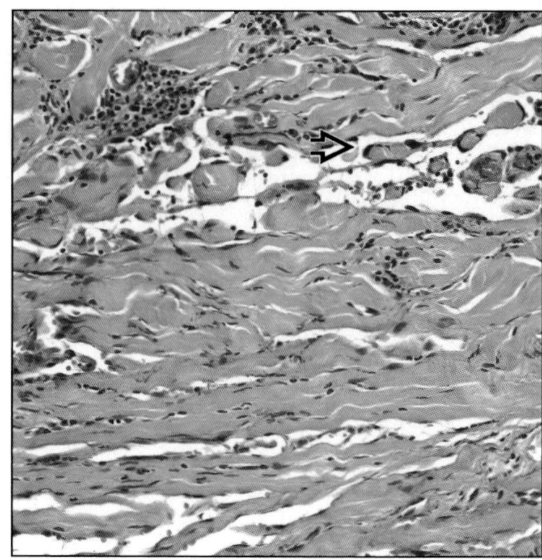

(Left) *Hematoxylin & eosin shows rosacea-like inflammatory changes. Note the anastomosing vascular spaces on the bottom of the slide.* ***(Right)*** *Hematoxylin & eosin shows higher power view with irregular-shaped and anastomosing vascular spaces lined by enlarged endothelial cells with enlarged and hyperchromatic nuclei ⇨.*

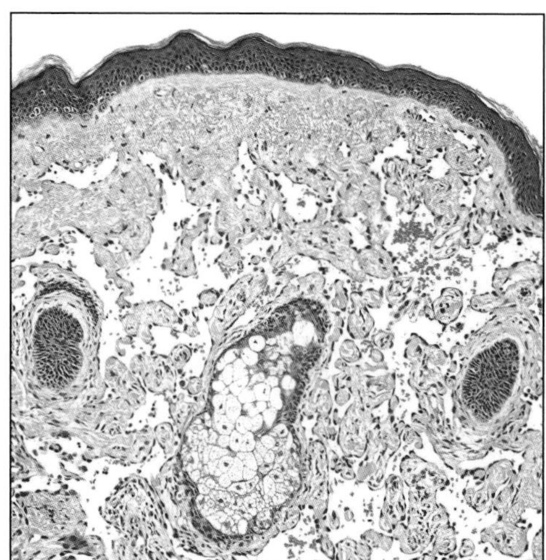

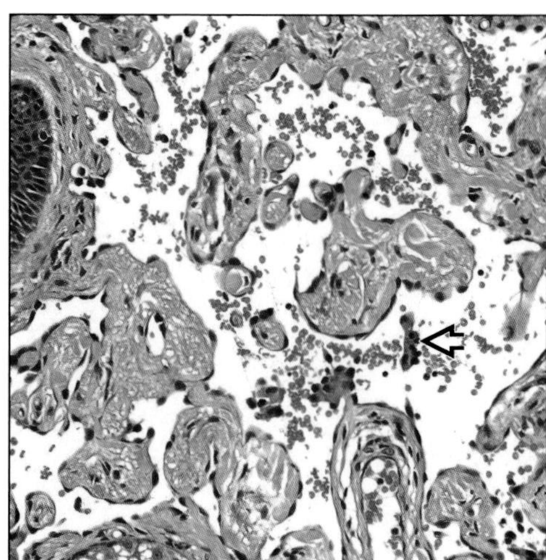

(Left) *Hematoxylin & eosin shows a case of well-differentiated cutaneous angiosarcoma arising in actinically damaged skin.* ***(Right)*** *Hematoxylin & eosin shows higher power view of well-differentiated cutaneous angiosarcoma. Note the enlarged endothelial cells, focal endothelial multilayering, and free-floating endothelial tumor cells ⇨.*

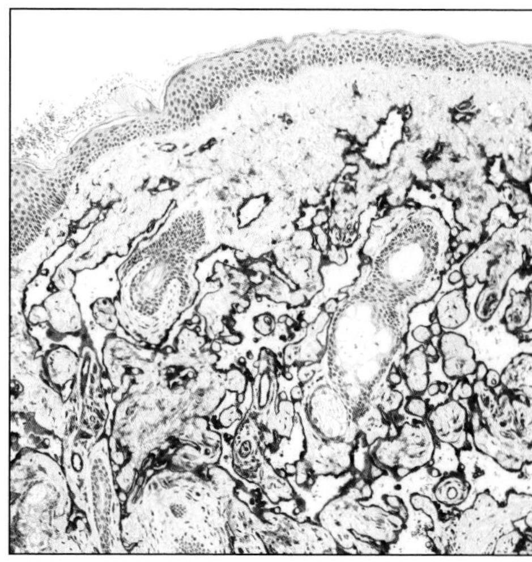

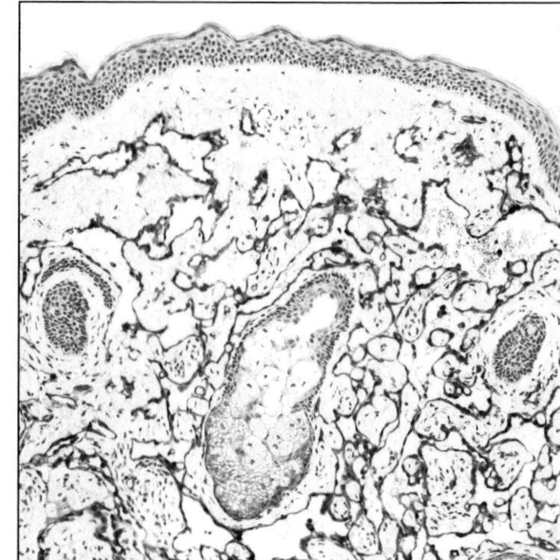

(Left) *CD31 shows positive immunostaining of well-differentiated cutaneous angiosarcoma. Anastomosing vascular spaces, enlarged endothelial cells, and focal endothelial multilayering are seen.* ***(Right)*** *Podoplanin shows positive immunostaining of neoplastic endothelial cells, a frequent finding in cutaneous angiosarcomas.*

Microscopic Features

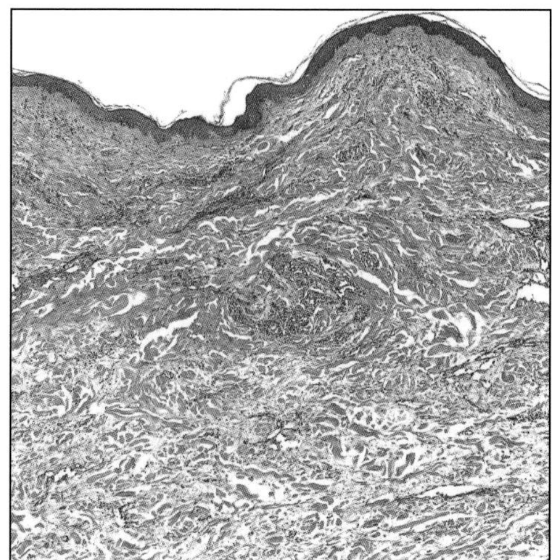

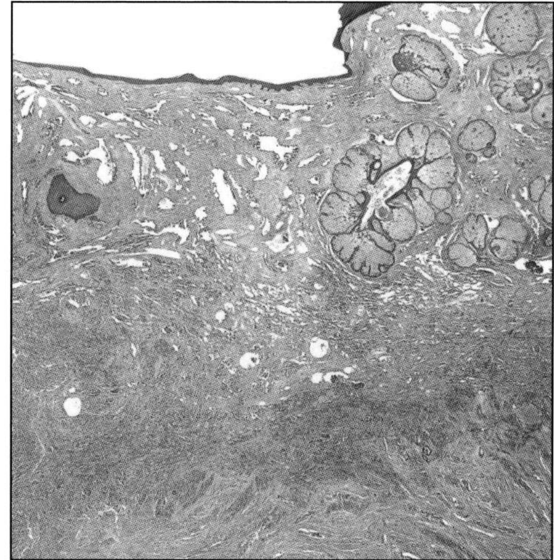

(Left) *Hematoxylin & eosin shows a case of post-irradiation cutaneous angiosarcoma. Note irregularly structured and anastomosing vascular spaces.* ***(Right)*** *Hematoxylin & eosin shows a cutaneous angiosarcoma with varying degrees of differentiation. Superficially, dilated vascular structures lined by atypical endothelial cells are seen, whereas in deeper parts of the specimen, cellular tumor areas are present.*

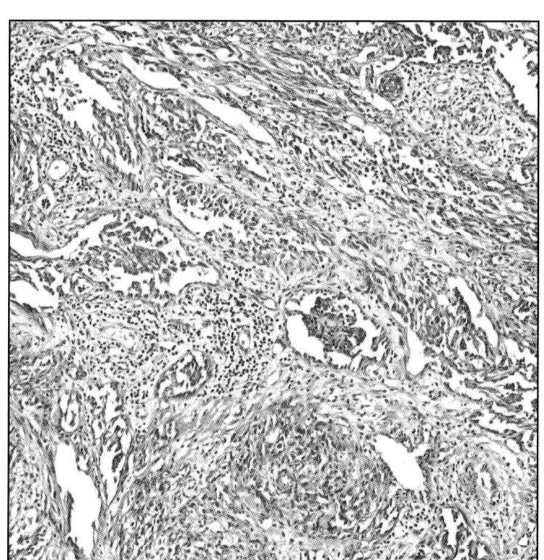

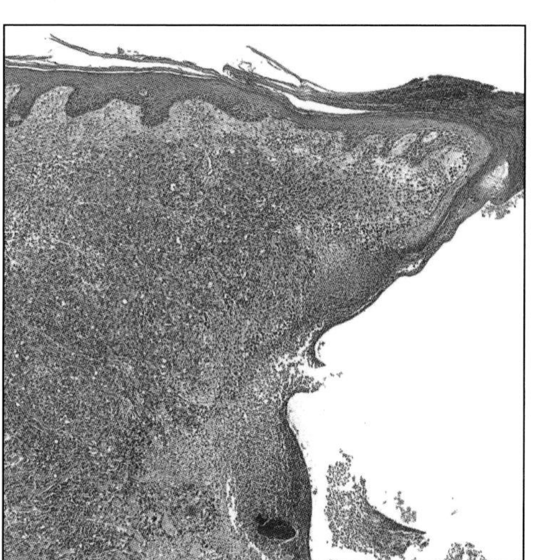

(Left) *Hematoxylin & eosin shows bridging and multilayering of atypical endothelial tumor cells that contain enlarged and hyperchromatic nuclei.* ***(Right)*** *Hematoxylin & eosin shows a rare example of ulcerated, predominantly epithelioid cutaneous angiosarcoma.*

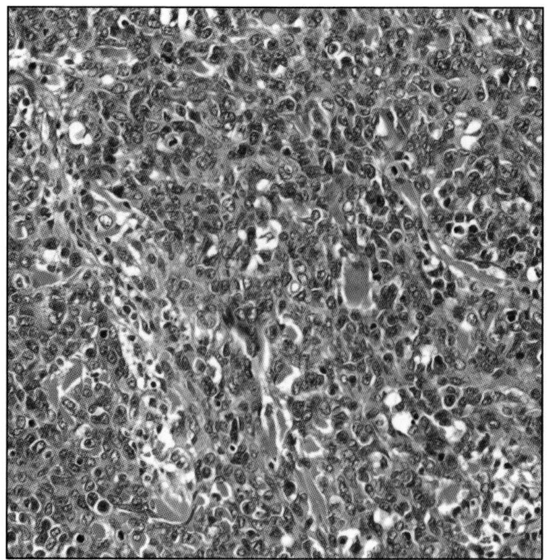

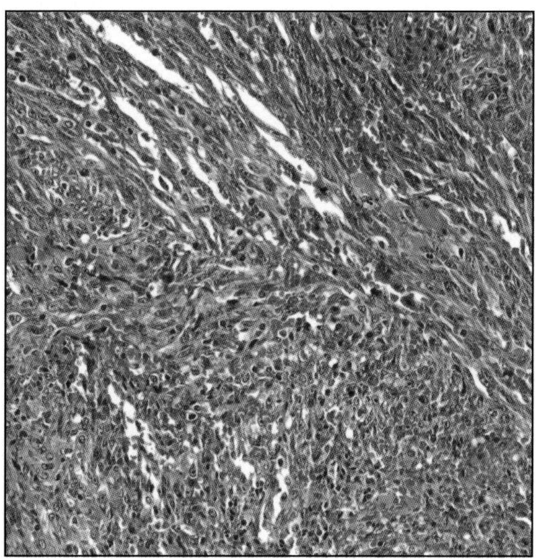

(Left) *Hematoxylin & eosin shows higher power view with sheets of enlarged epithelioid endothelial tumor cells.* ***(Right)*** *Hematoxylin & eosin shows a rare case of predominantly spindle cell cutaneous angiosarcoma.*

ANGIOSARCOMA OF SOFT TISSUE

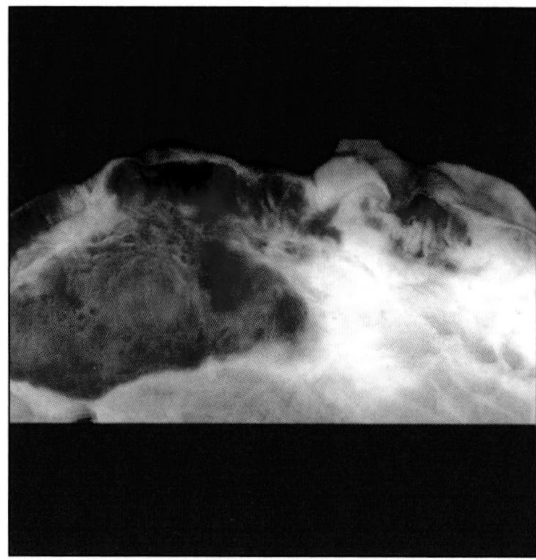

Gross pathology shows an ill-defined hemorrhagic neoplasm in deep soft tissue, a rare location for angiosarcoma.

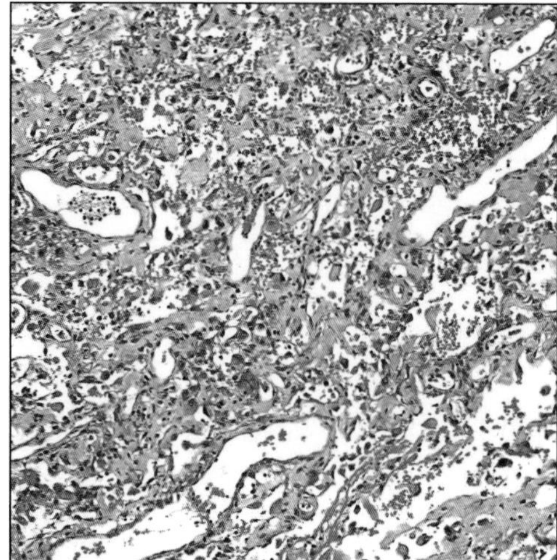

Hematoxylin & eosin shows anastomosing vascular structures lined by enlarged, atypical endothelial cells in this well-differentiated angiosarcoma.

TERMINOLOGY

Synonyms

- Hemangiosarcoma
- Hemangioblastoma
- Malignant hemangioendothelioma

Definitions

- Malignant mesenchymal neoplasm of cells recapitulating variably morphologic and functional features composed of endothelial cells

ETIOLOGY/PATHOGENESIS

Developmental Anomaly

- Develops rarely in association with genetic syndromes
  - Klippel-Trenaunay syndrome
  - Maffucci syndrome

Environmental Exposure

- Rarely develops adjacent to foreign material or synthetic vascular grafts

CLINICAL ISSUES

Epidemiology

- Incidence
  - Rare
    - < 1% of all sarcomas
  - More frequent in superficial locations
    - 1/4 of angiosarcomas arise in deep soft tissues
- Age
  - Occur at any age but most common in older adults
  - Very rare in childhood
- Gender
  - M > F

Site

- Deep soft tissues
- Lower extremities > upper extremities
- Trunk > head/neck region
- Significant proportion arises in abdomen and retroperitoneum
- Rarely multifocal

Presentation

- Slow growing
- Deep mass
- Usually large mass
- Hematologic abnormalities
- Thrombocytopenia may be present
- Arteriovenous shunting may be present
- Rarely arise in nonlipogenic component of dedifferentiated liposarcomas
- Rarely arise in benign or malignant nerve sheath tumors
- Very rarely arise in preexisting benign hemangioma

Treatment

- Surgical approaches
  - Aggressive surgical resection with wide tumor-free margins
- Adjuvant therapy
  - Response to chemotherapy
  - Inhibition of angiogenesis

Prognosis

- Poor prognosis irrespective of grade of malignancy
  - Local recurrence in 20-30%
  - Distant metastases in 50%
  - 5-year survival 20-30% at best

MACROSCOPIC FEATURES

General Features

- Infiltrating neoplasm
- Areas of hemorrhage

ANGIOSARCOMA OF SOFT TISSUE

Key Facts

Terminology

- Malignant mesenchymal neoplasm of cells recapitulating variably morphologic and functional features composed of endothelial cells

Clinical Issues

- Deep soft tissues
  - Lower extremities, followed by upper extremities
  - Trunk > head and neck
  - Significant proportion intraabdominal and retroperitoneal
- Rare (more frequent in superficial locations)
  - < 1% of all sarcomas
- Any age but most common in older adults
- Poor prognosis irrespective of grade of malignancy
  - 5-year survival 20-30% at best
- Aggressive surgical resection with wide tumor-free margins

Microscopic Pathology

- Irregular, anastomosing vascular spaces
- Variably pleomorphic endothelial tumor cells
- Endothelial multilayering and papillary formation
- Solid areas common
- No complete rim of actin(+) (myo)pericytes
- Often intracytoplasmic lumina
- Prominent nuclear atypia
- Numerous mitoses
- Expression of endothelial markers
- Epithelioid angiosarcomas occur relatively frequent in deep soft tissues
  - Solid sheets of large epithelioid cells in epithelioid angiosarcoma

MICROSCOPIC PATHOLOGY

Histologic Features

- Angiosarcoma
  - Usually no relationship to preexisting vessels
  - Irregular infiltrating vascular spaces
  - Anastomosing vascular spaces
  - Variably pleomorphic endothelial tumor cells
  - Endothelial multilayering
  - Endothelial papillary formations
  - Solid areas common
  - Neoplastic vascular structures encircled by reticulin fibers
  - No complete rim of actin(+) (myo)pericytes
  - Often intracytoplasmic lumina
  - Lumina may contain erythrocytes
  - Prominent nuclear atypia
  - Numerous mitoses
  - Areas of hemorrhage and necrosis may be present
  - Rare predominantly spindle cell morphology
  - Clear distinction between lymphatic and vascular differentiation remains problematic
- Epithelioid angiosarcoma
  - More frequent in deep soft tissues
  - Often rapid growth
  - Very aggressive clinical course
  - Solid sheets of large epithelioid cells
  - Tumor cells with abundant eosinophilic cytoplasm and large vesicular nuclei
  - Prominent cytologic atypia
  - Numerous mitoses
  - Often areas of tumor necrosis
- Rare granular cell variant
- Rare inflammatory variant

Predominant Pattern/Injury Type

- Diffuse

Predominant Cell/Compartment Type

- Endothelial

DIFFERENTIAL DIAGNOSIS

Hemangioma

- Lobular architecture
- Well-formed vascular structures
- No endothelial multilayering and papillary formation
- Usually complete rim of actin(+) (myo)pericytes
- No prominent cytologic atypia
- No/few mitoses of endothelial cells

Metastatic Malignant Melanoma

- No vascular spaces
- No intracytoplasmic vacuoles with erythrocytes
- Round tumor cells
- Vesicular nuclei with prominent nucleoli
- Endothelial immunohistochemical markers negative
- Melanocytic immunohistochemical markers positive
- Clinical features

Metastatic Carcinoma

- No vascular spaces
- Obvious epithelial structures
- Endothelial immunohistochemical markers negative
- Homogeneous expression of epithelial immunohistochemical markers
- Clinical features

Proximal-type Epithelioid Sarcoma

- No vascular structures
- Endothelial immunohistochemical markers negative
- Loss of INI1 expression
- Epithelioid and rhabdoid tumor cells

Malignant Myoepithelioma

- Often at least focally epithelial structures
- Often focal myxoid stromal changes
- Often expression of S100 protein
- Often expression of actins
- Endothelial immunohistochemical markers negative

Retiform Hemangioendothelioma

- Distal extremities
- Young patients

ANGIOSARCOMA OF SOFT TISSUE

Immunohistochemistry			
Antibody	Reactivity	Staining Pattern	Comment
CD31	Positive	Cell membrane & cytoplasm	
CD34	Positive	Cell membrane & cytoplasm	Not sensitive, may be negative
FLI-1	Positive	Nuclear	Not specific
Podoplanin	Positive	Cytoplasmic	Not specific
Actin-sm	Positive	Cytoplasmic	In some cases
CK-PAN	Positive	Cytoplasmic	In some cases (in 50% of epithelioid angiosarcoma)
SNF5	Positive	Nuclear	Consistently expressed
S100P	Negative		
EMA	Equivocal	Cell membrane & cytoplasm	In some cases

- Dermal/subcutaneous location
- Rete testis-like infiltrative pattern
- Hobnail cytomorphology of endothelial cells
- No prominent cytologic atypia
- Usually no multilayering
- Often focal lymphocytic infiltration

(Epithelioid) Gastrointestinal Stromal Tumor

- No vascular structures
- CD31(-)
- CD117(+)
- Characteristic molecular findings

Sclerosing (Pseudovascular) Rhabdomyosarcoma

- Scattered rhabdomyoblasts
- Prominent sclerosis
- Desmin(+)
- Scattered cells express myogenin
- No expression of endothelial immunohistochemical markers

Large Cell Anaplastic Lymphoma

- No expression of endothelial immunohistochemical markers
- Expression of lymphatic markers

DIAGNOSTIC CHECKLIST

Clinically Relevant Pathologic Features

- Gross appearance
- Age distribution

Pathologic Interpretation Pearls

- Irregular anastomosing vascular structures
- Atypical proliferating endothelial tumor cells
- No complete rim of actin(+) (myo)pericytes

SELECTED REFERENCES

1. Schlemmer M et al: Paclitaxel in patients with advanced angiosarcomas of soft tissue: a retrospective study of the EORTC soft tissue and bone sarcoma group. Eur J Cancer. 44(16):2433-6, 2008
2. Abraham JA et al: Treatment and outcome of 82 patients with angiosarcoma. Ann Surg Oncol. 14(6):1953-67, 2007
3. Fayette J et al: Angiosarcomas, a heterogeneous group of sarcomas with specific behavior depending on primary site: a retrospective study of 161 cases. Ann Oncol. 18(12):2030-6, 2007
4. Syed SP et al: Angiostatin receptor annexin II in vascular tumors including angiosarcoma. Hum Pathol. 38(3):508-13, 2007
5. Toro JR et al: Incidence patterns of soft tissue sarcomas, regardless of primary site, in the surveillance, epidemiology and end results program, 1978-2001: An analysis of 26,758 cases. Int J Cancer. 119(12):2922-30, 2006
6. Leowardi C et al: Malignant vascular tumors: clinical presentation, surgical therapy, and long-term prognosis. Ann Surg Oncol. 12(12):1090-101, 2005
7. Skubitz KM et al: Paclitaxel and pegylated-liposomal doxorubicin are both active in angiosarcoma. Cancer. 104(2):361-6, 2005
8. Rossi S et al: Utility of the immunohistochemical detection of FLI-1 expression in round cell and vascular neoplasm using a monoclonal antibody. Mod Pathol. 17(5):547-52, 2004
9. Fanburg-Smith JC et al: Oral and salivary gland angiosarcoma: a clinicopathologic study of 29 cases. Mod Pathol. 16(3):263-71, 2003
10. Ferrari A et al: Malignant vascular tumors in children and adolescents: a report from the Italian and German Soft Tissue Sarcoma Cooperative Group. Med Pediatr Oncol. 39(2):109-14, 2002
11. Rossi S et al: Angiosarcoma arising in hemangioma/vascular malformation: report of four cases and review of the literature. Am J Surg Pathol. 26(10):1319-29, 2002
12. Miettinen M et al: Distribution of keratins in normal endothelial cells and a spectrum of vascular tumors: implications in tumor diagnosis. Hum Pathol. 31(9):1062-7, 2000
13. Meis-Kindblom JM et al: Angiosarcoma of soft tissue: a study of 80 cases. Am J Surg Pathol. 22(6):683-97, 1998
14. Schuborg C et al: Cytogenetic analysis of four angiosarcomas from deep and superficial soft tissue. Cancer Genet Cytogenet. 100(1):52-6, 1998
15. Mark RJ et al: Angiosarcoma. A report of 67 patients and a review of the literature. Cancer. 77(11):2400-6, 1996
16. Naka N et al: Angiosarcoma in Japan. A review of 99 cases. Cancer. 75(4):989-96, 1995
17. Fletcher CD et al: Epithelioid angiosarcoma of deep soft tissue: a distinctive tumor readily mistaken for an epithelial neoplasm. Am J Surg Pathol. 15(10):915-24, 1991
18. Maddox JC et al: Angiosarcoma of skin and soft tissue: a study of forty-four cases. Cancer. 48(8):1907-21, 1981

Microscopic Features

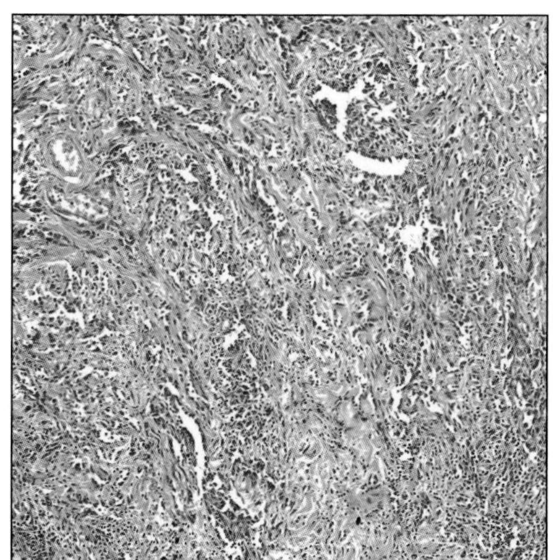

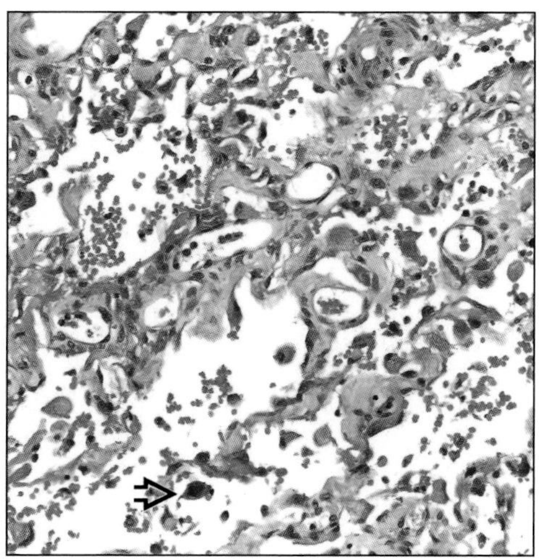

(Left) *Hematoxylin & eosin shows narrow and dilated vascular structures lined by atypical endothelial cells.* ***(Right)*** *Hematoxylin & eosin of this well-differentiated angiosarcoma shows enlarged endothelial cells with enlarged and hyperchromatic nuclei. Note the free-floating atypical endothelial cells ⇨, a frequent finding in well-differentiated lesions.*

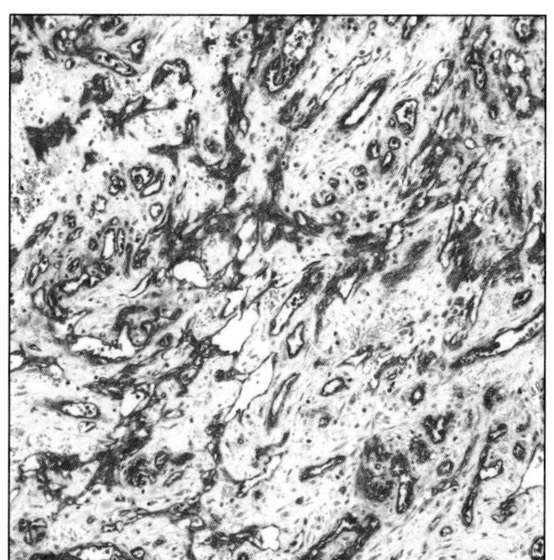

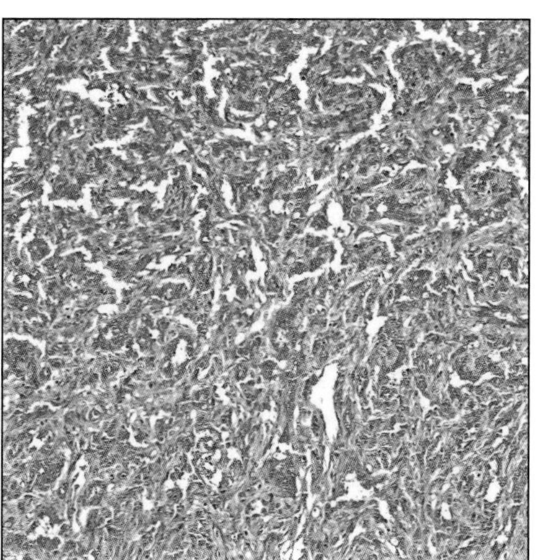

(Left) *CD31 immunostain shows anastomosing vascular structures lined by atypical endothelial cells.* ***(Right)*** *Hematoxylin & eosin shows irregularly shaped vascular spaces.*

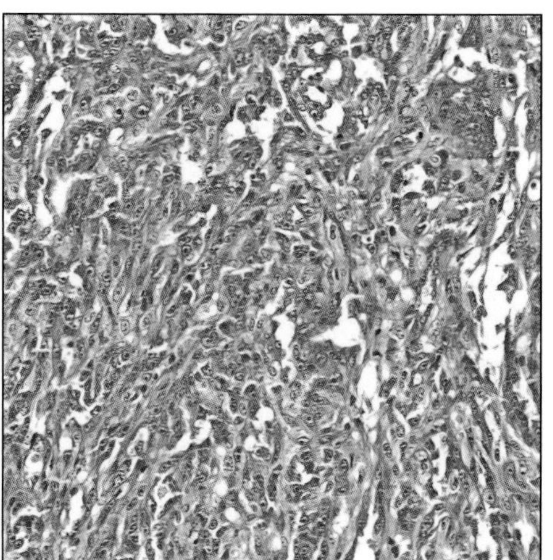

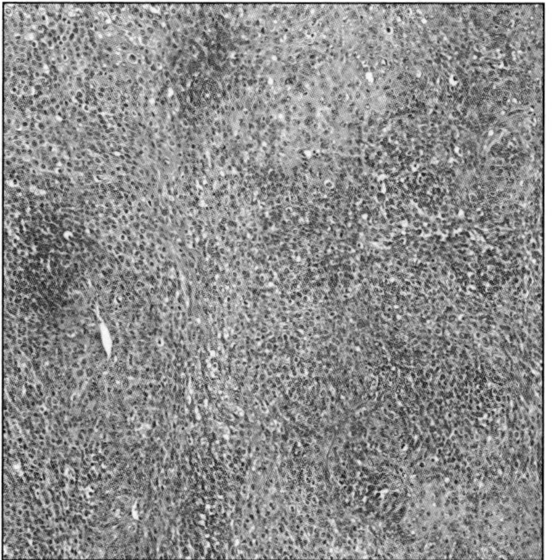

(Left) *Hematoxylin & eosin shows enlarged epithelioid tumor cells with enlarged vesicular nuclei.* ***(Right)*** *Hematoxylin & eosin of this epithelioid angiosarcoma shows sheets of atypical epithelioid tumor cells.*

ANGIOSARCOMA OF SOFT TISSUE

Microscopic Features

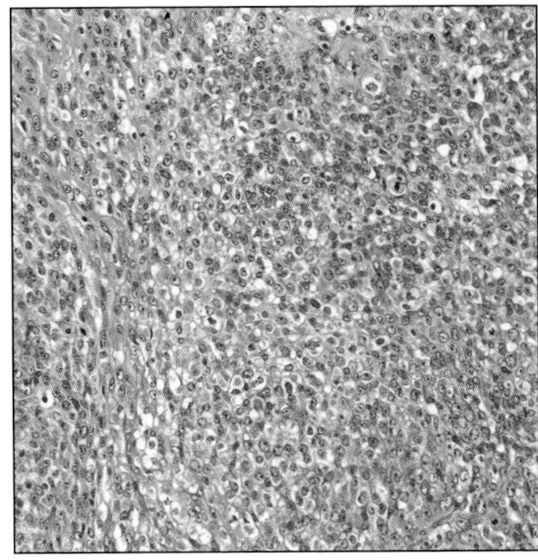
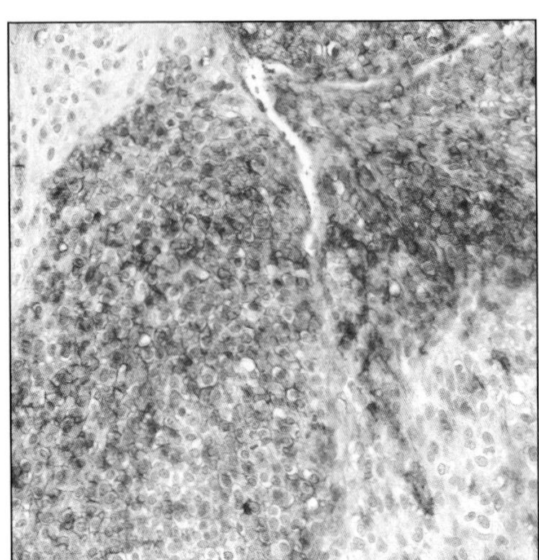

(Left) *Hematoxylin & eosin shows atypical epithelioid tumor cells with enlarged vesicular nuclei.* ***(Right)*** *CD31 immunostaining shows expression of this endothelial marker by epithelioid tumor cells.*

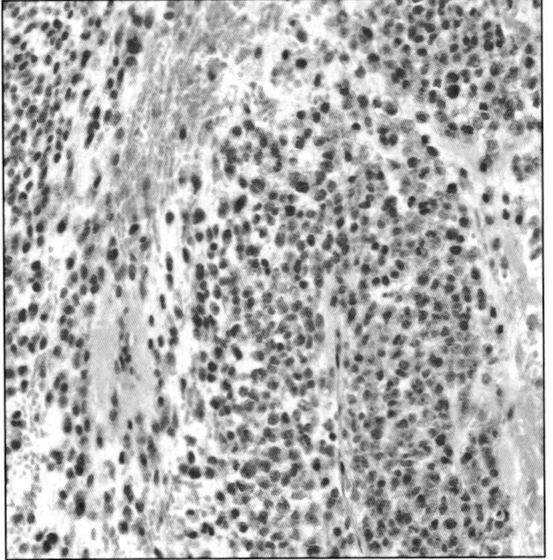
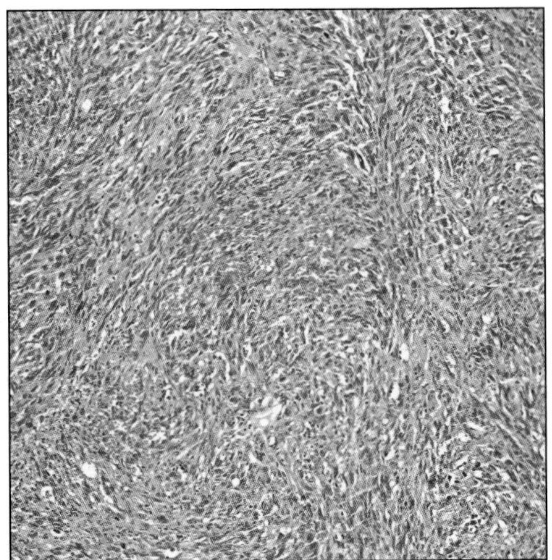

(Left) *FLI-1 immunostaining shows nuclear expression.* ***(Right)*** *Hematoxylin & eosin shows an example of angiosarcoma of soft tissue composed predominantly of spindle-shaped tumor cells.*

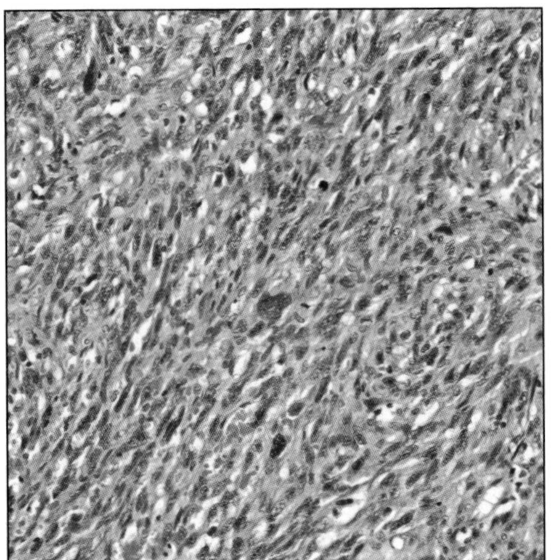
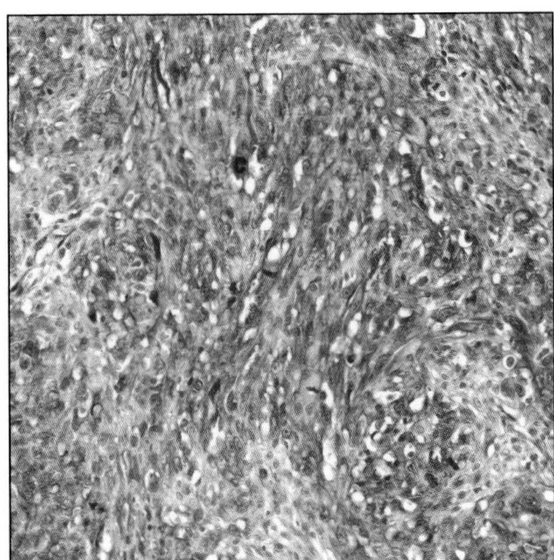

(Left) *Hematoxylin & eosin shows high-power view of spindle cell angiosarcoma. Note the striking cytologic atypia in contrast to Kaposi sarcoma.* ***(Right)*** *CD31 immunostaining confirms the endothelial line of differentiation of tumor cells in this spindle cell angiosarcoma.*

Microscopic Features

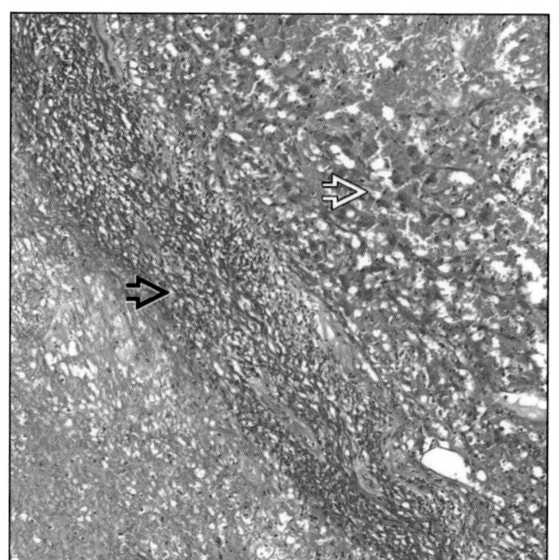

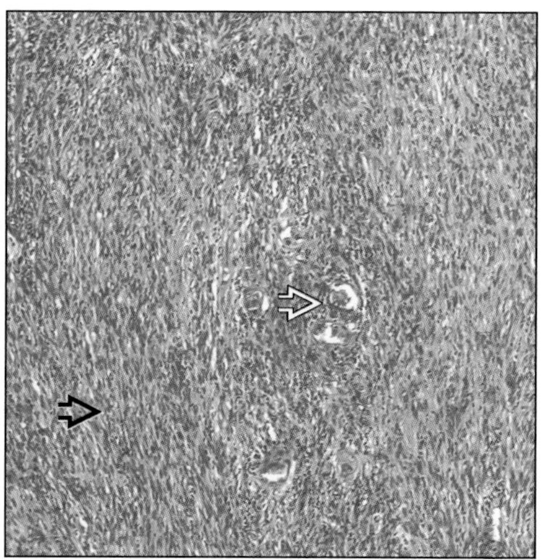

(Left) *Hematoxylin & eosin shows a rare example of angiosarcoma arising in low-grade malignant peripheral nerve sheath tumor. Note spindle cell areas ➪ & dilated, anastomosing vascular structures lined by atypical endothelial tumor cells ➡.* ***(Right)*** *Hematoxylin & eosin shows an area of angiosarcoma arising in a low-grade malignant peripheral nerve sheath tumor. Note spindle cell areas ➪ & atypical epithelioid endothelial tumor cells ➡.*

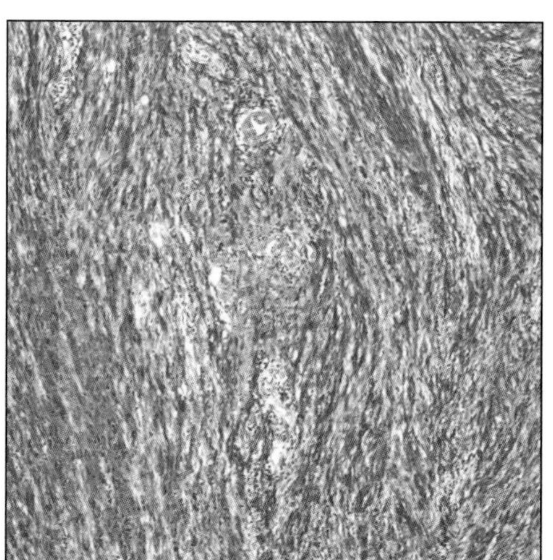

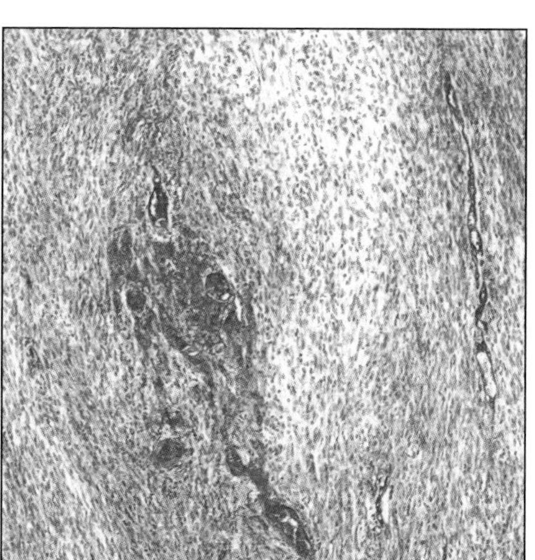

(Left) *S100P immunostaining shows expression by many (but not all) spindle-shaped tumor cells of the low-grade malignant peripheral nerve sheath tumor component.* ***(Right)*** *CD31 immunostaining shows expression by neoplastic cells of the angiosarcomatous component.*

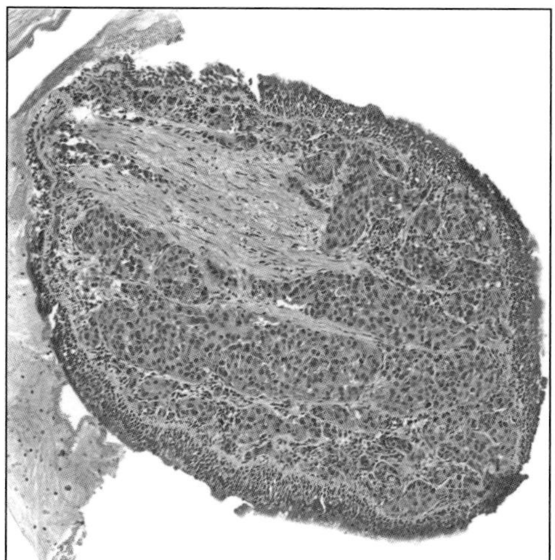

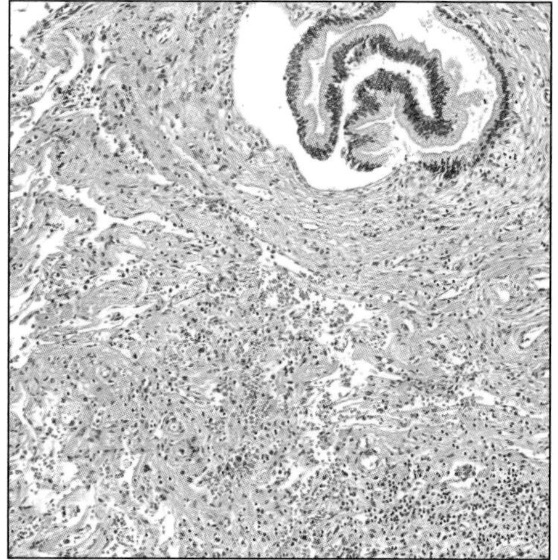

(Left) *Hematoxylin & eosin shows an example of pulmonary epithelioid angiosarcoma.* ***(Right)*** *Hematoxylin & eosin shows a well-differentiated angiosarcoma arising in the liver.*

Lesions of Uncertain Differentiation

Benign

Intermediate

Malignant

INTRAMUSCULAR MYXOMA

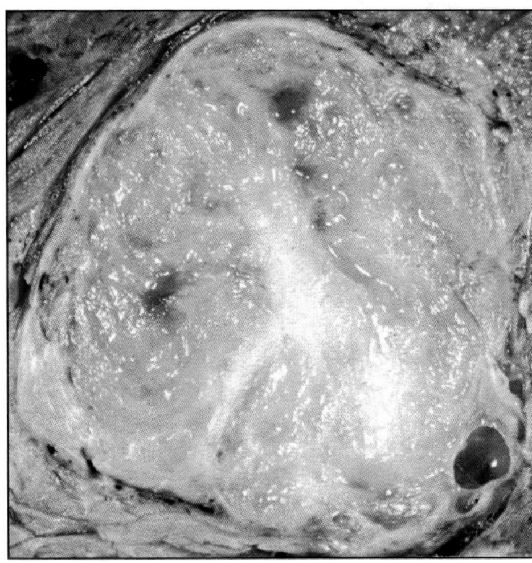

Gross image shows an intramuscular myxoma. This is a circumscribed and lobulated tumor with a white or glistening cut surface. Note the smooth interface with adjacent skeletal muscle.

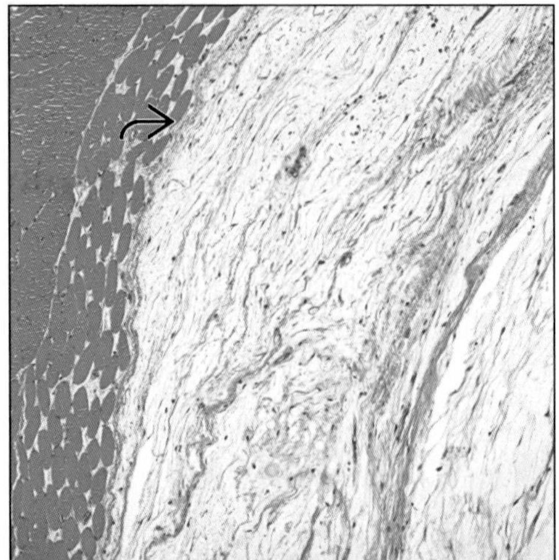

In this intramuscular myxoma, the lesion abuts skeletal muscle ⮫. The lesion is sparsely cellular; the constituent cells are small and bland and arranged in patternless distributions within the myxoid stroma.

TERMINOLOGY

Definitions

- Benign soft tissue tumor composed of bland fibroblasts embedded in abundant extracellular myxoid stroma
- Can sometimes be cellular
  - Cellular or hypercellular intramuscular myxoma

CLINICAL ISSUES

Epidemiology

- Age
  - Middle-aged adults
- Gender
  - Female predilection

Site

- Usually large muscles
  - Thigh
  - Buttock
  - Shoulder
  - Arm

Presentation

- Painless mass
- Associated with fibrous dysplasia of bone in Mazabraud syndrome
  - May have multiple lesions

Treatment

- Simple resection

Prognosis

- Typical intramuscular myxoma does not usually recur
- Cellular variant rarely recurs locally
- No metastases reported

MACROSCOPIC FEATURES

General Features

- Circumscribed
  - May infiltrate adjacent skeletal muscle on closer inspection
- Lobulated
- Gelatinous or more fibrous
  - Depending on amount of collagen or myxoid material
- Cystic spaces

Size

- Most < 10 cm in greatest dimension
  - Can measure up to 20 cm

MICROSCOPIC PATHOLOGY

Histologic Features

- Hypocellular
- Bland spindle or stellate cells
  - Patternless arrays
  - Small nuclei
  - Fibrillary cytoplasm
- Abundant extracellular myxoid stroma
- May contain microcystic spaces
  - Sometimes filled with pale eosinophilic material
- Small collagen bundles may be distributed in stroma
- Vasculature is sparse
- Frequently infiltrates between skeletal muscle fibers or bundles at periphery
- Cellular variant
  - Increased cellularity
  - Increased vascularity and collagen deposition
  - Cytologic features similar to the usual type
- No nuclear atypia, mitoses, or necrosis

Predominant Cell/Compartment Type

- Fibroblast

INTRAMUSCULAR MYXOMA

Key Facts

Terminology

- Benign soft tissue tumor composed of bland spindle to stellate fibroblasts within abundant extracellular myxoid matrix

Clinical Issues

- Middle-aged adults
  - Female predilection
- Site: Large muscles, such as thigh or shoulder

Macroscopic Features

- Largely circumscribed, gelatinous mass
  - May show skeletal muscle infiltration

Microscopic Pathology

- Hypocellular and hypovascular
- Spindle and stellate cells
- Patternless arrays
- Mitoses, atypia, and necrosis absent
- Cellular variant also exists: Cellular myxoma

ANCILLARY TESTS

Immunohistochemistry

- Variable expression of CD34 and actin
- Negative for S100 protein

Molecular Genetics

- Activating missense mutations at Arg 201 codon of gene encoding α subunit of Gs (*GNAS1*)
  - Recognized in fibrous dysplasia of bone
  - Mutations also detected in intramuscular myxomas, both ± fibrous dysplasia

DIFFERENTIAL DIAGNOSIS

Myxoid Neurofibroma

- "Buckled" or wavy nuclei
- S100 protein(+)

Low-Grade Fibromyxoid Sarcoma

- Bland, squared, or angulated nuclei with fine chromatin
- Collagenous as well as myxoid stroma
- May contain giant collagen rosettes
- Characteristic translocations

Myxofibrosarcoma

- Elderly patients
- Often distal and superficial (subcutis)
- More cellular
- Variable, often marked cytologic atypia
- Vascularity more pronounced

Myxoid Liposarcoma

- Greater cellularity
- Plexiform vascular pattern
- May contain lipoblasts
- Characteristic translocations

SELECTED REFERENCES

1. Faivre L et al: Mazabraud syndrome in two patients: clinical overlap with McCune-Albright syndrome. Am J Med Genet. 99(2):132-6, 2001
2. Okamoto S et al: Activating Gs(alpha) mutation in intramuscular myxomas with and without fibrous dysplasia of bone. Virchows Arch. 437(2):133-7, 2000
3. Nielsen GP et al: Intramuscular myxoma: a clinicopathologic study of 51 cases with emphasis on hypercellular and hypervascular variants. Am J Surg Pathol. 22(10):1222-7, 1998
4. Hashimoto H et al: Intramuscular myxoma. A clinicopathologic, immunohistochemical, and electron microscopic study. Cancer. 58(3):740-7, 1986
5. Miettinen M et al: Intramuscular myxoma--a clinicopathological study of twenty-three cases. Am J Clin Pathol. 84(3):265-72, 1985
6. Wirth WA et al: Multiple intramuscular myxomas. Another extraskeletal manifestation of fibrous dysplasia. Cancer. 27(5):1167-73, 1971
7. Enzinger FM: Intramuscular myxoma; a review and follow-up study of 34 cases. Am J Clin Pathol. 43:104-13, 1965

IMAGE GALLERY

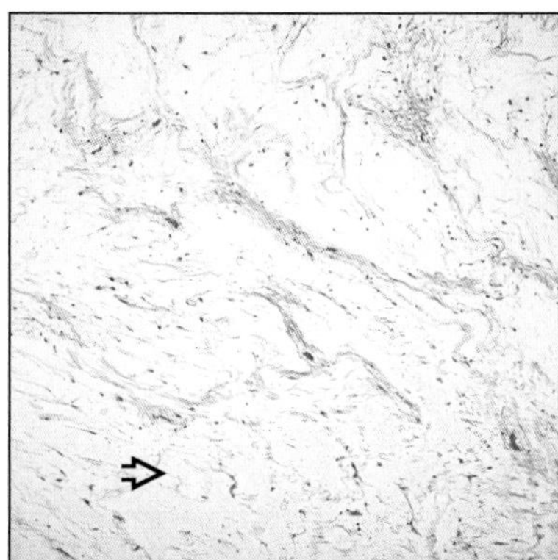

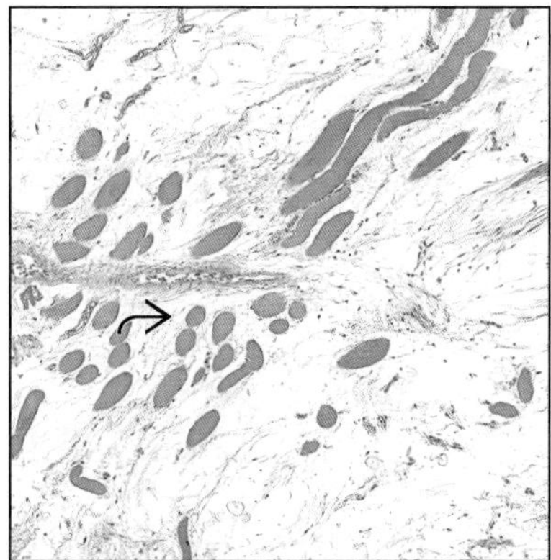

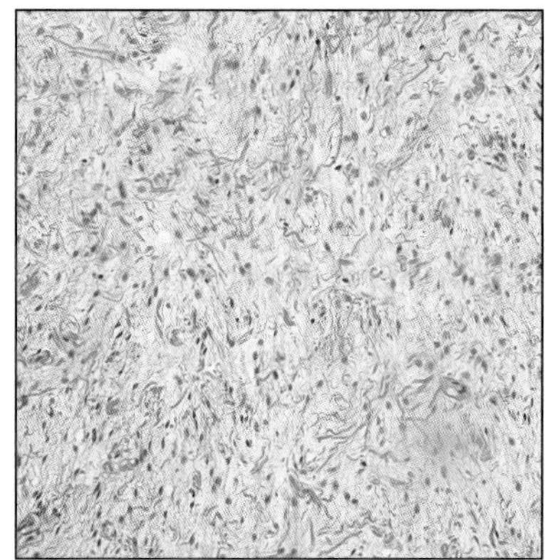

(Left) *The low-power view of this intramuscular myxoma shows a hypocellular lesion, composed of bland spindle to stellate cells within a notably hypovascular myxoid background* ⇨. ***(Center)*** *Lesions are grossly circumscribed, but infiltration between peripheral muscle fibers* ↷ *is often seen.* ***(Right)*** *In this cellular myxoma, the lesion shows greater cellularity than typical intramuscular myxoma. The cytomorphology remains similar, and no atypia is present within the spindle cells.*

JUXTAARTICULAR MYXOMA

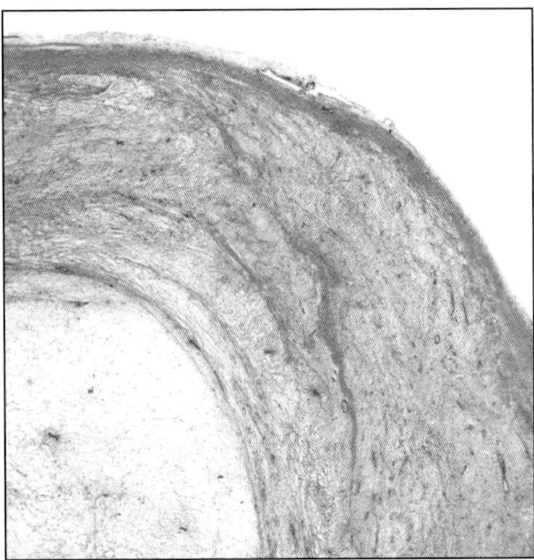

In this juxtaarticular myxoma, the lesion is circumscribed and composed of spindle to stellate fibroblast-like cells that are small and bland, within abundant myxoid stroma.

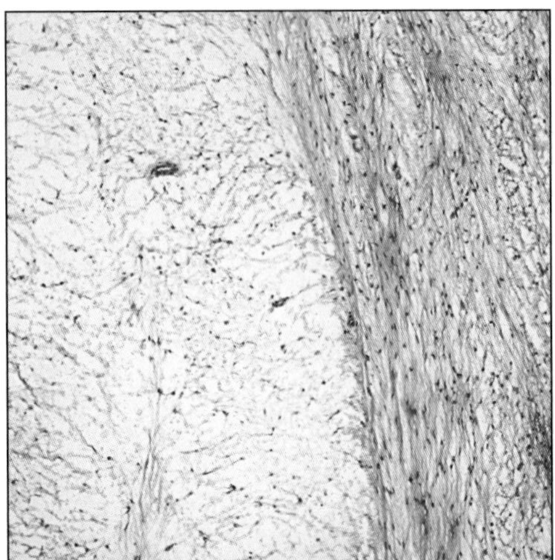

The lesion varies from sparsely cellular (right) to paucicellular (left). The cells are embedded in patternless distributions within stroma that is myxoid and hypovascular.

TERMINOLOGY

Abbreviations

- Juxtaarticular myxoma (JAM)

Definitions

- Benign lesion occurring in region of large joints, histologically similar to intramuscular myxoma

ETIOLOGY/PATHOGENESIS

Environmental Exposure

- Lesions have been associated with trauma
- May also occur adjacent to osteoarthritic joint

Genetic Abnormality

- Clonal chromosomal abnormalities shown by cytogenetic analysis in 1 case
  - Suggests that some lesions may be neoplastic rather than reactive

CLINICAL ISSUES

Epidemiology

- Age
  - Adults
    - Predominantly 3rd-5th decades
- Gender
  - M > F

Site

- Occurs adjacent to large joints
  - 90% occur around knee joint
  - Also shoulder, elbow, ankle, and hip
- Can involve periarticular tendons, ligaments, joint capsules, muscles, and subcutis

Presentation

- Painful or painless mass
  - Lesion duration varies

Prognosis

- Local recurrence in approximately 30%
- No malignant transformation reported

MACROSCOPIC FEATURES

General Features

- Myxoid, gelatinous cut surface
- May be cystic

Size

- Varies from < 1 cm to > 10 cm
- Mean size: 3.5 cm

MICROSCOPIC PATHOLOGY

Histologic Features

- Spindle or stellate fibroblast-like cells
  - Cytologically bland
- Myxoid stroma
  - Hypovascular
- May have areas of increased cellularity
- Mitotic figures rare or absent
- Cystic spaces present in many
  - Ganglion-like
  - Lined by fibrin or collagen
- Hemorrhage
- Hemosiderin deposition
- May have fibrin deposition
- Variable mild chronic inflammatory cell infiltrate
- Borders often ill defined, with infiltration of adjacent tissue

ANCILLARY TESTS

Immunohistochemistry

- Similar immunoprofile to intramuscular myxoma

JUXTAARTICULAR MYXOMA

Key Facts

Terminology
- Benign lesion occurring in region of large joints, with histologic features of myxoma

Etiology/Pathogenesis
- Some associated with trauma or occur adjacent to osteoarthritic joint
- Clonal chromosomal abnormalities in 1 case suggest that some lesions may be neoplastic

Clinical Issues
- 90% occur around knee joint
- Local recurrence in a proportion of cases

Microscopic Pathology
- Bland spindle or stellate fibroblast-like cells
- Hypovascular myxoid stroma
- Cystic spaces present in many
- Mitotic figures rare or absent

  - CD34(+) and actin-sm(+) in some cases

Cytogenetics
- Analysis of 1 case showed 2 distinct cytogenetically abnormal cell populations
  - Clonal chromosomal changes suggest that some examples are neoplastic not reactive

Molecular Genetics
- Lack Arg 201 mutations of *GNAS1* gene found in intramuscular myxoma
  - Genetically distinct from intramuscular myxoma

DIFFERENTIAL DIAGNOSIS

Superficial Angiomyxoma
- Trunk, head and neck, or vulvovaginal sites
- Prominent vasculature
- Can have neutrophilic infiltrate
- May contain admixed epithelial structures

Intramuscular Myxoma
- Most common in large muscles of lower limb
- Many contain mutations of *GNAS1* gene

Myxoid Neurofibroma
- Buckled, elongated nuclei
- S100 protein(+)

Aggressive Angiomyxoma
- Adult women
- Deep soft tissues of vulvovaginal region
- Numerous vessels of varying sizes

Myxofibrosarcoma
- Often subcutaneous location
- Greater cellularity
- Cellular atypia
- Prominent coarse vascularity in stroma

Low-Grade Fibromyxoid Sarcoma
- Greater cellularity
- May contain collagen rosettes
- Fibrous areas also prominent
- Characteristic translocations

SELECTED REFERENCES

1. Okamoto S et al: Juxta-articular myxoma and intramuscular myxoma are two distinct entities. Activating Gs alpha mutation at Arg 201 codon does not occur in juxta-articular myxoma. Virchows Arch. 440(1):12-5, 2002
2. Allen PW: Myxoma is not a single entity: a review of the concept of myxoma. Ann Diagn Pathol. 4(2):99-123, 2000
3. Okamoto S et al: Activating Gs(alpha) mutation in intramuscular myxomas with and without fibrous dysplasia of bone. Virchows Arch. 437(2):133-7, 2000
4. Sciot R et al: Clonal chromosomal changes in juxta-articular myxoma. Virchows Arch. 434(2):177-80, 1999
5. Meis JM et al: Juxta-articular myxoma: a clinical and pathologic study of 65 cases. Hum Pathol. 23(6):639-46, 1992

IMAGE GALLERY

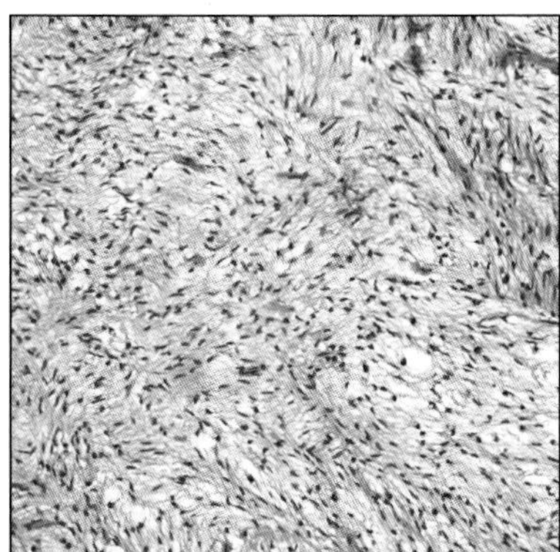
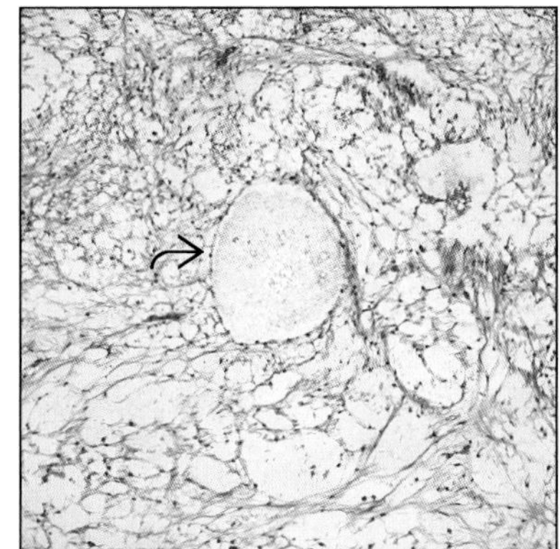
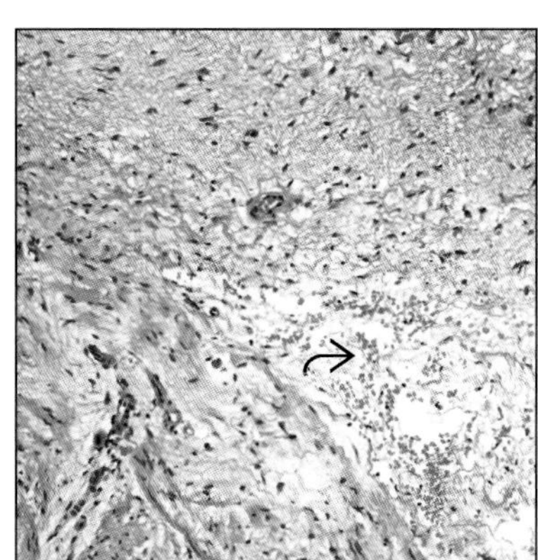

(Left) *In this juxtaarticular myxoma, the cells are spindle to stellate, with small hyperchromatic nuclei and fibrillary cytoplasm, and are embedded within myxoid or myxocollagenous stroma.* ***(Center)*** *Stromal cysts can be prominent features ⇨. The hypovascularity of the myxoid matrix is also notable.* ***(Right)*** *There is often hemorrhage ⇨, and there may be hemosiderin deposition and an interspersed inflammatory infiltrate.*

SUPERFICIAL ANGIOMYXOMA

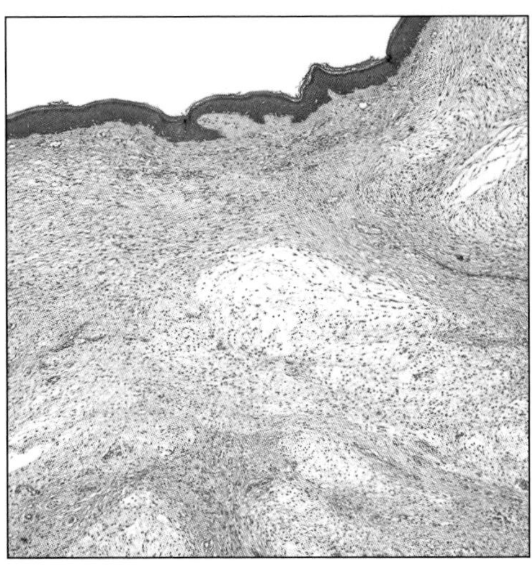

In this superficial angiomyxoma, the dermis shows an ill-defined lesion with prominent myxoid stroma. Lesions can also appear circumscribed.

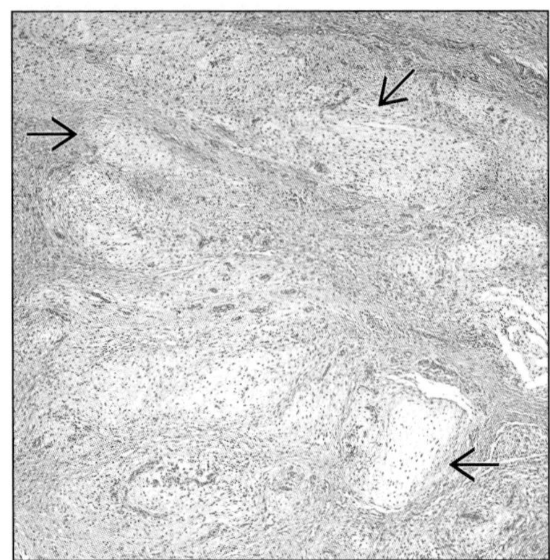

Superficial angiomyxoma has a multilobulated appearance ⇒ at low power and shows patternless distributions of spindle and stellate cells.

TERMINOLOGY

Synonyms

- Cutaneous myxoma

Definitions

- Benign, cutaneous myxoid lesion, associated in some cases with Carney complex

CLINICAL ISSUES

Epidemiology

- Age
  - Adults (mean: 3rd-5th decades)
    - Rarely congenital
- Gender
  - Slight male preponderance

Site

- Most common on trunk, head and neck, and lower extremities
- Smaller proportion occur in genital area
- Predilection for ear, eyelid, and nipple in Carney complex
- Rarely in oral cavity

Presentation

- Incidental, painless mass
- Papule, nodule, or polyp

Treatment

- Surgical approaches
  - Local excision with follow-up

Prognosis

- Can recur if incompletely excised
- Does not metastasize

MACROSCOPIC FEATURES

General Features

- Usually solitary
  - Can be multiple
    - Especially in Carney complex
- Usually circumscribed
- Gelatinous cut surface
- May contain keratinous debris

Size

- Mostly small (up to 5 cm)

MICROSCOPIC PATHOLOGY

Histologic Features

- Lobular and sparsely cellular
- Commonly in dermis
  - Can extend into subcutis and occasionally skeletal muscle
- Spindle and stellate cells in myxoid stroma
  - Minimal to mild atypia
  - Often bi- or multinucleated
- Mitoses rare
- Divided into poorly defined lobules by fibrous septa
- Vasculature may be prominent
  - Arborizing thin-walled vessels
- Sparse mixed inflammatory infiltrate
  - Neutrophils can be prominent
- Bland epithelial structures admixed in up to 25%
  - Epidermoid cysts
  - Strands of squamous epithelium
  - Buds of basaloid cells
  - Possibly represent entrapped adnexal structures
- Acellular mucin pools

SUPERFICIAL ANGIOMYXOMA

Key Facts

Terminology
- Benign, cutaneous myxoid lesion, associated in some cases with Carney complex

Clinical Issues
- Trunk, head and neck, lower extremities, and genital area

Microscopic Pathology
- Lobular and sparsely cellular
- Spindle and stellate cells in myxoid stroma
- Minimal to mild atypia
- Sparse inflammatory infiltrate
  - Neutrophils
- Vasculature may be prominent
- Admixed epithelial structures in some cases

Ancillary Tests
- CD34 expression
- Occasional actin-sm expression

ANCILLARY TESTS

Immunohistochemistry
- Immunoreactive for CD34
- Occasional SMA and muscle specific actin expression
- Negative for desmin, S100 protein, cytokeratin, and ER and PR

DIFFERENTIAL DIAGNOSIS

Digital Mucous Cyst
- Typically on dorsum of fingers
- Lacks lobular architecture and neutrophils

Dermal Nerve Sheath Myxoma
- Prominent lobular architecture
- Cells usually strongly S100 protein(+)
- Most are also GFAP(+)
- EMA reactivity in perineurial cells bordering tumor nodules

Myxoid Neurofibroma
- Buckled, elongated nuclei
- S100 protein(+)

Superficial Acral Fibromyxoma
- Acral extremities; often periungual
- Fibrous and myxoid stroma

Aggressive Angiomyxoma
- Usually pelvic and perineal regions of females
- Lesions larger, deeper, and invade surrounding tissues

Myxoid Liposarcoma
- Deeper location
- Curvilinear vascular pattern
- Lipoblasts often present
- Characteristic translocations

Low-Grade Myxofibrosarcoma
- Greater cellularity
- Cellular atypia
- Prominent coarse vascular pattern

Low-Grade Fibromyxoid Sarcoma
- Usually larger and deeper
- Prominent fibrous areas
- May contain giant collagen rosettes
- Characteristic translocations

SELECTED REFERENCES

1. Allen PW: Myxoma is not a single entity: a review of the concept of myxoma. Ann Diagn Pathol. 4(2):99-123, 2000
2. Calonje E et al: Superficial angiomyxoma: clinicopathologic analysis of a series of distinctive but poorly recognized cutaneous tumors with tendency for recurrence. Am J Surg Pathol. 23(8):910-7, 1999
3. Fetsch JF et al: Superficial angiomyxoma (cutaneous myxoma): a clinicopathologic study of 17 cases arising in the genital region. Int J Gynecol Pathol. 16(4):325-34, 1997

IMAGE GALLERY

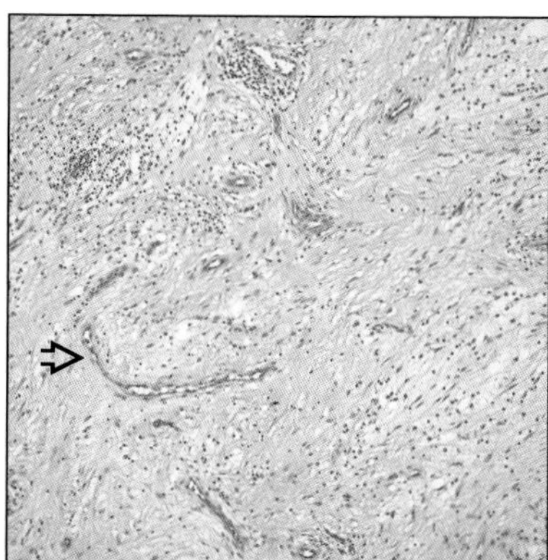
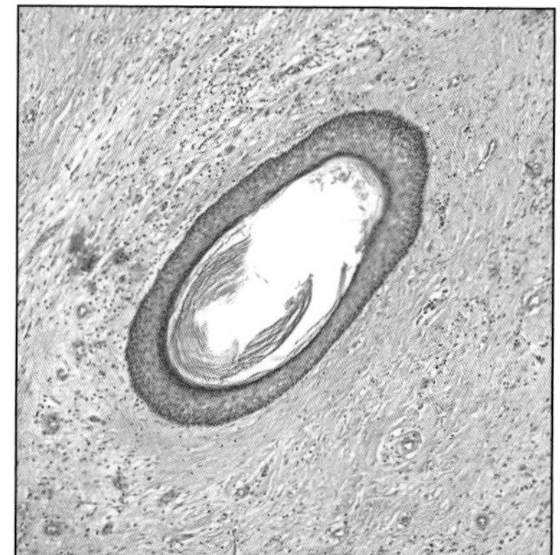
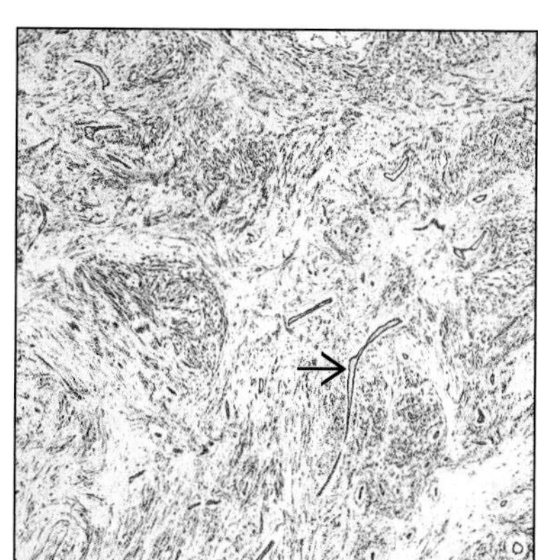

(Left) *This superficial angiomyxoma is sparsely cellular, with prominent myxoid or fibromyxoid stroma. Vasculature can be prominent ⇨. Inflammatory cells include neutrophils.* ***(Center)*** *Bland epithelial inclusions are often admixed. Here there is an island of squamous epithelium with keratin, which may represent an entrapped adnexal structure.* ***(Right)*** *There is strong expression of CD34 within spindle and stellate cells. Note also the prominent vasculature →.*

SUPERFICIAL ACRAL FIBROMYXOMA

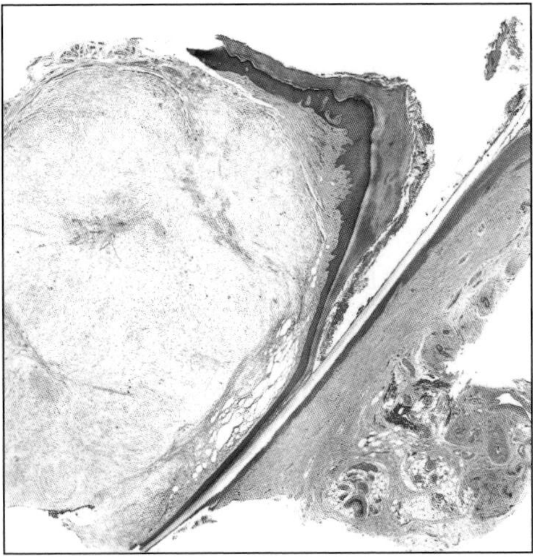

Hematoxylin & eosin shows a low-power view of a hypocellular dermal neoplasm in the nail bed region.

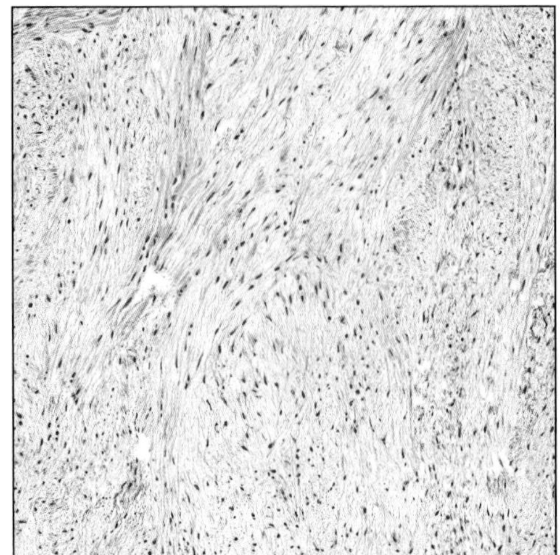

Hematoxylin & eosin shows relatively bland spindle-shaped tumor cells arranged in loose fascicles and set in a myxoid stroma.

TERMINOLOGY

Abbreviations

- Superficial acral fibromyxoma (SAF)

Definitions

- Benign fibroblastic neoplasm with predilection for hands and feet, especially nail bed region

ETIOLOGY/PATHOGENESIS

Environmental Exposure

- Previous trauma reported only rarely

CLINICAL ISSUES

Epidemiology

- Incidence
  - Rare
- Age
  - Mainly adults
- Gender
  - More frequent in males

Presentation

- Solitary mass
- Usually painless lesions
- Longstanding lesions
- Dermal subcutaneous neoplasms
- Arise usually on toe, finger, or palm of hand
- Majority of cases involve nail bed region
- Rare on heel

Natural History

- Local recurrences sometimes seen
- No reported case of metastasis or progression

Treatment

- Surgical approaches
  - Complete excision

Prognosis

- Biologically benign neoplasm
- Recurrences have been reported in up to 22%

MACROSCOPIC FEATURES

General Features

- Superficial lesions
- Lesions may appear dome-shaped, polypoid, or verrucoid

Size

- Usually < 5 cm

MICROSCOPIC PATHOLOGY

Histologic Features

- Moderately cellular
- Nodular, lobular, or infiltrative growth
- Dermal neoplasms with involvement of deeper structures in some cases
- Myxoid, myxocollagenous, or predominantly collagenous stroma
- Numerous blood vessels
- Rarely contains lipomatous component
- May contain inflammatory cells (mast cells)
- Minimal cytologic atypia
- Rare mitoses
- Increased cellularity and atypia
  - Have no prognostic influence

Predominant Pattern/Injury Type

- Storiform
- Fascicular

Predominant Cell/Compartment Type

- Spindle
  - Spindled and stellate fibroblast-like cells

SUPERFICIAL ACRAL FIBROMYXOMA

Key Facts

Terminology
- Benign fibroblastic neoplasm with predilection for hands and feet, especially nail bed region

Clinical Issues
- Solitary mass involving toe, finger, or palm of hand
- Significant number of cases involve nail region
- Dermal subcutaneous neoplasm
- Incidence: Rare
- Age: Mainly adults
- Treatment: Complete excision
- Prognosis
  - Biologically benign neoplasm
  - Local recurrences rare

Macroscopic Features
- Superficial lesions

Microscopic Pathology
- Dermal neoplasms with involvement of deeper structures in some cases
- Loose storiform &/or fascicular growth pattern
- Rare infiltrative growth
- Spindled and stellate fibroblast-like cells
- Rare multinucleated cells
- Moderately cellular
- Minimal cytologic atypia
- Rare mitoses
- Scattered inflammatory cells (mast cells)
- CD34 and EMA often positive

  - Multinucleated stromal cells may be present

DIFFERENTIAL DIAGNOSIS

Dermatofibroma
- Hyperplastic epidermis
- Stellate growth
- Mainly dermal lesions
- Spindled and histiocytoid cells
- Storiform growth
- Hyalinized collagenous stroma
- Rarely myxoid stroma
- CD34(-)
- EMA(-)

Dermatofibrosarcoma Protuberans
- Exophytic neoplasms on trunk or proximal parts of extremities
- Infiltrating, destructive neoplasms
- Numerous local recurrences
- Fibrosarcomatous progression
- Monotonous storiform growth pattern
- Diffuse infiltration of subcutaneous tissue
- Bland neuroid tumor cells
- Rarely myxoid
- Homogeneous CD34 expression
- Characteristic genetic changes

Acquired Digital Fibrokeratoma
- Hyperkeratotic lesion
- Normocellular connective tissue core

Sclerosing Perineurioma
- Small epithelioid and spindled cells
- Whorled (perivascular) growth pattern
- Myxohyaline stroma
- EMA(+)
- Claudin-1(+)

Superficial Angiomyxoma
- Lobular growth
- Blood vessels with slightly fibrosed walls
- Prominent myxoid stroma
- Perivascular neutrophils

Low-Grade Fibromyxoid Sarcoma
- Only rarely superficial
- Characteristic whorling growth pattern
- Varying myxoid and collagenous stroma
- May contain giant rosettes
- Bland spindled tumor cells
- Arcades of blood vessels
- Characteristic genetic changes
  - Translocation t(7;16)(q33;p11)
  - *FUS-CREB3L2* (or rarely *FUS-CREB3L1*) fusion gene

Acral Myxoinflammatory Fibroblastic Sarcoma
- Mainly subcutaneous
- Ill-defined, multinodular growth
- Contains large cells with large and pleomorphic nuclei containing prominent nucleoli
- Atypical spindle-shaped tumor cells
- Pseudolipoblasts sometimes present
- Prominent inflammatory infiltrate

Low-Grade Myxofibrosarcoma
- Multinodular neoplasm
- Atypical fibroblastic cells
- Enlarged, hyperchromatic nuclei
- May contain pseudolipoblasts
- Mitoses
- Prominent myxoid stroma
- Elongated curvilinear blood vessels

Myxoid Neurofibroma
- Elongated wrinkled nuclei
- Diffuse growth
- S100 protein(+)
- Axons sometimes detectable by immunostaining for neurofilaments

Myxoid Leiomyoma
- Eosinophilic tumor cells
- Fibrillary cytoplasm

SUPERFICIAL ACRAL FIBROMYXOMA

Immunohistochemistry

Antibody	Reactivity	Staining Pattern	Comment
CD34	Positive	Cytoplasmic	Positive in ~ 1/2 of the cases
EMA	Positive	Cytoplasmic	Positive in ~ 1/2 of the cases
CD10	Positive	Cytoplasmic	
CD99	Positive	Cytoplasmic	
Nestin	Positive		
S100	Negative		
Actin-sm	Negative		
CK-PAN	Negative		
Desmin	Negative		

- Cigar-shaped nuclei
- Expression of myogenic markers
  - SMA, desmin, H-caldesmon

Myxoid Leiomyosarcoma

- Eosinophilic tumor cells
- Enlarged, hyperchromatic nuclei
- Increased mitoses
- Expression of myogenic markers
  - SMA, desmin, H-caldesmon

Myxoid Epithelioid Sarcoma

- Locally aggressive neoplasm
- Numerous recurrences
- Numerous metastases
- Mainly composed of epithelioid tumor cells
- Granulomatous, nodular growth
- Loss of INI1 expression
- Expression of epithelial markers
  - Pancytokeratin, EMA

Myxoid Solitary Fibrous Tumor

- Rare in superficial location
- Varying cellularity
- Elongated spindled tumor cells with neuroid features
- Hemangiopericytoma-like vessels
- Keloid-like stromal hyalinizations

DIAGNOSTIC CHECKLIST

Clinically Relevant Pathologic Features

- Organ distribution
  - Often involvement of nail bed region

Pathologic Interpretation Pearls

- Spindled and stellate fibroblast-like tumor cells
- Absence of significant nuclear pleomorphism
- Fascicular or loose storiform growth pattern
- Varying myxoid/collagenous stroma
- CD34 and EMA often positive

SELECTED REFERENCES

1. Al-Daraji WI et al: Superficial acral fibromyxoma: a clinicopathological analysis of 32 tumors including 4 in the heel. J Cutan Pathol. 35(11):1020-6, 2008
2. Al-Daraji WI et al: Superficial acral fibromyxoma: report of two cases and discussion of the nomenclature. Dermatol Online J. 14(2):27, 2008
3. Lisovsky M et al: Apolipoprotein D in CD34-positive and CD34-negative cutaneous neoplasms: a useful marker in differentiating superficial acral fibromyxoma from dermatofibrosarcoma protuberans. Mod Pathol. 21(1):31-8, 2008
4. Misago N et al: Superficial acral fibromyxoma on the tip of the big toe: expression of CD10 and nestin. J Eur Acad Dermatol Venereol. 22(2):255-7, 2008
5. Oteo-Alvaro A et al: Superficial acral fibromyxoma of the toe, with erosion of the distal phalanx. A clinical report. Arch Orthop Trauma Surg. 128(3):271-4, 2008
6. Prescott RJ et al: Superficial acral fibromyxoma: a clinicopathological study of new 41 cases from the U.K.: should myxoma (NOS) and fibroma (NOS) continue as part of 21st-century reporting? Br J Dermatol. 159(6):1315-21, 2008
7. Tardío JC et al: Superficial acral fibromyxoma: report of 4 cases with CD10 expression and lipomatous component, two previously underrecognized features. Am J Dermatopathol. 30(5):431-5, 2008
8. Varikatt W et al: Superficial acral fibromyxoma: a report of two cases with radiological findings. Skeletal Radiol. 37(6):499-503, 2008
9. Mentzel T et al: Myxoid dermatofibrosarcoma protuberans: clinicopathologic, immunohistochemical, and molecular analysis of eight cases. Am J Dermatopathol. 29(5):443-8, 2007
10. Abou-Nukta F et al: Superficial acral fibromyxoma of the distal phalanx of the thumb. J Hand Surg [Br]. 31(6):619-20, 2006
11. McNiff JM et al: Cellular digital fibromas: distinctive CD34-positive lesions that may mimic dermatofibrosarcoma protuberans. J Cutan Pathol. 32(6):413-8, 2005
12. Perret AG et al: [Superficial angiomyxoma: report of four cases, including two subungueal tumors] Ann Pathol. 25(1):54-7, 2005
13. Quaba O et al: Superficial acral fibromyxoma. Br J Plast Surg. 58(4):561-4, 2005
14. André J et al: Superficial acral fibromyxoma: clinical and pathological features. Am J Dermatopathol. 26(6):472-4, 2004
15. Meyerle JH et al: Superficial acral fibromyxoma of the index finger. J Am Acad Dermatol. 50(1):134-6, 2004
16. Kazakov DV et al: Superficial acral fibromyxoma: report of two cases. Dermatology. 205(3):285-8, 2002
17. Fetsch JF et al: Superficial acral fibromyxoma: a clinicopathologic and immunohistochemical analysis of 37 cases of a distinctive soft tissue tumor with a predilection for the fingers and toes. Hum Pathol. 32(7):704-14, 2001

Microscopic Features

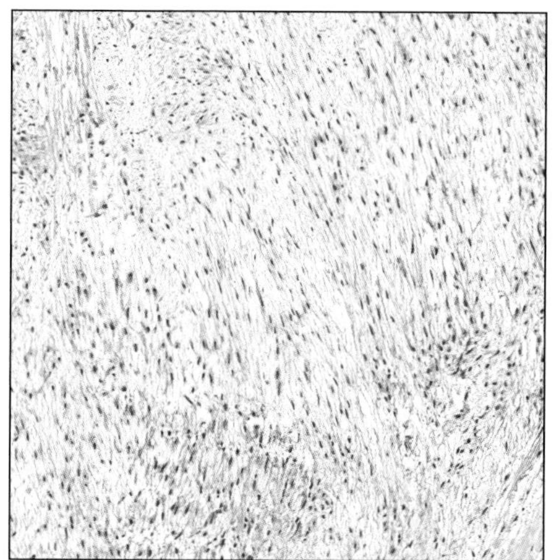

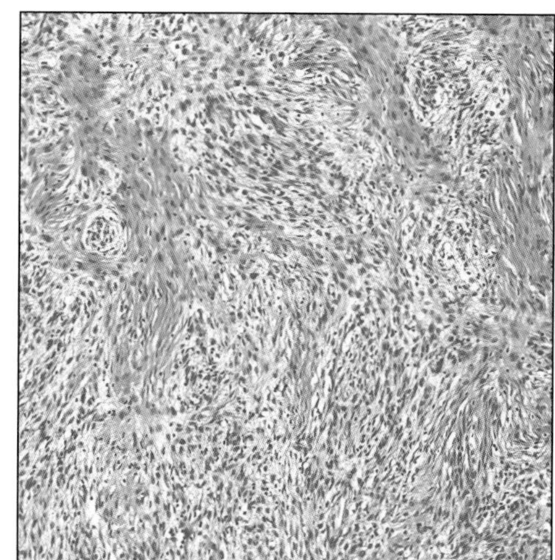

(Left) *Hematoxylin & eosin shows a predominantly myxoid spindle cell neoplasm with variable cellularity.* ***(Right)*** *Hematoxylin & eosin shows a more cellular lesion composed of spindled tumor cells set in a varying myxoid and collagenous stroma.*

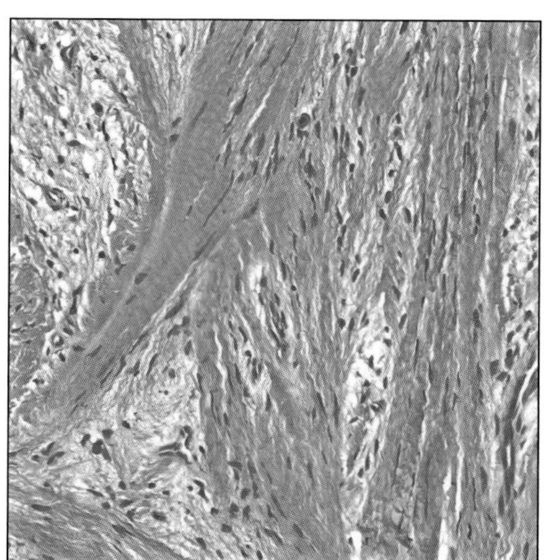

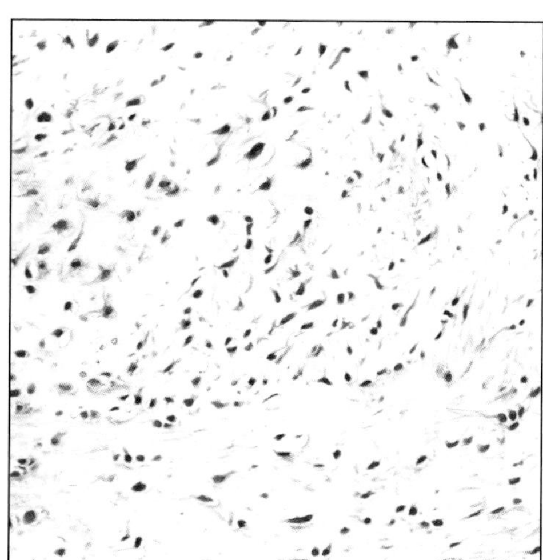

(Left) *High-power view shows bland spindled tumor cells with an ill-defined, pale, eosinophilic cytoplasm and elongated nuclei. Note the scattered mast cells and fibrous bands.* ***(Right)*** *Hematoxylin & eosin shows focal chondroid stromal changes in this example of superficial acral fibromyxoma.*

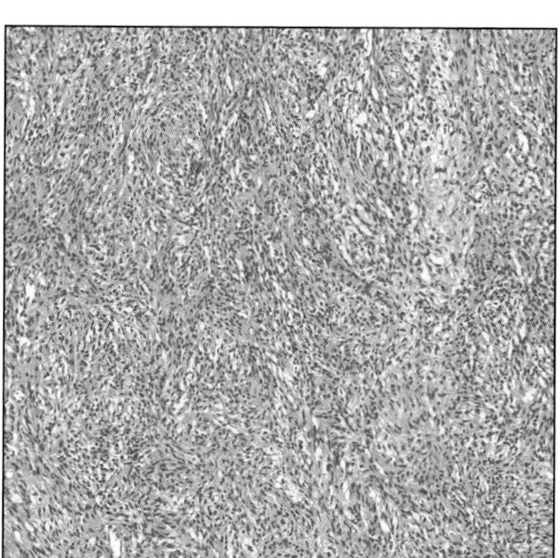

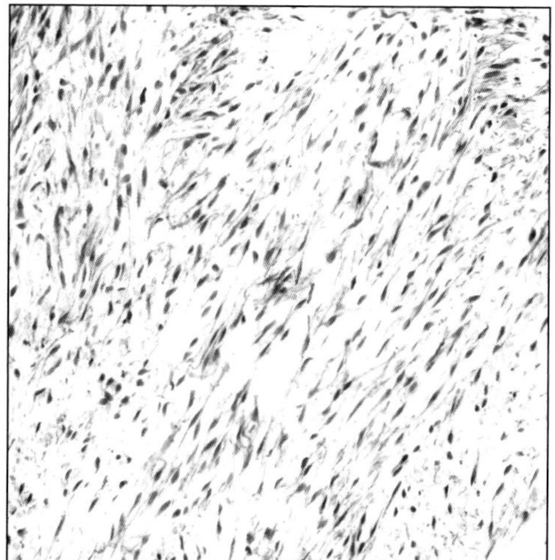

(Left) *Hematoxylin & eosin shows a markedly cellular superficial acral fibromyxoma with minimal stroma.* ***(Right)*** *Positive EMA shows predominantly cytoplasmic expression.*

HEMOSIDEROTIC FIBROHISTIOCYTIC LIPOMATOUS LESION

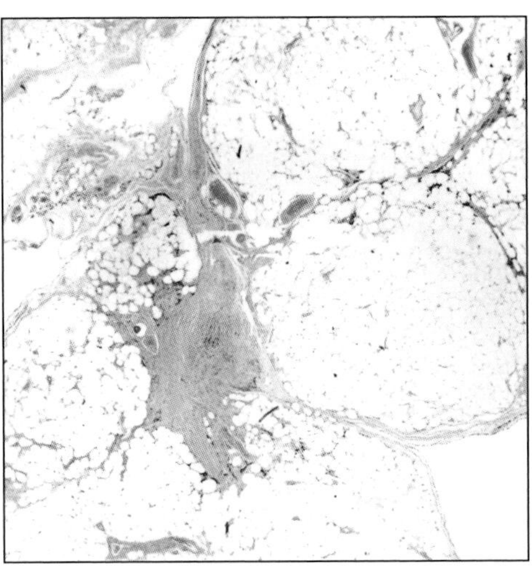

Hemosiderotic fibrohistiocytic lipomatous lesion (HFLL) is composed largely of homogeneous fat with septal proliferations. It is not a mass-like lesion.

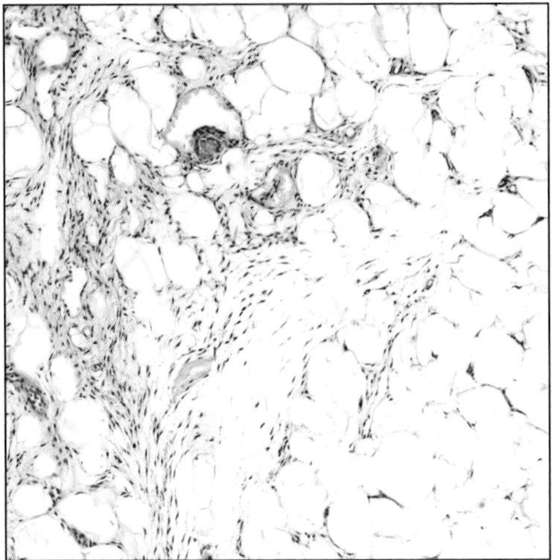

The septal proliferations are sometimes wispy, myxoid, spindled, inflamed, and hemosiderin-rich, as seen here.

TERMINOLOGY

Abbreviations

- Hemosiderotic fibrohistiocytic lipomatous lesion (HFLL)

Synonyms

- Hemosiderotic fibrolipomatous tumor is separate entity from pleomorphic hyalinizing angiectatic tumor (PHAT)

Definitions

- Benign, probably reactive, lesion that occurs in ankle region of adult women
  - Usually secondary to ill-fitting shoes or other trauma
  - Composed predominantly of fat with septal spindled, inflammatory, and hemosiderin changes

ETIOLOGY/PATHOGENESIS

Typical Cause

- Trauma or ill-fitting shoes

CLINICAL ISSUES

Epidemiology

- Incidence
  - Rare
    - Less than 0.2% (10/5,666 benign lipomatous tumors)
- Age
  - Adults
    - Range: 42-63 years
    - Median: 50 years
- Gender
  - 80% females

Site

- Foot and ankle (80%)
- Hand/cheek is rare

Presentation

- Subcutaneous mass

Treatment

- Complete excision for diagnosis

Prognosis

- Excellent, benign, probably reactive
- 50% recurrence in this rare entity

MACROSCOPIC FEATURES

General Features

- Fatty process with dark yellow-brown to white small nodularity

MICROSCOPIC PATHOLOGY

Histologic Features

- Subcutaneous lobules of homogeneous fat
- Predominantly septal spindled change
- Plump, but no significant pleomorphism
- Occasional floret-type and osteoclast-type giant cells
- No mitotic activity
- Myxoid change may be present
- Inflamed, including xanthoma cells, lymphocytes, plasma cells, and mast cells
- Hemosiderin (abundant iron pigment) always present
- No mass-like proliferation of spindled cells

Predominant Pattern/Injury Type

- Circumscribed

Predominant Cell/Compartment Type

- Fibrohistiocytic

HEMOSIDEROTIC FIBROHISTIOCYTIC LIPOMATOUS LESION

Key Facts

Terminology
- Benign, probably reactive, lesion that occurs in ankle region of adult females, usually secondary to ill-fitting shoes or other trauma
- Composed predominantly of fat with septal spindled, inflammatory, and hemosiderin changes

Clinical Issues
- Ankle
- Middle-aged females

Microscopic Pathology
- Subcutaneous
- Lobules of fat with homogeneous adipocytes
- Predominantly septal spindled change
- Plump but no significant pleomorphism
- Occasionally floret or osteoclast giant cells
- No mitotic activity
- Inflammation including xanthoma cells, plasma cells, mast cells

Immunohistochemistry
- Vimentin, CD34, calponin, lysozyme, CD68 positive
- S100, HMB-45, keratins, EMA, desmin, actin-sm, caldesmon negative

DIFFERENTIAL DIAGNOSIS

Fibrous Histiocytoma
- Dermal-based, solitary spindled mass
- Pushing, stellate periphery
- Rare involvement of subcutis in deep lesions
- Lack of mast cells

Acroangiodermatitis of Mali
- Distal lower extremity ulceration
- Vascular insufficiency
- Dermal vascular proliferation
- No fat
- Not subcutaneous, spindled, or hemosiderin-rich

Pleomorphic Hyalinizing Angiectatic Tumor of Soft Parts
- Ankle location, but occurs elsewhere
- No history of trauma
- Female predominance
- Solid mass, no fat
- Atypia, ectatic and hyalinized vessels, pseudoinclusion
- CD34(+)
- Low grade, malignant

Dermatofibrosarcoma Protuberans
- Infiltrates fat, but dermal/subcutaneous junction based
- Storiform growth pattern
- Monotonous spindled cells, no inflammation or hemosiderin
- CD34(+)
- Low grade, malignant

SELECTED REFERENCES

1. Browne TJ et al: Haemosiderotic fibrolipomatous tumour (so-called haemosiderotic fibrohistiocytic lipomatous tumour): analysis of 13 new cases in support of a distinct entity. Histopathology. 48(4):453-61, 2006
2. Kazakov DV et al: Hemosiderotic fibrohistiocytic lipomatous lesion: clinical correlation with venous stasis. Virchows Arch. 447(1):103-6, 2005
3. Michal M et al: Relationship between pleomorphic hyalinizing angiectatic tumor and nemosiderotic fibrohistiocytic lipomatous lesion. Am J Surg Pathol. 29(9):1256-7; author reply 1259, 2005
4. Folpe AL et al: Pleomorphic hyalinizing angiectatic tumor: analysis of 41 cases supporting evolution from a distinctive precursor lesion. Am J Surg Pathol. 28(11):1417-25, 2004
5. Guillou L et al: Newly described adipocytic lesions. Semin Diagn Pathol. 18(4):238-49, 2001
6. Marshall-Taylor C et al: Hemosiderotic fibrohistiocytic lipomatous lesion: ten cases of a previously undescribed fatty lesion of the foot/ankle. Mod Pathol. 13(11):1192-9, 2000

IMAGE GALLERY

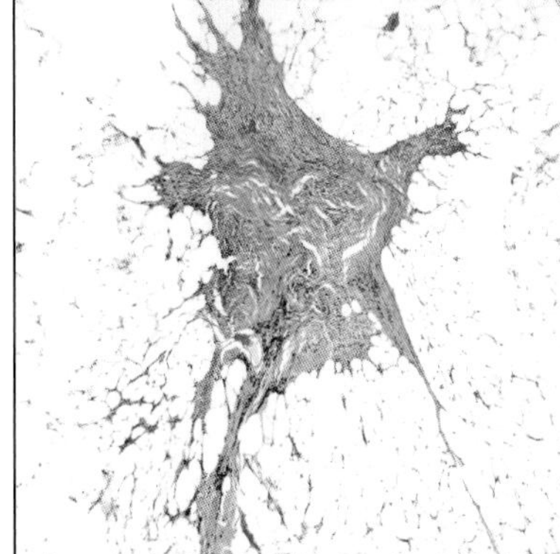

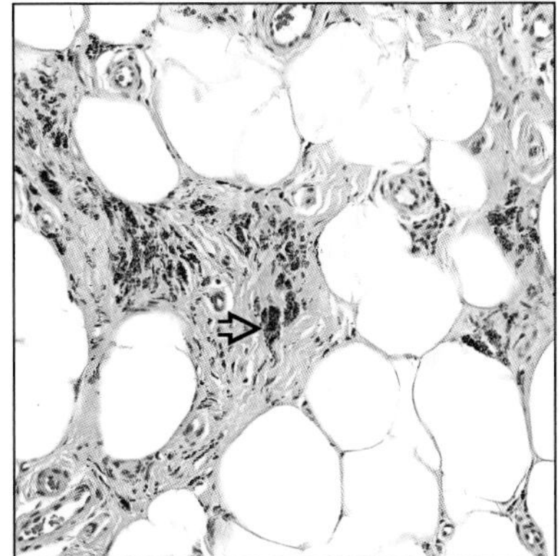

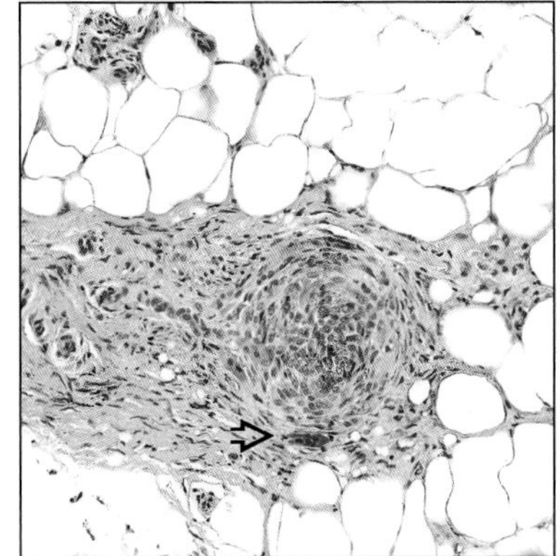

(Left) *At higher magnification, the spindled cells have hemosiderin pigment and resemble a reactive process.* ***(Center)*** *Note the admixture of the spindled cells with fat. There is no solid component, even in recurrences. Hemosiderin pigment is prominent ⇨.* ***(Right)*** *HFLL can have floret cells or even osteoclast-type giant cells, the latter demonstrated here ⇨.*

PLEOMORPHIC HYALINIZING ANGIECTATIC TUMOR

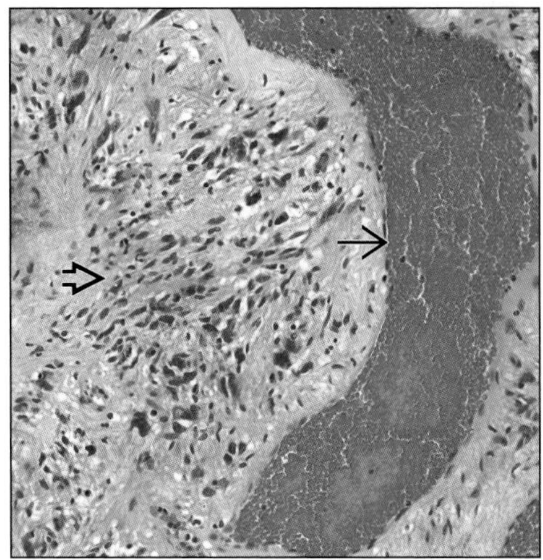

Pleomorphic spindle and polygonal cells ⇨ lie in fibrous stroma adjacent to an angiectatic thin-walled vessel →. The cells have hyperchromatic nuclei but lack prominent nucleoli and mitoses.

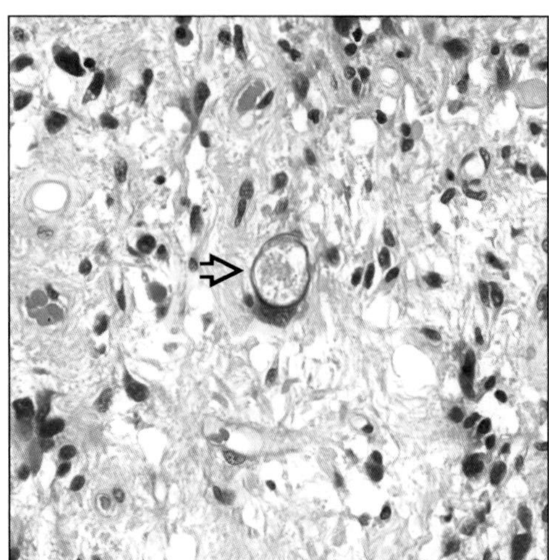

Prominent nuclear inclusions ⇨ are a feature of PHAT; they represent included cytoplasm. This appearance should not be misinterpreted as a signet ring adenocarcinoma cell.

TERMINOLOGY

Abbreviations

- Pleomorphic hyalinizing angiectatic tumor (PHAT)

Definitions

- Locally recurrent but nonmetastasizing tumor characterized by dilated vascular spaces and atypical spindle cells

ETIOLOGY/PATHOGENESIS

Neoplastic

- Early PHAT resembles hemosiderotic fibrohistiocytic lipomatous lesion

CLINICAL ISSUES

Epidemiology

- Age
  - Mostly adults; range: 10-79 years (median: 51 years)
- Gender
  - Slight female predominance

Site

- Subcutaneous
- Majority at ankle
- Leg, thigh, rarely other sites

Presentation

- Painless mass

Natural History

- Grows slowly, can persist following excision
- 1 case developed myxofibrosarcoma in recurrence

Prognosis

- About 1/3 recur locally following excision
- No metastases reported

MACROSCOPIC FEATURES

General Features

- Circumscribed
- Dark brown or red due to hemorrhage
- Discoloration extends into adjacent fat

Size

- Median: 6 cm; range: < 1 cm to 20 cm

MICROSCOPIC PATHOLOGY

Histologic Features

- Circumscribed but not encapsulated
- Angiectatic thin-walled vessels in clusters
  - Fibrinoid and hyaline material in vessel walls
- Spindle cells with hyperchromatic enlarged nuclei
  - Prominent intranuclear cytoplasmic inclusions
- Hemosiderin pigment in tumor cell cytoplasm
- Focal myxoid change
- No or minimal mitotic activity
- No necrosis

Predominant Pattern/Injury Type

- Hemorrhagic

Predominant Cell/Compartment Type

- Fibroblast

ANCILLARY TESTS

Electron Microscopy

- Transmission
  - Atypical cells appear fibroblastic
    - Cytoplasm has abundant vimentin-reactive intermediate filaments
    - Ganglion cell-like fibroblasts reported

PLEOMORPHIC HYALINIZING ANGIECTATIC TUMOR

Key Facts

Terminology
- Locally recurrent but nonmetastasizing tumor characterized by dilated vascular spaces and atypical spindle cells

Etiology/Pathogenesis
- Early PHAT resembles hemosiderotic fibrohistiocytic lipomatous lesion

Clinical Issues
- Subcutaneous
- Majority at ankle
- About 1/3 recur locally following excision

Macroscopic Features
- Circumscribed
- Dark brown or red due to hemorrhage

Microscopic Pathology
- Angiectatic thin-walled vessels in clusters
- Fibrinoid and hyaline material in vessel walls
- Spindle cells with hyperchromatic enlarged nuclei
- Prominent intranuclear cytoplasmic inclusions
- Hemosiderin pigment in tumor cell cytoplasm
- No or minimal mitotic activity
- No necrosis

Ancillary Tests
- CD34(+) in majority
- S100 protein(-)

Top Differential Diagnoses
- Schwannoma
- Angiomatoid fibrous histiocytoma

Immunohistochemistry

Antibody	Reactivity	Staining Pattern	Comment
CD34	Positive	Cell membrane	In over 50% of cases
CD99	Positive	Cell membrane & cytoplasm	Some examples
VEGF	Positive	Cytoplasmic	Some examples
Vimentin	Positive	Cytoplasmic	Stains intermediate filaments; nonspecific
S100	Negative	Not applicable	Excludes schwannoma
Desmin	Negative	Not applicable	

DIFFERENTIAL DIAGNOSIS

Schwannoma
- Encapsulated
- S100 protein diffusely positive

Aneurysmal Fibrous Histiocytoma
- Predominantly dermal lesion
- Features of regular or cellular cutaneous fibrous histiocytoma
- Absence of pleomorphic fibroblasts
- Hemosiderin in macrophages and multinucleated cells

Angiomatoid Fibrous Histiocytoma
- Fibrous and lymphoid cuff
- Sheets of histiocyte-like cells
- Pleomorphism rare
- Desmin(+)
- Specific translocations

Undifferentiated Pleomorphic Sarcoma
- Proximal location
- Pleomorphism more marked and diffuse
- Frequent and abnormal mitoses
- Necrosis

Angiosarcoma
- Hemorrhagic
- Spaces lined by atypical cells
- Solid areas with epithelioid morphology
- Immunoreactive for CD34, CD31, and FLI-1

DIAGNOSTIC CHECKLIST

Clinically Relevant Pathologic Features
- Location
  - Mostly ankle or lower leg
  - In subcutis

Pathologic Interpretation Pearls
- Nuclear features
  - Pleomorphism without mitoses
- No necrosis

SELECTED REFERENCES

1. Ke Q et al: Clinicopathologic features of pleomorphic hyalinizing angiectatic tumor of soft parts. Chin Med J (Engl). 120(10):876-81, 2007
2. Capovilla M et al: Pleomorphic hyalinizing angiectatic tumor of soft parts: ultrastructural analysis of a case with original features. Ultrastruct Pathol. 30(1):59-64, 2006
3. Luzar B et al: Hemosiderotic fibrohistiocytic lipomatous lesion: early pleomorphic hyalinizing angiectatic tumor? Pathol Int. 56(5):283-6, 2006
4. Suarez-Vilela D et al: Lipoblast-like cells in early pleomorphic hyalinizing angiectatic tumor. Am J Surg Pathol. 29(9):1257-9; author reply 1259, 2005
5. Folpe AL et al: Pleomorphic hyalinizing angiectatic tumor: analysis of 41 cases supporting evolution from a distinctive precursor lesion. Am J Surg Pathol. 28(11):1417-25, 2004
6. Smith ME et al: Pleomorphic hyalinizing angiectatic tumor of soft parts. A low-grade neoplasm resembling neurilemoma. Am J Surg Pathol. 20(1):21-9, 1996

PLEOMORPHIC HYALINIZING ANGIECTATIC TUMOR

Gross and Microscopic Features

(Left) *This pleomorphic hyalinizing angiectatic tumor is partially circumscribed → but focally extends into fat →. The tumor is reddish-brown due to a combination of old and recent hemorrhage.* ***(Right)*** *Pleomorphic hyalinizing angiectatic tumor shows large angiectatic spaces containing thrombus →, separated by cellular fibrous tissue →. The lesion infiltrates subcutaneous fat at the periphery →.*

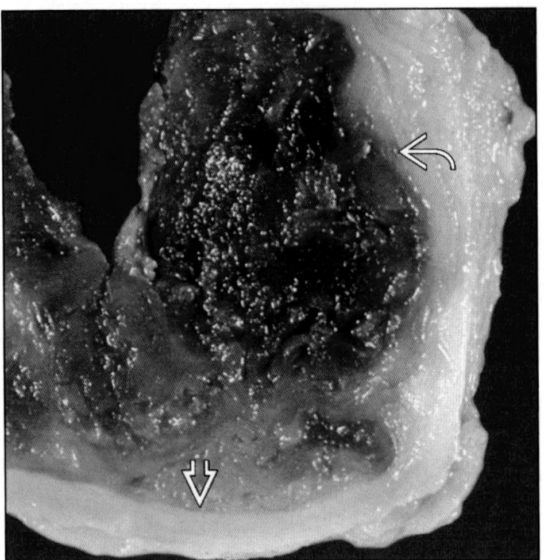

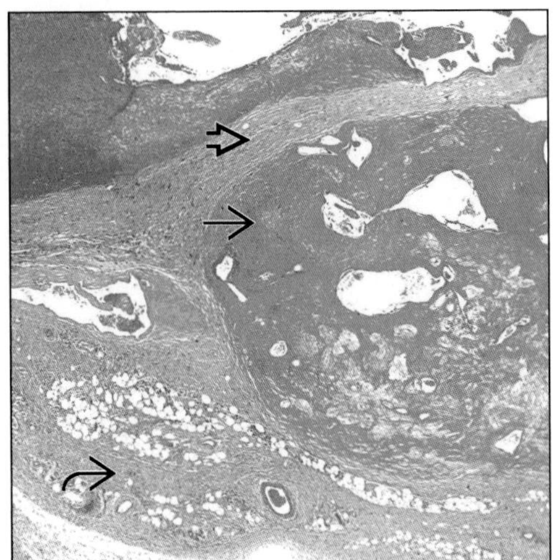

(Left) *This PHAT has dilated thin-walled vessels of varying size →, within variably cellular fibrous or myxoid stroma containing characteristic atypical cells →.* ***(Right)*** *This field shows a cluster of angiectatic blood vessels with variable caliber and irregular contours. The vessels have a periadventitial layer of extravasated fibrinoid material →.*

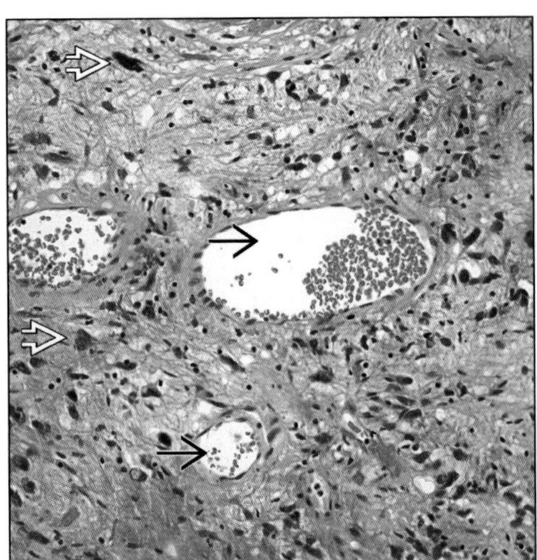

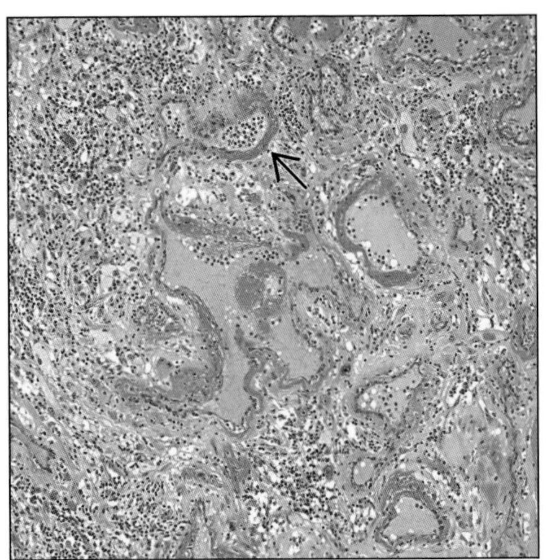

(Left) *This example of PHAT has thin-walled angiectatic vessels, some of which show fibrinoid material in parts of the wall and outside →. The pleomorphism of the lesion's stromal cells is evident at low magnification →.* ***(Right)*** *Higher magnification shows that fibrinoid material surrounds the vessel wall in a thin layer → and extends as a large deposit → into the adjacent stroma. This contains scattered inflammatory cells, but atypical stromal cells are absent.*

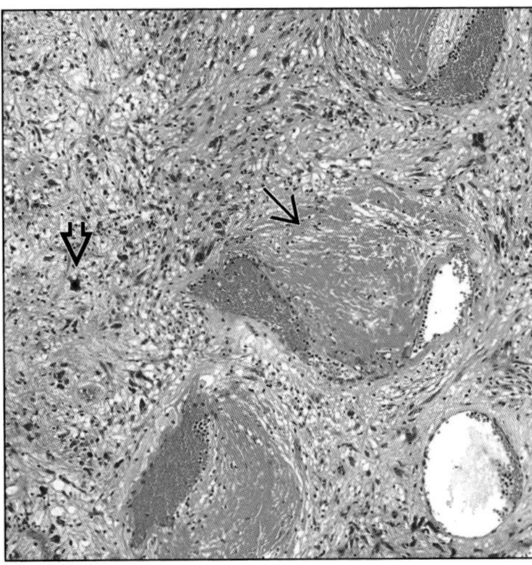

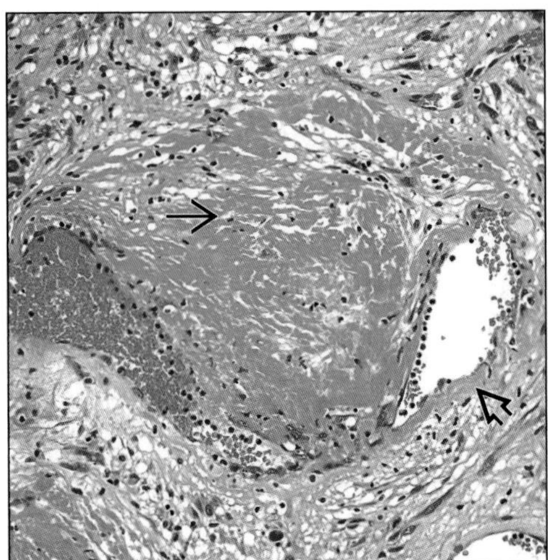

Microscopic Features

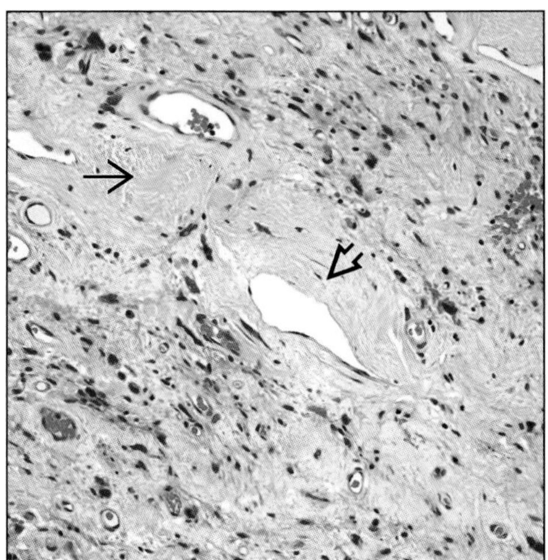

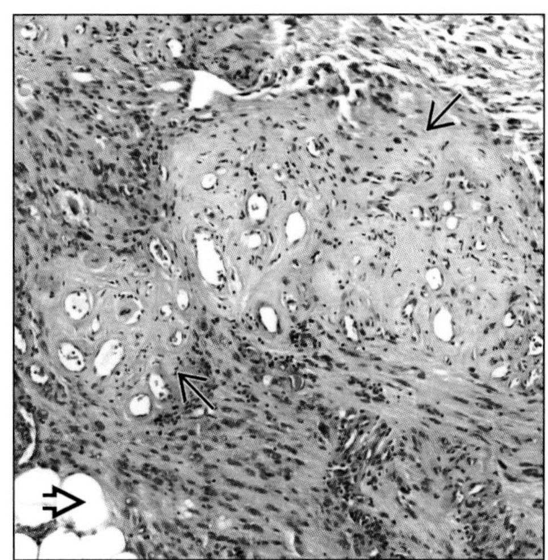

(Left) Perivascular ⇨ and interstitial → hyalinization are features of PHAT. A variable mixture of fibrinoid and collagenous material is usually seen. Presumably the hyalinization results from organization and fibrosis of the perivascular fibrinoid material. **(Right)** In this PHAT there are aggregates of angiectatic blood vessels with hyalinized walls that have fused →. This resembles the vascular changes in "ancient" schwannoma. Note the fatty tissue at the margin ⇨.

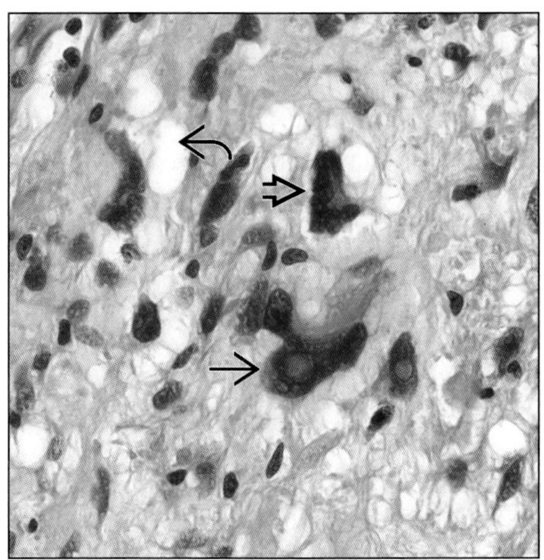

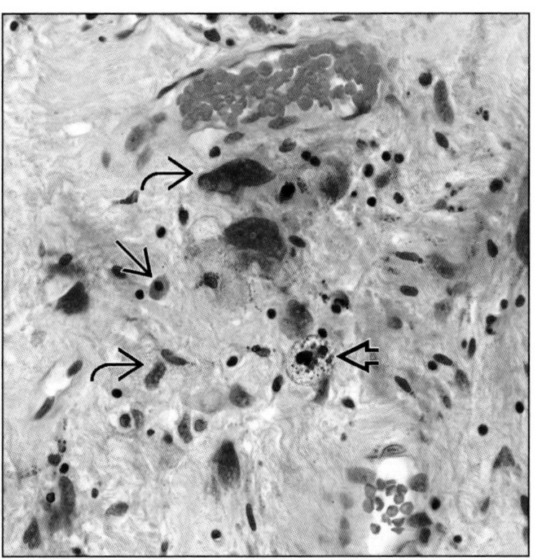

(Left) The atypical cells have enlarged hyperchromatic nuclei and can be multinucleated ⇨. Several nuclei have eosinophilic inclusions →. In this area, the stroma is myxoid and demonstrates microcyst formation ↷. **(Right)** The stroma in this example of PHAT contains lymphocytes, mast cells →, and hemosiderin pigment ⇨ in macrophages and tumor cells. Note the variation in size of the lesional spindle cells ↷.

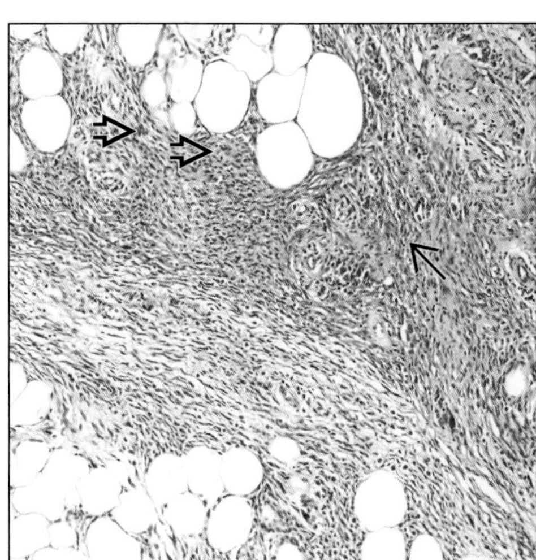

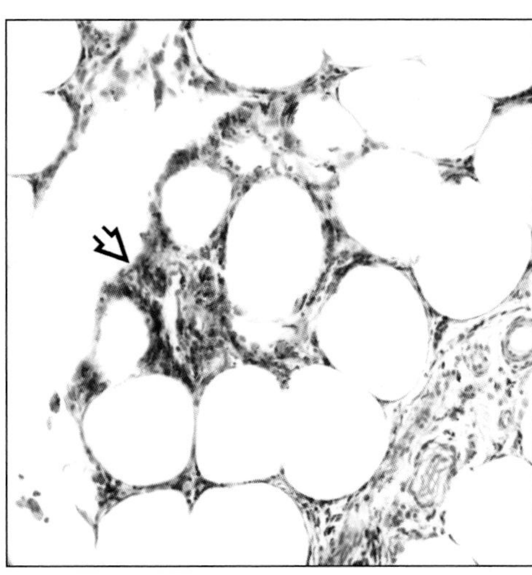

(Left) Early PHAT involving ankle resembles hemosiderotic fibrohistiocytic lipomatous tumor. A sheet of spindle cells with focal nuclear pleomorphism ⇨ infiltrates subcutaneous fat. There is abundant hemosiderin pigment →. **(Right)** An area of early PHAT shows heavy staining for iron pigment ⇨ with Perls stain. This is a characteristic feature of both PHAT and hemosiderotic fibrohistiocytic lipomatous lesions.

ECTOPIC HAMARTOMATOUS THYMOMA

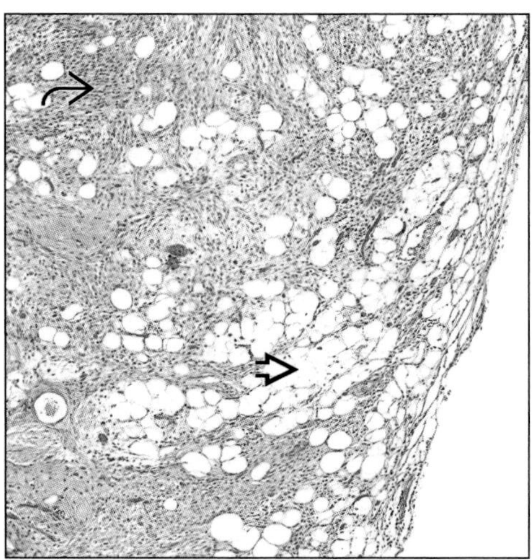

In this case of ectopic hamartomatous thymoma, the lesion is circumscribed, as is typical. The admixture of cellular elements ⮫ and mature adipose tissue ⇨ is discernible at low power.

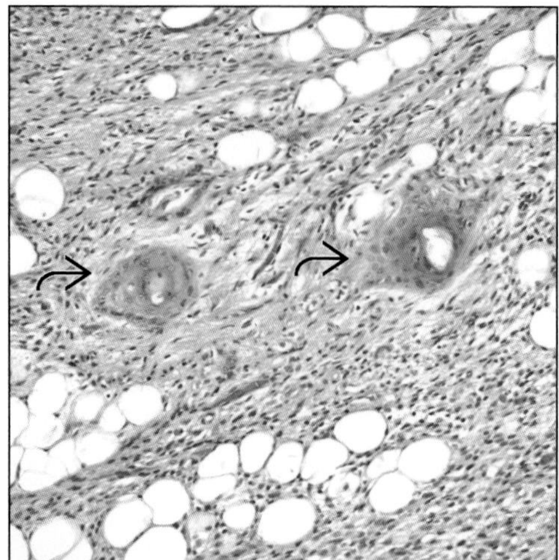

All 3 components are illustrated in this example. Mature fat is intermixed with sheets of bland spindle cells, and epithelial elements are interspersed, here, as squamous islands ⮫.

TERMINOLOGY

Abbreviations

- Ectopic hamartomatous thymoma (EHT)

Definitions

- Rare benign tumor composed of spindle, epithelial, and adipose tissue elements that occurs mainly in lower neck region of adult men

ETIOLOGY/PATHOGENESIS

Developmental Anomaly

- Suggested derivation from sequestered branchial epithelium
- Possible branchial anlage mixed tumor
- No evidence of true thymic differentiation

CLINICAL ISSUES

Epidemiology

- Age
  - Adults
- Gender
  - M > F

Site

- Lower neck
- Rarely presternal
- Deep soft tissue

Presentation

- Painless mass
  - Enlarging
  - May be of long duration
  - Clinical presentation and diagnostic imaging may suggest malignant lesion, such as sarcoma

Treatment

- Surgical approaches
  - Conservative surgical excision

Prognosis

- Most tumors do not recur after complete excision
- No metastases or tumor-related deaths described

MACROSCOPIC FEATURES

General Features

- Circumscribed, lobulated/multilobulated mass
- White to yellow, firm cut surface

MICROSCOPIC PATHOLOGY

Histologic Features

- Typically circumscribed
- Haphazard admixture of spindle cells, epithelial cells, and adipose tissue
  - All elements have benign cytological features
  - Proportion of each component varies
- Spindle cells
  - Sheets or short fascicles
  - Bland, elongated, sometimes tapering nuclei
  - Cytoplasm may be eosinophilic
- Epithelial cells
  - Solid, cystic, or glandular components
  - Squamous elements
  - Epithelial-lined cysts seen focally in many cases
  - Adenocarcinoma arising from EHT reported in 2 cases
- Adipose tissue
  - Mature type
    - Intermingled haphazardly
- Mitoses may be present but are rare
  - 0-7 mitoses per 50 high-power fields

ECTOPIC HAMARTOMATOUS THYMOMA

Key Facts

Terminology

- Rare benign tumor composed of spindle, epithelial, and adipose tissue elements that occurs mainly in lower neck region of adult men

Etiology/Pathogenesis

- Suggested derivation from sequestered branchial epithelium

Microscopic Pathology

- Typically circumscribed
- Haphazard admixture of spindle cells, epithelial cells, and adipose tissue
- Diffuse expression of cytokeratins, particularly of high molecular weight, in both spindle and epithelial components
- Can also express CD34, α-smooth muscle actin, and CD10

ANCILLARY TESTS

Immunohistochemistry

- Partial myoepithelial immunophenotype
  - Diffuse CK expression (particularly high molecular weight), in both spindle and epithelial components
    - e.g., CK5/6, CK14
  - Can also express α-smooth muscle actin and CD10
- CD34 can be positive in spindle cells
- S100 protein(-) and desmin(-)

DIFFERENTIAL DIAGNOSIS

Mixed Tumor of Skin Adnexal or Salivary Gland Origin

- Various anatomic sites
- Prominent chondromyxoid stroma in most cases
- In addition to cytokeratins, tumors also variably express S100 protein, GFAP, and calponin

Biphasic Synovial Sarcoma

- CK expression is focal, rather than diffuse and widespread
- CD34(-)
- Characteristic t(X;18)
  - Fusions between *SS18* and *SSX1, 2,* or *4*

Malignant Peripheral Nerve Sheath Tumor with Glandular Elements

- May originate from large nerve
- Focal nuclear expression of S100 protein in many cases
- Keratin expression very rare or absent

Sarcomatoid Carcinoma

- May have primary site elsewhere
- Dysplasia in overlying epithelium
- Nested architecture
- Nested reticulin pattern

SELECTED REFERENCES

1. Fetsch JF et al: Ectopic hamartomatous thymoma: a clinicopathologic and immunohistochemical analysis of 21 cases with data supporting reclassification as a branchial anlage mixed tumor. Am J Surg Pathol. 28(10):1360-70, 2004
2. Fukunaga M: Ectopic hamartomatous thymoma: a case report with immunohistochemical and ultrastructural studies. APMIS. 110(7-8):565-70, 2002
3. Marschall J et al: The sarcomatous guise of cervical ectopic hamartomatous thymoma. Head Neck. 24(8):800-4, 2002
4. Michal M et al: Pitfalls in the diagnosis of ectopic hamartomatous thymoma. Histopathology. 29(6):549-55, 1996
5. Rosai J et al: Ectopic hamartomatous thymoma. A distinctive benign lesion of lower neck. Am J Surg Pathol. 8(7):501-13, 1984

IMAGE GALLERY

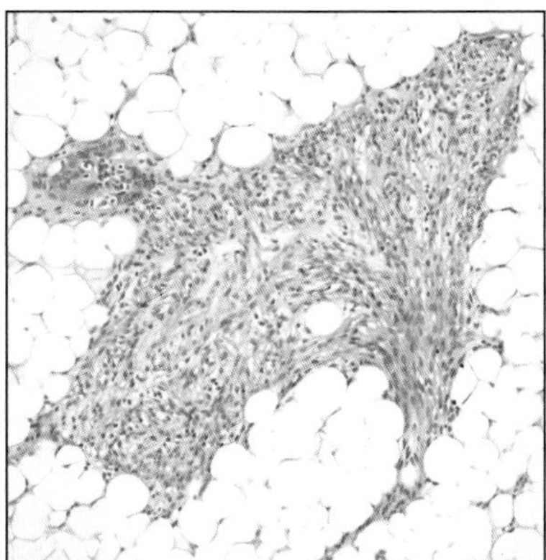

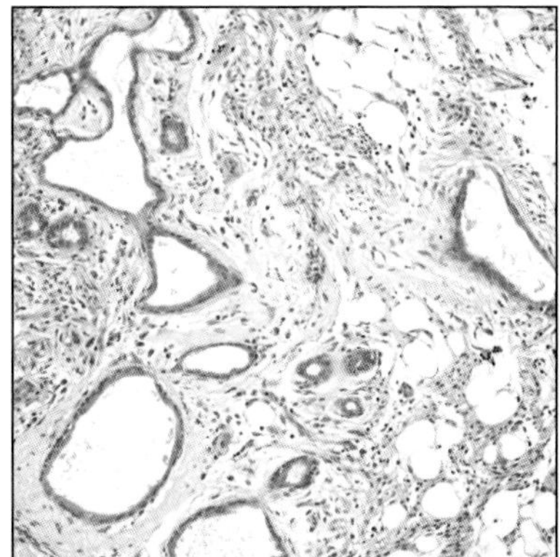

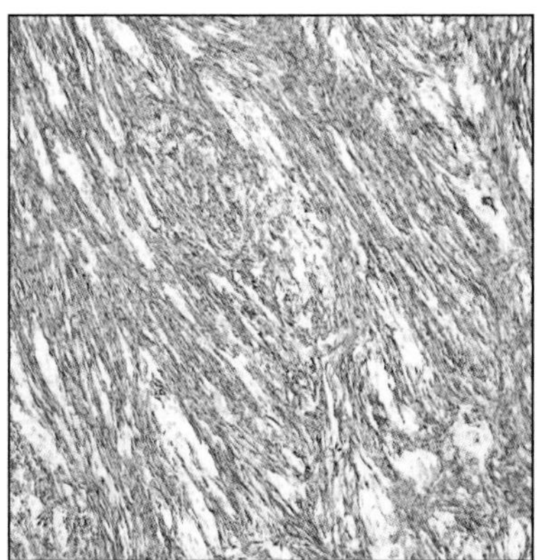

(Left) *In this case of ectopic hamartomatous thymoma, the spindle cells are bland, with ovoid nuclei and even chromatin. The proportions of spindle, epithelial, and fatty components can vary. This case has a predominant adipocytic component.* ***(Center)*** *The epithelial elements may be squamous, glandular, solid, or cystic. Here, they are present as dilated glandular structures.* ***(Right)*** *There is widespread expression of pancytokeratin, such as AE1/AE3, within the spindle cell component.*

PARAGANGLIOMA-LIKE DERMAL MELANOCYTIC TUMOR

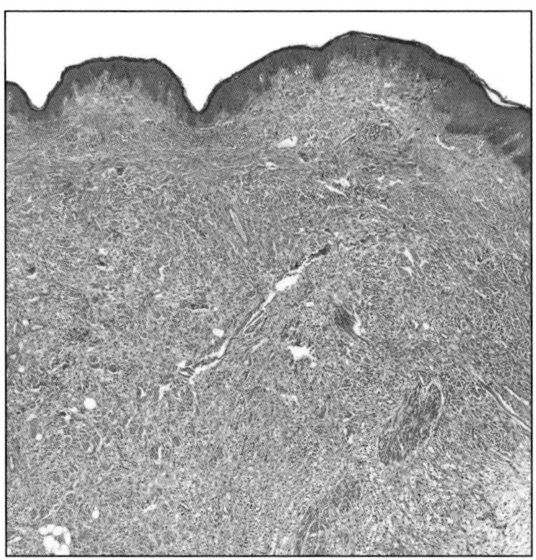

Histologic section shows a diffuse proliferation of clear cells located in the dermis. PDMTs are often a well-circumscribed but unencapsulated, dermal-based tumor that can extend into the subcutis.

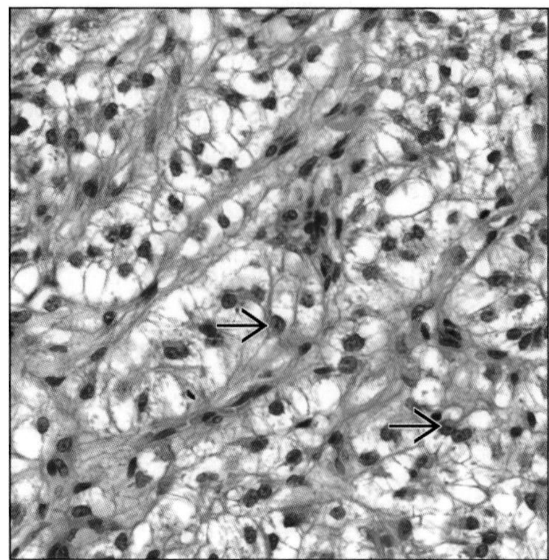

The tumor is composed of closely packed nests of cells with clear or granular cytoplasm and round to oval nuclei with small nucleoli ➔.

TERMINOLOGY

Abbreviations

- Paraganglioma-like dermal melanocytic tumor (PDMT)

Definitions

- Dermal-based low-grade melanocytic tumor with histologic similarities to paraganglioma

CLINICAL ISSUES

Epidemiology

- Incidence
  - Very rare tumors; only 10 cases reported to date
- Age
  - Typically occurs in young adults
    - Range: 18-53 years
    - Mean: 35 years
- Gender
  - More common in females

Site

- Usually on extremities
  - Mostly lower limb
    - Thigh, knee, lower leg

Presentation

- Dermal-based lesion
  - Clinically amelanotic in most cases

Treatment

- Surgical approaches
  - Complete excision should be recommended given the uncertain biologic potential of these tumors

Prognosis

- Local recurrences rare
- No metastases yet reported

MACROSCOPIC FEATURES

General Features

- Circumscribed dermal-based nodule

MICROSCOPIC PATHOLOGY

Histologic Features

- Nodular dermal-based melanocytic tumor
  - Relatively well-circumscribed, nonencapsulated, and symmetric-appearing nodular tumor
    - Focal infiltrative features at edges of tumor in some cases
- Typically composed of well-formed packets of bland pale to clear-staining oval-shaped cells, mimicking paraganglioma
  - Cells are surrounded by thin fibrous septa
  - Cells show moderate amounts of clear cytoplasm
  - Only focal, fine cytoplasmic melanin pigment may be found in some cases
- Mitotic activity may be present but is usually low (1-4/10 HPFs)

Cytologic Features

- Uniform oval to spindle-shaped nuclei
- Small nucleoli
- Abundant clear cytoplasm
- No high-grade cytologic atypia described

ANCILLARY TESTS

Immunohistochemistry

- Positive for S100 protein, variably so for Melan-A and HMB-45

Molecular Genetics

- *EWS* gene rearrangement absent

PARAGANGLIOMA-LIKE DERMAL MELANOCYTIC TUMOR

Key Facts

Terminology
- Paraganglioma-like dermal melanocytic tumor (PDMT)
- Rare dermal-based, low-grade melanocytic tumor with histologic similarities to paraganglioma

Microscopic Pathology
- Typically composed of packets of oval to spindle-shaped cells surrounded by thin fibrous septa
- Uniform nuclei, small nucleoli, clear cytoplasm

Ancillary Tests
- Positive for S100 protein, Melan-A and HMB-45 (variable)

Top Differential Diagnoses
- Clear cell/balloon cell melanoma
- Clear cell sarcoma
- Perivascular epithelioid cell tumor (PEComa)
- Primary dermal melanoma

DIFFERENTIAL DIAGNOSIS

Clear Cell/Balloon Cell Melanoma
- Atypical proliferation of melanocytes, often with overlying intraepidermal component
- Pagetoid spread and lentiginous hyperplasia in junctional component
- Dermal component shows greater cytologic atypia and mitotic activity than PDMT

Clear Cell Sarcoma of Soft Parts
- Typically in deep subcutis, may invade dermis
- Young adults, often on lower extremity
- Immunohistochemistry like that of PDMT
  - Multiple melanocytic markers typically expressed
- t(12;22), *EWS/ATF1* fusion

Perivascular Epithelioid Cell Tumor (PEComa)
- Rare tumors composed of nests and sheets of bland-appearing clear cells
- HMB-45(+) and weakly/focally for S100 (as in PDMT)
- SMA(+) and variably so for desmin and CK (unlike in PDMT)

Primary Dermal Melanoma
- Very rare variant of melanoma located in dermis &/or subcutaneous tissues
- Well-circumscribed, large, cellular nodule, which mimics metastatic melanoma in most cases
- Cytologic atypia, mitotic activity, sometimes necrosis
- S100 protein, Melan-A, and HMB-45 positive
- Lacks t(12;22), *EWS/ATF1* fusion

DIAGNOSTIC CHECKLIST

Clinically Relevant Pathologic Features
- Mitotic rate may be important if higher than usual

Pathologic Interpretation Pearls
- Dermal melanocytes in small nests in fibrous septa

SELECTED REFERENCES

1. Hantschke M et al: Cutaneous clear cell sarcoma: a clinicopathologic, immunohistochemical, and molecular analysis of 12 cases emphasizing its distinction from dermal melanoma. Am J Surg Pathol. 34(2):216-22, 2010
2. Cimpean AM et al: Paraganglioma-like dermal melanocytic tumor: a case report with particular features. Int J Clin Exp Pathol. 3(2):222-5, 2009
3. Walsh SN et al: PEComas: a review with emphasis on cutaneous lesions. Semin Diagn Pathol. 26(3):123-30, 2009
4. Cassarino DS et al: Primary dermal melanoma: distinct immunohistochemical findings and clinical outcome compared with nodular and metastatic melanoma. Arch Dermatol. 144(1):49-56, 2008
5. Sarma DP et al: Paraganglioma-like dermal melanocytic tumor: a case report. Cases J. 1(1):48, 2008
6. Deyrup AT et al: Paraganglioma-like dermal melanocytic tumor: a unique entity distinct from cellular blue nevus, clear cell sarcoma, and cutaneous melanoma. Am J Surg Pathol. 28(12):1579-86, 2004

IMAGE GALLERY

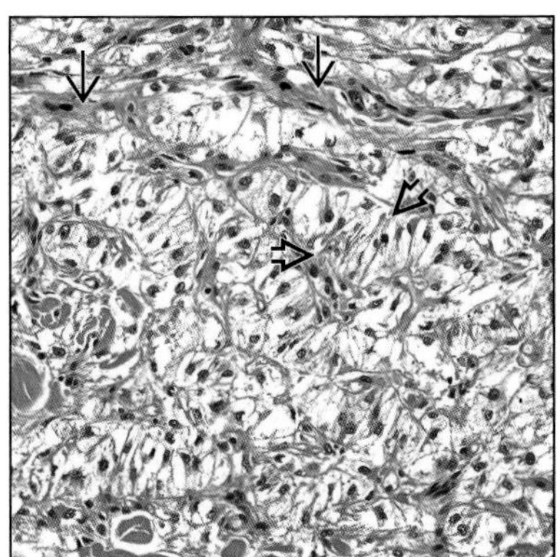

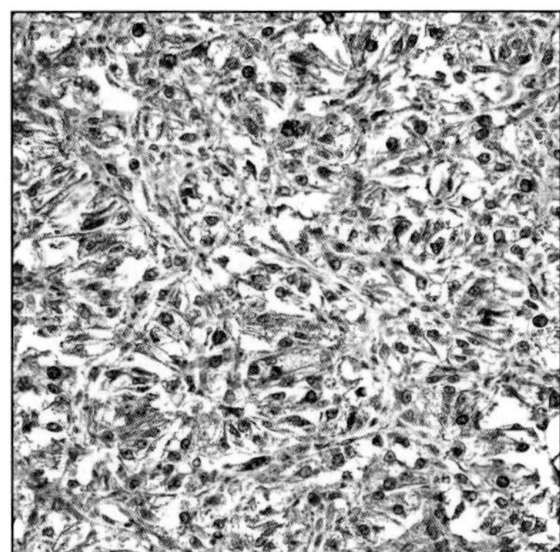

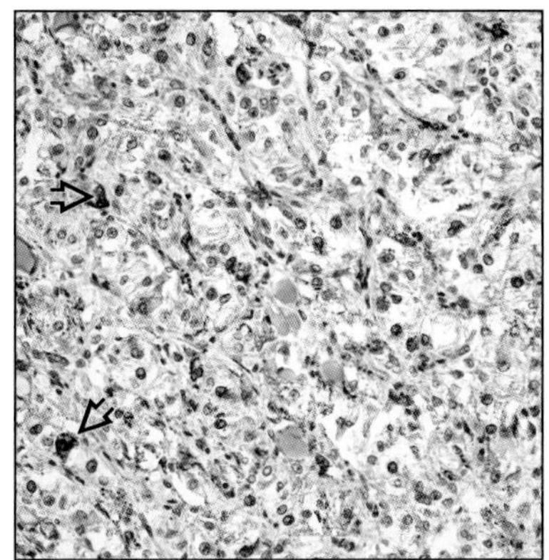

(Left) *The paraganglioma-like cell nests ⊳ are separated by delicate fibrous septa →.* ***(Center)*** *Immunostaining for S100 protein shows diffuse nuclear and cytoplasmic positivity. This helps distinguish PDMT from PEComa, which is usually negative or only very focally positive.* ***(Right)*** *Lesional cells show focal cytoplasmic positivity for HMB-45 ⊳.*

DERMAL CLEAR CELL MESENCHYMAL NEOPLASM

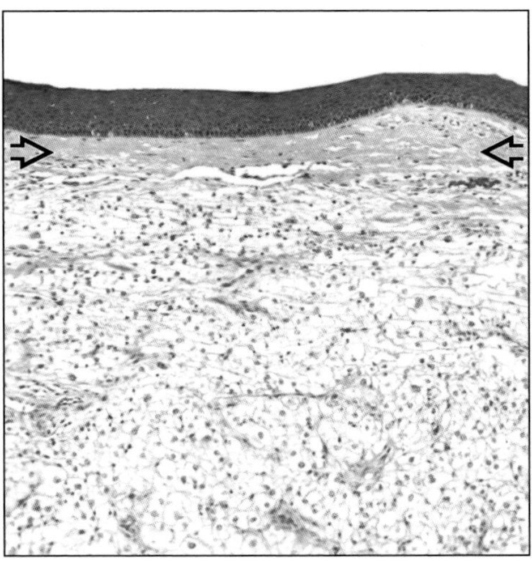

Low-power examination shows a dermal-based clear cell tumor with a thin Grenz zone ⇨ separating it from the overlying epidermis. (Courtesy A. Lazar, MD.)

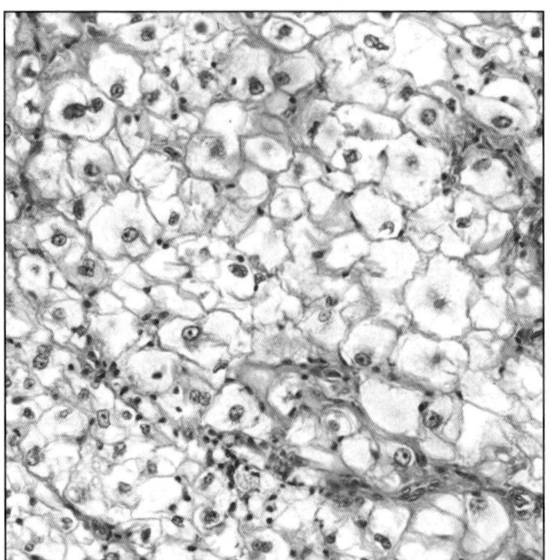

Higher magnification shows the relatively bland cytologic features of the large clear cells with vesicular nuclei and abundant clear cytoplasm. (Courtesy A. Lazar, MD.)

TERMINOLOGY

Abbreviations

- Dermal clear cell mesenchymal neoplasm (DCCMN)

Definitions

- Rare dermal-based clear cell tumor of unclear derivation

ETIOLOGY/PATHOGENESIS

Unknown

- Very rare tumors of unknown etiology

CLINICAL ISSUES

Epidemiology

- Age
  - Reported in adults over age 35

Site

- Most cases have occurred on lower extremities

Presentation

- Cutaneous nodule

Treatment

- Surgical approaches
  - Complete conservative excision should be encouraged

Prognosis

- Uncertain, given rarity of this tumor, but appears to be benign or low-grade tumor

MACROSCOPIC FEATURES

General Features

- Nonencapsulated, poorly circumscribed reticular dermal-based nodule

Size

- 0.5-3 cm in greatest dimension

MICROSCOPIC PATHOLOGY

Histologic Features

- Dermal-based tumor composed of nodules of large clear cells
  - Tumors may focally infiltrate subcutaneous adipose tissue
  - Lateral borders are typically poorly circumscribed, but deep border is smooth and rounded
- Cytologically, cells are usually bland-appearing with vesicular nuclei and abundant clear cytoplasm
  - Some cases may show cytologic atypia and pleomorphism, with increased numbers of mitoses

Predominant Pattern/Injury Type

- Clear cell

Predominant Cell/Compartment Type

- Mesenchymal

ANCILLARY TESTS

Immunohistochemistry

- Reportedly positive for CD63 in all cases
- Variable positivity for CD68 and vimentin
- Negative for CD34, FXIIIa, and melanocytic (S100, HMB-45, Melan-A), smooth muscle (actin-sm, desmin), and epithelial (cytokeratins) markers

DERMAL CLEAR CELL MESENCHYMAL NEOPLASM

Key Facts

Terminology
- Rare, dermal-based clear cell tumor of unknown derivation

Clinical Issues
- Cutaneous nodule
- Most cases have been reported on lower extremities
- Uncertain, given rarity of this tumor, but appear to be benign or low-grade tumors

Microscopic Pathology
- Clear cell proliferation
- Cytologically, cells are usually bland-appearing, with vesicular nuclei and abundant clear cytoplasm

Top Differential Diagnoses
- Clear cell sarcoma
- Clear cell fibrous papule
- Clear cell squamous cell carcinoma and trichilemmal carcinoma

DIFFERENTIAL DIAGNOSIS

Clear Cell Sarcoma
- Packets of atypical spindled clear cells surrounded by fibrous stroma
- Positive for S100 and other melanocytic markers, such as HMB-45, Melan-A, or tyrosinase
- Usually deep soft tissue tumor, may rarely involve dermis

Clear Cell Squamous Cell Carcinoma and Trichilemmal Carcinoma
- Should show more cytologic atypia and abundant mitoses than DCCMN
- Focal epidermal attachments and areas of keratinization and dyskeratotic cells often present
- Positive for cytokeratins, especially those of high molecular weight (CK5/6, CK903, etc.) and p63

Clear Cell Fibrous Papule
- More superficial, often in papillary dermis with dome-shaped appearance
- Cells may show staining for CD68 and FXIIIa

Paraganglioma-like Dermal Melanocytic Tumor
- Packets of cells with clear to eosinophilic-staining cytoplasm
- Melanocytic markers, including S100, HMB-45, and Melan-A, are positive

Perivascular Epithelioid Cell Tumor (PEComa)
- Rare soft tissue tumor, which may occasionally present in skin
- Tumor cells typically show clear, palely eosinophilic, or granular cytoplasm
- Immunoreactivity for melanocytic markers, especially HMB-45 and smooth muscle actin

DIAGNOSTIC CHECKLIST

Pathologic Interpretation Pearls
- Dermal-based proliferation composed of nodules of large clear cells

SELECTED REFERENCES

1. Gavino AC et al: Atypical distinctive dermal clear cell mesenchymal neoplasm arising in the scalp. J Cutan Pathol. 35(4):423-7, 2008
2. Liegl B et al: Primary cutaneous PEComa: distinctive clear cell lesions of skin. Am J Surg Pathol. 32(4):608-14, 2008
3. Cassarino DS et al: Cutaneous squamous cell carcinoma: a comprehensive clinicopathologic classification--part two. J Cutan Pathol. 33(4):261-79, 2006
4. Lee AN et al: Clear cell fibrous papule with NKI/C3 expression: clinical and histologic features in six cases. Am J Dermatopathol. 27(4):296-300, 2005

IMAGE GALLERY

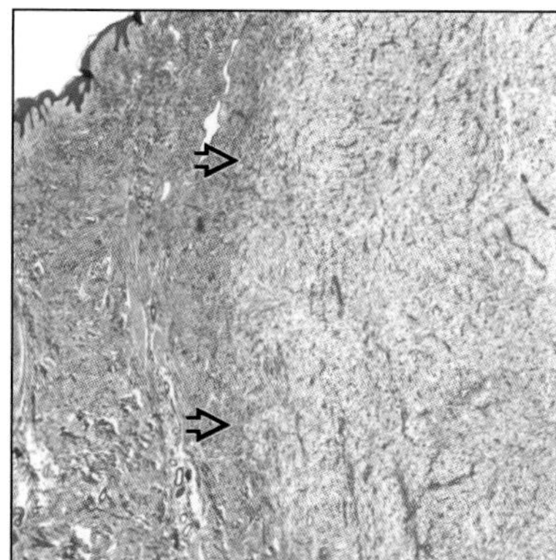

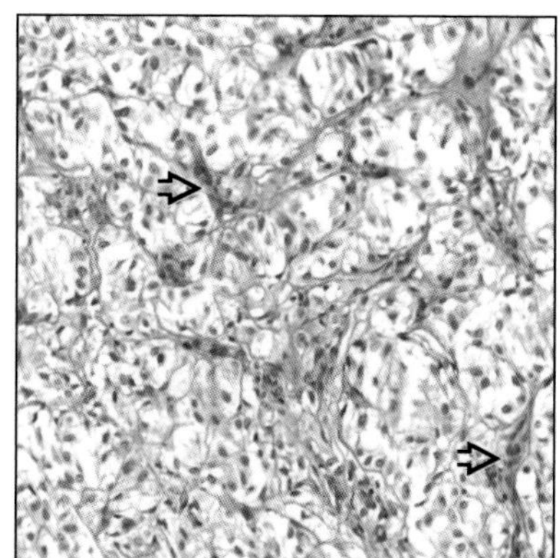

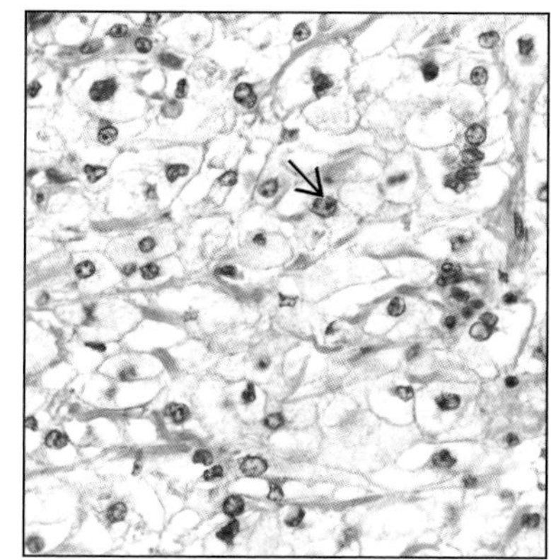

(Left) *Low-power examination of histologic section shows nonencapsulated lateral border ⮚ of the tumor. (Courtesy A. Lazar, MD.)* ***(Center)*** *Intermediate magnification shows vaguely nested appearance & numerous small caliber blood vessels ⮚ surrounding tumor cells. (Courtesy A. Lazar, MD.)* ***(Right)*** *Higher magnification shows relatively bland cytologic features of large clear cells, which show enlarged nuclei with vesicular chromatin & focally prominent nucleoli ⮚. Cytoplasm is predominantly clear to focally granular-appearing. (Courtesy A. Lazar, MD.)*

ANGIOMATOID FIBROUS HISTIOCYTOMA

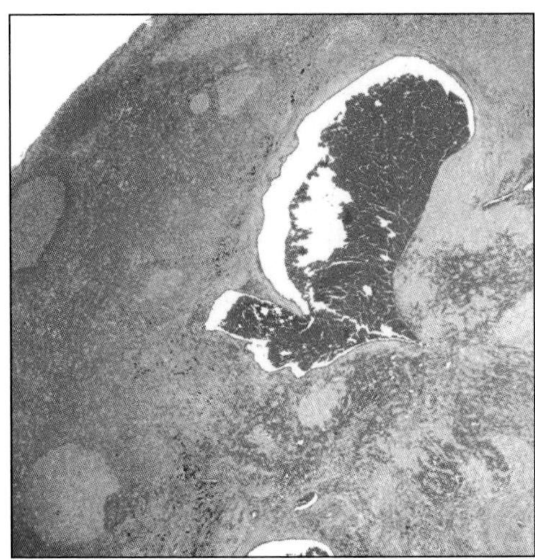

Hematoxylin & eosin shows a circumscribed lesion with a pronounced lymphoid cuff, including prominent germinal centers. This appearance may mimic that of a tumor metastatic to a lymph node.

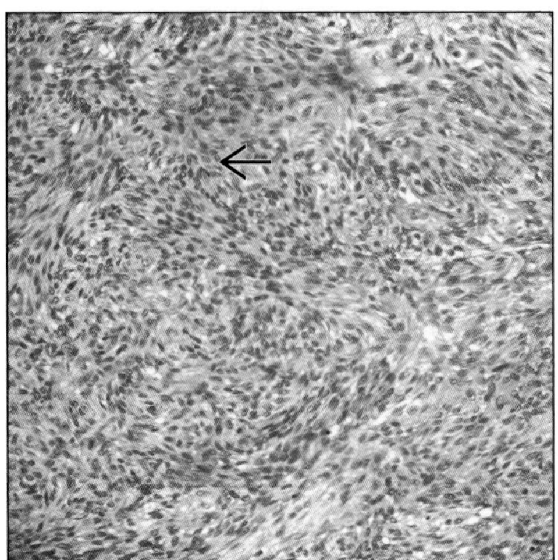

Hematoxylin & eosin shows cellular proliferations of spindle cells in loose fascicles and areas ⇒ with a storiform pattern. The cells have bland ovoid nuclei in this angiomatoid fibrous histiocytoma.

TERMINOLOGY

Abbreviations

- Angiomatoid fibrous histiocytoma (AFH)

Synonyms

- Originally angiomatoid "malignant" fibrous histiocytoma
  - Term "malignant" removed due to indolent behavior
  - Unrelated to malignant fibrous histiocytoma (MFH)/ pleomorphic sarcoma group of neoplasms

Definitions

- Rare neoplasm of intermediate biologic potential with 3 characteristic translocations

ETIOLOGY/PATHOGENESIS

Lineage Unknown

- Endothelial or histiocytic differentiation not proven
- Desmin expression suggests myoid or myofibroblastic differentiation
- Postulated nodal fibroblastic reticulum cell differentiation

CLINICAL ISSUES

Epidemiology

- Incidence
  - Rare
  - Accounts for approximately 0.3% of all soft tissue neoplasms
- Age
  - Infancy to 8th decade
  - Predominantly in children and young adults
- Gender
  - Slight female predilection

Site

- Extremities
- Trunk
- Head and neck
- 1 primary intracerebral case reported
- Usually superficial
  - Deep dermis and subcutis
- Few arise deeply

Presentation

- Slowly growing, painless mass
  - Usually small
    - Most often 2-4 cm
- Constitutional symptoms in subset
  - e.g., malaise, pyrexia, and anemia
  - Possible tumoral cytokine production

Treatment

- Surgical approaches
  - Wide excision
    - Usually curative
  - Radiotherapy and chemotherapy
    - For rare metastatic or unresectable tumors

Prognosis

- Excellent in most cases
  - Majority of lesions indolent
- Regional recurrence rate up to 15%
- Metastasis rate of approximately 1%
  - Rare cause of death
- No firm morphologic or clinical indicators of behavior
  - Infiltrative margin and deep location can predict recurrence

MACROSCOPIC FEATURES

General Features

- Firm
- Circumscribed
- Blood-filled cystic cavities

ANGIOMATOID FIBROUS HISTIOCYTOMA

Key Facts

Terminology
- Rare neoplasm of intermediate biologic potential
- Most often arises in extremities of children and young adults
- Histologically often confused with both benign and malignant lesions
- 3 characteristic translocations
  - 2 identical to those of clear cell sarcoma

Clinical Issues
- Slowly growing
- Mostly indolent
- 15% recur
- 1% metastasize

Microscopic Pathology
- Fibrous and lymphoplasmacytic cuff
  - Germinal centers
- Sheets of histiocyte-like and spindle cells
- Blood-filled spaces

Ancillary Tests
- Desmin positivity in 1/2 of cases
- Specific translocations

Top Differential Diagnoses
- Pleomorphic sarcoma (malignant fibrous histiocytoma)
- Aneurysmal benign fibrous histiocytoma
- Palisaded (intranodal) myofibroblastoma
- Kaposi sarcoma

Diagnostic Checklist
- Age distribution

Sections to Be Submitted
- Lesion should be thoroughly sampled
  - Features, such as lymphoid cuff, may only be present focally
- Small lesions should be submitted in entirety

MICROSCOPIC PATHOLOGY

Histologic Features
- Circumscribed
- Lobulated
- Fibrous pseudocapsule
  - Dense peripheral lymphoplasmacytic cuff in up to 80%
- Cellular tumor
  - Cells with bland, vesicular, ovoid to spindled nuclei
  - Sheets
  - Short fascicles
  - Occasional storiform patterns
  - Ovoid or spindle forms may predominate
  - Mitoses infrequent
- Hemorrhagic cavities
  - No endothelial lining
- Some show marked pleomorphism and mitotic activity
- Giant cells in some cases

Predominant Pattern/Injury Type
- Circumscribed
- Cystic, macroscopic

Predominant Cell/Compartment Type
- Mesenchymal

ANCILLARY TESTS

Immunohistochemistry
- Desmin positivity
  - Approximately half of cases
  - Strong cytoplasmic expression
  - Scattered desmin(+) cells may be present within lymphoid proliferation
  - Tumors negative for skeletal muscle markers
    - e.g., myogenin and MYOD1
- Epithelial membrane antigen (EMA)
  - Just under half of cases
- CD68
  - Frequent but nonspecific
- CD99
  - Frequent but nonspecific
- Very occasional "intermediate" CD34 expression reported
  - Usually negative
  - Other vascular endothelial markers also usually absent

Cytogenetics
- 3 characteristic translocations identified
  - t(2:22)(q33:q12)
    - *EWSR1-CREB1*
    - Most common
  - t(12:16)(q13:p11)
    - *FUS-ATF1*
  - t(12:22)(q13:q12)
    - *EWSR1-ATF1*
- Latter 2 translocations are identical to those of clear cell sarcoma (CCS)
  - CCS is morphologically and clinically distinct neoplasm
- No correlation between type of fusion gene and clinicopathologic features

In Situ Hybridization
- Translocated chromosomes can be identified by FISH
  - Frozen or paraffin-embedded material

PCR
- Fusion gene transcripts can be identified by RT-PCR
  - Frozen or paraffin-embedded material

Electron Microscopy
- No diagnostic ultrastructural findings

ANGIOMATOID FIBROUS HISTIOCYTOMA

DIFFERENTIAL DIAGNOSIS

Granulomatous Lesions
- Predisposing factors may be noted clinically
- Granulomas are usually dispersed and discrete
- Lack solid pattern of AFH
- Lack cystic hemorrhage
- CD68(+)
- Desmin(-)

Spindle Cell Hemangioma
- Poorly circumscribed
- Cavernous vascular spaces
  - Endothelial lining
- Epithelioid endothelial cells with vacuoles
- Spindle cells are SMA(+), desmin(-), and CD34(-)

Aneurysmal Benign Fibrous Histiocytoma
- Usually dermal
- Epidermal hyperplasia overlying lesion
- Tumor is not circumscribed
- Peripheral collagen bundles
- Mixed cell population
  - Giant cells
  - Siderophages
  - Chronic inflammatory cells
- Desmin(-)

Palisaded (Intranodal) Myofibroblastoma
- In lymph node
  - Majority in inguinal region in males
  - Occasionally in submandibular node
- Delicate spindle cells in fascicles
- Palisading
- Amianthoid fibers
- SMA(+)
- Desmin(-)

Inflammatory Pseudotumor of Lymph Node
- Lacks pseudovascular spaces
- Myofibroblastic differentiation
- Desmin(-)

Nodular Kaposi Sarcoma
- Predisposing factors
- Endothelial-lined spaces
- CD34(+), CD31(+), and D2-40(+)
- HHV8 positivity in nuclei

Myofibroma/Myofibromatosis
- May be multicentric
- Most common from birth to 2 years
- Most solitary examples in subcutaneous tissues of head and neck
- Biphasic pattern
- Myoid nodules
- Cellular areas with hemangiopericytic vascular pattern
- Spindle cell areas
- Desmin usually negative or focal

Nodular Fasciitis
- Superficial location
- Spindle and stellate fibroblasts with tissue culture appearance
- Related phenomena
  - e.g., extravasated erythrocytes, giant cells
- Smooth muscle actin(+)

Smooth Muscle Tumors
- Not lobulated
- Perpendicularly oriented or intersecting fascicles
- Blunt-ended nuclei
- Eosinophilic cytoplasm
- Express actins and H-caldesmon
- May express ER/PR

Nodal Metastasis
- Primary tumor site may be evident clinically
- True nodal architecture present
  - e.g., subcapsular and medullary sinuses
  - Well-organized germinal centers

Pleomorphic Sarcoma (Malignant Fibrous Histiocytoma)
- Older age group
- Deep soft tissue
- Spindle cells
- Polygonal cells
- Giant cells
- Marked diffuse pleomorphism
- Atypical mitoses
- Necrosis

Rhabdomyosarcoma
- Urogenital or head and neck sites in embryonal rhabdomyosarcoma
- Small round cells and at least focal alveolar pattern in alveolar rhabdomyosarcoma
- Pleomorphic rhabdomyoblasts may be present
- Nuclear expression of skeletal muscle markers
  - Myogenin
  - MYOD1

Epithelioid Sarcoma (Classic Type)
- Multinodular
- Bland epithelioid cells
  - Eosinophilic cytoplasm
  - Mitoses
- Spindle cells at periphery of nodule
- Central necrosis
- Lacks fibrous or lymphoid cuff
- Desmin(-)
- CK(+) and EMA(+)
- CD34(+) (50% of cases)
- SNF5(-) (90% of cases)

Extrarenal Rhabdoid Tumor
- Often infants and very young children
- Larger cells
  - Eccentric nuclei
  - Abundant cytoplasm
  - Hyaline inclusions
- Desmin(-)
- Keratin(+)
- SNF5(-)
  - Chromosome 22q deletions

ANGIOMATOID FIBROUS HISTIOCYTOMA

Immunohistochemistry

Antibody	Reactivity	Staining Pattern	Comment
Desmin	Positive	Cytoplasmic	50% of cases
EMA	Positive	Cell membrane	Almost 50% of cases
CD68	Positive	Cytoplasmic	Focal, nonspecific
CD99	Positive	Cell membrane	Nonspecific
Actin-HHF-35	Positive	Cytoplasmic	Focal in 14% of cases
Actin-sm	Positive	Cytoplasmic	Focal in 14% of cases
Caldesmon	Positive	Cytoplasmic	Positive in some cases
SNF5	Positive	Nuclear	
Myogenin	Negative	Not applicable	
MYOD1	Negative	Not applicable	
CD34	Negative	Not applicable	Very occasional faint staining
CD31	Negative	Not applicable	
AE1/AE3	Negative	Not applicable	
CK8/18/CAM5.2	Negative	Not applicable	
CD45	Negative	Not applicable	
CD30	Negative	Not applicable	
S100P	Negative	Not applicable	
CD117	Negative	Not applicable	
Calponin	Equivocal	Cytoplasmic	Occasional

DIAGNOSTIC CHECKLIST

Clinically Relevant Pathologic Features

- Age distribution
- Gross appearance

Pathologic Interpretation Pearls

- Tumor is circumscribed
- Lymphoid cuff, fibrous capsule, and hemorrhagic cavities
  - May be absent from any lesion
  - May be only present focally
- Several tumor blocks should be sampled in tumors with appropriate clinical setting
- Desmin(+)
- Myogenin(-)

SELECTED REFERENCES

1. Dunham C et al: Primary intracerebral angiomatoid fibrous histiocytoma: report of a case with a t(12;22)(q13;q12) causing type 1 fusion of the EWS and ATF-1 genes. Am J Surg Pathol. 32(3):478-84, 2008
2. Thway K: Angiomatoid fibrous histiocytoma: a review with recent genetic findings. Arch Pathol Lab Med. 132(2):273-7, 2008
3. Hallor KH et al: Fusion genes in angiomatoid fibrous histiocytoma. Cancer Lett. 251(1):158-63, 2007
4. Rossi S et al: EWSR1-CREB1 and EWSR1-ATF1 fusion genes in angiomatoid fibrous histiocytoma. Clin Cancer Res. 13(24):7322-8, 2007
5. Raddaoui E et al: Fusion of the FUS and ATF1 genes in a large, deep-seated angiomatoid fibrous histiocytoma. Diagn Mol Pathol. 11(3):157-62, 2002
6. Fanburg-Smith JC et al: Angiomatoid "malignant" fibrous histiocytoma: a clinicopathologic study of 158 cases and further exploration of the myoid phenotype. Hum Pathol. 30(11):1336-43, 1999
7. Morgan MB et al: Angiomatoid malignant fibrous histiocytoma revisited. An immunohistochemical and DNA ploidy analysis. Am J Dermatopathol. 19(3):223-7, 1997
8. Smith ME et al: Evaluation of CD68 and other histiocytic antigens in angiomatoid malignant fibrous histiocytoma. Am J Surg Pathol. 15(8):757-63, 1991
9. Costa MJ et al: Angiomatoid malignant fibrous histiocytoma. A follow-up study of 108 cases with evaluation of possible histologic predictors of outcome. Am J Surg Pathol. 14(12):1126-32, 1990
10. Pettinato G et al: Angiomatoid malignant fibrous histiocytoma: cytologic, immunohistochemical, ultrastructural, and flow cytometric study of 20 cases. Mod Pathol. 3(4):479-87, 1990
11. Kanter MH et al: Angiomatoid malignant fibrous histiocytoma. Cytology of fine-needle aspiration and its differential diagnosis. Arch Pathol Lab Med. 109(6):564-6, 1985
12. Kay S: Angiomatoid malignant fibrous histiocytoma. Report of two cases with ultrastructural observations of one case. Arch Pathol Lab Med. 109(10):934-7, 1985
13. Leu HJ et al: Angiomatoid malignant fibrous histiocytoma. Case report and electron microscopic findings. Virchows Arch A Pathol Anat Histol. 395(1):99-107, 1982
14. Sun CC et al: An ultrastructural study of angiomatoid fibrous histiocytoma. Cancer. 49(10):2103-11, 1982
15. Enzinger FM: Angiomatoid malignant fibrous histiocytoma: a distinct fibrohistiocytic tumor of children and young adults simulating a vascular neoplasm. Cancer. 44(6):2147-57, 1979

ANGIOMATOID FIBROUS HISTIOCYTOMA

Microscopic Features

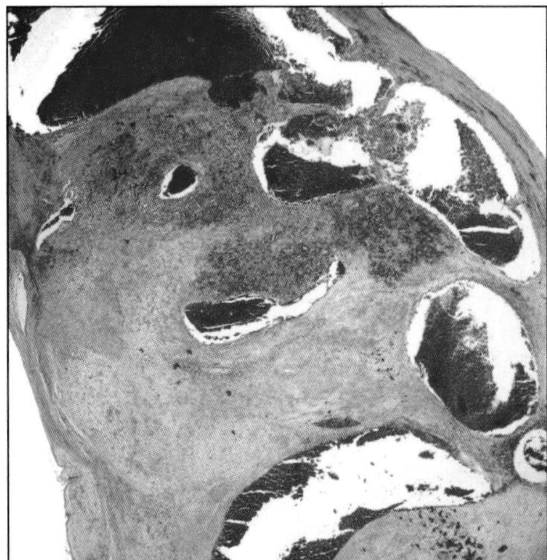

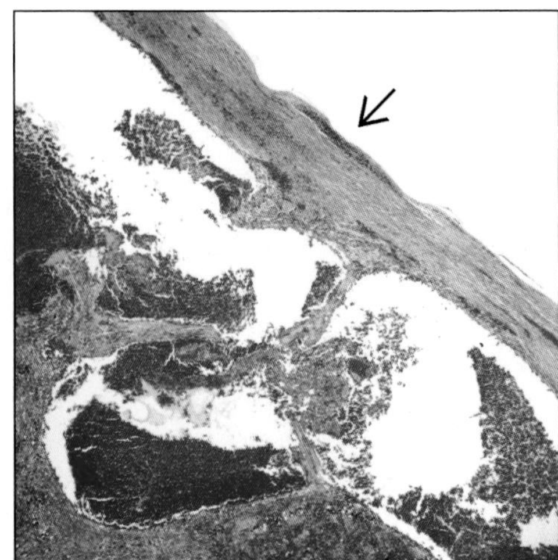

(Left) *Hematoxylin & eosin shows a circumscribed nodular lesion with prominent cavernous blood-filled spaces, adjacent to solid cellular lesional areas. This is a typical appearance of angiomatoid fibrous histiocytoma.* ***(Right)*** *Hematoxylin & eosin shows a thick fibrous capsule. The lymphoid cuff may be sparse ⇒, as shown here, or entirely absent. While angiomatoid fibrous histiocytoma is usually encapsulated, a small number of cases are focally infiltrative.*

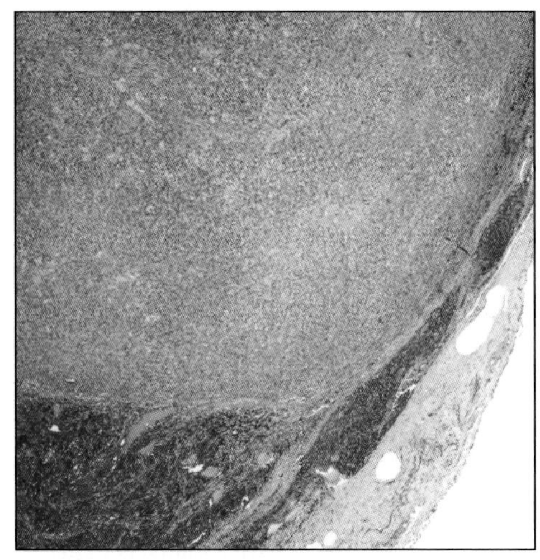

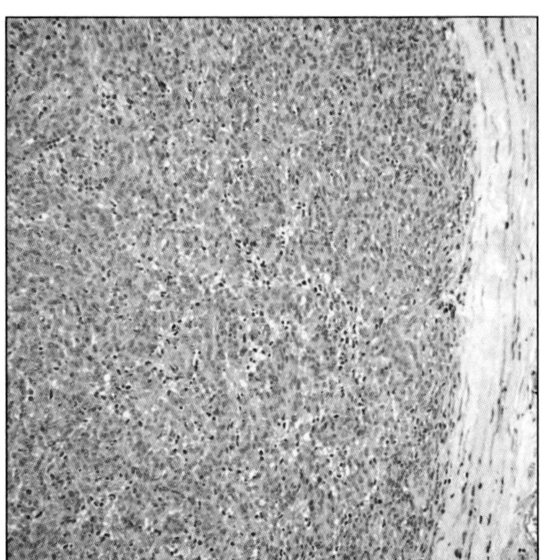

(Left) *Hematoxylin & eosin shows a tumor with a lymphoid cuff and fibrous capsule. This example has a predominantly solid growth pattern, but there is hemorrhage at lower left.* ***(Right)*** *Hematoxylin & eosin shows a tumor with solid morphology. Note absence of peripheral lymphoid cuff and hemorrhagic cavity formation. These variants of AFH may be difficult to distinguish from other neoplasms, and a high index of clinical suspicion is required for diagnosis.*

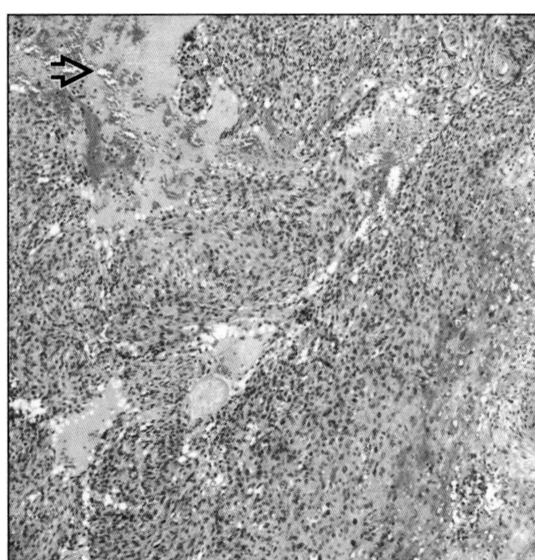

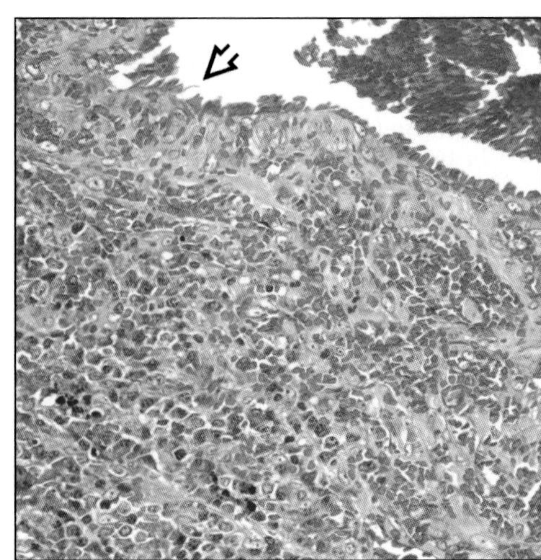

(Left) *Hematoxylin & eosin shows multiple nodules of spindle and ovoid cells next to irregularly shaped foci of hemorrhage and fibrin deposition ⇨.* ***(Right)*** *Hematoxylin & eosin shows hemosiderin deposition and a lymphoplasmacytic infiltrate. The hemorrhagic cavities are lined by tumoral cells ⇨ and lack a vascular endothelial layer, making immunostaining for CD34 or CD31 negative here.*

Microscopic Features and Ancillary Techniques

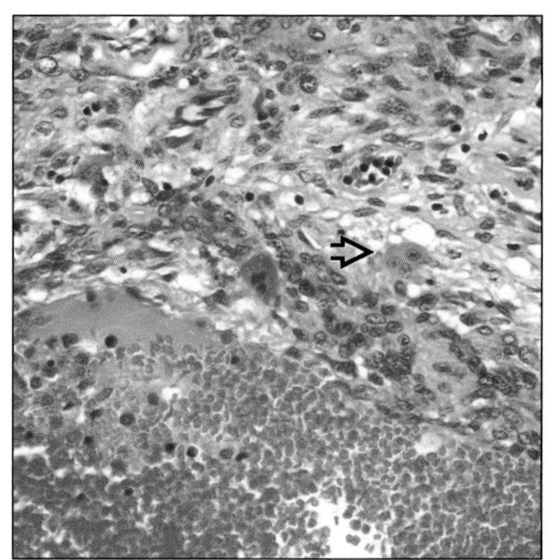

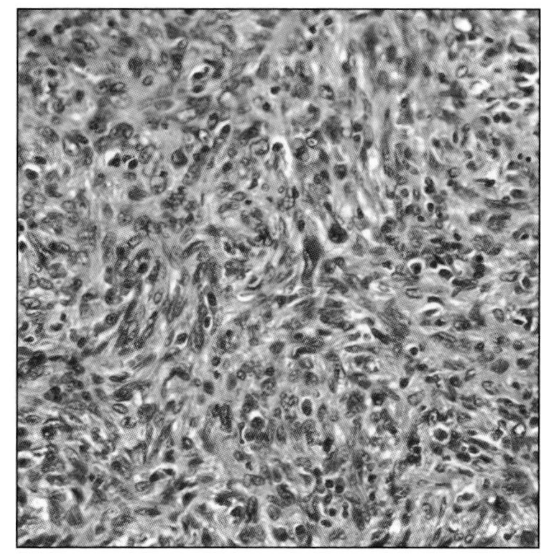

(Left) *Hematoxylin & eosin shows a higher power view of the cavity-tumoral interface. Occasional giant cells ⇨ are dispersed among the lesional cells. These are a feature in a small number of cases.* ***(Right)*** *Hematoxylin & eosin shows dense storiform fascicles of spindle cells. Pleomorphism is minimal. Note the infiltrate of lymphocytes scattered throughout. The appearances here somewhat resemble those of cutaneous fibrous histiocytoma.*

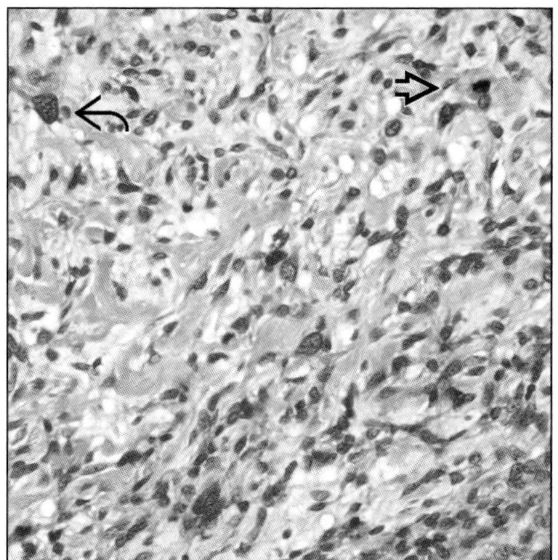

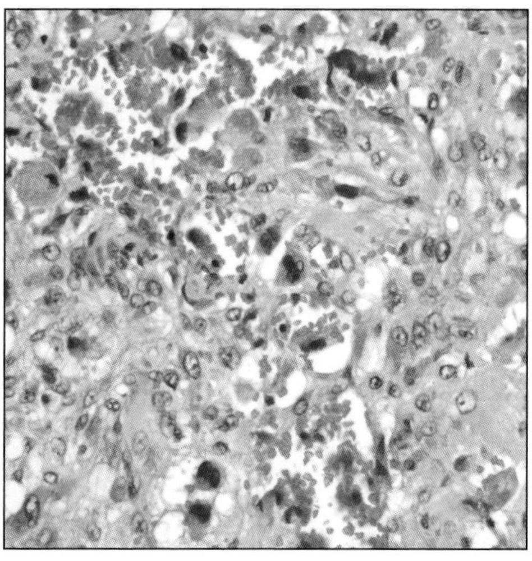

(Left) *Hematoxylin & eosin shows an example of angiomatoid fibrous histiocytoma with occasional atypical nuclei ↗ and a mitotic figure ⇨. Note the stromal fibrosis.* ***(Right)*** *Hematoxylin & eosin shows angiomatoid fibrous histiocytoma with focal but pronounced cellular atypia, seen in a number of cases. The hemorrhagic channels are irregular, and the appearances can mimic Kaposi sarcoma or angiosarcoma.*

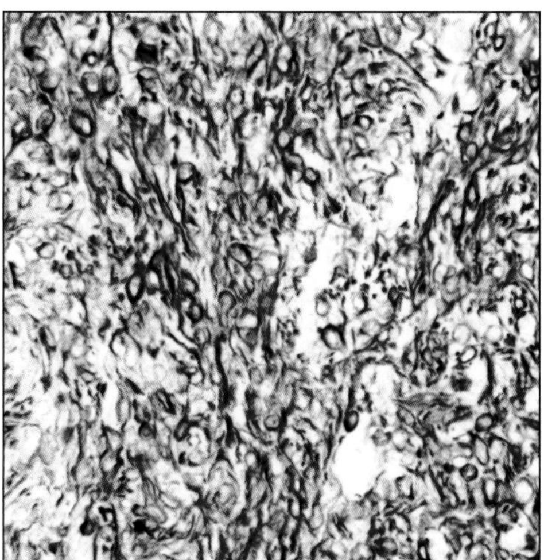

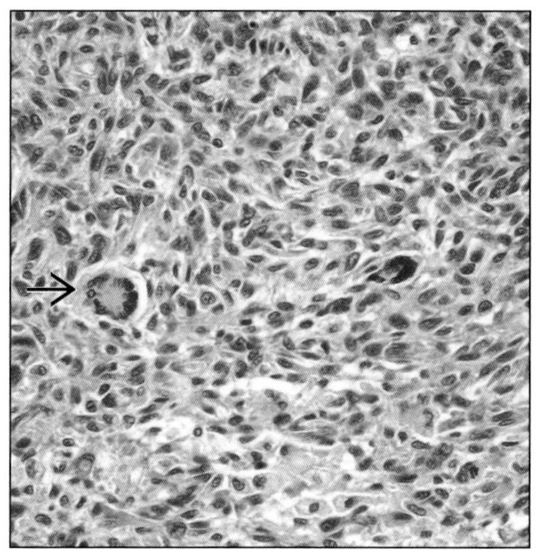

(Left) *Desmin shows strong cytoplasmic positivity in angiomatoid fibrous histiocytoma. This can be diffuse, as here, but is more often focal. Immunoreactivity for desmin is found in about 50% of cases & is a useful diagnostic finding.* ***(Right)*** *Hematoxylin & eosin shows angiomatoid fibrous histiocytoma with multinucleated giant cells. One has a Touton giant cell-like appearance →. The morphology suggests these are probably neoplastic rather than reactive osteoclast-like cells.*

OSSIFYING FIBROMYXOID TUMOR

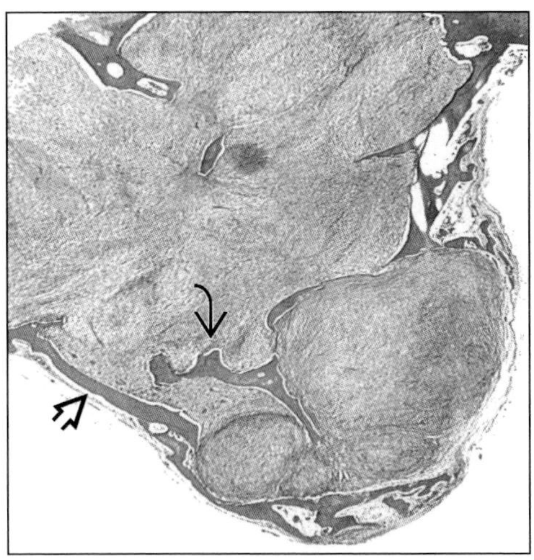

Hematoxylin & eosin shows an ossifying fibromyxoid tumor with variable cellularity and a rim of mature bone ⇨ with septal extensions ⇨ into the tumor mass.

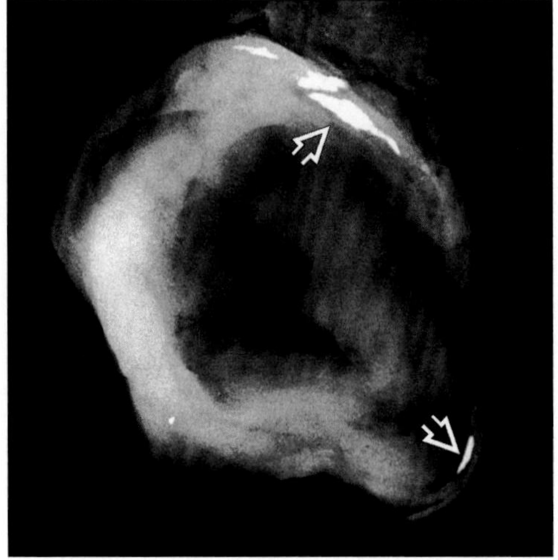

Specimen radiograph shows focal ossification ⇨ in the capsule of an ossifying fibromyxoid tumor.

TERMINOLOGY

Abbreviations

- Ossifying fibromyxoid tumor (OFMT)

Synonyms

- Ossifying fibromyxoid tumor of soft parts

Definitions

- Encapsulated tumor of small polygonal cells in fibromyxoid stroma with metaplastic ossification
- Majority benign; rare atypical or malignant variants

ETIOLOGY/PATHOGENESIS

Differentiation

- Various lineages suggested
  - Neural (Schwann cell), chondroid, myoepithelial

CLINICAL ISSUES

Epidemiology

- Incidence
  - Rare
- Age
  - 2nd-8th decades
    - Mean 50 years, rare in childhood
- Gender
  - M:F = 2:1

Site

- Mostly subcutaneous
  - Extremities, head and neck
    - Also trunk, retroperitoneum, mediastinum

Presentation

- Painless mass

Treatment

- Surgical approaches
  - Local excision

Prognosis

- Local recurrence in 22-27%, often after many years
- Very rarely cases metastasize to lung

IMAGE FINDINGS

Specimen Radiographic Findings

- Partial rim of bone around tumor

MACROSCOPIC FEATURES

General Features

- Circumscribed firm pale tumor, rarely cystic
  - Bone may be apparent on attempted slicing

Size

- Up to 17 cm (mean: 4 cm)

MICROSCOPIC PATHOLOGY

Histologic Features

- Well-defined thick fibrous capsule, extends as septa
- Rarely plexiform: Main lesion and satellite nodules
- Ovoid (rarely spindled) uniform cells in cords, nests, or sheets
  - Rounded uniform nuclei, small distinct nucleoli
  - Rare mitoses
  - Pale cytoplasm, distinct cell boundaries
- Stroma fibromyxoid, rarely hyaline
- Partial rim of bone in 60-80%
  - Ossification extends into tumor along septa
  - Occasionally cartilage is seen
- Atypical variant
  - Mitoses > 2 per 50 high-power fields
  - Increased cellularity, high nuclear grade
  - Necrosis, intratumoral osteoid formation

OSSIFYING FIBROMYXOID TUMOR

Key Facts

Terminology
- Encapsulated tumor of small polygonal cells in fibromyxoid stroma with metaplastic ossification
- Majority benign
- Occasional atypical or malignant variants

Etiology/Pathogenesis
- Schwann cell, chondroid, and myoepithelial lineages variously suggested

Clinical Issues
- Most common in extremities
- Mostly subcutaneous
- Local recurrence in up to 27% of cases, often after long interval
- Rare cases metastasize to lung
- Extremities, head and neck

Microscopic Pathology
- Well-defined thick fibrous capsule
- Ovoid (rarely spindled) uniform cells in cords, small nests, or sheets
- Partial rim of bone in 60-80%
- Atypical variant
  - Mitoses > 2 per 50 high-power fields
  - High nuclear grade
  - Intratumoral osteoid formation, necrosis

Ancillary Tests
- S100 protein typically positive
- GFAP, desmin, SMA, cytokeratin sometimes positive
- Ultrastructure shows external lamina and interdigitating cell processes
- No consistent genetic abnormalities

Predominant Pattern/Injury Type
- Fibromyxoid

Predominant Cell/Compartment Type
- Mesenchymal

ANCILLARY TESTS

Cytogenetics
- Inconsistent findings in 3 cases
  - t(3;11)(p21;p15) with various deletions
  - t(11;19)(q11;q13) with changes in chromosomes 1 and 3
  - Unbalanced translocation involving 6p and 14q

Electron Microscopy
- Transmission
  - Findings suggest nerve sheath differentiation
    - Interdigitating cytoplasmic processes
    - Discontinuous thick external lamina

DIFFERENTIAL DIAGNOSIS

Schwannoma
- Also has distinct capsule
- Often has neural connection
- Epithelioid variant has larger cells, more cytoplasm
- Lacks bone formation
- Strong diffuse S100 protein positivity

Myoepithelioma
- Wider range of patterns
- CK(+) and S100 protein(+)
- Myofilaments and junctions on electron microscopy

Glomus Tumor
- Nonencapsulated
- Cells arranged around blood vessels
- S100 protein(-) and GFAP(-)
- SMA(+) and H-caldesmon(+)

Extraskeletal Myxoid Chondrosarcoma
- Nonencapsulated
- Larger cells with eosinophilic cytoplasm
- Glycogen in cytoplasm, stroma hyaluronidase-resistant
- Specific translocations t(9;22)(q22;q12), t(9;17)(q22;q11), t(9;15)(q22;q21)
- Electron microscopy shows microtubular aggregates

DIAGNOSTIC CHECKLIST

Pathologic Interpretation Pearls
- Capsule with bone formation highly characteristic
- Distinctive glomus-like cells
- S100 protein positivity

SELECTED REFERENCES

1. Miettinen M et al: Ossifying fibromyxoid tumor of soft parts--a clinicopathologic and immunohistochemical study of 104 cases with long-term follow-up and a critical review of the literature. Am J Surg Pathol. 32(7):996-1005, 2008
2. Folpe AL et al: Ossifying fibromyxoid tumor of soft parts: a clinicopathologic study of 70 cases with emphasis on atypical and malignant variants. Am J Surg Pathol. 27(4):421-31, 2003
3. Zámecník M et al: Ossifying fibromyxoid tumor of soft parts: a report of 17 cases with emphasis on unusual histological features. Ann Diagn Pathol. 1(2):73-81, 1997
4. Kilpatrick SE et al: Atypical and malignant variants of ossifying fibromyxoid tumor. Clinicopathologic analysis of six cases. Am J Surg Pathol. 19(9):1039-46, 1995
5. Fisher C et al: Ossifying fibromyxoid tumor of soft parts with stromal cyst formation and ribosome-lamella complexes. Ultrastruct Pathol. 18(6):593-600, 1994
6. Schofield JB et al: Ossifying fibromyxoid tumour of soft parts: immunohistochemical and ultrastructural analysis. Histopathology. 22(2):101-12, 1993
7. Enzinger FM et al: Ossifying fibromyxoid tumor of soft parts. A clinicopathological analysis of 59 cases. Am J Surg Pathol. 13(10):817-27, 1989

OSSIFYING FIBROMYXOID TUMOR

Gross and Microscopic Features

(Left) Gross pathology shows pale pink-gray cut surface with shallow cysts ➪. This is a rare finding in ossifying fibromyxoid tumor. The cysts are lined by tumor cells, contain clear fluid, and are of no prognostic significance. ***(Right)*** *Hematoxylin & eosin shows a tumor within a thick fibrous capsule →, which contains a small focus of mature bone ➪. Note sharp demarcation of the tumor from surrounding soft tissue.*

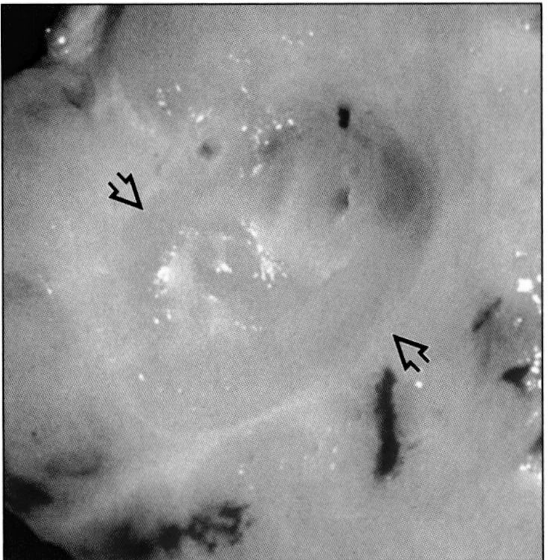

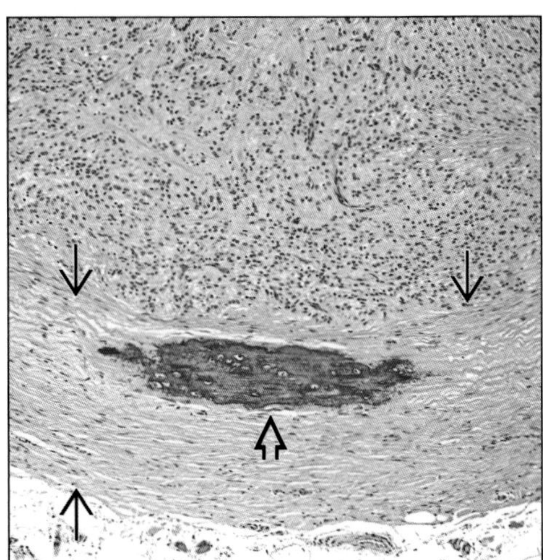

(Left) *Hematoxylin & eosin shows branching cords of tumor cells within fibrous stroma with focal myxoid change.* ***(Right)*** *Hematoxylin & eosin shows higher magnification of tumor cells, which have ovoid uniform nuclei and small amounts of eosinophilic cytoplasm. Note that the cords are 1 cell wide.*

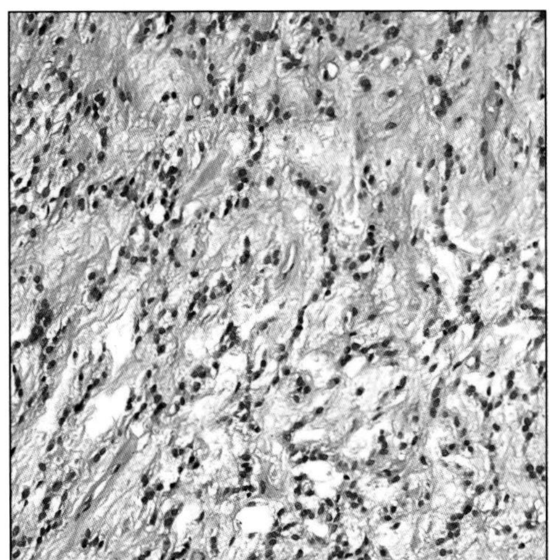

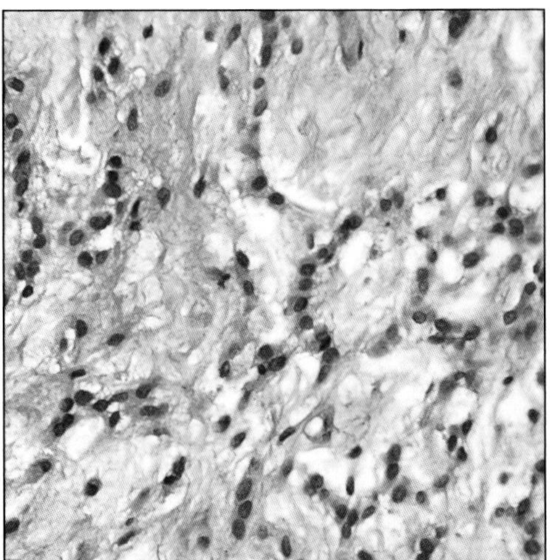

(Left) *Hematoxylin & eosin shows tumor cells forming a patternless sheet. Note slight variation in nuclear size (not amounting to high-grade change), small nucleoli, and distinct cell boundaries.* ***(Right)*** *Hematoxylin & eosin shows ossifying fibromyxoid tumor with stromal sclerosis, forming a pattern of small nests or groups of lesional cells.*

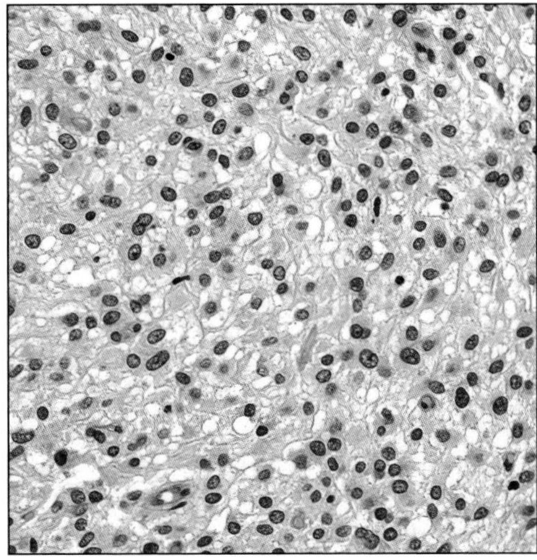

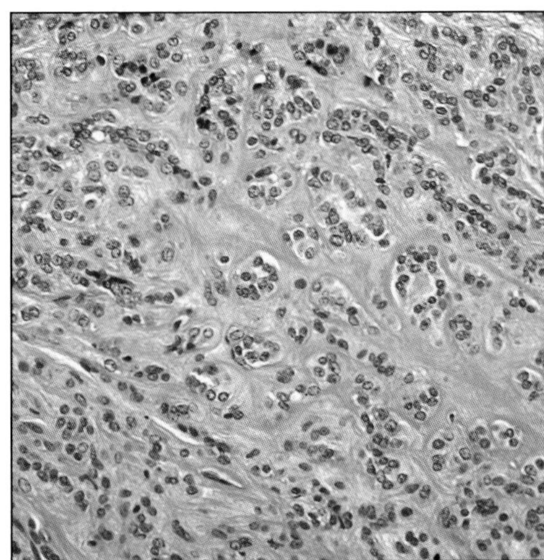

Variant Microscopic Features and Immunohistochemistry

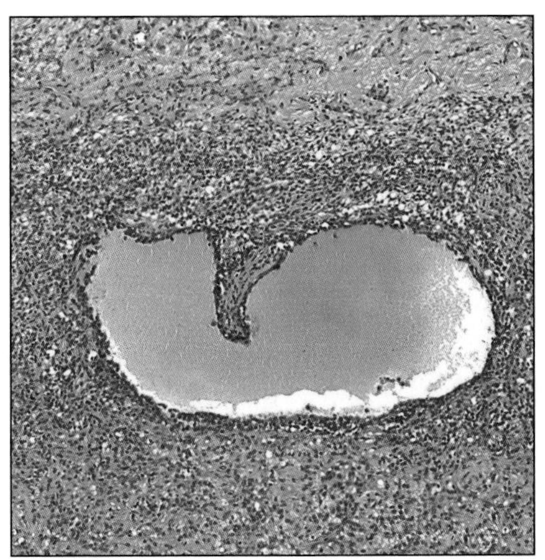

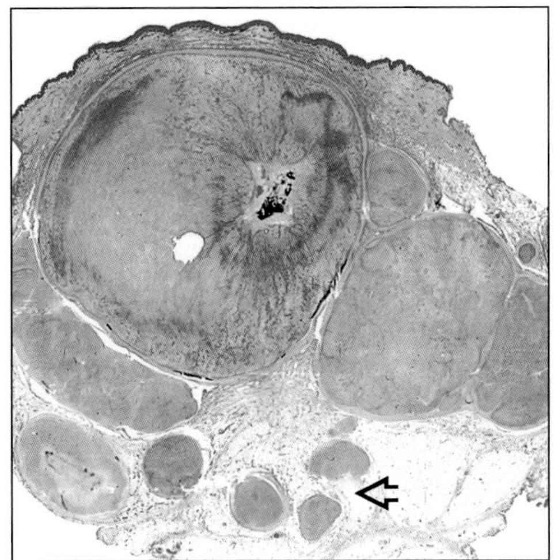

(Left) Hematoxylin & eosin shows a rare microcystic change. The cyst contains proteinaceous fluid. Note the condensation of cells at the edge of the cystic space. The cysts form in the stroma and lack an endothelial or epithelial lining ***(Right)*** Hematoxylin & eosin shows dermis and subcutis infiltrated by ossifying fibromyxoid tumor in a plexiform or multinodular pattern. There are 2 or 3 main nodules with several smaller ones extending into subcutaneous fat ⇨.

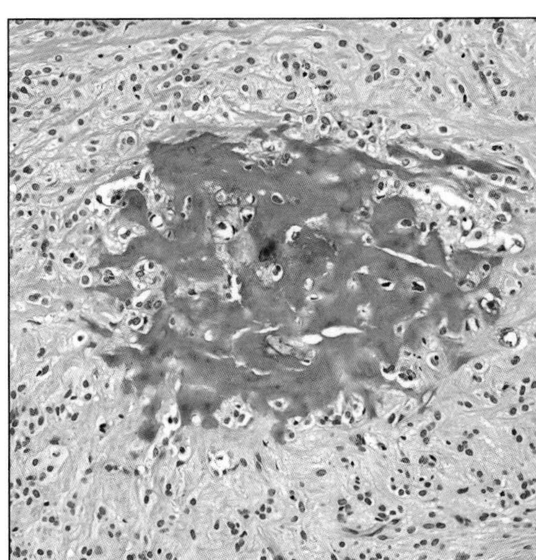

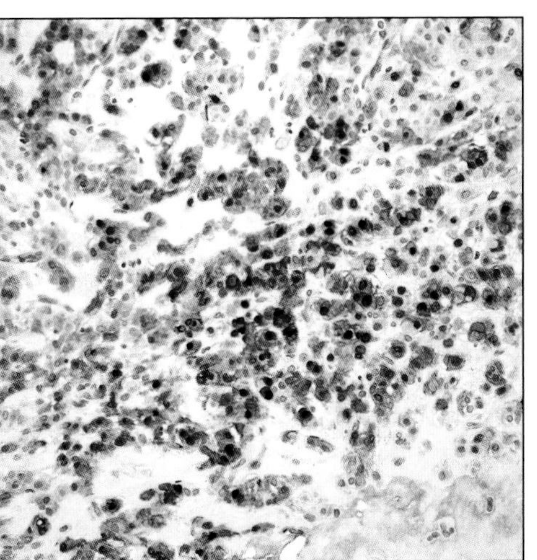

(Left) Hematoxylin & eosin shows intratumoral ossification, an unusual finding. Osteoid formation within the substance of the tumor can be a feature of the atypical variant. ***(Right)*** Positive S100 protein shows diffuse nuclear positivity. This is seen in the majority of ossifying fibromyxoid tumors, though not all.

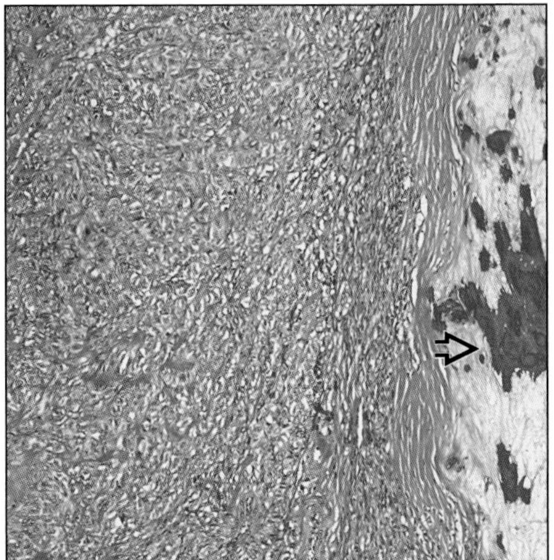

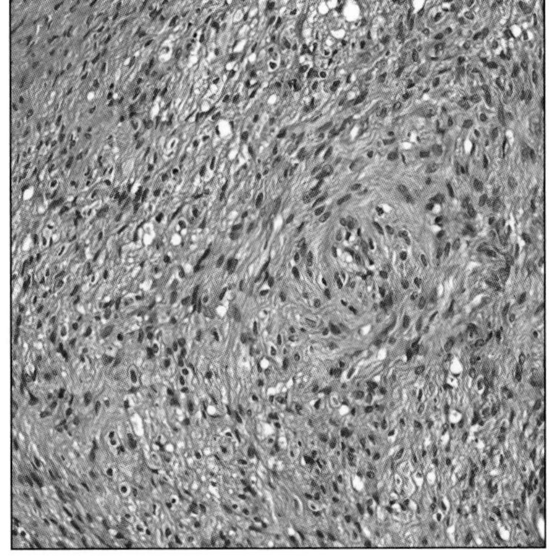

(Left) Hematoxylin & eosin shows an atypical variant of ossifying fibromyxoid tumor, with sheets of cells with enlarged atypical nuclei. Note the capsule with irregular bone formation ⇨. ***(Right)*** Hematoxylin & eosin shows rare spindling of tumor cells. Other parts of this tumor were more cellular with mitotic activity and resembled spindle cell sarcoma. This is a very unusual variant.

PHOSPHATURIC MESENCHYMAL TUMOR

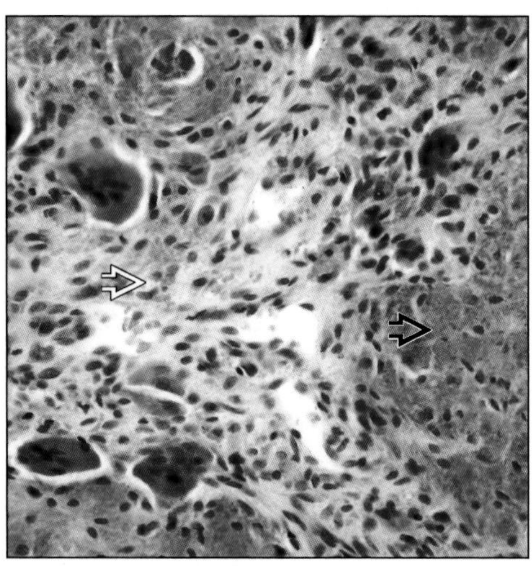

Hematoxylin & eosin shows an admixture of multinucleated giant cells, spindle cells, flocculent grumous ("grungy") material ➡, and hemosiderin ➡.

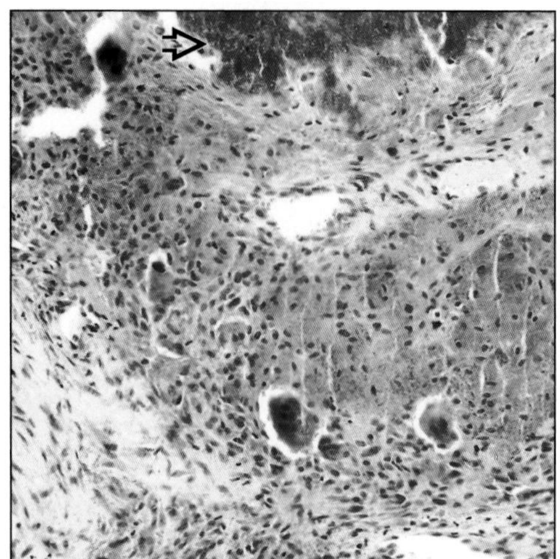

Hematoxylin & eosin shows another area of the neoplasm, with more prominent mineralization ➡.

TERMINOLOGY

Abbreviations

- Phosphaturic mesenchymal tumor (PMT)
- Phosphaturic mesenchymal tumor (mixed connective tissue variant) PMT-MCT

Synonyms

- Osteomalacia-associated mesenchymal tumor

Definitions

- Rare distinctive mesenchymal neoplasm associated with oncogenic osteomalacia
  - Syndrome of osteomalacia due to phosphate wasting

CLINICAL ISSUES

Epidemiology

- Incidence
  - Rare: Only 9 cases from archives of Armed Forces Institute of Pathology
- Age
  - Middle-aged adults (range: 3-73 years)
- Gender
  - No predilection
- Ethnicity
  - No predominance

Presentation

- Osteomalacia and phosphaturia accompanied by bone or soft tissue tumor
  - Soft tissue and bone each ~ 50% of cases
- Soft tissue PMT location
  - Most common in thigh followed by foot
- Bone PMT location
  - No site predilection

Prognosis

- Complete excision cures intractable oncogenic osteomalacia
- Most PMTs behave in benign fashion
  - Those with cytologically malignant features have behaved as malignant neoplasms

MACROSCOPIC FEATURES

Size

- Soft tissue: 2-14 cm
- Bone: 2-4 cm

MICROSCOPIC PATHOLOGY

Histologic Features

- Well-marginated at low magnification
- Spindled to stellate neoplastic cells
- Normochromatic small nuclei
- Indistinct nucleoli
- Minimal mitotic activity (< 1/10 HPF)
- Low cellularity
- Matrix production
  - Myxochondroid with variable hyalinization and flocculent mineralization
  - Microcystic change
  - Osteoid-like matrix
- Elaborate microvasculature
  - "Staghorn," delicate capillaries, and thick-walled vessels all present
- Osteoclast-like cells
- Adipose tissue component
- Rare cytologically malignant subset
  - High cellularity, high nuclear grade, > 5 mitoses/10 HPF

ANCILLARY TESTS

Immunohistochemistry

- Cells express FGF-23 (cytoplasmic) but not CD34, S100 protein, desmin, or cytokeratin

Key Facts

Terminology

- Synonym: Osteomalacia-associated mesenchymal tumor
- Definition: Rare distinctive mesenchymal neoplasm associated with oncogenic osteomalacia

Clinical Issues

- Complete excision cures intractable oncogenic osteomalacia
- Most neoplasms behave in benign fashion

Microscopic Pathology

- Spindled to stellate neoplastic cells
- Elaborate microvasculature
- Matrix production
- Myxochondroid with variable hyalinization and flocculent mineralization
- Osteoclast-like cells
- Adipose tissue component

PCR

- Amplification of *FGF23*

DIFFERENTIAL DIAGNOSIS

Other Tumor Types associated with Oncogenic Osteomalacia

- Metastatic carcinomas
- Sinonasal hemangiopericytoma
- Osteosarcomas
- Hemangiomas of bone
- All easily distinguished histologically

Hemangiopericytoma

- Uniformly distributed branching vessels
- Uniform round to ovoid cells
- CD34 labeling
- Devoid of matrix

Chondroma

- Lacks bland spindle cells
- No fat

Giant Cell Tumor of Soft Tissue and Bone

- Can have osteoclastic cells, fibrohistiocytic features, and woven bone
- Lacks spindle cells and matrix

Mesenchymal Chondrosarcoma

- Overtly malignant
- Round blue cells, hemangiopericytoma-like vascularity, foci of mature-appearing cartilage

SELECTED REFERENCES

1. Bahrami A et al: RT-PCR analysis for FGF23 using paraffin sections in the diagnosis of phosphaturic mesenchymal tumors with and without known tumor induced osteomalacia. Am J Surg Pathol. 33(9):1348-54, 2009
2. Folpe AL et al: Most osteomalacia-associated mesenchymal tumors are a single histopathologic entity: an analysis of 32 cases and a comprehensive review of the literature. Am J Surg Pathol. 28(1):1-30, 2004
3. Wilkins GE et al: Oncogenic osteomalacia: evidence for a humoral phosphaturic factor. J Clin Endocrinol Metab. 80(5):1628-34, 1995
4. Park YK et al: Oncogenic osteomalacia: a clinicopathologic study of 17 bone lesions. J Korean Med Sci. 9(4):289-98, 1994
5. Stone MD et al: A neuroendocrine cause of oncogenic osteomalacia. J Pathol. 167(2):181-5, 1992
6. Schultze G et al: [Oncogenic hypophosphatemic osteomalacia] Dtsch Med Wochenschr. 114(27):1073-8, 1989
7. Weidner N et al: Phosphaturic mesenchymal tumors. A polymorphous group causing osteomalacia or rickets. Cancer. 59(8):1442-54, 1987
8. Stone E et al: Oncogenic osteomalacia associated with a mesenchymal chondrosarcoma. Clin Invest Med. 7(3):179-85, 1984
9. Daniels RA et al: Tumorous phosphaturic osteomalacia. Report of a case associated with multiple hemangiomas of bone. Am J Med. 67(1):155-9, 1979

IMAGE GALLERY

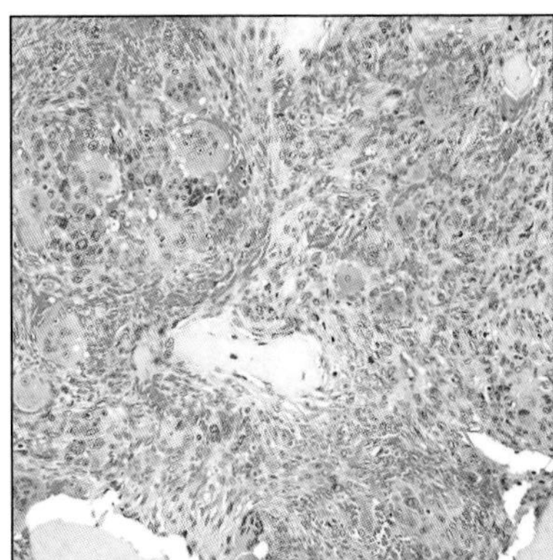

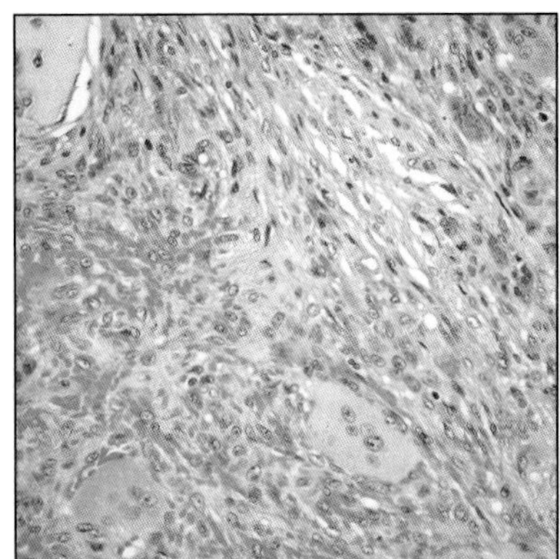

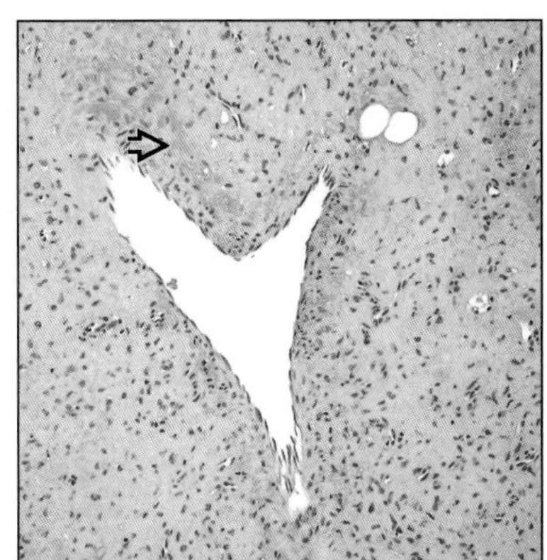

*(**Left**) Hematoxylin & eosin shows another example of phosphaturic mesenchymal tumor, this one with a more prominent hemangiopericytoma-like vascular pattern. (**Center**) Hematoxylin & eosin shows a prominent spindle cell zone in the tumor. (**Right**) Hematoxylin & eosin shows another phosphaturic mesenchymal tumor. This one lacks giant cells but has a hemangiopericytoma-like vascular pattern and more subtle flocculent grumous ("grungy") material ⇨ than other examples.*

EXTRASKELETAL MYXOID CHONDROSARCOMA

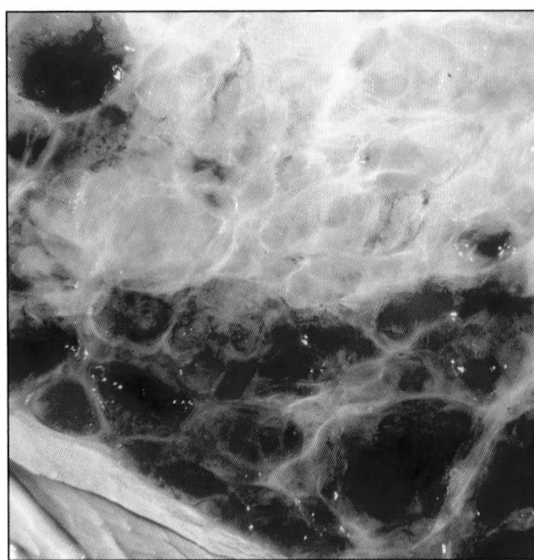

Characteristic gross appearance of an extraskeletal myxoid chondrosarcoma (EMC) displays well-defined lobular architecture, gelatinous yellow cut surface, and intralesional hemorrhage.

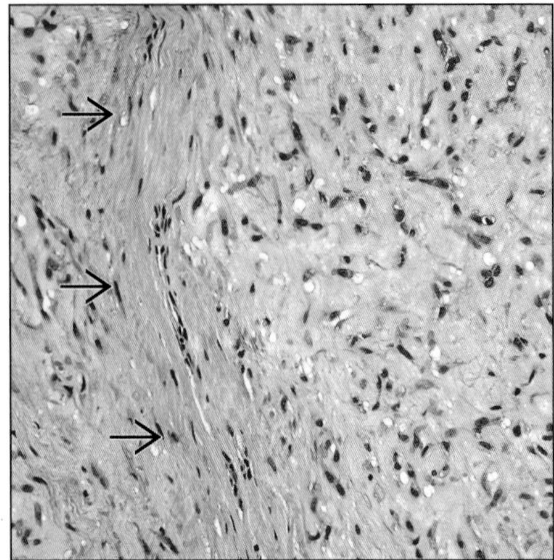

Microscopically, EMC has a lobular architecture defined by thick fibrous bands ⇒ that divide it into myxoid lobules containing cords of interconnecting uniform cells.

TERMINOLOGY

Abbreviations

- Extraskeletal myxoid chondrosarcoma (EMC)

Synonyms

- Chordoid sarcoma

Definitions

- Soft tissue sarcoma of uncertain differentiation with abundant myxoid matrix, multilobular architecture, and uniform cells in cords, clusters, and fine networks

CLINICAL ISSUES

Epidemiology

- Incidence
  - Rare, < 3% of soft tissue sarcomas
- Age
  - Median: 50 years; range: 5-90 years; rare in children
- Gender
  - M:F = 2:1

Site

- Extremities; lower extremity most common
- Rare in abdomen, pelvis, retroperitoneum, head and neck, cranium, and pleura

Presentation

- Deep mass
- Large tumors can ulcerate or impair range of motion
- 13% present with pulmonary metastases

Treatment

- Surgical approaches
  - Wide local excision
- Drugs
  - Poor response to chemotherapy

Prognosis

- High recurrence rate
  - Local (30-50%)
  - Metastases (35-45%), usually pulmonary
- Often prolonged course
- Old age, large size, and proximal location (but not grade) are adverse prognostic factors

MACROSCOPIC FEATURES

General Features

- Well demarcated; contained by pseudocapsule
- Gelatinous lobules separated by fibrous septa
- Cystic areas, hemorrhage, and necrosis common

Size

- Usually large; median: 7 cm; range: 1-30 cm

MICROSCOPIC PATHOLOGY

Histologic Features

- Conventional EMC
  - Multilobular architecture with fibrous septa, abundant pale blue myxoid matrix; true hyaline cartilage rarely if ever present
  - Uniform cells with eosinophilic cytoplasm and round to spindle-shaped nuclei arranged in cords, clusters, or fine networks with low mitotic rate
  - Necrosis, acute hemorrhage, and hemosiderosis common
- Cellular/poorly differentiated EMC
  - Densely cellular, often with little myxoid matrix
  - Large epithelioid or rhabdoid cells
  - Nonmyxoid spindle cell areas (dedifferentiation)

Predominant Pattern/Injury Type

- Myxoid

Predominant Cell/Compartment Type

- Spindle and epithelioid

EXTRASKELETAL MYXOID CHONDROSARCOMA

Key Facts

Terminology
- Soft tissue sarcoma of uncertain differentiation with abundant myxoid matrix, multilobular architecture, and uniform cells in cords, clusters, and fine networks

Clinical Issues
- Median age: 50 years old; M:F = 2:1
- Lower extremity most common
- High rate of local and distant recurrence
- Poor response to chemotherapy

Macroscopic Features
- Gelatinous lobules separated by thick fibrous septa
- Cystic areas, hemorrhage, and necrosis common

Microscopic Pathology
- Abundant myxoid matrix; true hyaline cartilage rarely if ever present
- Cells interconnect to form cords, clusters, or fine networks
- Cellular variant with minimal myxoid matrix

Ancillary Tests
- Positive for S100 but variable and inconsistent
- Cytogenetics, t(9;22)(q22;q12.2) most common
- Break-apart FISH for *EWSR1*

Top Differential Diagnoses
- Chordoma
- Parachordoma/myoepithelioma
- Soft tissue chondroma
- Myxofibrosarcoma, epithelioid variant

ANCILLARY TESTS

Immunohistochemistry
- Positive for S100 but variable and inconsistent
- Minority of cases positive for cytokeratin &/or EMA
- Negative for brachyury and podoplanin; usually negative for CD117
- Tumors with rhabdoid features negative for SNF5

Cytogenetics
- t(9;22)(q22;q12.2) most common; t(9;17)(q22;q11.2)

In Situ Hybridization
- Break-apart FISH for *EWSR1* diagnostically useful

Electron Microscopy
- Transmission
  - Intracisternal bundles of parallel microtubules
  - Rhabdoid cells with perinuclear whorls of intermediate filaments

DIFFERENTIAL DIAGNOSIS

Chordoma
- Larger cells with more abundant cytoplasm, including physaliferous cells
- Positive for cytokeratin, EMA, S100, and brachyury
- Affects sacrum, clivus, vertebral bodies

Parachordoma/Myoepithelioma
- Most are histologically benign
- Positive for cytokeratin and S100; minority positive for actin-sm

Soft Tissue Chondroma
- May have lobular myxoid architecture and interconnecting cells
- True hyaline cartilage, often heavily calcified
- Predilection for hands and feet

Myxofibrosarcoma, Epithelioid Variant
- High-grade pleomorphic cytology
- Prominent curvilinear blood vessels
- Usually admixed with conventional myxofibrosarcoma
- Negative for S100

Epithelioid GIST
- May have abundant myxoid matrix and cell cords
- Positive for CD117 and CD34
- Origin from gastric wall

Myxoid Mesothelioma
- Epithelioid mesothelioma with abundant myxoid matrix
- Hyaluronidase-sensitive mucin
- Positive for cytokeratin, calretinin, WT1
- Pleural tumor

Chordoid Meningioma
- Usually admixed with conventional meningioma
- Positive for EMA and podoplanin

Sarcomatoid Carcinoma with Myxoid Stroma
- High-grade cytology
- Positive for cytokeratin

SELECTED REFERENCES

1. Drilon AD et al: Extraskeletal myxoid chondrosarcoma: a retrospective review from 2 referral centers emphasizing long-term outcomes with surgery and chemotherapy. Cancer. 113(12):3364-71, 2008
2. Meis-Kindblom JM et al: Extraskeletal myxoid chondrosarcoma: a reappraisal of its morphologic spectrum and prognostic factors based on 117 cases. Am J Surg Pathol. 23(6):636-50, 1999

EXTRASKELETAL MYXOID CHONDROSARCOMA

Gross, Radiographic, and Microscopic Features

*(**Left**) Grossly, most EMCs form large, demarcated tumors with a well-defined lobular pattern created by thick fibrous septa that divide it into gelatinous lobules. Necrosis, intratumoral hemorrhage, and cyst formation are often present, as shown here. (**Right**) Axial T2-weighted MR discloses a large, deep-seated EMC of the thigh with heterogeneous hyperintense signal and well-defined lobular architecture.*

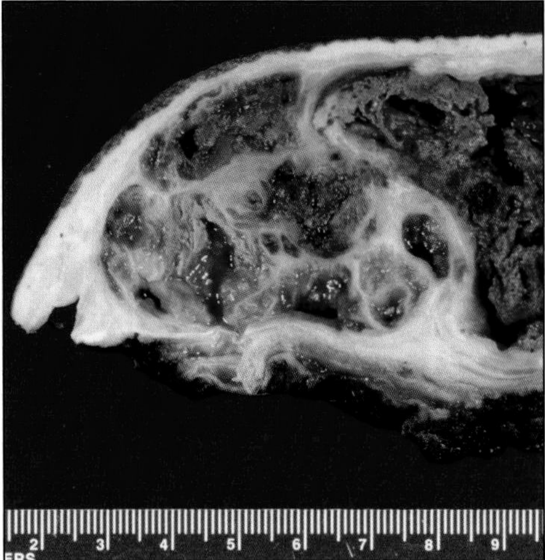

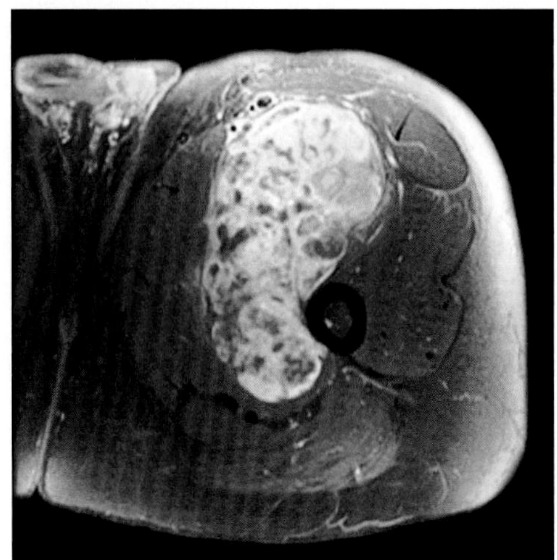

*(**Left**) This low-power image highlights the lobular growth pattern of EMC, characterized by thick fibrous bands →. Areas of acute hemorrhage ⇨, hemosiderosis ➡, and scarring ↷ are common, as are necrosis and cyst formation (not shown). (**Right**) The neoplastic cells in an EMC interconnect to form cord, clusters, and cribriform structures within a background of myxoid matrix. True hyaline cartilage is virtually never seen. Note the thick fibrous band ⇨.*

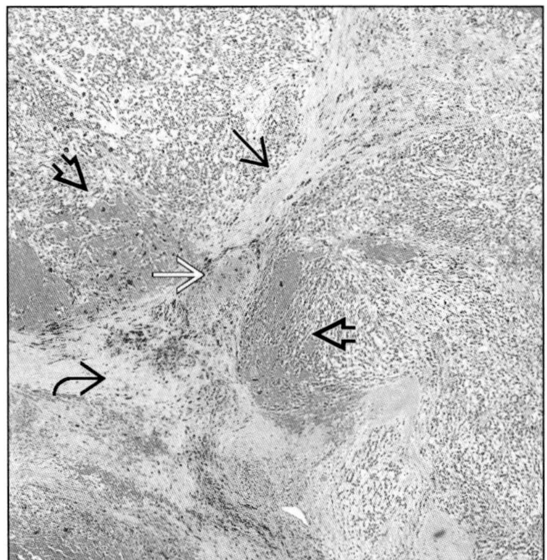

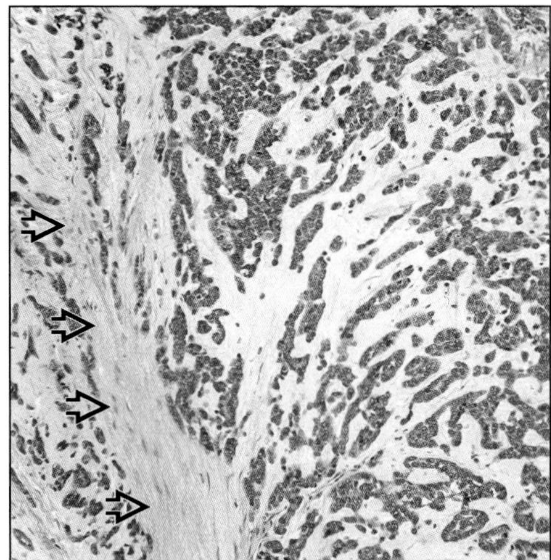

*(**Left**) A conventional EMC is typically composed of uniform cells with round to oval nuclei and wisps of eosinophilic cytoplasm that interconnect with each other. (**Right**) Spindle cell differentiation is common in EMC, and the amount varies from focal to diffuse. Note the interconnecting cell pattern forming cords and fine networks.*

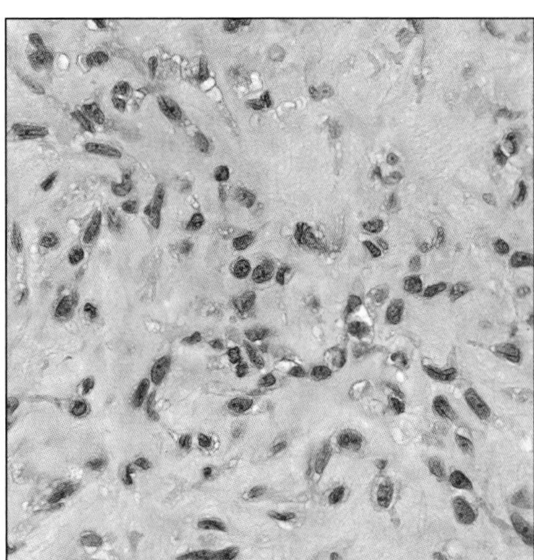

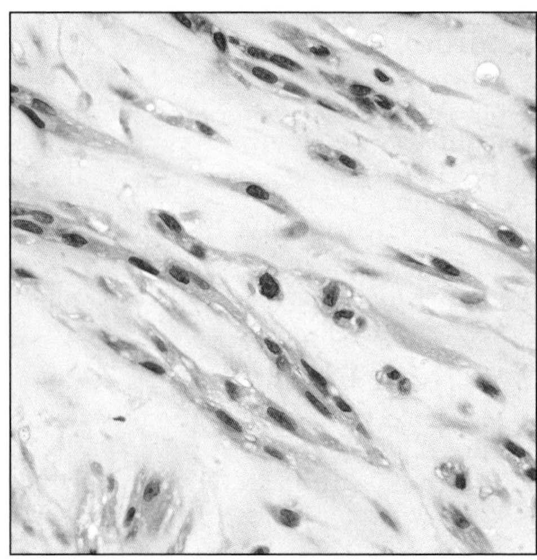

Microscopic Features and Ancillary Techniques

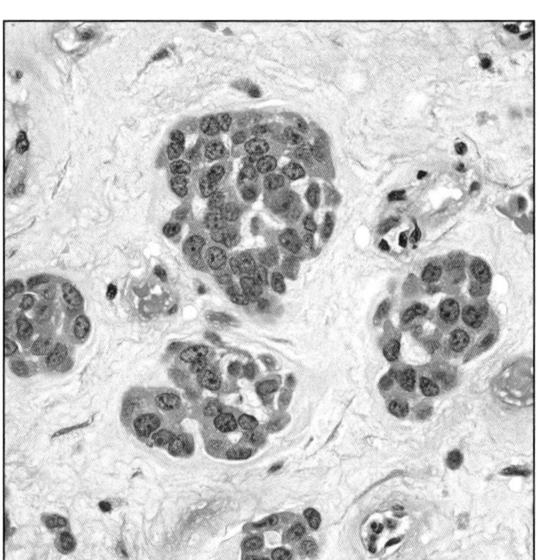

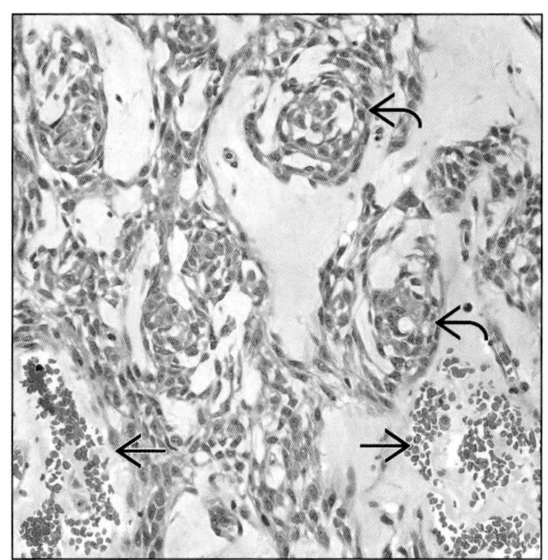

(Left) *The neoplastic cells in an EMC can form rounded cohesive clusters. Note the epithelioid cytology with densely eosinophilic cytoplasm and abundant pale blue myxoid matrix.* ***(Right)*** *This EMC has a complex reticular architecture characterized by cohesive arrays of epithelioid and spindle cells forming cribriform and whorling ⮳ patterns. Note the acute hemorrhage at the bottom ⮕.*

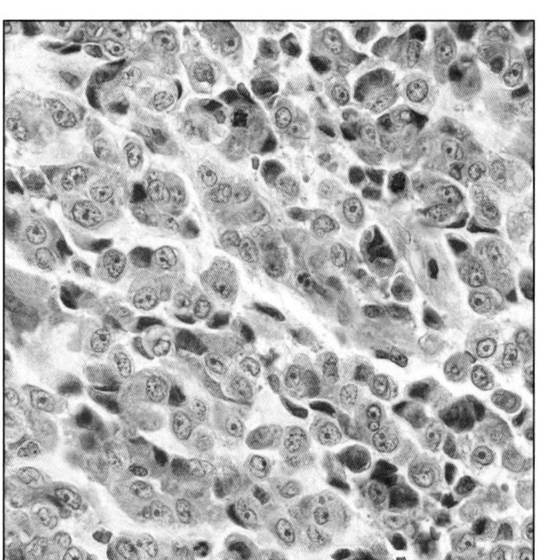

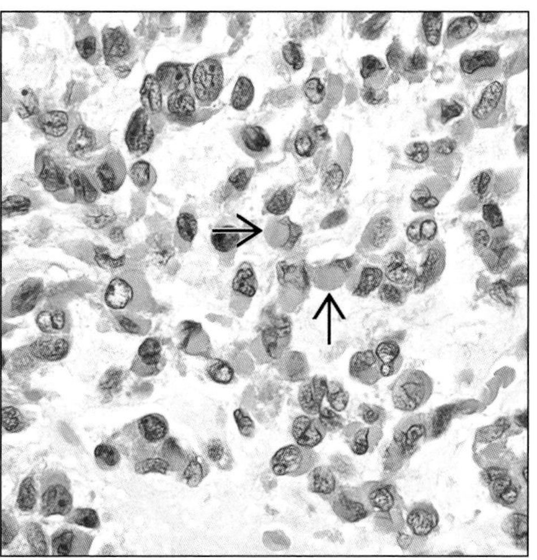

(Left) *Cellular EMC is characterized by sheets of cells with little or no intervening matrix. These tumors often have large epithelioid cells with vesicular nuclei, prominent nucleoli, and brisk mitotic activity. Histologic grade is generally not regarded as a prognostic variable in an EMC.* ***(Right)*** *Rhabdoid cells with eccentric eosinophilic cytoplasm and perinuclear hyalin globules ⮕ can be found in an EMC. As in rhabdoid tumor, these cells are negative for SNF5.*

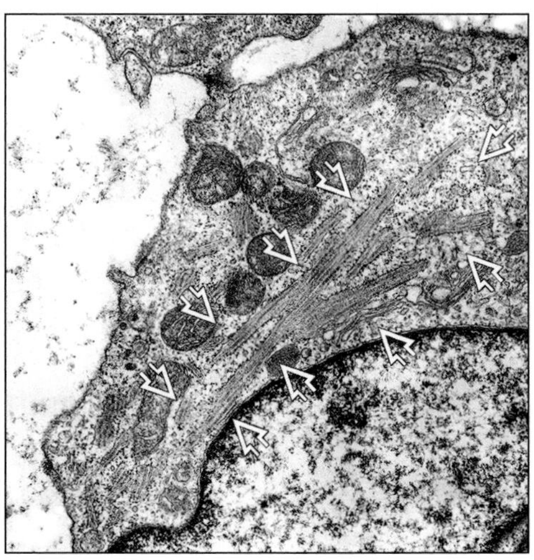

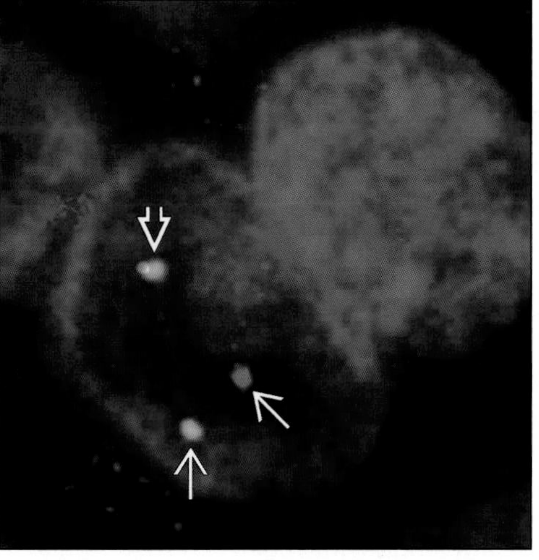

(Left) *Electron micrograph depicts parallel bundles of microtubules ⮕ within the cisternal compartment of an EMC, a highly characteristic feature found only in a minority of cases. Rhabdoid cells in an EMC have perinuclear whorls of intermediate filaments (not shown).* ***(Right)*** *Break-apart FISH for EWSR1 is a useful diagnostic test for EMC. This immunofluorescence image depicts a normal allele with fused red and green signals ⮕ and a broken apart allele ⮕.*

SYNOVIAL SARCOMA

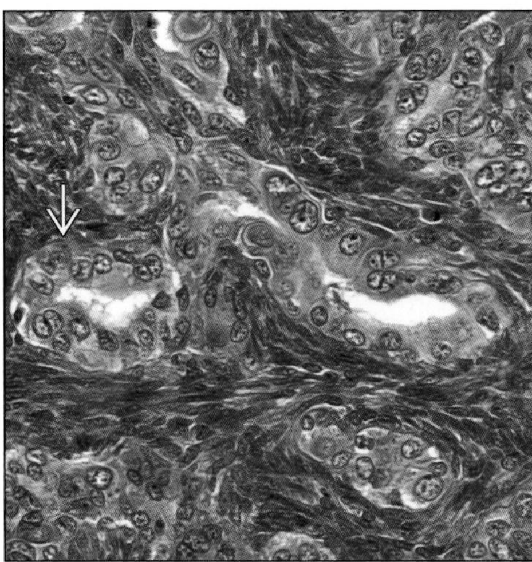

Hematoxylin & eosin shows a biphasic synovial sarcoma (SS) with irregular-shaped glandular structures ➔ dispersed in a spindle cell component. The epithelial cell nuclei are rounded and uniform.

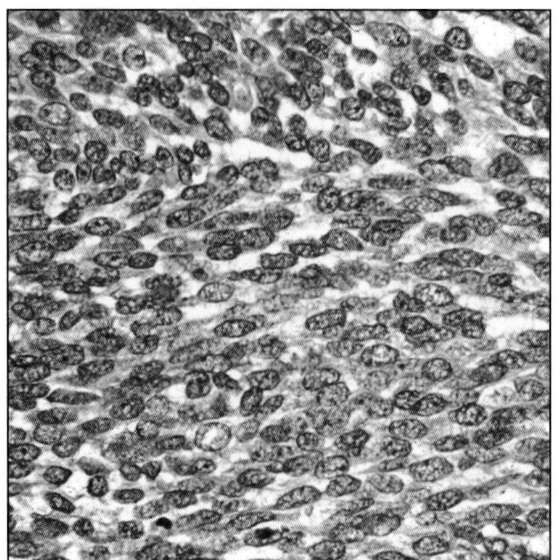

Hematoxylin & eosin shows monophasic SS composed of irregular small short or ovoid spindle cells with apparently overlapping vesicular nuclei. Note the absence of nuclear pleomorphism.

TERMINOLOGY

Abbreviations

- Synovial sarcoma (SS)

Synonyms

- Terms no longer commonly used
  - Synovial cell sarcoma
  - Malignant synovioma

Definitions

- Mesenchymal spindle cell tumor with variable epithelial differentiation, including gland formation
  - Characterized by specific chromosomal translocation t(X;18)(p11;q11)
- Name is historical accident
  - Tumor does not arise from or differentiate toward synovium

ETIOLOGY/PATHOGENESIS

Environmental Exposure

- Very rare examples arise in field of prior irradiation
- 1 case reported at site of metal prosthetic implant

Acquired Genetic Abnormality

- Translocation between chromosomes X and 18

CLINICAL ISSUES

Epidemiology

- Incidence
  - 5-10% of all soft tissue sarcomas
  - Can occur in any anatomic location; rare in joints
  - 90% in extremities
    - Most common around knee region
    - In periarticular soft tissue and tendon sheaths
  - Subset in head and neck
    - Parapharynx, oral cavity, tonsil
  - Rare subsets
    - Abdominal wall
    - Retroperitoneum/omentum
    - Mediastinum
    - Intravascular, intraneural
- Age
  - Majority in young adults 15-35 years
  - Rare over age of 50
- Gender
  - More frequent in males

Presentation

- Slow growing
- Deep mass, with local pressure effects
- Painful mass
  - > 1/2 of cases
- Painless mass
  - < 1/2 of cases

Natural History

- Can be present for long period: 2-20 years
- Local recurrence frequent especially if inadequate resection
- Metastasis in 45% of cases
  - Lung (95%)
    - Late metastases can appear after many years
  - Bone
  - Lymph nodes (10%)

Treatment

- Options, risks, complications
  - Based on
    - Size, location of primary tumor, and stage
- Adjuvant therapy
  - Preoperative irradiation for large or initially unresectable primary tumor
  - Chemotherapy for disseminated disease
    - Ifosfamide or doxorubicin
    - Combination chemotherapy
- Surgical approaches
  - Local excision of primary tumor with clear margin

SYNOVIAL SARCOMA

Key Facts

Terminology

- Name is historical accident, as tumor does not arise from or differentiate toward synovium
- Mesenchymal spindle cell tumor with variable epithelial differentiation, including gland formation
  - Characterized by specific chromosomal translocation t(X;18)(p11;q11)

Clinical Issues

- Accounts for 5-10% of all soft tissue sarcomas
- Can occur in any anatomic location
- Majority in young adults 15-35 years
- More frequent in males
- Presence of biphasic pattern does not influence behavior
- Poorly differentiated histology worsens prognosis

Image Findings

- Scattered calcifications

Microscopic Pathology

- Sheets of uniform small spindle cells with ovoid nuclei and scanty cytoplasm
  - If pleomorphic, consider other diagnoses
- Focal epithelial differentiation
  - Glandular structures
  - Solid cords or nests
- Never low-grade tumor

Ancillary Tests

- Epithelial markers focally positive
- If CD34(+), consider other diagnoses
- Identification of t(X;18)(p11.q11) and *SS18-SSX* fusions diagnostic

---

    - Limb sparing
    - Amputation rarely required
  - Excision of recurrences
    - Limb sparing where possible
    - Radical, including amputation
  - Pulmonary metastasectomy for small numbers of metastases

Prognosis

- 5-year survival (50-85%)
- Presence of biphasic pattern does not influence behavior
- Favorable prognostic factors
  - Small tumor size (< 5 cm)
  - Young age, especially childhood
  - Calcifying/ossifying variant (not in all series)
  - Possibly tumors with *SSX2* gene rearrangement (not in all series)
- Adverse prognostic factors
  - Age > 40 years
  - Large tumor size (> 5 cm)
  - Poorly differentiated histology

IMAGE FINDINGS

General Features

- Best diagnostic clue
  - Scattered calcifications
  - Circumscribed mass
- Location
  - 1st consideration for tumors around knee
- Size
  - Variable
    - Usually > 5 cm in diameter
    - Can be very small
    - Rarely > 10 cm, though up to 15 cm described
- Morphology
  - Circumscribed

Specimen Radiographic Findings

- Small scattered calcifications

MACROSCOPIC FEATURES

General Features

- Circumscribed tan tumor mass
- Soft cut surface
- Cysts occasionally seen
  - Smooth walled
  - Contain mucoid fluid or blood
- Focal necrosis and hemorrhage in poorly differentiated tumors

Sections to Be Submitted

- Sample margins and representative sections of tumor

Size

- Wide range from minute (< 1 cm) to 15 cm diameter

MICROSCOPIC PATHOLOGY

Histologic Features

- Sheets of uniform small spindle cells with ovoid nuclei and scanty cytoplasm
- Focal epithelial differentiation
  - Glandular structures
  - Solid cords or nests
- Intercellular stroma minimal except in
  - Occasional hyalinizing monophasic SS
  - Calcifying variants
  - Recurrences after irradiation

Lymphatic/Vascular Invasion

- Rarely

Margins

- Infiltrative microscopically, pseudocapsule of adjacent tissue

Lymph Nodes

- Metastases in up to 10% of cases

Predominant Pattern/Injury Type

- Fascicular
  - Herringbone

- Sheets
- Ill-defined palisading occasionally seen
- Hemangiopericytic pattern common, especially in poorly differentiated SS

Predominant Cell/Compartment Type

- Spindle and epithelioid
- Small round

Grade

- Either grade II or III; never grade I

ANCILLARY TESTS

Cytology

- Diagnosis can be made on cell-rich aspirates
  - Biphasic pattern rarely seen
  - Monophasic SS
    - Cellular clusters
    - Hyperchromatic, overlapping short ovoid nuclei
    - Inconspicuous nucleoli
    - Scanty cytoplasm
    - Mast cells, calcifications

Flow Cytometry

- Not routinely used for diagnosis or prognosis
- About 2/3 diploid, 1/3 aneuploid; some have intratumoral heterogeneity

Cytogenetics

- > 90% of SS have balanced reciprocal translocation
  - t(X;18)(p11.q11)
  - *SSX* gene on chromosome X fuses to *SS18* gene (formerly termed *SYT*) on chromosome 18
    - Commonly exon 10 of *SS18* gene is fused to exon 6 of *SSX* gene
  - *SSX* gene has 5 variants
    - *SSX1*, *SSX2*, and very rarely *SSX4* undergo rearrangement
  - Results in SS18-SSX fusion protein (unknown function)
- Additional rare abnormalities include t(X;20)(p11;q13)

In Situ Hybridization

- Translocated chromosomes can be identified by FISH

PCR

- Fusion transcripts can be identified by RT-PCR
- Sensitivity in paraffin material
  - Improves with laboratory's experience
  - ↓ with time since fixation and processing

Gene Expression Profiling

- Has identified unsuspected genes activated in SS
  - e.g., *TLE1* (transducin-like enhancer of split)
    - In 95% of synovial sarcomas
    - Rare in other sarcoma types

Electron Microscopy

- Transmission
  - Biphasic SS
    - Glands enclosed in continuous external lamina
    - Junctional complexes, surface microvilli, tonofilaments
  - Monophasic SS
    - Cells closely packed with rare, poorly formed intercellular junctions
    - Rare intercellular spaces with few microvilli
    - Rare fragments of external lamina
    - Variable rough endoplasmic reticulum sometimes resembling fibroblast

DIFFERENTIAL DIAGNOSIS

Malignant Peripheral Nerve Sheath Tumor

- Association with neurofibromatosis type 1
- Alternating myxoid and cellular areas
- Nuclei wavy, buckled, or arrowhead-shaped
- S100 protein in 67% of cases
- Epithelial markers usually absent; CK19(-)

Spindle Cell Carcinoma

- Relationship to epithelial surface
- Dysplasia or in situ carcinoma in overlying epithelium
- Nuclear pleomorphism
- Cytokeratin positivity can be diffuse rather than focal

Leiomyosarcoma

- Relationship to vein
- Fascicles arranged at abrupt right angles
- Nontapered cell shape
- Elongated parallel-sided nuclei with blunt ends
- Paranuclear vacuoles
- Eosinophilic cytoplasm with longitudinal fibrils
- Can be pleomorphic
- Desmin, smooth muscle actin, H-caldesmon positive
- Cytokeratin, EMA rarely expressed

Spindle Cell Rhabdomyosarcoma

- Focal rhabdomyoblastic differentiation
- Desmin(+), myogenin(+)

Solitary Fibrous Tumor

- Hemangiopericytic pattern usually peripheral
- So-called "patternless" pattern
  - Random orientation of cells
- Diffuse or focal collagenization
- CD34(+)

Ewing Sarcoma/PNET

- Lacks hemangiopericytic pattern
- Uniform sheets of cells without spindle cell or epithelial areas
- Nuclei rounded
  - Do not appear to overlap
- Reticulin fibers are typically
  - Absent between cells
  - Around blood vessels only
- CD99 diffusely positive with membrane staining
- Cytokeratin sometimes positive
  - Often with paranuclear dot distribution
- CD56(-)
- Different translocations
  - (11;22)(q24;q12) with *FLI1-EWS* fusion gene most common
  - Others fuse *EWS* with different gene partners

SYNOVIAL SARCOMA

Immunohistochemistry			
Antibody	**Reactivity**	**Staining Pattern**	**Comment**
EMA	Positive	Cell membrane	In 70-100% of MSS, focal
CK-PAN	Positive	Cytoplasmic	In 90% of MSS, focal
Bcl-2	Positive	Cytoplasmic	In 98% of cases, diffuse
CD56	Positive	Cytoplasmic	In 80% of cases
CD99	Positive	Cell membrane	In 66% of cases, focal
S100	Positive	Nuclear	In 40% of cases, focal
Calretinin	Positive	Nuclear	In 40% of cases, focal
β-catenin	Positive	Nuclear	In 40% of cases, diffuse
FLI-1	Positive	Nuclear	In 22% of cases
TLE1	Positive	Nuclear	In 95% of cases
CD34	Negative		Very focally positive in < 5% of cases

Alveolar Rhabdomyosarcoma

- Solid variant can mimic poorly differentiated SS
- Immunohistochemical positivity for
  - Desmin in cytoplasm
  - Myogenin in nuclei
- Specific translocations
  - (1;13)(p36;q14) with *PAX7-FKHR* fusion gene
  - (2;13)(q35;q14) with *PAX3-FKHR* fusion gene

Epithelioid Sarcoma

- Classical type superficially located
- Proximal type pleomorphic: Resembles carcinoma or melanoma
- Not biphasic; epithelioid and spindle cells merge
- Cells have more cytoplasm
- Epithelial markers diffusely positive
- CD34 is positive in 50%
- INI1 is negative in 90% of cases
- Lacks t(X;18)

DIAGNOSTIC CHECKLIST

Clinically Relevant Pathologic Features

- Age distribution
- Organ distribution
  - Most common site is around knee
  - Can arise at any anatomical site
- Symptom time frame
  - Unusually among sarcomas, can be present for several years before presentation

Pathologic Interpretation Pearls

- Biphasic pattern distinctive
- Monophasic SS has sheets of uniform spindle cells
  - CK positivity is focal (single cells) not diffuse
  - EMA positivity is focal (single cells) not diffuse
  - CD34 almost always negative
  - Bcl-2 almost always positive
  - TLE1 very sensitive marker
- Pleomorphism very rare
- Poorly differentiated SS has nested reticulin pattern
- Genetic findings are specific and diagnostic

SELECTED REFERENCES

1. Terry J et al: TLE1 as a diagnostic immunohistochemical marker for synovial sarcoma emerging from gene expression profiling studies. Am J Surg Pathol. 31(2):240-6, 2007
2. Michal M et al: Minute synovial sarcomas of the hands and feet: a clinicopathologic study of 21 tumors less than 1 cm. Am J Surg Pathol. 30(6):721-6, 2006
3. Ferrari A et al: Synovial sarcoma: a retrospective analysis of 271 patients of all ages treated at a single institution. Cancer. 101(3):627-34, 2004
4. Guillou L et al: Histologic grade, but not SYT-SSX fusion type, is an important prognostic factor in patients with synovial sarcoma: a multicenter, retrospective analysis. J Clin Oncol. 22(20):4040-50, 2004
5. Akerman M et al: Fine-needle aspiration of synovial sarcoma: criteria for diagnosis: retrospective reexamination of 37 cases, including ancillary diagnostics. A Scandinavian Sarcoma Group study. Diagn Cytopathol. 28(5):232-8, 2003
6. Chan JA et al: Synovial sarcoma in older patients: clinicopathological analysis of 32 cases with emphasis on unusual histological features. Histopathology. 43(1):72-83, 2003
7. Coindre JM et al: Should molecular testing be required for diagnosing synovial sarcoma? A prospective study of 204 cases. Cancer. 98(12):2700-7, 2003
8. Ladanyi M et al: Impact of SYT-SSX fusion type on the clinical behavior of synovial sarcoma: a multi-institutional retrospective study of 243 patients. Cancer Res. 62(1):135-40, 2002
9. Pelmus M et al: Monophasic fibrous and poorly differentiated synovial sarcoma: immunohistochemical reassessment of 60 t(X;18)(SYT-SSX)-positive cases. Am J Surg Pathol. 26(11):1434-40, 2002
10. Spillane AJ et al: Synovial sarcoma: a clinicopathologic, staging, and prognostic assessment. J Clin Oncol. 18(22):3794-803, 2000
11. Krane JF et al: Myxoid synovial sarcoma: an underappreciated morphologic subset. Mod Pathol. 12(5):456-62, 1999
12. van de Rijn M et al: Poorly differentiated synovial sarcoma: an analysis of clinical, pathologic, and molecular genetic features. Am J Surg Pathol. 23(1):106-12, 1999
13. Fisher C: Synovial sarcoma. Ann Diagn Pathol. 2(6):401-21, 1998
14. Smith ME et al: Synovial sarcoma lack synovial differentiation. Histopathology. 26(3):279-81, 1995

SYNOVIAL SARCOMA

Gross and Microscopic Features

*(**Left**) Gross pathology specimen shows a circumscribed tumor located in skeletal muscle beneath the deep fascia ➔. The cut surface of the tumor is tan and displays focal hemorrhage. (**Right**) Hematoxylin & eosin shows a biphasic synovial sarcoma forming a papillary structure within a cystic space. The papilla has a core of neoplastic spindle cells and a surface layer of epithelial cells. This differs from cystadenocarcinoma in having a spindle cell component.*

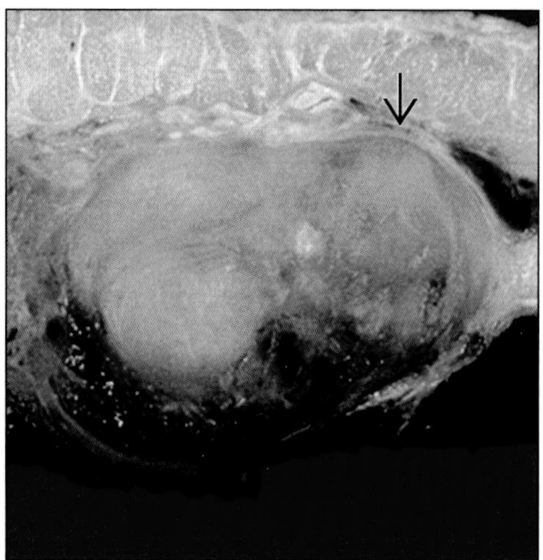

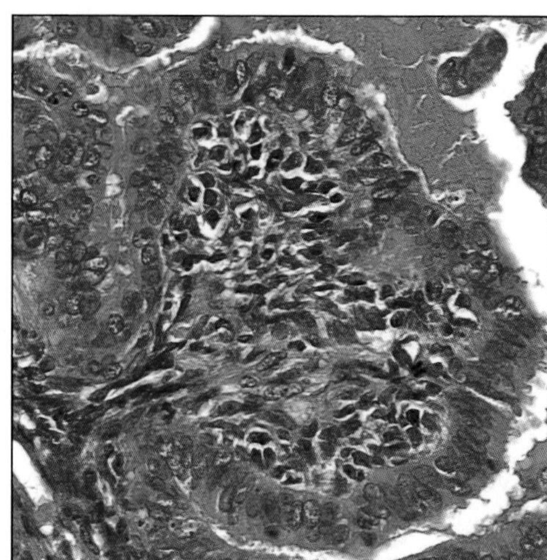

*(**Left**) Hematoxylin & eosin shows a biphasic synovial sarcoma in which the epithelial component forms solid nests with an occasional tiny glandular lumen ➔. (**Right**) Hematoxylin & eosin shows a biphasic synovial sarcoma in which the epithelial component forms solid cords of cells ➲ permeating between areas of spindle cell tumor.*

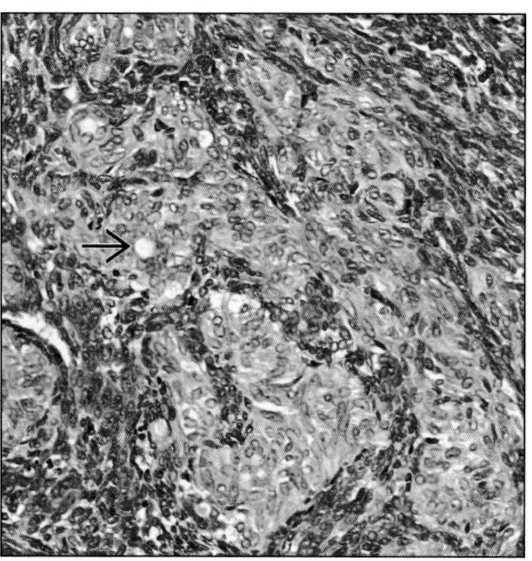

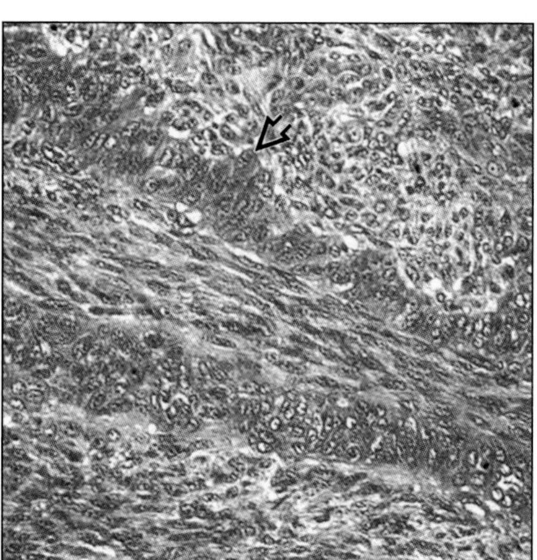

*(**Left**) Hematoxylin & eosin shows a monophasic synovial sarcoma with sheets and ill-defined fascicles of uniform ovoid cells with occasional mitotic figures. The cytoplasm is barely discernible. Note the absence of intervening stroma between the cells. (**Right**) Hematoxylin & eosin shows a variant of monophasic synovial sarcoma with more elongated single cells. Note that the nuclei are uniform and crowded or overlapping and that the cytoplasm is very scanty. Scattered mast cells are seen.*

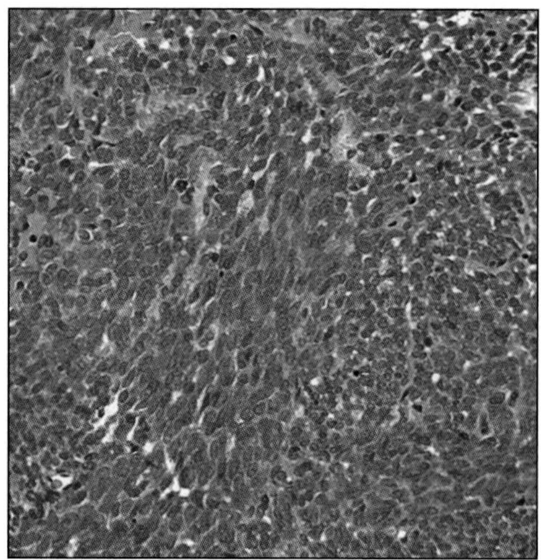

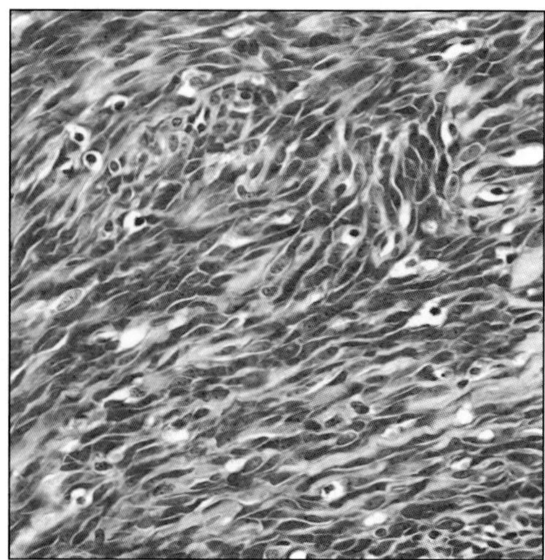

Variant Microscopic Features

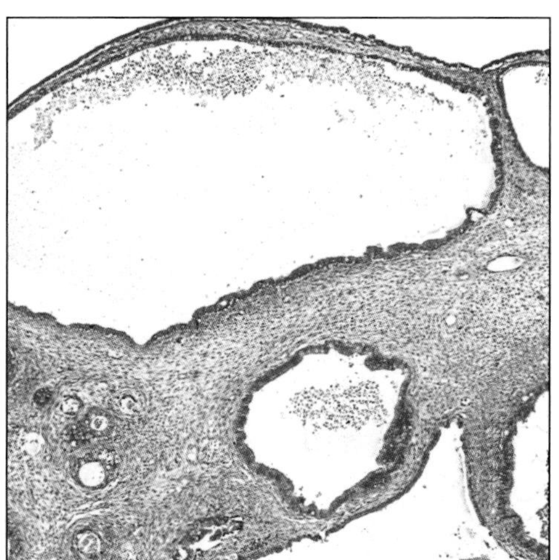

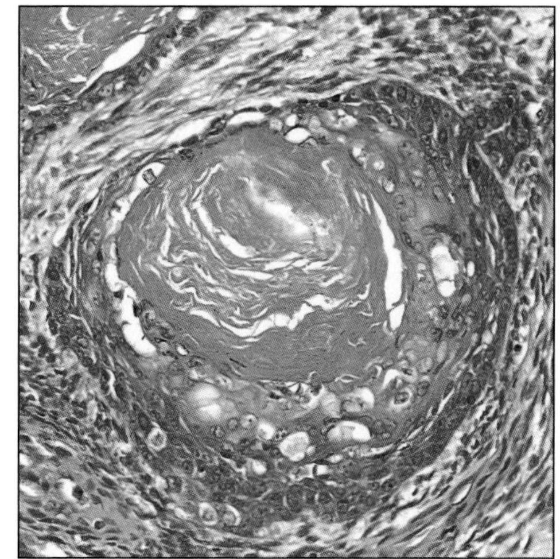

(Left) *Hematoxylin & eosin shows SS with predominantly glandular differentiation. Markedly dilated glands contain mucin, and a spindle cell component is seen between the glands. Variant can be confused with carcinoma or teratoma, requiring genetic analysis for diagnosis.* ***(Right)*** *Hematoxylin & eosin shows squamous metaplasia with central keratinization in the epithelial component. This is a rare finding in biphasic SS. Squamous cell carcinoma lacks a uniform spindle component.*

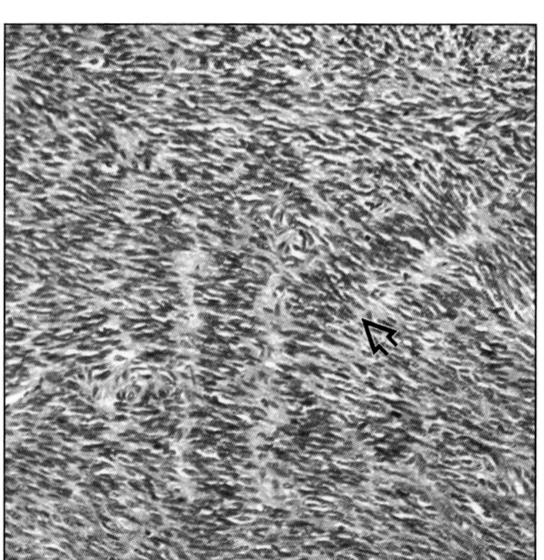

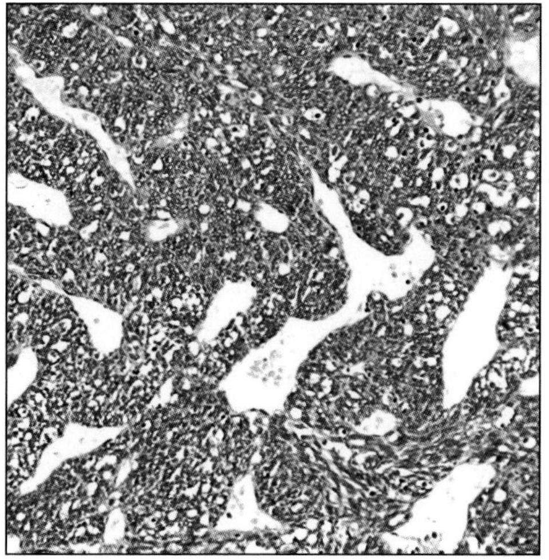

(Left) *Hematoxylin & eosin shows ill-defined palisading formed by aligned nuclei ⇨ in poorly differentiated SS. This feature can also be seen in smooth muscle and nerve sheath tumors.* ***(Right)*** *Hematoxylin & eosin shows a hemangiopericytic pattern of irregularly dilated thin-walled vessels, some with "staghorn" outline. This is characteristic of poorly differentiated synovial sarcoma, but it can also be seen in numerous other types of benign or malignant soft tissue tumors.*

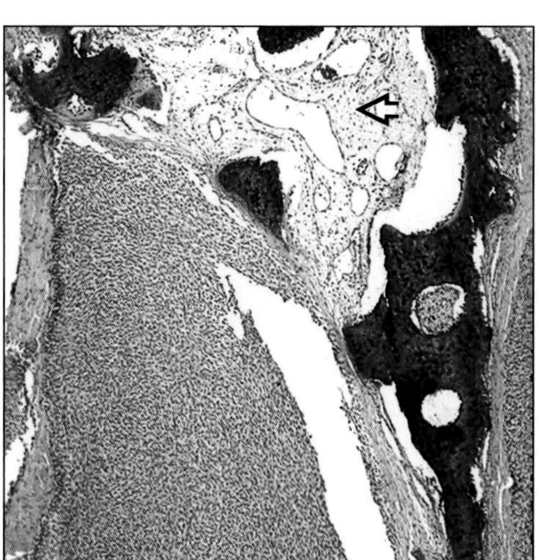

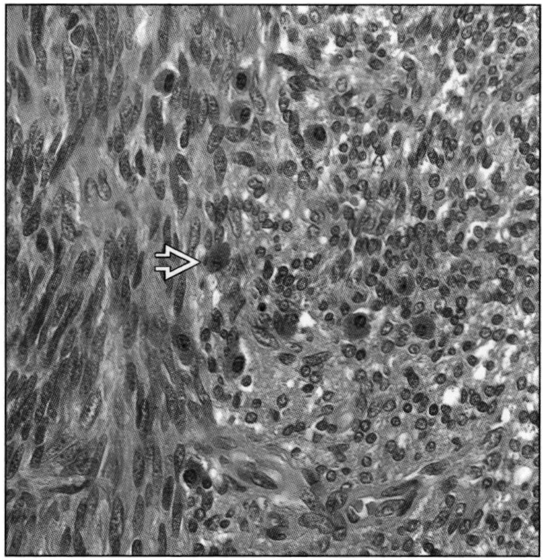

(Left) *Hematoxylin & eosin shows metaplastic bone formation with vascular fibrous tissue ⇨ in marrow space in the stroma of this monophasic SS. This differs from ossifying SS, in which the ossification forms within the tumor rather than in the stroma.* ***(Right)*** *Hematoxylin & eosin shows numerous mast cells ➡, which are often a prominent feature in the spindle component of synovial sarcoma. These can be seen clearly here, and they can also be highlighted by immunostaining for CD117.*

SYNOVIAL SARCOMA

Morphologic Subtypes

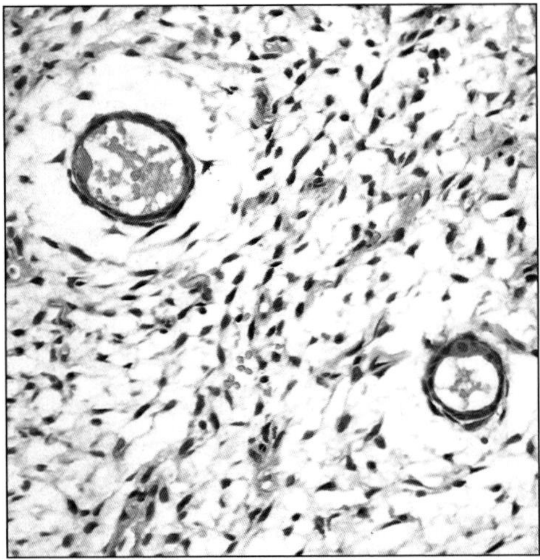

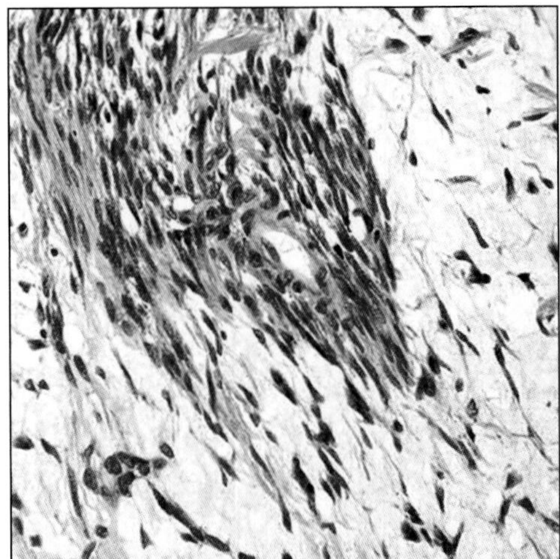

(Left) *Hematoxylin & eosin shows a biphasic myxoid synovial sarcoma with glands containing mucin and lined by flattened cells. Note periglandular clear zone and spindle cells dispersed in myxoid stroma. This pattern is very rare. This tumor occurred in the abdomen and had t(X;18) and rearranged SSX1 gene.* ***(Right)*** *Hematoxylin & eosin shows monophasic myxoid synovial sarcoma. This is also difficult to recognize, but the presence of the more typical cellular areas facilitates diagnosis.*

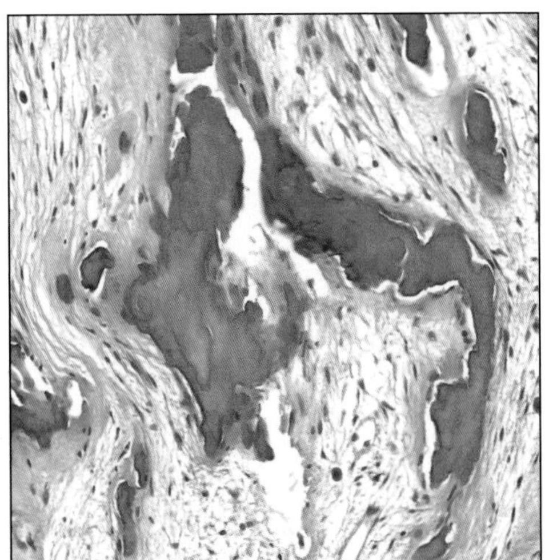

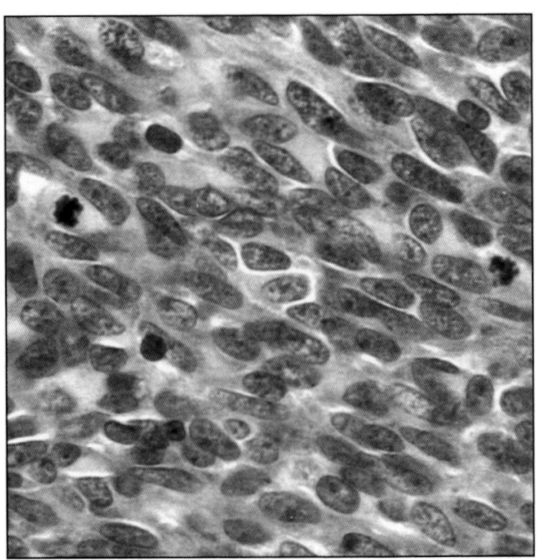

(Left) *Hematoxylin & eosin shows a calcifying/ossifying SS. Irregular foci of calcification occur in both monophasic and biphasic SS. The spindle cells are sparse & bland and can be easily overlooked or dismissed as benign, but they are focally cytokeratin(+) and EMA(+).* ***(Right)*** *Hematoxylin & eosin shows a poorly differentiated SS composed of rounded cells with scanty cytoplasm and indistinct cell boundaries, overlapping nuclei, and mitotic figures.*

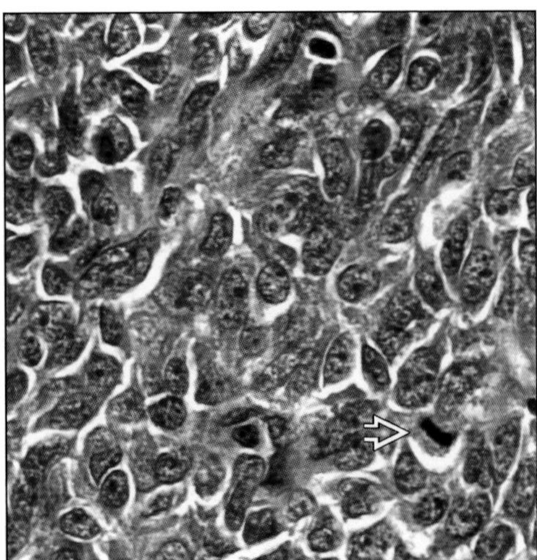

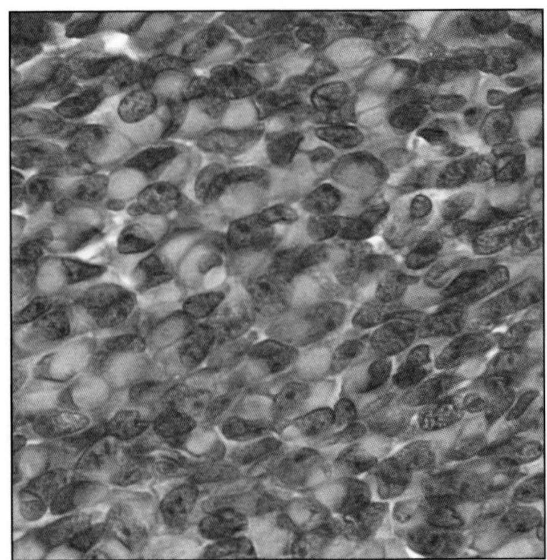

(Left) *Hematoxylin & eosin shows a poorly differentiated synovial sarcoma composed of small round cells with moderate amounts of cytoplasm. Note the mitotic activity ⇨.* ***(Right)*** *Hematoxylin & eosin shows rhabdoid cells, with displacement of nuclei by abundant eosinophilic cytoplasm. Electron microscopy shows whorls of intermediate filaments that are composed mainly of vimentin and sometimes of keratin.*

Ancillary Techniques

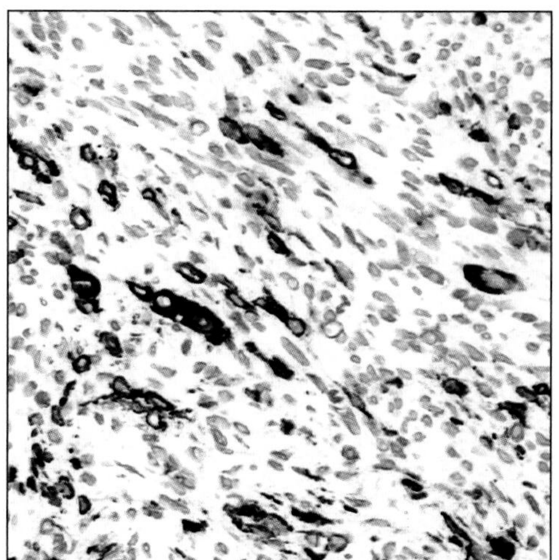

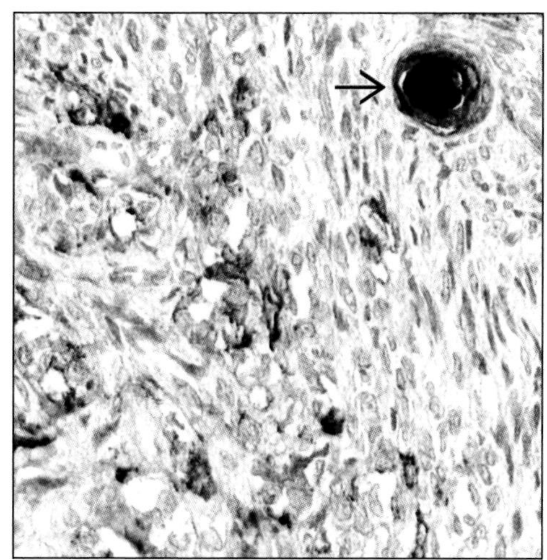

(Left) *CK-PAN shows cytoplasmic staining in scattered individual spindle cells of monophasic SS. Diffuse cytokeratin positivity would be more suggestive of sarcomatoid carcinoma.* ***(Right)*** *EMA shows membranous staining of occasional individual cells. A small epithelial nest is highlighted ⇒. As with cytokeratin, diffuse EMA positivity should prompt consideration of other tumor types.*

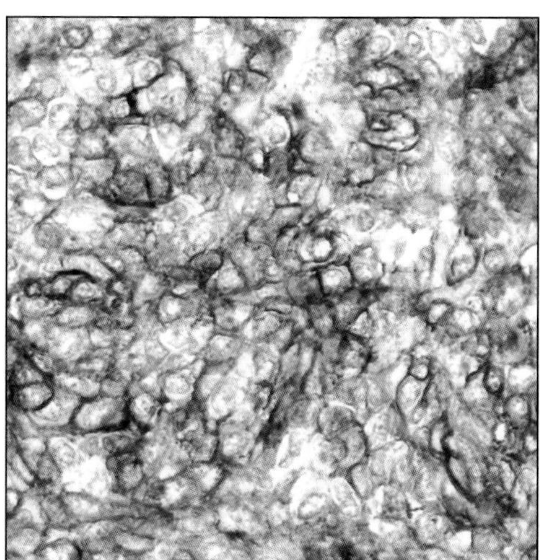

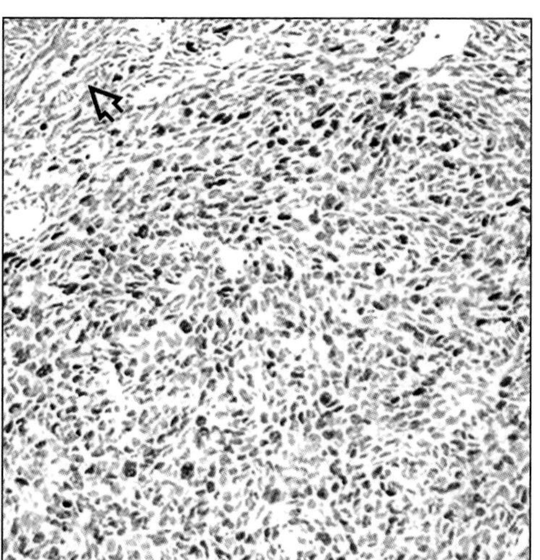

(Left) *CD99 shows diffuse membranous staining in this poorly differentiated SS. The distinction from Ewing sarcoma, which can also express CK and EMA, can require genetic analysis.* ***(Right)*** *Positive Ki-67 shows a high level of proliferative activity in areas of poorly differentiated synovial sarcoma, manifested as positive nuclear staining. A lower level of proliferative activity is seen in adjacent spindle cell focus ⇨.*

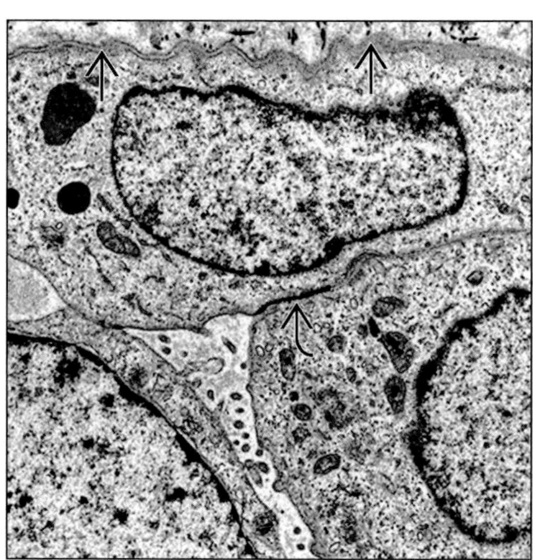

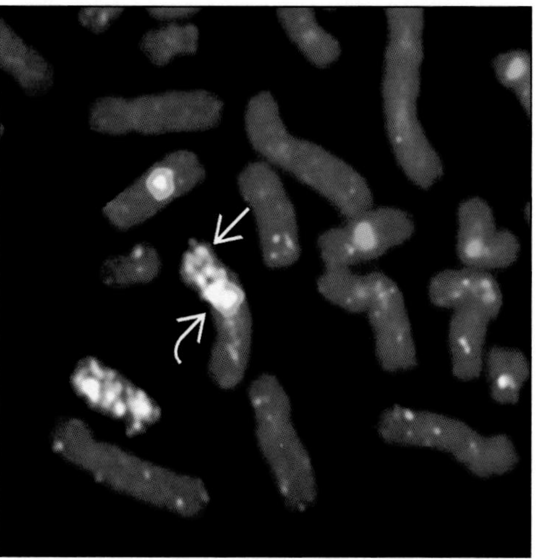

(Left) *Electron micrograph shows a glandular structure enclosed within external lamina ⇒. Cells surround a space with microvillous processes, bounded by intercellular junctions ⇗.* ***(Right)*** *FISH shows translocation. A portion of chromosome 18 (stained pink) ➡ is joined to centromere of chromosome X (white) ➡. A further portion of chromosome 18 is also shown.*

EPITHELIOID SARCOMA

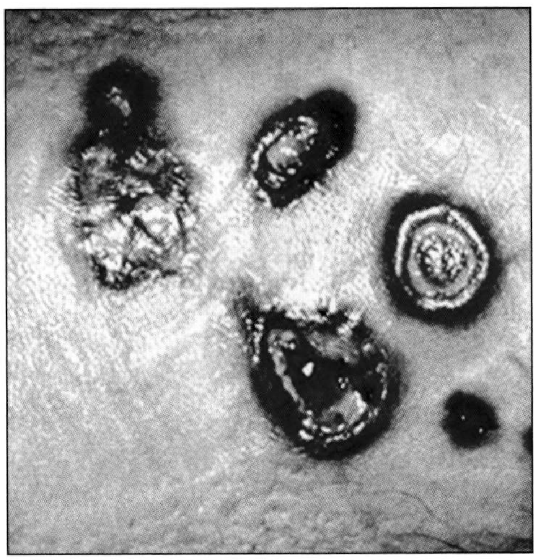

Clinical photograph shows several rounded lesions with raised red margins and central "targetoid" ulceration on the forearm of a 23-year-old man. Nonhealing ulcers are typical of epithelioid sarcoma.

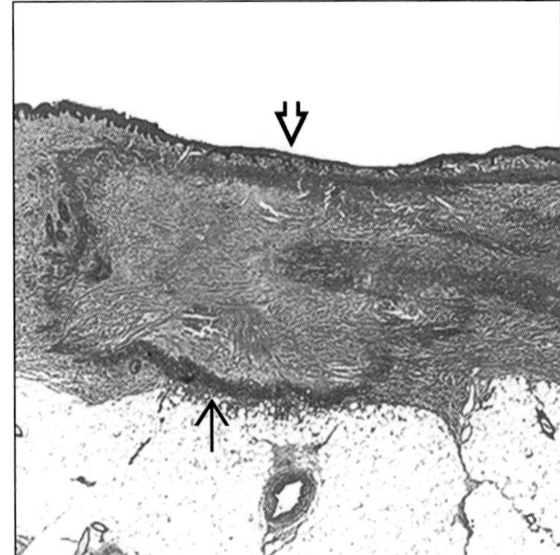

Hematoxylin & eosin shows skin with an irregularly shaped dermal lesion. Note the cellular rim ➔ and the necrobiotic central zone. The epidermis shows thinning and ulceration ➔ over the lesion.

TERMINOLOGY

Abbreviations

- Epithelioid sarcoma (ES)

Synonyms

- Epithelioid cell sarcoma (no longer recommended)

Definitions

- Malignant mesenchymal tumor resembling carcinoma or granuloma, which shows predominantly epithelial but also mesenchymal differentiation
- ES occurs in classical and proximal (aggressive, large cell, or rhabdoid) forms

ETIOLOGY/PATHOGENESIS

Genetic Factors

- Some cases have abnormalities of chromosome 22q
- Rare association with neurofibromatosis type 2

CLINICAL ISSUES

Epidemiology

- Incidence
    - Rare
        - Accounts for about 1% of all soft tissue sarcomas
    - Classic ES
        - Most common in distal extremities, especially hand and forearm
        - Head and neck
        - Penis, vulva
    - Proximal ES
        - Proximal limb girdle
        - Axial locations: Perineum, pelvis, mediastinum
        - Trunk: Chest wall
- Age
    - Any age
    - Classic ES
        - Mostly 2nd-4th decades
    - Proximal ES
        - Median age 40 years (range 13-80 years)
- Gender
    - More frequent in males

Presentation

- Slow growing
- Subcutaneous mass
- Ulcer
    - Classic ES
        - Dermal or subcutaneous nodule
        - Nonhealing ulcer
    - Proximal ES
        - Subcutaneous or deep mass
        - Can appear more rapidly

Natural History

- Classic ES
    - Persistent and multiple recurrences
        - Successive lesions often recur and extend more proximally in limb
    - Eventual metastasis
        - To regional lymph nodes
        - Via blood to lungs, bone, brain, and soft tissue, notably scalp
- Proximal ES
    - Rapidly growing, locally aggressive mass with high mortality

Treatment

- Options, risks, complications
    - Mainly surgical
- Surgical approaches
    - Adequate local excision
        - Amputation for intractable recurrences
- Adjuvant therapy
    - No specific effective therapy

Prognosis

- Classic ES

EPITHELIOID SARCOMA

Key Facts

Terminology

- Malignant mesenchymal tumor resembling carcinoma or granuloma
  - Shows predominantly epithelial but also mesenchymal differentiation
  - Occurs in classical and proximal aggressive forms

Etiology/Pathogenesis

- Some cases have abnormalities of chromosome 22q

Clinical Issues

- Most common in distal extremities, especially hand and forearm
- More frequent in males
- Subcutaneous nonhealing ulcer or deep mass
- High-grade sarcoma
  - Persistent and multiple recurrences
  - 50% metastasize

Macroscopic Features

- Raised "sealing-wax" margins around ulcer

Microscopic Pathology

- Central necrosis
- Transition to spindle cells at periphery
- Nuclei bland or mildly atypical, resembles granuloma

Ancillary Tests

- CK(+) and EMA(+)
- CD34(+) in 50% of cases
- S100 protein(-), desmin(-) and INI1(-)

Diagnostic Checklist

- Granulomatous lesion: Look for CK positivity

  - > 70% recur
  - 30-50% metastasize
  - 5-year survival (70%), 10-year survival (40%)
- Proximal ES
  - 65% local recurrence
  - 45-75% metastasize
  - 5-year survival (35-65%)
- Favorable prognostic factors
  - Young age at 1st diagnosis
  - Female sex
  - Primary tumor < 2 cm diameter
- Adverse prognostic factors
  - Proximal location
  - Amount of necrosis
  - Vascular invasion
  - Inadequate local excision

MACROSCOPIC FEATURES

General Features

- Classic ES
  - Ulcerated skin nodule
  - Raised "sealing-wax" margins
- Proximal ES
  - Multinodular mass
  - Hemorrhage and necrosis

Size

- Classic ES: 0.2 cm to > 5 cm diameter
- Proximal ES: Up to 20 cm diameter

MICROSCOPIC PATHOLOGY

Histologic Features

- Classic ES
  - Small dermal/subcutaneous nodules with central necrosis
  - Epithelioid cells, spindled at periphery
  - Mildly atypical nuclei, eosinophilic cytoplasm
  - Rare multinucleated osteoclast-like cells
  - Rare myxoid change
  - Calcification in 20%, rare stromal bone formation
  - Occasional hemorrhage ("angiomatoid" or angiosarcoma-like variant)
- Proximal ES
  - Multiple large nodules with necrosis
  - Large polygonal cells
  - Vesicular nuclei, prominent eosinophilic nucleoli
  - Abundant cytoplasm, rhabdoid cytomorphology
- Rare fibroma-like variant of ES
  - Hypocellularity, fibrous stroma
  - Storiform pattern
  - Bland spindle or polygonal cells with indistinct cell boundaries
  - Affinity for involving bone

Lymphatic/Vascular Invasion

- In 10% of ES

Margins

- Irregular, infiltrative

Lymph Nodes

- 30% of metastases are to lymph nodes

Predominant Pattern/Injury Type

- Multinodular
  - Central necrosis

Predominant Cell/Compartment Type

- Mesenchymal, epithelioid
- Mesenchymal, spindle

ANCILLARY TESTS

Flow Cytometry

- Can be diploid or polypoid

Cytogenetics

- Chromosome 22q deletions
  - Classical ES: Inconsistent t(8;22)(q22;q11)
  - Proximal ES: t(10;22) in 2 cases
- Abnormalities in 18q11 region described

EPITHELIOID SARCOMA

Immunohistochemistry

Antibody	Reactivity	Staining Pattern	Comment
CK-PAN	Positive	Cytoplasmic	In 95% of cases, diffuse
CK7	Positive	Cytoplasmic	In 22% of cases, focal
CK20	Positive	Cytoplasmic	In 13% of cases, focal
CK8/18/CAM5.2	Positive	Cytoplasmic	In 94% of cases
CK19	Positive	Cytoplasmic	In 72% of cases
CK5/6	Positive	Cytoplasmic	In 30% of cases, focal
EMA	Positive	Cell membrane	In 98% of cases, diffuse
CD34	Positive	Cell membrane	In 52% of cases
CD99	Positive	Cell membrane & cytoplasm	In 25% of cases
Actin-sm	Positive	Cytoplasmic	In 17% of cases in spindle cells
Cyclin-D1	Positive	Nuclear	In 96% of cases
CD31	Negative	Cell membrane & cytoplasm	Very occasional cytoplasmic positivity
S100	Negative		
Desmin	Negative	Cytoplasmic	Very occasionally, proximal variant is positive
SNF5	Negative	Nuclear	Positive in about 7% of cases
FLI-1	Negative		

Electron Microscopy

- Transmission
  - Varies between cases; not all features in any 1 tumor
    - Surface microvilli, junctions, tonofilaments
    - Subplasmalemmal thin filaments, rare fibronexus

DIFFERENTIAL DIAGNOSIS

Granuloma Annulare

- Cells smaller, cytoplasm less eosinophilic
- No spindle cells at periphery of nodule
- Epithelial markers absent

Carcinoma

- In situ component
- Usually more pleomorphic than classical ES
- CK5/6(+) and INI1(+), CD34(-)

Melanoma

- Junctional component
- Larger more pleomorphic cells than classic ES
- S100 protein(+) and INI1(+), HMB-45 and Melan-A variable

Rhabdomyosarcoma

- More infiltrative than nodular when in skin
- Desmin(+), myogenin(+), MYOD1(+)

Epithelioid Hemangioendothelioma

- Cords of cells
- Intracytoplasmic lumina
- Myxoid/chondromyxoid stroma
- CD31(+), CD34(+), FVIIIRAg(+), INI1(+)

Epithelioid Sarcoma-like Hemangioendothelioma

- Sheets of bland cells with intracytoplasmic lumina
- Keratin(+) but EMA(-)
- CD31(+) but CD34(-)

Epithelioid Angiosarcoma

- Sheets of pleomorphic epithelioid cells + hemorrhage
- Foci of vasoformation
- INI1(+), FLI-1(+), variable for CD31, CD34, FVIIIRAg

Clear Cell Sarcoma

- Deep subcutis, related to tendon sheaths
- Nests of uniform polygonal cells
- Clear or granular cytoplasm
- Round uniform nuclei, basophilic nucleoli
- S100 protein(+), HMB-45(+), Melan-A(+)
- Specific translocation t(11;22)

DIAGNOSTIC CHECKLIST

Clinically Relevant Pathologic Features

- Ulcerated granulomatous lesion with CK positivity

Pathologic Interpretation Pearls

- Coexpression of CK, EMA, and CD34, absence of INI1

GRADING

High Grade

- High-grade sarcoma

SELECTED REFERENCES

1. Fisher C: Epithelioid sarcoma of Enzinger. Adv Anat Pathol. 13(3):114-21, 2006
2. Miettinen M et al: Epithelioid sarcoma: an immunohistochemical analysis of 112 classical and variant cases and a discussion of the differential diagnosis. Hum Pathol. 30(8):934-42, 1999
3. Guillou L et al: "Proximal-type" epithelioid sarcoma, a distinctive aggressive neoplasm showing rhabdoid features. Clinicopathologic, immunohistochemical, and ultrastructural study of a series. Am J Surg Pathol. 21(2):130-46, 1997

Microscopic Features

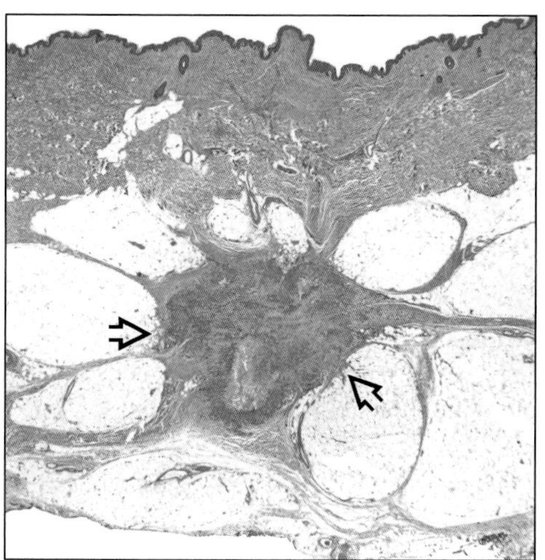

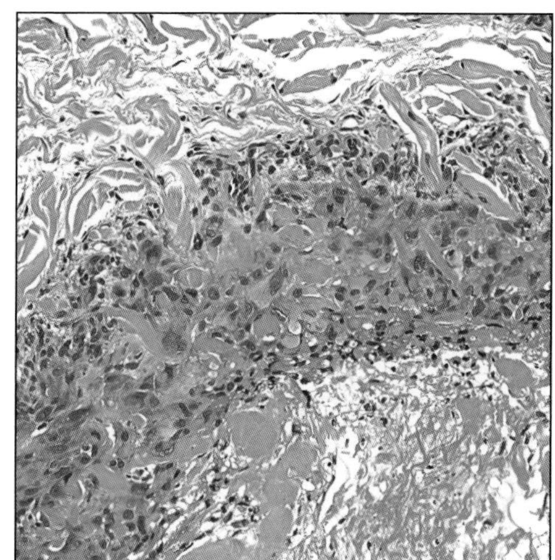

(Left) *Hematoxylin & eosin shows a subcutaneous nodule of epithelioid sarcoma ⇨. Note the lack of circumscription, incipient extension along the interlobular septa, and the central focus of necrosis. The overlying skin is intact.* ***(Right)*** *Hematoxylin & eosin shows the cellular rim of the tumor nodule. The cells show distinctive cytoplasmic eosinophilia and uneven distribution of nuclei. Spindle cells are often seen at the periphery of tumor nodules in ES but are not prominent here.*

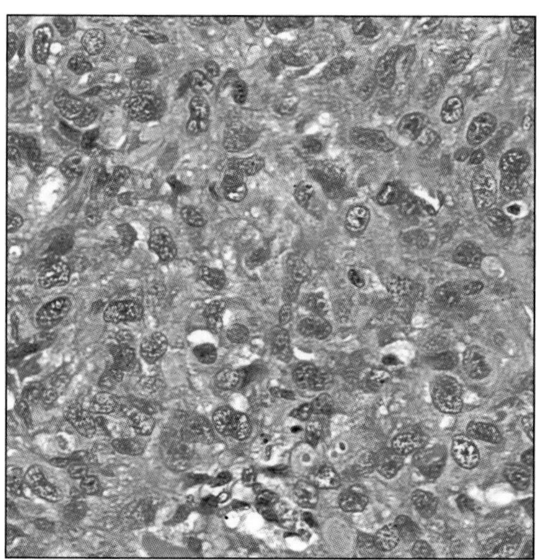

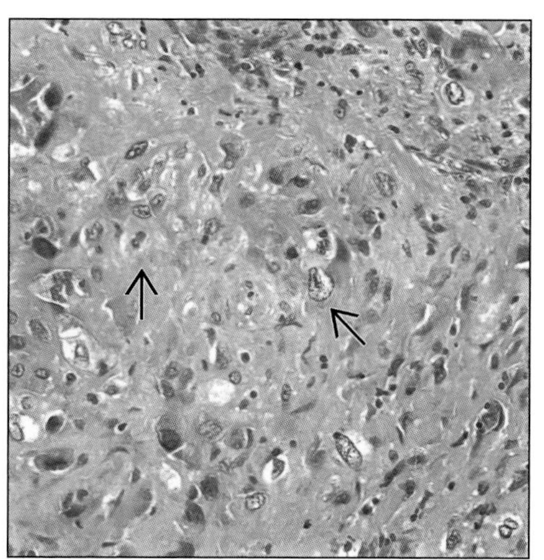

(Left) *Hematoxylin & eosin shows cytomorphology of epithelioid sarcoma. The cells have mildly pleomorphic vesicular nuclei, moderate amounts of cytoplasm, and indistinct margins.* ***(Right)*** *Hematoxylin & eosin shows recurrent epithelioid sarcoma at the site of a previous surgery. Neoplastic cells → are scattered within the fibrous tissue. Knowledge of the patient's history and high suspicion are needed to identify the tumor. Cytokeratin immunostaining is diagnostic.*

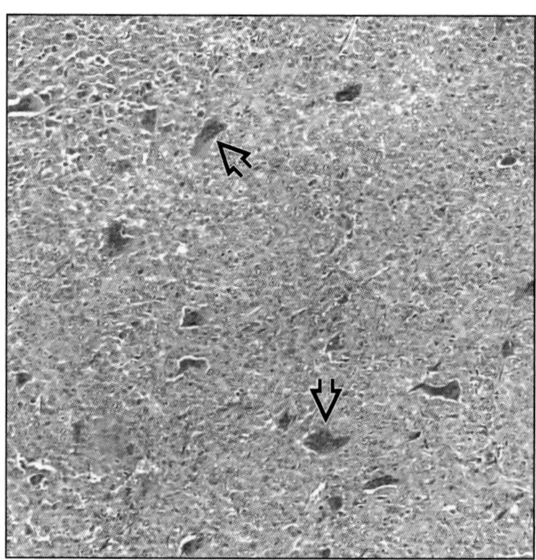

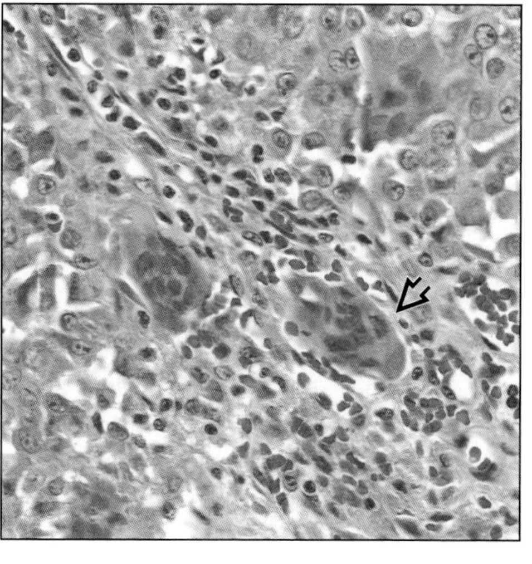

(Left) *Hematoxylin & eosin shows an unusual example of epithelioid sarcoma containing osteoclast-like giant cells ⇨ scattered within a sheet of tumor cells. This is usually a focal finding.* ***(Right)*** *Hematoxylin & eosin shows higher magnification of multinucleated (osteoclast-like) cells ⇨ that are reactive, though not neoplastic, and are immunoreactive for CD68. Tumor cells express CK, EMA, and CD34, unlike tendon sheath-type giant cell tumor.*

EPITHELIOID SARCOMA

Variant Microscopic Features

*(**Left**) Low-power photomicrograph of proximal epithelioid sarcoma shows a lobulated, highly cellular tumor with irregular margins and geographic central necrosis. The tumor ulcerates at skin surface. (**Right**) Hematoxylin & eosin shows a tumor composed of large polygonal cells in discohesive nodules with a focus of necrosis ⇨. Note that this deposit of tumor is circumscribed but not encapsulated. There is scant adjacent inflammation.*

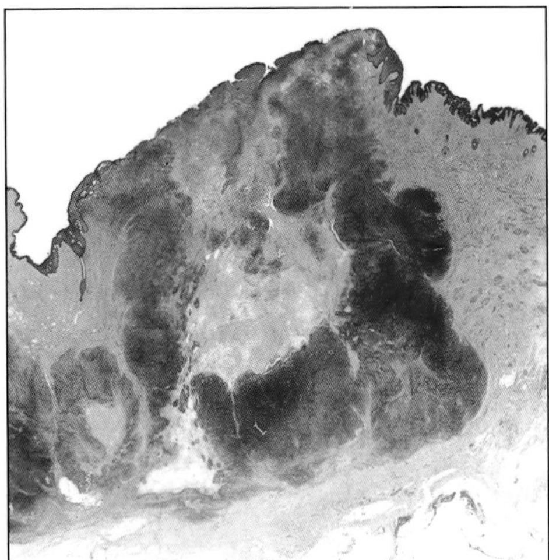

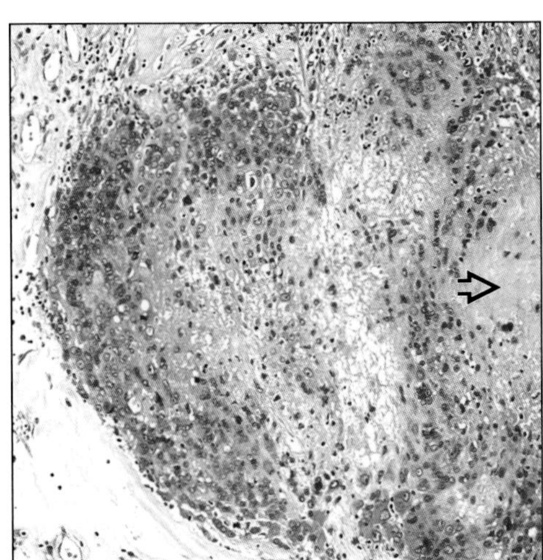

*(**Left**) Hematoxylin & eosin shows unevenly distributed cells in proximal epithelioid sarcoma with rounded, vesicular nuclei and prominent eosinophilic nucleoli. The cells are larger than those of classic epithelioid sarcoma. (**Right**) Hematoxylin & eosin shows proximal epithelioid sarcoma with prominent rhabdoid morphology →. The cells have abundant eosinophilic cytoplasm and eccentric displacement of nuclei. The cytoplasm contains vimentin and cytokeratin intermediate filaments.*

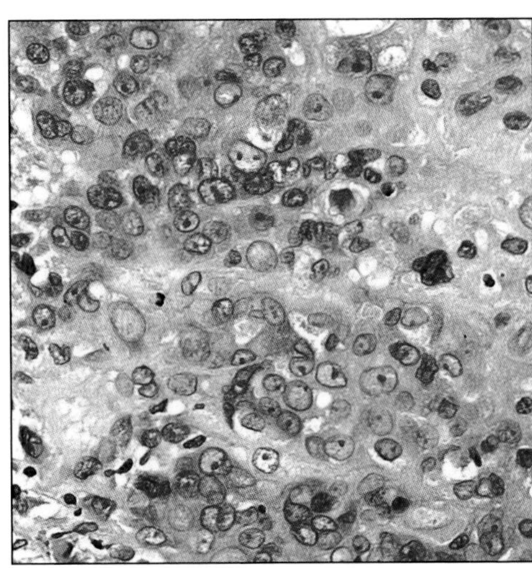

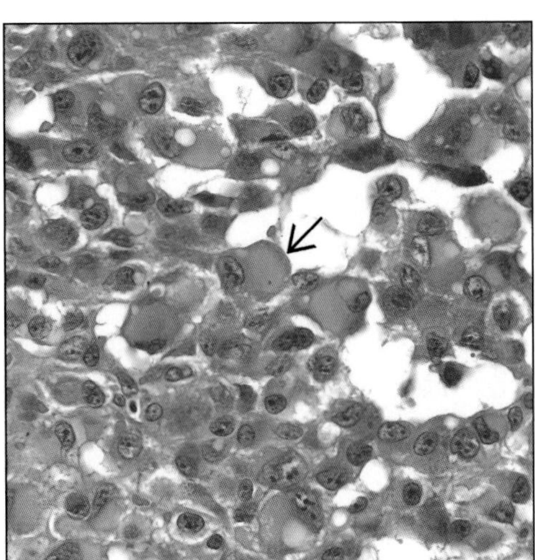

*(**Left**) Hematoxylin & eosin shows dilated vascular spaces with hemorrhage imparting pseudoangiosarcomatous (angiosarcoma-like) appearance. This change is usually focal rather than diffuse but can cause diagnostic difficulty in a biopsy specimen, especially when it is CD34(+). (**Right**) Hematoxylin & eosin shows a very rare finding of myxoid change in an epithelioid sarcoma. Unlike in mucinous adenocarcinoma, the mucin is stromal and extracellular.*

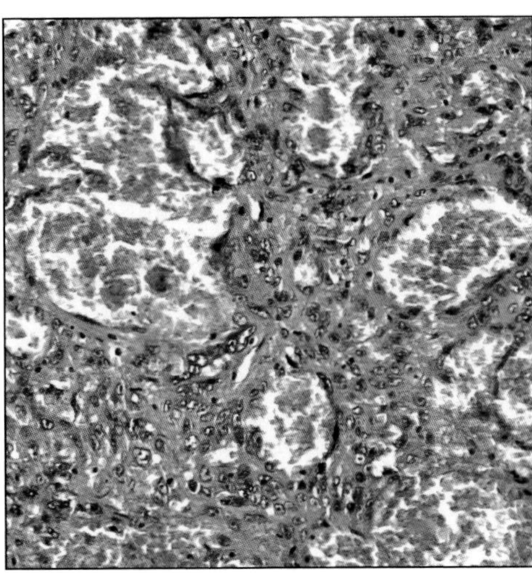

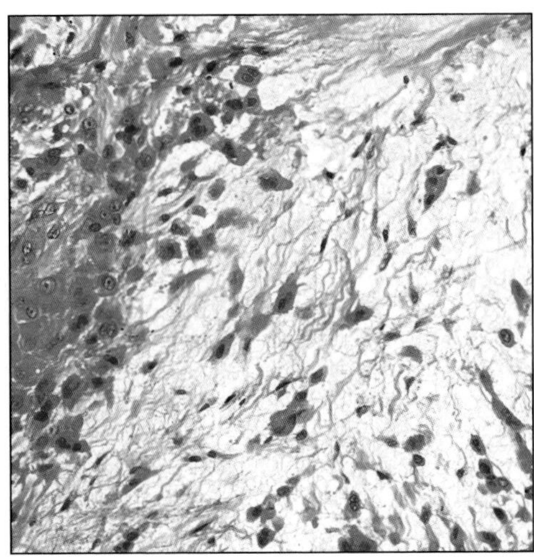

Variant Microscopic Features and Ancillary Techniques

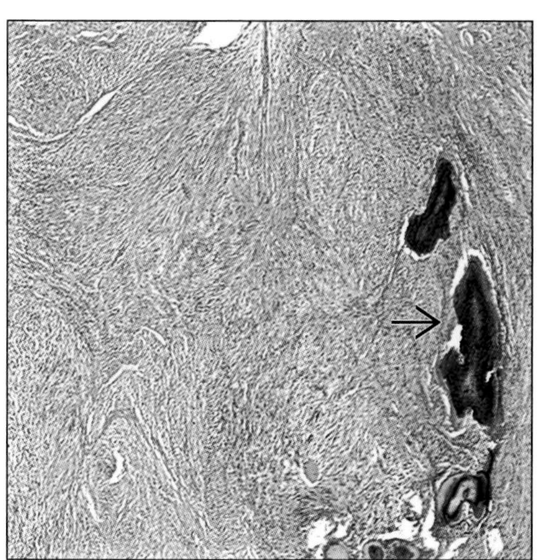

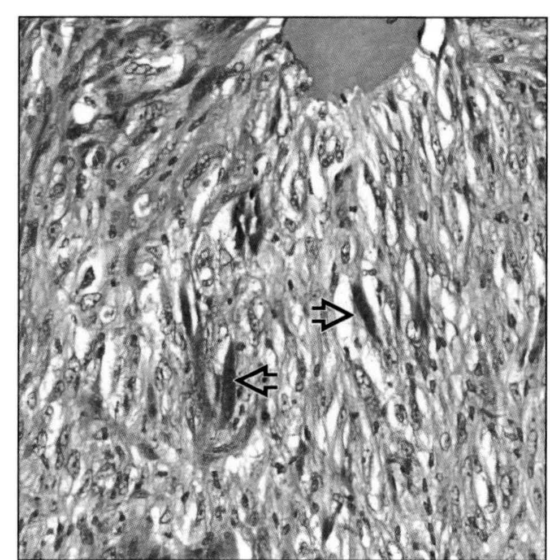

(Left) Hematoxylin & eosin shows fibroma-like variant with peripheral foci of metaplastic bone formation ➔. This rare feature is also occasionally found in typical epithelioid sarcoma. **(Right)** Hematoxylin & eosin shows fibroma-like variant of epithelioid sarcoma with spindle cells in fibrous stroma. Note focal nuclear enlargement and hyperchromasia ➔. This variant can have a storiform pattern resembling fibrous histiocytoma but differs in expressing CK and EMA.

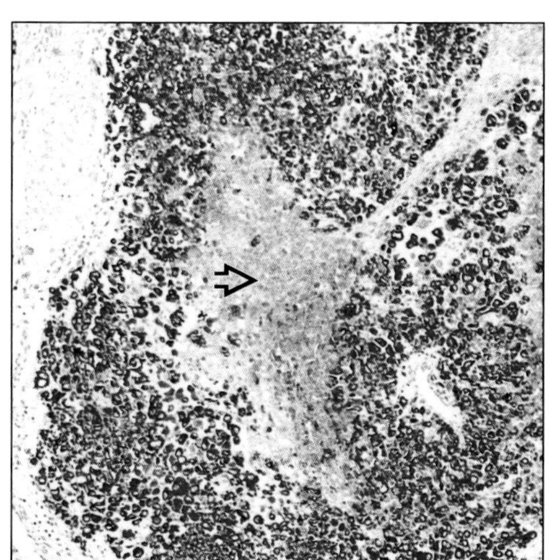

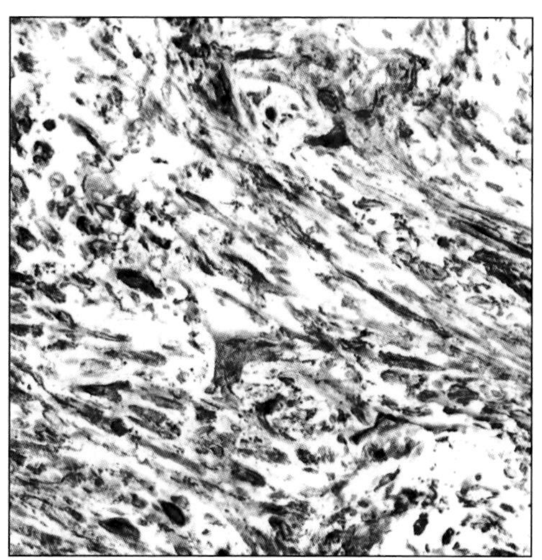

(Left) AE1/AE3 shows classic epithelioid sarcoma with diffuse positivity in lesional cells surrounding necrotic zone ➔. This staining pattern is typical of epithelioid sarcoma and excludes nonneoplastic granulomatous lesions. **(Right)** AE1/AE3 shows widespread positivity in spindle cells of fibroma-like variant of epithelioid sarcoma. These cells also express EMA and are CD34 positive (50%). Principal differential diagnosis is spindle cell carcinoma, which is CD34(-).

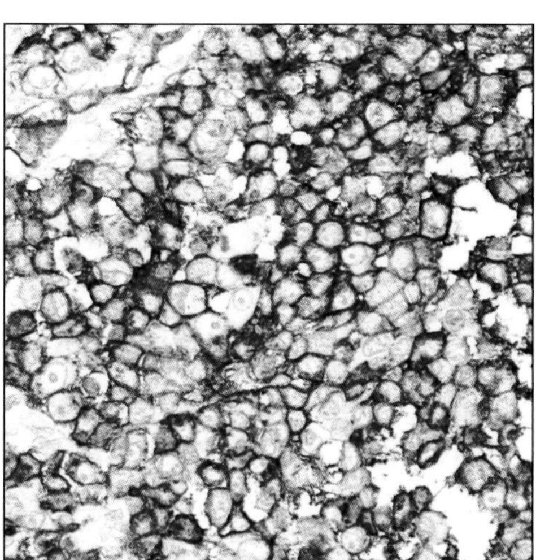

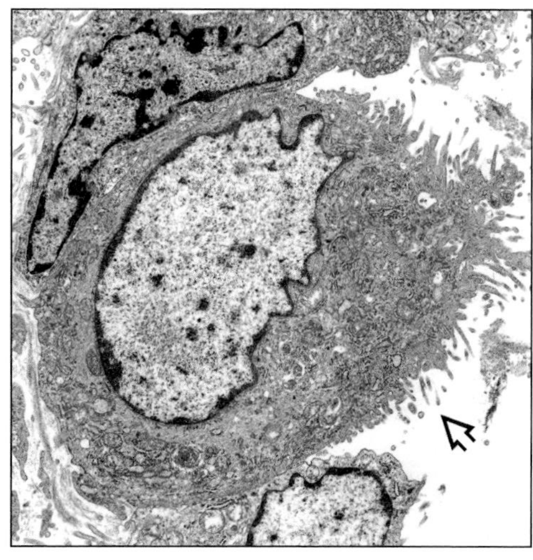

(Left) CD34 shows membranous immunoreactivity on lesional cells, found in about 1/2 of ES cases. The distribution of staining is diffuse in this classical ES, but it is often focal. Absence of CD31 and FLI-1 help to exclude angiosarcoma. **(Right)** Electron micrograph shows tumor cell with numerous surface microvillous projections ➔. This is a feature of epithelial differentiation. Other features sometimes seen are intercellular junctions and cytoplasmic tonofilaments.

EXTRARENAL RHABDOID TUMOR

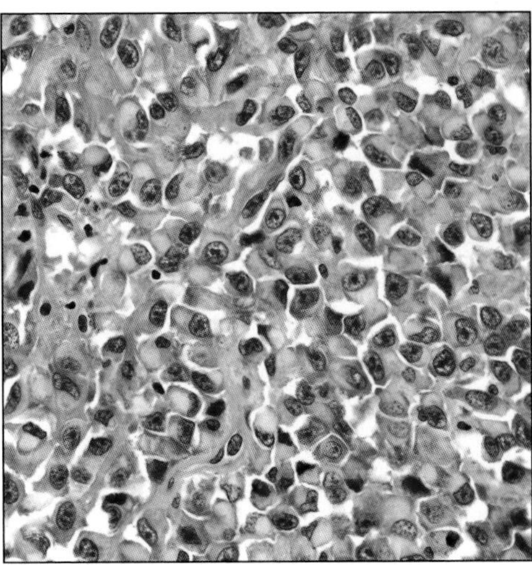

Hematoxylin & eosin shows sheets of rhabdoid cells without architecture. The cells have amphophilic cytoplasm and eccentric rounded nuclei with large nucleoli and are often discohesive, as seen here.

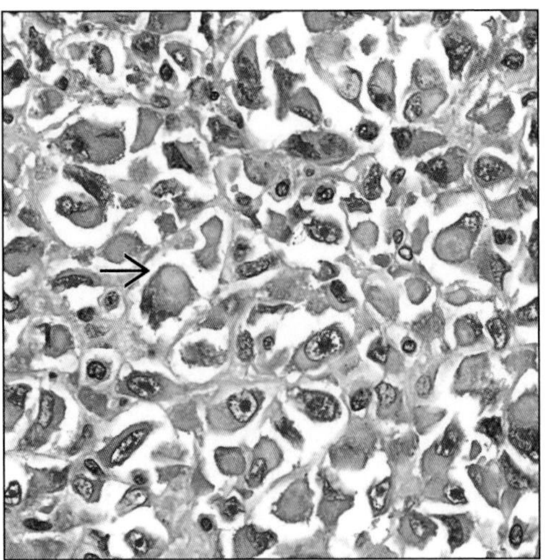

Hematoxylin & eosin shows cell detail, with abundant cytoplasm containing pale-staining inclusions ⇒. These are composed of cytokeratin- and vimentin-intermediate filaments. Note the prominent nucleoli.

TERMINOLOGY

Abbreviations

- Extrarenal rhabdoid tumor (ERT)

Synonyms

- Malignant rhabdoid tumor
- Atypical teratoid/rhabdoid tumor: Term for similar neoplasm in central nervous system

Definitions

- Rare malignant neoplasm of characteristic polygonal cells
  - Large nuclei with prominent nucleoli
  - Abundant eosinophilic cytoplasm, which displaces nucleus to 1 side
- Requires exclusion of specific tumor types with occasional rhabdoid cytomorphology
  - Extraskeletal myxoid chondrosarcoma
  - Leiomyosarcoma
  - Myoepithelial tumor
  - Gastrointestinal stromal tumor
  - Endometrial stromal sarcoma
  - Synovial sarcoma
  - Mesothelioma
  - Carcinoma
  - Melanoma
- Can be pure or form part of specific tumor type (composite ERT)

ETIOLOGY/PATHOGENESIS

Genetic Factors

- Some have abnormalities of chromosome 22q11.2
- Some patients have germline mutations of *hSNF5/ SMARCB1* gene
- Some associated with myofibroma- or hamartoma-like cutaneous lesions
- Rarely multiple

CLINICAL ISSUES

Epidemiology

- Incidence
  - Rare
- Age
  - Majority in childhood, including congenitally
  - Rare examples in adults after all mimics excluded

Site

- Deep soft tissue or skin
  - Axial and paraxial, cervical or paravertebral regions, vulva, perineum
  - Thigh, limb girdles
- Viscera
  - GI tract, liver, heart, bladder, brain

Presentation

- Rapidly growing mass, occasionally ulcerates

Natural History

- Aggressive with frequent local recurrence and metastasis

Treatment

- Surgical approaches
  - Excision where feasible
- Drugs
  - Chemotherapy
    - Rarely effective

Prognosis

- Very poor

MACROSCOPIC FEATURES

General Features

- Multinodular, nonencapsulated, poorly circumscribed
- Pale or tan, with hemorrhage and necrosis

EXTRARENAL RHABDOID TUMOR

Key Facts

Terminology
- Malignant neoplasm of polygonal cells with characteristic large cytoplasmic inclusion and eccentric large nucleus
- Requires exclusion of specific tumor types with rhabdoid cytomorphology
- Can be component of other tumors as composite rhabdoid tumor

Clinical Issues
- Majority in childhood, including congenitally
- Deep soft tissue or skin
- Visceral locations
- Aggressive with frequent local recurrence and metastasis
- Prognosis very poor

Microscopic Pathology
- Polygonal cells in discohesive sheets

Ancillary Tests
- Most cases express cytokeratin or epithelial membrane antigen
- Absence of immunoreactivity for INI1 is diagnostically useful
- CD34(-)
- Chromosome 22q11.2 deletions
- Ultrastructurally, large cytoplasmic inclusion comprising whorl of intermediate filaments 8-10 microns in diameter

Diagnostic Checklist
- Exclude specific tumor subtype with rhabdoid cell morphology

Size
- Up to 5 cm or more at presentation

MICROSCOPIC PATHOLOGY

Histologic Features
- Highly cellular
- Polygonal cells in discohesive sheets
  - Rounded vesicular nuclei
  - Prominent nucleoli
  - Frequent and abnormal mitoses
  - Eccentric eosinophilic cytoplasm
- Occasional small round cell component
- Rare osteoclast-like giant cells
- Rare myxoid change

Predominant Pattern/Injury Type
- Sheets

Predominant Cell/Compartment Type
- Rhabdoid

ANCILLARY TESTS

Histochemistry
- Periodic acid-Schiff with diastase digestion
  - Reactivity: Positive
  - Staining pattern
    - Cytoplasmic inclusion

Immunohistochemistry
- Most cases express cytokeratin or epithelial membrane antigen
- Some express CD99 and neuroendocrine markers
- Absence of immunoreactivity for INI1 is diagnostically useful

Cytogenetics
- Chromosome 22q11.2 monosomy or deletions
  - Site of *hSN5/SMARCB1* tumor suppressor gene, which often shows homozygous deletion or mutation
    - Component of SWI/SNF chromatin remodeling complex
    - Gene product is INI1 (BAF47), negative in ERT
  - Rarely translocations between 22q and 1p, 6p, 11p, or 18q

Electron Microscopy
- Transmission
  - Cytoplasmic inclusion has whorls of intermediate filaments
    - 8-10 microns in diameter
    - Composed mostly of cytokeratin with some vimentin
  - Whorl entraps lipid droplets, mitochondria

DIFFERENTIAL DIAGNOSIS

Melanoma
- S100 protein(+) in almost all cases
- HMB-45, Melan-A positivity in many cases
- INI1(+) in nuclei

Epithelioid Sarcoma (Proximal Variant)
- Can be closely similar morphologically
- INI1 also negative in 80-93% of cases
- Immunophenotype overlaps, but CD34(+) in 50% of cases
- Dysadherin(+)
- Frequency of *SMARCB1/INI1* gene alteration at DNA level < in ERT
- Prognosis relatively better

Rhabdomyosarcoma
- Strap-shaped or polygonal cells
- Cytoplasmic immunoreactivity for desmin
- Nuclear immunoreactivity for myogenin

Extraskeletal Myxoid Chondrosarcoma
- More often in extremities

EXTRARENAL RHABDOID TUMOR

Immunohistochemistry

Antibody	Reactivity	Staining Pattern	Comment
Vimentin	Positive	Cytoplasmic inclusion	
AE1/AE3	Positive	Cytoplasmic inclusion	In 80% of cases
CK8/18/CAM5.2	Positive	Cytoplasmic inclusion	Nearly all cases
EMA	Positive	Cell membrane & cytoplasm	
CD99	Positive	Cell membrane	Some examples
Synaptophysin	Positive	Cytoplasmic	Some examples
SNF5	Negative		Diagnostically useful
Desmin	Negative		Occasional examples are focally positive
HMB-45	Negative		
Dysadherin	Negative		Positive in proximal epithelioid sarcoma
CD34	Equivocal		
S100P	Equivocal	Nuclear & cytoplasmic	Occasional examples

- Cells in cords
- Nuclei smaller, lack large nucleoli
  - Can sometimes have focal rhabdoid morphology
- Prominent myxoid stroma
- Lacks cytokeratin
- Specific translocations
- More indolent clinical course

Carcinomas

- Organ based
  - Can be metastatic in soft issue, but primary site usually evident
- Variable morphology
- Specific marker expression
  - Cytokeratins, EMA
  - Thyroglobulin, PSA
- Nuclear immunoreactivity for INI1

Myoepithelioma

- Can have rhabdoid cytoplasmic morphology
- Lack large vesicular nuclei with prominent nucleoli
- Positive myoepithelial markers
  - Calponin, p63, CD10, H-caldesmon, podoplanin

Synovial Sarcoma

- Biphasic morphology diagnostic
- Spindle cells short with uniform nuclei and scanty cytoplasm
  - Rhabdoid cells seen focally in rare examples
- Epithelial marker expression only focal
- Nuclear immunoreactivity for INI1

DIAGNOSTIC CHECKLIST

Clinically Relevant Pathologic Features

- Cytoplasmic features
- Nuclear features

Pathologic Interpretation Pearls

- Exclude specific sarcoma subtype with rhabdoid cell morphology

SELECTED REFERENCES

1. Argenta PA et al: Proximal-type epithelioid sarcoma vs. malignant rhabdoid tumor of the vulva: a case report, review of the literature, and an argument for consolidation. Gynecol Oncol. 107(1):130-5, 2007
2. Kohashi K et al: Highly aggressive behavior of malignant rhabdoid tumor: a special reference to SMARCB1/INI1 gene alterations using molecular genetic analysis including quantitative real-time PCR. J Cancer Res Clin Oncol. 133(11):817-24, 2007
3. Biegel JA: Molecular genetics of atypical teratoid/rhabdoid tumor. Neurosurg Focus. 20(1):E11, 2006
4. Izumi T et al: Prognostic significance of dysadherin expression in epithelioid sarcoma and its diagnostic utility in distinguishing epithelioid sarcoma from malignant rhabdoid tumor. Mod Pathol. 19(6):820-31, 2006
5. Oda Y et al: Extrarenal rhabdoid tumors of soft tissue: clinicopathological and molecular genetic review and distinction from other soft-tissue sarcomas with rhabdoid features. Pathol Int. 56(6):287-95, 2006
6. Tekkök IH et al: Primary malignant rhabdoid tumor of the central nervous system--a comprehensive review. J Neurooncol. 73(3):241-52, 2005
7. Higashino K et al: Malignant rhabdoid tumor shows a unique neural differentiation as distinct from neuroblastoma. Cancer Sci. 94(1):37-42, 2003
8. Yoshida S et al: Malignant rhabdoid tumor shows incomplete neural characteristics as revealed by expression of SNARE complex. J Neurosci Res. 69(5):642-52, 2002
9. Duvdevani M et al: Pure rhabdoid tumor of the bladder. J Urol. 166(6):2337, 2001
10. Ogino S et al: Malignant rhabdoid tumor: A phenotype? An entity?--A controversy revisited. Adv Anat Pathol. 7(3):181-90, 2000
11. White FV et al: Congenital disseminated malignant rhabdoid tumor: a distinct clinicopathologic entity demonstrating abnormalities of chromosome 22q11. Am J Surg Pathol. 23(3):249-56, 1999
12. Fanburg-Smith JC et al: Extrarenal rhabdoid tumors of soft tissue: a clinicopathologic and immunohistochemical study of 18 cases. Ann Diagn Pathol. 2(6):351-62, 1998
13. Bhattacharjee M et al: Primary malignant rhabdoid tumor of the central nervous system. Ultrastruct Pathol. 21(4):361-8, 1997
14. Wick MR et al: Malignant rhabdoid tumors: a clinicopathologic review and conceptual discussion. Semin Diagn Pathol. 12(3):233-48, 1995

Microscopic Features and Ancillary Techniques

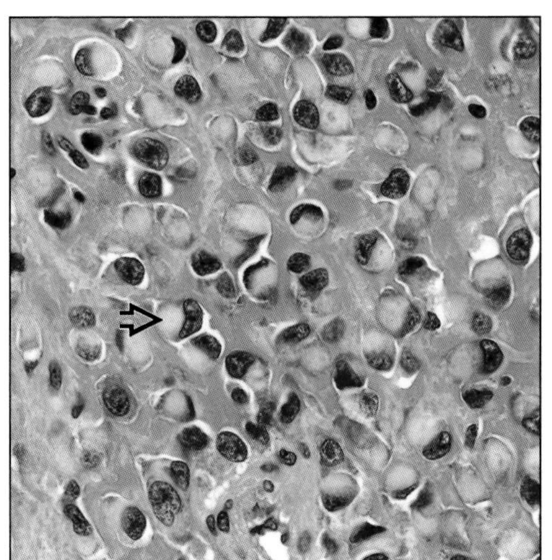

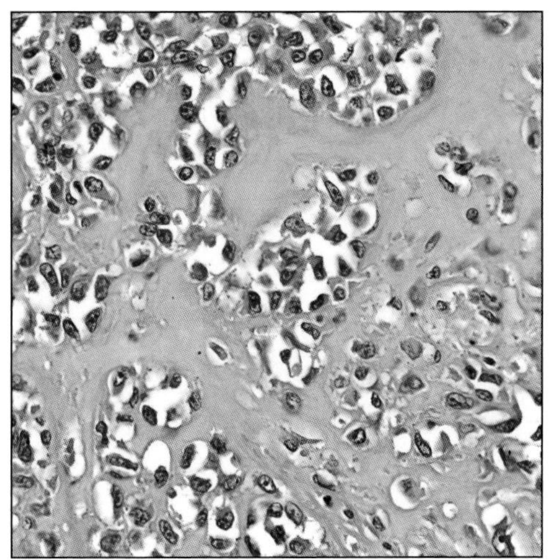

(Left) *Hematoxylin & eosin shows the area of a malignant rhabdoid tumor with uniform cells. Note that the nuclei are indented by the cytoplasmic inclusions ⇨. Cells here resemble signet ring adenocarcinoma.* ***(Right)*** *Hematoxylin & eosin shows stroma sclerosis, which divides the tumor into nests. This can be confused with alveolar soft part sarcoma, which has more delicate fibrous septa, lacks rhabdoid features, & is cytokeratin(-). Other parts of this tumor were more typical of ERT.*

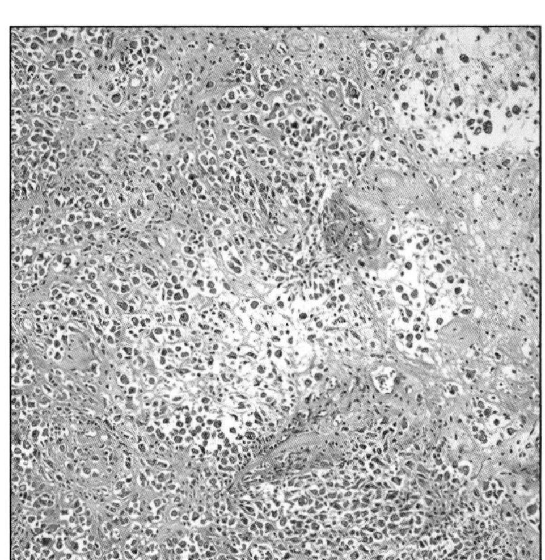

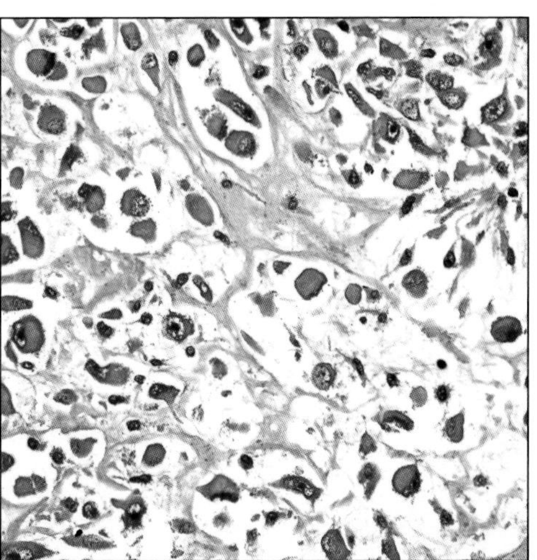

(Left) *Hematoxylin & eosin shows ill-defined nodules of myxoid stromal change, with decreased cellularity in these areas. This is a rare feature of malignant extrarenal rhabdoid tumors, which are usually focal and unlikely to be diagnostically confused with other myxoid neoplasms.* ***(Right)*** *Hematoxylin & eosin shows focal myxoid stroma with marked discohesion of cells. The stromal mucin stains with Alcian blue, but intracellular mucin stains (e.g., mucicarmine) are negative.*

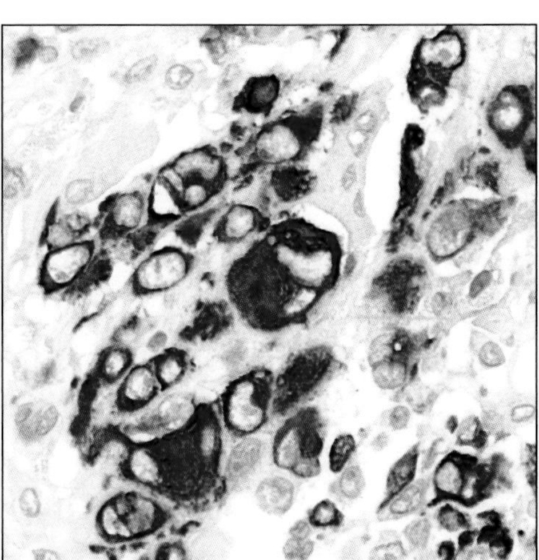

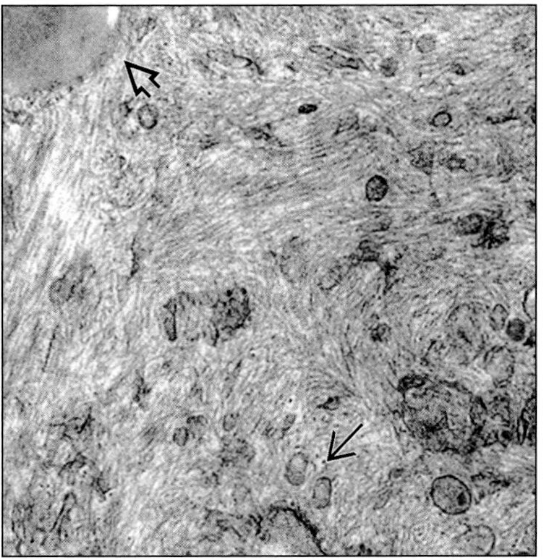

(Left) *Positive CK8/18/CAM5.2 shows cytokeratin in cytoplasm, with accentuation in intermediate filaments of paranuclear inclusion. A similar pattern is demonstrated by immunohistochemical staining for vimentin.* ***(Right)*** *Electron micrograph shows features of globoid hyaline cytoplasmic inclusion. There are whorls of intermediate filaments about 10 microns in diameter, with entrapped mitochondria → and part of a lipid droplet ⇨.*

ALVEOLAR SOFT PART SARCOMA

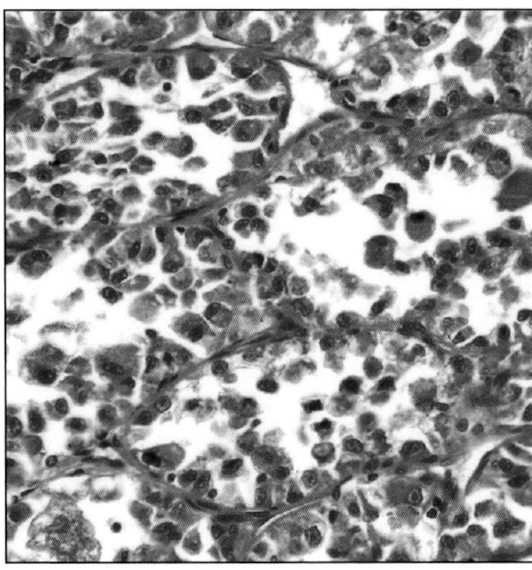

Hematoxylin & eosin shows a typical example of alveolar soft part sarcoma with an alveolar pattern, mostly seen in older patients. The cells are polygonal and appear to slough into the "alveolar space."

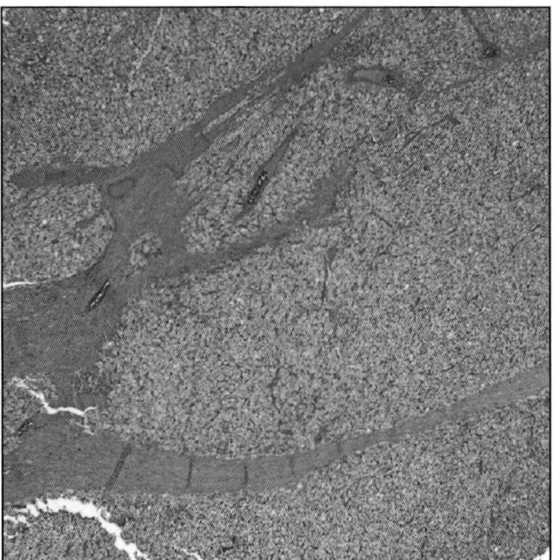

Hematoxylin & eosin shows alveolar soft part sarcoma with a solid growth pattern separated with thick, fibrous septa. This pattern is common in the tongue and ophthalmic region of younger patients.

TERMINOLOGY

Abbreviations

- Alveolar soft part sarcoma (ASPS)

Definitions

- Malignant soft tissue tumor of uncertain phenotype that mainly affects young adults and children
- Clustering alveolar-like growth pattern, separated by fibrous septa

CLINICAL ISSUES

Presentation

- Painless mass
- Intramuscular
- Hemorrhage
- Lymphatic invasion

Prognosis

- Deceptively indolent course
- Distant metastasis to lung, bone, and brain present in 25%
- Late recurrence and metastasis common
- ~ 60% of patients have distant metastases
- 5-year survival rate is 65%

MICROSCOPIC PATHOLOGY

Histologic Features

- Solid type: Most common in infants in tongue and eye
  - Solid pattern
    - Sheets of polygonal cells
    - Separated by fibrous septa
- Alveolar type: More common than solid type, usually buttocks, thigh in older child
  - Alveolar pattern
    - Polygonal cells separated into nests by fibrovascular septa
    - Cells slough into center of "alveolus"
- Eosinophilic cytoplasm
- Eccentric nuclei with prominent nucleoli
- Cytologic atypia rare
- Mitotic activity low
- High vascularity
- Vascular/lymphatic invasion almost always present
- Metastases to lung, bone, and brain
  - Lung metastases hard to separate from alveoli
  - See hemorrhage and tumor

Predominant Pattern/Injury Type

- Organoid

Predominant Cell/Compartment Type

- Polygonal

Histochemistry

- PAS(+), diastase-resistant granular to crystalline cytoplasmic material, varies from few to all cells

Immunohistochemistry

- Vimentin(-)
- Desmin focally positive
- MYOD1(-) (always cytoplasmic)
- HMB-45(-) and S100(-)
- Keratin(-), CD34(-)

Molecular

- TFE3(+) by immunohistochemistry, unbalanced translocation (X;17) by cytogenetics
- *TFE3* gene is on Xp11.2 chromosome
- *ASPL* gene is on 17q25

DIFFERENTIAL DIAGNOSIS

Myomelanocytic Tumors

- Similar cell clustering
- Lymphatic invasion not present
- Positive for HMB-45 and desmin
- Negative for TFE3 at AFIP labs

Key Facts

Terminology

- Alveolar soft part sarcoma (ASPS)
  - Malignant soft tissue tumor of uncertain phenotype that mainly affects young adults and children
  - Clustering alveolar-like growth pattern, separated by fibrous septa

Clinical Issues

- Intramuscular
- Hemorrhage
- Lymphatic invasion
- Deceptively indolent course
- Distant metastasis
  - To lung bone and brain
  - Present in 25%

Microscopic Pathology

- Solid type: Most common in infants in tongue and eye
- Alveolar type: More common than solid type, usually buttocks, thigh in older child
- High vascularity
- PAS(+), diastase-resistant granular to crystalline cytoplasmic material, varies from few to all cells
- Vimentin(-), desmin focally positive, MYOD1(-) (always cytoplasmic)
- S100, keratins, CD34 all negative
- TFE3(+)

Diagnostic Checklist

- PAS(+) diastase-resistant granular to crystalline material is present in all cases (< 5-100% of cells)

Paraganglioma

- Usually benign endocrine tumor
- Similar zellballen pattern
- More atypia than ASPS
- S100-protein(+) sustentacular cells and chromogranin(+)
- Negative for cytoplasmic granules/crystals and TFE3

Rhabdomyoma

- Benign skeletal muscle tumor
- Large polygonal cells and spider cells, no atypia
- Desmin and myoregulatory protein positive
- Negative for cytoplasmic granules/crystals and TFE3

Granular Cell Tumor

- Nerve sheath tumor
- More granularity of cytoplasm
- Lacks diffuse prominent nucleoli and mitotic activity, unless malignant
- Contains cytoplasmic globules with surrounding clear halo
- Cytoplasmic material positive for KP1
- Tumor strongly positive for S100 protein, unlike ASPS
- Negative for TFE3

Hibernoma

- Benign brown fat tumor
- Composed of large cells with multiple cytoplasmic vacuoles and sometimes eosinophilia
- No polygonal cells or prominent nucleoli
- No grouping into clusters
- Absence of mitoses
- S100 protein(+)

Clear Cell Sarcoma

- Clusters of epithelioid to spindled cells with prominent nucleoli
- HMB-45 strongly positive

DIAGNOSTIC CHECKLIST

Clinically Relevant Pathologic Features

- Painless mass
- Tissue distribution
  - Tongue, eye, solid type found in young child
  - Buttocks, thigh is alveolar type found in older child
- Highly vascular, so hemorrhage is common
- Lymphatic invasion almost always present; therefore, be aware of late metastases

Pathologic Interpretation Pearls

- Always intramuscular
- Alveolar spaces are separated by fibrovascular septa
- Always lymphovascular invasion
- PAS(+) diastase-resistant granular to crystalline material is present in all cases (< 5-100% of cells)
- Vimentin(-), MYOD1 cytoplasmic staining (negative intranuclear)
- TFE3(+) by immunohistochemistry, unbalanced translocation (X;17) by cytogenetics
- *TFE3* gene is on Xp11.2 chromosome and *ASPL* gene is on 17q25

SELECTED REFERENCES

1. Bodi I et al: Meningeal alveolar soft part sarcoma confirmed by characteristic ASPCR1-TFE3 fusion. Neuropathology. 29(4):460-5, 2009
2. Tsuda M et al: TFE3 fusions activate MET signaling by transcriptional up-regulation, defining another class of tumors as candidates for therapeutic MET inhibition. Cancer Res. 67(3):919-29, 2007
3. Folpe AL et al: Alveolar soft-part sarcoma: a review and update. J Clin Pathol. 59(11):1127-32, 2006
4. Fanburg-Smith JC et al: Lingual alveolar soft part sarcoma; 14 cases: novel clinical and morphological observations. Histopathology. 45(5):526-37, 2004
5. Ladanyi M et al: The precrystalline cytoplasmic granules of alveolar soft part sarcoma contain monocarboxylate transporter 1 and CD147. Am J Pathol. 160(4):1215-21, 2002
6. Ordóñez NG: Alveolar soft part sarcoma: a review and update. Adv Anat Pathol. 6(3):125-39, 1999

ALVEOLAR SOFT PART SARCOMA

Radiographic, Gross, and Microscopic Features

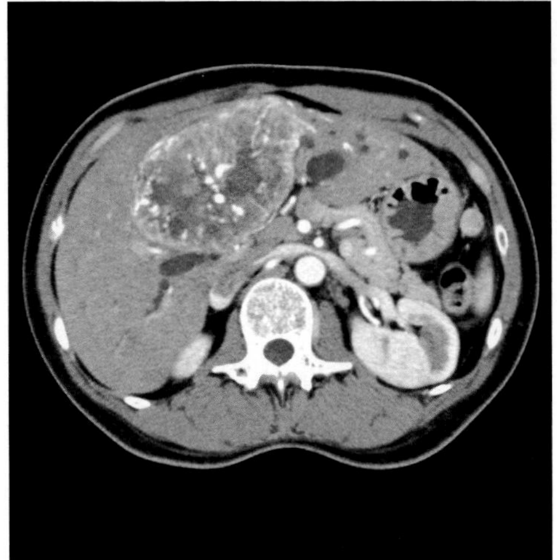

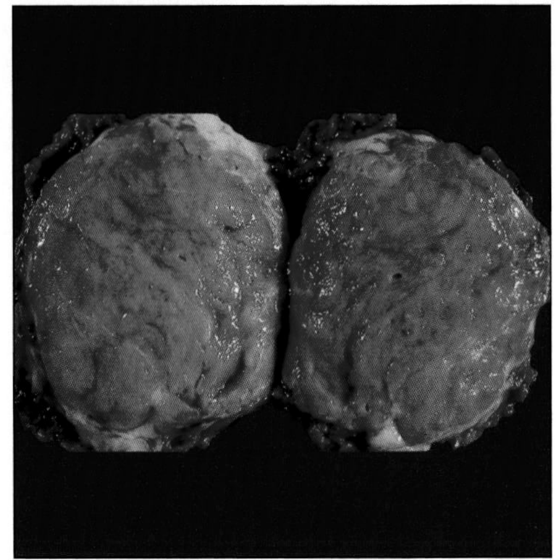

(Left) *CT illustrates an exceedingly rare example of an intrahepatic alveolar soft part sarcoma.* ***(Right)*** *Gross photograph shows a more typical alveolar soft part sarcoma arising in the buttock. This is a well-delineated intramuscular mass with a fleshy firm tan/hemorrhagic cut surface. Note the increase in vascularity within the tumor.*

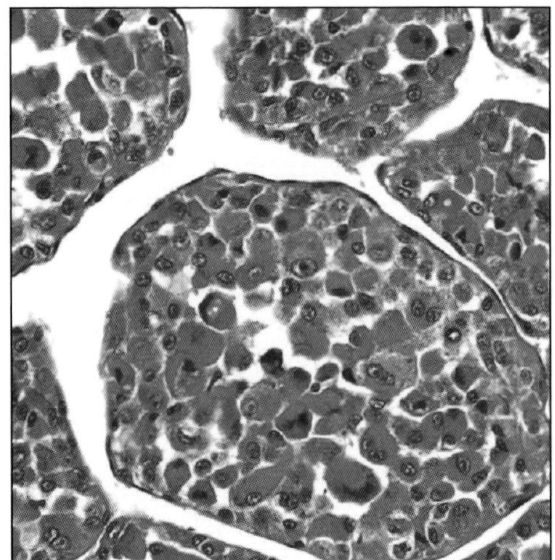

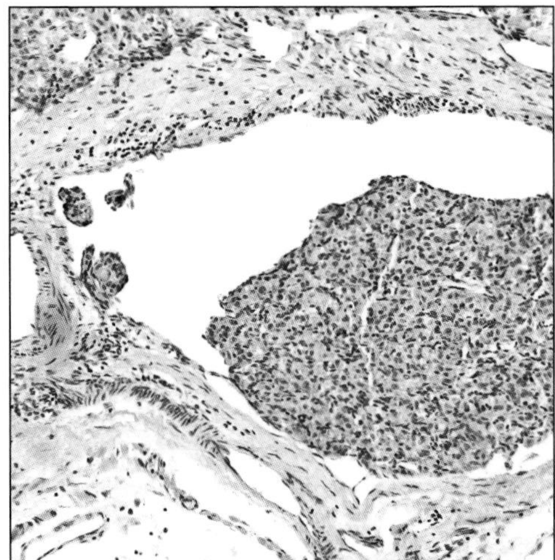

(Left) *Hematoxylin & eosin shows a high magnification on 1 alveolus that demonstrates large polygonal cells with eosinophilic cytoplasm, eccentric nuclei, and prominent nucleoli.* ***(Right)*** *Hematoxylin & eosin shows lymphatic invasion, a very common finding in alveolar soft part sarcoma.*

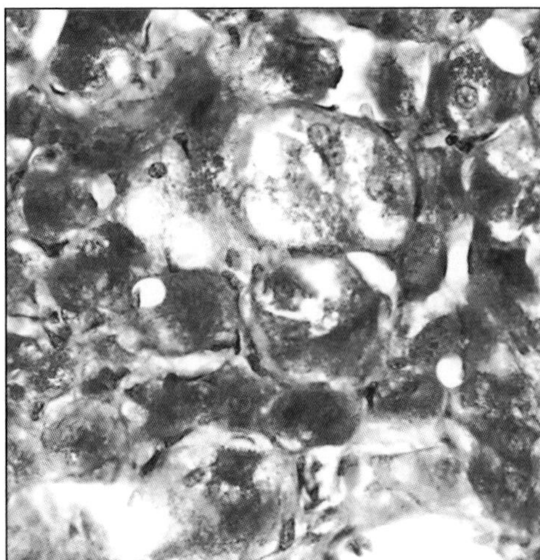

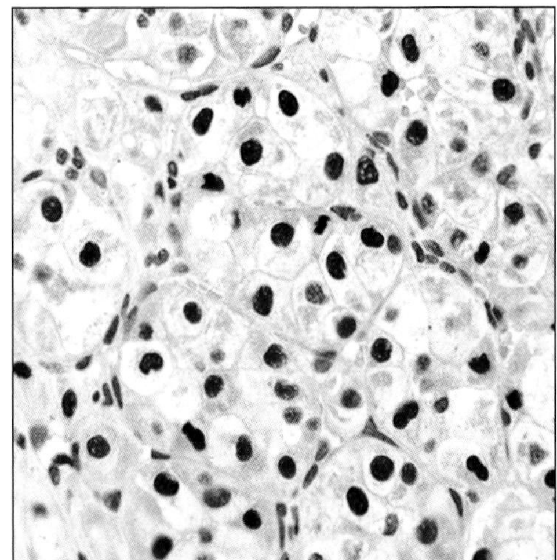

(Left) *Periodic acid-Schiff with diastase digestion shows abundant granular or crystalline cytoplasmic PAS(+) diastase-resistant material.* ***(Right)*** *Positive TFE3 by immunohistochemistry is the gold standard in the diagnosis of ASPS. This is an immunohistochemical marker for a molecular event.*

Microscopic and Immunohistochemical Features

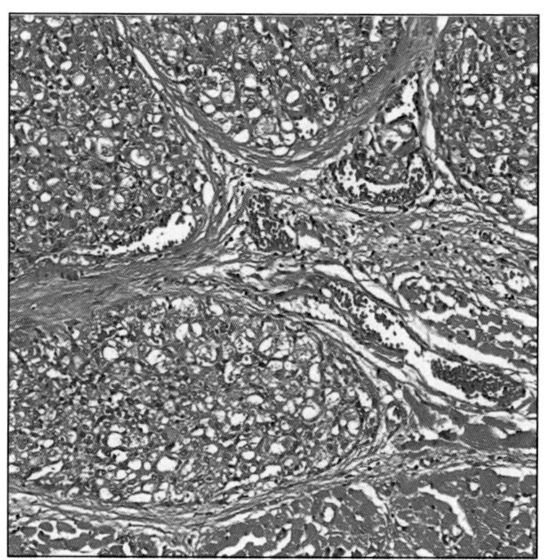

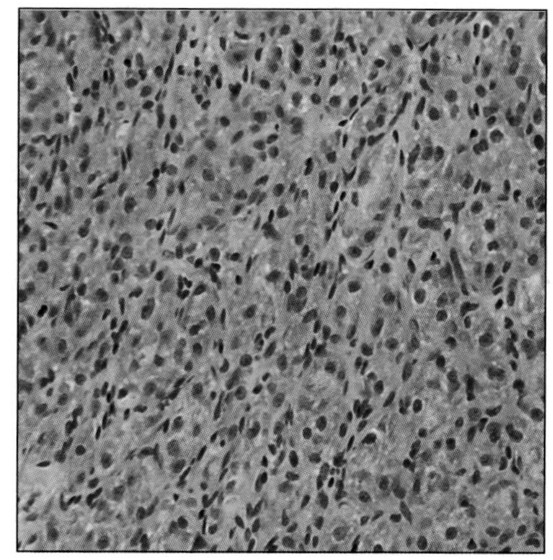

(Left) *Alveolar soft part sarcoma is always an intramuscular tumor, as demonstrated here. The image also shows broad bands of fibrous tissue separating lobules, even in solid forms.* ***(Right)*** *Hematoxylin & eosin shows an example of a solid ASPS. It is found more readily in young children in the tongue or eye. The tumor seems to become more alveolar as the child gets older.*

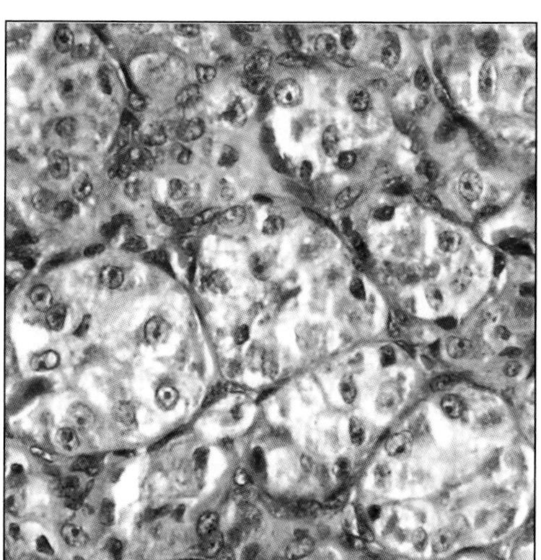

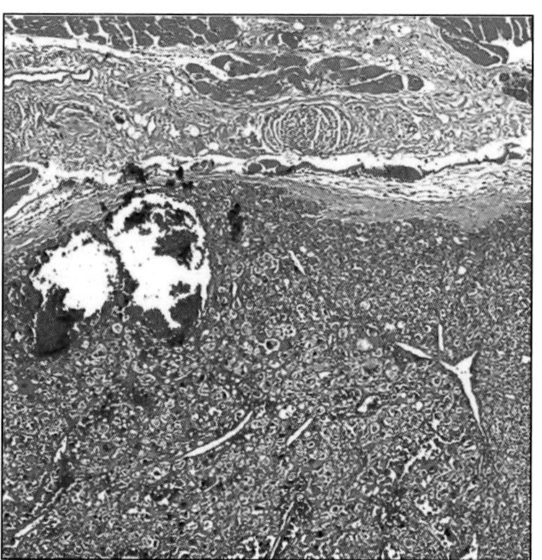

(Left) *Hematoxylin & eosin shows ASPS in the tongue of an older child, demonstrating a more alveolar pattern.* ***(Right)*** *Hematoxylin & eosin shows that ASPS is notably vascular. This is also observed clinically, radiologically, and grossly. Hemorrhage may occur during surgery. This lesion also has pleomorphism.*

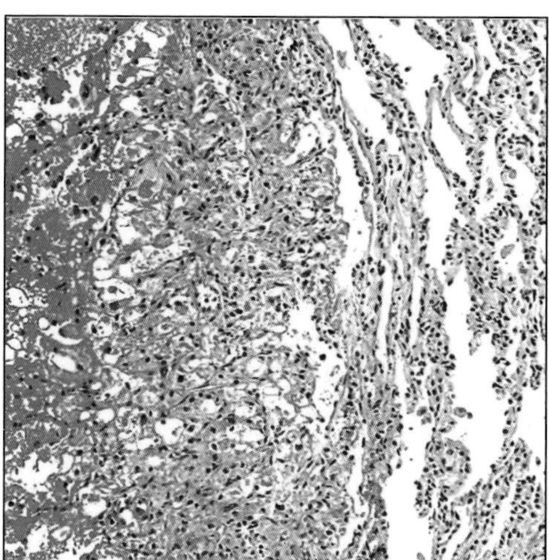

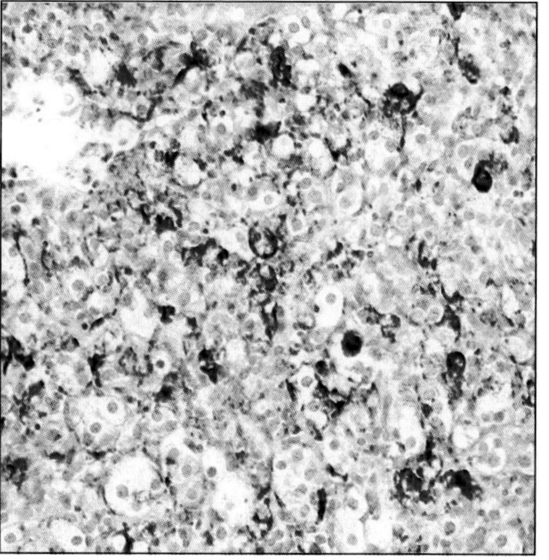

(Left) *Hematoxylin & eosin shows a lung metastasis of ASPS, which may be hard to separate from the alveolar pattern of a normal lung. However, there is hemorrhage and a tumor present within the alveoli.* ***(Right)*** *Negative MYOD1 shows no nuclear staining, only cytoplasmic staining. This was initially misinterpreted as positive for MYOD1, leading to the incorrect assumption that this tumor was of the skeletal muscle phenotype.*

CLEAR CELL SARCOMA

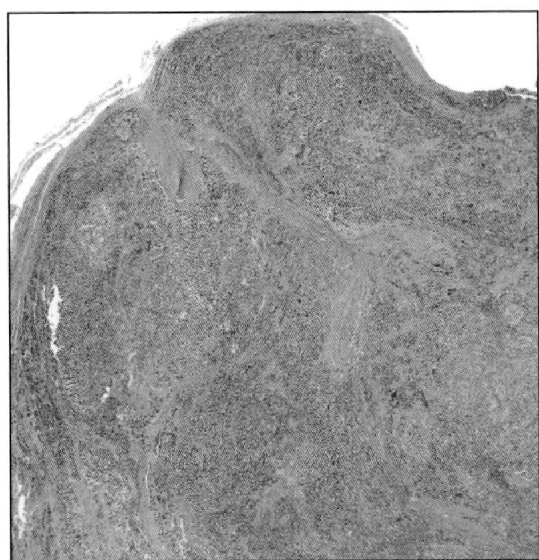

Hematoxylin & eosin shows a lobulated ("packeted") appearance of nests of neoplastic cells in a tendon or aponeurosis.

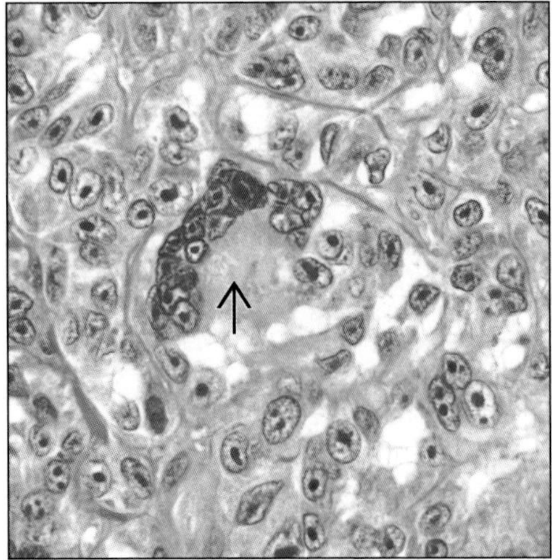

Hematoxylin & eosin shows monotonous cells, each with a uniform enlarged nucleus. A wreath-like tumor giant cell ➔ is present in the center of the field.

TERMINOLOGY

Abbreviations

- Clear cell sarcoma (CCS)

Synonyms

- Malignant melanoma of soft parts

Definitions

- Sarcoma showing melanocytic differentiation
  - Different from clear cell sarcoma of kidney

CLINICAL ISSUES

Epidemiology

- Incidence
  - Rare
- Age
  - Young adults (3rd or 4th decade)
- Gender
  - Slight female predominance

Presentation

- Painless mass
- Usually affects extremities (> 90%)
  - Foot most common site
- Often attached to tendon or aponeurosis
- No associated skin lesions
  - Important in separating CCS from melanoma
- Occasional visceral examples
  - GI tract most common visceral site
    - Ileum most common GI site

Prognosis

- Behaves as high-grade sarcoma
  - 5-year survival (50-65%)
- Metastasizes to lymph nodes and lung
- Differs from behavior of melanoma despite overlapping features
  - For example, 1 cm clear cell sarcoma may have good prognosis while 1 cm melanoma likely to be lethal
  - Metastatic pattern that of sarcoma

MACROSCOPIC FEATURES

Size

- 2-6 cm; median size: 2.5-3.5 cm
- Lobulated gray-white masses

MICROSCOPIC PATHOLOGY

Histologic Features

- Monotonous clear to spindled cells arranged in nests/packets usually infiltrating tendon sheath
  - Abundant glycogen can be detected by PAS or PAS with diastase
- Prominent uniform nucleoli
- Most cases lack necrosis
- Scattered wreath-like tumor giant cells
- Occasional melanin pigment
- Rare cases have nuclear pleomorphism
- Most cases have few mitoses

ANCILLARY TESTS

Immunohistochemistry

- Profile like that of melanoma in most cases
  - Occasional synaptophysin, CD56, epithelial membrane antigen, cytokeratin AE1/AE3, CD34
  - Negative α-smooth muscle actin, desmin, and cytokeratin CAM5.2

Cytogenetics

- t(12;22)(q13;q12)
  - Most soft tissue cases
- t(2;22)(q13;q12)
  - Often in gastrointestinal cases

CLEAR CELL SARCOMA

Key Facts

Terminology
- Sarcoma showing melanocytic differentiation
- Malignant melanoma of soft parts

Clinical Issues
- Young adults (3rd or 4th decade)
- Usually affects extremities (> 90%)
  - Foot most common site
- Behaves as high-grade sarcoma
- Metastasizes to lymph nodes and lung
- Often attached to tendon or aponeurosis
- Occasional visceral examples
  - Ileum most common GI site

Microscopic Pathology
- Monotonous clear to spindled cells arranged in nests/packets usually infiltrating tendon sheath
- Prominent uniform nucleoli
- Scattered wreath-like tumor giant cells
- Most cases have few mitoses

Ancillary Tests
- Immunohistochemical profile like that of melanoma in most cases
- t(12;22)(q13;q12)
  - *EWS-ATF1* fusion (detectable by PCR)
- *EWS-CREB1* fusion: Often in gastrointestinal CCS (lacks melanocytic differentiation)
  - Cases express S100 protein but not melanocytic markers
  - Same transcripts found in angiomatoid fibrous histiocytoma (different morphology, excellent prognosis)

PCR
- Useful for diagnosis in unusual cases
  - *EWS-ATF1* fusion (detectable by PCR)
    - Found in 90% of soft tissue cases
  - Alternate *EWS-CREB1* fusion
    - Same transcripts found in angiomatoid fibrous histiocytoma (which has different morphology and prognosis)
    - Noted in gastrointestinal CCS that lack melanocytic differentiation
    - Cases express S100 protein but not melanocytic markers
  - Melanocyte-specific splice form of MITF transcript found in examples with melanocytic differentiation

Gene Expression Profiling
- Has overlap with cutaneous melanoma profile

DIFFERENTIAL DIAGNOSIS

Melanoma
- Association with skin
- Prominent nuclear pleomorphism
  - Prominent nucleoli, intranuclear inclusions
- Single cell infiltration
- Spindle cell examples often have inconspicuous nucleoli
  - Express S100 protein but not specific melanocytic markers
- Epithelioid melanomas express S100 protein and melanocytic markers
- Many (up to 40%) express CD117
  - Subset with *CKIT* mutations
- Most have complex karyotypes rather than characteristic translocation
- Metastases to any site in body
- Some have *BRAF* mutations

Epithelioid Sarcoma
- Distal extremities
  - Hands and feet
- Epithelioid cells arranged around central necrotic zones in dermis
  - So-called proximal type has sheets of overtly malignant epithelioid cells
- Prominent eosinophilic cytoplasm
- Express CAM 5.2, AE1/3, often CD34(+)
  - CK5/6(-), S100 protein(-), loss of *INI1*
- No characteristic translocation
  - No characteristic gene fusion product
- Bi-allelic loss of *INI1* gene

Tenosynovial Giant Cell Tumor
- Also called giant cell tumor of tendon sheath (GCTTS) when localized
  - Infiltrative (diffuse) form termed pigmented villonodular tenosynovitis
- Usually in fingers
- Female predominance
- Lobulated nests of histiocytoid cells
- Background lymphoplasmacytic cells, giant cells, foam cells, hemosiderin
- CD68(+)
  - Negative S100 protein, keratins, melanocytic markers
- Occasionally locally destructive, especially diffuse form

Schwannoma
- Common in head and neck, deep soft tissue, retroperitoneum, posterior mediastinum
- Well-marginated tumors
- Spindled, palisaded cellular (Antoni A) foci and myxoid (Antoni B) areas
- Thick-walled vessels, foam cells, hemosiderin deposition
- Strong S100 protein
  - Negative melanocytic markers, variable CD34, negative keratins
- Benign with negligible risk for malignant degeneration
- *NF2* gene alterations

Malignant Peripheral Nerve Sheath Tumor
- Some arise in association with neurofibroma

CLEAR CELL SARCOMA

Immunohistochemistry

Antibody	Reactivity	Staining Pattern	Comment
S100	Positive	Nuclear & cytoplasmic	Nearly all cases
HMB-45	Positive	Cytoplasmic	About 80%
Mart-1	Positive	Cytoplasmic	
MITF	Positive	Nuclear	Stains virtually all cases with melanocytic differentiation
CD117	Positive	Cell membrane & cytoplasm	About 15%
CD57	Positive	Cytoplasmic	
Bcl-2	Positive	Cytoplasmic	

- Especially in neurofibromatosis type 1 patients
- Deep large soft tissue lesions, usually of proximal extremities
- Fibrosarcoma-like growth pattern, occasionally palisading
- Bullet-shaped nuclei
  - Inconspicuous nucleoli
- Usually only focal S100 protein expression, no melanocytic differentiation
  - Exception is epithelioid malignant peripheral nerve sheath tumor
    - Prominent nucleoli, strong S100 protein, negative melanocytic markers
- Some with skeletal muscle differentiation (Triton tumors)
- No characteristic translocation or gene fusion product

PEComa (Perivascular Epithelioid Cell Neoplasms)

- Encompass angiomyolipoma, clear cell "sugar" tumor of lung, lymphangiomyomatosis, clear cell myelomelanocytic tumor of falciform ligament
- Nests of epithelioid cells, some with clear cell features
- Spindle cells with smooth muscle features
- Some with fat component (angiomyolipoma)
- Express smooth muscle markers and melanocytic markers
  - But not keratins or S100 protein

DIAGNOSTIC CHECKLIST

Clinically Relevant Pathologic Features

- Metastatic distribution
  - To lymph nodes and lungs
    - Contrasts to multiorgan pattern in melanoma

Pathologic Interpretation Pearls

- Consider clear cell sarcoma before diagnosing tenosynovial giant cell tumor (giant cell tumor of tendon sheath) in foot

SELECTED REFERENCES

1. Clark MA et al: Clear cell sarcoma (melanoma of soft parts): The Royal Marsden Hospital experience. Eur J Surg Oncol. 34(7):800-4, 2008
2. Hisaoka M et al: Clear cell sarcoma of soft tissue: a clinicopathologic, immunohistochemical, and molecular analysis of 33 cases. Am J Surg Pathol. 32(3):452-60, 2008
3. Lyle PL et al: Gastrointestinal melanoma or clear cell sarcoma? Molecular evaluation of 7 cases previously diagnosed as malignant melanoma. Am J Surg Pathol. 32(6):858-66, 2008
4. Antonescu CR et al: EWS-CREB1: a recurrent variant fusion in clear cell sarcoma--association with gastrointestinal location and absence of melanocytic differentiation. Clin Cancer Res. 12(18):5356-62, 2006
5. Segal NH et al: Classification of clear-cell sarcoma as a subtype of melanoma by genomic profiling. J Clin Oncol. 21(9):1775-81, 2003
6. Antonescu CR et al: Molecular diagnosis of clear cell sarcoma: detection of EWS-ATF1 and MITF-M transcripts and histopathological and ultrastructural analysis of 12 cases. J Mol Diagn. 4(1):44-52, 2002
7. Granter SR et al: Clear cell sarcoma shows immunoreactivity for microphthalmia transcription factor: further evidence for melanocytic differentiation. Mod Pathol. 14(1):6-9, 2001
8. Rubin BP et al: Clear cell sarcoma of soft parts: report of a case primary in the kidney with cytogenetic confirmation. Am J Surg Pathol. 23(5):589-94, 1999
9. Donner LR et al: Clear cell sarcoma of the ileum: the crucial role of cytogenetics for the diagnosis. Am J Surg Pathol. 22(1):121-4, 1998
10. Lucas DR et al: Clear cell sarcoma of soft tissues. Mayo Clinic experience with 35 cases. Am J Surg Pathol. 16(12):1197-204, 1992
11. Montgomery E et al: Clear cell sarcoma of tendons and aponeuroses. A clinicopathologic study of 58 cases with analysis of prognostic factors. Int J Surg Pathol. 1:89-100, 1992
12. Reeves BR et al: Translocation t(12;22)(q13;q13) is a nonrandom rearrangement in clear cell sarcoma. Cancer Genet Cytogenet. 64(2):101-3, 1992
13. Pavlidis NA et al: Clear-cell sarcoma of tendons and aponeuroses: a clinicopathologic study. Presentation of six additional cases with review of the literature. Cancer. 54(7):1412-7, 1984
14. Chung EB et al: Malignant melanoma of soft parts. A reassessment of clear cell sarcoma. Am J Surg Pathol. 7(5):405-13, 1983
15. Enzinger FM: Clear-cell sarcoma of tendons and aponeuroses. An analysis of 21 cases. Cancer. 18:1163-74, 1965

Microscopic Features

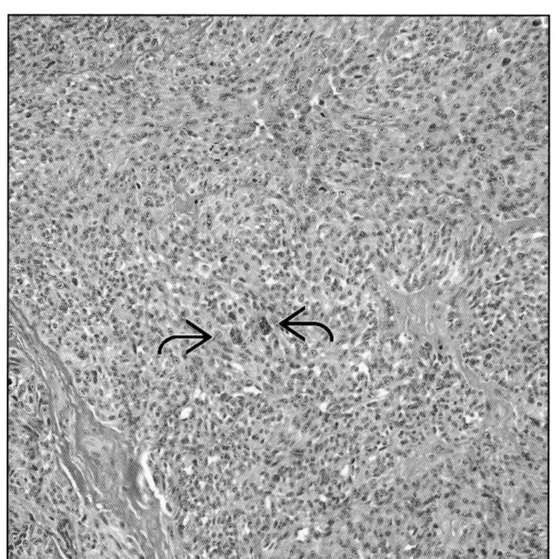

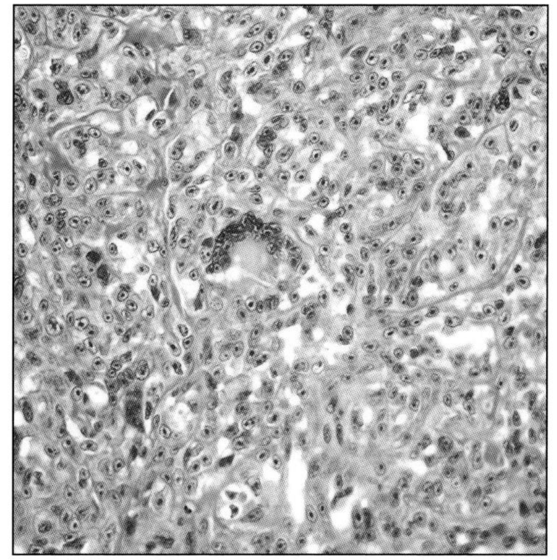

*(**Left**) Hematoxylin & eosin at intermediate magnification shows a clear cell sarcoma, featuring a packeted arrangement of neoplastic cells separated by collagenous bands. Scattered giant cells ⮫ are seen in this field, a finding that sometimes leads to a misdiagnosis of tenosynovial giant cell tumor (GCTTS). This lesion differs from GCTTS by lacking an inflammatory cell component. (**Right**) Hematoxylin & eosin shows monotonous neoplastic cells.*

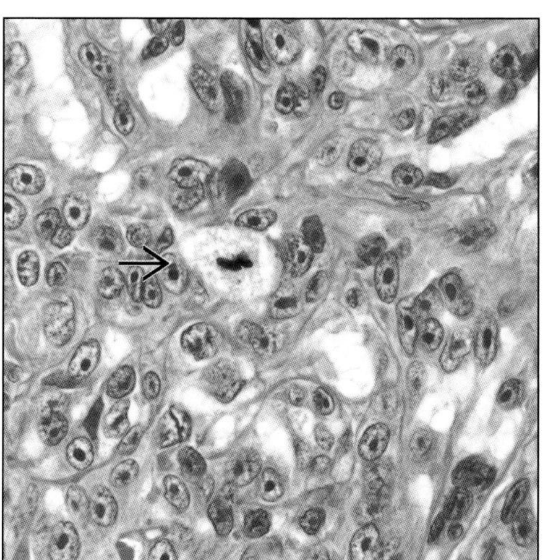

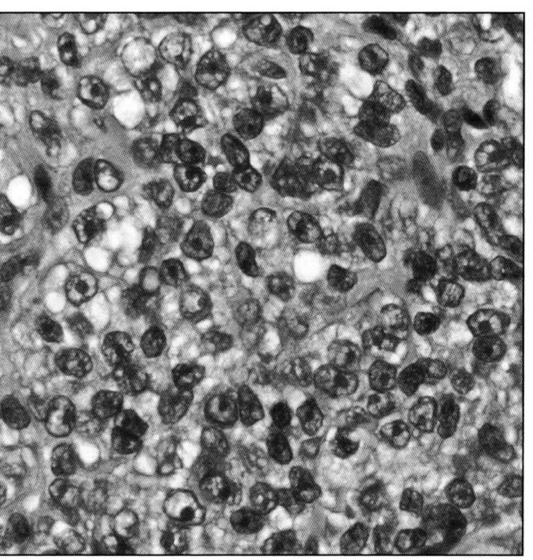

*(**Left**) Hematoxylin & eosin shows a (typical) mitosis → in a clear cell sarcoma. Atypical mitoses are not identified in these tumors, as they have a characteristic translocation rather than chromosomal instability. (**Right**) Hematoxylin & eosin shows another clear cell sarcoma, this one with smaller cells than depicted in the previous image. The cells retain their monotonous appearance and prominent nucleoli.*

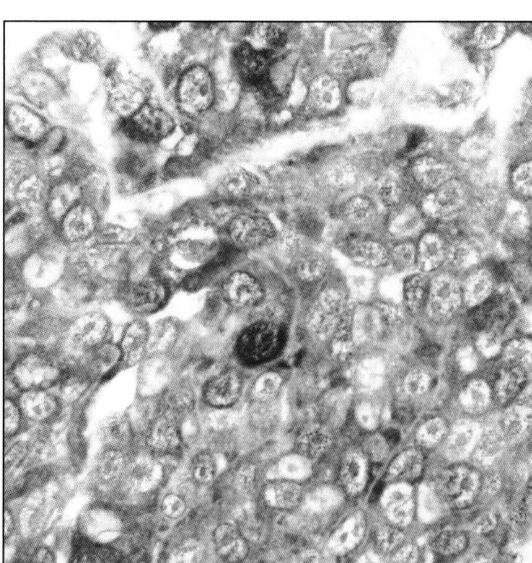

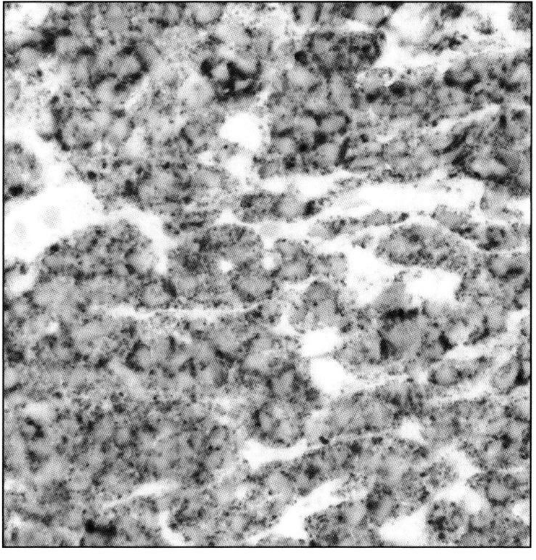

*(**Left**) S100 shows nuclear and cytoplasmic labeling in most clear cell sarcomas. (**Right**) HMB-45 shows cytoplasmic labeling in most clear cell sarcomas of soft tissue, although melanocytic markers are often negative in clear cell sarcomas of the gastrointestinal tract.*

CLEAR CELL SARCOMA

Microscopic Features

*(**Left**) Periodic acid-Schiff shows abundant glycogen (sensitive to diastase digestion) in many clear cell sarcomas. (**Right**) CD117 shows labeling in this particular clear cell sarcoma of soft tissue, although most clear sarcomas are CD117(-). Note the membranous and cytoplasmic pattern.*

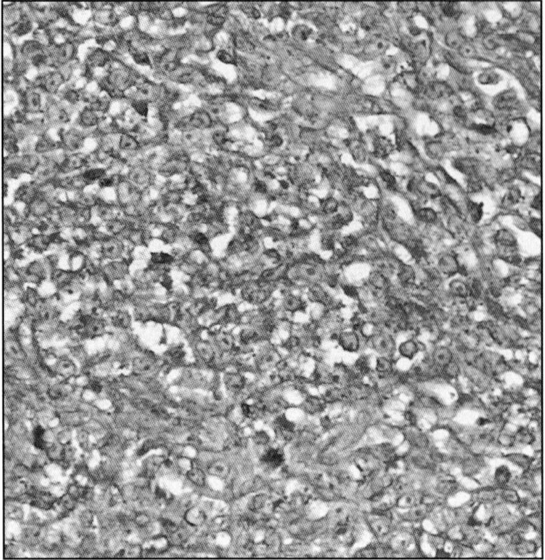

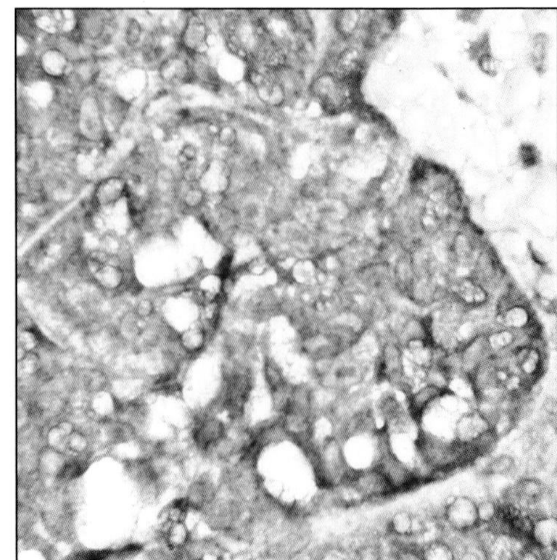

*(**Left**) Hematoxylin & eosin shows low magnification of a small intestinal clear cell sarcoma. The lesion is centered on the muscularis propria and retains the packeted appearance of soft tissue examples. (**Right**) Hematoxylin & eosin shows nodules of clear cell sarcoma of the gastrointestinal tract. The cells are highly uniform and have a clear appearance at low magnification.*

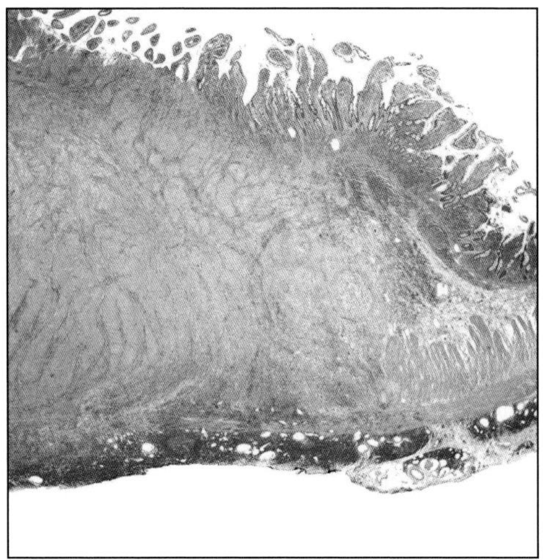

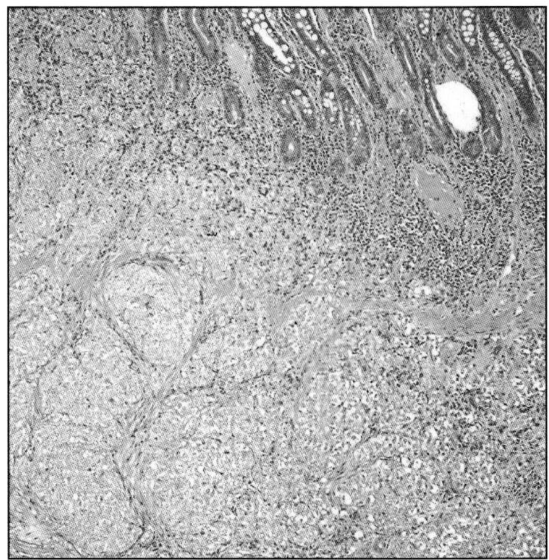

*(**Left**) Hematoxylin & eosin shows the cytologic features of a gastrointestinal tract clear cell sarcoma, displaying monotonous nuclei, many of which have prominent nucleoli. (**Right**) S100 shows strong labeling in a gastrointestinal tract clear cell sarcoma. In contrast to examples in soft tissue, gastrointestinal examples often lack melanocytic differentiation and have alternate gene rearrangements.*

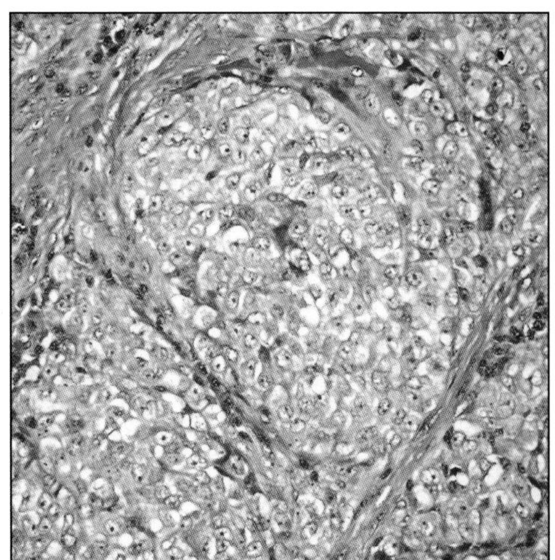

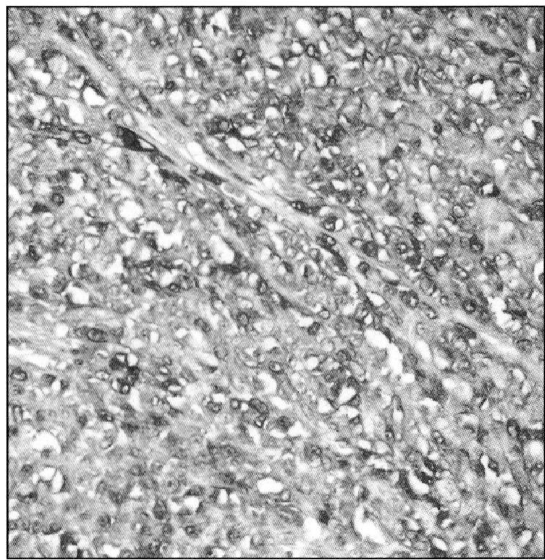

Differential Diagnosis

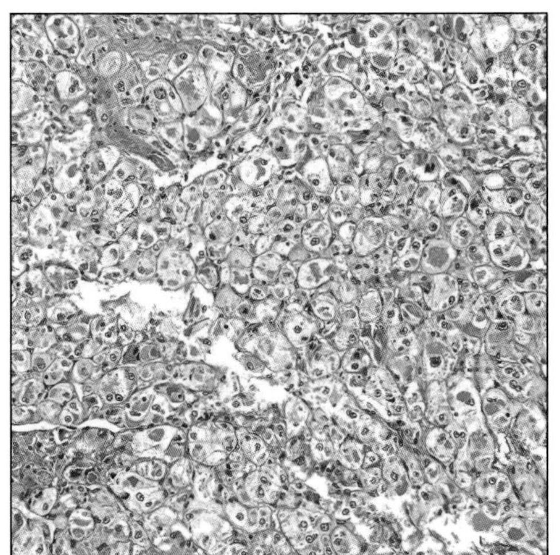
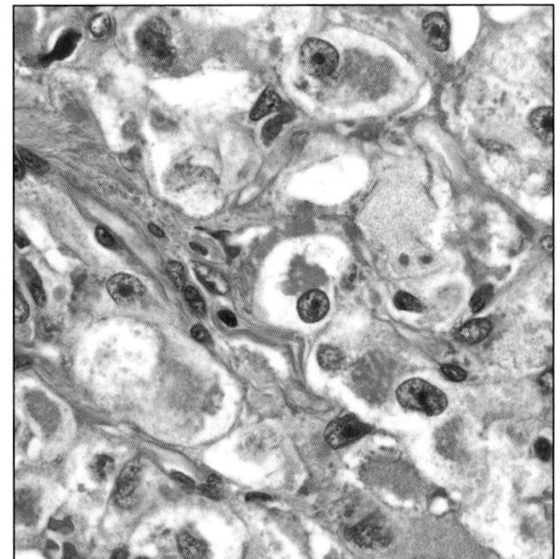

(Left) *Hematoxylin & eosin shows an alveolar soft part sarcoma. It is more richly vascularized than clear cell sarcoma with vessels separating small nests of cells (alveolar pattern).* ***(Right)*** *Hematoxylin & eosin shows the classic cytologic features of alveolar soft part sarcoma. Note that there are uniform nuclei and prominent nucleoli. There is more abundant cytoplasm in these cells than in those of clear cell sarcoma.*

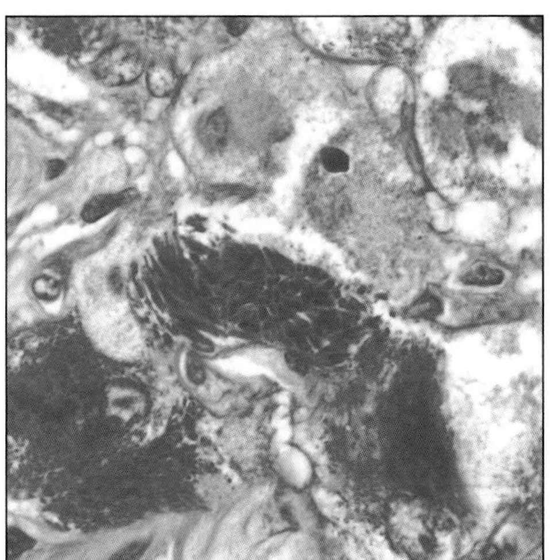
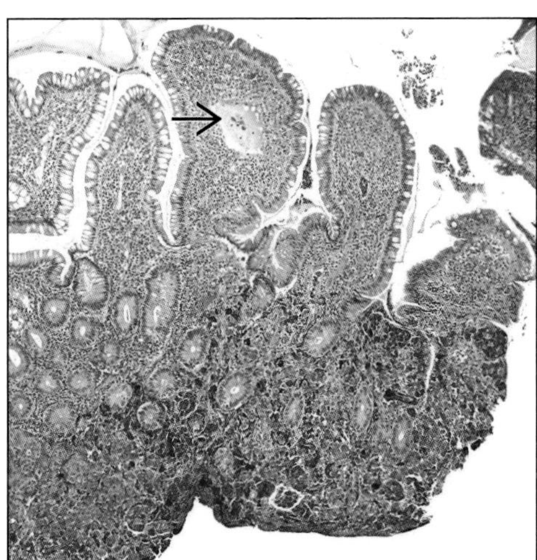

(Left) *Periodic acid-Schiff shows striking cytoplasmic crystals in this alveolar soft part sarcoma.* ***(Right)*** *Hematoxylin & eosin shows metastatic melanoma involving the duodenum. This example is pigmented. The cells are arranged in sheets. Note the tumor cells in lacteals* ⇒.

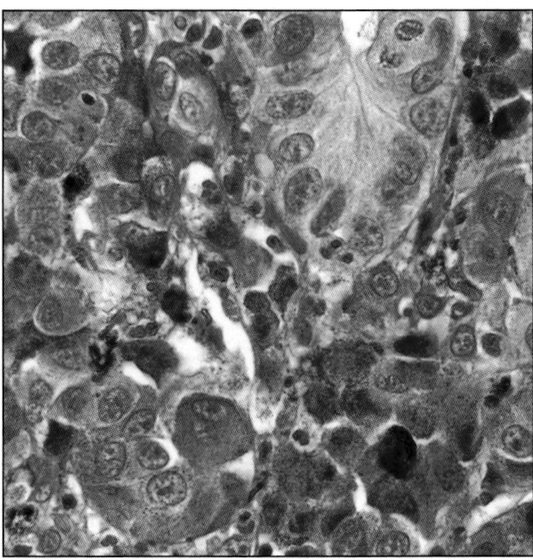
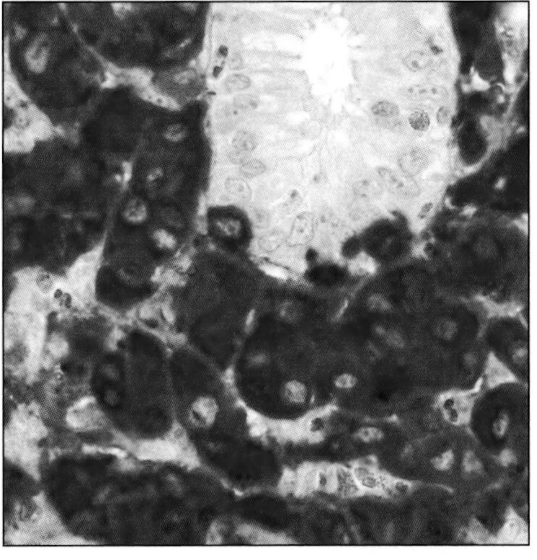

(Left) *Hematoxylin & eosin shows the pleomorphic cytologic features and single cell infiltrative pattern of a melanoma. Most melanomas can be separated from clear cell sarcomas by noting nuclear pleomorphism in melanomas.* ***(Right)*** *Mart-1 shows strong labeling in a melanoma metastatic to the gastrointestinal tract. Melanocytic markers tend to be absent in primary gastrointestinal tract clear cell sarcomas.*

DESMOPLASTIC SMALL ROUND CELL TUMOR

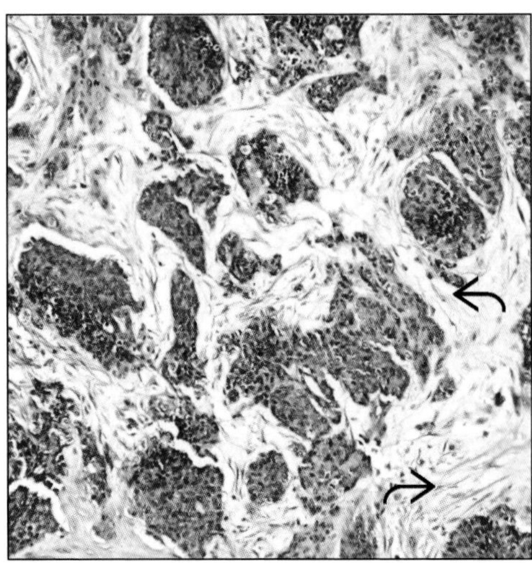

In desmoplastic small round cell tumor, islands of neoplastic cells proliferate in dense desmoplastic stroma. The tumor cells are markedly hyperchromatic in contrast to the stromal myofibroblasts ⇗.

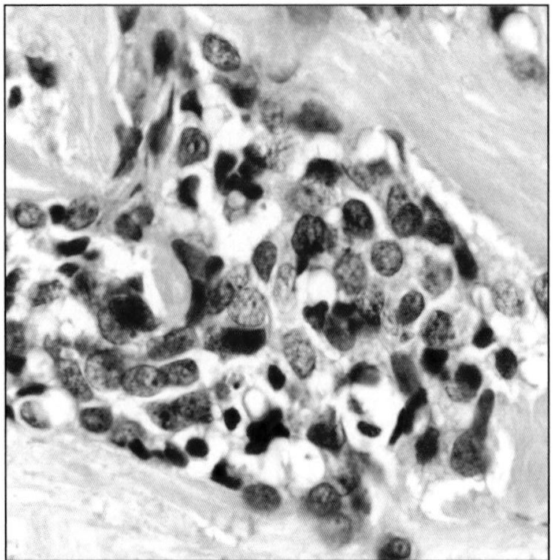

The neoplastic cells in desmoplastic round cell tumor are quite uniform, a feature of sarcomas with balanced reciprocal translocations. Nucleoli are inconspicuous, and cytoplasm is scanty.

TERMINOLOGY

Abbreviations

- Desmoplastic small round cell tumor (DSRCT)

Synonyms

- Desmoplastic small round cell tumor with divergent differentiation
- Polyphenotypic small round cell tumor
- Desmoplastic primitive neuroectodermal tumor
- Intraabdominal desmoplastic small round cell tumor

Definitions

- Primitive malignant neoplasm arising in serosal surfaces with distinctive histology composed of primitive small round blue cells embedded in abundant desmoplastic stroma

CLINICAL ISSUES

Presentation

- Male predilection
- Pain and weight loss
- Most common in children and young adults (2nd or 3rd decade; median age: 20 years)
- Most commonly present in peritoneal cavity
  - Also reported in paratesticular region, ovary, thoracic cavity, lung, central nervous system, and head and neck

Treatment

- Surgical excision
- Chemotherapy

Prognosis

- Poor prognosis
  - Nearly uniformly fatal
- Frequent local recurrence; rarely metastasizes
- Median survival is 24 months

MACROSCOPIC FEATURES

General Features

- Large, bulky tumors (> 10 cm in greatest dimension)
- May also grow in multinodular fashion
- Firm homogeneous cut surface
- Hemorrhage and necrosis

MICROSCOPIC PATHOLOGY

Histologic Features

- Nests, trabeculae, or sheets of small round blue cells embedded in abundant desmoplastic fibrous stroma
- Nests may display peripheral palisading of tumor cells
- Rosette-like structures

Cytologic Features

- Small to intermediate-sized round to oval cells with scant cytoplasm
- Round to oval, hyperchromatic nuclei
- Small nucleoli
- High mitotic rate, with typical mitoses (translocation sarcoma)

ANCILLARY TESTS

Immunohistochemistry

- Staining pattern is polyphenotypic
- Vimentin, cytokeratin, desmin, EMA, and WT1 consistently stain tumor cells in ~ 90% of cases
- Staining pattern for desmin and vimentin is characteristically dot-like and paranuclear
- May also show focal positivity for CD56, NSE, chromogranin, synaptophysin, and S100 protein

Cytogenetics

- Shows t(11:22)(p13;q12), similar to Ewing sarcoma/PNET

DESMOPLASTIC SMALL ROUND CELL TUMOR

Key Facts

Clinical Issues
- Most common in children and young adults
  - Median age: 20 years
- Male predilection
- Large abdominal mass on chest x-rays and CT scans
- Poor prognosis
- Median survival is 24 months

Macroscopic Features
- Large, bulky tumors (> 10 cm in greatest dimension)

Microscopic Pathology
- Nests, trabeculae, or sheets of uniform small round cells embedded in abundant desmoplastic fibrous stroma
- Rosette-like structures
- Small to intermediate-sized round to oval cells with scant cytoplasm
- High mitotic index, often with atypical (abnormal) mitoses
- Immunohistochemically polyphenotypic
- Vimentin, keratin, desmin, EMA, and WT1 consistently positive in tumor cells in approximately 90% of cases
  - Staining pattern for desmin and vimentin is characteristically dot-like and paranuclear
- May also show focal positivity for CD56, NSE, chromogranin, synaptophysin, and S100 protein
- Genetically shows t(11:22)(p13;q12), similar to Ewing sarcoma/PNET
  - Differs from Ewing sarcoma as rearranged gene on chromosome 11 is *WT1* rather than *FLI1*

- Unlike Ewing sarcoma, site on chromosome 11 is *WT1* gene rather than *FLI1* gene
  - The 2 genes (*EWS* and *WT1*) are rearranged and functionally fused
  - *EWS* breakpoint in introns 7-10
  - *WT1* breakpoint between exons 7 and 8
- *EWS-WT1* chimera encodes a novel transcription factor detectable by PCR as a diagnostic test
- Rare hybrid tumors have *EWS-ERG* fusion

DIFFERENTIAL DIAGNOSIS

Peripheral Neuroectodermal Tumor (PNET)/ Ewing Sarcoma
- Similar cell population in both, but prominent desmoplastic stroma is not seen in PNET
- Lacks strong expression of polyphenotypic markers, such as desmin, cytokeratin, and WT1
- Strongly positive for CD99 in most cases; CD99 is seen only in 20% of cases of DSRCT
- Translocation in PNET is t(11:22)(p24;q12); translocation in DSRCT is t(11:22)(p13;q12)

Metastatic Neuroendocrine Carcinoma
- Lacks prominent desmoplastic stroma separating tumor cell nests
- Has distinctive "smudged" or "salt & pepper" chromatin pattern
- Positive for neuroendocrine markers, such as chromogranin, CD56, and synaptophysin
- Does not express EMA, desmin, or WT1

Malignant Lymphoma
- Discohesive pattern of growth without striking desmoplasia
- Express CD45 and variety of other lymphoid markers, e.g., CD3, CD20, CD30, CD43, but not keratin, desmin, or WT1
- Lymphoblastic lymphoma in children and adolescents shows nuclear positivity for TdT and is positive for CD99

Alveolar Rhabdomyosarcoma
- Multinucleated cells, some pleomorphism
- Diffuse positivity for desmin and myogenin

DIAGNOSTIC CHECKLIST

Clinically Relevant Pathologic Features
- Preferentially affects children and young adults, although it can affect older patients

Pathologic Interpretation Pearls
- Nests of small round blue cells surrounded by abundant desmoplastic fibrous stroma
- Primitive appearance of tumor cells
- High mitotic activity and areas of tumor cell necrosis
- Distinctive pattern of immunohistochemical staining: CK, EMA, vimentin, desmin, and WT1 positive
- Dot-like, paranuclear (Golgi-zone) staining for vimentin and desmin
- Specific cytogenetic translocation: t(11:22)(p13;q12)

SELECTED REFERENCES

1. Lae ME et al: Desmoplastic small round cell tumor: a clinicopathologic, immunohistochemical, and molecular study of 32 tumors. Am J Surg Pathol. 26(7):823-35, 2002
2. Ordóñez NG: Desmoplastic small round cell tumor: I: a histopathologic study of 39 cases with emphasis on unusual histological patterns. Am J Surg Pathol. 22(11):1303-13, 1998
3. Ordóñez NG: Desmoplastic small round cell tumor: II: an ultrastructural and immunohistochemical study with emphasis on new immunohistochemical markers. Am J Surg Pathol. 22(11):1314-27, 1998
4. Ladanyi M et al: Fusion of the EWS and WT1 genes in the desmoplastic small round cell tumor. Cancer Res. 54(11):2837-40, 1994
5. Gerald WL et al: Intra-abdominal desmoplastic small round-cell tumor. Report of 19 cases of a distinctive type of high-grade polyphenotypic malignancy affecting young individuals. Am J Surg Pathol. 15(6):499-513, 1991

DESMOPLASTIC SMALL ROUND CELL TUMOR

Microscopic Features

(Left) It is not unusual to encounter comedo-type necrosis in desmoplastic small round cell tumor. Together with the lesion's characteristic keratin expression, this pattern can cause diagnostic confusion with carcinomas. Note, however, that the lesional cells lack pleomorphism. ***(Right)*** *Although this desmoplastic small round cell tumor has the characteristic desmoplastic stroma, it is unusual in featuring multinucleated cells ⇒, a finding suggestive of alveolar rhabdomyosarcoma.*

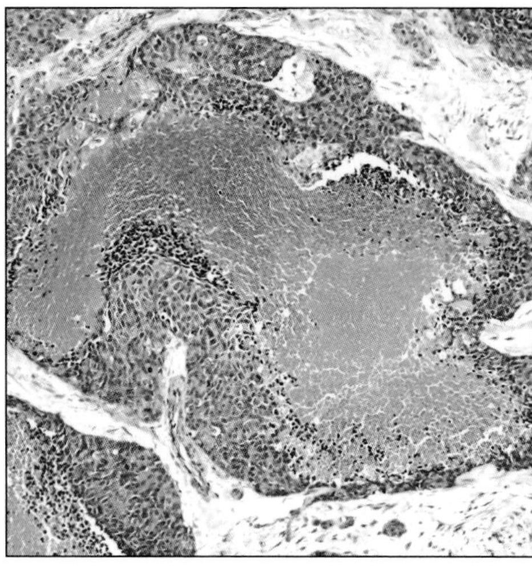

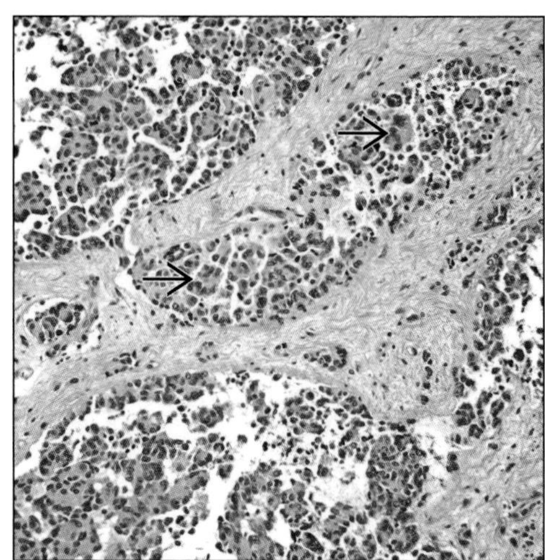

(Left) This desmoplastic round cell sarcoma has a spindled pattern. Note the absence of nuclear pleomorphism. ***(Right)*** *H&E shows clear cell pattern in a desmoplastic small round cell tumor. An erythrocyte ⇒ in the center of the field can be used as a size indicator; the proliferating cells have relatively small nuclei with very uniform rather than pleomorphic features, an appearance that belies the aggressive nature of these lesions.*

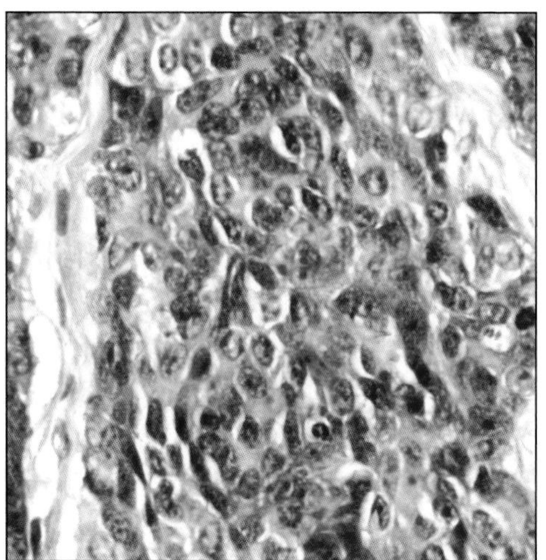

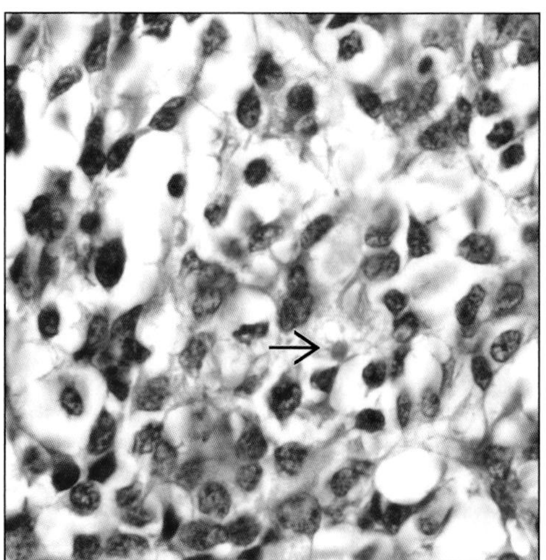

(Left) The nuclei in this desmoplastic small round cell tumor are arranged in a rare rosette pattern ⇨. There was a typical desmoplastic stroma elsewhere in the neoplasm, but in this focus it appears myxoid ⇒. ***(Right)*** *The cells in this desmoplastic small round cell tumor are somewhat spindled, and the eosinophilic cytoplasm appears syncytial. The tumor cells have small nuclei that are about twice the size of the erythrocyte in the upper left hand corner of the field ↗.*

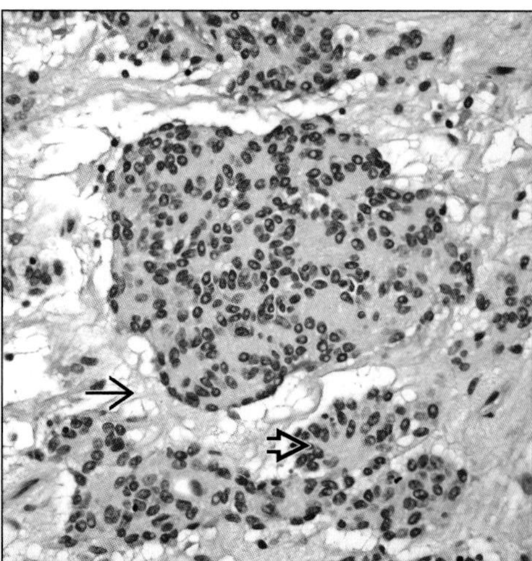

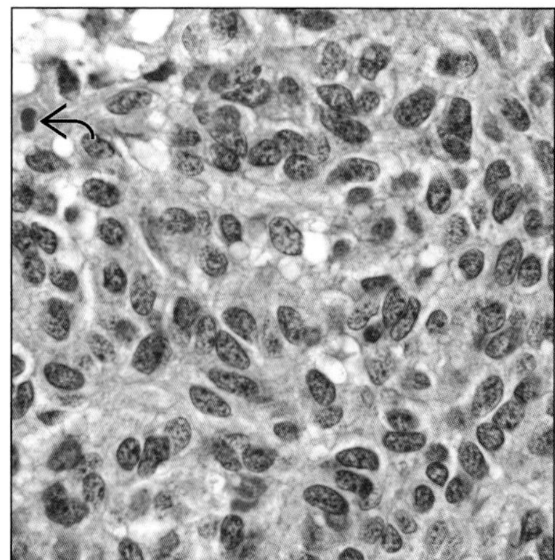

Immunohistochemical Features

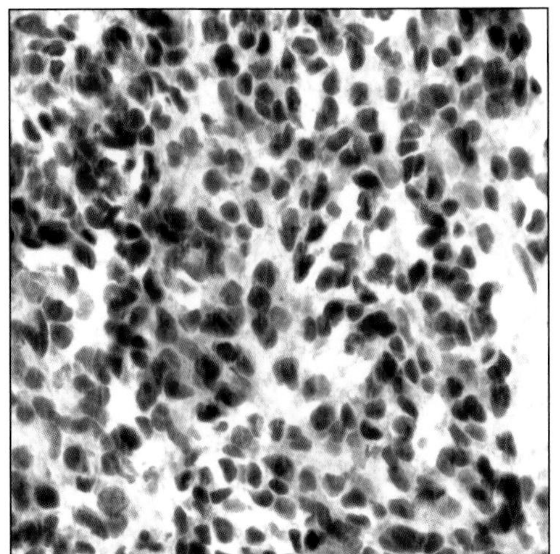

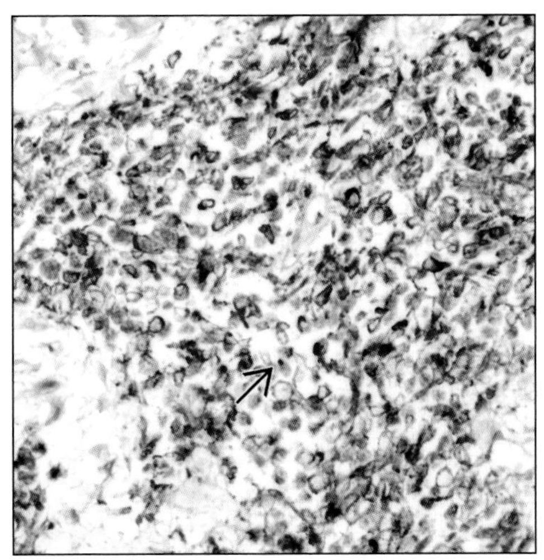

(Left) *Desmoplastic small round cell tumors display strong nuclear labeling for WT1 in most cases. This helps distinguish it from Ewing sarcoma and alveolar rhabdomyosarcoma (which can have cytoplasmic positivity).* ***(Right)*** *Immunohistochemical staining of desmoplastic small round cell tumor for cytokeratin shows cytoplasmic positivity in the majority of the tumor cells, with a paranuclear dot pattern in some* ⇒.

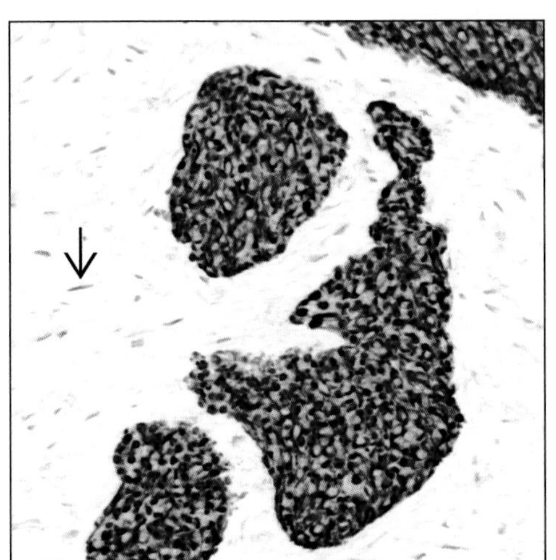

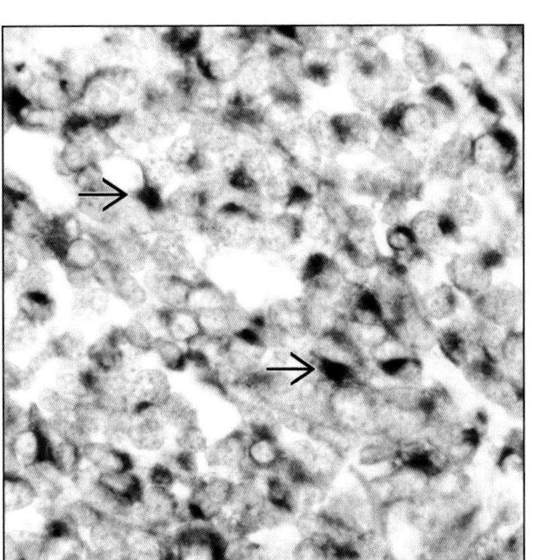

(Left) *Desmin expression is a characteristic feature of desmoplastic small round cell tumor, present in over 90% of cases. In this example, the staining is diffuse and highlights the tumor islands. The spindle cells in the stroma* ⇒ *are negative.* ***(Right)*** *Immunostaining for desmin in desmoplastic small round cell tumor typically shows a punctate (dot) paranuclear pattern* ⇒*. These neoplasms do not express myogenin, a feature that is useful for excluding alveolar rhabdomyosarcoma.*

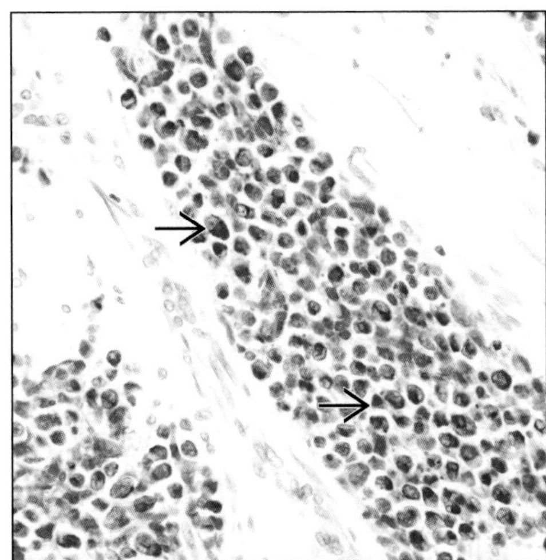

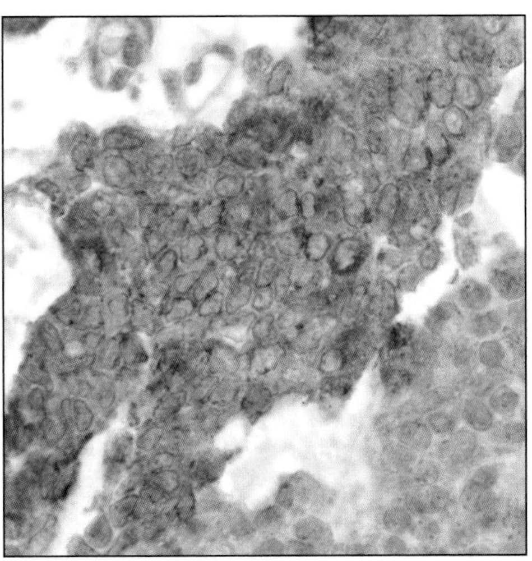

(Left) *Immunohistochemical staining of desmoplastic small round cell tumor for vimentin shows the majority of the tumor cells are positive for this marker and display a distinctive dot-like, paranuclear (Golgi zone) staining pattern* ⇒*.* ***(Right)*** *CD99 is usually negative in desmoplastic round cell tumors, but weak cytoplasmic staining is seen in some cases. This differs from the strong membranous staining of Ewing sarcoma, but cytogenetic studies can be required to make the diagnosis.*

PECOMA

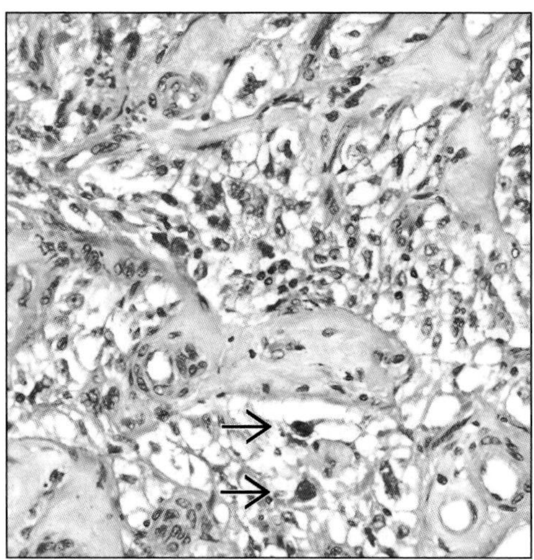

Hematoxylin & eosin shows a PEComa with epithelioid cells proliferating around vessels. There are scattered large nuclei ⇒ in this field but no mitoses.

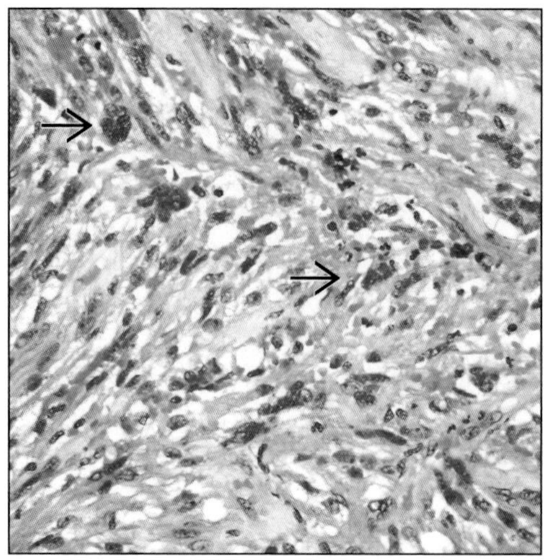

Hematoxylin & eosin shows a more myoid portion of a PEComa with more prominent cytoplasmic eosinophilia than in the previous image. This example also has scattered pleomorphic nuclei ⇒.

TERMINOLOGY

Abbreviations

- Perivascular epithelioid cell (PEC)
- Thus neoplasms are termed "PEComa"

Synonyms

- Extrapulmonary sugar tumor
- Perivascular epithelioid cell tumor
- Monotypic epithelioid angiomyolipoma

Definitions

- Mesenchymal neoplasms composed of distinctive perivascular epithelioid cells (PEC) category includes
  - Angiomyolipoma (AML)
  - Clear cell "sugar" tumor of lung (CCST)
  - Lymphangioleiomyomatosis (LAM)
  - Clear cell myomelanocytic tumor of falciform ligament/ligamentum teres (CCMMT)
- In many respects, PEComas are simply angiomyolipomas without fat
- Subset displays overt histologic features of malignancy and malignant clinical behavior

ETIOLOGY/PATHOGENESIS

Association with Tuberous Sclerosis

- Genetic alterations of tuberous sclerosis complex (TSC), losses of *TSC1* (9q34) or *TSC2* (16p13.3) genes
- Autosomal dominant
- Benign tumors of brain (most common), kidneys, heart, eyes, lungs, and skin
  - Name comes from characteristic tuber or potato-like nodules in brain, which calcify with age and become hard or sclerotic
- AML, CCST, and LAM are associated with tuberous sclerosis but not other types

CLINICAL ISSUES

Epidemiology

- Incidence
  - AML, CCST, LAM are rare
    - Other PEComas extremely rare
- Age
  - CCMMT typically encountered in girls in late childhood
  - Most others seen in adults 50-60 years old
  - AML detected in younger patients in setting of tuberous sclerosis
- Gender
  - Marked overall female predominance

Site

- Reported in multiple sites
  - Kidney, liver, falciform ligament, deep soft tissues of extremities, skin, uterus, vulva, heart, gallbladder, gastrointestinal tract

Presentation

- CCMMT presents as painful abdominal mass
- Uterine examples manifest as uterine bleeding
- Most other categories of PEComas present as painless masses
- Brain tumors in patients with tuberous sclerosis present with seizures, developmental delay, behavioral problems

Treatment

- Surgical excision

Prognosis

- Most are benign
  - Rare documented examples of malignancy
    - Usually not in AML, LAM, or CCST types
    - Malignant examples behave as aggressive sarcomas

PECOMA

Key Facts

Terminology

- PEComa is abbreviation for neoplasms with perivascular epithelioid cell differentiation
- Mesenchymal neoplasms composed of distinctive perivascular epithelioid cells
  - Includes angiomyolipoma (AML), clear cell "sugar" tumor of lung (CCST), lymphangioleiomyomatosis (LAM), clear cell myomelanocytic tumor of falciform ligament/ligamentum teres (CCMMT)
  - In many respects, PEComas are simply angiomyolipomas without fat

Etiology/Pathogenesis

- AML, CCST, and LAM are associated with tuberous sclerosis but not other types

Clinical Issues

- Most are benign

Microscopic Pathology

- PECs consist of epithelioid to spindled cells arranged around vessels extending outward radially
- Clear to granular, lightly eosinophilic cytoplasm and round to oval nuclei with small nucleoli
- Myoid component with densely eosinophilic cytoplasm
- Adipose tissue component present in lesions termed AML

MICROSCOPIC PATHOLOGY

Histologic Features

- PECs consist of epithelioid to spindled cells arranged around vessels extending outward radially
  - Clear to granular, lightly eosinophilic cytoplasm and round to oval nuclei with small nucleoli
  - Lesions are richly vascular
  - Small arching vessels divide tumor into packets (similar to pattern in renal cell carcinoma)
- Myoid component with densely eosinophilic cytoplasm
  - Nuclei less rounded than those of true smooth muscle
- Adipose tissue component present in lesions termed AML
- CCMMT is almost exclusively spindle cell lesion
  - Uniform, moderate-sized cells set in elaborate lace-like vasculature

Rare Malignant Examples

- Criteria for malignancy
  - Infiltrative growth
  - Marked hypercellularity
  - Nuclear enlargement and hyperchromasia
  - Numerous &/or atypical mitotic figures
  - Necrosis

DIFFERENTIAL DIAGNOSIS

Renal Cell Carcinoma

- Clear epithelial cells and rich vascular pattern
  - Sarcomatoid examples overtly high-grade neoplasms
- Usually displays epithelial markers by immunohistochemistry
- Lacks adipose tissue component

Hepatocellular Carcinoma

- Large atypical cells with opaque eosinophilic cytoplasm, rich vascularity
- Usually has marked nuclear pleomorphism
- Expresses epithelial markers (CAM5.2), sometimes Hep-Par1
  - Canalicular pattern on immunolabeling with CD10 or polyclonal CEA
- No adipose tissue component
- Some examples have cytoplasmic bile

True Smooth Muscle Tumors

- Perpendicularly oriented fascicles of spindle cells with brightly eosinophilic cytoplasm and blunt-ended nuclei
  - Criteria for malignancy site specific and related to mitotic activity and nuclear atypia
- Intensely eosinophilic cytoplasm
- Usually lack adipose tissue component
  - Exception is myolipoma
- Lack PEC differentiation
  - Most smooth muscle tumors lack melanocytic antigens and express desmin
- Lack rich vascular pattern (although some leiomyosarcomas arise in association with vessels)
- Some examples are associated with Epstein-Barr virus

Well-Differentiated Liposarcoma

- Shows fat punctuated by atypical nuclei
  - Fibrous septa containing enlarged hyperchromatic nuclei
  - Can have areas of dedifferentiation to high-grade sarcoma
    - Overt high-grade spindle cell sarcoma with numerous mitoses and atypical nuclei
- Most examples not richly vascular
- Show nuclear MDM2 or CDK4 immunolabeling
  - Negative melanocytic markers

Gastrointestinal Stromal Tumor

- Epithelioid or spindle cell neoplasms usually involving muscularis propria of gastrointestinal tract
  - Cytoplasmic vacuoles common
  - Cytoplasm eosinophilic
  - Uniform nuclei
  - CD117 immunolabeling and *KIT* mutations in most cases

PECOMA

Immunohistochemistry

Antibody	Reactivity	Staining Pattern	Comment
HMB-45	Positive	Cytoplasmic	
Mart-1	Positive	Cytoplasmic	
Tyrosinase	Positive	Cytoplasmic	
MITF	Positive	Nuclear	
α1-antichymotrypsin	Positive	Cytoplasmic	
HCAD	Positive	Cytoplasmic	
Calponin	Positive	Cytoplasmic	
CD117	Positive	Cell membrane & cytoplasm	
S100	Negative		
CK-PAN	Negative		
Desmin	Equivocal	Cytoplasmic	Often weak and focal

    - Variable immunolabeling with smooth muscle markers
    - Usually negative for melanocytic markers (some have focal Melan-A)
- Lack adipose tissue component and clear cells
- Vessels inconspicuous

Clear Cell Sarcoma

- Usually involves feet and hands of young adults
- Consists of highly uniform cells with clear cytoplasm and uniform nuclei with single large nucleolus
  - Packeted arrangement with groups of cells separated by slender connective tissue septa
- Most examples express S100 protein
- Soft tissue examples express melanocytic markers
  - Subset of visceral examples express only S100 protein but not melanocytic markers
    - This relates to *EWS-CREB1* fusion in visceral examples (in contrast with *EWS-ATF1* fusion in other cases)
- Lack CD117 expression
- No adipose tissue component of myoid component
- Vessels inconspicuous

Melanoma

- Can be spindled to epithelioid
- Marked cytologic atypia with prominent nucleoli is rule
- Some cases display melanin pigment
- Large lesions highly aggressive clinically
- Label with S100 protein
  - Melanocytic markers expressed in most classic examples, negative in spindled lesions
- Vessels inconspicuous

Intramuscular Hemangioma

- Capillary or cavernous vascular lesion
- Often has abundant overgrowth of mature adipose tissue
- No spindle cell component
- No immunolabeling with melanocytic markers

SELECTED REFERENCES

1. Sukov WR et al: Perivascular epithelioid cell tumor (PEComa) of the urinary bladder: report of 3 cases and review of the literature. Am J Surg Pathol. 33(2):304-8, 2009
2. Hornick JL et al: Sclerosing PEComa: clinicopathologic analysis of a distinctive variant with a predilection for the retroperitoneum. Am J Surg Pathol. 32(4):493-501, 2008
3. Liegl B et al: Primary cutaneous PEComa: distinctive clear cell lesions of skin. Am J Surg Pathol. 32(4):608-14, 2008
4. Martignoni G et al: PEComas: the past, the present and the future. Virchows Arch. 452(2):119-32, 2008
5. Fine SW et al: Angiomyolipoma with epithelial cysts (AMLEC): a distinct cystic variant of angiomyolipoma. Am J Surg Pathol. 30(5):593-9, 2006
6. Folpe AL et al: Perivascular epithelioid cell neoplasms of soft tissue and gynecologic origin: a clinicopathologic study of 26 cases and review of the literature. Am J Surg Pathol. 29(12):1558-75, 2005
7. Harris GC et al: Malignant perivascular epithelioid cell tumour ("PEComa") of soft tissue: a unique case. Am J Surg Pathol. 28(12):1655-8, 2004
8. Vang R et al: Perivascular epithelioid cell tumor ('PEComa') of the uterus: a subset of HMB-45-positive epithelioid mesenchymal neoplasms with an uncertain relationship to pure smooth muscle tumors. Am J Surg Pathol. 26(1):1-13, 2002
9. Folpe AL et al: Clear cell myomelanocytic tumor of the falciform ligament/ligamentum teres: a novel member of the perivascular epithelioid clear cell family of tumors with a predilection for children and young adults. Am J Surg Pathol. 24(9):1239-46, 2000
10. L'Hostis H et al: Renal angiomyolipoma: a clinicopathologic, immunohistochemical, and follow-up study of 46 cases. Am J Surg Pathol. 23(9):1011-20, 1999
11. Tsui WM et al: Hepatic angiomyolipoma: a clinicopathologic study of 30 cases and delineation of unusual morphologic variants. Am J Surg Pathol. 23(1):34-48, 1999
12. Pea M et al: Apparent renal cell carcinomas in tuberous sclerosis are heterogeneous: the identification of malignant epithelioid angiomyolipoma. Am J Surg Pathol. 22(2):180-7, 1998
13. Eble JN et al: Epithelioid angiomyolipoma of the kidney: a report of five cases with a prominent and diagnostically confusing epithelioid smooth muscle component. Am J Surg Pathol. 21(10):1123-30, 1997

PECOMA

Microscopic Features

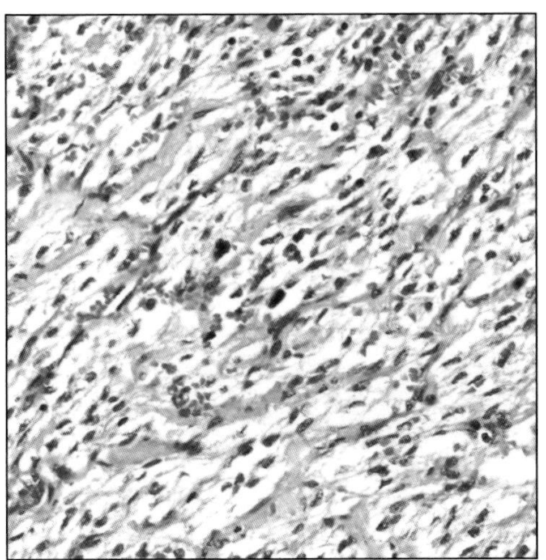

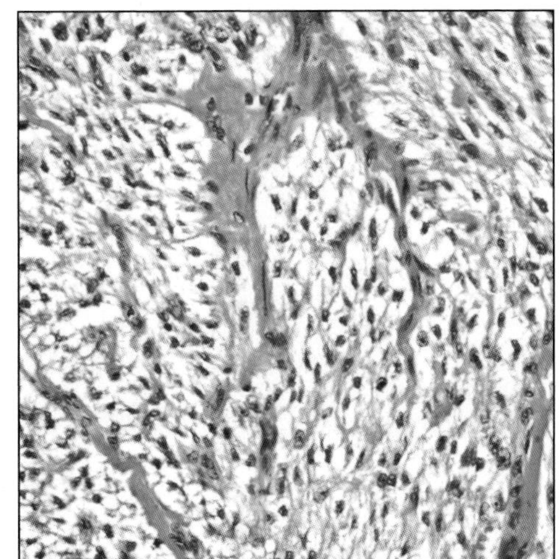

(Left) *Hematoxylin & eosin shows a clear cell pattern in PEComa with numerous fibrovascular channels between spindled to epithelioid clear cells.* ***(Right)*** *Hematoxylin & eosin shows a "packeted" appearance formed by fibrovascular separations between bundles of proliferating cells. This pattern is reminiscent of that of renal cell carcinoma or clear cell sarcoma.*

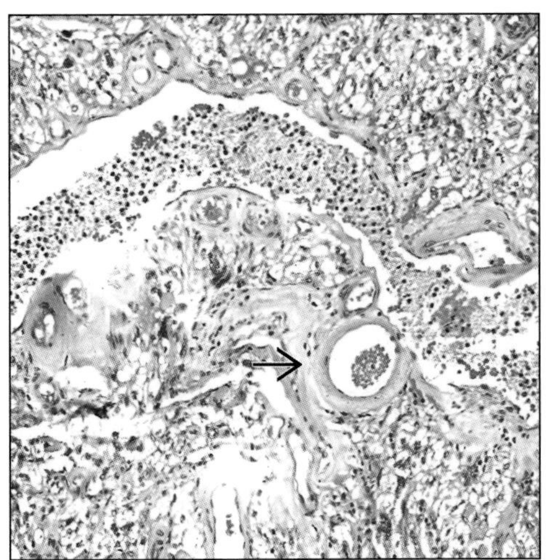

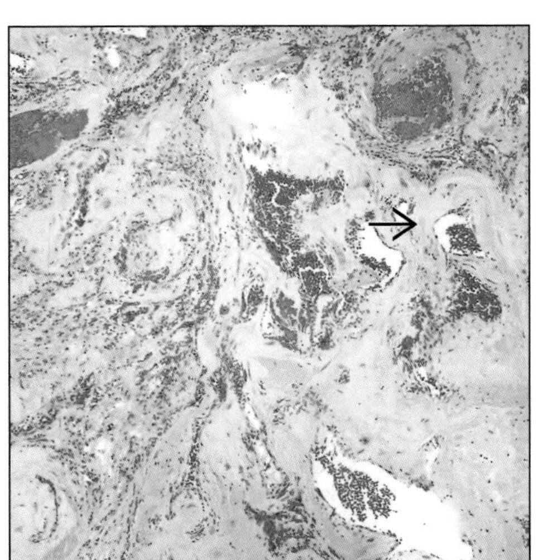

(Left) *Hematoxylin & eosin shows the lesional cells surrounding disorganized, medium-sized vessels ⇒.* ***(Right)*** *Hematoxylin & eosin shows the central portion of a renal PEComa. Large thick vessels ⇒ form the epicenter of the lesion.*

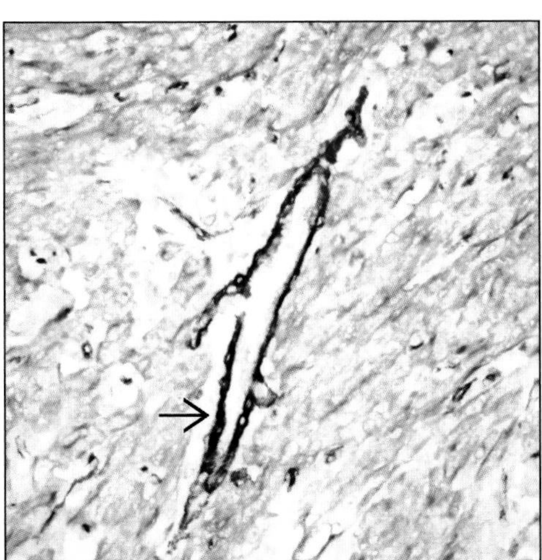

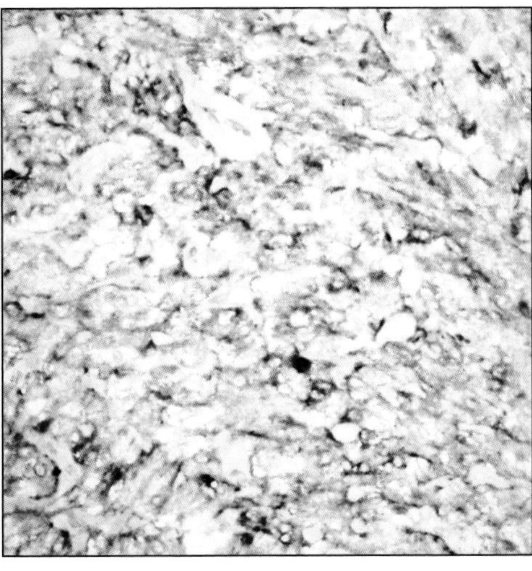

(Left) *Actin-HHF-35 shows cytoplasmic labeling in a PEComa. Note that the internal control (vessel wall ⇒) labels more intensely.* ***(Right)*** *HMB-45 shows cytoplasmic expression in PEComa. These lesions also express other markers of melanocytic differentiation, as well as CD117, but lack S100 protein and keratin expression.*

INTIMAL SARCOMA

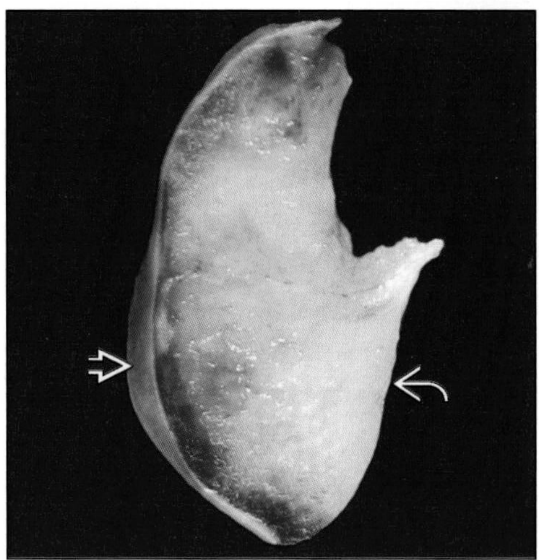

This pulmonary artery sarcoma adheres to the vessel wall ➲ and extends along a large part of its circumference. The bulk of the tumor lies within the arterial lumen ➦.

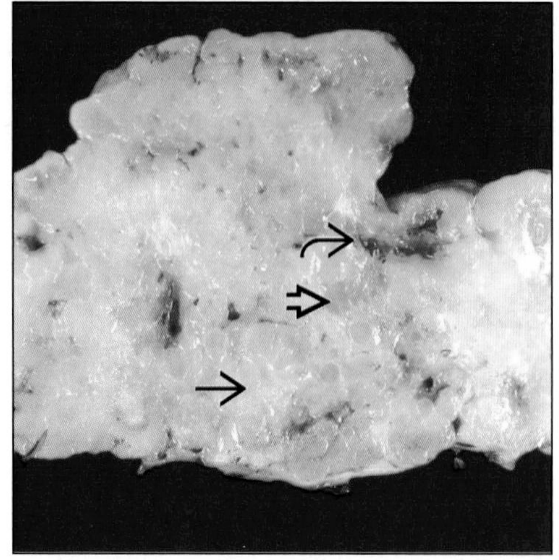

Intimal sarcoma often has a gelatinous appearance ➙ reflecting marked myxoid stromal change within the tumor. Foci of hemorrhage ➦ and necrosis ➲ are also seen.

TERMINOLOGY

Definitions

- Malignant neoplasm arising from intimal aspect of large blood vessels

ETIOLOGY/PATHOGENESIS

Environmental Exposure

- Rare association with Dacron prosthetic graft

CLINICAL ISSUES

Epidemiology

- Incidence
  - Rare
- Age
  - Older adults
- Gender
  - Either sex
    - Pulmonary vessel tumor more common in females

Site

- Pulmonary trunk or pulmonary artery
  - Can extend to pulmonary valve or right ventricle
- Descending thoracic or lower abdominal aorta

Presentation

- Symptoms due to obstruction by mass
- Embolic phenomena in lung, liver, bone
- Many found incidentally at autopsy

Treatment

- Surgical approaches
  - Excision where feasible
- Adjuvant therapy
  - Chemotherapy for inoperable or disseminated diseases

Prognosis

- Poor; 80% of patients diagnosed dead in 1 year

MACROSCOPIC FEATURES

General Features

- Intravascular, polypoid
- Adherent to vessel wall
  - Can extend along intimal aspect
- Myxoid, hemorrhagic, or fibrous areas

MICROSCOPIC PATHOLOGY

Histologic Features

- Variable cellularity
- Pleomorphic spindle, polygonal, and multinucleated cells
- Frequent mitoses
- Focal myxoid stroma is common
- Necrosis often a feature
- Specific differentiation sometimes identifiable focally (especially in pulmonary arterial tumors)
  - Rhabdomyosarcoma
  - Osteosarcoma
  - Angiosarcoma

ANCILLARY TESTS

Molecular Genetics

- Amplification of *MDM2*, *SAS*, and *CDK4* in 1 case

DIFFERENTIAL DIAGNOSIS

Cardiac (Atrial) Myxoma

- Pedunculated lesion mostly in left atrium
- Arises from interatrial septum
- Bland spindle cells

INTIMAL SARCOMA

Key Facts

Terminology
- Malignant neoplasm arising from intimal aspect of large blood vessels

Clinical Issues
- Pulmonary trunk or pulmonary artery
- Descending thoracic or lower abdominal aorta
- Can be found incidentally at autopsy
- Poor prognosis

Macroscopic Features
- Intravascular, polypoid

Microscopic Pathology
- Pleomorphic spindle, polygonal, and multinucleated cells
- Focal myxoid stroma is common
- Necrosis often a feature
- Specific differentiation sometimes identifiable focally (especially in pulmonary arterial tumors)

Immunohistochemistry

Antibody	Reactivity	Staining Pattern	Comment
Actin-sm	Positive	Cytoplasmic	Subplasmalemmal (myofibroblastic), variable
CD31	Positive	Cell membrane	Seen focally in many; widespread positivity indicates angiosarcoma; also stains macrophages
Desmin	Positive	Cytoplasmic	Can be focally positive; also in rhabdomyosarcomatous component
CD34	Positive	Cell membrane	Can be focal; widespread positivity raises possibility of angiosarcoma
CK-PAN	Negative	Cytoplasmic	Any positivity raises possibility of carcinoma
S100	Negative	Not applicable	

- Myxoid stroma

Primary Cardiac Sarcomas
- Similar range of patterns
- Involve myocardium

Leiomyosarcoma
- Fascicular architecture
- Cells have blunt-ended nuclei, eosinophilic cytoplasm
- SMA, desmin, H-caldesmon positive

Metastatic Carcinoma
- Primary site elsewhere
- At least focal CK and EMA positivity
- Other markers expressed, e.g., TTF-1

Metastatic Melanoma
- Primary site elsewhere
- S100 protein(+)
- HMB-45 and Melan-A confirmatory when positive

SELECTED REFERENCES

1. Scheidl S et al: Intimal sarcoma of the pulmonary valve. Ann Thorac Surg. 89(4):e25-7, 2010
2. Timmers L et al: Intimal sarcoma of the pulmonary artery: a report of two cases. Acta Cardiol. 64(5):677-9, 2009
3. Zhang H et al: Cytogenetic and molecular cytogenetic findings of intimal sarcoma. Cancer Genet Cytogenet. 179(2):146-9, 2007
4. Alexander JJ et al: Primary intimal sarcoma of the aorta associated with a dacron graft and resulting in arterial rupture. Vasc Endovascular Surg. 40(6):509-15, 2006
5. Sebenik M et al: Undifferentiated intimal sarcoma of large systemic blood vessels: report of 14 cases with immunohistochemical profile and review of the literature. Am J Surg Pathol. 29(9):1184-93, 2005

IMAGE GALLERY

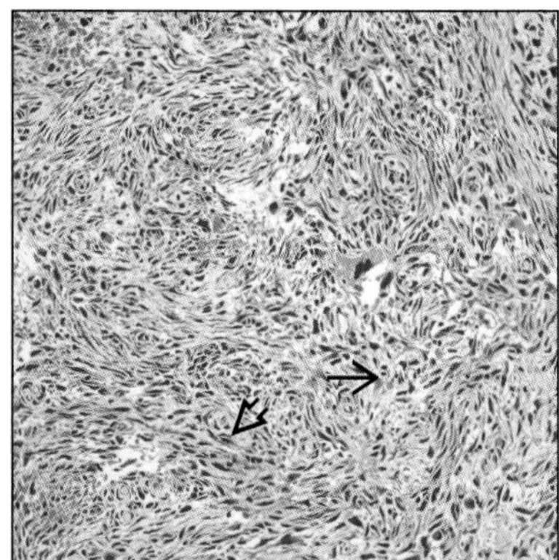

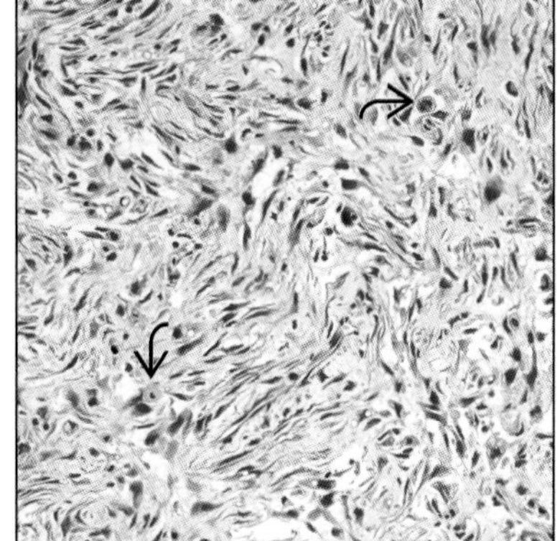

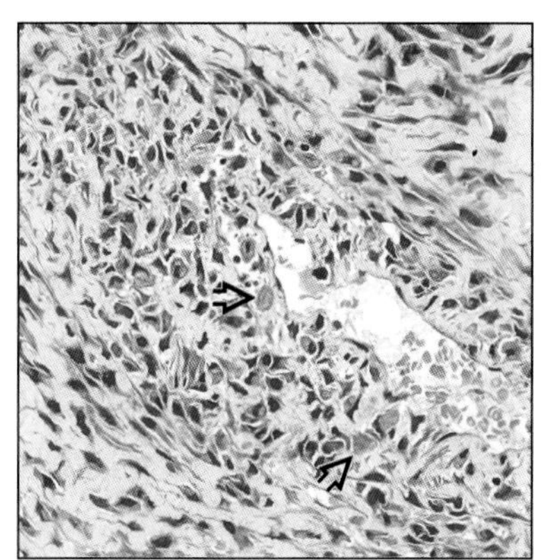

(Left) *This intimal sarcoma has fascicular* ⇨ *and storiform* ⇨ *areas. Note focally marked nuclear pleomorphism.* ***(Center)*** *Focal myxoid change imparts resemblance to myxofibrosarcoma. Abnormal mitoses are seen* ⇨. ***(Right)*** *This field shows plump tumor cells with abundant eosinophilic cytoplasm* ⇨*, resembling rhabdomyoblastic differentiation. However, desmin and myogenin are negative and SMA is positive, indicating myofibroblastic differentiation.*

Other Lesions

Benign

Malignant

Examination of GIST Specimens

AMYLOIDOMA

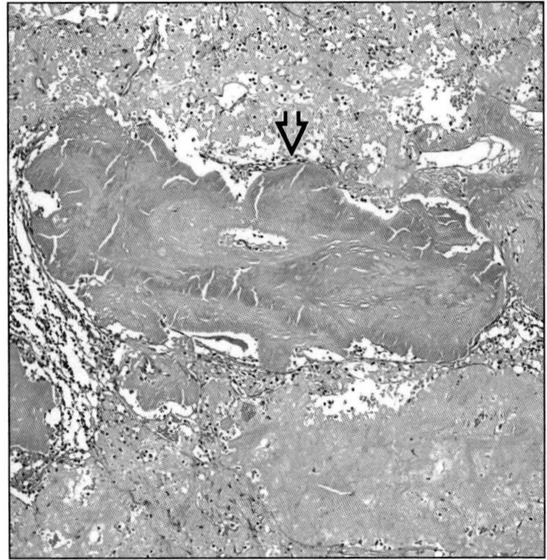

Hematoxylin & eosin shows irregular-shaped amyloid deposits ⇨ with adjacent stroma containing inflammatory cells.

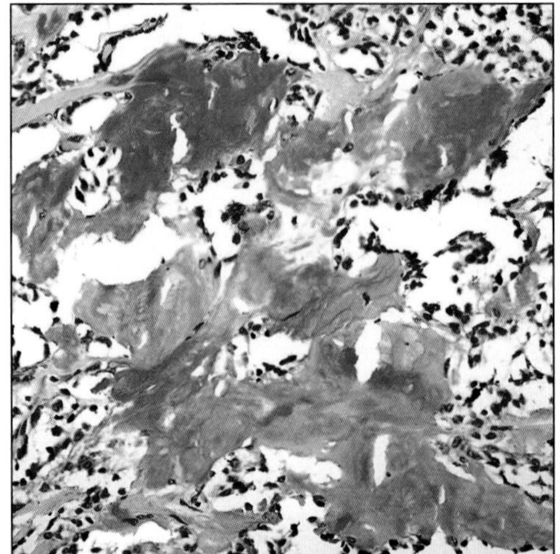

Congo red stain shows the intense red (congophilic) coloration of amyloid. Note the slight variation in staining intensity and the angulated shape and distinct demarcation of the deposits.

TERMINOLOGY

Synonyms

- Tumoral amyloidosis

Definitions

- Solitary localized tumor-like deposit of amyloid in absence of systemic amyloidosis

ETIOLOGY/PATHOGENESIS

Idiopathic

- No associated disease

Immune Dyscrasias

- Myeloma, plasmacytoid lymphoma
- AL (light chain) amyloid
  - Green birefringence resistant to pre-treatment with potassium permanganate

Long-term Hemodialysis

- β2 microglobulin deposition

Chronic Inflammation

- Rheumatoid arthritis
- Osteomyelitis
- Tuberculosis
- AA amyloid (associated with serum amyloid A protein)
  - Green birefringence removed by pre-treatment with permanganate

CLINICAL ISSUES

Epidemiology

- Incidence
  - Rare
  - Extremities, mostly leg
  - Mediastinum, abdomen, viscera
- Age
  - Usually older adults
- Gender
  - Male or female

Presentation

- Painless mass

Treatment

- Surgical approaches
  - Excision

Prognosis

- Benign lesion
- Relates to prognosis of underlying condition

MACROSCOPIC FEATURES

General Features

- Lobulated firm mass
- Pale waxy cut surface

MICROSCOPIC PATHOLOGY

Histologic Features

- Amorphous acellular eosinophilic material
- Vessel walls involved
- Plasma cell and lymphocytic infiltrate
- Multinucleated giant cells
- Metaplastic bone or cartilage
- Microcalcification

ANCILLARY TESTS

Histochemistry

- Congo red
  - Reactivity: Positive
  - Staining pattern
    - Stromal matrix
    - Apple-green areas in polarized light

AMYLOIDOMA

Key Facts

Terminology
- Solitary localized tumor-like deposit of amyloid in absence of systemic amyloidosis

Macroscopic Features
- Pale waxy cut surface

Microscopic Pathology
- Amorphous acellular eosinophilic material
- Adjacent lymphoplasmacytic infiltrate

Ancillary Tests
- Congo red
  - Apple-green areas in polarized light
  - AL amyloid is permanganate resistant

Top Differential Diagnoses
- Elastofibroma
- Amianthoid fibers
- Fibrin deposits
- Tumoral calcinosis

  - In AL amyloid, persists after pre-treatment with permanganate
- PAS-diastase
  - Reactivity: Positive

Electron Microscopy
- Transmission
  - Nonbranching fibrils 70-100 nm in diameter

DIFFERENTIAL DIAGNOSIS

Elastofibroma
- Scapular location
- Elastic stain shows fragmented and globular fibers
- Congo red(-)

Amianthoid Fibers
- Part of a neoplasm
- Stellate shape
- Lighter staining at periphery

Fibrin
- Fibrillary
- Associated red cells and neutrophils
- Trichrome(+)
- Congo red(-)

Tumoral Calcinosis
- Fibroblastic proliferation
- Calcification

SELECTED REFERENCES

1. Pasternak S et al: Soft tissue amyloidoma of the extremities: report of a case and review of the literature. Am J Dermatopathol. 29(2):152-5, 2007
2. Bardin RL et al: Soft tissue amyloidoma of the extremities: a case report and review of the literature. Arch Pathol Lab Med. 128(11):1270-3, 2004
3. Yin H et al: Soft tissue amyloidoma with features of plasmacytoma: a case report and review. Arch Pathol Lab Med. 126(8):969-71, 2002
4. Romagnoli S et al: Amyloid tumour (amyloidoma) of the leg: histology, immunohistochemistry and electron microscopy. Histopathology. 35(2):188-9, 1999
5. Sidoni A et al: Amyloid tumours in the soft tissues of the legs. Case report and review of the literature. Virchows Arch. 432(6):563-6, 1998
6. Yokoo H et al: Primary localized amyloid tumor of the breast with osseous metaplasia. Pathol Int. 48(7):545-8, 1998
7. Pambuccian SE et al: Amyloidoma of bone, a plasma cell/plasmacytoid neoplasm. Report of three cases and review of the literature. Am J Surg Pathol. 21(2):179-86, 1997
8. Tom Y et al: Bilateral beta 2-microglobulin amyloidomas of the buttocks in a long-term hemodialysis patient. Arch Pathol Lab Med. 118(6):651-3, 1994
9. Krishnan J et al: Tumoral presentation of amyloidosis (amyloidomas) in soft tissues. A report of 14 cases. Am J Clin Pathol. 100(2):135-44, 1993
10. Weiss SW: Tumoral amyloidosis of soft tissue (amyloidoma). New approaches to an old problem. Am J Clin Pathol. 100(2):91, 1993

IMAGE GALLERY

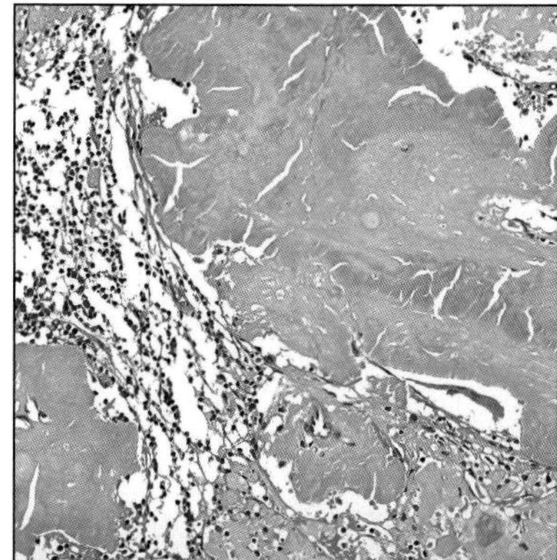

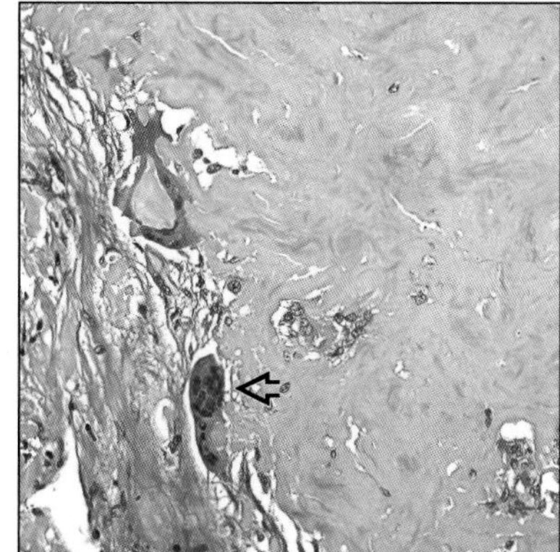

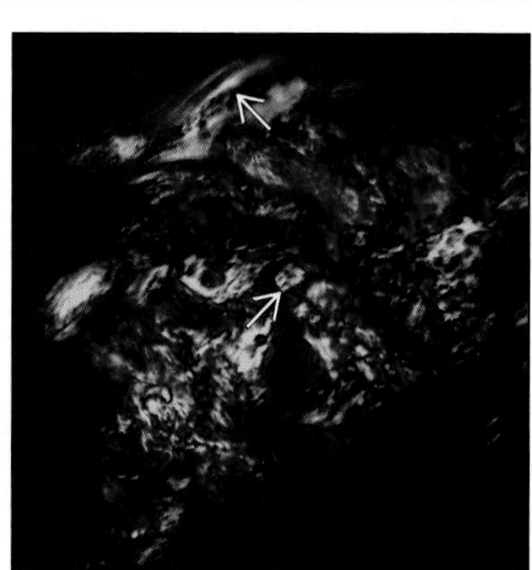

(Left) *Hematoxylin & eosin shows amorphous nature of the amyloid deposit. Note well-defined edge, absence of cells, and artifactual cracking. There is a lymphoplasmacytic infiltrate in the adjacent stroma.* ***(Center)*** *Hematoxylin & eosin shows multinucleated (foreign body-type) giant cell reaction ⇨ at the periphery of the focus of amyloid.* ***(Right)*** *Congo red shows apple-green birefringence ➡ with polarized light. This is typically focal, and other colors that can be seen are nonspecific.*

MYCOBACTERIAL PSEUDOTUMOR

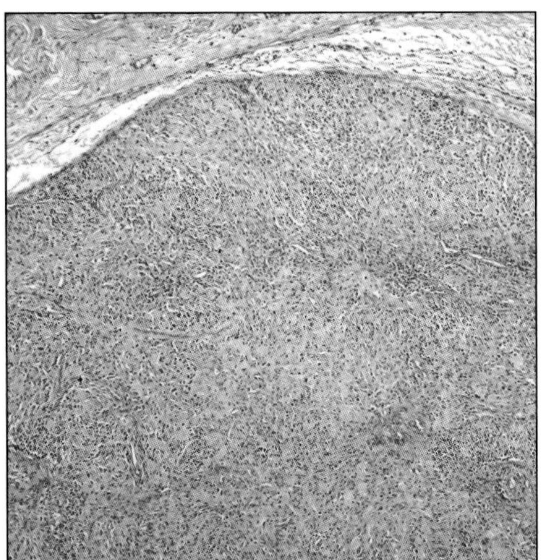

Hematoxylin & eosin at low magnification of a mycobacterial spindle cell tumor shows a loosely lobulated proliferation of epithelioid cells with a background of lymphoplasmacytic cells.

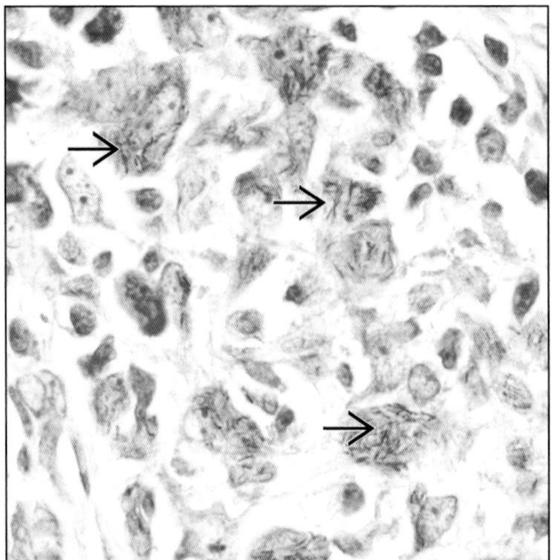

Acid-fast bacteria stain highlights numerous organisms in the proliferating spindled histiocytes ⇒. The diagnosis is easy to make as long as it is considered.

TERMINOLOGY

Definitions

- Exuberant spindle cell lesion, usually involving lymph nodes, induced by mycobacteria

CLINICAL ISSUES

Presentation

- Immunocompromised patients
  - Majority have AIDS
    - Often also have evidence of systemic infection with *Mycobacterium avium complex* organisms
  - Examples reported in individuals with immune comprise from entities other than AIDS
    - e.g., lupus on long-term steroid treatment
  - Seldom encountered in USA recently since many patients are better treated for their HIV disease
    - Reports peaked in early 1990s

Treatment

- Drugs
  - Antimycobacterial drugs

Prognosis

- Good after treatment of infection

MACROSCOPIC FEATURES

General Features

- Firm white lesions
- Size: 2-5 cm
- Multinodular

MICROSCOPIC PATHOLOGY

Histologic Features

- Multinodular appearance at low magnification
- Spindle cells arranged in loose storiform pattern
- Scattered mitoses
- Admixed lymphocytes and plasma cells
  - Occasional neutrophils
  - Occasional multinucleated histiocytes
- Mycobacteria can be seen on PAS and acid-fast stains

Predominant Cell/Compartment Type

- Hematopoietic, histiocytic

ANCILLARY TESTS

Histochemistry

- Aci bacteria
  - Reactivity: Positive
  - Staining pattern
    - Cytoplasmic inclusion
- PAS-diastase
  - Reactivity: Positive
  - Staining pattern
    - Cytoplasmic inclusion

DIFFERENTIAL DIAGNOSIS

Kaposi Sarcoma

- Displays more atypical spindle cells
- Hyaline globules, hemosiderin
- No acid-fast organisms on Ziehl-Neelsen stain
  - However, rare lesions also show mycobacteria
- Immunoreactive for HHV8, CD34, CD31

Fibrous Histiocytoma

- Peripheral collagen trapping (rather than lobulated low-power appearance with well-marginated borders)
- Immunoreactive for CD68, Factor XIII
- PAS(-)
- Acid-fast organisms absent

MYCOBACTERIAL PSEUDOTUMOR

Key Facts

Terminology

- Exuberant spindle cell lesion, usually involving lymph nodes, induced by mycobacteria

Clinical Issues

- Immunocompromised patients
- Majority have AIDS and often also have evidence of systemic infection with *Mycobacterium avium complex* organisms

Microscopic Pathology

- Spindle cells and admixed lymphocytes and plasma cells
- Occasional multinucleated histiocytes
- Delicate mycobacterial forms can be seen on both PAS and acid-fast stains

Immunohistochemistry

Antibody	Reactivity	Staining Pattern	Comment
S100	Positive	Nuclear & cytoplasmic	Sometimes focal
CD68	Positive	Cytoplasmic	
FXIIIA	Negative		
Actin-HHF-35	Negative		Occasional staining can be seen in reactive myofibroblasts
Desmin	Negative		
HHV8	Negative		It is important to exclude Kaposi sarcoma in immunosuppressed population
CD31	Negative		
CD34	Negative		

Palisaded Myofibroblastoma of Lymph Node

- Palisaded or purely spindled rather than storiform
- Lacks inflammatory background
- Spindle cells are actin(+)

DIAGNOSTIC CHECKLIST

Pathologic Interpretation Pearls

- Worth considering in inflammatory spindle cell tumors in immunocompromised persons

SELECTED REFERENCES

1. Shiomi T et al: Mycobacterial spindle cell pseudotumor of the skin. J Cutan Pathol. 34(4):346-51, 2007
2. Logani S et al: Spindle cell tumors associated with mycobacteria in lymph nodes of HIV-positive patients: 'Kaposi sarcoma with mycobacteria' and 'mycobacterial pseudotumor'. Am J Surg Pathol. 23(6):656-61, 1999
3. Morrison A et al: Mycobacterial spindle cell pseudotumor of the brain: a case report and review of the literature. Am J Surg Pathol. 23(10):1294-9, 1999
4. Suster S et al: Mycobacterial spindle-cell pseudotumor of the spleen. Am J Clin Pathol. 101(4):539-42, 1994
5. Chen KT: Mycobacterial spindle cell pseudotumor of lymph nodes. Am J Surg Pathol. 16(3):276-81, 1992
6. Weiss SW et al: Palisaded myofibroblastoma. A benign mesenchymal tumor of lymph node. Am J Surg Pathol. 13(5):341-6, 1989
7. Wood C et al: Pseudotumor resulting from atypical mycobacterial infection: a "histoid" variety of Mycobacterium avium-intracellulare complex infection. Am J Clin Pathol. 83(4):524-7, 1985

IMAGE GALLERY

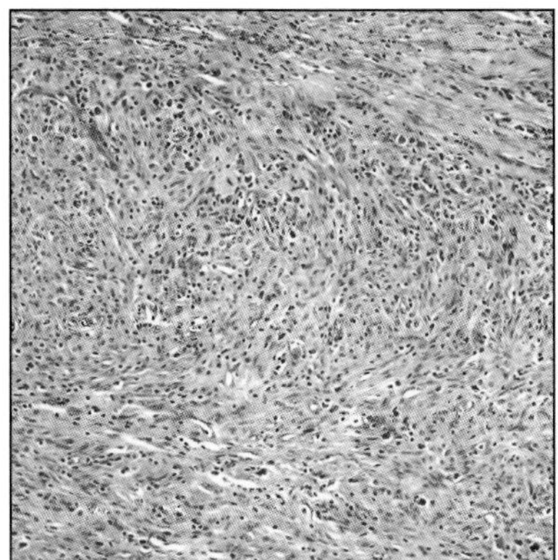

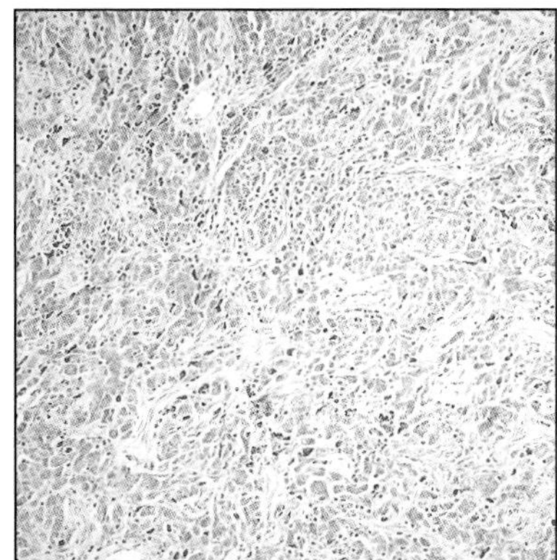

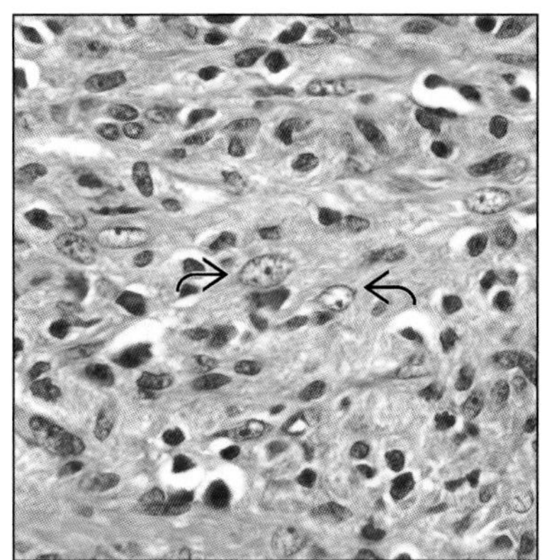

(Left) *At intermediate magnification, the proliferating cells are not particularly hyperchromatic, a feature that should prompt consideration of a reactive rather than neoplastic process.* ***(Center)*** *Acid-fast bacteria stains organisms that are so plentiful that a red hue is imparted even at low magnification.* ***(Right)*** *Note the bland cytologic features of the spindled histiocytes ⮫ in this mycobacterial spindle cell tumor.*

SILICONE REACTION

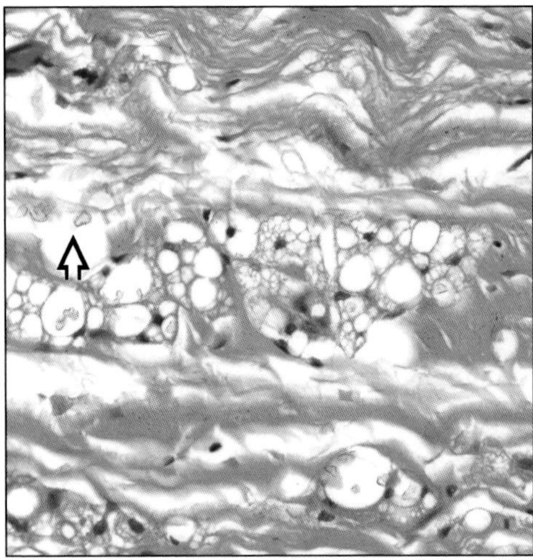

Hematoxylin & eosin shows fibrous reaction around a breast implant. There are clusters of univacuolated or multivacuolated cells, some containing refractile material ⇨.

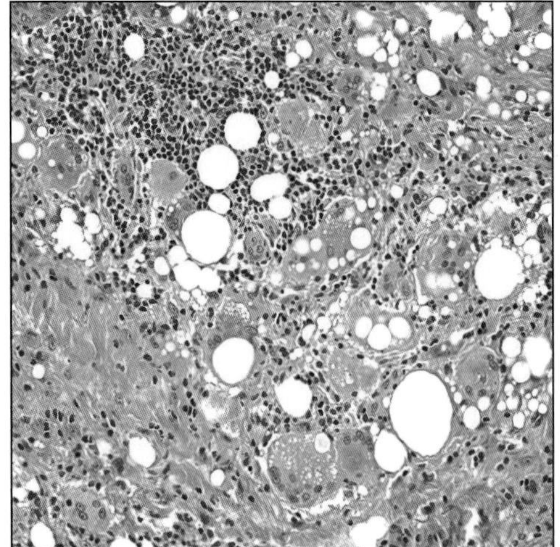

Hematoxylin & eosin shows a multinucleated giant cell and lymphocytic reaction around variable-sized cystic spaces in the fibrous tissue.

TERMINOLOGY

Synonyms

- Silicone granuloma

Definitions

- Tissue reaction to silicone (dimethylpolysiloxane) implant, liquid silicone, or silicone gel

ETIOLOGY/PATHOGENESIS

Iatrogenic

- Leakage from prosthetic implant in breast
  - Spontaneous
  - Following trauma, including compression mammography
- Cosmetic injection
  - Face
    - Nose, lips
  - Earlobes
  - Abdominal wall
  - Genitalia

Arthroplasty

- Temporomandibular joint
- Carpal and metacarpophalangeal joints

CLINICAL ISSUES

Presentation

- Painful or painless mass
  - Usually appears within 12 months of injection
  - Can occur up to several years later
- Silicone can migrate along tissue planes
  - Soft tissue lesion remote from injection site
  - Involvement of regional lymph nodes
    - Reaction in axillary node following breast implant

Treatment

- Surgical approaches
  - Excision of affected area

Prognosis

- Excellent

MICROSCOPIC PATHOLOGY

Histologic Features

- Vacuolated macrophages resembling lipoblasts
  - Usually in subcutis
  - Arranged around "empty" cyst-like spaces of variable size
  - Refractile content
- Foreign body giant cells
- Chronic inflammation
- Fibrosis especially around breast implant
- Calcification around some longstanding implants

Predominant Cell/Compartment Type

- Histiocyte/macrophage

DIFFERENTIAL DIAGNOSIS

Lipoblasts

- Clinical context
  - No history of silicone injection
  - Rare in usual sites of cosmetic enhancement
- Fewer in number
- Larger vacuoles
- More indented nucleus
- Lacks giant cell and inflammatory reaction
- S100 protein(+)
- Can be indistinguishable

Fat Necrosis

- History of trauma
- Macrophages with finely granular cytoplasm

SILICONE REACTION

Key Facts

Terminology

- Tissue reaction to silicone (dimethylpolysiloxane) implant, liquid silicone, or silicone gel

Etiology/Pathogenesis

- Leakage from prosthetic implant in breast
- Cosmetic injection

Clinical Issues

- Silicone can migrate along tissue planes
- Lesion can appear up to several years after injection

Microscopic Pathology

- Vacuolated macrophages resembling lipoblasts
  - Refractile contents
  - Arranged around "empty" cyst-like spaces of variable size
- Foreign body giant cells
- Fibrosis especially around breast implant
- Calcification around some longstanding implants

- Nuclei not indented
- Multinucleated giant cells
- Variable-sized fat spaces

Malakoplakia

- Mostly in urinary tract
- Associated with immunocompromise
- Eosinophilic cytoplasm
- Michaelis-Gutman bodies
  - Laminated, iron containing

Rosai Dorfman Disease

- Sheets of macrophages
- Nuclear atypia
- Emperipolesis
  - Phagocytosis of lymphocytes
- S100 protein(+), CD1a(-)

Liposarcoma

- No nuclear atypia

DIAGNOSTIC CHECKLIST

Clinically Relevant Pathologic Features

- Organ distribution

Pathologic Interpretation Pearls

- History of silicone injection
- Cystic spaces
- Vacuolated macrophages
- Granulomatous inflammation and fibrosis

SELECTED REFERENCES

1. Jung DH et al: Gross and pathologic analysis of long-term silicone implants inserted into the human body for augmentation rhinoplasty: 221 revision cases. Plast Reconstr Surg. 120(7):1997-2003, 2007
2. Jeng CJ et al: Vulvar siliconoma migrating from injected silicone breast augmentation. BJOG. 112(12):1659-60, 2005
3. Ficarra G et al: Silicone granuloma of the facial tissues: a report of seven cases. Oral Surg Oral Med Oral Pathol Oral Radiol Endod. 94(1):65-73, 2002
4. Bigatà X et al: Adverse granulomatous reaction after cosmetic dermal silicone injection. Dermatol Surg. 27(2):198-200, 2001
5. van Diest PJ et al: Pathology of silicone leakage from breast implants. J Clin Pathol. 51(7):493-7, 1998
6. Weiss SW: Lipomatous tumors. Monogr Pathol. 38:207-39, 1996
7. Wassermann RJ et al: Debilitating silicone granuloma of the penis and scrotum. Ann Plast Surg. 35(5):505-9; discussion 509-10, 1995
8. Amemiya T et al: Granuloma after augmentation of the eyelids with liquid silicone: an electron microscopic study. Ophthal Plast Reconstr Surg. 10(1):51-6, 1994
9. Williams CW: Silicone gel granuloma following compressive mammography. Aesthetic Plast Surg. 15(1):49-51, 1991
10. Dolwick MF et al: Silicone-induced foreign body reaction and lymphadenopathy after temporomandibular joint arthroplasty. Oral Surg Oral Med Oral Pathol. 59(5):449-52, 1985

IMAGE GALLERY

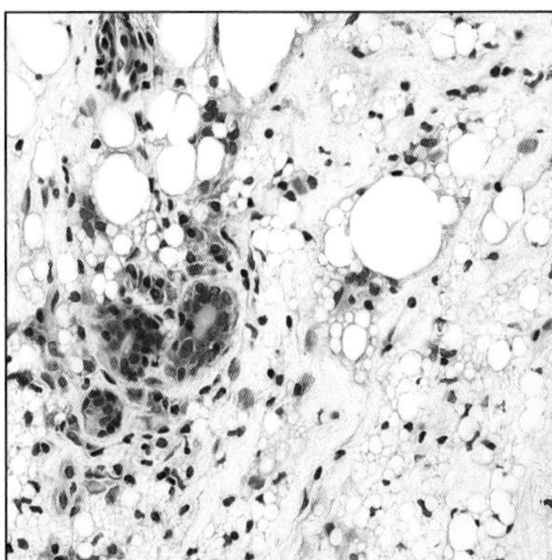
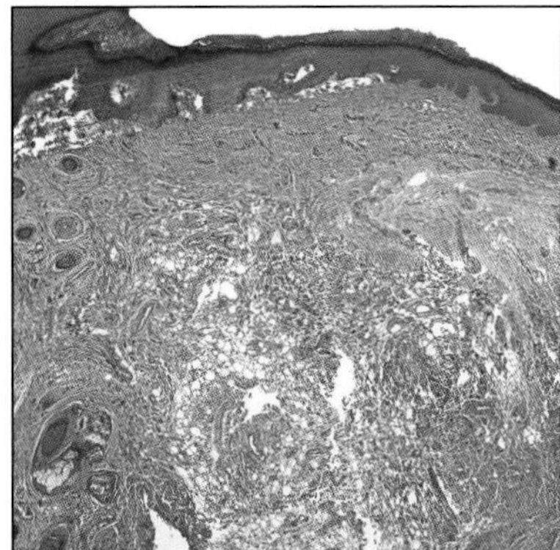
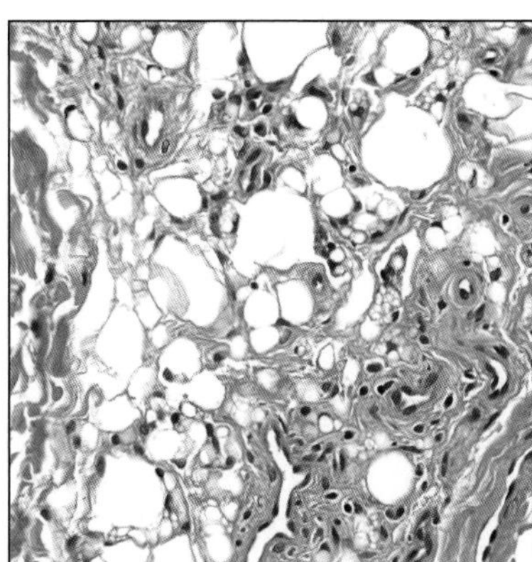

(Left) *Hematoxylin & eosin shows clusters of vacuolated cells of varying size in a myxohyaline stroma with patchy inflammation. This is a reaction in the breast tissue adjacent to an implant.* ***(Center)*** *Hematoxylin & eosin shows ill-defined microcysts in the fibrous tissue in the dermis and subcutis following a silicone injection for cosmetic enhancement.* ***(Right)*** *Hematoxylin & eosin shows variable-sized cystic spaces and univacuolated and multivacuolated cells in the dermis following a silicone injection.*

POLYVINYLPYRROLIDONE STORAGE DISEASE

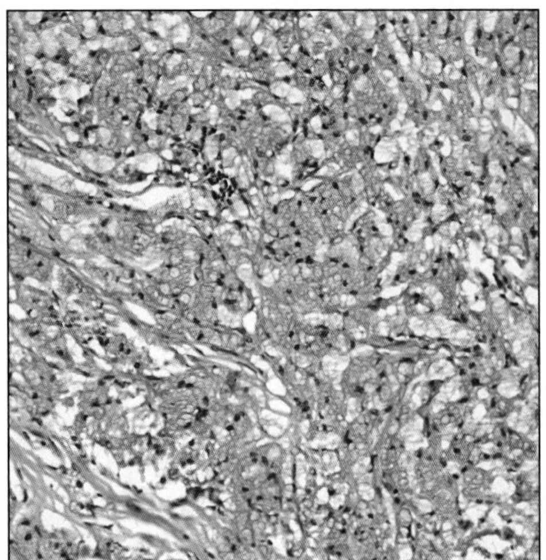

This is a low magnification image of PVP storage disease showing soft tissue infiltrated by sheets and nests of uniform macrophages containing basophilic material in the cytoplasm.

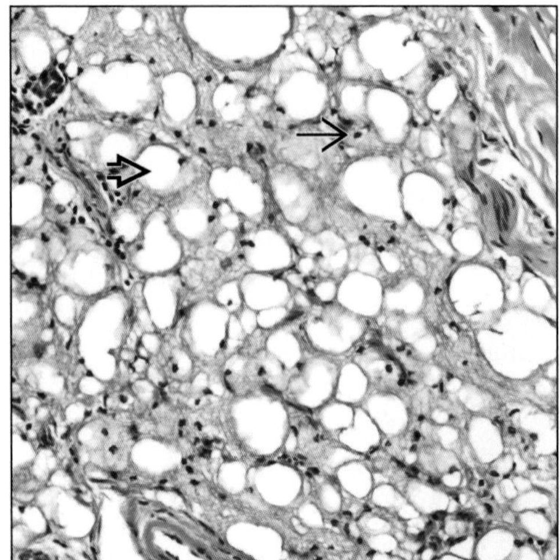

Hematoxylin & eosin shows histiocytic infiltrate with "bubbly" basophilic cytoplasm containing PVP and circular spaces ⇒. The nuclei → are small and lack atypia and mitotic activity

TERMINOLOGY

Abbreviations

- Polyvinylpyrrolidone (PVP) storage disease

Synonyms

- Mucicarminophilic histiocytosis
- Polyvinylpyrrolidone granuloma

Definitions

- Phagocytic foreign body-type reactive condition in which PVP is deposited and retained in tissue

ETIOLOGY/PATHOGENESIS

Causes

- Synthesized during World War II, used intravenously as plasma expander
- PVP found in aerosol hair sprays, adhesives, and lithographic solutions, and cosmetics, including shaving products, plastics, and inks
- Used to improve clarity and stability of wine and fruit juice
- Used as component in oral medications and Betadine

CLINICAL ISSUES

Epidemiology

- Incidence
  - Associated with IV drug use

Site

- Skin, bone marrow, lung

Presentation

- Skin rash
  - Localized reactions may present as induration at injection site
  - Plaques, erythematosus nodules, and purpuric to brown macules
  - Found during work-up for gastrointestinal bleeding in Munchausen syndrome
- Anemia
  - Due to marrow involvement, bony destruction

Treatment

- Prevent additional administration of high molecular weight PVP
- No effective treatment for removal of high molecular weight PVP

Prognosis

- Depending on amount of PVP accumulation, PVP storage disease may be incidental finding
- Can lead to severe irreversible anemia when there is bone marrow involvement
- Pulmonary angiothrombotic granulomatosis involving PVP (crospovidone) may lead to cor pulmonale and death

MICROSCOPIC PATHOLOGY

Histologic Features

- Microscopic
  - Blue-gray bubbly histiocyte with bubbly cytoplasmic contents, no pleomorphism
  - Multinucleated giant cells, foam cells, and granulomas present
  - Blue-gray material in extracellular pools as well as within histiocyte cytoplasm
- Histochemistry
  - Mucicarmine red, Congo red, Sirius red and colloidal iron positive
  - PAS, Alcian blue, and Giemsa negative
- Immunohistochemistry
  - Keratin(-), S100(-), and CD1a(-)
  - CD68(+), CD163(+)

POLYVINYLPYRROLIDONE STORAGE DISEASE

Key Facts

Etiology/Pathogenesis

- PVP storage disease is phagocytic foreign body-type reactive condition
- Found in aerosol hair sprays, adhesives, lithographic solutions, shaving products, plastics
- Used to improve clarity and stability of wine and fruit juice; used in oral medications and Betadine
- Presents as skin rash with nodules and macules, untreatable anemia due to bone marrow involvement

Microscopic Pathology

- Histiocytes with blue-gray, bubbly cytoplasm, in small groups or large sheets
- No nuclear atypia or mitotic activity
- Giant cells may be present
- PAS, Alcian blue, and Giemsa negative
- Mucicarmine, Congo red, Sirius red, and colloidal iron positive
- CD68(+), CD163(+)

Predominant Pattern/Injury Type

- Inflammatory

Predominant Cell/Compartment Type

- Mesenchymal, fibrohistiocytic

DIFFERENTIAL DIAGNOSIS

Signet Ring Cell Adenocarcinoma

- Signet ring cells look like PVP-containing histiocytes
- Positive for mucicarmine and cytokeratin
- Negative for PAS

Myxofibrosarcoma

- Presence of mitotic activity, cytologic activity, and prominent vasculature
- Positive for Alcian blue

Sea Blue Histiocytosis

- Histiocytic proliferation
- Primary or secondary in hematologic/systemic disorders
- Blue with Giemsa; PAS(+)

DIAGNOSTIC CHECKLIST

Clinically Relevant Pathologic Features

- May present as subcutaneous masses
- Material may be present at injection site
- Tissue distribution
  - Skin, bone marrow
  - Can be extensive

Pathologic Interpretation Pearls

- Histiocytes with blue-gray, bubbly cytoplasm, in small groups or large sheets, giant cells
- Nuclear pleomorphism, mitoses, necrosis are absent
- Cytokeratins(-), CD68(+)

SELECTED REFERENCES

1. Ganesan S et al: Embolized crospovidone (poly[N-vinyl-2-pyrrolidone]) in the lungs of intravenous drug users. Mod Pathol. 16(4):286-92, 2003
2. Groisman GM et al: Mucicarminophilic histiocytosis (benign signet-ring cells) and hyperplastic mesothelial cells: two mimics of metastatic carcinoma within a single lymph node. Arch Pathol Lab Med. 122(3):282-4, 1998
3. Kuo TT et al: Cutaneous involvement in polyvinylpyrrolidone storage disease: a clinicopathologic study of five patients, including two patients with severe anemia. Am J Surg Pathol. 21(11):1361-7, 1997
4. Hizawa K et al: Subcutaneous pseudosarcomatous polyvinylpyrrolidone granuloma. Am J Surg Pathol. 8(5):393-8, 1984
5. Kuo TT et al: Mucicarminophilic histiocytosis. A polyvinylpyrrolidone (PVP) storage disease simulating signet-ring cell carcinoma. Am J Surg Pathol. 8(6):419-28, 1984
6. Bubis JJ et al: Storage of polyvinylpyrrolidone mimicking a congenital mucolipid storage disease in a patient with Munchausen's syndrome. Isr J Med Sci. 11(10):999-1004, 1975

IMAGE GALLERY

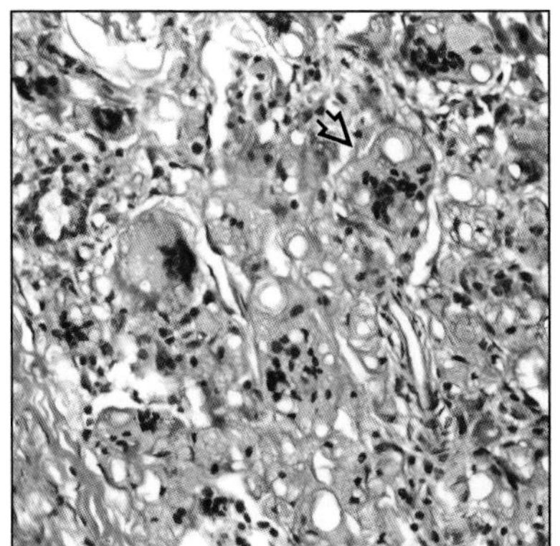

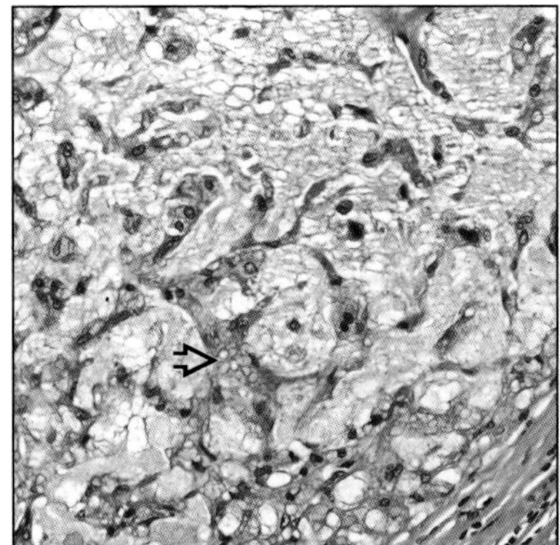

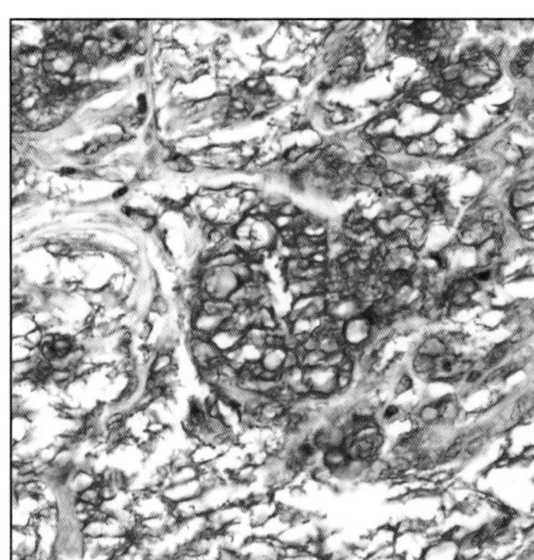

(Left) *Hematoxylin & eosin shows multinucleated histiocytes with abundant cytoplasm ⇨.* ***(Center)*** *Hematoxylin & eosin shows basophilic bubbly material (PVP), largely extracellular but also within histiocytes ⇨, here mimicking myxofibrosarcoma or extraskeletal myxoid chondrosarcoma.* ***(Right)*** *Mucicarmine shows positivity in PVP. The term "mucicarminophilic histiocytosis" has been applied to this condition, which can resemble adenocarcinoma but lacks epithelial markers.*

CRYSTAL-STORING HISTIOCYTOSIS

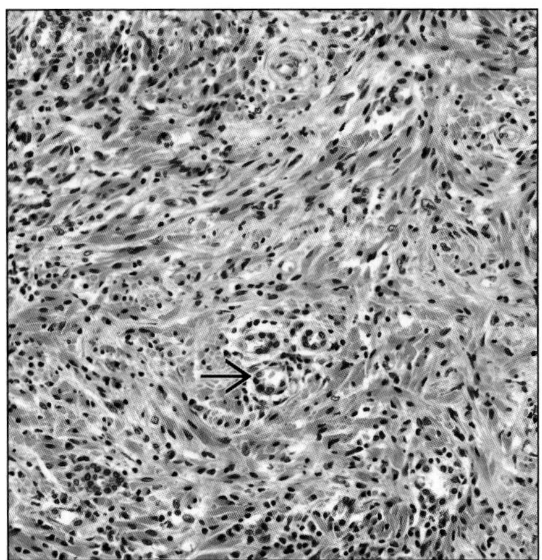

Crystal-storing histiocytosis involving the lung of a patient with myeloma displays sheets of polygonal or spindled histiocytes that infiltrate inflamed loosely fibrous stroma, separating lung structures ⇒.

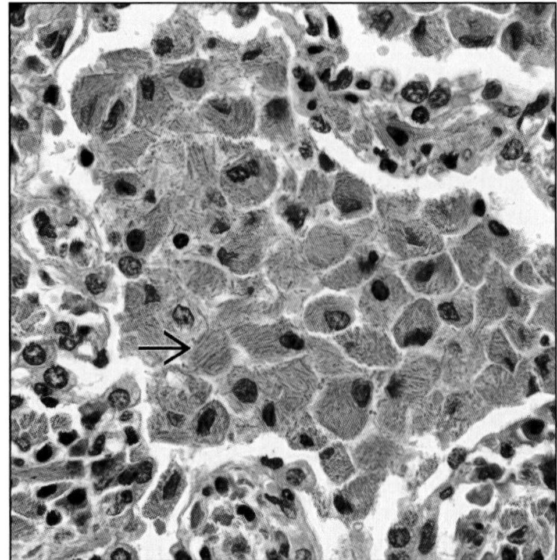

Higher magnification shows aggregate of large polygonal histiocytes. The eosinophilic cytoplasm is distended by sheaves of crystalline structures ⇒.

TERMINOLOGY

Abbreviations

- Crystal-storing histiocytosis (CSH)

Definitions

- Soft tissue aggregate of macrophages containing crystalline material

ETIOLOGY/PATHOGENESIS

Paraneoplastic Phenomenon

- In B-cell lymphoreticular neoplasia
  - Lymphoplasmacytoid lymphoma
  - Chronic lymphocytic leukemia
  - Extranodal marginal zone lymphoma
  - MALT lymphoma
  - Plasma cell dyscrasias
    - Monoclonal gammopathy
    - Myeloma
- Mastocytosis

Inflammatory Disease

- Eosinophilic colitis

Iatrogenic

- Treatment of lepromatous leprosy with clofazimine

Pathogenesis

- Crystals are formed
  - Immunoglobulins
  - Charcot-Leyden crystals
    - Derived from cytoplasmic granules of eosinophils
  - Clofazimine
- Crystals are phagocytosed by macrophages
- Macrophages aggregate to form ill-defined mass
  - Infiltrate adjacent tissues

CLINICAL ISSUES

Epidemiology

- Incidence
  - Very rare
- Age
  - Older age groups
- Gender
  - Male or female

Site

- Soft tissue
- Viscera
  - Heart, lung, kidney
- Can be generalized

Presentation

- Incidental finding

Prognosis

- Related to prognosis of underlying disease

MICROSCOPIC PATHOLOGY

Histologic Features

- Sheets of rounded or epithelioid histiocytes
- Can be spindled or angulated
- Occasionally multinucleated
- Eosinophilic cytoplasm
  - Clusters of elongated crystals
- Adjacent mild fibrosis
- Chronic inflammation
- Associated lymphoid neoplasm

Predominant Pattern/Injury Type

- Inflammatory, chronic

Predominant Cell/Compartment Type

- Hematopoietic, histiocytic

CRYSTAL-STORING HISTIOCYTOSIS

Key Facts

Terminology
- Soft tissue aggregate of macrophages containing crystalline material

Etiology/Pathogenesis
- In low-grade B-cell lymphomas
- Monoclonal gammopathy
- Myeloma
- Eosinophilic colitis
- Treatment of lepromatous leprosy with clofazimine

Clinical Issues
- Site: Soft tissue, viscera
- Can be generalized

Microscopic Pathology
- Sheets of rounded or epithelioid histiocytes
- Can be spindled or angulated
- Eosinophilic cytoplasm
- Clusters of elongated crystals
- Lesional cells are CD68(+)

ANCILLARY TESTS

Immunohistochemistry
- Lesional cells are CD68(+)

Electron Microscopy
- Transmission
  - Immunoglobulin crystals
    - Elongated, polygonal or trapezoidal
    - Variable width
    - Periodicity of 450-600 nm
  - Charcot-Leyden crystals
    - Up to 50 microns in length
    - Paired hexagonal pyramids
  - Clofazimine crystals
    - Dissolve in processing, crystal-shaped spaces

DIFFERENTIAL DIAGNOSIS

Rhabdomyoma
- Well-defined tumor mass
- Cytoplasm is granular
- Immunoreactive for desmin and myogenin

Mycobacterial Pseudotumor
- Associated with immunocompromise
- Abundant acid-fast bacilli

Granular Cell Histiocytosis
- Site of previous surgery
- Granular cytoplasm
- Absence of crystals

Polyvinylpyrrolidone Granuloma
- Bubbly blue-gray cytoplasm
- Foreign body giant cells
- Congo red(+)

Malakoplakia
- Urinary tract
- Associated with chronic infection
- Michaelis-Gutmann bodies
  - Demonstrable by von Kossa stain

SELECTED REFERENCES

1. Wang CW et al: Histiocytic lesions and proliferations in the lung. Semin Diagn Pathol. 24(3):162-82, 2007
2. Pais AV et al: Intra-abdominal, crystal-storing histiocytosis due to clofazimine in a patient with lepromatous leprosy and concurrent carcinoma of the colon. Lepr Rev. 75(2):171-6, 2004
3. Sukpanichnant S et al: Clofazimine-induced crystal-storing histiocytosis producing chronic abdominal pain in a leprosy patient. Am J Surg Pathol. 24(1):129-35, 2000
4. Jones D et al: Crystal-storing histiocytosis: a disorder occurring in plasmacytic tumors expressing immunoglobulin kappa light chain. Hum Pathol. 30(12):1441-8, 1999
5. Llobet M et al: Massive crystal-storing histiocytosis associated with low-grade malignant B-cell lymphoma of MALT-type of the parotid gland. Diagn Cytopathol. 17(2):148-52, 1997

IMAGE GALLERY

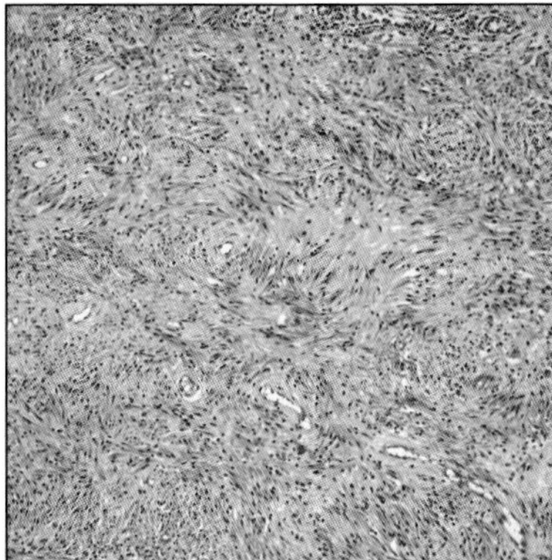

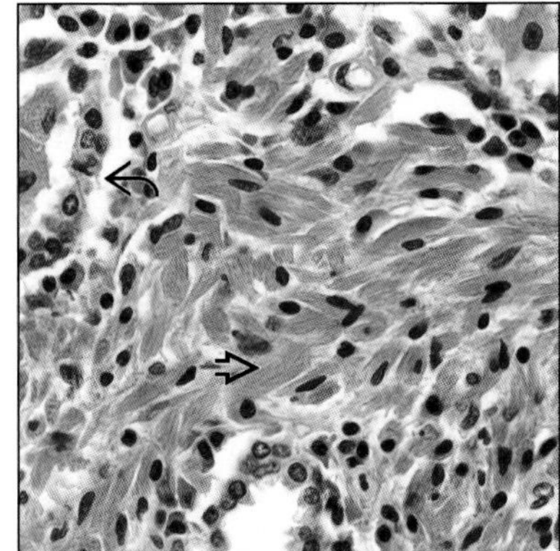

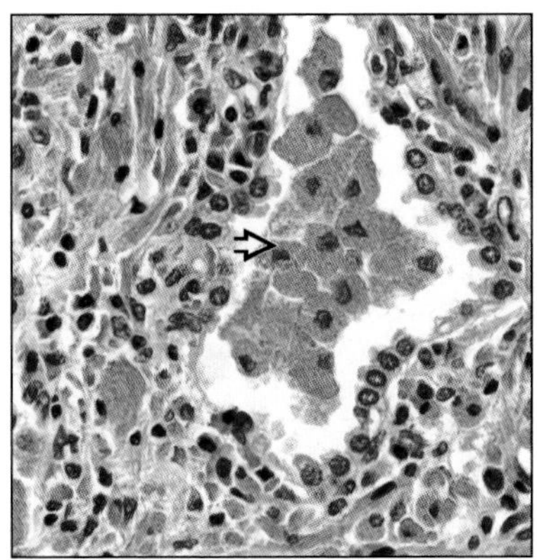

(Left) *Predominantly spindle-shaped lesional macrophages are dispersed in a loosely collagenous stroma with a mild chronic inflammatory infiltrate.* ***(Center)*** *In this lung lesion, the histiocytic cells infiltrate between bronchioles ⇗. The cells are elongated or spindle-shaped, with eosinophilic cytoplasm in which slender needle-like crystals can be discerned ⇒.* ***(Right)*** *A bronchiole with a cluster of large polygonal lesional cells in the lumen ⇒ is shown.*

GRANULAR HISTIOCYTIC REACTON

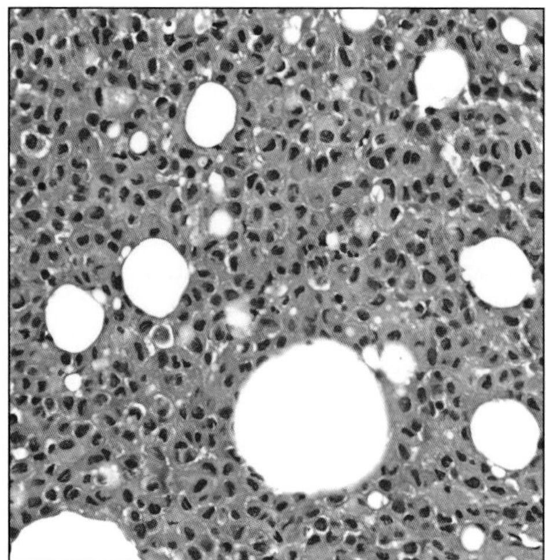

Hematoxylin & eosin shows sheets of granular histiocytes in a woman who had previously undergone abdominal surgery.

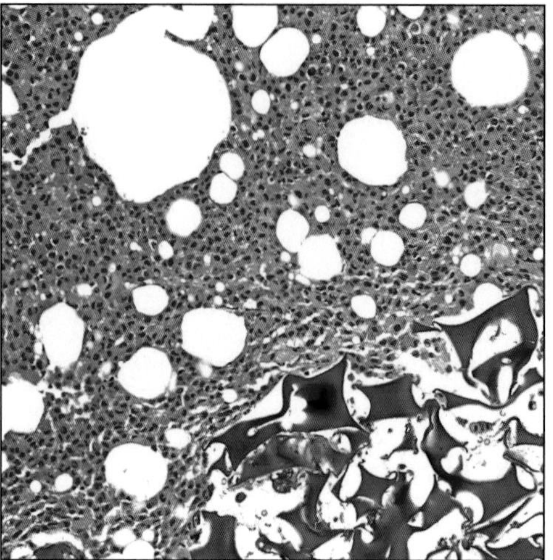

Hematoxylin & eosin shows sheets of granular histiocytes around iatrogenic hemostasis material from a previous surgery.

TERMINOLOGY

Abbreviations

- Granular histiocytic reaction (GHR)

Synonyms

- Reactive granular cells
- Postsurgical granular reactions

Definitions

- Post-surgery collections of histiocytes with granular cytoplasm
  - Collect at site of surgical trauma

CLINICAL ISSUES

Epidemiology

- Incidence
  - Rare
- Age
  - Usually adults
- Gender
  - F > M

Site

- Usually abdomen
  - Has occurred in thyroid and other locations

Presentation

- Deep mass

Natural History

- Incidental finding
- No progression of disease

Prognosis

- Histiocytes are reactive; disease is self-limited

MACROSCOPIC FEATURES

General Features

- May observe scar from original surgery

MICROSCOPIC PATHOLOGY

Histologic Features

- Microscopic
  - Fringe of histiocytes around core of granular/ amorphous material
  - Histiocytes with granular, eosinophilic cytoplasm

Predominant Pattern/Injury Type

- Inflammatory

Predominant Cell/Compartment Type

- Mesenchymal, fibrohistiocytic

ANCILLARY TESTS

Histochemistry

- Acid fast with Ziehl-Neelsen stain
- Autofluorescent

DIFFERENTIAL DIAGNOSIS

Rosai-Dorfman Disease

- Large polygonal histiocytes with emperipolesis
- Marked lymphoplasmacytic response
- Reactivity for S100

Langerhans Cell Histiocytosis

- Unusual in soft tissue
- Reniform, embryo-like histiocytes
- Scattered eosinophils
- CD1a(+) and S100(+)

GRANULAR HISTIOCYTIC REACTON

Key Facts

Terminology
- Post-surgery collections of histiocytes with granular cytoplasm collecting at site of surgical trauma

Microscopic Pathology
- Histiocytes with granular, eosinophilic cytoplasm
- Fringe of histiocytes around core of granular/ amorphous material
- Autofluorescent
- Acid fast with Ziehl-Neelsen stain

Top Differential Diagnoses
- Granular cell tumor
- Rosai-Dorfman disease
- Langerhans cell histiocytosis

Diagnostic Checklist
- CD163(+), CD68(+)
- Negative for S100 and other markers
- Sheets of granular histiocytes without atypia or mitotic activity

Granular Cell Tumor
- S100(+)
- Cytoplasmic globules with surrounding halos
- CD68(+) in globules
- Lysosomes by EM

Ankle-type Fibrous Histiocytoma
- Predominantly histiocytoid cells
- Embedded in fibrous tissue
- Mass-like process

Granular Smooth Muscle Tumors
- Spindled
- Interlacing fascicles
- Actin-sm(+) and desmin(+)

Granular Melanoma
- Atypical with prominent nucleoli
- Mitotic activity
- S100(+) and HMB-45(+)

Plasmacytoma with Granular Features
- Sheets of dysplastic monoclonal plasma cells
- May have sequelae of multiple myeloma
- Stain for κ light chain or λ light chain and CD138, CD38

DIAGNOSTIC CHECKLIST

Clinically Relevant Pathologic Features
- Cytoplasmic features
- Nuclear features
- Tissue distribution
- Mostly found in abdomen
  - Women
    - After surgery
- Sheets of histiocytes with granular cytoplasm
- Tissue distribution at site of previous surgery
- Usually found incidentally in re-excision surgical specimen

Pathologic Interpretation Pearls
- Sheets of granular histiocytes without atypia or mitotic activity
- Often granular amorphous material present
- Not diagnostic of other histiocytic or granular entities
- CD163(+), CD68(+)
- Negative for S100
- Negative for CK-PAN
- Negative for desmin

SELECTED REFERENCES

1. Dudorkinová D et al: [Histiocytic reaction in the lymph nodes after total hip joint endoprosthesis surgery] Cesk Patol. 33(2):53-6, 1997
2. Hicks DG et al: Granular histiocytosis of pelvic lymph nodes following total hip arthroplasty. The presence of wear debris, cytokine production, and immunologically activated macrophages. J Bone Joint Surg Am. 78(4):482-96, 1996

IMAGE GALLERY

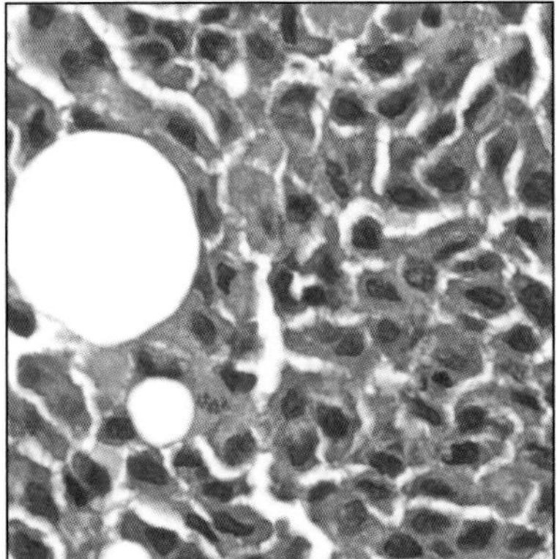

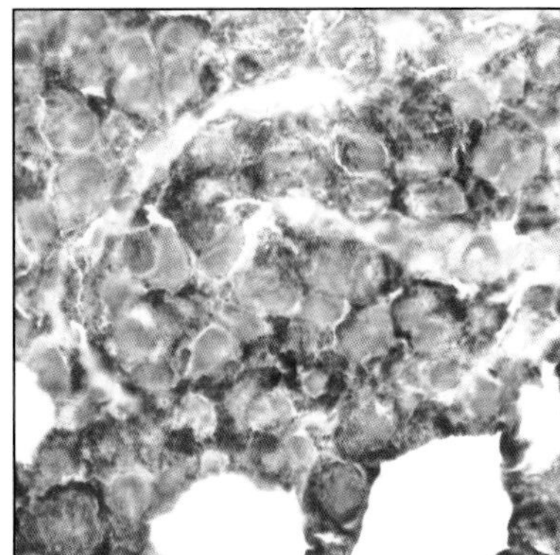

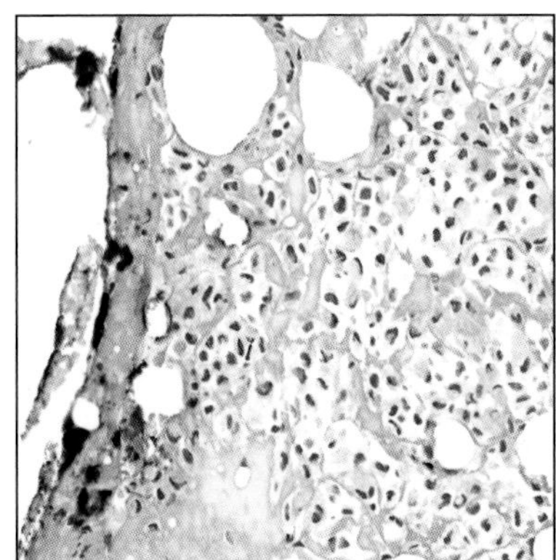

(Left) *Hematoxylin & eosin shows higher magnification of sheets of granular histiocytes with eccentric cytoplasm and bland nuclei.* ***(Center)*** *CD163 shows positive histiocytes in granular histiocytic reaction.* ***(Right)*** *CK-PAN shows keratin(-) granular histiocytic reaction. Staining is present in preexisting normal mesothelial lining.*

TUMORAL CALCINOSIS

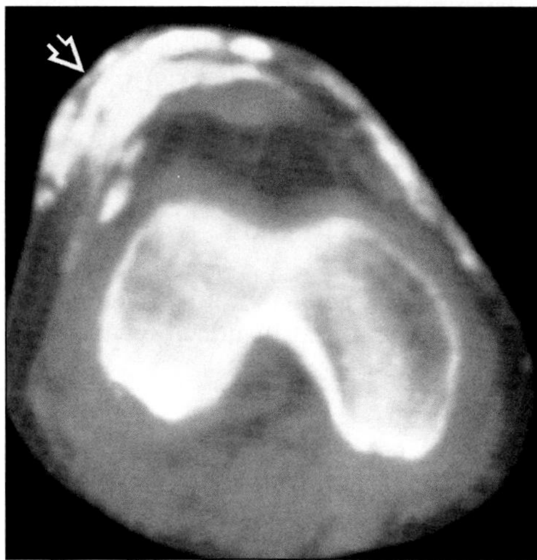

CT scan of knee in a patient with tumoral calcinosis shows amorphous, dense subcutaneous extraarticular calcification ➨. The differential diagnosis includes renal osteodystrophy and collagen vascular disease.

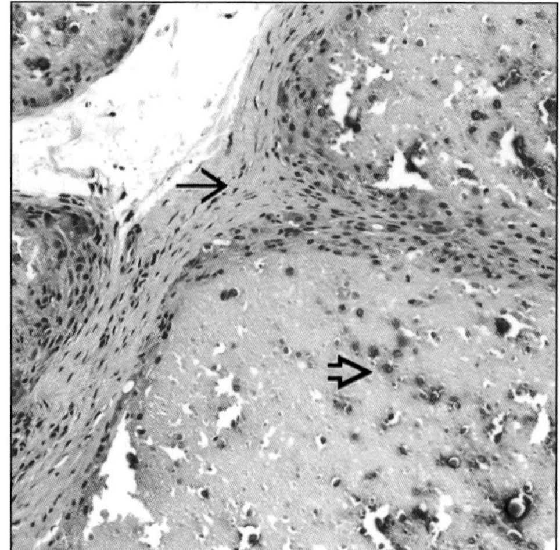

Multilocular cystic lesion of tumoral calcinosis demonstrates cysts separated by fibrous septa →. The cysts contain basophilic amorphous material with small foci of granular calcification ➨.

TERMINOLOGY

Synonyms

- Lipid calcinosis
- Calcifying collagenolysis
- Tumoral lipocalcinosis

Definitions

- Extraskeletal soft tissue calcification with granulomatous response

ETIOLOGY/PATHOGENESIS

Etiology Theories

- Inborn error of phosphorus metabolism

Associated Conditions

- Hyperphosphatemia

Genetics

- Most cases sporadic
- Some familial
  - Autosomal recessive
  - Mutations in *GALNT3*, *FGF23*, or *KL* genes
    - Some hyperphosphatemic
  - Normophosphatemic patients show mutations in *SAMD9* gene

CLINICAL ISSUES

Epidemiology

- Age
  - Most cases < 20 years
  - Rarely > 50 years
- Gender
  - M = F
- Ethnicity
  - More common in black Africans

Site

- In subcutis around large joints
  - Hip, buttock, thigh
  - Shoulder
- Occasionally spine, smaller joints, skin
- Often multiple
  - Can be bilateral or symmetrical
- Subset of similar lesions in distal extremities
  - Digits, ankle, foot, wrist
  - Some associated with scleroderma
  - Normophosphatemic

Presentation

- Painless subcutaneous mass
  - Attached to deep fascia and tendons
  - Unrelated to bone
  - Rarely ulcerates
- Slowly growing

Laboratory Tests

- Serum calcium and alkaline phosphatase normal
- Mild hyperphosphatemia
- Elevated serum 1, 25-dihydroxy-vitamin D

Prognosis

- Benign
- Slow expansion
- Can recur/regrow if incompletely excised

IMAGE FINDINGS

MR Findings

- Fluid level
- Peripheral rim of higher signal intensity on T2, enhances with contrast

CT Findings

- Area of dense periarticular calcification
- Radiolucent septations
- No bony abnormalities

TUMORAL CALCINOSIS

Key Facts

Terminology
- Extraskeletal soft tissue calcification with granulomatous response

Clinical Issues
- Most cases < 20 years
- Some familial
- In subcutis around large joints

Macroscopic Features
- Poorly defined, infiltrative, multilocular cyst

Microscopic Pathology
- Amorphous granular material (hydroxyapatite crystals)
- Surrounding histiocytes with granulation tissue in early stage
- Later irregular calcification, calcospherites

MACROSCOPIC FEATURES

General Features
- Poorly defined, infiltrative, multilocular cyst
- Cyst content white-yellow fluid or semisolid

Size
- Up to 30 cm, can be small, incidental finding

MICROSCOPIC PATHOLOGY

Histologic Features
- Amorphous granular material (hydroxyapatite crystals)
- Surrounding histiocytes with granulation tissue in early stage
  - Multinucleated giant cells, fibroblasts
- Dense fibrous tissue in cyst wall
- Later irregular calcification, calcospherites

DIFFERENTIAL DIAGNOSIS

Secondary Hyperparathyroidism, Chronic Renal Disease
- Older patients
- Associated disease, abnormal serum chemistry
- Deposits in viscera, blood vessels

Milk Alkali Syndrome
- Clinical history, hypercalcemia

Calcified Soft Tissue Chondroma
- Extremity lesion, usually digits
- Component of hyaline cartilage

Gout
- Birefringent needle-like crystals

DIAGNOSTIC CHECKLIST

Clinically Relevant Pathologic Features
- Exclude other causes of soft tissue calcification

Pathologic Interpretation Pearls
- No neoplastic cells in lesion

SELECTED REFERENCES

1. Chaabane S et al: Idiopathic tumoral calcinosis. Acta Orthop Belg. 74(6):837-45, 2008
2. Ozcelik C et al: Tumoral calcinosis of the hand. Orthopedics. 31(11):1145, 2008
3. Laskin WB et al: Calcareous lesions of the distal extremities resembling tumoral calcinosis (tumoral calcinosislike lesions): clinicopathologic study of 43 cases emphasizing a pathogenesis-based approach to classification. Am J Surg Pathol. 31(1):15-25, 2007
4. Specktor P et al: Hyperphosphatemic familial tumoral calcinosis caused by a mutation in GALNT3 in a European kindred. J Hum Genet. 51(5):487-90, 2006
5. Möckel G et al: Tumoral calcinosis revisited: pathophysiology and treatment. Rheumatol Int. 25(1):55-9, 2005

IMAGE GALLERY

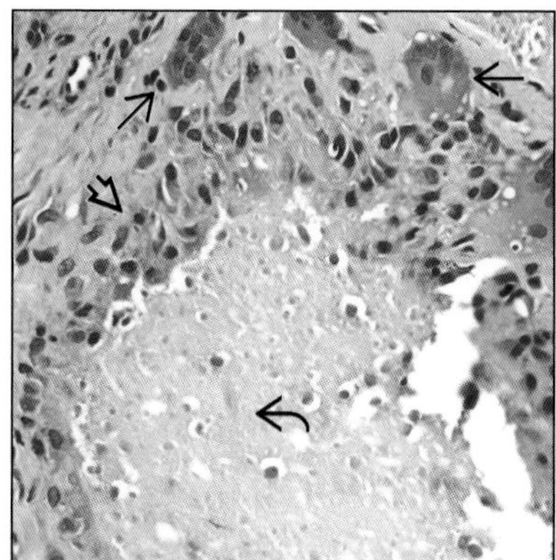

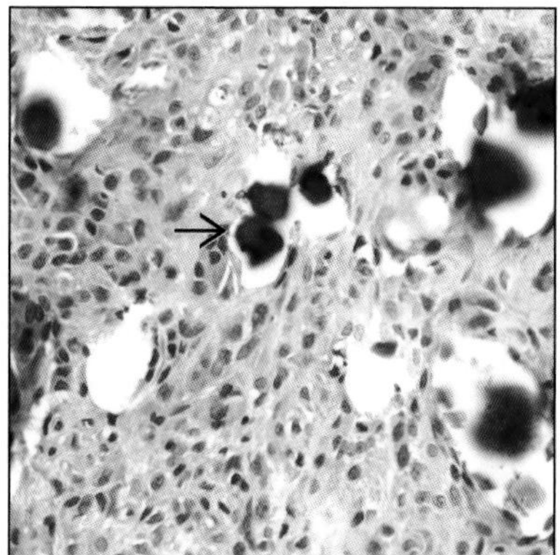

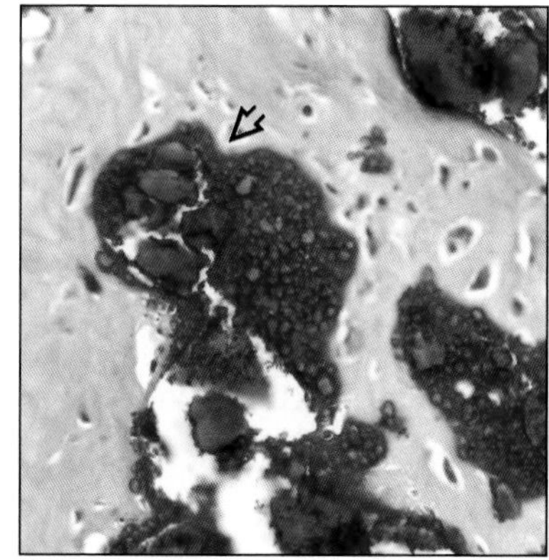

(Left) *Early lesion of tumoral calcinosis shows amorphous debris ➢ within fibrous lining containing macrophages ➢ and multinucleated giant cells ➔. This lesion has not yet become calcified.* ***(Center)*** *This lesion has rounded microscopic deposits of calcium (calcospherites) ➔ in fibrous tissue containing aggregates of histiocytes.* ***(Right)*** *Older lesion of tumoral calcinosis shows irregular masses of calcification ➢ within sparsely cellular fibrous tissue.*

ROSAI-DORFMAN DISEASE OF SOFT TISSUE

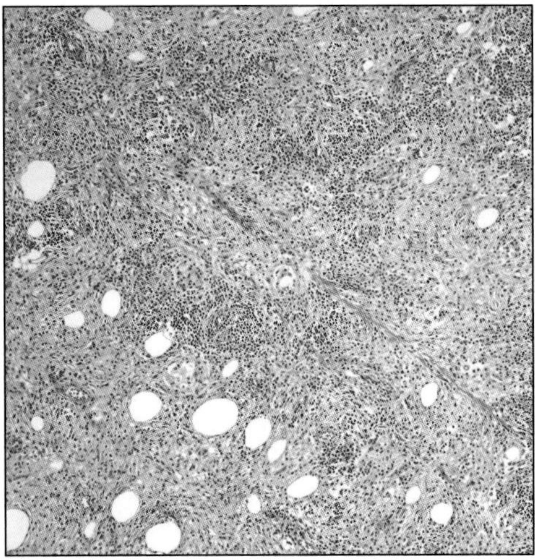

Low-power image of extranodal (soft tissue) Rosai-Dorfman disease shows proliferating histiocytes that are spindled, infiltrating fat. Lymphoid aggregates are present.

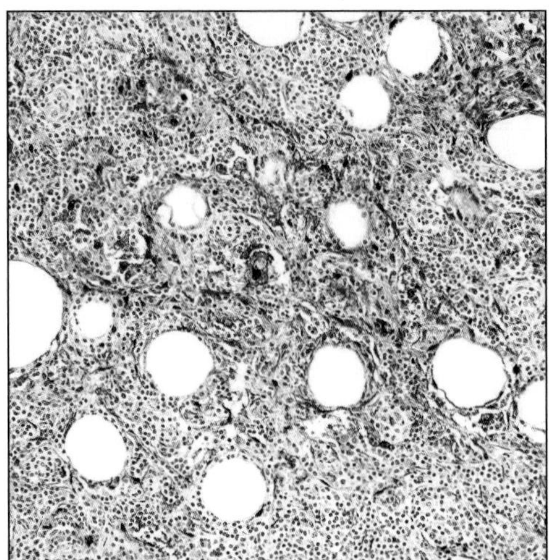

S100 protein shows labeling of the proliferating histiocytes. The staining pattern is not diffuse and must be correlated with the morphology. Some labeled cells are dendritic cells.

TERMINOLOGY

Abbreviations

- Rosai-Dorfman disease (RDD)

Synonyms

- Sinus histiocytosis with massive lymphadenopathy (SHML)
  - Applies to disease involving lymph nodes

Definitions

- Rare, acquired, nonmalignant proliferation of distinctive histiocytes that presents with lymphadenopathy or extranodal disease
  - Lesional histiocytes contain variable numbers of intact lymphocytes within cytoplasm
    - Phenomenon referred to as lymphophagocytosis or emperipolesis
  - Primarily in children and young adults

ETIOLOGY/PATHOGENESIS

Exuberant Hematopoietic Response to Undetermined Immunologic Trigger

- Association with autoimmune lymphoproliferative syndrome has been described
  - Inherited disorder of lymphocyte-programmed cell death with mutations in death receptor genes that specifically eliminate apoptosis in lymphocyte subsets
  - Occurs primarily in early childhood
  - May represent acquired disorder of deregulation of apoptotic signaling pathways
- Various infections associated with cases of RDD/SHML, but none proven as etiologic infectious agent
  - Parvovirus
  - Epstein-Barr virus
  - HHV6

CLINICAL ISSUES

Presentation

- Varies with site
  - Painless lymphadenopathy is most frequent presenting symptom
    - Involves cervical region in up to 90% of patients
- 30-45% of patients have at least 1 site of extranodal involvement as well as lymph node involvement
  - Hepatosplenomegaly uncommon
- ~ 25% of patients have extranodal disease only
- Skin and soft tissue most common extranodal site
- Approximate frequency of extranodal sites
  - Skin and soft tissue (16%)
  - Nasal cavity and paranasal sinuses (16%)
  - Eye, orbit, and ocular adnexa (11%)
  - Bone (11%)
  - Salivary gland (7%)
  - Central nervous system (7%)
  - Oral cavity (4%)
  - Kidney and genitourinary tract (3%)
  - Respiratory tract (3%)
  - Liver (1%)
  - Tonsil (1%)
  - Breast (< 1%)
  - Gastrointestinal tract (< 1%)
  - Heart (< 1%)
- Simultaneous involvement of multiple extranodal sites not unusual
- Involvement of kidney, lower respiratory tract, and liver associated with worse clinical outcome (as is number of extranodal sites)

Treatment

- Most patients require little intervention

Prognosis

- Most patients have complete and spontaneous remission

ROSAI-DORFMAN DISEASE OF SOFT TISSUE

Key Facts

Terminology

- Lesional histiocytes contain variable numbers of intact lymphocytes within their cytoplasm
  - Phenomenon referred to as lymphophagocytosis or emperipolesis
- Synonym: Sinus histiocytosis with massive lymphadenopathy (term for disease involving lymph nodes)

Clinical Issues

- Painless lymphadenopathy most frequent presenting symptom
- Skin and soft tissue most common extranodal site
- Poor prognosis correlates with widespread dissemination
  - Involves kidneys, lower respiratory tract, liver, and immunologic abnormalities or anemia
- Most patients have complete and spontaneous remission
  - Some may experience recurrent or persistent but stable lymphadenopathy

Microscopic Pathology

- RDD of soft tissue has more subtle histologic features than its lymph node counterpart
  - Emperipolesis less conspicuous
  - Proliferating histiocytes frequently spindled
  - Majority of lesions label with S100 protein
  - Vague storiform pattern
  - Scattered lymphoplasmacytic aggregates

Top Differential Diagnoses

- Histiocytic lymphoma
- Langerhans cell histiocytosis

- Some may experience recurrent or persistent but stable lymphadenopathy
- In very few cases, disease follows aggressive course and may be fatal
  - Poor prognosis correlates with widespread dissemination, involvement of kidneys, lower respiratory tract, liver, and immunologic abnormalities or anemia

MACROSCOPIC FEATURES

General Features

- In soft tissues and other extranodal sites
  - Firm, poorly marginated lesion
- In lymph nodes
  - Firm, massively enlarged lymph nodes

MICROSCOPIC PATHOLOGY

Histologic Features

- In lymph nodes, as per name "sinus histiocytosis with massive lymphadenopathy"
  - Expanded sinuses contain histiocytic cells with abundant cytoplasm, sometimes multinucleated
  - Emperipolesis a striking feature
  - Lesional cells S100 protein reactive
- Majority of lesions label with S100 protein
- RDD of soft tissue has more subtle histologic features than its lymph node counterpart
  - Emperipolesis less conspicuous
  - Proliferating histiocytes frequently spindled
  - Abundant associated collagen deposition
  - Vague storiform pattern
  - Scattered lymphoplasmacytic aggregates
  - Mild cytologic atypia

Predominant Cell/Compartment Type

- Hematopoietic, histiocytic

DIFFERENTIAL DIAGNOSIS

Histiocytic Lymphoma

- Marked cytologic atypia
- Expresses host of histiocytic markers but not S100 protein
- Aggressive clinical course

Langerhans Cell Histiocytosis

- Cells with nuclear grooves, backdrop of eosinophils
- Expresses both S100 protein and CD1a

Various Disorders Featuring Granulomas

- Mycobacterial infection
  - Granulomas composed of S100 protein(-) cells
  - No emperipolesis
  - Organisms can be detected by culture/special stains
- Chronic granulomatous disease (CGD)
  - Rare primary inherited immunodeficiency (incidence 1:200,000 in USA)
  - Affects phagocytes (neutrophils & macrophages) that contain nicotinamide adenine dinucleotide phosphate (reduced NADPH) oxidase enzyme
    - Generates superoxide required for killing micro-organisms
  - Dysfunction of NADPH oxidase in CGD results in ineffective respiratory burst in phagocytes
    - Unable to kill and digest certain bacteria and fungi, predisposing patients to infections
  - Functional diagnosis of CGD
    - Demonstrate absence/marked reduction in phagocytic respiratory burst to form superoxides, using tests such as nitroblue tetrazolium (NBT) reduction
    - Neutrophils stimulated with phorbol myristate acetate and incubated with yellow dye NBT
    - Normal phagocytes reduce this to dark pigment formazan, with mixed NBT(+) and NBT(-) cells denoting carrier status
  - Features loose collections of pigmented histiocytes typically in lung and GI tract with variable granuloma formation

ROSAI-DORFMAN DISEASE OF SOFT TISSUE

Immunohistochemistry

Antibody	Reactivity	Staining Pattern	Comment
S100	Positive	Nuclear & cytoplasmic	Intracytoplasmic hematopoietic cells negative
CD68	Positive	Cytoplasmic	
CD1a	Negative		RDD is a non-Langerhans cell histiocytosis

- S100 protein stain(-)
- Malakoplakia
  - Acquired granulomatous disorder (1st described by Michaelis & Gutmann)
  - Believed to result from acquired bacteriocidal defect in macrophages
    - Occurring mostly in immunosuppressed patients or in setting of autoimmune disease
  - Usually in bladder or GI tract
  - Collections of histiocytes
    - S100 protein(-)
  - Contain targetoid inclusions that stain with von Kossa stain
    - Believed to reflect concretions of phagocytosed bacteria

Malignant Fibrous Histiocytoma (High-Grade Pleomorphic Undifferentiated Sarcoma)

- Composed of highly pleomorphic spindle cells
- Negative S100 protein
- Emperipolesis not a typical feature

Sarcoidosis

- Features granulomas but not emperipolesis
- Histiocytes lack S100 protein labeling

Follicular Dendritic Cell Tumor/Sarcoma

- Oval to spindle cells with eosinophilic cytoplasm, sheets & fascicles, focal storiform pattern & whorls like those seen in meningioma
- Oval or elongated nuclei with thin nuclear membranes, inconspicuous or small eosinophilic nucleoli, and clear or dispersed chromatin
- Tumor cells intimately admixed with small lymphocytes, with prominent perivascular cuffing
- Multinucleate cell common
- Necrosis, marked cellular atypia, high mitotic rate, &/ or abnormal mitoses common
- Expresses CD21, CD35, podoplanin (D2-40), S100 protein

Juvenile Xanthogranuloma

- Non-Langerhans cell histiocytosis
- Cutaneous form most common
  - Nodules often develop shortly after birth
  - Most common site head and neck followed by trunk and extremities
  - Many nodules regress spontaneously
- Rare deep cases
  - Skeletal muscle, parenchymal organs
- No association with lipid metabolism disorders
- Histiocytic cells with variable giant cells, lipid
- Background inflammatory cells, often many eosinophils
- CD68(+), CD31(+), S100 protein(-), CD1a(-)

SELECTED REFERENCES

1. Gaitonde S: Multifocal, extranodal sinus histiocytosis with massive lymphadenopathy: an overview. Arch Pathol Lab Med. 131(7):1117-21, 2007
2. Mehraein Y et al: Parvovirus B19 detected in Rosai-Dorfman disease in nodal and extranodal manifestations. J Clin Pathol. 59(12):1320-6, 2006
3. Wang KH et al: Cutaneous Rosai-Dorfman disease: clinicopathological profiles, spectrum and evolution of 21 lesions in six patients. Br J Dermatol. 154(2):277-86, 2006
4. Maric I et al: Histologic features of sinus histiocytosis with massive lymphadenopathy in patients with autoimmune lymphoproliferative syndrome. Am J Surg Pathol. 29(7):903-11, 2005
5. Rodriguez-Galindo C et al: Extranodal Rosai-Dorfman disease in children. J Pediatr Hematol Oncol. 26(1):19-24, 2004
6. Anders RA et al: Rosai-Dorfman disease presenting in the gastrointestinal tract. Arch Pathol Lab Med. 127(2):E74-5, 2003
7. Sneller MC et al: Autoimmune lymphoproliferative syndrome. Curr Opin Rheumatol. 15(4):417-21, 2003
8. Andriko JA et al: Rosai-Dorfman disease isolated to the central nervous system: a report of 11 cases. Mod Pathol. 14(3):172-8, 2001
9. Lauwers GY et al: The digestive system manifestations of Rosai-Dorfman disease (sinus histiocytosis with massive lymphadenopathy): review of 11 cases. Hum Pathol. 31(3):380-5, 2000
10. Green I et al: Breast involvement by extranodal Rosai-Dorfman disease: report of seven cases. Am J Surg Pathol. 21(6):664-8, 1997
11. Levine PH et al: Detection of human herpesvirus 6 in tissues involved by sinus histiocytosis with massive lymphadenopathy (Rosai-Dorfman disease). J Infect Dis. 166(2):291-5, 1992
12. Montgomery EA et al: Rosai-Dorfman disease of soft tissue. Am J Surg Pathol. 16(2):122-9, 1992
13. Eisen RN et al: Immunophenotypic characterization of sinus histiocytosis with massive lymphadenopathy (Rosai-Dorfman disease). Semin Diagn Pathol. 7(1):74-82, 1990
14. Foucar E et al: Sinus histiocytosis with massive lymphadenopathy (Rosai-Dorfman disease): review of the entity. Semin Diagn Pathol. 7(1):19-73, 1990
15. Foucar E et al: Sinus histiocytosis with massive lymphadenopathy. An analysis of 14 deaths occurring in a patient registry. Cancer. 54(9):1834-40, 1984
16. Walker PD et al: The osseous manifestations of sinus histiocytosis with massive lymphadenopathy. Am J Clin Pathol. 75(2):131-9, 1981
17. Rosai J et al: Sinus histiocytosis with massive lymphadenopathy. A newly recognized benign clinicopathological entity. Arch Pathol. 87(1):63-70, 1969

Microscopic Features and Differential Diagnosis

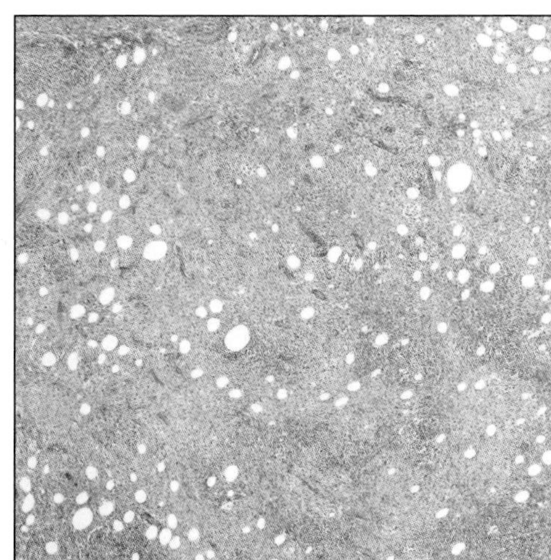

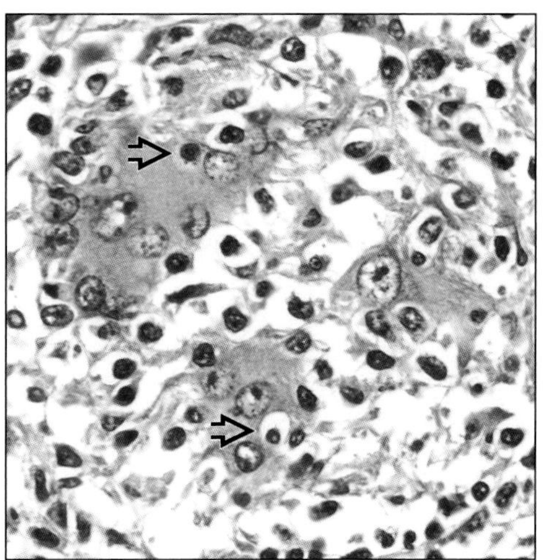

(Left) Hematoxylin & eosin shows a low-magnification view of a case of soft tissue Rosai-Dorfman disease. Note the scattered lymphoid aggregates arranged throughout the lesion in a random distribution. **(Right)** Hematoxylin & eosin shows the key microscopic feature of Rosai-Dorfman disease, namely striking emperipolesis by the proliferating histiocytes. The cytoplasmic lymphocytes are fully intact ➡.

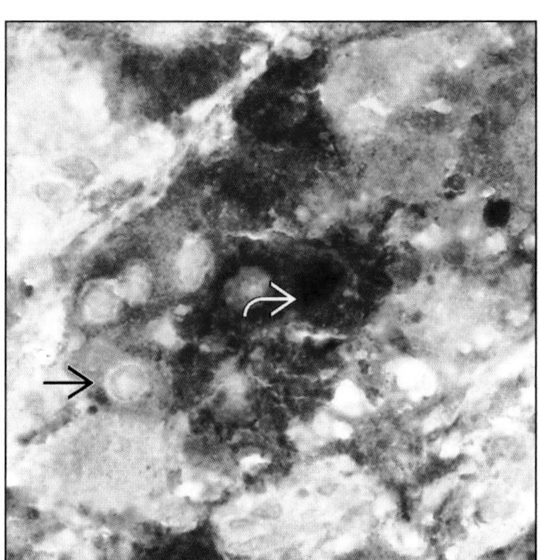

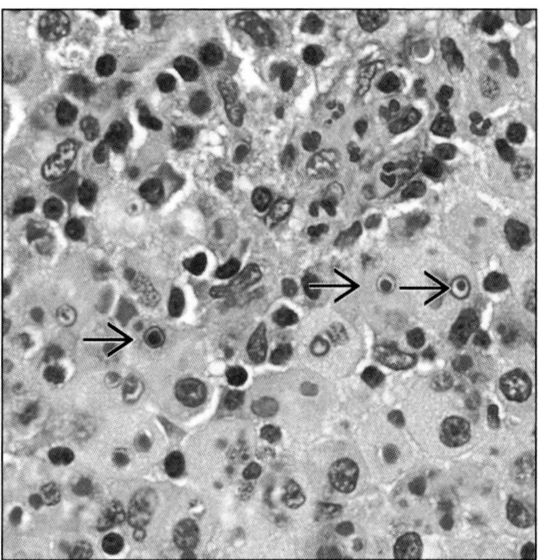

(Left) S100 shows nuclear ➡ and cytoplasmic labeling in the histiocytes. Note that the engulfed lymphocytes in the field do not express S100 protein. They are are undamaged and surrounded by a "halo" ➡. The S100 stain sometimes accentuates this emperipolesis. **(Right)** Hematoxylin & eosin shows an example of malakoplakia. There are several Michaelis-Gutmann bodies indicated ➡. These consist of incompletely eradicated engulfed bacteria.

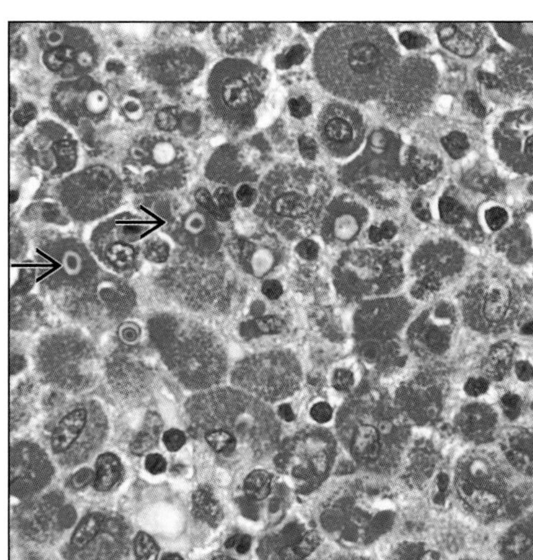

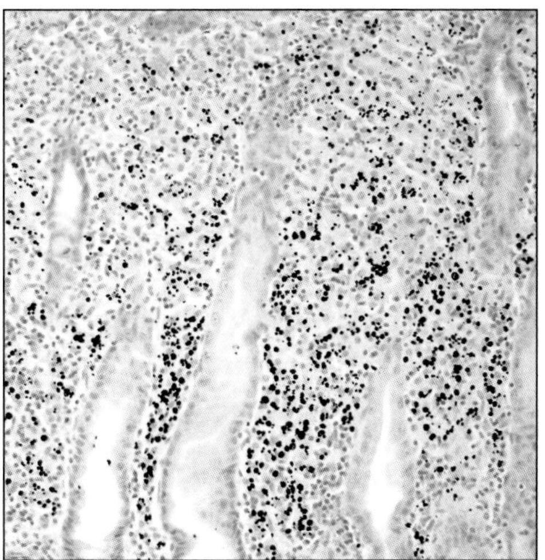

(Left) Periodic acid-Schiff with diastase digestion shows that, in malakoplakia, Michaelis-Gutmann are PAS(-) ➡ despite weak staining in the histiocyte cytoplasm. **(Right)** Von Kossa stain highlights the Michaelis-Gutmann bodies in malakoplakia. In this dramatic example, the bodies are numerous; most cases display fewer Michaelis-Gutmann bodies.

GASTROINTESTINAL STROMAL TUMOR

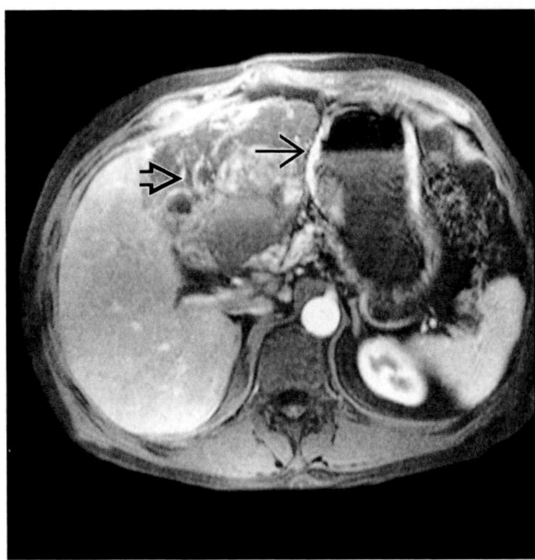

Radiologic image shows a large gastric stromal tumor ➭. The lesion compresses the liver but arises in association with the gastric wall →.

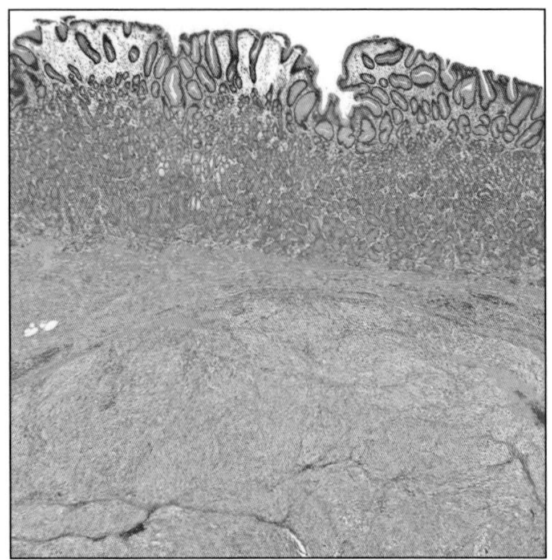

At low magnification, this gastric GIST involves the muscularis propria of the gastric body. The lesion is lobulated and well marginated.

TERMINOLOGY

Abbreviations

- Gastrointestinal stromal tumor (GIST)

Synonyms

- Gastrointestinal smooth muscle tumors (used interchangeably in the literature before year 2000)
- Gastrointestinal autonomic nerve tumor
  - Now subsumed under GIST
  - Dense core neurosecretory granules on ultrastructure, variable S100 protein, and neuron-specific enolase labeling

Definitions

- Generally CD117(+) *KIT* or *PDGFRA* mutation-driven mesenchymal tumors, usually of GI tract with characteristic histologic features
  - Spindle cells
  - Epithelioid cells
  - Pleomorphic morphology (rare)
- Familial cases
  - Germline mutations of *KIT* gene, autosomal dominant
- Neurofibromatosis type 1 (NF1)
  - Interaction between *KIT* gene product and *NF1* gene product
  - Tumors have CD117 immunolabeling but no *KIT* gene mutations
- Carney triad
  - Epithelioid gastric GISTs
  - Paraganglioma
  - Pulmonary chondroma
  - Lack *KIT* and *PDGFRA* mutations
  - Lack succinate dehydrogenase B expression (in contrast to most GISTs)

CLINICAL ISSUES

Epidemiology

- Incidence
  - 14.5/1,000,000 in Sweden, 11/1,000,000 in Iceland, about 4,500 new cases per year in USA
  - Clinically silent lesions (studied in gastroesophageal resections for carcinomas) are common (10%)
    - Suggests that most lesions remain clinically insignificant and do not progress
- Age
  - Median age: 60 years; tumors rare in children and young adults
    - Familial examples present in middle age
    - Carney triad cases may present in childhood
    - Mean age for NF1-associated lesions: 49 years
- Gender
  - No predilection in most series
  - May be slight male predilection
  - Strong female predilection in Carney triad-associated cases
- Ethnicity
  - Overrepresentation of malignant examples reported in African-Americans

Site

- Stomach most common site (60%)
  - All Carney triad cases are in stomach
- Jejunum and ileum (30%)
  - NF1-associated lesions tend to occur in small bowel
- Duodenum (5%)
- Colorectum (< 5%)
- Esophagus and appendix (rare)
- Primary extraintestinal (mesentery, omentum, retroperitoneum) is rare
  - Most lesions in mesentery are considered metastases/direct spread from GI tract
  - Lesions of omentum considered as contiguous with stomach

GASTROINTESTINAL STROMAL TUMOR

Key Facts

Terminology
- Generally Kit (CD117) positive or *KIT* or *PDGFRA* mutation-driven mesenchymal tumors usually of gastrointestinal tract with characteristic histologic features

Clinical Issues
- Molecular prognostication for GISTs
- Not indicated for all cases
- Best reserved for patients with advanced disease or disease refractory to treatment
- Both simple clinicopathologic features and molecular testing are prognostic
- Simple algorithms a function of size and mitotic counts
- Site is important risk factor
- 20-25% of gastric GISTs are malignant
- 40-50% of small intestinal GISTs are malignant
- Molecular analysis to determine likelihood of response to treatment
- *KIT* exon 11 (most common mutation type): Complete remission 6%, partial response 61%, stable disease 25%, progressive disease 3%
- *KIT* and *PDGFRA* wild type: Partial response 23%, stable disease 50%, progressive disease 19%

Microscopic Pathology
- Uniform spindle cells or epithelioid cells arranged in lobules
- Nuclear pleomorphism is rare
- Eosinophilic cytoplasm
- Cytoplasmic vacuoles common

- Reflected in American Joint Committee on Cancer (AJCC)/TNM 7th edition staging schemes

Presentation
- Gastrointestinal bleeding
  - Most common presentation
- GI obstruction
- Abdominal pain
- Incidental
  - During surgery, imaging studies, or endoscopy

Treatment
- Surgical approaches
  - Complete resection, regardless of site
- Drugs
  - Imatinib mesylate (Gleevec): Inhibits tyrosine kinases (such as Kit)
  - Newer drugs
    - Used for acquired resistance to imatinib (attributed to secondary *KIT* or *PDGFRA* mutations) or initial lack of response
    - Sunitinib malate (SU11248): Used for patients with *KIT* exon 9 mutations, others
    - Additional drugs in development

Prognosis
- Both simple clinicopathologic features and molecular testing are prognostic
  - Simple algorithms are function of size and mitotic counts
  - Site is important risk factor
    - 20-25% of gastric GISTs are malignant
    - 40-50% of small intestinal GISTs are malignant
- Small bowel criteria often applied for other sites of GISTs
- Molecular prognostication for GISTs
  - Not indicated for all cases
    - Best reserved for patients with advanced disease or disease refractory to treatment
- GISTs in patients with Carney triad have a high likelihood of metastases (about half)
  - Lymph node metastases in about 1/3

MACROSCOPIC FEATURES

General Features
- Usually well-marginated lesions with their epicenter in muscularis propria

MICROSCOPIC PATHOLOGY

Histologic Features
- Uniform spindle cells or epithelioid cells arranged in lobules
  - Nuclear pleomorphism is uncommon
  - Occasional cases show "dedifferentiated" pattern with bland areas and high-grade areas in same neoplasm
    - Reports of skeletal muscle differentiation in post-treatment lesions
  - Some cases have multinucleated cells
  - Some examples with nuclear palisading
    - Reminiscent of nerve sheath tumor pattern
  - Carney triad cases typically epithelioid
- Eosinophilic cytoplasm
- Cytoplasmic vacuoles common
- Minimal inflammation
- Inconspicuous vessels
- Can have myxoid or myxochondroid background
- Some cases have cystic spaces
- "Skeinoid" fibers in small bowel examples
  - Coarse, wire-like, haphazardly arranged collagen bundles
- Occasional extension into mucosa
  - Poor prognostic factor
- Tumor necrosis uncommon
  - Poor prognostic factor

Cytologic Features
- Uniform spindle cells on aspirates
- Performing immunolabeling on aspiration samples can be diagnostic

GASTROINTESTINAL STROMAL TUMOR

ANCILLARY TESTS

Immunohistochemistry

- Usually CD117(+)
  - Additional more specific markers
    - Protein kinase C theta (PKC-θ)
    - DOG1 (deleted on GIST 1)
  - Data accumulating on PDGFRA antibodies

DIFFERENTIAL DIAGNOSIS

Solitary Fibrous Tumor

- Vanishingly rare in GI tract
  - Classically encountered in pleura
- Spindle cell lesion, hemangiopericytoma-like vascular pattern
  - Uniform angulated cells in "patternless" pattern
  - Minimal inflammation
- CD34(+), Bcl-2(+), CD117(-)
- No *KIT* mutations
- Usually benign
  - Some malignant examples

Gastrointestinal Schwannoma

- Usually in muscularis propria of stomach
  - Spindle cells with focal palisading
  - May have infiltrative pattern
  - Minimal vascular changes
  - Negligible mitotic activity
- Prominent lymphoid cuff
- Intralesional lymphoplasmacytic inflammation
- S100(+), CD117(-)
- No *KIT* mutations
  - Differs from somatic soft tissue schwannoma by lacking *NF2* mutations
- Benign

Mesenteric Fibromatosis

- Epicenter in mesentery with extension into muscularis propria
- Infiltrative growth pattern
  - Poorly marginated
- Pale cells, abundant collagen, prominent small vessels
  - Mesenteric examples have ectatic thin-walled vessels
  - Mesenteric examples can have storiform pattern
  - Lesional cells have eosinophilic cytoplasm, delicate nuclear membranes, small uniform nucleoli
- Usually CD34(-), some cases have cytoplasmic CD117, nuclear β-catenin (GISTs lack nuclear β-catenin)
- β-catenin and *APC* gene mutations
- No *KIT* mutations
- Benign but prone to local recurrences

Gastrointestinal Leiomyoma

- Usually in esophagus or in association with colonic muscularis mucosae
  - Esophagus lesions often in muscularis propria
- Brightly eosinophilic cells with blunt-ended nuclei
  - No mitotic activity
  - Hypocellular
- Desmin(+), actin(+), CD117(-)
- No *KIT* mutations
- Benign

Gastrointestinal Leiomyosarcoma

- Brightly eosinophilic cells with blunt-ended nuclei
- Perpendicularly oriented fascicles
- Nuclear pleomorphism
  - Mitotic activity
  - Paranuclear vacuoles (similar to those in GIST but less abundant)
- Desmin(+), actin(+), CD117(-)
- No *KIT* mutations
- Malignant
  - Often high grade with aggressive behavior

Melanoma

- Metastases tend to spread to small bowel
  - Can be detected in lacteals on mucosal biopsy specimens
  - Occasional anal and esophageal primaries
- Typically more pleomorphic than GIST
  - May be pigmented
  - Intranuclear cytoplasmic invaginations (pseudoinclusions)
- CD117 often positive, but also S100 protein, other melanocytic markers
  - Spindle cell melanomas often lack "specific" melanocytic immunohistochemical markers
- About 20% of mucosal melanomas have *KIT* mutations and respond to treatment
- Aggressive lesions

Clear Cell Sarcoma of GI Tract

- Usually in small bowel
- Lobules of uniform spindle cells with prominent nucleoli
- S100(+), most CD117(-)
- t(12;22), *EWS-ATF1* fusion or *EWS-CREB1* fusion
  - Cases with *EWS-CREB1* fusion lack melanocytic differentiation and do not label with "melanoma markers"
  - Some cases require molecular confirmation to exclude melanoma
- High-grade sarcoma

Inflammatory Fibroid Polyp

- Submucosal based
- Bland proliferating cells
  - Characteristic "whorling" pattern around blood vessels
  - Scattered lesional giant cells
  - Numerous background eosinophils
- CD34(+), CD117(-)
- *PDGFRA* mutations, no *KIT* mutations
- Benign

Gastrointestinal Glomus Tumor

- Nearly always in stomach
- Adults
- Found in muscularis propria
- Uniform round cells proliferating around blood vessels
- Bland chromatin
- Actin(+), desmin(-), CD117(-)
- No *KIT* mutations
- Usually benign

- Rare reports of malignant behavior

Dedifferentiated Liposarcoma

- Large retroperitoneal masses of older adults
- Can involve mesentery and extend into muscularis propria of GI tract
- Undifferentiated sarcoma component
  - High-grade spindle cell sarcoma
- Component with adipocytic differentiation
  - Fat punctuated by enlarged hyperchromatic nuclei
    - Lipoblasts can be encountered but not necessary for diagnosis
- Nuclear immunolabeling with MDM2, CDK4
- MDM2 amplification
- Malignant, high grade

Endometrial Stromal Sarcoma

- Older women
- Classically involve uterus
  - Extrauterine examples can involve GI tract
- Uniform spindle cells with scant cytoplasm
- CD10(+), ER(+), PR(+), CD117(+/-), S100 protein(-)
- Malignant, usually low grade

DIAGNOSTIC CHECKLIST

Pathologic Interpretation Pearls

- If considering GIST diagnosis when confronted with pleomorphic mesenchymal neoplasm in GI tract, consider alternative diagnoses first
- CD117 immunolabeling is well known in other GI tract lesions, so panel approach to immunolabeling is important
  - Some CD117 reactive neoplasms
    - Fibromatosis
    - Dedifferentiated liposarcoma
    - Angiosarcoma
    - Melanoma
    - Carcinomas (especially small cell carcinoma)

SELECTED REFERENCES

1. Gill AJ et al: Immunohistochemistry for SDHB divides gastrointestinal stromal tumors (GISTs) into 2 distinct types. Am J Surg Pathol. 34(5):636-44, 2010
2. Information on sending samples for KIT mutational analysis: http://www.amptestdirectory.org. Accessed February 17, 2010
3. Antonescu CR: Targeted therapies in gastrointestinal stromal tumors. Semin Diagn Pathol. 25(4):295-303, 2008
4. Blanke CD et al: Long-term results from a randomized phase II trial of standard- versus higher-dose imatinib mesylate for patients with unresectable or metastatic gastrointestinal stromal tumors expressing KIT. J Clin Oncol. 26(4):620-5, 2008
5. Espinosa I et al: A novel monoclonal antibody against DOG1 is a sensitive and specific marker for gastrointestinal stromal tumors. Am J Surg Pathol. 32(2):210-8, 2008
6. Guler ML et al: Expression of melanoma antigens in epithelioid gastrointestinal stromal tumors: a potential diagnostic pitfall. Arch Pathol Lab Med. 132(8):1302-6, 2008
7. Heinrich MC et al: Primary and secondary kinase genotypes correlate with the biological and clinical activity of sunitinib in imatinib-resistant gastrointestinal stromal tumor. J Clin Oncol. 26(33):5352-9, 2008
8. Lasota J et al: Clinical significance of oncogenic KIT and PDGFRA mutations in gastrointestinal stromal tumours. Histopathology. 53(3):245-66, 2008
9. Abraham SC et al: "Seedling" mesenchymal tumors (gastrointestinal stromal tumors and leiomyomas) are common incidental tumors of the esophagogastric junction. Am J Surg Pathol. 31(11):1629-35, 2007
10. Joensuu H: Sunitinib for imatinib-resistant GIST. Lancet. 368(9544):1303-4, 2006
11. Miettinen M et al: Gastrointestinal stromal tumors in patients with neurofibromatosis 1: a clinicopathologic and molecular genetic study of 45 cases. Am J Surg Pathol. 30(1):90-6, 2006
12. Miettinen M et al: Gastrointestinal stromal tumors of the jejunum and ileum: a clinicopathologic, immunohistochemical, and molecular genetic study of 906 cases before imatinib with long-term follow-up. Am J Surg Pathol. 30(4):477-89, 2006
13. Miettinen M et al: Gastrointestinal stromal tumors: review on morphology, molecular pathology, prognosis, and differential diagnosis. Arch Pathol Lab Med. 130(10):1466-78, 2006
14. Miettinen M et al: Gastrointestinal stromal tumors of the stomach in children and young adults: a clinicopathologic, immunohistochemical, and molecular genetic study of 44 cases with long-term follow-up and review of the literature. Am J Surg Pathol. 29(10):1373-81, 2005
15. Miettinen M et al: Gastrointestinal stromal tumors of the stomach: a clinicopathologic, immunohistochemical, and molecular genetic study of 1765 cases with long-term follow-up. Am J Surg Pathol. 29(1):52-68, 2005
16. Tran T et al: The epidemiology of malignant gastrointestinal stromal tumors: an analysis of 1,458 cases from 1992 to 2000. Am J Gastroenterol. 100(1):162-8, 2005
17. Miettinen M et al: Gastrointestinal stromal tumors, intramural leiomyomas, and leiomyosarcomas in the duodenum: a clinicopathologic, immunohistochemical, and molecular genetic study of 167 cases. Am J Surg Pathol. 27(5):625-41, 2003
18. Fletcher CD et al: Diagnosis of gastrointestinal stromal tumors: A consensus approach. Hum Pathol. 33(5):459-65, 2002
19. Joensuu H et al: Effect of the tyrosine kinase inhibitor STI571 in a patient with a metastatic gastrointestinal stromal tumor. N Engl J Med. 344(14):1052-6, 2001
20. Miettinen M et al: Gastrointestinal stromal tumors, intramural leiomyomas, and leiomyosarcomas in the rectum and anus: a clinicopathologic, immunohistochemical, and molecular genetic study of 144 cases. Am J Surg Pathol. 25(9):1121-33, 2001
21. Miettinen M et al: Gastrointestinal stromal tumors and leiomyosarcomas in the colon: a clinicopathologic, immunohistochemical, and molecular genetic study of 44 cases. Am J Surg Pathol. 24(10):1339-52, 2000
22. Emory TS et al: Prognosis of gastrointestinal smooth-muscle (stromal) tumors: dependence on anatomic site. Am J Surg Pathol. 23(1):82-7, 1999
23. Hirota S et al: Gain-of-function mutations of c-kit in human gastrointestinal stromal tumors. Science. 279(5350):577-80, 1998
24. Kindblom LG et al: Gastrointestinal pacemaker cell tumor (GIPACT): gastrointestinal stromal tumors show phenotypic characteristics of the interstitial cells of Cajal. Am J Pathol. 152(5):1259-69, 1998

GASTROINTESTINAL STROMAL TUMOR

Clinical Prognostication for GISTs from Largest Series (Untreated with Imatinib)

Size	Mitoses/50 HPF	Metastases	Risk
Gastric GISTs			
≤ 2 cm	≤ 5	None	None to negligible
> 2 and ≤ 5 cm	≤ 5	2%	Low
> 5 and ≤ 10 cm	≤ 5	4%	Low
> 10 cm	≤ 5	12%	Intermediate
≤ 2 cm	> 5	None	Low
> 2 and ≤ 5 cm	> 5	16%	Intermediate
> 5 and ≤ 10 cm	> 5	55%	High
> 10 cm	> 5	88%	High
Small Bowel GISTs			
≤ 2 cm	≤ 5	None	None to negligible
> 2 and ≤ 5 cm	≤ 5	4%	Low
> 5 and ≤ 10 cm	≤ 5	24%	Intermediate
> 10 cm	≤5	52%	High
≤ 2 cm	> 5	50%	High
> 2 and ≤ 5 cm	> 5	85%	High
> 10 cm	> 5	90%	High

Molecular Prognostication for GISTs

Mutation	Site	Prognosis	Likelihood of Response to Treatment
KIT exon 9	Typical of small bowel GISTs	Not prognostic marker	Poor response to imatinib, improved by high dose treatment. Sunitinib malate (SU11248) can be used
KIT exon 11 deletions and substitutions	Found in all sites	May indicate poor prognosis	Complete remission (6%); partial response (61%); stable disease (25%); progressive disease (3%)
KIT exon 11 duplications	Gastric	May indicate improved prognosis	
KIT exon 13 mutations	All sites	May indicate poor prognosis in gastric GISTs	Partial response, all cases (rare)
KIT exon 17 mutations	Small bowel	No prognostic significance	Variable, depending on specific mutation
PDGFRA exon 12 deletions and substitutions	Gastric	May indicate good prognosis	Most respond to imatinib
PDGFRA exon 14 substitutions	Gastric	May indicate good prognosis	No data available
PDGFRA exon 18 deletions and substitutions	Gastric	May indicate good prognosis	Variable and mutation specific
KIT and *PDGFRA* wild type	Typical of NF1 and Carney triad tumors	No prognostic significance	Partial response (23%); stable disease (50%); progressive disease (19%)

Microscopic Features

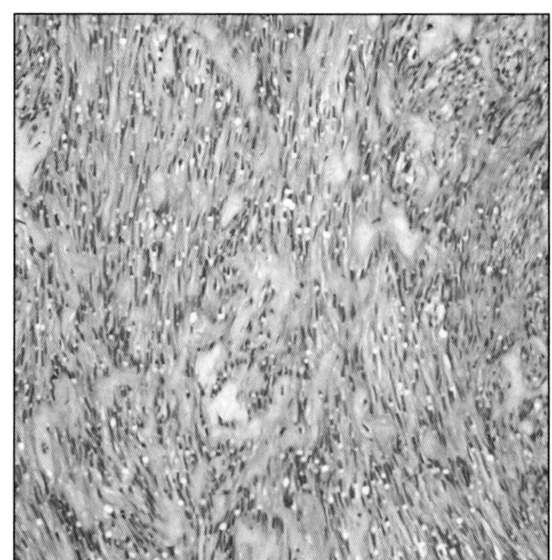

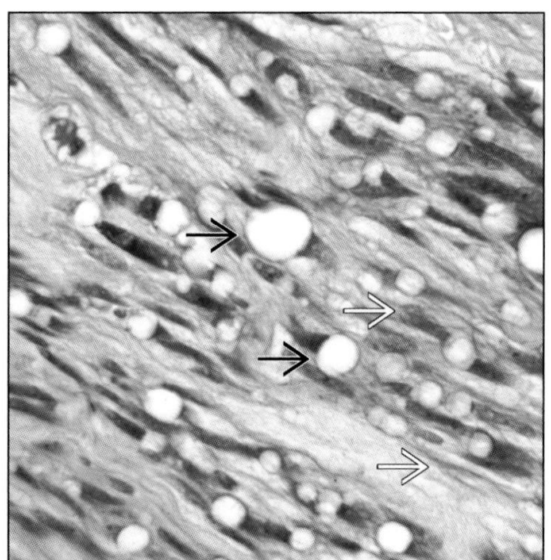

(Left) *In this image of a spindle cell gastric GIST, even at low magnification, paranuclear vacuoles, usually associated with benign behavior, are numerous.* ***(Right)*** *This image is taken at high magnification of a gastric GIST. In addition to prominent paranuclear vacuoles* ⇨*, note the brightly eosinophilic fibrillary cytoplasm* ➡*, both features reminiscent of smooth muscle differentiation. Such features led early authors to regard GISTs as smooth muscle neoplasms.*

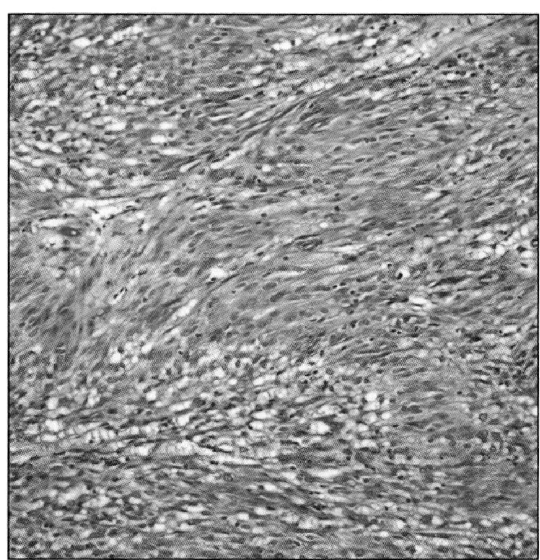

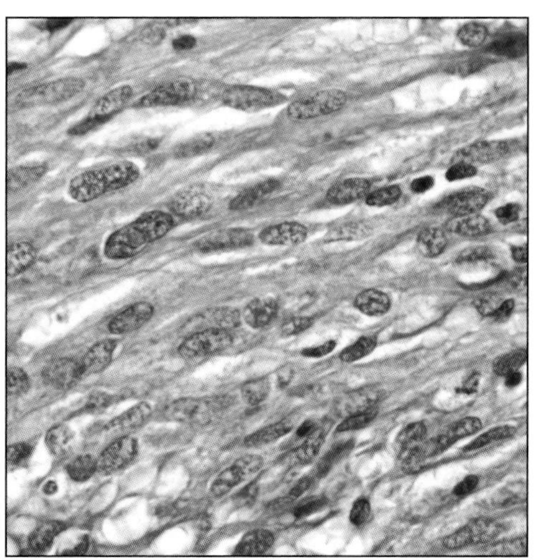

(Left) *This spindle cell gastric GIST has high cellularity and would be expected to have a high mitotic rate. Such appearances are often associated with an unfavorable outcome.* ***(Right)*** *The lesional cells in this gastric GIST are very uniform, a feature of tumors associated with characteristic mutations. The chromatin is slightly coarse but paler than that in leiomyosarcomas, and nucleoli are inconspicuous.*

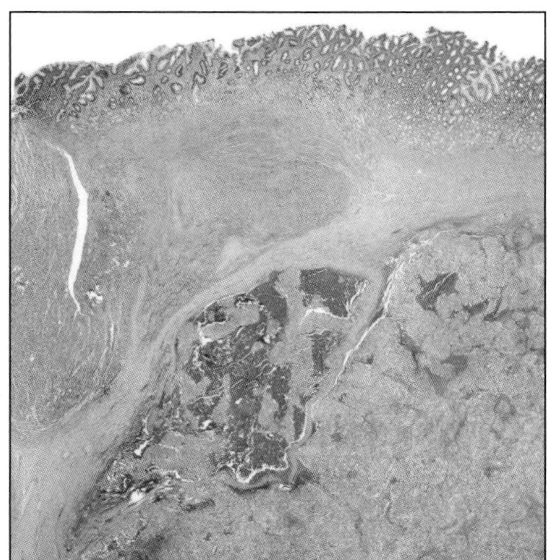

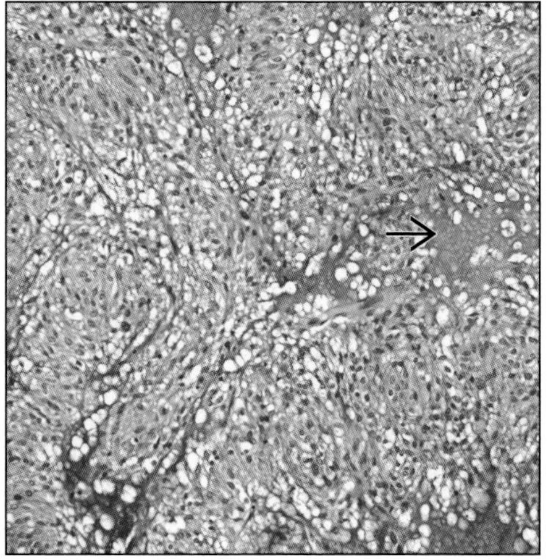

(Left) *This is an epithelioid gastric GIST with a lobulated appearance. It is centered in the muscularis propria. Most GISTs do not involve the mucosa. When they do, this feature suggests malignancy.* ***(Right)*** *This image shows an epithelioid GIST at intermediate magnification. There is a chondroid background* ⇨*, and the tumor cells have numerous cytoplasmic vacuoles. Epithelioid gastric GISTs, such as this, may be CD117(-) and have PDGFRA mutations.*

GASTROINTESTINAL STROMAL TUMOR

Microscopic and Gross Features

(Left) *This epithelioid gastric GIST tumor has uniform tumor cells with prominent vacuoles. The cellularity of this lesion is relatively low, such that there is minimal nuclear overlap. Patients whose tumors have such features typically have a favorable outcome.* ***(Right)*** *Several tiny ("seedling") GISTs ⮫ near the gastroesophageal junction are seen in this resection specimen. These were found incidentally in a resection performed for a separate gastric carcinoma.*

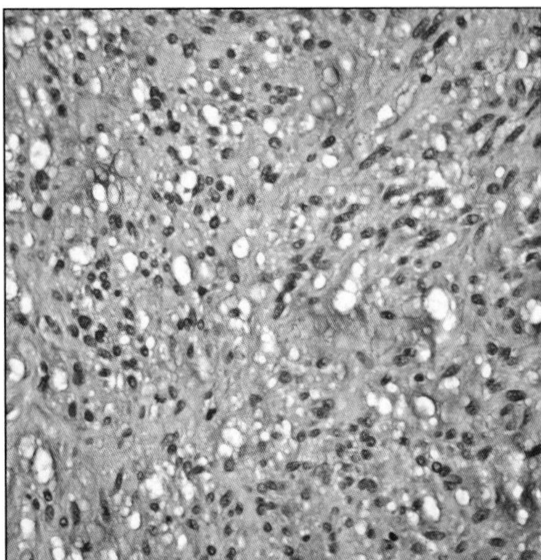

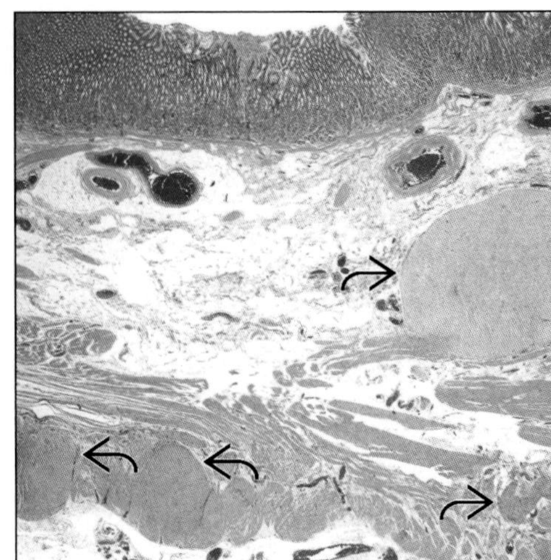

(Left) *Note the cytologic features of this epithelioid gastric GIST. The nuclei are uniform without prominent nucleoli, and there is a chondromyxoid background.* ***(Right)*** *CD34 shows prominent staining in "seedling" GISTs that were detected incidentally in a gastroesophageal resection specimen performed for a carcinoma. Such "seedling" GISTs are commonly found in such specimens if they are sought.*

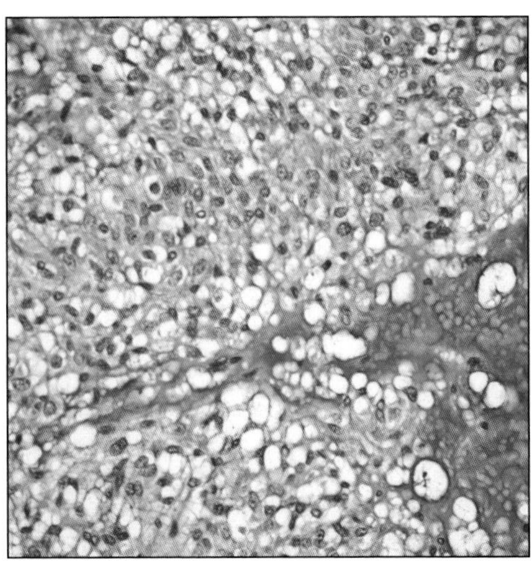

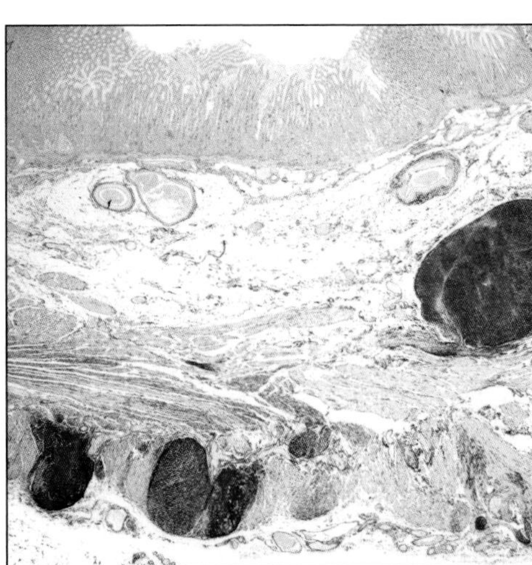

(Left) *CD117 shows labeling in "seedling" GISTs →. Such incidental tumors are very common, suggesting that most GISTs do not progress to clinically significant lesions.* ***(Right)*** *This gross photograph shows a small intestinal GIST. The bulk of the tumor is in the muscularis propria, but the lesion has extended into the submucosa and was diagnosed by mucosal biopsy. Note the overlying mucosa ⇨, which is eroded in places.*

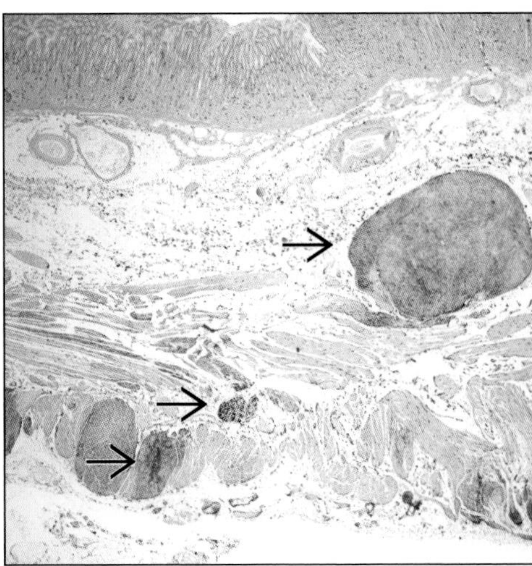

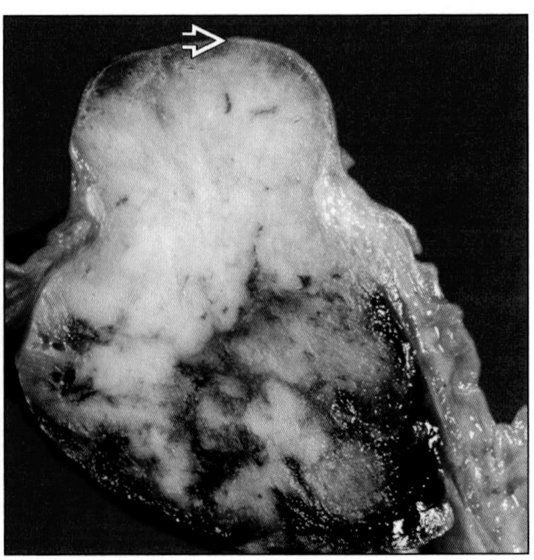

Microscopic Features

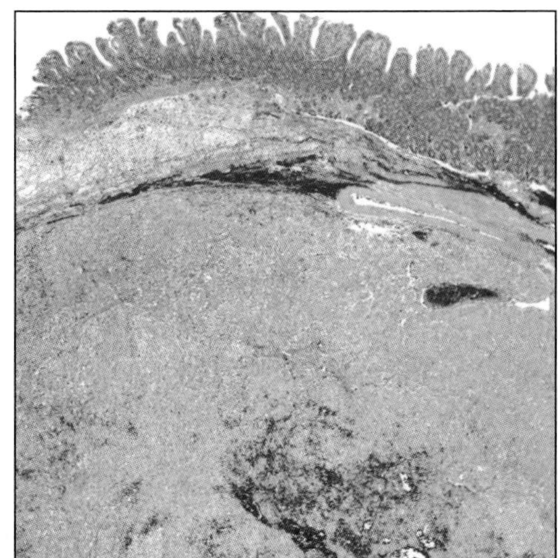

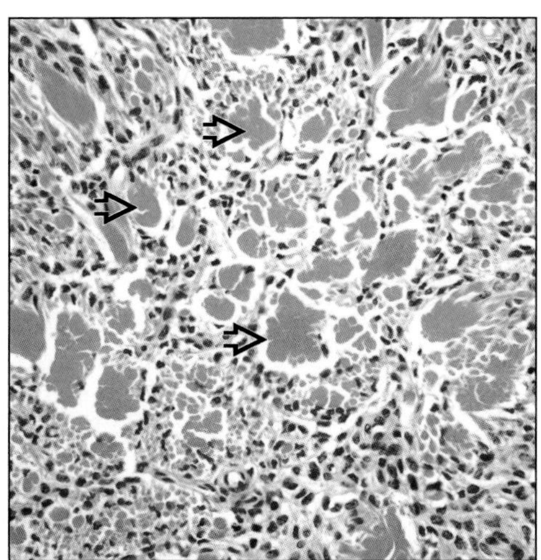

(Left) *This image shows a small intestinal GIST at low magnification. The lesion has extended into the submucosa, and the overlying mucosa appears inflamed.* ***(Right)*** *Prominent "skeinoid" fibers ⇨ consist of thick ropy matrix deposited between tumor cells. These are principally found in small bowel GISTs, where they are associated with a favorable outcome. They can be highlighted with periodic acid-Schiff (PAS) stains.*

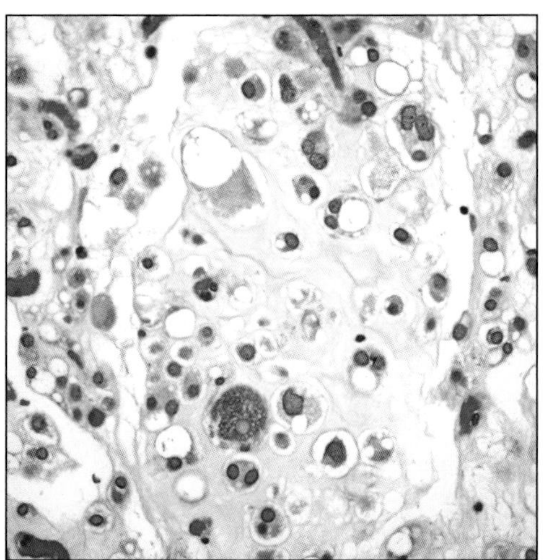

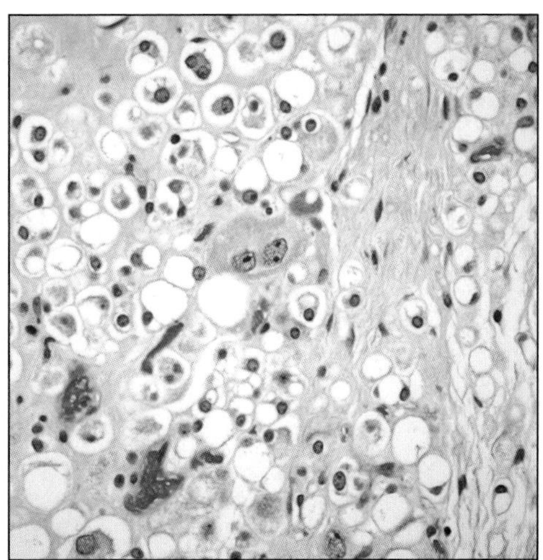

(Left) *This image shows nuclear pleomorphism in an extraintestinal epithelioid GIST. Nuclear pleomorphism is unusual in GISTs, and its presence should prompt other diagnostic considerations. Mesenteric GISTs often behave aggressively.* ***(Right)*** *This image shows striking cytoplasmic vacuoles in an extraintestinal epithelioid GIST. Cases such as this should be addressed as diagnoses of exclusion with an appropriate immunolabeling panel to exclude carcinoma.*

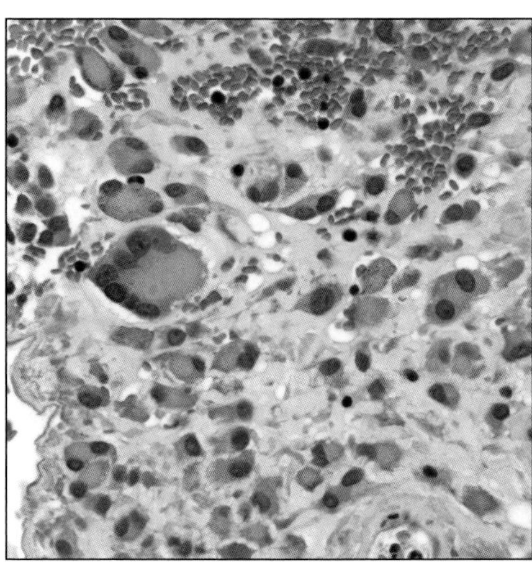

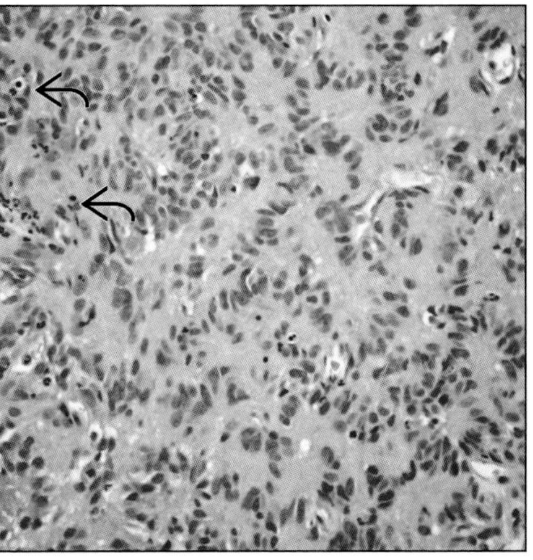

(Left) *This image shows peculiar tumor giant cells and plasmacytoid features in a GIST, a variant pattern.* ***(Right)*** *This small intestinal GIST has an unusual palisaded pattern, similar to that encountered in nerve sheath tumors. This lesion displayed foci of individual tumor cell necrosis ⇗. On immunolabeling, it was strongly CD117 reactive. The patient presented with liver metastases; this lesion proved lethal.*

GASTROINTESTINAL STROMAL TUMOR

Microscopic Features and Ancillary Techniques

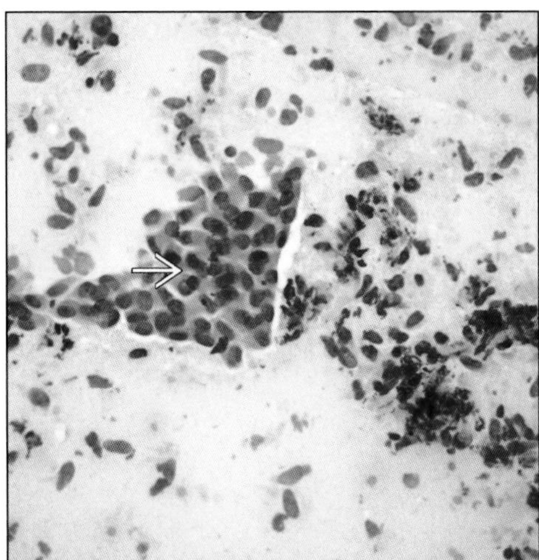

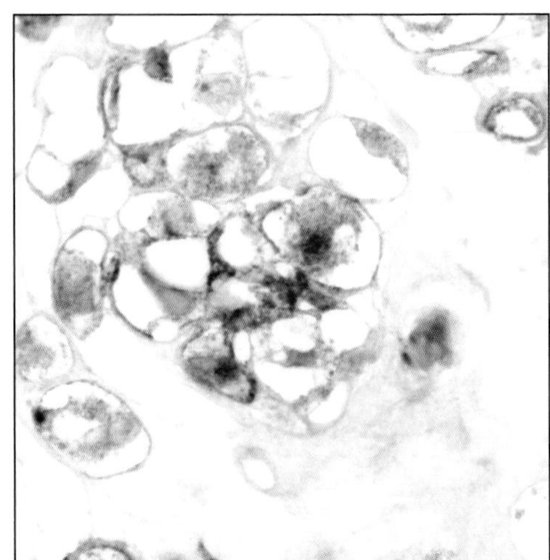

(Left) *This smear was prepared from an aspiration biopsy specimen of a malignant gastric GIST and stained with hematoxylin and eosin. There is a fragment of gastric mucosa* ➡*. The lesional cells do not have specific diagnostic features, although their uniformity suggests GIST; the diagnosis was made by performing immunohistochemistry on cell block material in this case.* ***(Right)*** *CD117 shows both Golgi zone and membranous labeling in this extraintestinal epithelioid GIST.*

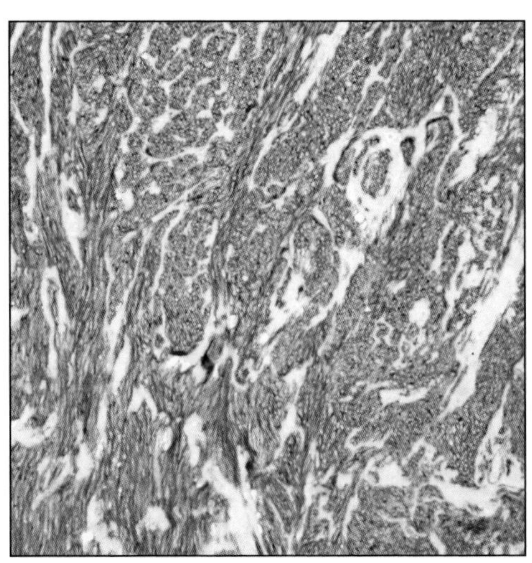

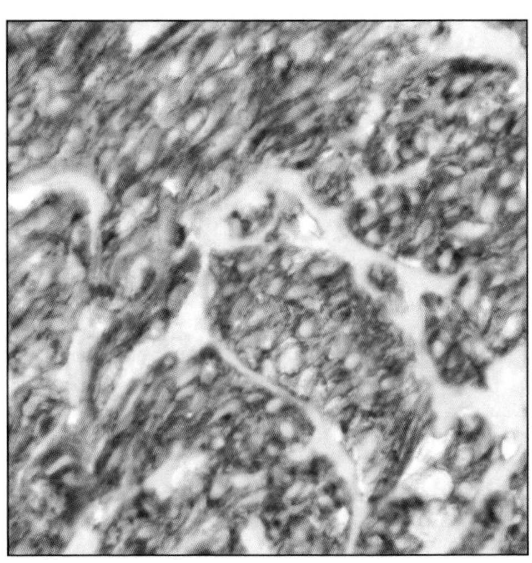

(Left) *CD117 shows strong diffuse labeling in a gastric spindle cell GIST.* ***(Right)*** *CD117 shows membranous and cytoplasmic labeling in a gastric spindle cell GIST. CD117 is extremely useful in confirming an impression of GIST but is is not specific for GIST; for example, melanomas commonly express CD117 in a membranous pattern. Staining with DOG1 can be used to label CD117(-) GISTs. Generally it is prudent to use a panel approach to immunostaining GISTs.*

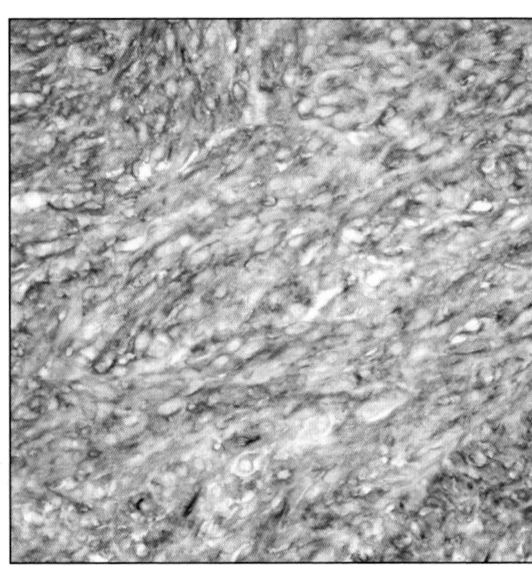

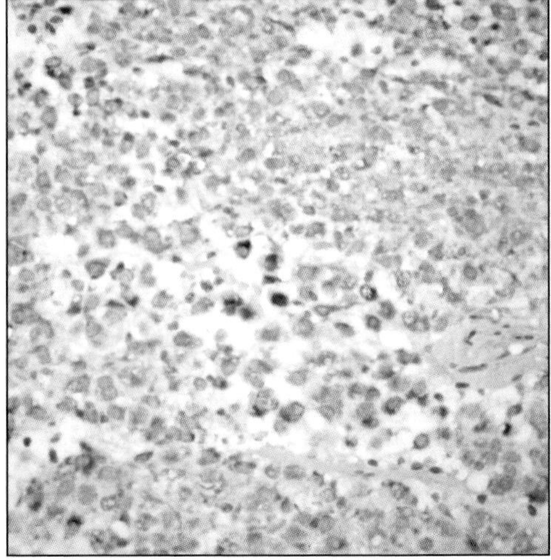

(Left) *CD34 shows cytoplasmic labeling in a gastric spindle cell GIST. About 80% of gastric GISTs express CD34, more than those in the small bowel (about 60%).* ***(Right)*** *Melan-A shows aberrant labeling in an epithelioid gastric GIST, a common finding that should not be misinterpreted as evidence of melanoma. Melanomas can express CD117, so pathologists must use caution interpreting immunolabeling patterns. Most melanomas are CD34(-), whereas most epithelioid GISTs are CD34(+).*

Differential Diagnosis

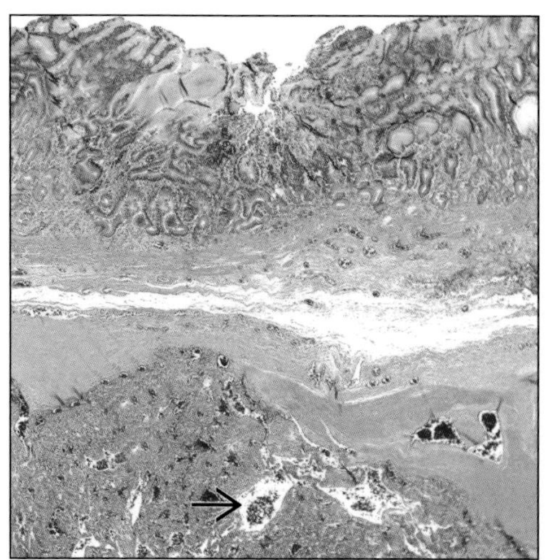

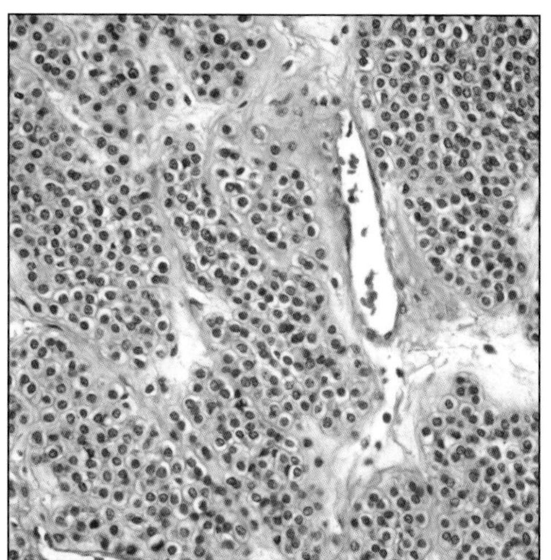

(Left) *This glomus tumor involves the muscularis propria of the stomach, a typical location for gastrointestinal glomus tumors. Most are benign, and all lack KIT mutations. Note the prominent vessels in the lesion ➔.* ***(Right)*** *At high magnification, the lesional cells of glomus tumor are perfectly round and there are prominent intercellular borders. Glomus tumors are richly vascular. The vast majority of gastrointestinal glomus tumors are benign.*

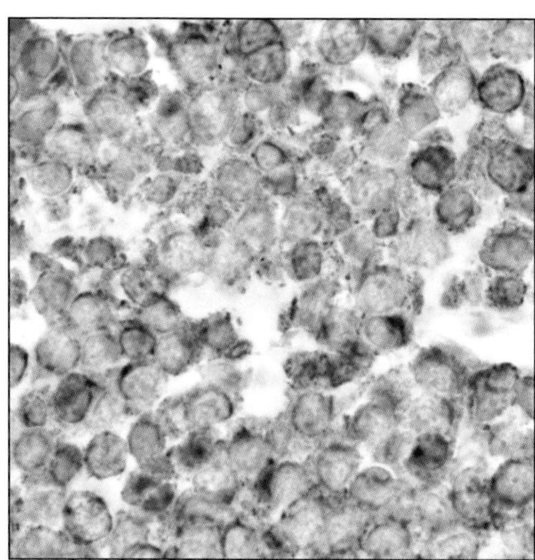

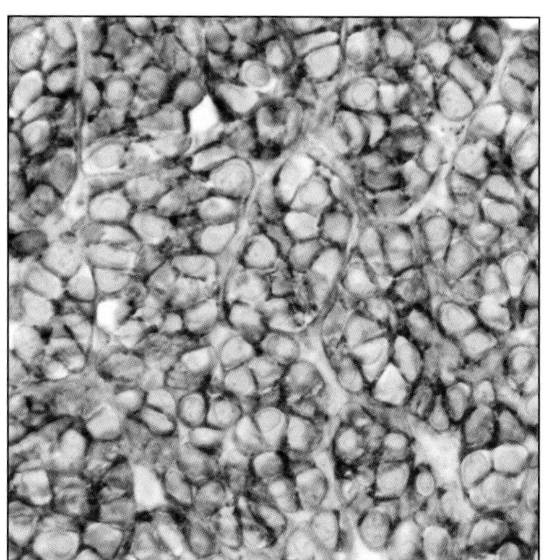

(Left) *Glomus tumors consistently express smooth muscle actin but lack desmin since they are modified smooth muscle cells. They are negative for CD117. They occasionally express synaptophysin, suggesting a neuroendocrine neoplasm, but keratins are negative.* ***(Right)*** *Stains that delineate basement membrane consistently show a net-like pattern in glomus tumors. This is a collagen type IV immunostain, but a similar pattern would be encountered using laminin stains.*

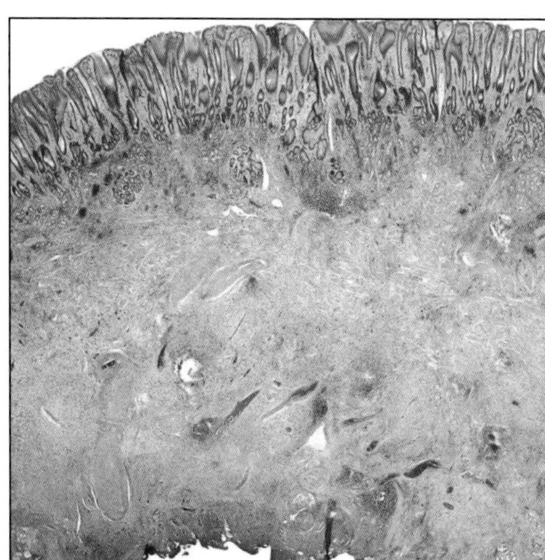

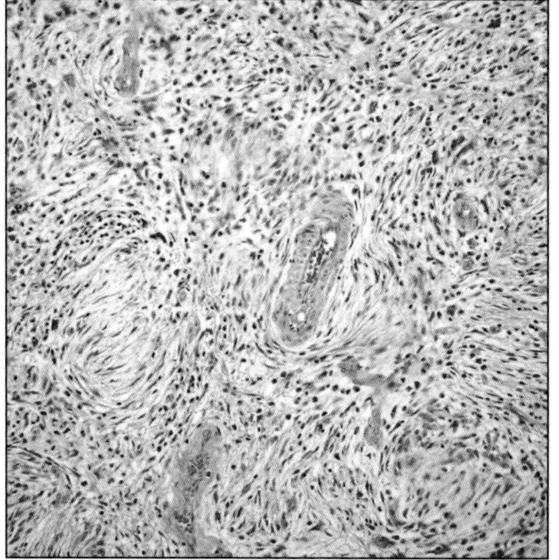

(Left) *Inflammatory fibroid polyp, like GIST, can harbor PDGFRA mutations but it has different morphology and is always benign. This lesion is centered in the submucosa of the antrum, the typical location for these tumors.* ***(Right)*** *At intermediate magnification, inflammatory fibroid polyp shows spindle cells that are arranged in a whorled configuration encircling blood vessels in a manner resembling onion skin. There is an eosinophil-rich inflammatory backdrop.*

FOLLICULAR DENDRITIC CELL SARCOMA

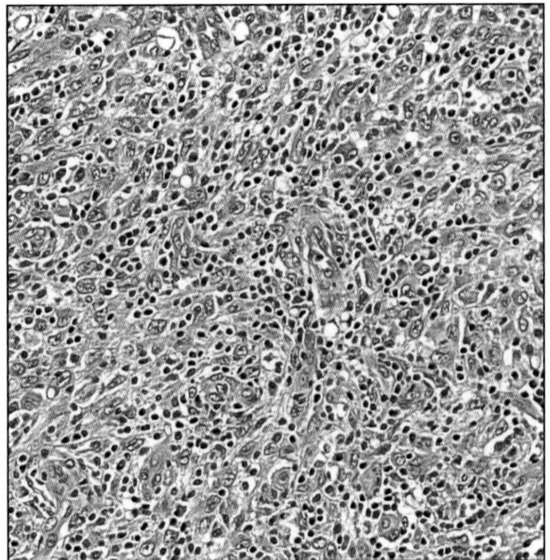

Hematoxylin & eosin shows sheets of ovoid tumor cells with admixed adherent lymphocytes and prominent blood vessels.

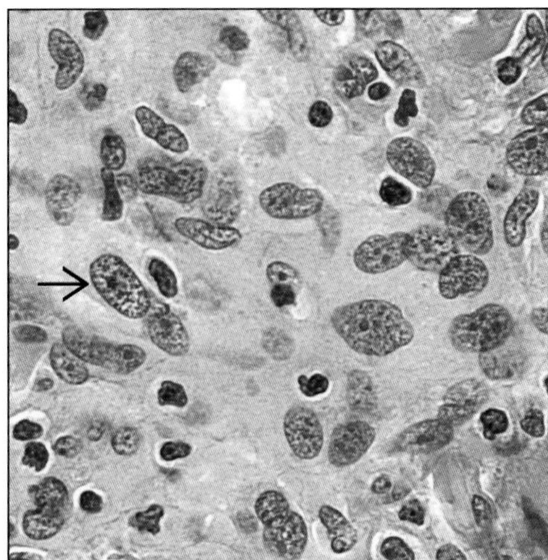

Hematoxylin & eosin shows neoplastic cells that have distinctive oval nuclei with speckled chromatin, small nucleoli, and prominent nuclear membrane ⇒. Indistinct cell margins give syncytial look.

TERMINOLOGY

Abbreviations

- Follicular dendritic cell sarcoma (FDCS)

Synonyms

- Dendritic reticulum cell sarcoma

Definitions

- Malignant tumor of follicular dendritic cells
  - Antigen-trapping cells of accessory immune system
  - Normally in germinal center of lymph node

ETIOLOGY/PATHOGENESIS

Varied Etiologies

- Most cases arise de novo
- 10-15% arise in hyaline-vascular-type Castleman disease
  - Antecedent dendritic cell hyperplasia and dysplasia
- Inflammatory pseudotumor-like variant is associated with EBV

CLINICAL ISSUES

Epidemiology

- Age
  - Young and middle-aged adults
- Gender
  - Slight female predominance

Site

- Majority involve lymph nodes
  - Neck, mediastinum
  - Spleen, tonsil
  - Liver
- Inflammatory pseudotumor-like variant
  - Females, in liver or spleen
- Over 1/3 arise in extranodal sites
  - GI tract: Stomach, colon
  - Mesentery, mesocolon, mediastinum
  - Head and neck: Pharynx, palate
  - Soft tissue sites: Neck, axilla, breast

Presentation

- Painless mass

Natural History

- Local recurrence
- Can metastasize to lymph nodes and lung

Treatment

- Surgical approaches
  - Adequate local excision
- Drugs
  - Chemotherapy for recurrent or metastatic disease

Prognosis

- Among extranodal cases
  - 43% recur locally
  - Late relapse common
  - At least 7% die of disease
  - 5-year recurrence-free survival is 27%

MACROSCOPIC FEATURES

General Features

- Firm white mass; rarely hemorrhage or necrosis

Size

- Up to 20 cm maximum dimension in reported cases

MICROSCOPIC PATHOLOGY

Histologic Features

- Ovoid cells in sheets, fascicles, or storiform whorls
- Long cell processes
- Nuclei distinctive
  - Dispersed, speckled chromatin with nucleolus

FOLLICULAR DENDRITIC CELL SARCOMA

Key Facts

Terminology
- Malignant tumor of follicular dendritic cells

Clinical Issues
- Over 1/3 arise in extranodal sites
- Can metastasize to lymph nodes and lung
- 43% recur locally

Microscopic Pathology
- Ovoid cells in sheets, fascicles, or storiform whorls
- Nuclei distinctive
  - Dispersed, speckled chromatin, small nucleolus
  - Prominent nuclear membrane
- Long cell processes
- Lymphocytes adherent to cell bodies and processes
- Rarely dense mixed chronic inflammatory infiltrate
  - Scattered neoplastic cells

Ancillary Tests
- Immunoreactive for
  - CD21 and CD35 (best used as cocktail)
  - CD23, podoplanin, fascin, clusterin, EGFR
  - S100 protein in 40%
  - EMA in 80%, desmoplakin in 60%
- EM shows interdigitating processes with desmosomes

Top Differential Diagnoses
- Lymphoepithelial carcinoma
  - Cytokeratin(+)
- Interdigitating reticulum cell sarcoma
  - Lacks follicular dendritic cell markers
- Anaplastic large cell lymphoma
  - CD30(+), CD45(+)
- Spindle cell sarcomas: Relevant markers positive

  - Prominent nuclear membrane
- Lymphocytes adherent to cell bodies and processes
- Multinucleated cells
- Mitoses and atypia sometimes
- Necrosis in rare examples

Predominant Cell/Compartment Type
- Mesenchymal, spindle

Inflammatory Pseudotumor-like Variant
- Dense mixed chronic inflammatory infiltrate
- Scattered neoplastic cells

Myxoid Variant
- Marked myxoid stroma
- Cells separated, lymphocytes remain adherent

ANCILLARY TESTS

Immunohistochemistry
- Positive for
  - CD21 (complement C3d receptor) and CD35 (C3b receptor) (best used as cocktail)
  - CD23, podoplanin, fascin, clusterin, EGFR
  - S100 protein in 40%
  - EMA in 80%, desmoplakin in 60%
  - EBER in inflammatory pseudotumor-like variant
- Negative for
  - CD45, CD30, cytokeratins, desmin

Electron Microscopy
- EM shows interdigitating processes with desmosomes

DIFFERENTIAL DIAGNOSIS

Lymphoepithelial Carcinoma
- Syncytial growth pattern
- Cytokeratin positivity

Interdigitating Reticulum Cell Sarcoma
- More pleomorphic
- S100 protein(+)
- Lacks follicular dendritic cell markers
- EM shows processes but no desmosomes

Anaplastic Large Cell Lymphoma
- CD30(+); lacks follicular dendritic cell markers

Spindle Cell Sarcomas
- Nuclear morphology differs
- Panel of markers identifies specific types
- Absence of CD21, CD35

SELECTED REFERENCES

1. Padilla-Rodríguez AL et al: Intra-abdominal follicular dendritic cell sarcoma with marked pleomorphic features and aberrant expression of neuroendocrine markers: report of a case with immunohistochemical analysis. Appl Immunohistochem Mol Morphol. 15(3):346-52, 2007
2. Soriano AO et al: Follicular dendritic cell sarcoma: a report of 14 cases and a review of the literature. Am J Hematol. 82(8):725-8, 2007
3. Shia J et al: Extranodal follicular dendritic cell sarcoma: clinical, pathologic, and histogenetic characteristics of an underrecognized disease entity. Virchows Arch. 449(2):148-58, 2006
4. Grogg KL et al: A survey of clusterin and fascin expression in sarcomas and spindle cell neoplasms: strong clusterin immunostaining is highly specific for follicular dendritic cell tumor. Mod Pathol. 18(2):260-6, 2005
5. Biddle DA et al: Extranodal follicular dendritic cell sarcoma of the head and neck region: three new cases, with a review of the literature. Mod Pathol. 15(1):50-8, 2002
6. Chan AC et al: Development of follicular dendritic cell sarcoma in hyaline-vascular Castleman's disease of the nasopharynx: tracing its evolution by sequential biopsies. Histopathology. 38(6):510-8, 2001
7. Fisher C et al: Myxoid variant of follicular dendritic cell sarcoma arising in the breast. Ann Diagn Pathol. 3(2):92-8, 1999
8. Arber DA et al: Detection of Epstein-Barr Virus in inflammatory pseudotumor. Semin Diagn Pathol. 15(2):155-60, 1998
9. Chan JK et al: Follicular dendritic cell sarcoma. Clinicopathologic analysis of 17 cases suggesting a malignant potential higher than currently recognized. Cancer. 79(2):294-313, 1997

FOLLICULAR DENDRITIC CELL SARCOMA

Microscopic Features

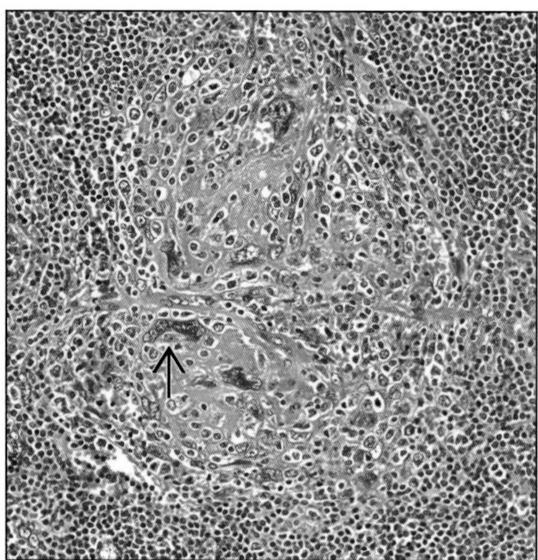

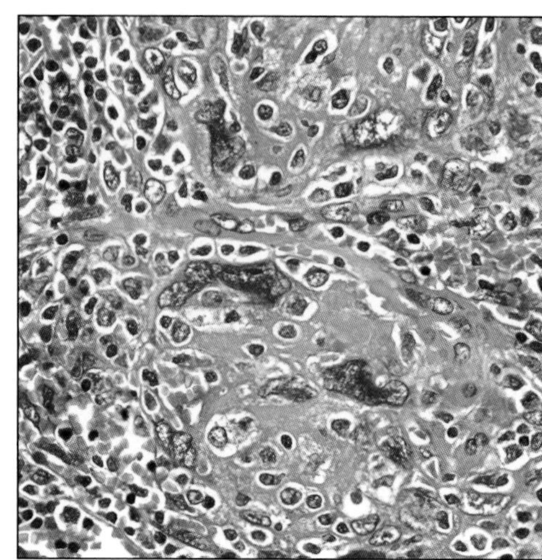

(Left) *Hematoxylin & eosin shows dendritic cell dysplasia in lymph node in hyaline-vascular-type of Castleman disease (angiofollicular hyperplasia). Atypical cells ⇒ are scattered within abnormal follicle.* ***(Right)*** *Hematoxylin & eosin shows dysplastic dendritic cells that display enlarged, irregular-shaped nuclei with coarse chromatin and nucleoli.*

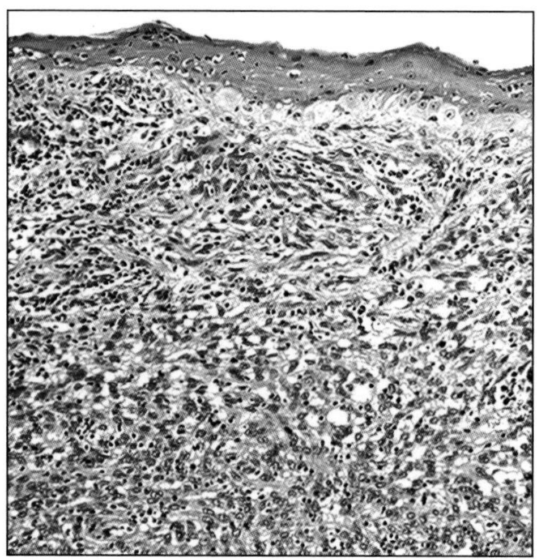

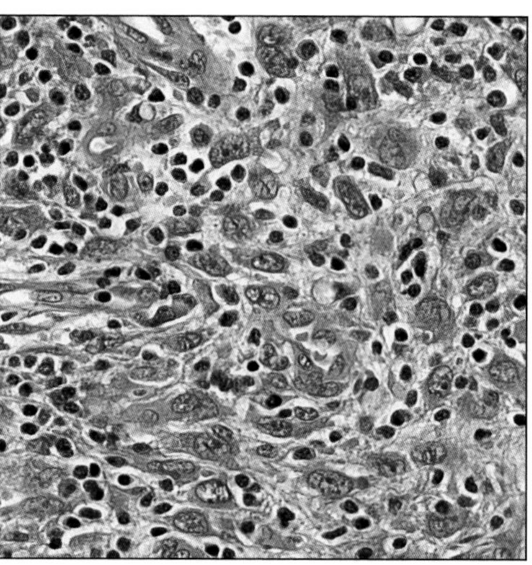

(Left) *Hematoxylin & eosin shows follicular dendritic cell sarcoma in the pharynx. The tumor is poorly circumscribed and infiltrates beneath squamous epithelium. This patient presented with difficulty swallowing and was found to have a large pharyngeal polyp.* ***(Right)*** *Hematoxylin & eosin shows uniform tumor cells with closely related infiltrating mature lymphocytes. The lymphocytes are considered as reactive rather than neoplastic and comprise a mixture of T and B cells.*

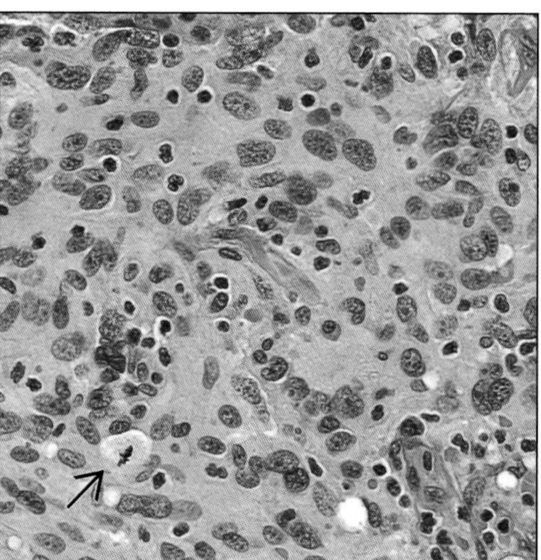

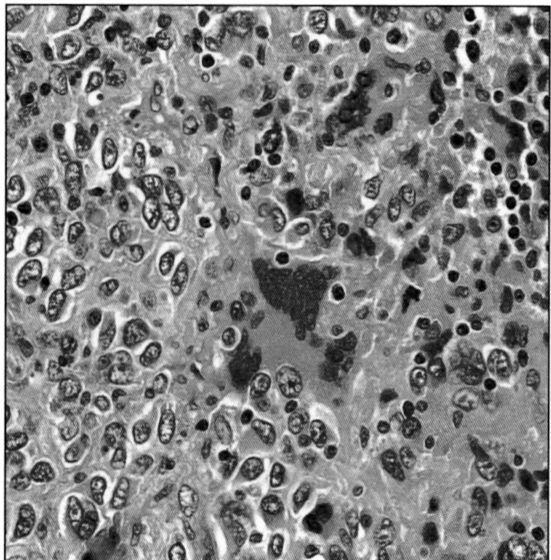

(Left) *Hematoxylin & eosin shows an area with only sparse lymphocytes. Cells appear syncytial, and tumor cell nuclei are separated or focally appear to overlap. Note mitotic figure ⇒.* ***(Right)*** *Hematoxylin & eosin shows multinucleated giant cells, which are sometimes a feature of follicular dendritic cell sarcoma (FDCS).*

Microscopic Features and Ancillary Techniques

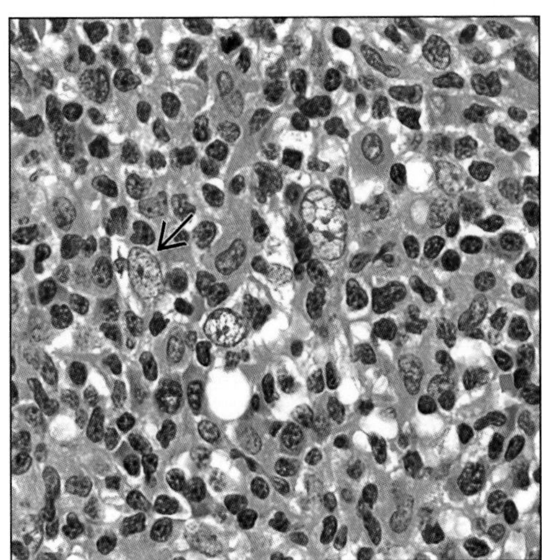

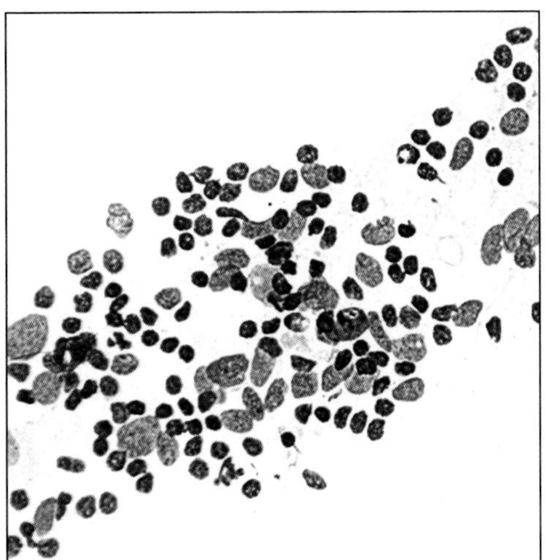

(Left) *Hematoxylin & eosin shows inflammatory pseudotumor-like (EBV-associated) variant of FDCS. Neoplastic cells* ➔ *are sparse in dense mixed chronic inflammation. Immunohistochemistry is required for diagnosis.* ***(Right)*** *Diff-Quik shows fine needle aspirate with neoplastic cells that demonstrate the typical speckled chromatin pattern of FDCS. Note the lymphocytes that accompany the aspirated tumor cells.*

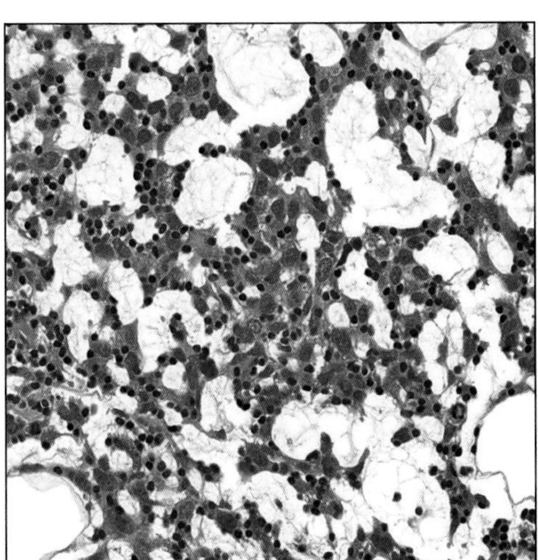

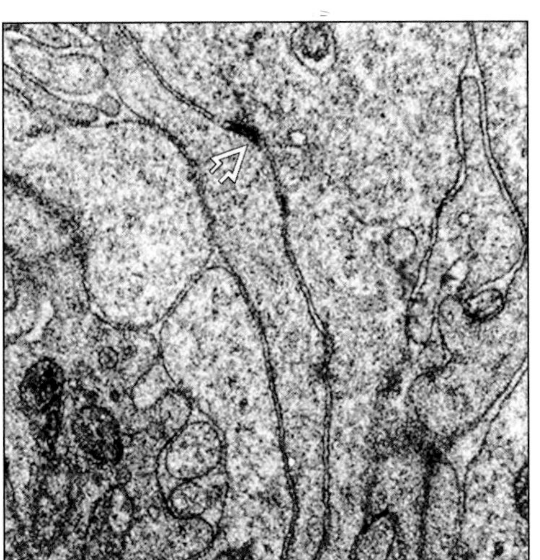

(Left) *Hematoxylin & eosin shows myxoid variant of FDCS. Cells are separated by prominent myxoid stroma. The lymphocytes mostly remain adherent to tumor cells. This tumor arose in the breast of a 41-year-old woman and metastasized to axillary lymph nodes several years later.* ***(Right)*** *TEM shows elongated interdigitating cell processes with occasional intercellular desmosome-like junctions* ➯.

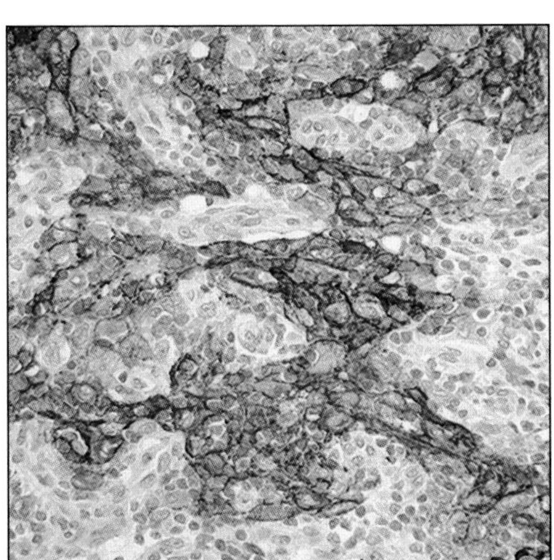

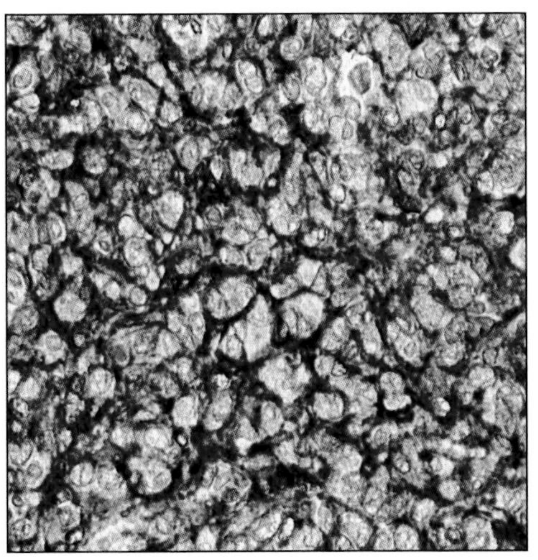

(Left) *Positive CD21 shows immunoreactivity on cell bodies and processes of infiltrating neoplastic cells.* ***(Right)*** *Positive CD21 shows membranous pattern of staining tumor cells, which form a sheet in this example.*

INTERDIGITATING RETICULUM CELL SARCOMA

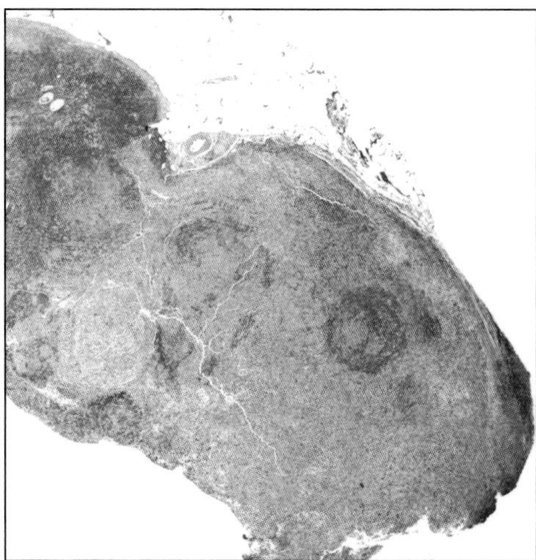

Interdigitating dendritic cell sarcoma subtotally replacing lymph node shows that the neoplasm tends to spare lymphoid follicles. The neoplasm was S100 protein(+).

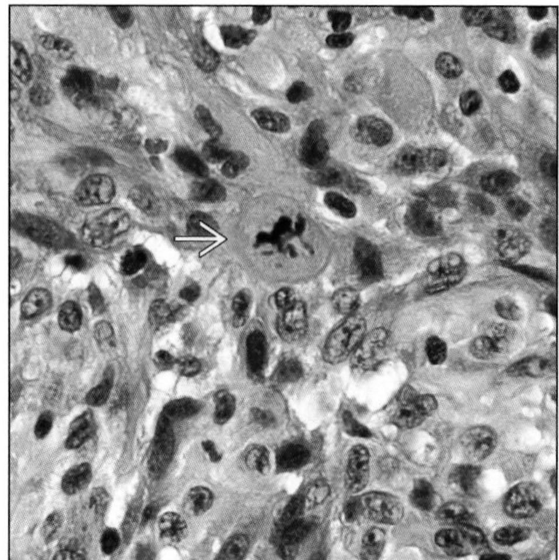

Interdigitating dendritic cell sarcoma involving lymph node shows that the neoplastic cells are spindled and epithelioid with abundant eosinophilic cytoplasm. A mitotic figure is present ➔.

TERMINOLOGY

Synonyms

- Interdigitating dendritic cell (IDC) tumor
- Interdigitating dendritic reticulum cell sarcoma

Definitions

- Neoplastic proliferation of cells with immunophenotype similar to normal IDCs

ETIOLOGY/PATHOGENESIS

Postulated Normal Cell Counterpart is IDC

- Antigen-presenting cell involved in T-cell immunity
- Derived from CD34(+) lymphoid/myeloid progenitor cell in bone marrow that homes to lymph node
- Normally found in
  - T-cell regions of lymph node
  - Periarteriolar lymphoid sheaths
  - Interfollicular areas of extranodal lymphoid tissue

Concept of "Transdifferentiation"

- Rare patients with histiocytic neoplasms also have clonally related B-cell lymphoma
  - Usually B-cell lymphoma precedes histiocytic neoplasm
    - IDC sarcoma and follicular lymphoma
    - Histiocytic sarcoma and follicular lymphoma
    - IDC sarcoma and chronic lymphocytic leukemia/small lymphocytic lymphoma
    - Histiocytic sarcoma and splenic marginal zone lymphoma
  - Histiocytic neoplasms associated with follicular lymphoma share
    - t(14;18)(q32;q21)/*BCL2-IgH* &/or identical *IgH* gene rearrangements
  - Histiocytic tumors and nonfollicular B-cell lymphomas share identical *IgH* gene rearrangements
- B-cell lymphoma might transform to histiocytic phenotype via "transdifferentiation"
  - Possibly due to loss of key components of B-cell differentiation

CLINICAL ISSUES

Epidemiology

- Incidence
  - Very rare
- Age
  - Most patients are adults; median: 6th-7th decade
  - Youngest patient reported was 2 years old
- Gender
  - Male to female ratio = 1.2:1

Site

- Lymph node
  - Most commonly a single lymph node is involved
  - Cervical, axillary, or inguinal lymph node groups most often affected
- Extranodal sites can be involved
  - Skin and soft tissue most common
  - Liver and spleen
  - Gastrointestinal tract, lung, kidney
  - Bone marrow is involved in < 20% of patients

Presentation

- Slow-growing, asymptomatic mass is most common
- Systemic symptoms occur in subset
  - Fever, night sweats, fatigue
- Some have IDC sarcoma and another hematopoietic neoplasm including
  - Chronic lymphocytic leukemia/small lymphocytic lymphoma
  - Mycosis fungoides
  - Acute lymphoblastic leukemia (mostly of T-cell lineage)
- Some have IDC sarcoma and carcinoma
  - Most common types: Breast, stomach, liver, colon

INTERDIGITATING RETICULUM CELL SARCOMA

Key Facts

Clinical Issues
- Wide age range
- Single lymph nodes most commonly involved
  - Cervical, axillary, or inguinal groups
  - Slow-growing, asymptomatic mass
- Rare cases associated with B- or T-cell lymphomas or leukemias

Microscopic Pathology
- Partial or complete replacement of lymph node architecture
- Sheets, whorls, nests, or fascicles
- Spindle-shaped or epithelioid cells
- Cytologic atypia can be mild or prominent

Ancillary Tests
- Immunohistochemistry
  - S100 strongly positive
  - Fascin(+)
  - CD68, CD45, lysozyme variable
- Molecular genetics
  - HUMARA has shown clonality in small subset of cases tested
  - Antigen receptor genes are usually in germline configuration
  - No chromosomal translocations
  - IDC sarcoma in patients with follicular lymphoma carry *IgH* rearrangements and t(14;18)/*IgH-BCL2*

Top Differential Diagnoses
- Langerhans cell sarcoma
- Follicular dendritic cell sarcoma
- Histiocytic sarcoma
- Melanoma

Treatment
- Surgical resection and radiation therapy for patients with localized disease
- No current established chemotherapy regimen
  - ABVD (doxorubicin, bleomycin, vincristine, and dacarbazine) and other regimens have been used
    - Many patients initially respond but relapse, and death is common in this subset of patients

Prognosis
- Variable clinical course
  - 40-50% of patients develop disseminated disease with poor outcome

IMAGE FINDINGS

Radiographic Findings
- Lymphadenopathy
- Positron emission tomography (PET) often shows increased fluorodeoxyglucose (FDG) uptake

MACROSCOPIC FEATURES

General Features
- Hemorrhage and necrosis can be present

Size
- Variable; range: 1-6 cm in most studies
- Lobulated mass with firm cut surface

MICROSCOPIC PATHOLOGY

Histologic Features
- Partial or complete replacement of lymph node architecture
  - Paracortical pattern in cases of partial involvement
    - Spares lymphoid follicles
  - Sinusoidal pattern of involvement can be prominent
- Sheets, whorls, nests, or fascicles
- Spindle-shaped or epithelioid cells
  - Vesicular nuclei; nucleoli can be small or prominent
  - Abundant eosinophilic cytoplasm with indistinct cell borders
- Cytologic atypia can be mild or prominent
  - Mitotic rate is variable; usually high in cases with marked atypia
- Inflammatory cells are common in background
  - Small lymphocytes present; usually T cells
  - Eosinophils and plasma cells (+/-)
- Hemophagocytosis is uncommon but has been reported

Cytologic Features
- Difficult diagnosis to establish by fine needle aspiration (FNA)
- Neoplastic cells in FNA smears are cytologically similar to those observed in tissue sections

ANCILLARY TESTS

Cytogenetics
- No recurrent cytogenetic abnormalities have been reported

In Situ Hybridization
- Epstein-Barr virus encoded RNA (EBER) is negative

Molecular Genetics
- Human androgen receptor assay (HUMARA) has shown clonality in small subset of cases tested
- In accord with origin from IDC
  - Antigen receptor genes are usually in germline configuration
  - No chromosomal translocations
- IDC sarcoma in patients with follicular lymphoma share
  - Monoclonal *IgH* rearrangements and t(14;18)(q32;q21)/*IgH-BCL2*

Electron Microscopy
- Transmission

INTERDIGITATING RETICULUM CELL SARCOMA

Immunohistochemistry

Antibody	Reactivity	Staining Pattern	Comment
S100	Positive	Nuclear & cytoplasmic	
CD11c	Positive	Cell membrane	
HLA-DR	Positive	Cell membrane	
Fascin	Positive	Cytoplasmic	
Vimentin	Positive	Cytoplasmic	
CD1a	Negative	Cell membrane	Occasional cases are positive
CD20	Negative	Cell membrane	
CD3	Negative	Cell membrane	
CD21	Negative	Cell membrane & cytoplasm	
CD35	Negative	Cell membrane & cytoplasm	
CD23	Negative	Cell membrane & cytoplasm	
CD30	Negative	Cell membrane	
CD68	Equivocal	Cytoplasmic	Positive in about 60% of cases
CD45	Equivocal	Cell membrane	Positive in about 60% of cases
CD4	Equivocal	Cell membrane	Positive in some cases
Lysozyme	Equivocal	Cytoplasmic	Positive in some cases

- Long, complex interdigitating cell processes and irregularly shaped nuclei
- No Birbeck granules, well-formed desmosomes, or melanosomes

DIFFERENTIAL DIAGNOSIS

Langerhans Cell Sarcoma

- Most commonly occurs in extranodal sites (e.g., skin, bone)
- Neoplastic IDC and Langerhans cells are cytologically similar
- Mitotic rate is usually high
- S100(+)
- CD1a(+) and langerin(+) (can be focal)
- Electron microscopy shows Birbeck granules

Follicular Dendritic Cell Sarcoma

- Commonly more spindled than IDC sarcoma
- Nuclear pseudoinclusions
- Binucleated, squared off follicular dendritic cells
- Reactive small lymphocytes of B-cell lineage
- Clusterin(+), fascin(+), and EGFR(+)
- CD21(+), CD23(+), CD35(+) in many cases
- S100(+) and EMA(+) in some
- Electron microscopy shows desmosomes

Histiocytic Sarcoma

- Tumor cells typically epithelioid without spindling
- CD68(+) and CD163(+)
- Lysozyme(+) and S100(+) in some

Metastatic Melanoma

- More pleomorphic, more necrosis
- History of primary neoplasm elsewhere
- HMB-45, Melan-A, tyrosinase variably positive

Malignant Peripheral Nerve Sheath Tumor

- Often related to nerve or neurofibroma
- S100 protein focally positive
  - Diffuse in epithelioid MPNST
    - Prominent nucleoli, INI negative (50%)

Metastatic Carcinoma

- Cells more cohesive
- More pleomorphic, more necrosis
- History of primary carcinoma elsewhere
- CK(+) and EMA(+), S100 in some

SELECTED REFERENCES

1. Orii T et al: Differential immunophenotypic analysis of dendritic cell tumours. J Clin Pathol. 63(6):497-503, 2010
2. Wang E et al: Histiocytic sarcoma arising in indolent small B-cell lymphoma: report of two cases with molecular/genetic evidence suggestive of a 'transdifferentiation' during the clonal evolution. Leuk Lymphoma. 51(5):802-12, 2010
3. Zhang D: Histiocytic sarcoma arising from lymphomas via transdifferentiation pathway during clonal evolution. Leuk Lymphoma. 51(5):739-40, 2010
4. Fraser CR et al: Transformation of chronic lymphocytic leukemia/small lymphocytic lymphoma to interdigitating dendritic cell sarcoma: evidence for transdifferentiation of the lymphoma clone. Am J Clin Pathol. 132(6):928-39, 2009
5. Feldman AL et al: Clonally related follicular lymphomas and histiocytic/dendritic cell sarcomas: evidence for transdifferentiation of the follicular lymphoma clone. Blood. 111(12):5433-9, 2008
6. Pileri SA et al: Tumours of histiocytes and accessory dendritic cells: an immunohistochemical approach to classification from the International Lymphoma Study Group based on 61 cases. Histopathology. 41(1):1-29, 2002
7. Gaertner EM et al: Interdigitating dendritic cell sarcoma. A report of four cases and review of the literature. Am J Clin Pathol. 115(4):589-97, 2001

Microscopic Features

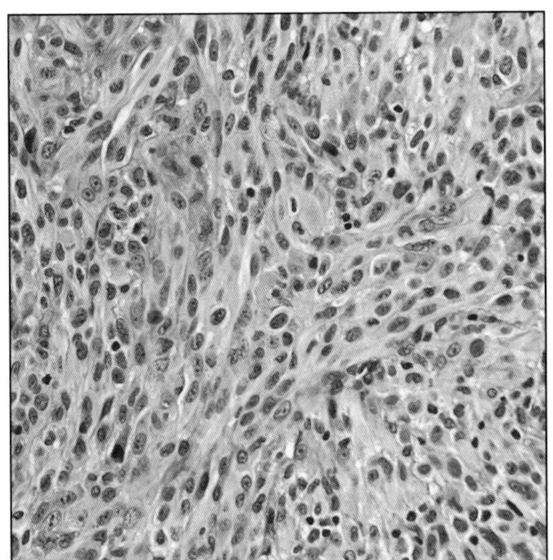

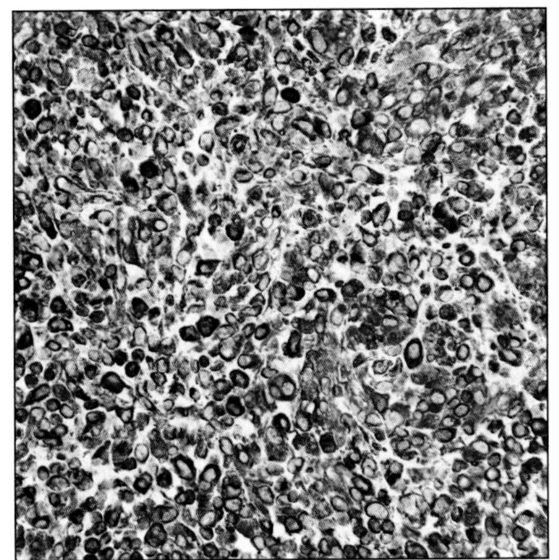

(Left) *Interdigitating dendritic cell (IDC) sarcoma replacing lymph node shows the neoplastic cells have abundant eosinophilic cytoplasm and are of spindle shape in this field, forming a storiform pattern. This case of IDC sarcoma showed mild to moderate atypia and had a relatively low mitotic rate.* ***(Right)*** *Interdigitating dendritic cell sarcoma replacing lymph node shows strong expression of vimentin. The neoplastic cells were also positive for S100 protein (not shown).*

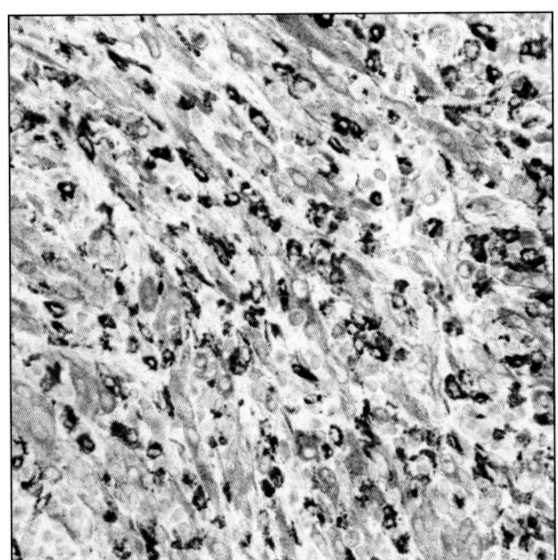

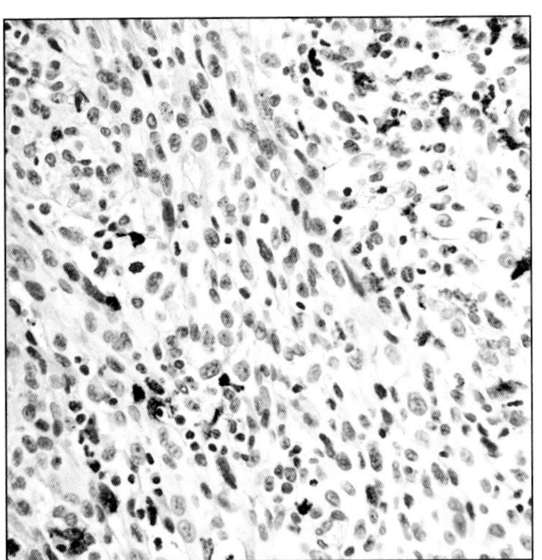

(Left) *Interdigitating dendritic cell sarcoma replacing lymph node shows moderate and variable expression of the lysosomal antigen CD68. The neoplastic cells were also positive for S100 protein (not shown).* ***(Right)*** *Interdigitating dendritic cell sarcoma replacing lymph node shows that the neoplastic cells are negative for CD45/LCA. Small reactive lymphocytes in the background are positive. This neoplasm was positive for S100 protein (not shown).*

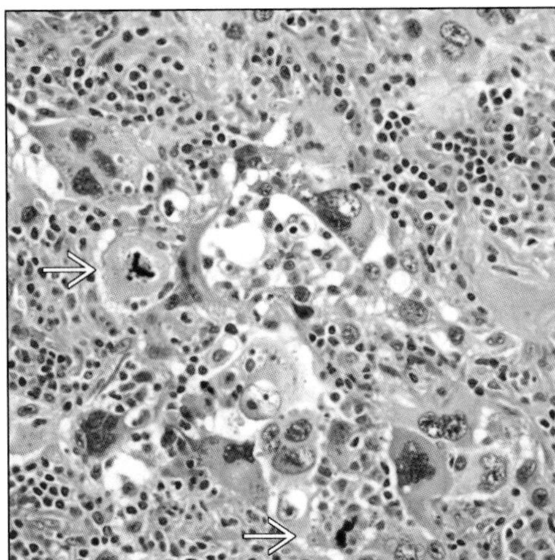

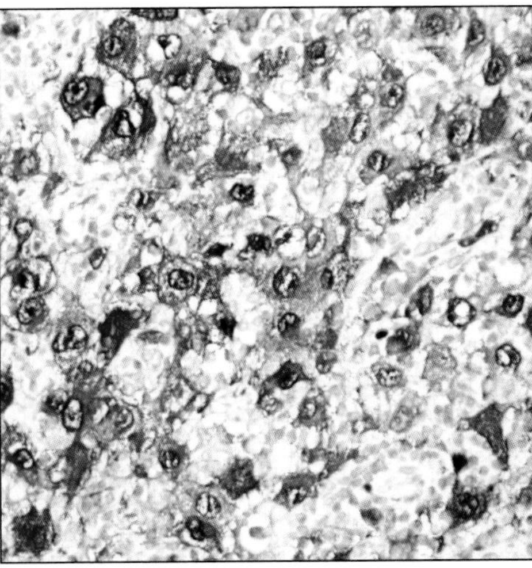

(Left) *The neoplastic cells in this case of IDC sarcoma involving lymph node show marked nuclear atypia and abundant eosinophilic cytoplasm and are oval to round in shape. This case of IDC sarcoma showed marked atypia and had a high mitotic rate, with 2 mitotic figures ➔ in this field.* ***(Right)*** *Interdigitating dendritic cell sarcoma involving lymph node shows the neoplastic cells strongly express S100 protein.*

LYMPHOMA OF SOFT TISSUE

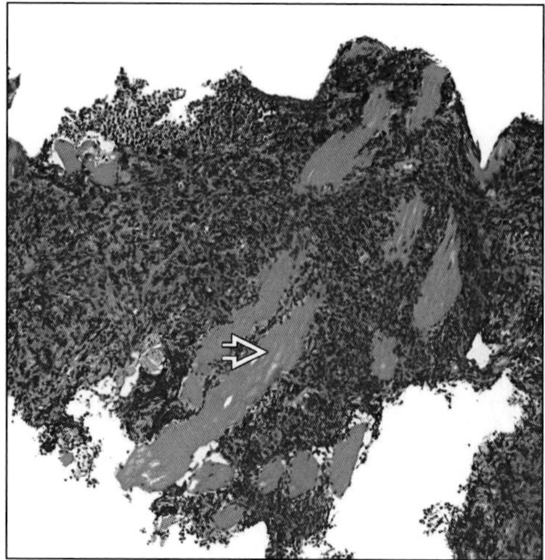

This core biopsy specimen shows skeletal muscle ➡ involved by lymphoma, which is composed of sheets of monotonous round cells. The pattern of infiltration between muscle fibers is characteristic of lymphoma.

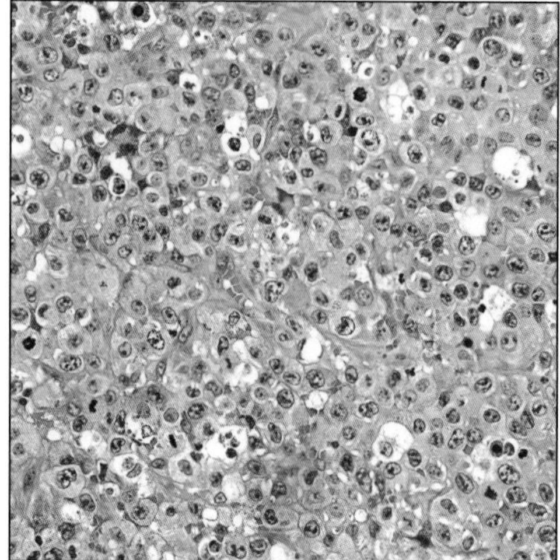

This anaplastic large cell lymphoma is composed of sheets of atypical polygonal cells. In soft tissue, this can be mistaken for pleomorphic sarcoma as well as pleomorphic neoplasms of other lineages.

TERMINOLOGY

Definitions

- Group of malignant neoplasms of lymphoreticular system that arise in soft tissue as a primary site, without evidence of lymph node or skin involvement

ETIOLOGY/PATHOGENESIS

Lymphomas Can Develop Secondary to

- Chronic inflammation and autoimmune mechanisms
  - e.g., lymphoma of mucosa-associated lymphoid tissue
- Immunocompromise

CLINICAL ISSUES

Epidemiology

- Incidence
  - Prevalence of true extranodal soft tissue lymphoma is low
- Gender
  - M = F

Site

- Virtually any soft tissue site
  - Exclude lymphadenopathy at other sites

Presentation

- Suddenly enlarging mass
  - Systemic symptoms may be present

Treatment

- Chemotherapy &/or radiotherapy
- Surgical excision not indicated

MICROSCOPIC PATHOLOGY

Histologic Features

- Soft tissue lymphomas are most commonly large cell lymphomas with B-cell phenotype
  - Infiltrative sheets of medium to large cells
    - Ovoid nuclei
    - Moderate amounts of amphophilic cytoplasm
    - Variably prominent nucleoli
    - Heterogeneous population of smaller lymphoid cells may be intermixed
- Other types include
  - Small cell lymphomas
  - Lymphoblastic lymphoma/leukemia
  - Anaplastic large cell lymphoma

ANCILLARY TESTS

Immunohistochemistry

- Most express CD45
- Approximately 80-85% of lymphoid neoplasms originate from B cells
  - CD20, CD79-α, etc.
- Relevant markers for other types
  - CD30, ALK, CD3, TdT, and other lymphoid markers

DIFFERENTIAL DIAGNOSIS

Ewing Sarcoma

- Lymphoblastic lymphoma can also be CD99(+), FLI-1(+), and CD45(-)
- TdT(-)
- Characteristic translocations involving fusions between *EWSR1* and *ETS* family of genes

Alveolar Rhabdomyosarcoma

- Characteristic nested pattern resembling pulmonary alveoli, present at least focally in most tumors

LYMPHOMA OF SOFT TISSUE

Key Facts

Terminology
- Group of malignant neoplasms of lymphoreticular system that arise in soft tissue as a primary site, without evidence of lymph node or skin involvement

Clinical Issues
- Virtually any soft tissue site
  - Prevalence of true extranodal soft tissue lymphoma is low
  - Therefore, important to exclude dissemination from other sites
- Systemic symptoms may be present

Ancillary Tests
- Most express CD45
- Approximately 80-85% of lymphoid neoplasms originate from B cells

- Diffuse expression of desmin and myogenic markers
- Characteristic translocations between *FOXO1* and *PAX3/7*

Desmoplastic Small Round Cell Tumor
- Intraabdominal and peritoneal sites
- Predilection for young adult males
- Polyphenotypic immunoprofile
  - May express desmin, keratins, and neural markers as well as nuclear WT1 (carboxy terminal)
- Characteristic translocation between *EWSR1* and *WT1*

Poorly Differentiated Synovial Sarcoma
- Focal expression of cytokeratins and EMA
- TLE1(+) in nuclei
- Translocations involving *SS18 (SYT)* and *SSX*

Pleomorphic Undifferentiated Sarcoma
- Absence of hematolymphoid markers

Neuroblastoma
- Diffuse NB84 expression
- Expression of various neural markers

Epithelioid Sarcoma
- Expression of cytokeratin, EMA, and CD34
- INI1(-); chromosome 22q deletions

Sclerosing Epithelioid Fibrosarcoma
- Negative for hematolymphoid markers

Malignant Rhabdoid Tumor
- Expression of cytokeratin and EMA
- INI1(-); chromosome 22q deletions

Small Cell Carcinoma
- Primary site may be evident
- Nuclear moulding
- CK (dot) and neuroendocrine marker expression
- TTF-1 in some

Merkel Cell Carcinoma
- Expression of pancytokeratin
- Dot cytoplasmic expression of CK20
- Neuroendocrine markers positive

Chloroma/Granulocytic Sarcoma
- Patient may have history of, or present simultaneously with, acute myeloid leukemia
- Eosinophilic myelocytes interspersed
- Expresses CD117, CD34, and myeloperoxidase

SELECTED REFERENCES

1. Knowles B et al: Extra-nodal lymphoma presenting as a mimic of soft-tissue sarcoma. ANZ J Surg. 73(1-2):26-30, 2003
2. Salamao DR et al: Lymphoma in soft tissue: a clinicopathologic study of 19 cases. Hum Pathol. 27(3):253-7, 1996
3. Lanham GR et al: Malignant lymphoma. A study of 75 cases presenting in soft tissue. Am J Surg Pathol. 13(1):1-10, 1989
4. Travis WD et al: Primary extranodal soft tissue lymphoma of the extremities. Am J Surg Pathol. 11(5):359-66, 1987

IMAGE GALLERY

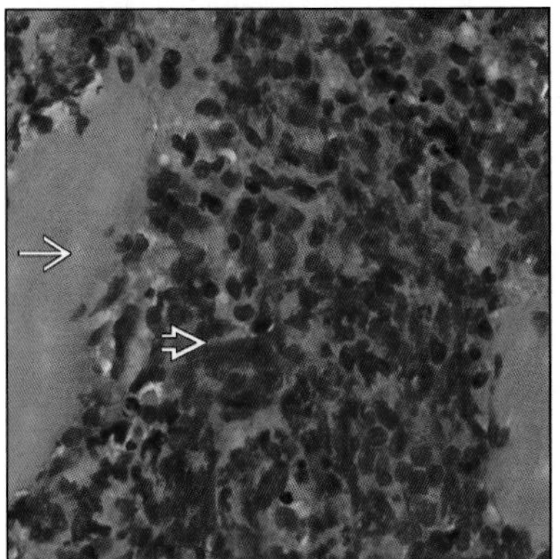

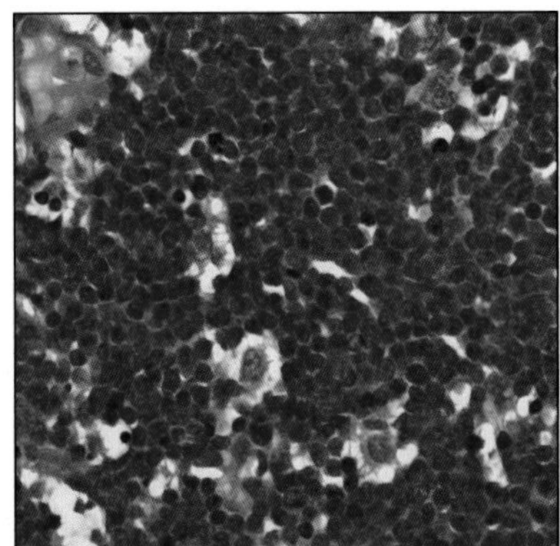

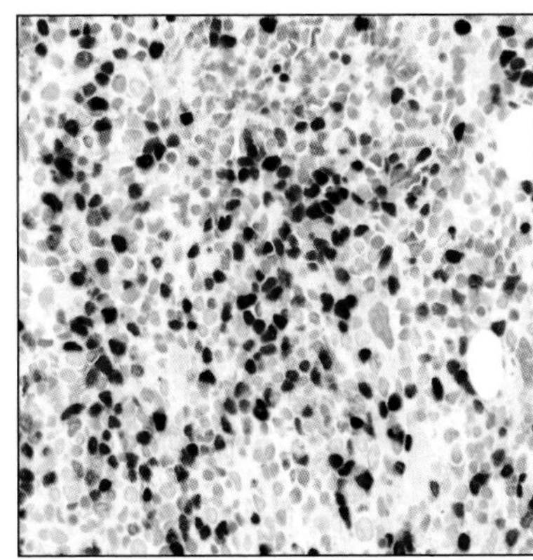

(Left) *High-power view shows diffuse large B-cell lymphoma infiltrating skeletal muscle ➡. The cells exhibit prominent crush artifact ➡, typical of many lymphoid neoplasms in soft tissue sites.* ***(Center)*** *Precursor T-cell acute lymphoblastic lymphoma (ALL) shows sheets of small, monotonous lymphoid blasts that resemble round cell tumors, such as Ewing sarcoma or poorly differentiated synovial sarcoma.* ***(Right)*** *TdT shows strong nuclear expression in precursor T-cell ALL.*

ENDOMETRIAL STROMAL SARCOMA

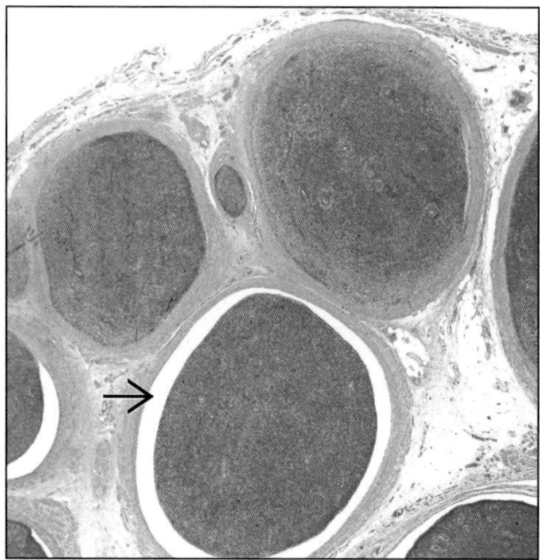

At low power, endometrial stromal sarcoma is a multilobulated, highly cellular tumor composed of islands of ovoid cells with scant cytoplasm, some in vessels ➔.

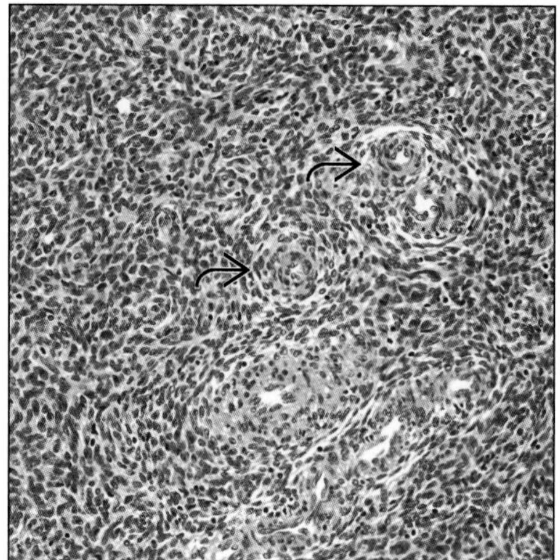

The constituent cells are present in solid sheets. They show minimal atypia. Tumor cells are arranged around a prominent capillary network ➔.

TERMINOLOGY

Abbreviations

- Endometrial stromal sarcoma (ESS)

Synonyms

- Low-grade endometrial stromal sarcoma
- Endolymphatic stromal myosis

Definitions

- Malignant mesenchymal tumor composed of cells that resemble those of proliferative endometrium
- Previous division of ESS into low-grade and high-grade categories has fallen out of favor
  - Term ESS is applied to tumors formerly referred to as "low-grade stromal sarcoma"
  - High-grade/undifferentiated stromal sarcoma is now thought to be unrelated to low-grade ESS

CLINICAL ISSUES

Epidemiology

- Age
  - Peak incidence in 4th-5th decades

Site

- Tumors arise from endometrium
  - Most limited to uterine corpus
  - May extend to parametria or abdomen
- Some arise in extrauterine sites
  - Origin in endometriosis postulated
- Can present as intraabdominal soft tissue tumor

Presentation

- Painful or painless intraabdominal mass
- Abdominal distension

Prognosis

- Recur in approximately 1/3
- Distant metastases and death in smaller percentage

MACROSCOPIC FEATURES

General Features

- Solid, white to tan cut surface
- May show cystic change
- Hemorrhage and necrosis

MICROSCOPIC PATHOLOGY

Histologic Features

- Can be polypoid or infiltrative
- Sheets of small cells
  - Resemble endometrial cells in proliferative phase
  - Ovoid or round vesicular nuclei
  - Scanty cytoplasm
  - Minimal nuclear atypia, but mitotically active
- Extrauterine spread in vessels
- Plexiform vascular pattern
- Stroma can be focally fibrous or myxoid
- Some show focal smooth muscle differentiation
- Can resemble patterns seen in sex cord stromal tumors
- Residual or associated endometriosis in some cases

ANCILLARY TESTS

Immunohistochemistry

- Diffuse CD10 expression
- Diffuse nuclear ER and PR positivity
- Desmin and SMA focally positive
- H-caldesmon(-)
- CK rarely focally positive
- β-catenin(+) in nuclei (40%)

Molecular Genetics

- > 60% have recurrent t(7;17)(p15; q21) with *JAZF1-JJAZ1* gene fusion
- Some have t(6;7)(p21;p22) with *JAZF1-PHF1* gene fusion

ENDOMETRIAL STROMAL SARCOMA

Key Facts

Terminology

- Malignant tumor composed of cells that resemble those of proliferative endometrium

Clinical Issues

- Peak incidence in 4th-5th decades
- Can present as intraabdominal soft tissue tumor
  - Extends from uterus or arises in endometriosis
- Mass or abdominal distension
- Wide differential diagnosis

Microscopic Pathology

- Sheets of uniform ovoid cells
- Minimal nuclear atypia
- Minimal cytoplasm
- Plexiform vascular pattern
- Associated endometriosis in some cases
- Focal smooth muscle differentiation in some
- Diffuse CD10, ER, and PR expression
- > 60% have t(7;17)(p15;q21) translocation

DIFFERENTIAL DIAGNOSIS

Synovial Sarcoma

- Can be biphasic
- Short ovoid nuclei with overlapping nuclei
- CK(+), EMA(+), TLE1(+)
- t(X;18) and *SS18-SSX* fusion genes

Lymphoma

- Presence of lymphoid markers

Ewing Sarcoma

- Younger age group
- Sheets of rounded cells
- CD99(+)
- Various rearrangements involving *EWSR1* gene

Desmoplastic Small Round Cell Tumor

- Adolescent age group
- Islands of small cells in desmoplastic stroma
- CK(+), desmin(+), neural markers(+), and WT1(+)
- t(11;22) with *EWSR1-WT1* gene fusion

Smooth Muscle Neoplasm

- Spindle cells with blunt-ended nuclei
- Diffuse desmin and SMA expression
- H-caldesmon(+)

Solitary Fibrous Tumor

- Cellular and fibrous areas
- Hemangiopericytomatous pattern
- Diffuse CD34 expression

Gastrointestinal Stromal Tumor

- Longer spindle cells or epithelioid cells
- Diffuse CD117 or DOG1 positivity
- May express CD34, H-caldesmon

SELECTED REFERENCES

1. Adegboyega PA et al: Immunohistochemical profiling of cytokeratin expression by endometrial stroma sarcoma. Hum Pathol. 39(10):1459-64, 2008
2. Nucci MR et al: Molecular analysis of the JAZF1-JJAZ1 gene fusion by RT-PCR and fluorescence in situ hybridization in endometrial stromal neoplasms. Am J Surg Pathol. 31(1):65-70, 2007
3. Huang HY et al: Molecular detection of JAZF1-JJAZ1 gene fusion in endometrial stromal neoplasms with classic and variant histology: evidence for genetic heterogeneity. Am J Surg Pathol. 28(2):224-32, 2004
4. Oliva E et al: Endometrial stromal tumors: an update on a group of tumors with a protean phenotype. Adv Anat Pathol. 7(5):257-81, 2000
5. Fukunaga M et al: Extrauterine low-grade endometrial stromal sarcoma: report of three cases. Pathol Int. 48(4):297-302, 1998
6. Chang KL et al: Primary extrauterine endometrial stromal neoplasms: a clinicopathologic study of 20 cases and a review of the literature. Int J Gynecol Pathol. 12(4):282-96, 1993
7. Baiocchi G et al: Endometrioid stromal sarcomas arising from ovarian and extraovarian endometriosis: report of two cases and review of the literature. Gynecol Oncol. 36(1):147-51, 1990

IMAGE GALLERY

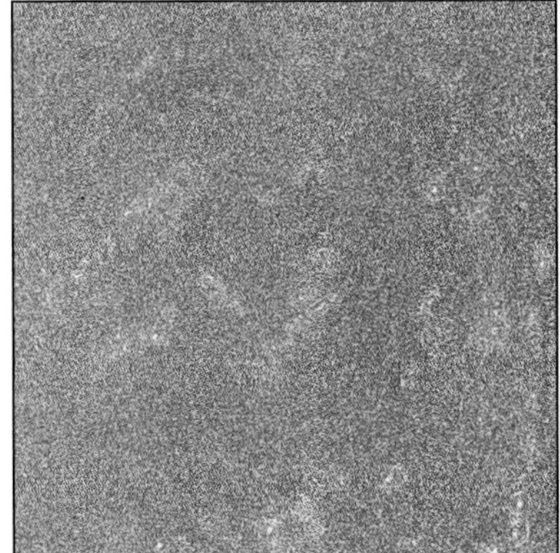
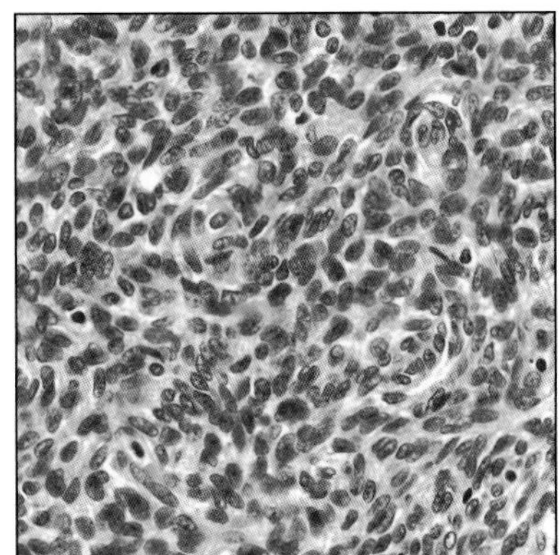
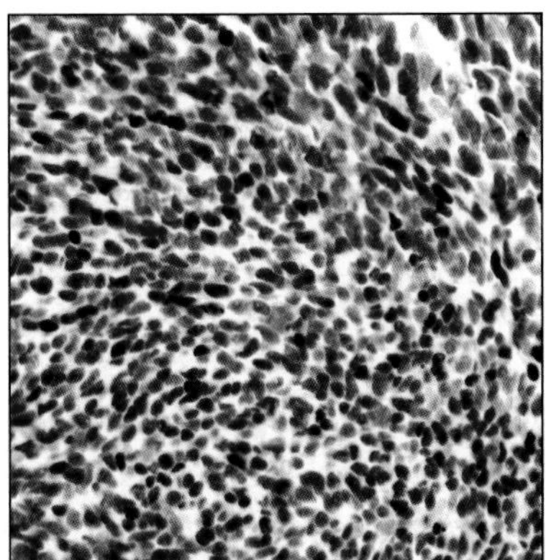

(Left) *At low power, endometrial stromal sarcoma is seen to be composed of sheets of monotonous ovoid to slightly spindled cells.* ***(Center)*** *At higher power, the cells contain bland, vesicular nuclei and small amounts of amphophilic cytoplasm. The mitotic index can be high, although this is not thought to alter prognosis. The stroma here is fibrous, but it can also be myxoid.* ***(Right)*** *There is diffuse and strong nuclear expression of estrogen receptor in almost every tumor cell.*

PROTOCOL FOR THE EXAMINATION OF GIST SPECIMENS

Gastrointestinal Stromal Tumor (GIST): Biopsy

Surgical Pathology Cancer Case Summary (Checklist)

Procedure

____ Core needle biopsy
____ Endoscopic biopsy
____ Other (specify): ____________________________
____ Not specified

**Specimen Size*

*Greatest dimension: _________ cm
*Additional dimensions: _________ x _________ cm
*Cannot be determined

Tumor Site

Specify: ____________________________
____ Not specified

**Tumor Size*

*Greatest dimension: _________ cm
*Additional dimensions: _________ x _________ cm
*____ Cannot be determined

GIST Subtype

____ Spindle cell
____ Epithelioid
____ Mixed
____ Other (specify): ____________________________

Mitotic Rate

Specify: _________ /50 high-power fields (HPF)

**Necrosis*

*____ Not identified
*____ Present
*Extent: _________ %
*____ Cannot be determined

Histologic Grade

____ GX: Grade cannot be assessed
____ G1: Low grade; mitotic rate ≤ 5/50 HPF
____ G2: High grade; mitotic rate > 5/50 HPF

Risk Assessment

____ None
____ Very low risk
____ Low risk
____ Intermediate risk
____ High risk
____ Overtly metastatic
____ Cannot be determined

Distant Metastasis

____ Cannot be assessed
____ Distant metastasis
Specify site(s), if known: ____________________________

Additional Pathologic Findings

Specify: ____________________________

Ancillary Studies (select all that apply)

Immunohistochemical studies

___ KIT (CD117)

___ Positive

___ Negative

___ Others (specify): ___________________________

___ Not performed

Molecular genetic studies (e.g., KIT or PDGFRA mutational analysis)

___ Submitted for analysis; results pending

___ Performed, see separate report: ___________________________

___ Performed

Specify method(s) and results: ___________________________

___ Not performed

Pre-biopsy Treatment (select all that apply)

___ No therapy

___ Systemic therapy performed

Specify type: ___________________________

___ Therapy performed, type not specified

___ Unknown

****Treatment Effect***

*Specify percentage of viable tumor: _________ %

**Data elements with asterisks are not required. However, these elements may be clinically important but are not yet validated or regularly used in patient management. Adapted with permission from College of American Pathologists, "Protocol for the Examination of Specimens from Patients with Gastrointestinal Stromal Tumor." Web posting date February 2010, www.cap.org.*

Gastrointestinal Stromal Tumor (GIST): Resection

Surgical Pathology Cancer Case Summary (Checklist)

Procedure

___ Excisional biopsy

___ Resection

Specify type (e.g., partial gastrectomy): ___________________________

___ Metastasectomy

___ Other (specify): ___________________________

___ Not specified

Tumor Site

Specify (if known): ___________________________

___ Not specified

Tumor Size

Greatest dimension: _________ cm

*Additional dimensions: _________ x _________ cm

___ Cannot be determined

Tumor Focality

___ Unifocal

___ Multifocal

Specify number of tumors: _________

Specify size of tumors: ___________________________

GIST Subtype

___ Spindle cell

___ Epithelioid

___ Mixed

___ Other (specify): ___________________________

Mitotic Rate

Specify: _________ /50 HPF

****Necrosis***

*___ Not identified

PROTOCOL FOR THE EXAMINATION OF GIST SPECIMENS

*___ Present

*Extent: _________ %

*___ Cannot be determined

Histologic Grade

___ GX: Grade cannot be assessed

___ G1: Low grade; mitotic rate ≤ 5/50 HPF

___ G2: High grade; mitotic rate > 5/50 HPF

Risk Assessment

___ None

___ Very low risk

___ Intermediate risk

___ High risk

___ Overtly malignant/metastatic

___ Cannot be determined

Margins

___ Cannot be assessed

___ Negative for GIST

Distance of tumor from closest margin: _________ cm

___ Margin(s) positive for GIST

Specify margin(s): ___________________________

Pathologic Staging (pTNM)

TNM descriptors (required only if applicable) (select all that apply)

___ m (multiple)

___ r (recurrent)

___ y (post-treatment)

Primary tumor (pT)

___ pTX: Primary tumor cannot be assessed

___ pT0: No evidence for primary tumor

___ pT1: Tumor ≤ 2 cm

___ pT2: Tumor > 2 cm but ≤ 5 cm

___ pT3: Tumor > 5 cm but ≤ 10 cm

___ pT4: Tumor > 10 cm in greatest dimension

Regional lymph nodes (pN)

___ Not applicable

___ pM1: Distant metastasis

*Specify site(s) if known: ___________________________

**Additional Pathologic Findings*

*Specify: ___________________________

Ancillary Studies (select all that apply)

Immunohistochemical studies

___ KIT (CD117)

___ Positive

___ Negative

___ Others (specify): ___________________________

___ Not performed

Molecular genetic studies (e.g., KIT or PDGFRA mutational analysis)

___ Submitted for analysis; results pending

___ Performed, see separate report: ___________________________

___ Performed

Specify method(s) and results: ___________________________

___ Not performed

PROTOCOL FOR THE EXAMINATION OF GIST SPECIMENS

Pre-resection Treatment (select all that apply)

____ No therapy

____ Previous biopsy or surgery

Specify: ______________________________

____ Systemic therapy performed

Specify type: ______________________________

____ Therapy performed, type not specified

____ Unknown

**Treatment Effect*

*Specify percentage of viable tumor: __________ %

**Data elements with asterisks are not required. However, these elements may be clinically important but are not yet validated or regularly used in patient management. Adapted with permission from College of American Pathologists, "Protocol for the Examination of Specimens from Patients with Gastrointestinal Stromal Tumor." Web posting date February 2010, www.cap.org.*

GIST Staging

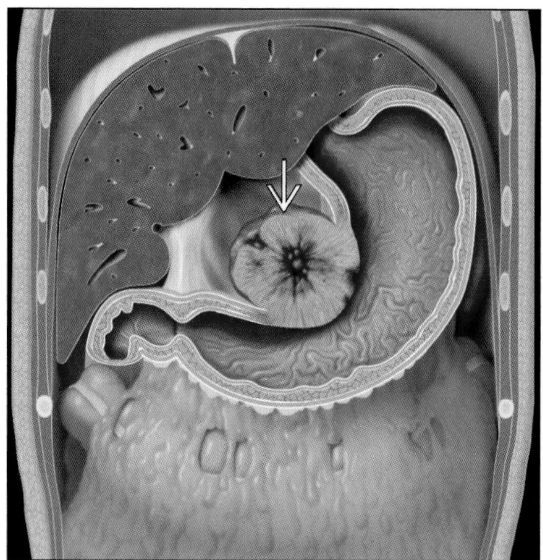

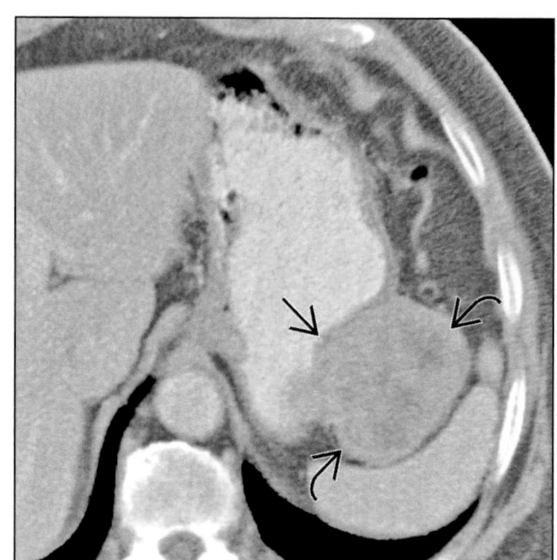

(Left) *Coronal graphic shows a gastric GIST ➡ involving the lesser curve of the stomach. Precise staging would be based on tumor size and grade in the absence of nodal or metastatic disease.* ***(Right)*** *Axial contrast-enhanced CT shows a heterogeneous GIST along the greater curve of the stomach. There is a small intraluminal component ➡ and a larger exophytic component ➦. This was an AJCC stage IIIA lesion based on size and high tumor grade.*

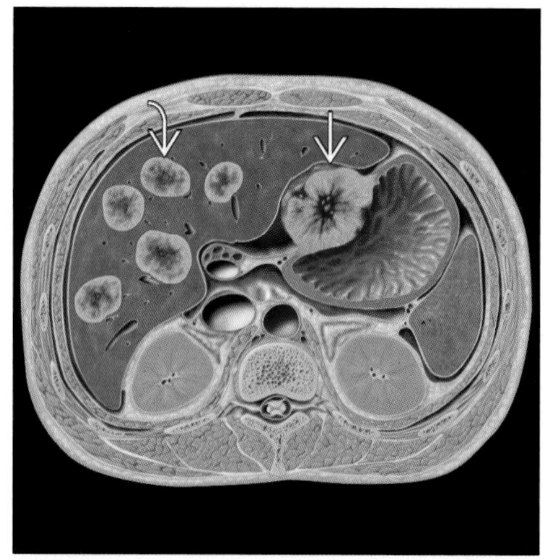

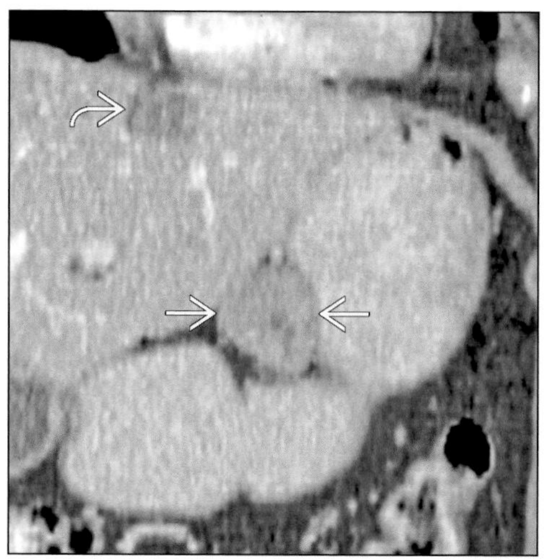

(Left) *Axial graphic shows a gastric GIST ➡ with solid hepatic metastases ➦. The presence of metastases makes this an AJCC stage IV lesion.* ***(Right)*** *Coronal contrast-enhanced CT shows a gastric GIST ➡ along the lesser curvature. A solitary liver metastasis ➦ is noted as well, making this AJCC stage IV disease.*

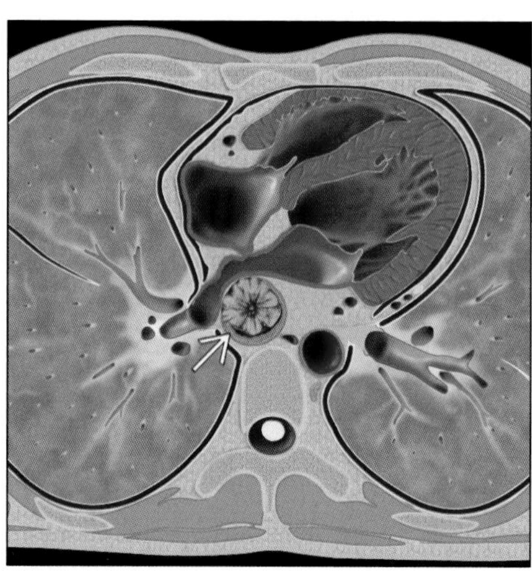

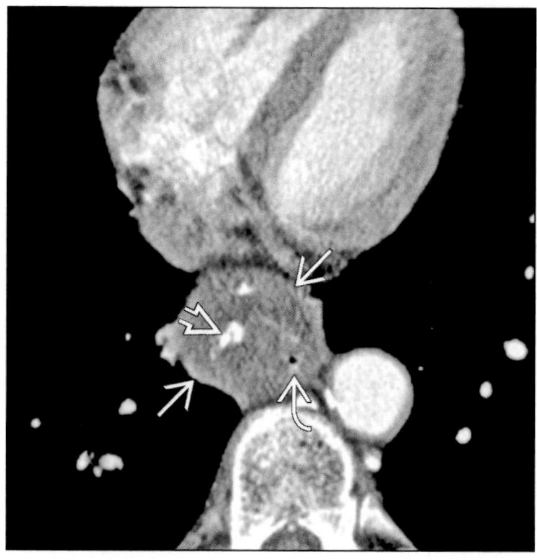

(Left) *Axial graphic shows mid-esophageal GIST ➡. The staging and grouping for small bowel GISTs would be used in this case. Precise staging is based on the lesion size and grade.* ***(Right)*** *Axial contrast-enhanced CT shows a GIST ➡ arising from the mid-esophagus. GISTs may occasionally show calcification ⇨. The eccentric nature of the mass, with displacement of the esophageal lumen ➦, suggests a mural origin.*

GIST Staging

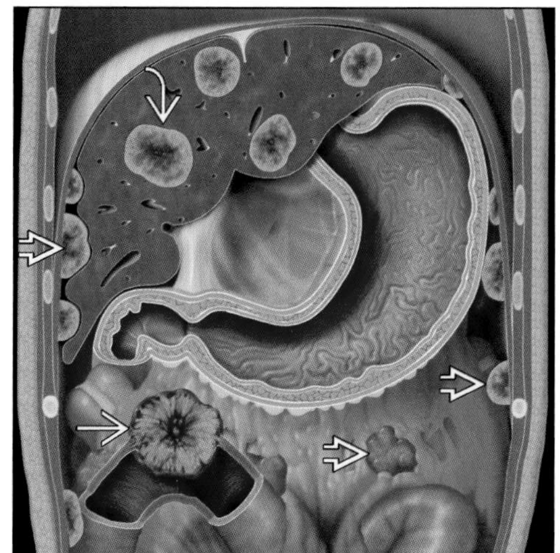

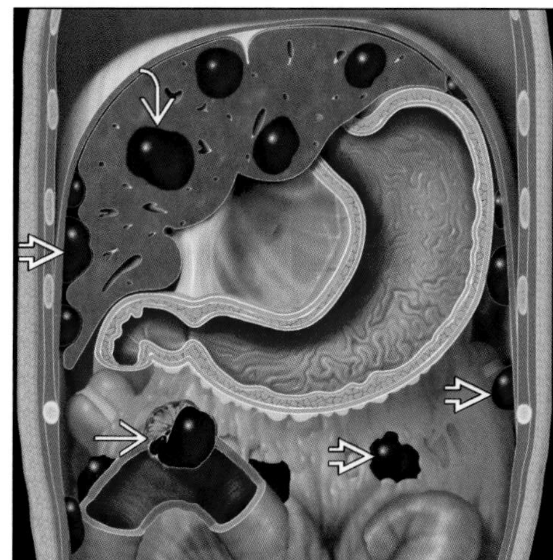

(Left) *Coronal graphic shows a small bowel GIST ➔ with hepatic ➔ and peritoneal ➔ metastases. This is an AJCC stage IV lesion.* ***(Right)*** *Coronal graphic shows a decrease in size and more cystic nature of primary small bowel GIST ➔ as well as hepatic ➔ and peritoneal ➔ metastases. This indicates a response to therapy.*

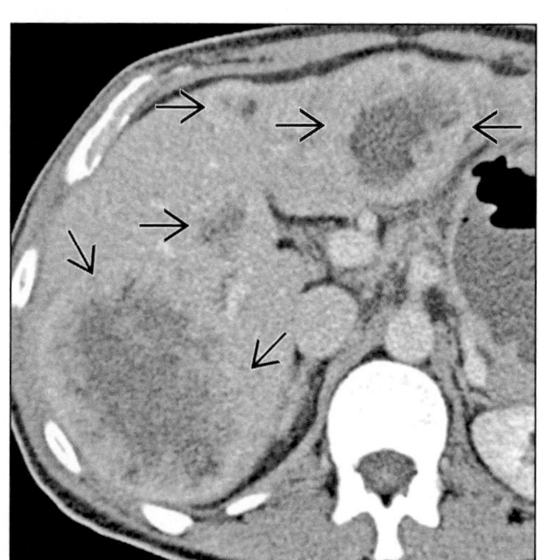

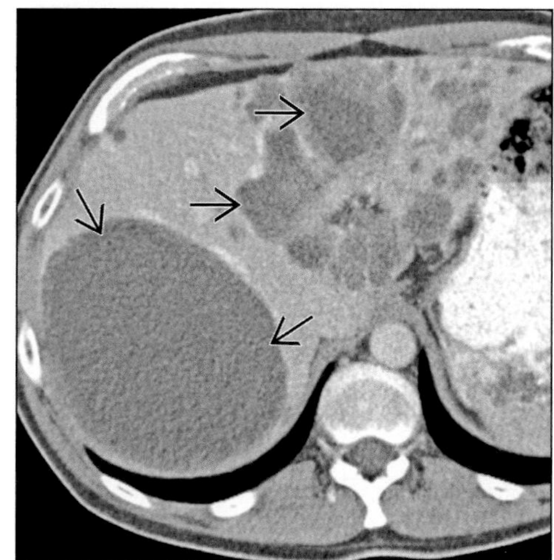

(Left) *Axial contrast-enhanced CT shows several necrotic masses with thick enhancing rims ➔ within the liver, representing metastases in a patient with GIST.* ***(Right)*** *Axial contrast-enhanced CT in the same patient after therapy with imatinib mesylate shows a decrease in density of the metastases ➔, consistent with response to therapy.*

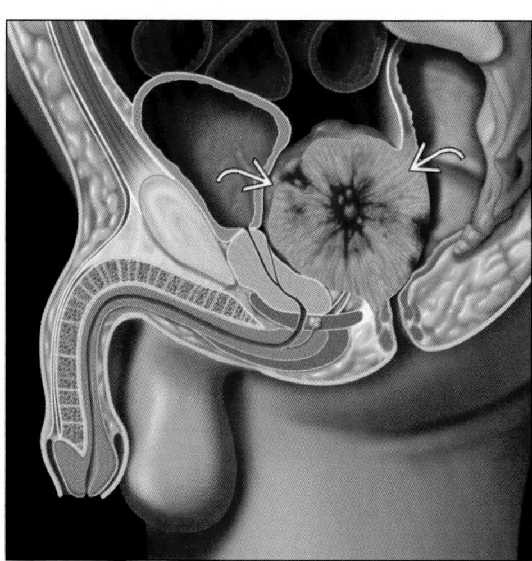

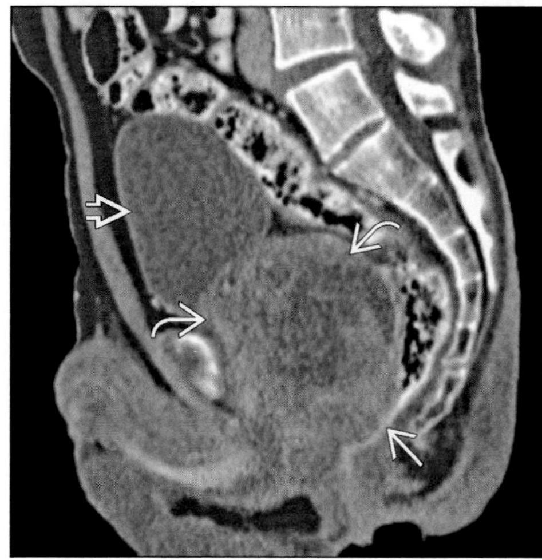

(Left) *Sagittal graphic shows a rectal GIST ➔. The staging and grouping for small bowel GISTs would be used in this case. Precise staging is based on lesion size and grade.* ***(Right)*** *Sagittal contrast-enhanced CT demonstrates the relationship of the rectal GIST ➔ to the adjacent pelvic organs. The GIST elevates the bladder ➔ and compresses the rectum ➔. The size was > 10 cm; therefore, this is a pT4 tumor.*

Antibody Index

ANTIBODY INDEX

Antibodies Discussed

Antibody Name/Symbol	Antibody Description	Clones/Alternative Names
34βE12	cytokeratin, high molecular weight (34βE12-; CK1, 5, 10, 14)	MA-903, CK903, high molecular weight keratin
α1-antichymotrypsin	alpha 1 antichromotripsin	A1ACT
α1-antitrypsin	alpha 1 antitrypsin	A1AT
β-catenin	Beta catenin; involved in regulation of cell adhesion and in signal transduction through Wnt pathway	B-catenin, Clone 14, E-5, RB-9035-Po, 17C2, 5H10, B-CATEN-MEM (beta catenin, membrane), B-CATEN-CYT, B-CATEN-NUC
κ light chain	kappa light chain	KAPPA
λ light chain	lambda light chain	LAMBDA
Actin-HHF-35	actin, muscle (HHF35)	MSA, HHF-35
Actin-sm	actin, smooth muscle	SMA, ASM-1, CGA7, 1A4, HUC1-1
AE1/AE3	AE1/AE3; mixture of 2 anti-cytokeratin clones that detect a variety of both high and low molecular weight cytokeratins	
AE13	AE13 (pilar-type keratin)	
ALK1	anaplastic lymphoma kinase-1	5A4, ALK, ALKC,
Androgen receptor	dihydrotestosterone receptor, nuclear receptor subfamily 3 group C member 4	AR441, F39.4.1, AR-N20, AR27
Aromatase	key enzyme in steroidogenesis with important roles in sexual differentiation, oestrogen biosynthesis, fertility, and carcinogenesis	SM1671P, ARO1, CPV, CYAR, CYP19, CYP19A1, CYPXIX
Bcl-2	B-cell CLL/lymphoma 2; suppresses apoptosis in a variety of cell systems	ONCL2, BCL2/100/D5, 124, 124.3
Caldesmon	actin interacting and calmodulin binding protein found in smooth muscle and other cell types	CAD, CALD1, Caldesmon 1 isoform [1-5], CDM, HCAD, LCAD, MGC21352, NAG22
Calponin	thin filament associated protein that is implicated in regulation and modulation of smooth muscle contraction	N3, 26A11, CALP, CNN1, SMCC, Sm Calp
Calretinin	29 kDa calcium binding protein that is expressed in central and peripheral nervous system and in many normal and pathological tissues	DAK-CALRET, 5A5, CAL 3F5, DC8, AB149
Caveolin-1		CAV-1, caveolin, VIP 21, CAV
CD1a	T-cell surface glycoprotein	JPM30, CD1A, O10, NA1/34
CD3	T-cell receptor	F7238, A0452, CD3-P, CD3-M, SP7, PS1
CD4	T-cell surface glycoprotein, L3T4	IF6, 1290, 4B12, CD4, 1F6, CD04
CD10	neutral endopeptidase, CALLA	CALLA, neprilysin, neutral endopeptidase, NEP
CD11c	integrin alpha X chain protein	LEU-M5
CD163	macrophage hemoglobin scavenging system	Hemoglobin scavenger receptor, 3A6, ALCAM
CD20	membrane spanning 4-domains of B lymphocytes	FB1, B1, L26, MS4A1
CD21	CR2, complement component receptor 2, Epstein-Barr virus receptor	IF8
CD23	Fc ϵ RII, low-affinity IgE receptor, IGEBF	1B12, MHM6, BU38
CD30	tumor necrosis factor receptor SF8	BER-H2, KI-1, TNFRSF8
CD31	platelet endothelial cell adhesion molecule	JC/70, JC/70A, PECAM-1
CD34	Hematopoietic progenitor cell antigen	MY10, IOM34, QBEND10, 8G12, 1309, HPCA-1, HPCA, NU-4A1, TUK4, clone 581, BI-3C5
CD35	erythrocyte complement receptor 1, immune adherence receptor, C3b/C4b receptor	CR1, BER-MAC-DRC, TO5, CD35, E11
CD38	acute lymphoblastic leukemia cell antigen, T10	CD38, SPC32, VS38, T10
CD45	leukocyte common antigen	PD7/26, 1.22/4.14, T29/33, CD45RB, RP2/18, CD45, PD7, 2D1, 2B11+PD7/26, LCA
CD56	NCAM (neural cellular adhesion molecule)	MAB 735, ERIC-1, 25-KD11, 123C3, 24-MB2, BC56C04, 1B6, 14-MAB735, NCC-LU-243, MOC-1, NCAM, LEU-19, 25KD11
CD57	β-1,3-glucuronyltransferase 1 (glucuronosyltransferase P)	LEU-7, NK1, HNK-1, TB01, B3GAT1
CD63	tetraspan intracellular granule protein	NKI/C3, basophil activation test in allergy
CD68	cytoplasmic granule protein of monocytes, macrophages	CD68, PG-M1, KP-1
CD99	cell surface glycoprotein for migration, T cell adhesion, MIC2	CD99-MEMB, MIC2, 12E7, HBA71, O13, P30/32MIC2, M3601

ANTIBODY INDEX

CD117	C-Kit; tyrosine-protein kinase activity	C-19 (C-KIT), 104D2, 2E4, C-KIT, A4502, H300, CMA-767
CDK4	Cyclin dependent kinase 4	C-22, CDK4, DCS-31
CEA-M	carcinoembryonic antigen, monoclonal	CEA-B18, CEA-D14, CEA-GOLD 1, T84.6, CEA-GOLD 2, CEA 11, CEA-GOLD 3, CEA 27, CEA-GOLD 4, CEA 41, CEA-GOLD 5, T84.1, CEA-M, A5B7, CEJ065, IL-7, T84.66, TF3H8-1, 0062, D14, alpha-7, PARLAM 1, ZC23, CEM010, A115, COL-1, AF4, 12.140.10, 11-7, M773, CEA-M431_31, CEJO65, mCEA
Chromogranin-A	Pituitary secretory protein I	PHE-5, PHE5, E001, DAK-A3, LK2H10, CGA, CHGA, SP1
CK5/6	cytokeratin 5/6; high molecular weight cytokeratins	D5/16 B4
CK7	cytokeratin 7; low molecular weight cytokeratin	K72.7, KS7.18, OVTL 12/30, LDS-68, CK 07
CK8/18/CAM5.2	cytokeratin 8/18 (CAM 5.2); simple epithelial-type cytokeratins	CAM 5.2, KER 10.11, NCL-5D3, keratin-LMW, cytokeratin 8/18-LMW
CK14	cytokeratin 14; high molecular weight cytokeratin	LL002
CK19	cytokeratin 19; low molecular weight cytokeratin	BA17, RCK108, LP2K, B170, A53-BA2, CK 19, KS19.1, 170.2.14
CK20	cytokeratin 20; low molecular weight cytokeratin	KS20.8
CK-HMW-NOS	cytokeratin, high molecular weight, not otherwise specified	keratin-HMW
CK-PAN	cytokeratin-pan (AE1/AE3/LP34); cocktail of high and low molecular weight cytokeratins	keratin pan, MAK-6, K576, LU-5, KL-1, KC-8, MNF 116, pankeratin, pancytokeratin
CLA	cutaneous lymphocyte antigen	CLA-HECA452
Claudin-1	senescence-associated epithelial membrane protein	JAD.8
Clusterin	clusterin, alpha chain specific	41D, E5
Collagen IV	major constituent of the basement membranes along with laminins, proteoglycans and enactins	CIV22, COL4A[1-5], collagen α-1(IV)chain
Cyclin-D1	protein with important cell cycle regulatory functions	Bcl-1 (Cyclin D1), A-12, PRAD1, AM29, DCS-6, SP4, 5D4, D1GM, P2D11F11, CCND1Cyl-1
Desmin	class III intermediate filaments found in muscle cells	M760, DE-R-11, D33, DE5, DE-U-10, ZC18
DOG1	transmembrane protein 16A	DOG 1.1, DOG1 (TMEM16A)
Dysadherin	cancer-associated cell membrane glycoprotein	NCC-M53
EGFR	v-erb-b1 erythroblastic leukemia viral gene,epidermal growth factor receptor	2-18C9, EGFR1, EGFR PHRMDX, NCL-R1, H11, C-ERBB-1, E30, EGFR.113, 31G7, 3C6, 2-18C9
EMA/MUC1	epithelial membrane antigen	EMA, GP1.4, 214D4, MC5, E29, MUC1, LICR-LON-M8, BC3, DF3, VU3D1, MUSEII, RD-1, MA695, MA552, PS2P446, 115D8, MUC1, MAM6, CA15.3, MUC01
EpCAM/BER-EP4/CD326	epithelial cell adhesion molecule	AUA1, VU-1D9, EPCAM, C10, HEA125, BER-EP4
ERP	estrogen receptor protein	1D5, 6F11, SP1, 15D, H222, TE111, ER, ER1D5, NCLER611, NCL-ER-LH2, PGP-1A6
Fascin	singed-like protein	55K2, FAN1, Fascin 1, FSCN1, p55, SNL, singed like protein antibody
FGF-23	fibroblast growth factor 23	
FLI1	Friend leukemia virus integration 1	GI146-222, SC356,FLK-1,FLT-1
FN1	fibronectin	FN1, A0245, CIG
FVIIIRAg	factor VIII-related-antigen	F8/86, von Willebrand factor
FXIIIA	factor XIIIA (fibrin stabilizing factor)	factor XIIIa
GFAP	glial fibrillary acidic protein	6F2, M761, GA-51, GFP-8A
GH	growth hormone	HGH
GLUT1	glucose transporter 1	
HCAD	H-caldesmon (high molecular weight caldesmon)	H-CD
Hep-Par1	hepatocyte paraffin 1	OCH1E5.2.10, HEPPAR-1
HHV8	human herpes virus 8, human herpesvirus-8 latent nuclear antigen 1	13B10
HLA-DR	human leukocyte antigen DR	DK22, LN3, TAL.1B5, LK8D3
HMB-45	melanoma antibody	LB39 AA, CMM1, CMM, DNS, FAMMM, MART1, Melan-A, MLM, tyrosinase
HMGA1	high mobility group chromatin protein A1	
HMGA2	high mobility group chromatin protein A2	HMGI-C
IGF-2	insulin-like growth factor 2	W2-H1
IgG	immunoglobulin G	

ANTIBODY INDEX

IL-15	interleukin 15	
Inhibin-α	inhibin alpha	
Ki-67	Ki-67 (MIB-1); marker of cell proliferation	MMI, KI88, IVAK-2, MIB1
LEP	leptin	
Lysozyme	1,4-beta-N-acetylmuramidase C	Lyz, LZM, Ec 3.2.1.17
LYVE-1	lymph vessel endothelial hyaluronan receptor 1	
MAC387	macrophage antibody	MAC387
Mart-1	mart-1 clone of Melan A	
MDM2	murine double minute oncogene (mdm2)	HDM2, IF2, 2A10, 1B10, SMP14, murine double minute 2
Mesothelin	pre-pro-megakaryocyte-potentiating factor	5B2, CAK1, MPF, MSLN, SMR
MITF	microphthalmia-associated transcription factor	34CA5, D5, C5+D5
MK	neurite growth promoting factor 2	MIDKINE, G2a
MOC-31	lung cancer marker	
MT	metallothionein	CLONE E9
myc	myelocytomatosis viral oncogene	C-MYC, 9E10, 9E11, 1-262, c-myc
MYOD1	myogenic differentiation 1	5.8A, 5.2F
Myogenin	myogenic factor 4; Class C basic helix-loop-helix protein 3	F5D, MYF3, MYF4, LO26, bHLHc3, cb553, MYF4, MYOG
Myosin-fast	fast skeletal myosin antibody	MY-32, A1 catalytic, A2 catalytic, Alkali myosin light chain 1 (or 3), DKFZp778C0757, MGC13450, MLC1F, MLC3F, MRLC2, MYL1 protein, MYLPF
NB84	neuroblastoma	
Nestin	neural stem cell marker	10C2
NFP	neurofilament H/M phosphorylated protein	TPNFP-1A3, SMI31, SMI33, NFP, SMI32, TA-51, 2F11
NGFR	nerve growth factor receptor	
NSE	neuron specific enolase	BSS/H14
Osteocalcin	bone gamma carboxyglutamate gla protein osteocalcin antibody	OC-1, OC, PMF1, BGLAP, BGP
p27	cyclin dependent kinase inhibitor 1B	P27_KIP1, 57, 1B4, DCS-72.F6, SX53G8, K25020, DCS72, KIP-1
p53	p53 tumor suppressor gene protein	DO7, 21N, BP53-12-1, AB6, CM1, PAB1801, DO1, BP53-11, PAB240, RSP53, MU195, PAB1801
p63	tumor protein p63	4A4, H-137, 7JUL
PDGF-B	granulin, PC cell-derived growth factor (progranulin)	
PGP9.5	protein gene product 9.5	31A3,13C4
Podoplanin	Lymphatic endothelial marker	D2-40 clone, D2-40, M2A
PRP	progesterone receptor protein	10A9, PGR-1A6, KD68, PGR-ICA, PR, PRP-P, PRI, 1A6, 1AR, HPRA3, PGR-636, 636, PR88, NCL-PGR
PSA	prostate specific antigen	PSA-M, ER-PR8, PSA-P, F5
PTEN	phosphatase and tensin homolog	PN37
Rb	retinoblastoma-associated protein	3C8, 3H9, PRB1, G3-245, RB1, RB-WL 1, RB-1, 1F8, PRB
S100		S100 protein, A6, 15E2E2, Z311, 4C4.9
S100-pla	S100 placental	S100P, S100PL, S0084, 16
SCC	small cell carcinoma	F2H7C
SMM	myosin heavy chain smooth muscle	SMHC, ID8, SM_MYOSIN_H, HSM-V, SMMS-1
SNF5	member of SWI/SNF chromatin remodeling complex	BAF47/SNF5, INI1
SOX9	SRY (sex-determining region Y)-box 9 protein	CMD1, CMPD1
SV40	simian virus 40	
Synaptophysin	major synaptic vesicle protein P38 antibody	SVP38, SY38, SNP-88, SYP, SYPH, Sypl, Syn p38
TdT	terminal deoxynucleotidyl transferase	SEN 28
TFE3	transcription factor E3	
Thrombomodulin	fetomodulin; CD antigen CD141	1009, 15C8, CD141, fetomodulin, THBD, THRM, TM
TLE1	transducer like enhancer 1	
TRAP	tartrate resistant acid phosphatase	26E5, TRAP, 9C5
TTF-1	transcription termination factor	8G7G3/1, SPT-24, SC-13040

ANTIBODY INDEX

VEGF	vascular endothelial growth factor	JH121, 26503.11, VPF, VPF/VEGF, VEGF-A, VEGF-C, RP 077, VEGFR-1, RP 076, VEGFR-2, 9D9, VEGFR-3, FLT-4
Vimentin	major subunit protein of the intermediate filaments of mesenchymal cells	43BE8, 3B4, V10, V9, VIM-3B4, VIM
WT1	Wilms tumor gene-01	6F-H2, C-19

INDEX

A

INDEX

INDEX

B

C

INDEX

D

INDEX

E

INDEX

F

INDEX

INDEX

INDEX

INDEX

G

INDEX

INDEX

INDEX

INDEX

INDEX

L

INDEX

INDEX

M

INDEX

INDEX

INDEX

INDEX

INDEX

INDEX

INDEX

R

INDEX

INDEX

S

INDEX

INDEX

INDEX

INDEX

W

X